REGIONAL ANESTHESIA AND ACUTE PAIN MEDICINE

ANESTHESIOLOGY: A PROBLEM-BASED LEARNING APPROACH

Series Editor: Magdalena Anitescu, MD

Published and Forthcoming Titles

Pain Management, edited by Magdalena Anitescu

Anesthesiology, edited by Tracey Straker and Shobana Rajan

Pediatric Anesthesia, edited by Kirk Lalwani, Ira Todd Cohen, Ellen Y. Choi, and Vidya T. Raman

Neuroanesthesia, edited by David E. Traul and Irene P. Osborn

Cardiac Anesthesia, edited by Mohammed M. Minhaj

Critical Care, edited by Taylor Johnston and Steven Miller

Perioperative Care, edited by Deborah Richman and Debra Pulley

Regional Anesthesia and Acute Pain Medicine, edited by Nabil Elkassabany and Eman Nada

REGIONAL ANESTHESIA AND ACUTE PAIN MEDICINE

A PROBLEM-BASED LEARNING APPROACH

EDITED BY

Nabil Elkassabany and Eman Nada

OXFORD
UNIVERSITY PRESS

OXFORD
UNIVERSITY PRESS

Oxford University Press is a department of the University of Oxford. It furthers the University's objective of excellence in research, scholarship, and education by publishing worldwide. Oxford is a registered trade mark of Oxford University Press in the UK and certain other countries.

Published in the United States of America by Oxford University Press
198 Madison Avenue, New York, NY 10016, United States of America.

CIP data is on file at the Library of Congress
ISBN 978–0–19–751851–9

DOI: 10.1093/med/9780197518519.001.0001

Printed by Integrated Books International, United States of America

We dedicate this book to our late parents, family, teachers, and mentors for their continued support and care, and to the entire regional anesthesia and acute pain medicine community

CONTENTS

CONTRIBUTORS

Daniel Abraham, MD
Assistant Professor
Department of Anesthesiology and Critical Care
University of Pennsylvania
Philadelphia, PA, USA

Sanjib Das Adhikary, MBBS, MD
Professor of Anesthesiology, Orthopedics, & Rehabilitation
Vice Chair for Research and Innovation
Division Director for Orthopedic Anesthesia, & Regional Anesthesia and Acute Pain Medicine
Department of Anesthesiology & Perioperative Medicine
Penn State College of Medicine
Hershey, PA, USA

José Eduardo De Aguilar-Nascimento, TCBC-MT
Professor
Titular do Departamento de Cirurgia da Faculdade de Medicina da
Universidade Federal De Mato Grosso
Várzea Grande, Cuiabá, MT, BR

Davies G. Agyekum, MD, PhD
Anesthesiologist
Department of Anesthesiology
Newton-Wellesley Hospital
Newton, MA, USA

Sanchit Ahuja, MD
Fellow
Department of Cardiothoracic Anesthesia
Anesthesiology Institute
Cleveland Clinic
Cleveland, OH, USA

Michael Akerman, MD
Assistant Professor
Department of Anesthesiology
Cornell Medical Center
New York, NY, USA

Brenton Alexander, MD
Attending Physician
Department of Regional Anesthesiology and Acute Pain Management
University of California, San Diego
San Diego, CA, USA

Ariel Anderson, MD
Clinical Instructor of Anesthesiology Keck School of Medicine
University of Southern California
Los Angeles, CA, USA

Gustavo Angaramo, MD
Associate Professor of Anesthesiology and Critical Care
Director of Regional Anesthesia Division
Director of Peri-operative Units
University of Massachusetts Medical School
Worcester, MA, USA

Alberto E. Ardon, MD, MPH
Assistant Professor
Department of Anesthesiology and Perioperative Medicine
Mayo Clinic
Jacksonville, FL, USA

Ignacio Badiola, MD
Assistant Professor of Anesthesiology and Critical Care
Department of Anesthesiology and Critical Care
Perelman School of Medicine
University of Pennsylvania
Philadelphia, PA, USA

Neil Batta
Resident in Physical Medicine and Rehabilitation
Interventional Pain Management
NeoSpine
Gig Harbor, WA, USA

Himani V. Bhatt, DO, MPA, FASE, FASA
Associate Professor of Anesthesiology
Perioperative and Pain Medicine
Director, Division of Cardiac Anesthesiology
Mount Sinai Morningside Medical Center
Associate Professor of Cardiovascular Surgery
Icahn School of Medicine at Mount Sinai
Director, Division of Cardiac Anesthesiology
Mount Sinai St. Luke's Hospital
New York, NY, USA

Derek Blankenship, MD
Anesthesiologist
Anne Burnett Marion School of Medicine at Texas Christian University Baylor Scott &White All Saints Medical Center
NorthStar Anesthesia
Irving, TX, USA

Shelly B. Borden, MD
Clinical Anesthesiologist
William S. Middleton Memorial Veterans Hospital
Madison, WI, USA

Mitchell Cahan, MD
Chairman, Department of Surgery
Mount Auburn Hospital
Vice Chairman
Roberta and Stephen R. Weiner Department of Surgery
Beth Israel Deaconess Medical Center
Professor of Surgery (Adjunct)
Department of Surgery
University of Massachusetts Chan Medical School
Worcester, MA, USA

Franklin Chiao, MD, MS, MBA, LAc, FASA
Director of Acute Pain Management
Medical Director
Westchester Medical Center
New York, NY, USA

Simon Chin, MD
Clinical Assistant Professor
Department of Surgery
Donald and Barbara Zucker School of Medicine at Hofstra/Northwell
Hempstead, NY, USA

Iris Chu, MD
Assistant Professor
Department of Anesthesiology
Geisel School of Medicine at Dartmouth College
Dartmouth-Hitchcock
Lebanon, NH, USA

Peter Dienhart, MD
Assistant Professor
Department of Anesthesiology
Ohio State University Wexner Medical Center
Columbus, OH, USA

Osemeke Edobor, MD
Anesthesiologist
Department of Anesthesiology
Morristown Medical Center
Atlantic Health System
Morristown, New Jersey, USA

Nabil Elkassabany, MD, MSCE
Professor and Vice Chair of Clinical Operations
Department of Anesthesiology
University of Virginia
Charlottesville, VA, USA

Dalia Elmofty, MD
Associate Professor
Department of Anesthesia and Critical Care
University of Chicago
Chicago, IL, USA

Shimon Gabriel Farkas, MD
Staff Anesthesiologist
United Anesthesia Services PC
Paoli, PA, USA

Mohamed Fayed, MD
Resident
Henry Ford Health System
Detroit, Michigan, USA

Colin Feduska MD
Assistant Professor
Department of Anesthesiology and Critical Care
University of Pennsylvania
Philadelphia, PA, USA

Michael Feduska, MD
Assistant Professor
Department of Anesthesiology and Critical Care
University of Pennsylvania
Philadelphia, PA, USA

Arthur Formanek, MD
Instructor
Brigham and Women's Hospital
Harvard Medical School
Boston, MA, USA

Rodney Gabriel, MD
Chief of Department of Regional Anesthesiology and Acute Pain Management
University of California, San Diego
San Diego, CA, USA

Robert Gaiser, MD
Professor
Department of Anesthesiology
Yale University
New Haven, CT, USA

Veena Graff, MD, MS
Assistant Professor
Department of Anesthesiology and Critical Care
Perelman School of Medicine, University of Pennsylvania
Philadelphia, PA, USA

Taras Grosh, MD
Assistant Professor
Department of Anesthesiology and Critical Care
Perelman School of Medicine, University of Pennsylvania
Hospital of the University of Pennsylvania
Philadelphia, PA, USA

Thomas Halaszynski, DMD, MD, MBA
Professor
Department of of Anesthesiology
Yale University
New Haven, CT, USA

H. David Hardman, MD, MBA, FASA
Professor
Department of Anesthesiology
University of North Carolina
Chapel Hill, NC, USA

N. Robert Harvey, MD
Assistant Professor
Department of Anesthesia and Perioperative Medicine
Medical University of South Carolina
Charleston, SC, USA

Erik Helander, MD
Fellow
Department of Anesthesiology
University of Florida College of Medicine
Gainesville, FL, USA

Balazs Horvath, MD, FASA
Associate Professor
Department of of Anesthesiology
University of Minnesota
M Health Fairview University of Minnesota Masonic Children's Hospital
Minneapolis, MN, USA

Stephanie Huang, MD
Assistant Professor
Department of Clinical Anesthesiology and Critical Care
Perelman School of Medicine, University of Pennsylvania
Philadelphia, PA, USA

Mohamed Ibrahim, MD, PhD
Assistant Professor
Obstetric Anesthesiology Fellowship Program Director
University of Texas Medical Branch
Galveston, TX, USA

Luiz Eduardo Imbelloni
Professor of Anesthesiology
Director
Institute for Regional Anesthesia Hospital de Base-FAMERP
São José do Rio Preto, SP, Brazil

Samiat Jinadu, MD
Assistant Professor
Department of Anesthesiology and Perioperative Medicine, School of Medicine
Oregon Health and Science University
Portland, OR, USA

Janet Jira, MD
Regional Anesthesiologist
Long Island Jewish Medical Center
New Hyde Park, NY, USA

James Kim, MD
Assistant Professor
Department of Anesthesiology and Critical Care
University of Pennsylvania Health System
Philadelphia, PA, USA

Lisa L. Klesius, MD
Assistant Professor
Division Chief of Regional Anesthesia and Acute Pain Medicine
Department of Anesthesiology
University of Wisconsin School of Medicine and Public Health
Madison, WI, USA

Benjamin Kloesel, MD, MSBS
Assistant Professor
Department of of Anesthesiology
University of Minnesota
M Health Fairview University of Minnesota Masonic Children's Hospital
Minneapolis, MN, USA

Lynn Kohan, MD, MS
Associate Professor
Department of of Anesthesiology
University of Virginia
Charlottesville, VA, USA

Sree Kolli, MD
Staff Anesthesiologist
Department of Anesthesiology, Acute Pain and Regional Anesthesia
Cleveland Clinic
Cleveland, OH, USA

Sandra L. Kopp, MD
Professor of Anesthesiology
Department of Anesthesiology and Perioperative Medicine
Mayo Clinic
Rochester, MN, USA

Michael Kushelev, MD
Assistant Professor
Department of Anesthesiology
Ohio State University Wexner Medical Center
Columbus, OH, USA

Yan Lai, MD, MPH, FASA
Assistant Professor
Department of Anesthesiology
Icahn School of Medicine
Mount Sinai Medical Center
New York, NY, USA

Alina Lazar, MD
Assistant Professor
Department of Anesthesia and Critical Care
University of Chicago
Chicago, IL, USA

Bradley H. Lee, MD
Assistant Attending Anesthesiologist
Hospital for Special Surgery Clinical Instructor of Anesthesiology
Weill Cornell Medical College Department of Anesthesiology
Critical Care and Pain Management Hospital for Special Surgery
New York, NY, USA

Linda Thi Le-Wendling
Associate Professor
Department of Anesthesiology
University of Florida
Florida, FL, USA

Philipp Lirk, MD, MSc, PhD
Associate Professor of Anaesthesia
Department of Anesthesiology, Perioperative and Pain Medicine
Brigham and Women's Hospital
Harvard Medical School
Boston, MA, USA

Jiabin Liu, MD PhD
Associate Attending Anesthesiologist
Hospital for Special Surgery
Clinical Associate Professor
Department of Anesthesiology
Weill Cornell Medical College
New York, NY, USA

Gustavo A. Lozada, MD, MSEd
Clinical Director of Longwood
Massachusetts Eye and Ear
Instructor, Harvard Medical School
Boston, MA, USA

Choopong Luansritisakul, MD
Staff Anesthesiologist
Department of Anesthesiology
Siriraj Hospital
Mahidol University
Bangkok, Thailand

Alvaro Andres Macias, MD
Chief of Anesthesia
Massachusetts Eye and Ear
Assistant Professor
Harvard Medical School
Boston, MA, USA

Marko Mamic, MD
DuPage Valley Anesthesiologists
Department of Anesthesiology
Naperville, IL, USA

Caroline Martinello, MD
Assistant Professor
Department of Anesthesiology
University of Arkansas for Medical Sciences
Little Rock, AR, USA

Jennifer Matos, MD
Assistant Professor
Department of Anesthesia and Perioperative Medicine
Medical University of South Carolina
Charleston, SC, USA

Robert L. McClain, MD
Assistant Professor
Department of Anesthesiology and Perioperative Medicine
Mayo Clinic
Jacksonville, FL, USA

Jamie-Lee Metesky, MD
Assistant Professor
Department of Anesthesiology, Perioperative & Pain Medicine
Mount Sinai Morningside and Mount Sinai West
New York, NY, USA

Jill M. Mhyre, MD
The Dola S. Thompson Professor and Chair
Department of Anesthesiology
University of Arkansas for Medical Sciences
Little Rock, AR, USA

Jeffrey J. Mojica, DO
Clinical Assistant Professor
Department of Anesthesiology
Sidney Kimmel Medical College at Thomas Jefferson University
Philadelphia, PA, USA

Eman Nada, MD, PhD
Associate Professor
Chief of Regional Anesthesia
Department of Anesthesiology
Renaissance School of Medicine
Stony Brook University
Stony Brook, NY, USA

Joseph M. Neal, MD
Emeritus Anesthesiology Faculty
Affiliate Investigator (Benaroya Research Institute)
Virginia Mason Medical Center
Seattle, WA, USA

Mark D. Neuman, MD, MSc
Associate Professor
Department of Anesthesiology and Critical Care
Perelman School of Medicine
University of Pennsylvania
Philadelphia, PA, USA

Maryam Nilforoshan, MD
Assistant Professor
Department of Anesthesiology and Critical Care
Perelman School of Medicine
University of Pennsylvania
Philadelphia, PA, USA

Olga "Kiki" Nin, MD
Clinical Associate Professor
Medical Director
Department of Anesthesiology
Medical Director Florida Surgical center
Florida Surgical Center
University of Florida College of Medicine
Gainesville, FL, USA

Ryan Norman
Fellow
Regional Anesthesiology and Acute Pain Medicine
Massachusetts General Hospital
Harvard Medical School
Boston, MA, USA

Jason B. Ochroch, MD
Assistant Professor
Department of Anesthesiology and Critical Care
Perelman School of Medicine, University of Pennsylvania
Philadelphia, PA, USA

Archana O'Neill, MD
Instructor in Anaesthesia
Department of Anesthesiology, Perioperative and Pain Medicine
Brigham and Women's Hospital
Harvard Medical School
Boston, MA, USA

Amberly Orr, MD
Pain Fellow
Department of Anesthesia and Critical Care
University of Chicago
Chicago, IL, USA

Melissa Brooks Peterson, MD
Associate Professor
Department of Pediatric Anesthesiology
Children's Hospital Colorado
University of Colorado, Anschutz Medical Campus
Aurora, CO, USA

Victor Polshin, MD
Anesthesiologist at Beth-Israel Deaconess Medical Center
Instructor
Harvard Medical School
Boston, MA, USA

Steven B. Porter, MD
Assistant Professor
Department of Anesthesiology and Perioperative Medicine
Mayo Clinic
Jacksonville, FL, USA

Yatish Ranganath, MD
Associate Professor
Division Chief | Regional Anesthesia & Acute Pain Medicine
Department of Anesthesia
Indiana University School of Medicine
Indianapolis, IN, USA

Shanthi Reddy, MD
Anesthesiologist
University of Virginia Health System
Valley Anesthesiology Consultants
Phoenix, AZ, USA

Meg A. Rosenblatt, MD, FASA
Professor of Anesthesiology and Orthopedics
Chair of the Department of Anesthesiology, Perioperative & Pain Medicine
Mount Sinai Morningside and West Hospitals
New York, NY, USA

Engy T. Said, MD
Clinical Associate Professor of Anesthesiology
Division of Regional Anesthesia & Acute Pain
University of California, San Diego
San Diego, CA, USA

Francis V. Salinas, MD
Staff Anesthesiologist
Medical Director
Interventional Platform Swedish Issaquah Hospital
Issaquah, WA, USA

Lauren Sayre, MD
Anesthesiologist
Department of Anesthesiology
Seven Hills Anesthesia, St. Elizabeth Division
Edgewood, KY, USA

Eric S. Schwenk, MD
Associate Professor
Department of Anesthesiology and Orthopedic Surgery
Sidney Kimmel Medical College at Thomas Jefferson University
Philadelphia, PA, USA

Ali N. Shariat, MD
Assistant Professor
Department of Anesthesiology
Perioperative and Pain Medicine
Mount Sinai Morningside Medical Center
Icahn School of Medicine at Mount Sinai
New York, NY, USA

Stanislav Sidash, MD
Assistant Professor
Department of Anesthesiology
Geisel School of Medicine
Dartmouth-Hitchcock Medical Center
Lebanon, NH, USA

Lauren Steffel, MD
Acting Assistant Professor
Department of Anesthesiology
University of Washington
Veterans Affairs Puget Sound Health Care System
Seattle, WA, USA

Cameron Sumner, MD
Anesthesiologist at US Anesthesia Partners
Denver, CO, USA

Reda Tolba, MD
Clinical Professor
Department of Anesthesiology
Cleveland Clinic Lerner College of Medicine, Cleveland
Chair of department of Pain Management, Cleveland Clinic
Abu Dhabi, UAE

Rakesh Vadhera, MD, FRCA, FFARCSI
Professor of Anesthesiology and Director of Obstetric Anesthesia
University of Texas, UTMB
Galveston, TX, USA

Manuel C. Vallejo, MD, DMD
Designated Institutional Official
Associate Dean
Professor of Medical Education, Anesthesiology, Obstetrics and Gynecology
Department of Anesthesiology
West Virginia University School of Medicine
Morgantown, WV, USA

Kamen V. Vlassakov, MD
Chief, Regional and Orthopedic Anesthesiology
Brigham and Women's Hospital
Assistant Professor
Department of Anesthesiology, Perioperative and Pain Medicine
Harvard Medical School
Boston, MA, USA

Richa Wardhan, MD
Associate Professor
Department of Anesthesiology
College of Medicine-University of Florida
Gainesville, FL, USA

Dennis J. Warfield Jr., MD
Assistant Professor of Anesthesiology
Department of Anesthesiology & Perioperative Medicine
Penn State College of Medicine
Hershey, PA, USA

Sean Washek, DO
Clinical Instructor of Anesthesiology
Sidney Kimmel Medical College at Thomas Jefferson University
Philadelphia, PA, USA

Leah Margalit Winters Webb, MD
Assistant Professor
Department of Pediatric Anesthesiology
Children's Hospital Colorado
University of Colorado, Anschutz Medical Campus
Aurora, CO, USA

Matthew Williams, MD
Assistant Professor
Department of Anesthesiology
University of Arkansas for Medical Sciences
Little Rock, AR, USA

Sylvia H. Wilson, MD
Associate Professor
Department of Anesthesia and Perioperative Medicine
Medical University of South Carolina
Charleston, SC, USA

Yury Zasimovich, MD
Assistant Professor
Department of Anesthesiology
University of Florida College of Medicine
Gainesville, FL, USA

Nantthasorn Zinboonyahgoon, MD
Associate Professor
Department of Anesthesiology
Siriraj Hospital
Mahidol University
Bangkok, Thailand

SECTION 1

GENERAL CONSIDERATIONS

Jinlei Li

1.

TOPOGRAPHIC ANATOMY AND PHYSIOLOGIC CONSIDERATIONS

N. Robert Harvey and Sylvia H. Wilson

STEM CASE AND KEY QUESTIONS

A 62-year-old 100-kg male is involved in a motor vehicle collision and sustains bilateral T5–8 rib fractures, a right radius fracture, a small right pneumothorax, and multiple lower extremity lacerations. The intensive care team contacts the regional acute pain service to assist with pain management for the patient's numerous injuries. Specifically, he is hypoventilating and splinting from his four rib fractures. The intensive care team is concerned that the patient will require intubation soon if his rib fracture pain is not promptly controlled.

(1) WHAT SURFACE LANDMARKS MAY ASSIST WITH SELECTING THE OPTIMAL THORACIC LEVEL FOR EPIDURAL ANALGESIA?

As this patient has T5–8 rib fractures, the inferior angles of the scapula are marked to identify T7 spinous process. You then palpate one interspace above and mark the T6–T7 interspace. This anatomic level is further verified by palpating the spinous process at the vertebral prominence at C7. You then palpate down the spine to confirm the previously marked T6–T7 interspace. Last, you palpate the patient's iliac crest as a marker for the L4 spinous process and L4–L5 interspace. The spine is then palpated cephalad to again confirm the T6–T7 interspace. With the T6–T7 interspace confirmed, the patient is prepped and draped for epidural placement.

(2) WHAT IS THE NEURAXIAL ANATOMY TRANSVERSED WITH EPIDURAL PLACEMENT?

Following placement of a subcutaneous local anesthetic (LA) skin wheal, a 17-gauge Tuohy is advanced through the skin, subcutaneous fat, supraspinous ligament, and interspinous ligament. As an increased resistance is noted, a glass syringe with saline is connected to the Tuohy needle and a loss of resistance technique is used to advance the needle through the ligamentum flavum. The saline suddenly is easy to inject at 6 cm and the epidural space is identified. An epidural catheter is easily threaded into the epidural space and the Tuohy needle is removed. As the loss of resistance was noted at 6 cm, the catheter is secured at 11 cm using a sterile, clear, occlusive dressing.

(3) WHAT FACTORS IMPACT THE NEURAXIAL BLOCK HEIGHT?

After negative catheter aspiration for blood and cerebrospinal fluid (CSF), a 3 ml test dose (lidocaine 1.5% with epinephrine 5μg/ml) is administered. The patient's heart rate is stable (70–73 bpm) and he denies perioral numbness, a metallic taste, or any heaviness is his lower extremities or gluteal region. You note that the patient is over 60 years old and an average height at 5′8″. Since the patient has been hemodynamically stable (blood pressure 112/71), he is bolused with 5 ml of 0.15% bupivacaine in two divided aliquots. Vital signs are assessed every 5 minutes and the patient remains hemodynamically stable. A continuous LA infusion (bupivacaine 0.1%) is started at a rate of 6 ml/h.

(4) WHAT SURFACE ANATOMY WOULD INDICATE THE EPIDURAL IS COVERING THE APPROPRIATE DERMATOMES? WHAT METHODS ARE USED TO EVALUATE BLOCK COVERAGE?

After epidural catheter placement and dosing, the patient reports reduced pain at both rest (1/10 from 6/10) and with deep inspiration (3/10 from 10/10). On a physical exam, he has bilateral decreased temperature sensation to ice from the skin at his nipple line to the skin superior to his umbilicus. He maintains normal handgrip, hip flexor, and quadricep muscle strength bilaterally. Last, the patient is able to demonstrate 1500 ml inspiratory volumes consistently using a bedside incentive spirometer with reasonable comfort.

(5) WHAT ARE OTHER REGIONAL ANESTHETIC OPTIONS FOR POLY-TRAUMA PATIENTS?

Now that the patient's pain is well controlled, he asks what regional anesthetic options are possible for his multiple lacerations and fractured radius. As he has multiple injuries in several anatomic areas, you are concerned that performing regional techniques to cover all of his injuries would lead to LA toxicity. You recommend starting systemic non-opioid analgesic medications. You prescribe a combination of scheduled oral acetaminophen, oral gabapentin, and intravenous ketorolac with breakthrough tramadol for moderate pain and oxycodone for severe pain. You assure him that the regional and acute pain service will continue to follow him while his epidural is in place and can reassess his analgesic regimen daily. You also discuss brachial plexus blocks for his radius fracture if oral therapy fails, as this is the area causing the most discomfort now that his ribs are anesthetized.[1]

(6) DESCRIBE THE USE OF LOCAL ANESTHETICS FOR ANALGESIC VERSUS ANESTHETIC BLOCKS.

The patient requires open reduction and internal fixation of his radius fracture the next day. He and his surgeon both wish to avoid general anesthesia given his numerous rib fractures and small pneumothorax. However, he is doing well with his epidural and systemic regimen and does not think he needs an indwelling perineural catheter. You agree and place a single injection, brachial plexus block (axillary approach) for surgical anesthesia using 20 ml of ropivacaine 0.5%. A medical student asks why ropivacaine 0.5% was chosen rather than ropivacaine 0.2% or 1.0% or lidocaine 1.5%. You explain that ropivacaine 0.5% will provide surgical anesthesia coupled with postoperative analgesia for approximately 6–12 hours. Conversely, ropivacaine 0.2% would provide some postoperative analgesia but would not provide a block dense enough to deliver surgical anesthesia. Ropivacaine 1.0% would also provide surgical anesthesia with postoperative pain control, but this patient is also receiving an epidural infusion of LA. Total LA dose delivered to a patient must be considered, especially in patients receiving multiple regional anesthetic techniques. While lidocaine 1.5% could also provide surgical anesthesia, the anesthetic effects would only last 1–2 hours. Thus, lidocaine would provide dense surgical anesthesia, but without the benefit of postoperative pain control for the patient.

DISCUSSION

Comprehension of the relationship between surface anatomy and nervous system is one of the most essential building blocks for regional anesthesia procedures and assessment. Neuraxial techniques, in particular, are an excellent way to understand this relationship.

NEURAXIAL TECHNIQUES

Neuraxial anesthesia has been a common regional technique for over five decades and involves the injection of medicines into the epidural and/or subarachnoid space. Thus epidural, spinal, and combined spinal epidural (CSE) anesthesia represent the different types of regional neuraxial techniques. Neuraxial blocks may be used as the primary anesthetic (e.g., lower extremity arthroplasty or cesarean delivery), to minimize postoperative pain (e.g., esophagectomy or ventral hernia repair), or for analgesia separate from a surgical or interventional procedure (e.g., rib fractures or labor analgesia).

Neuraxial Anatomy

Detailed knowledge of anatomical layers, bones, and ligaments superficial to and surrounding the neuraxis is paramount to avoid complications, expedite procedures, and trouble-shoot techniques in complicated patients. The spine is made up of 24 true (unfused) vertebrae and 9 fused vertebrae (sacral and coccygeal). The first 7 vertebrae are termed cervical and are located in the neck. The next 12 are thoracic and attach to the ribs. The remaining 5 vertebrae are found in the lumbar region. Of note, the spine curves in a convex manner (lordosis) at the cervical and lumbar levels, while it is concave (kyphosis) in the thoracic and sacral portions. Notably, the spinal cord, originating from the foramen magnum, terminates (conus medullaris) at approximately L1 in adults but at L3 in newborns and infants. As neuraxial procedures at the lumbar level have the advantage of being below the conus medullaris, this is an important consideration.

Below the skin and subcutaneous fat, several ligaments provide stability to the vertebral column superficial to the meninges and spinal cord. These are commonly presented in a superficial to deep manner. First, the supraspinous ligament spans the tips of the spinous processes. Between the spinous processes runs the interspinous ligament, which fuses with the supraspinous ligament posteriorly (superficial) and the ligamentum flavum anteriorly (deep). Deep to the ligamentum flavum lie the meninges: dura mater, arachnoid mater, and pia mater (superficial to deep). The epidural space is a potential space deep to the ligamentum flavum and superficial to the dura mater. The subarachnoid space is deep to the arachnoid mater and contains CSF. Notably, further stability to the spine is provided by the anterior and posterior longitudinal ligaments that surround the anterior and posterior vertebral bodies, respectively. These ligaments are not encountered with neuraxial block placement.[2]

Surface Anatomy

As delivery of neuraxial LA to a targeted group of dermatomes can lower drug requirements and medication related side effects, knowledge of surface and dermatomal anatomy is essential for neuraxial procedures. Dermatomes are skin areas that are mainly supplied by sensory (afferent) nerve fibers from a single dorsal spinal nerve root. While dermatomes will be discussed in more detail with neuraxial block assessment, the dermatomes impacted by pain must be considered when selecting a needle insertion site for a neuraxial procedure to deliver analgesia to the appropriate area. While ultrasonography of the neuraxis has experienced growing popularity, neuraxial procedures are classically performed with palpation of surface landmarks and are considered "blind techniques." Consequently, surface landmarks along the posterior spine remain essential to recognize the optimal site for needle insertion.

Four key surface landmarks are utilized to identify the appropriate level to perform neuraxial procedures (Table 1.1). The bony knob palpated in the distal neck is known as the vertebral prominence and represents the C7 spinous process.

Table 1.1 NEURAXIAL LEVELS AND CORRESPONDING ANATOMIC SURFACE LANDMARKS

LEVEL	SURFACE ANATOMY
C7	Vertebral prominence
T7	Inferior angle of scapula
L4	Iliac crest
S2	Posterior, superior iliac spine

While, this landmark is consistent, it can be challenging to palpate in the obese and morbidly obese patient populations. The inferior angle of the scapula represents the T7 spinous process and most commonly establishes the correct interspace for thoracic epidural placement. However, studies have shown that there is patient variability, and the inferior angle of the scapula may also correspond to T6 spinous process (25%), T8 spinous process (18%), and less commonly to T4 spinous process (1%), T5 spinous process (1%), or T9 spinous process (1%).[3] In the lumbar region, the line between iliac crests is termed the intercristal line or Tuffier's line. This landmark corresponds to the level of the L4 spinous process or L4–L5 interspace and is employed for lumbar epidural placement. However, similar to the thoracic spine, anatomic variability is possible and should be anticipated in parturients. In a 2011 study of 45 pregnant women, the intercristal line was noted by ultrasonography to be above the L4–L5 interspace in 100% of subjects. While the intercristal line most often corresponded to immediately below the L2–L3 interspace, it ranged from immediately above the L1–L2 to immediately cephalad to the L4–L5 interspace.[4] Last, a line drawn between the posterior superior iliac spines represents the level of the S2 and the caudal limit of the dural sac for adult patients. When a targeted area of analgesia is required at an interspace other than these four sites, these surface landmarks are first marked and then the spinous processes palpated either cephalad or caudad to identify the desired interspace for needle insertion. Given the anatomic variability between patients, it is advisable to utilize more than one surface landmark when identifying a neuraxial level for needle placement (Figure 1.1).

Neuraxial Block Placement

The midline approach for neuraxial blocks is a popular technique, and the needle transverses several layers before reaching the epidural and subarachnoid spaces. All neuraxial techniques begin with identification of the correct interspace, aseptic preparation of the skin, sterile drape placement, and placement of an LA skin wheal over the intended needle insertion site. For epidural placement, a 17–18 gauge Tuohy needle is inserted at the skin and passed through the subcutaneous fat, supraspinous ligament, interspinous ligament, and ligamentum flavum. Notably, once the needle reaches the interspinous ligament, it often becomes anchored and remains in place without external support. Next, the ligamentum flavum generally conveys an increased resistance, like pushing through a rubber eraser. Since this indicates the ligamentous layer just superficial to the epidural space, the Tuohy is advanced slowly, using a loss of resistance technique to saline or air. Loss of resistance signals entering the epidural space, a potential space between the ligamentum flavum and the dura.[5] After the epidural space is identified, a catheter (19–20 gauge based on the Tuohy size) is threaded. The catheter is often secured 4–5 cm deeper than the depth where the loss of resistance was encountered. This allows for some movement of the epidural catheter as the patient moves, while preserving the catheter in the epidural space. As epidural placement is a "blind" technique, it is important to ensure that the epidural catheter has not been inadvertently threaded into a blood vessel or into the subarachnoid space. This is accomplished with a "test dose" that is most often composed of lidocaine and epinephrine.[6] Intravascular injection of lidocaine is associated with perioral numbness or a metallic taste, while intravascular injection of 10–15 μg epinephrine raises the heart rate 10–15 beats per minute. Conversely, a subarachnoid injection results in heaviness or numbness in the proximal lower extremities or gluteal regions. Patients should be queried for these signs or symptoms and the heart rate should be monitored for changes. Any change in patient sensation or hemodynamics should prompt procedure cessation and further investigation. After a negative test dose, the epidural catheter may be bolused to achieve the desired anesthesia or analgesia. Since dosing of the epidural is likely to cause hemodynamic changes (e.g., hypotension), it is essential that heart rate and blood pressure monitoring occur during this time period and immediately after. In obstetric anesthesia, fetal heart tone monitoring is also advisable.[7]

In a midline-approach subarachnoid block or spinal, the needle is advanced through the same layers as described with epidural placement, but then further advanced through the dura until CSF returns freely.[5] Medication is then injected into the CSF. Common spinal needles are divided into blunt needles (e.g., Whitacre, Sprotte, and Gertie Marx) and cutting needles (e.g., Quincke). Because the dura is punctured in a subarachnoid block, this places the patient at risk for postdural puncture headache (PDPH). While the risk of PDPH is lower with blunt needles, it is also significantly lowered by a smaller needle gauge. As a result, spinal needles are typically 24–27 gauge. To a greater extreme than in epidural anesthesia, hypotension should be anticipated and expected with subarachnoid blocks. Common strategies to mitigate the hypotensive response include co-loading of intravenous fluids at the start of block placement and the initiation of vasopressors (e.g., phenylephrine or norepinephrine) upon successful intrathecal medication injection.[8]

Neuraxial techniques can also be combined. A CSE block allows providers to place a spinal prior to epidural placement. If a CSE is planned, the Tuohy is first placed in the epidural space as described above. The Tuohy then remains in place and an appropriately sized spinal needle (26–27 gauge based on the size and design of the Tuohy needle) is inserted into the Tuohy needle, through the dura, and into the subarachnoid space. Free CSF confirms position, and medications are injected. Following medication injection, the spinal needle is removed but the Tuohy needle left in place. The epidural

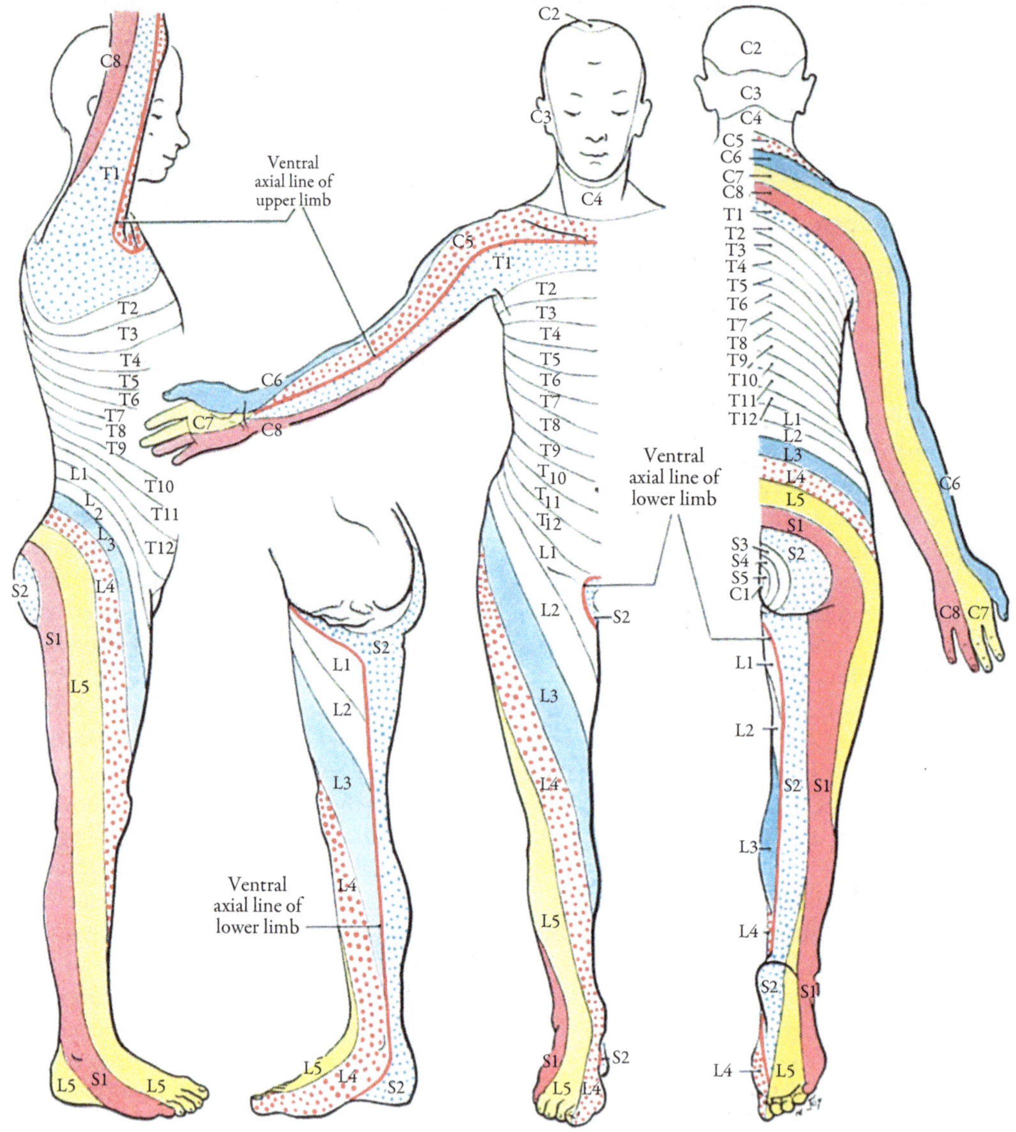

Figure 1.1. Dermatomes.
Grant's Atlas, 1962. Wikipedia, public common domain. Accessed May 8, 2021. https://en.wikipedia.org/wiki/Dermatome_(anatomy)#/media/File:Grant_1962_663.png.

catheter is then threaded and secured as with epidural placement. CSE permits multiple options, as a small LA dose or only opiates may be injected into the CSF to expedite analgesia. Additionally, spinal anesthetic may be placed and the epidural catheter threaded to provide continued anesthesia if the subarachnoid block resolves. A more recent variation of the CSE is a dural puncture epidural (DPE).[8] In this technique, the Tuohy is placed in the epidural space and the dura punctured with the spinal needle, similar to the CSE; however, no medications are injected into the CSF. The spinal needle is removed and the epidural catheter placed, secured, and dosed. Despite the absence of injection of intrathecal medications, DPE has been associated with more rapid onset of labor analgesia and improved block quality (e.g., bilateral coverage and density) compared to a labor epidural without DPE. While DPE does not provide as rapid analgesia as CSE, it is associated with fewer side effects, including less maternal hypotension and fetal bradycardia.[9]

For patients with narrow intervertebral spaces or who have difficulty with flexed positioning, alternatives to the midline approach may be useful. In the paramedian approach, the needle is inserted 1 cm lateral and 1 cm caudal to the traditional midline insertion site. The needle is then advanced in a cephalo-medial direction until loss of resistance is obtained and epidural space identified. With the paramedian technique, the ligamentum flavum is the first ligament encountered, as the needle does not pass through the supraspinous or interspinous ligaments. This technique may also be utilized for spinal anesthesia with the needle advanced until CSF flow is encountered, identifying the subarachnoid space. In the Taylor approach, the paramedian technique is used to enter the L5–S1 interspace. The skin is anesthetized 1 cm medial and 1 cm caudal to the posterior superior iliac spine. The needle is advanced in a cephalo-medial direction at approximately a 55-degree angle. This approach is advantageous since it requires minimal patient flexion; however, it is technically complicated.[10]

Neuraxial Local Anesthetic Spread

Selection of LA type, concentration, and dose depends on the need for analgesia versus surgical anesthesia and block duration required. LA are classified into two main groups: esters and amides (Table 1.2).[10] Amides are metabolized by the liver and generally have longer durations than esters, which are metabolized by pseudocholinesterase. Ester LAs include benzocaine, chloroprocaine, procaine, and tetracaine. Amide LAs include bupivacaine, levobupivacaine, lidocaine, mepivacaine, prilocaine, and ropivacaine.

LAs inhibit nerve conduction by binding with intracellular voltage-gated sodium channels in a reversible fashion. The greatest binding affinity of LAs occurs when the sodium channel is in the open state. When the sodium channel closes, the blinding affinity is the lowest.

For onset, LAs must become unionized and permeate the nerve lipid bilayer to reach the intracellular sodium channels. Thus, speed of onset is related to lipid solubility and pKa. Local anesthetics with a pKa closer to physiologic pH more rapidly reach a unionized state. However, an increased amount of the unionized form can also be achieved with a larger drug dose and to expedite anesthetic onset. A classic example of this is the administration of 20 ml of 3% chloroprocaine (pK_a 8.7) by epidural catheter for emergent cesarean delivery rather than 20 ml of 2% lidocaine (pK_a 7.9) with epinephrine. Despite having a pK_a farther from physiologic pH, chloroprocaine provides a more rapid onset for surgical anesthesia since a 600 mg dose is delivered, compared to a 400 mg dose of lidocaine. Additionally, as lipid-soluble drugs more rapidly cross the nerve cell membrane, the most significant factor in determining potency is lipid solubility or hydrophobicity. More lipophilic molecules are also highly protein bound in the bloodstream, increasing duration of block. Notably, duration is also related to metabolism as esters are rapidly metabolized by pseudocholinesterase and amides more slowly metabolized by the liver.

Understanding neuraxial medication spread is important when administering medications as either a bolus or infusion. Several factors impact the spread of LAs in the epidural and subarachnoid spaces. Consequently, the area anesthetized may vary between patients.

Factors that impact neuraxial spread or block height may be categorized as drug factors, patient factors, and positioning. Above all other factors, the total mass of LA seems to be the most significant factor in determining the extent of sensory, sympathetic, and motor neural blockade. Patient factors resulting in increased neuraxial spread include age and gravity. In lumbar epidurals, several studies have reported spread 3–8 segments higher in patients over 60 years old compared with patients under 40 years old.[11,12] Conversely, in thoracic epidurals, patients over 60 years old consistently have decreased epidural dose requirements (40% less) coupled with increased hemodynamic instability, compared with patients under 40 years old.[13,14] Similarly, parturients require decreased LA doses compared to non-pregnant patients. As increased abdominal pressure results in engorged epidural veins, it is theorized that this explains the decreased neuraxial dose requirements for pregnant patients. However, weight (obesity) does not impact LA spread, and height only impacts spread for extremely short (increased spread) or extremely tall (decreased spread) subjects. Notably, the number of segments blocked does not differ significantly by insertion site (e.g., high thoracic, mid-thoracic, low thoracic, or lumbar) when age and gravity are considered. While the supine and sitting positions do not impact block height when dosing lumbar epidurals, the head-down position (15 degrees) results in an increased block height when dosing lumbar epidurals. In the same way, a sensory block of 0–3 segments produces greater results on the dependent side when epidurals are dosed in the lateral position. No differences are noted in block height for thoracic epidurals, regardless of patient position.[15]

Similar to epidural anesthesia, LA spread, or block height, is also impacted by drug factors, positioning, and patient factors for spinal anesthesia. The primary drug factors impacting block height are dose, baricity, and positioning. Increased LA dose correlates with greater block height. Patient position impacts block spread depending on the baricity utilized. Hyperbaric solutions spread with gravity to more dependent regions, while isobaric injectates spread evenly, and hypobaric

Table 1.2 LOCAL ANESTHETICS FREQUENTLY USED FOR REGIONAL ANESTHESIA[11]

CLASS	PKA	MAX DOSE PLAIN (MG/KG)	MAX DOSE EPINEPHRINE (MG/KG)	ONSET (MINUTES)	DURATION (HOURS)
Ester					
Chloroprocaine	8.7	10	15	5–10	0.5–1.5
Amide					
Bupivacaine	8.1	2.5	2.5	10–15	6–12+
Levobupivacaine	8.1	2.5	2.5	10–15	6–12+
Lidocaine	7.9	5	7	5–10	2–4
Mepivacaine	7.6	5	7	5–10	2–4
Ropivacaine	8.1	2.5	6	10–20	6–12+

injectates spread against gravity. Isobaric solutions are generally not affected by positioning. Conversely, hyperbaric solutions lead to cephalad spread in the Trendelenburg position, but result in a saddle block if the patient is left sitting upright. The opposite occurs with hypobaric solutions, and a lateral position results in denser blockade of the non-dependent side. Neuraxial spread may be increased by patient factors including advanced age and pregnancy. As with epidurals, height is generally a factor only for patients at extreme ends of the spectrum. Scoliosis does not affect blockade spread; however, kyphosis may alter the spread of hyperbaric injectates in supine patients. Injection into the epidural space following a spinal anesthetic (as with a CSE) also appears to increase block height.[2]

Surface Anatomy and Dermatomes for Neuraxial Analgesic Assessment

Dermatomes are skin areas innervated by sensory (afferent) nerve fibers from a single spinal nerve. After epidural or subarachnoid block placement and dosing, loss of sensation must be assessed by dermatomal markers. The relationship between dermatomes and surface landmarks is useful to assess adequate analgesia or anesthesia. For neuraxial block assessment, sensory changes are assessed along dermatomal distributions in a systematic fashion. At the cephalad end and extremes of a block (e.g., cheek, or shoulder of a patient with a mid-thoracic epidural), sensation should be intact and patients should not be able to discern a differential block. Studies have shown that blocks do not terminate completely over the course of one dermatome. Instead, patients report a change in sensation or fading of the block over the course of two dermatomes with the complete loss of cold sensation often extending slightly cephalad by 1–2 dermatomes compared to the loss of light touch and pinprick.[16]

Several dermatomal markers are important for block assessment and for prevention or evaluation of potentially adverse events (Table 1.3). In terms of neuraxial block assessment, the nipple line (T4), xiphoid process (T6), and umbilicus (T10) are commonly used to assess thoracic epidural analgesia. In obstetric anesthesia, the xiphoid process (T6) and umbilicus (T10) are also frequently used to assess adequate anesthesia for cesarean delivery (T6) and labor analgesia (T10), respectively. Remarkably, obstetric analgesia almost exclusively involves lumbar neuraxial techniques, but uses both increased LA volumes combined with the decreased LA requirements needed for parturients to obtain thoracic level anesthesia and analgesia. In regard to adverse event diagnosis, numbness in the hands (C6–C8) or at the level of the sternal notch (C4) likely indicates high neuraxial blockade at or near the level of the phrenic nerve (C3–C5) or cardioaccelerator fibers (T1–T4). These signs and symptoms necessitate prompt diagnosis and changes in management or even interventions to prevent adverse events. Similarly, numbness over the upper thigh (L2–L3) or patella (L4) in patients ambulating with epidural

Table 1.3 DERMATOMES, CORRESPONDING SURFACE LANDMARKS, AND OTHER SIGNIFICANT INDICATIONS[2]

DERMATOME	SURFACE ANATOMY	BLOCK SIGNIFICANCE
C4	Sternal notch	Phrenic nerve likely compromised
C5	Lateral antecubital fossa	Evaluate for phrenic nerve compromise
C6	Thumb	Evaluate for phrenic nerve compromise
C7	Middle finger	Cardioaccelerator fiber blocked
C8	Little finger	Cardioaccelerator fiber blocked
T1	Medial antecubital fossa	Likely some cardioaccelerator fibers blocked
T2	Manubrium	Likely some cardioaccelerator fibers blocked
T3	Axillary apex	
T4	Nipple line	
T6	Xiphoid process	Splanchnic fibers may be blocked (T5–L1)
T10	Umbilicus	Sympathetic nervous system block restricted to lower extremities
T12	Inguinal ligament	No sympathetic nervous system block
L1–2	Anterior, superior thigh	
L4	Patella and medial malleolus	
L5	Third metatarsal	
S1	Little toe	

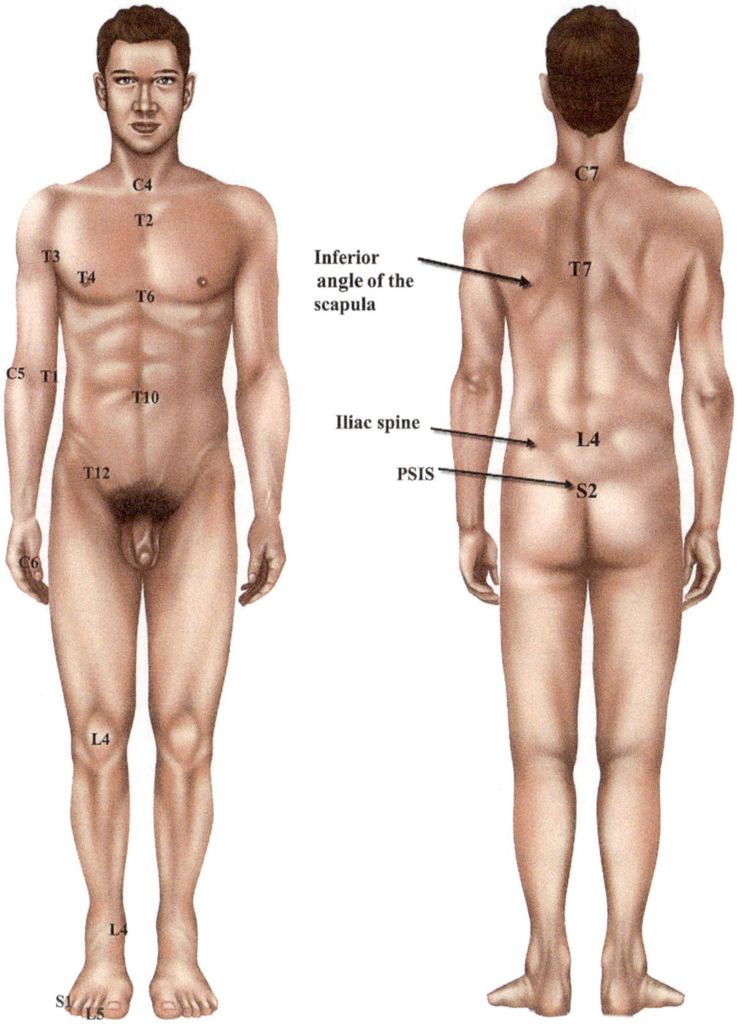

Figure 1.2. Surface anatomy landmarks in relation to dermatomal coverage in neuraxial blocks.

analgesia may indicate a need to decrease the epidural infusion rate to prevent a patient fall. For these reasons and others, dermatomal block distributions should be assessed after neuraxial block placement until block resolution and for the duration of epidural catheter maintenance. Dermatome levels may also be used to assess the density of brachial plexus (C5–T1) or individual peripheral nerve blocks (Figures 1.1 and 1.2).

PERIPHERAL NERVE ANATOMY AND FIBER TYPES

As all regional techniques are commonly evaluated by asking the patient to discern peripheral sensory changes to light touch, cold, or pinprick, it is important to review basic peripheral nerve anatomy and nerve fiber types.

Peripheral nerves refer to the parts of spinal nerves distal to the nerve roots. Each spinal nerve is covered with an outer layer of protective epineurium and contains several fascicles covered by perineurium. Each fascicle is composed of afferent (sensory) and efferent (motor) nerve fibers (axons) with variable sympathetic input. Axons are further encircled by connective tissue containing glial cells termed *endoneurium*. Each fascicle also contains capillaries and fibroblasts. Nerves have a high metabolic activity and may require reliable blood flow. Peripheral nerves' blood supply arises from collateral arterial branches of adjacent arteries that contribute to the vasa nervorum and anastomose to provide an uninterrupted circulation along the course of the nerve. Myelin, derived from Schwann cells, further insulates nerve axons and increases conduction velocity by forcing current to flow through periodic breaks in the myelin sheath termed *nodes of Ranvier*, creating saltatory conduction. LAs block nerve conduction reliably if at least three successive nodes of Ranvier are exposed to adequate concentrations of an LA. Thus, increased concentrations of LAs result in progressive interruption of autonomic, sensory, and motor impulses. Furthermore, LAs placed around a given peripheral nerve diffuse to block the outer fascicles first, before diffusing to the core bundles toward the center of the nerve. As outer fascicles correlate with more proximal sites, proximal structures become anesthetized prior to the more distal areas that correlate with the central nerve fibers.

Peripheral nerves are classified based on function, size, and conduction velocity (Table 1.4). Increased nerve diameter

Table 1.4 NERVE FIBER TYPES[17]

FIBER TYPE	SIZE	CONDUCTION VELOCITY	FUNCTION
A-α and A-β	2–33 microns	30–120 m/sec	Motor and proprioception
A-γ fibers	3–6 micron	15–35 m/sec	Muscle tone
A-δ fibers	1–4 micron	5–25 m/sec	Pain, touch, and temperature
B-fibers	<3micron	3–15 m/sec	Preganglionic sympathetic fibers
C-fibers	0.3–1.3 micron	2 m/sec	Postganglionic sympathetic; afferent sensory (autonomics, pain, and temperature)

and the presence of myelin, which acts as an insulator and promotes saltatory conduction, both increase conduction velocity. The largest myelinated fibers, A-fibers, are able to conduct motor and sensory signals at high speeds. The fastest and largest of these are A-α and A-β fibers, which conduct proprioception and motor signals. A-γ fibers are slightly smaller and supply muscle tone by innervating the muscle spindle. Last, A-δ fibers convey afferent information concerning pain, touch, and temperature. Notably, light touch is mediated by A-β fibers, whereas pinprick and cold are both mediated by A-δ fibers.[17] Nerve fibers carrying autonomic information, B- and C-fibers, are smaller than A-fibers. B-fibers are preganglionic sympathetic fibers and the smallest myelinated nerves. The smallest of all fibers are C-fibers, which are unmyelinated and carry postganglionic sympathetic and afferent sensory information. Note that while A-δ fibers and C-fibers respond to pain, A-δ fibers respond to early, superficial pain and require a rapid response. Conversely, C-fibers react to late, intense noxious stimuli that may be chemical, mechanical, or thermal.[17]

PERIPHERAL NERVE BLOCKS

Regional anesthesia can provide significant analgesia to patients both in and out of the operating room. In addition to neuraxial blocks, common regional techniques include plexus blocks, selective peripheral nerves blocks, and plane blocks.

BRACHIAL PLEXUS

The brachial plexus provides motor and sensory information to and from the upper extremity, back, and chest. Formed from the spinal nerve roots of C5–T1, the plexus is organized into roots, trunks, divisions, cords, and branches. The spinal nerve roots pass through the intervertebral foramina to form the superior (C5–C6), middle (C7), and inferior (C8–T1) trunks. The long thoracic nerve is also formed from contributions from C5–C7 nerve roots, while the subclavian and suprascapular nerves arise from the superior trunk. The cords then form from anterior and posterior divisions from the three trunks. The lateral cord arises from the anterior divisions of the superior and middle trunks, while the medial cord is formed by the anterior division of the inferior trunk. The posterior cord is formed by the contributions from the posterior divisions of all three trunks. The lateral cord further divides into the musculocutaneous, lateral root of the median and lateral pectoral nerves. The medial cord gives rise to the ulnar, medial root of the median, medial pectoral, medial antebrachial cutaneous, and medial brachial cutaneous nerves. Finally, the posterior cord gives off the radial, axillary, thoracodorsal, inferior subscapular, and superior subscapular nerves[2] (Figure 1.3).

Approaches to brachial plexus blocks are generally described by their anatomical block location. The interscalene approach blocks roots C5–C7 between the anterior and middle scalene muscles. In the supraclavicular approach, the block is placed above the clavicle as the trunks-divisions lie lateral to the subclavian artery just above the first rib. The infraclavicular approach blocks the cords below the clavicle as they surround the infraclavicular artery. Finally, the axillary approach involves LA injection at the level of the axilla as the median, ulnar, and radial nerves surround the axillary artery, while the musculocutaneous nerve is superior-lateral in the muscular plane between the biceps and the coracobrachialis muscles.[18]

LUMBAR PLEXUS AND SACRAL PLEXUS

The lumbar and sacral plexuses are closely related, with each giving contribution to the other with high variability.

The lumbar plexus is formed from spinal nerve roots of L1–L5. Iliohypogastric and ilioinguinal nerves arise from T12–L1, while the genitofemoral nerve is formed by L1–L2 and the lateral femoral cutaneous nerve of the thigh from L2–L3. Both the obturator and femoral nerves receive contributions from L2–L4. The lumbar plexus is commonly blocked for hip and proximal leg procedures, although the gluteal and posterior thigh regions will be spared as these arise from the sacral plexus. The femoral nerve and its distal branch, the saphenous nerve, are often blocked for knee analgesia. Notably, the saphenous nerve is the only branch of the lumbar plexus that innervates areas below the knee. This sensory branch covers the medial leg and ankle and must be blocked for medial ankle coverage[2] (Figure 1.4).

The sacral plexus is formed by the spinal nerve roots of S1–S5, with contribution from L4–L5 in the form of the

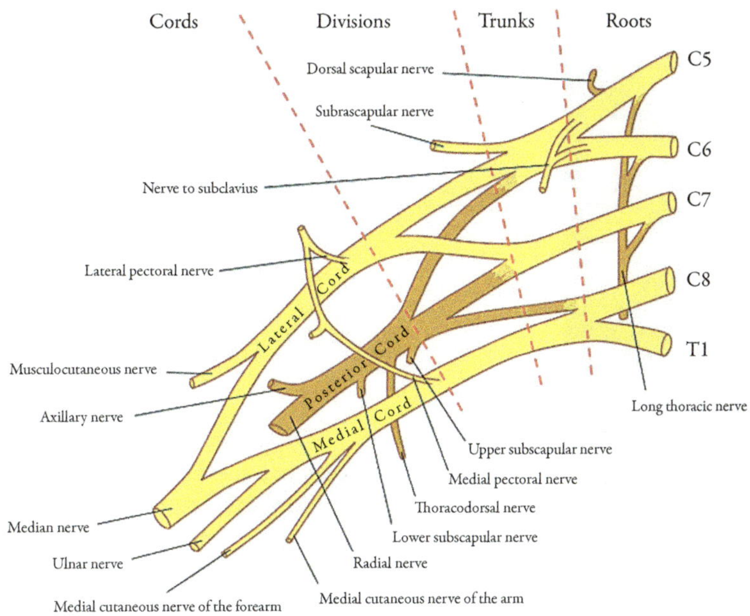

Figure 1.3. Brachial plexus anatomy illustration.
Modified by Mattopaedia from the 1918 edition of *Gray's Anatomy*. Wikipedia Public Domian. Accessed May 8, 2021. https://en.wikipedia.org/wiki/File.

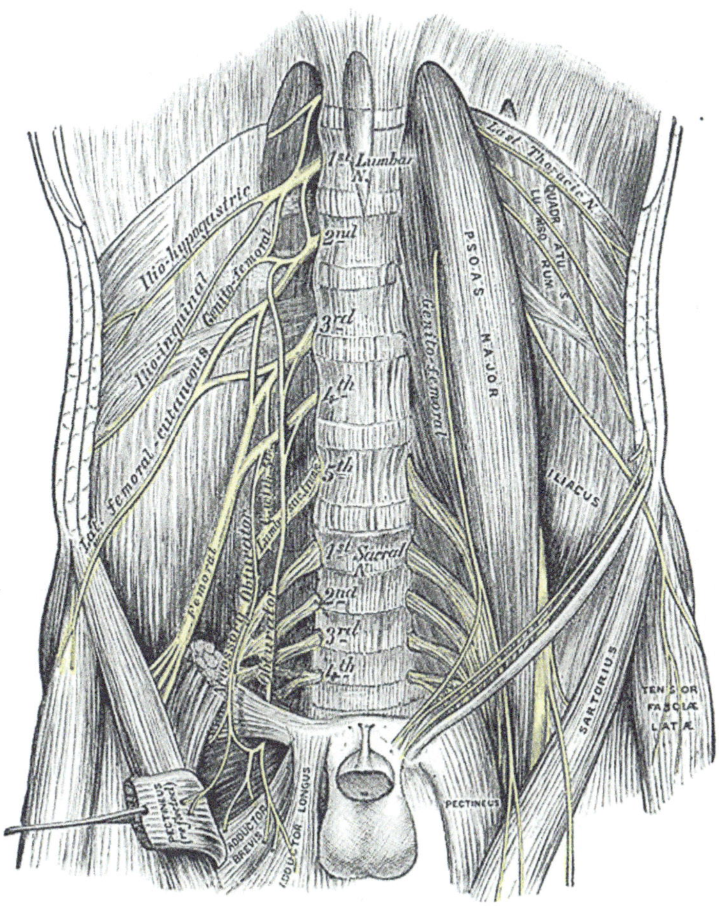

Figure 1.4. Lumbar plexus anatomy.
Henry Gray, *Anatomy of the Human Body* (1918). Wikipedia Public Domain. Accessed May 8, 2021. https://en.wikipedia.org/wiki/Radiation-induced_lumbar_plexopathy#/media/File:Gray823.png.

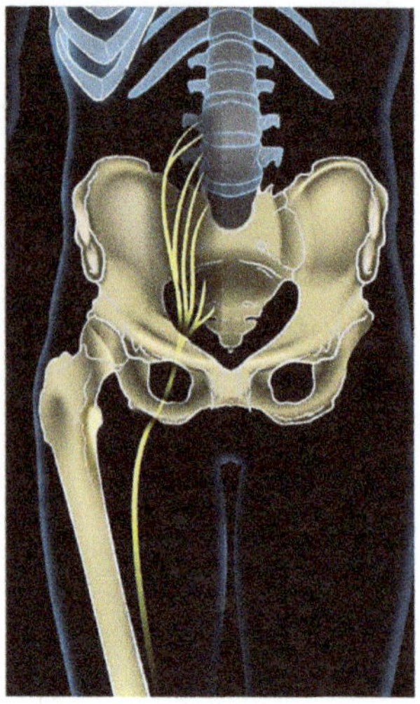

Figure 1.5. Sacral plexus and sciatic nerve.
Wikimedia Commons. Accessed May 8, 2021. https://en.wikipedia.org/wiki/Sciatic_nerve#/media/File:Sciatic_nerve2.jpg.

lumbosacral trunk (Figure 1.5). The largest and longest nerve in the body, the sciatic nerve (L4–S3), arises from the sacral plexus and later divides into the common fibular (peroneal) and tibial nerves proximal to the popliteal fossa. Notably, the sciatic nerve innervates the entire lower leg and foot below the knee, with the exception of the medial leg and ankle which is innervated by the saphenous nerve, a branch of the femoral nerve. Other major nerves arising from the sacral plexus include superior gluteal (L4–S1), inferior gluteal (L5–S2), and posterior femoral cutaneous (S1–S3) nerves. Nerves to quadratus femoris (L4–S1), inferior gemellus (L4–S1), obturator internus (L5–S2), superior gemellus (L5–S2), and piriformis (S1–S2) also arise from the sacral plexus. The sciatic nerve is commonly blocked for anesthesia and analgesia. While the Labat and parasacral approaches cover the sciatic nerve and additional portions of the sacral plexus, the popliteal approach is quite popular for superficial location and ease of block placement.[2]

SELECTIVE PERIPHERAL NERVE BLOCKS

Selective peripheral nerve block may be used to target analgesia for a specific nerve. This may be preferred in order to preserve proximal motor function. Adductor canal blocks are commonly used to target the saphenous nerve and achieve knee analgesia while minimizing the quadriceps weakness observed with a femoral nerve block. Alternatively, selective peripheral nerve blocks may be chosen to augment a plexus block that is not sufficient. For example, a distal median nerve block at the elbow may be used to supplement a brachial plexus block if analgesia is inadequate in the median distribution.

PLANE BLOCKS

Plane blocks are a more recent regional phenomenon. They involve injection of LA into an intramuscular plane rather than directing the injection in the area of a specific nerve or group of nerves. Types include serratus anterior plane (SAP), pectoralis (PEC I and II), transverse abdominis plane (TAP), quadratus lumborum (QL), and erector spinae (ESP) blocks, to name a few. Generally, these blocks are easily taught and performed with less risk of nerve injury as they deliver LA in an intramuscular plane. Conversely, since LAs are not delivered in a targeted fashion near the neuraxis, a plexus, or a target peripheral nerve, the analgesic impact may not be as profound. However, plane blocks may offer a reasonable alternative for analgesia to patients who are not candidates for deeper plexus or neuraxial techniques.

BLOCK SELECTION

Regional anesthesia techniques are chosen based on patient and surgical factors. Patient factors include comorbidities or anticoagulation status. In cases of anticoagulation, certain regional techniques may still be appropriate while others are contraindicated. Surgical factors must also be evaluated. These factors include the location of surgery and the need for neurologic assessment in the postoperative period.

LOCAL ANESTHESIA INFILTRATION

LA infiltration may also be performed by a surgeon during a surgical procedure for postoperative analgesia, intraoperative analgesia, or to supplement a regional technique. Advantages of infiltration include low cost, technical ease compared to other regional techniques, less motor blockade than other regional techniques, and relative lack of contraindications. Disadvantages include a short duration of analgesia, need for a high volume of LA, inadequate analgesia in areas without complete infiltration, and possible toxicity to surrounding structures. Notably, the high LA volume required may inhibit the use of other regional anesthesia options postoperatively and possibly increase the risk of local anesthetic systemic toxicity (LAST). Finally, infiltration may be ineffective at surgical sites with ongoing infections due to the decreased pH of the surrounding tissues rendering the LAs ineffective.[19]

RISKS OF REGIONAL ANESTHESIA PROCEDURES

Adverse outcomes for regional anesthesia are rare but can be catastrophic for patients; therefore, informed consent is essential. The most common risks include infection, bleeding, reactions to medications, and injury to structures below the skin. Infectious risks can range from a superficial cellulitis at the skin to an epidural abscess or meningitis.[20] Bleeding risks must be assessed by the type of block and the patient's coagulation status. The American Society of Regional Anesthesia and other societies have published guidelines to assist with decision-making for patients with altered coagulation.[21,22] These guidelines should be reviewed and understood prior to offering patients any regional technique. Reactions to medications for regional anesthesia can vary from the expected hypotension with spinal anesthesia to an unintentional high spinal or LAST. The knowledge to diagnose and treat these must be in the repertoire of every regional anesthesiologist. Specific to LAST, intralipid should be immediately available at any site where regional anesthesia is administered, and treatment guidelines with a checklist should be on every regional supply cart.[23] Finally, needle insertion can result in trauma to structures below the skin including muscles, blood vessels, and nerves. Dural puncture with epidural insertion can lead to post-dural puncture headache. Although neural injury is rare, any nerve injury, even transiently, can cause emotional distress to the patient, and the risk must be discussed prior to block placement.

REGIONAL ANESTHESIA VERSUS ANALGESIA

The decision whether to place an analgesic versus an anesthetic block depends on surgical procedure, contraindications, and patient-specific factors.[24] Some procedures are well tolerated under a regional anesthesia technique, while others are not. Similarly, a need for early neurological assessment in the immediate postoperative period may make some regional techniques less desirable. Additionally, patient factors may impede or complicate the ability to perform a regional block. While individual patient anatomy may make some regional blocks more challenging, ultrasonography may assist with patient-specific anatomical evaluation. However, certain comorbidities may be contraindicated with specific regional blocks (e.g., spinal anesthesia in a patient with severe aortic stenosis or patients taking potent anticoagulants). Occasionally, low patient weights may limit total LA dose, making surgical blocks unattainable. This may occur more often in the extreme geriatric and pediatric populations. In these cases, regional analgesia for postoperative pain control should still be considered and discussed in cases where surgical anesthesia is not possible or contraindicated.

Analgesic blocks often utilize decreased concentrations of LAs (e.g., ropivacaine 0.2% for analgesia rather than 0.5% for surgical anesthesia). They provide pain relief and decreased sensation, but do not provide sufficient block density for a surgical procedure.[17] In situations in which peripheral or neuraxial techniques are contraindicated, systemic analgesic medications and infiltration of LA at the surgical site may attenuate patient discomfort.

CONCLUSIONS

- A detailed understanding of anatomy is essential prior to performing any regional technique.
- Assessment of both neuraxial and peripheral nerve blocks require comprehension of dermatomal distributions and peripheral nerve innervation.
- Patient factors and procedure factors must both be accounted for when selecting a regional technique to ensure adequate anesthesia and analgesia and minimize patient risk.

REFERENCES

1. Capdevila M, Ramin S, Capdevila X. Regional anesthesia and analgesia after surgery in ICU. *Curr Opin Crit Care.* 2017;23(5):430–439.
2. Miller RD. *Miller's Anesthesia.* 8th ed. Philadelphia, PA: Elsevier/Saunders; 2015.
3. Ambulkar R, Patil V, Doctor JR, Desai M, Shetty N, Agarwal V. Accuracy of ultrasound imaging versus manual palpation for locating the intervertebral level. *J Anaesthesiol Clin Pharmacol.* 2017;33(3):348–352.
4. Margarido CB, Mikhael R, Arzola C, Balki M, Carvalho JC. The intercristal line determined by palpation is not a reliable anatomical landmark for neuraxial anesthesia. *Can J Anaesth.* 2011;58(3):262–266.
5. Chin KJ, Karmakar MK, Peng P. Ultrasonography of the adult thoracic and lumbar spine for central neuraxial blockade. *Anesthesiology.* 2011;114(6):1459–1485.
6. Guay J. The epidural test dose: a review. *Anesth Analg.* 2006;102(3):921–929.
7. Lappen JR, Myers SA, Bolden N, Mercer BM, Chien EKS. Maternal pulse pressure and the risk of postepidural complications: a randomized controlled trial. *Obstet Gynecol.* 2017;130(6):1366–1376.
8. Fitzgerald JP, Fedoruk KA, Jadin SM, Carvalho B, Halpern SH. Prevention of hypotension after spinal anaesthesia for caesarean section: a systematic review and network meta-analysis of randomised controlled trials. *Anaesthesia.* 2020 Jan;75(1):109–121.
9. Wilson SH, Wolf BJ, Bingham K, et al. Labor analgesia onset with dural puncture epidural versus traditional epidural using a 26-gauge Whitacre needle and 0.125% bupivacaine bolus: a randomized clinical trial. *Anesth Analg.* 2018;126(2):545–551.
10. Taylor JA. Lumbosacral subarachnoid tap. *J Urol.* 1940;43(4):561.
11. Wilson SH, Anderson MA. Local anesthetics and regional anesthesia. In: Reves JG, SR Barnett, JR McSwain, GA Rooke, eds. *Geriatric Anesthesiology.* 3rd ed. New York: Springer Science+Business Media; 2018:303–319.
12. Simon MJ, Veering BT, Stienstra R, van Kleef JW, Burm AG. The effects of age on neural blockade and hemodynamic changes after epidural anesthesia with ropivacaine. *Anesth Analg.* 2002;94(5):1325–1330.
13. Hoyle J, Yentis SM. Assessing the height of block for caesarean section over the past three decades: trends from the literature. *Anaesthesia.* 2015;70(4):421–428.
14. Wink J, Wolterbeek R, Aarts LP, Koster SC, Versteegh MI, Veering BT. Upper thoracic epidural anaesthesia: effects of age on neural blockade and cardiovascular parameters. *Acta Anaesthesiol Scand.* 2013;57(6):767–775.
15. Yokoyama M, Hanazaki M, Fujii H, et al. Correlation between the distribution of contrast medium and the extent of blockade during epidural anesthesia. *Anesthesiology.* 2004;100(6):1504–1510.
16. Camorcia M, Capogna G. Sensory assessment of epidural block for Caesarean section: a systematic comparison of pinprick, cold and touch sensation. *Eur J Anaesthesiol.* 2006;23(7):611–617.
17. Curatolo M, Petersen-Felix S, Arendt-Nielsen L. Sensory assessment of regional analgesia in humans: a review of methods and applications. *Anesthesiology.* 2000;93(6):1517–1530.
18. Mian A, Chaudry I, Huang R, Rizk E, Tubbs RS, Loukas M. Brachial plexus anesthesia: a review of the relevant anatomy, complications, and anatomical variations. *Clin Anat.* 2014;27(2):210–221.
19. Moiniche S, Mikkelsen S, Wetterslev J, Dahl JB. A qualitative systematic review of incisional local anaesthesia for postoperative pain relief after abdominal operations. *Br J Anaesth.* 1998;81(3):377–383.
20. Practice advisory for the prevention, diagnosis, and management of infectious complications associated with neuraxial techniques: an updated report by the American Society of Anesthesiologists Task Force on Infectious Complications Associated with Neuraxial Techniques and the American Society of Regional Anesthesia and Pain Medicine. *Anesthesiology.* 2017;126(4):585–601.

21. Horlocker TT, Vandermeuelen E, Kopp SL, Gogarten W, Leffert LR, Benzon HT. Regional anesthesia in the patient receiving antithrombotic or thrombolytic therapy: American Society of Regional Anesthesia and Pain Medicine evidence-based guidelines (fourth edition). *Reg Anesth Pain Med.* 2018;43(3):263–309.
22. Leffert L, Butwick A, Carvalho B, et al. The Society for Obstetric Anesthesia and Perinatology consensus statement on the anesthetic management of pregnant and postpartum women receiving thromboprophylaxis or higher dose anticoagulants. *Anesth Analg.* 2018;126(3):928–944.
23. Neal JM, Woodward CM, Harrison TK. The American Society of Regional Anesthesia and Pain Medicine checklist for managing local anesthetic systemic toxicity: 2017 version. *Reg Anesth Pain Med.* 2018;43(2):150–153.
24. Bonnet F, Marret E. Influence of anaesthetic and analgesic techniques on outcome after surgery. *Br J Anaesth.* 2005;95(1):52–58.

REVIEW QUESTIONS

(1) What surface landmark is most often used to guide the needle insertion site for thoracic epidural placement?

A. Vertebral prominence
B. Nipple line
C. Scapular ridge
D. Inferior tip of scapula

(2) Which dermatome typically corresponds to the umbilicus?

A. T4
B. T6
C. T10
D. L2

(3) Decreased sensation to cold over the patella would indicate blockade of which nerve root?

A. T1
B. T12
C. L4
D. S3

(4) Through which ligament does the Tuohy needle pass just prior to entering the epidural space?

A. Supraspinous
B. Interspinous
C. Ligamentum flavum
D. Anterior cruciate

(5) Which nerve fibers exhibit the fastest conduction velocities?

A. Large myelinated
B. Large unmyelinated
C. Small myelinated
D. Small unmyelinated

(6) Which nerve root does NOT contribute to the brachial plexus?

A. C5
B. C6
C. T1
D. T2

(7) Which nerve arises from the lumbar plexus and provides innervation in the lower leg, below the knee?

A. Iliohypogastric
B. Ilioinguinal
C. Lateral femoral cutaneous
D. Saphenous

(8) At what pK_a will local anesthetics most rapidly cross the lipid bilayer?

A. 6.5
B. 7.0
C. 7.5
D. 8.0

(9) Hypobaric bupivacaine is injected in the subarachnoid space at the L3–4 interspace. If the patient lays in left lateral position (left side down), which of the following directions describes the predominant direction of local anesthetic spread?

A. Caudad
B. Cephalad
C. Left
D. Right

(10) Regional anesthesia by brachial plexus block is planned for open repair of a metacarpal fracture. Which of the following best describes is the lowest concentration of ropivacaine to provide surgical anesthesia?

A. 1.0%
B. 0.5%
C. 0.375%
D. 0.25%

ANSWERS

(1) **D.** The tips of the scapulae are often used as the landmark to place thoracic epidurals, as they most commonly align with the T7 interspace. Interspaces may be palpated and counted up or down, depending on the desired level for epidural placement. The vertebral prominence is at C7, and this landmark may be helpful to confirm a level counted from the tips of the scapulae. The nipple line is associated with the T4 dermatome, but is of limited utility in neuraxial placement due to its anterior location. The scapular ridge or spine of the scapula is aligned with T3 at the root of the spine of the scapula; however, this landmark may be more difficult to palpate and may vary more with patient positioning or movement.

Reference

Ambulkar R, Patil V, Doctor JR, Desai M, Shetty N, Agarwal V. Accuracy of ultrasound imaging versus manual palpation for locating the intervertebral level. *J Anaesthesiol Clin Pharmacol.* 2017;33(3):348–352.

(2) **C.** The umbilicus corresponds to the T10 dermatome. T4 corresponds to the nipple, T6 corresponds to the xiphoid process, and L2 corresponds to the anterior thigh.

Reference

Miller RD. *Miller's Anesthesia.* 8th ed. Philadelphia, PA: Elsevier/Saunders; 2015.

(3) **C.** Decreased sensation to cold over the patella would correspond to blockade of the L4 nerve fibers. T1 corresponds to the antecubital fossa. T12 corresponds between the umbilicus at T10 and the groin (L1). S3 corresponds to the peri-anal area.

Reference

Miller RD. *Miller's Anesthesia.* 8th ed. Philadelphia, PA: Elsevier/Saunders; 2015.

(4) **C.** The ligamentum flavum is the tough ligament passed through just before entering the epidural space, often known for a distinct increase in resistance just before encountering the loss of resistance of the epidural space. The supraspinous ligament runs along the tips of the spinous processes. The interspinous ligament runs between the spinous processes and is firm enough to anchor the Tuohy needle without requiring external support. The anterior cruciate ligament is in the knee.

Reference

Chin KJ, Karmakar MK, Peng P. Ultrasonography of the adult thoracic and lumbar spine for central neuraxial blockade. *Anesthesiology.* 2011;114(6):1459–1485.

(5) **A.** Large myelinated fibers exhibit the highest conduction velocities, 30–120 m/sec. The largest are the A-(fibers and the A-β fibers which carry motor and proprioception information. Factors increasing conduction velocity include large fiber size and the presence of myelin. Myelin acts as an insulator, allowing the conduction to skip from myelin cell to myelin cell, resulting in saltatory conduction.

Reference

Curatolo M, Petersen-Felix S, Arendt-Nielsen L. Sensory assessment of regional analgesia in humans: a review of methods and applications. *Anesthesiology.* 2000;93(6):1517–1530.

(6) **D.** T2 does not contribute to the brachial plexus. T2 gives sensation to the chest wall, axilla, and the medial upper arm. The brachial plexus is formed by contributions from C5, C6, C7, C8, and T1.

Reference

Miller RD. *Miller's Anesthesia.* 8th ed. Philadelphia, PA: Elsevier/Saunders; 2015.

(7) **D.** The lower leg is innervated (both motor and sensory) exclusively by branches of the sciatic nerve, except for the medial portion. The saphenous nerve, an extension of the femoral nerve below the knee, provides sensory input to the medial lower leg and ankle. It does not have motor input.

Reference

Miller RD. *Miller's Anesthesia.* 8th ed. Philadelphia, PA: Elsevier/Saunders; 2015.

(8) **C.** Local anesthetics with a pK_a closest to physiologic pH, 7.4, will demonstrate the most rapid onset. Local anesthetics must cross the lipid bilayer of the cell to reach their site of action, the Na^+ channels. A pK_a close to the physiologic pH allows the LA to convert to its un-ionized state more rapidly.

Reference

Wilson SH, Anderson MA. Local anesthetics and regional anesthesia. In. Reves JG, SR Barnett, JR McSwain, GA Rooke, ed. *Geriatric anesthesiology.* 3rd ed. New York: Springer Science+Business Media; 2018:303–319.

(9) **D.** Local anesthetic movement within the CSF is determined by baricity. Hypobaric solutions are less dense than the surrounding CSF, and thus will move against gravity. In this patient, the left side is down so the hypobaric bupivacaine will move against gravity to the right side (up side).

Reference

Miller RD. *Miller's Anesthesia.* 8th ed. Philadelphia, PA: Elsevier/Saunders; 2015.

(10) **B.** Analgesic blocks utilize a lower concentration of local anesthetic to provide pain relief, but are not dense enough to tolerate surgical procedures. Increasing concentration of local anesthetic increases the density of the block, allowing for surgical manipulation. A concentration of 0.5% ropivacaine would provide adequate density for an anesthetic block. A 1% ropivacaine solution would increase likelihood of neurotoxicity and also for a potential LAST reaction.

Reference

Curatolo M, Petersen-Felix S, Arendt-Nielsen L. Sensory assessment of regional analgesia in humans: a review of methods and applications. *Anesthesiology.* 2000;93(6):1517–1530.

2.

PERIOPERATIVE CONSIDERATIONS FOR SUCCESS OF REGIONAL ANESTHESIA

Richa Wardhan and Janet Jira

STEM CASE AND KEY QUESTIONS

A 65-year-old patient with a history of hypertension, hypercholesterolemia, diabetes, and osteoarthritis presents to the hospital for a right below-knee amputation. Patient has been seen by the preoperative anesthesia clinic and in agreement with the surgeon is expecting to receive a general anesthetic for surgery with sciatic nerve catheter and a femoral nerve catheter for postoperative pain management.

(1) WHAT ARE THE KEY ELEMENTS IN PREPARING A PATIENT FOR A PERIPHERAL NERVE BLOCK FOR POSTOPERATIVE PAIN MANAGEMENT?

When patients receive timely information regarding nerve blocks at the surgeon's office, they are less likely to be apprehensive on the day of surgery. Discussion regarding the nerve block should start at the surgeon's office.

The patient should be scheduled to arrive an hour to two hours in advance if the perineural catheter is to be placed. Arrival of the patient earlier than the scheduled time for their surgery provides the extra time needed to place the nerve block.

An organized acute pain team is key in accomplishing the goals of pain management without placing excessive strain on the infrastructure. A well-established acute pain team includes anesthesiologists, surgeons, nurses, and physical therapists.[1]

A succinct time-out checklist prior to nerve block placement is helpful in preventing mistakes and complications. The critical items on a nerve block time-out sheet should include the site of surgery, updated and valid surgical and anesthesia consents, and allergies. The "Safe Surgery Saves Lives" project developed by the World Health Organization (WHO) designed a 19-item perioperative surgical checklist to minimize the risk of adverse events during non-cardiac surgery. It advises practitioners to address surgical issues orally at three time points: "sign-in," "time-out," and "sign out." Studies using this checklist have shown a significant decrease in both surgery-related complications and patient deaths.[2]

A dedicated, supportive, and trained nursing staff is the mainstay of a block procedure. Sedation administered safety increases patient satisfaction and block success. Deep sedation or general anesthesia in adults adds risk of unintended intraneural injection without the patient having the ability to communicate pain/paresthesia when the needle is placed in the wrong location.[3]

(2) WHAT DOCUMENTS ARE WARRANTED IN ORDER TO SAFELY CONDUCT A REGIONAL ANESTHETIC PREOPERATIVELY?

History and physical examination (H&P) from the surgeon, a preoperative note from the anesthesiologist, a surgical consent, and an anesthesiology consent should all be available and accurate prior to proceeding with a nerve block procedure preoperatively. The procedure should absolutely not commence without surgical and anesthesia (verbal or written) consent. Informed consent is a legal requirement before performance of any medical/surgical procedure, except for emergency situations. Proceeding with an elective procedure without consent constitutes assault.[4] Nerve blocks are almost never an emergency procedure; therefore the proceduralist is ethically and legally obligated to obtain consent. In obtaining consent it is important to ensure that the patient is competent and has adequate decision-making capacity.

Consent can be written or verbal. A written consent serves as evidence that consent was obtained, assuming that the patient had adequate capacity and information and there was no coercion.[4]

Elements of consent include *capacity*, *disclosure*, and *voluntariness*:[5]

- *Capacity* refers to the patient's ability to understand information offered to them and to make decisions regarding their care.
- *Disclosure* is the process by which physicians describe the procedure in terms that are comprehensible to the patient, including alternatives and their associated benefits and risks.
- *Voluntariness* demands that a patient is allowed to consent or dissent without any coercion, allowing for patient autonomy.

It is worth noting that there is broad variability in consent requirements across various institutions.[4] For instance, at our institution the anesthesia team obtains a written anesthesia consent separate from the surgical consent. At some institutions, a written anesthesia consent is not required; by signing the surgical consent it is implied that the patient also consents for anesthesia as it is necessary for surgery.[5,6] In such cases, even though a written consent is not needed, it is important that the anesthesiologist discuss the anesthesia plan, including its associated benefits, risks, and alternatives, with the patient to afford the patient an opportunity to participate in decision-making as far as the anesthetic plan is concerned.

(3) HOW IMPORTANT IS PATIENT SELECTION FOR A PERINEURAL PROCEDURE? SHOULD ONE CONSIDER DEEP SEDATION OR GENERAL ANESTHESIA FOR IT?

To deeply sedate versus not is a complex yet controversial topic in the field of regional anesthesia. While paresthesia may be directly related to the patient's anxiety, caution is advised in deeply sedating patients, especially during neuraxial or close to neuraxis blocks (spinal, epidural, lumbar plexus, and interscalene blocks). Deep sedation inhibits early recognition of intravascular or intraneuraxial injection. The American Society of Regional Anesthesia's (ASRA's) practice advisory on neurological complications suggests that regional anesthetic or pain blocks should not be performed in adults with concurrent general anesthesia or heavy sedation except in those circumstances when the physician and patient conclude that benefit clearly outweighs risk.[7]

Reassuring the patient is paramount in this situation. At our institute, we describe light sedation as being comfortable and unconcerned while the procedure is in progress. Most patients are instantly reassured upon hearing this. If the patient continues to request general anesthesia, then risk and benefits should be weighed. If the block is "non-essential" and primarily used for postoperative pain management, then it should be omitted even if it means that the patient will need to be admitted overnight for pain management.

(4) WHAT AGENTS CAN BE USED FOR INTRAVENOUS SEDATION TO A PATIENT FOR SAFE PLACEMENT OF A PERINEURAL BLOCK?

The choice of sedation agents is influenced by the patient's baseline mental status and medical comorbidities. At our institution we use midazolam and alfentanil for patients who are relatively healthy, with no severe cardiopulmonary compromise. Both have relatively quick onsets and short durations of action, which makes them perfect for nerve block procedures. These agents are titrated to patient comfort while ensuring adequate spontaneous respirations and hemodynamic profile.

In case the patient becomes disinhibited, or is uncooperative, deeper sedation with anesthetic agents such as propofol/ketamine becomes necessary. Before administering deep sedation, we have to ascertain the presence of airway management equipment, and an anesthesiologist, in addition to the block proceduralist, capable of managing the airway and ensuring adequate oxygenation, ventilation, and stable hemodynamics.

DISCUSSION

NERVE STIMULATION

A nerve stimulator is used to localize a nerve prior to local anesthetic or catheter insertion. The ability of a nerve stimulator to elicit a motor response depends on the distance of the stimulus from the nerve, and the intensity and duration of the current used.[8] A motor response can only be elicited with a stimulating current of low intensity (0.1 mA) when the needle is in contact with the nerve, whereas a current of a much higher intensity (2.5 mA) is required to stimulate the nerve when the needle is approximately 2.5 cm away.[8] An accurate current in the range of electrical output now recommended for peripheral perineurals is 0.1–0.5 mA for best outcomes.[9]

The frequency of the stimulating current varies between 1 and 5 Hz. Longer pauses are required between stimuli at 1 versus 2 Hz or more. Therefore, the needle should be advanced slowly when using a stimulator with a 1-Hz frequency in order to avoid missing or impaling the nerve.[10] Maximum voltage output of around 1 mA is enough for most patients to elicit a motor response. However, patients with nerve conduction issues, especially those with diabetes, may require higher voltage to evoke a response.

Knowing the equipment has the most impact on the overall success of a block. Nerve stimulation and ultrasound together or independently of each other are most commonly used to perform perineural injection. Understanding the basic principles behind it is vital.

If the nerve stimulator adequately but it still fails to illicit a motor response, other reasons for failure to illicit a response should be considered, as discussed in the following.

Nerve Conduction Issues

Patients with diabetes suffer from chronic hyperglycemia, which induces inflammation and oxidative stress, causing micro vascular changes, ischemia, and decreased axonal conduction velocity. The electric stimulation threshold of the nerve is markedly increased, whereby the risk for needle trauma in stimulator-guided perineural is theoretically elevated.[11] Patients with vascular disease have similar pathophysiological changes where prolonged ischemia to the nerve may increase the threshold for nerve stimulation.

Patient Size

Caution should be advised in thin patients when administering the local anesthetic to the skin prior to introducing the perineural needle. Femoral nerves can be as shallow as 1 cm in such patients, and deeper deposition of the local anesthetic to the skin can block the nerve, preventing nerve stimulation.

ULTRASOUND

An ultrasound wave is a form of acoustic energy, which is generated when multiple piezoelectric crystals inside a transducer (i.e., the probe) vibrate at high frequency in response to an alternating current.[12]

The degree to which the ultrasound waves reflect off a structure and return to the probe determines the signal intensity. Structures that strongly reflect ultrasound, called echogenic, generate large signal intensities and appear whiter or hyper-echoic (e.g., pleura). In contrast, hypo-echoic structures weakly reflect ultrasound and appear darker (e.g., vessels).[12]

Broadly there are two types of probes:

Linear or high-frequency probe: high-frequency transducer probes emit high-energy sound waves (10–15 MHz) that have low tissue penetration but permit high-resolution imaging of superficial structures.[13]

Curvilinear or low-frequency probe: low-frequency probes (e.g., 2–5 MHz) emit low-energy sound waves that allow for deeper tissue penetration but at the cost of fine resolution. Curved array probes afford a wider field of vision compared to linear array probes. Curved array probes are most useful when the areas of interest lie far apart from one another but at a similar depth.[14]

There are two approaches to needle entry when using an ultrasound. *In plane* refers to imaging the nerve in the longitudinal view (i.e., when the probe is oriented in parallel plane with the needle shaft), and *out of plane* is imaging the nerve in transverse view (when the probe is oriented perpendicular to the needle shaft). In-plane or longitudinal view is preferred because it is safer and more precise since the entire needle shaft can be visualized as it is manipulated to avoid vessels or pleura on approach to the target nerve.[13]

If the ultrasound visualization is poor, it is usually from attenuation. Attenuation is the diminution of acoustic energy as a wave passes through tissue. Energy loss mainly occurs due to conversion of some of the acoustic energy into heat. Attenuation results in a very poor and dark picture. Two maneuvers can help remedy this. The first one is artificially increased (or decreased) by adjusting the gain control higher. Second, most machines offer the operator the ability to control gain independently at specified depth intervals. This is known as *time gain compensation*. This can be increased as the depth of penetration increases in order to compensate for the corresponding loss of signal intensity.[12]

The next step is to obtain the best needle visualization under ultrasound. Several maneuvers can lead to success when it comes to visualization of the needle under an ultrasound.

Step 1: Holding and stabilizing the probe is the first step. The operator's hand (ulnar side) should be resting on the patient for support, as shown in Figure 2.1.A. This will enable finer adjustment and promote better grip on the transducer. If not done properly, as shown is the position illustrated in (Figure 2.1.B), it will predispose to instability and fatigue.

Applying firm pressure on the body part compresses the structures underneath and brings deeper structures in view, especially when using a high-resolution probe.

Step 2: Alignment of the needle to the probe and avoid tilting the probe. Needle-probe position is critical to visualize the shaft of the needle in the in-plane approach. The thickness of the ultrasound beam is in millimeters, which does not make the process any simpler, thus the freehand technique requires bimanual coordination in 3 dimensions while looking at a 2-dimensional image on the ultrasound screen.[15]

As much as possible, the probe should be placed perpendicular to the skin surface. This is usually not a problem with most blocks, but in some situations like an ultrasound guided paravertebral block, tilting the probe may be the only way to visualize the target.

Once the probe is 90 degrees to the skin, the needle should be aligned in the center of the thickness of the probe, as shown in Figure 2.2. If the target is shallower and the needle is still not visible, sliding the probe across the needle shaft is the most

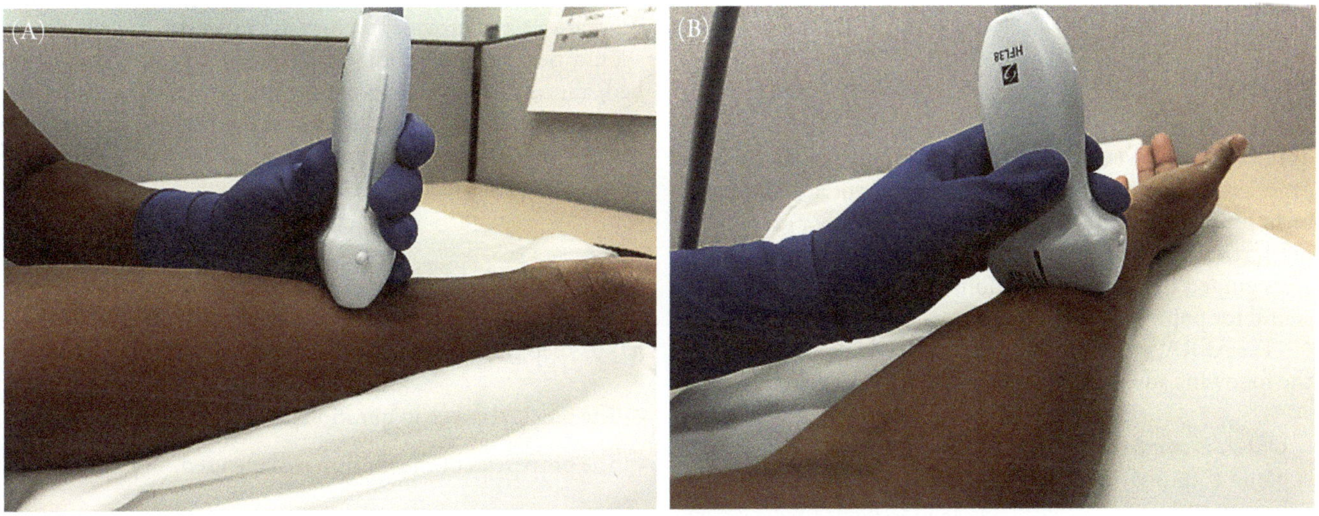

Figure 2.1. A and B: operator's hand/wrist (ulnar side) should be resting on the patient for support, as shown in (A), to enable finer adjustment and promote better grip on the transducer. The hand position illustrated in (B) will predispose to instability and fatigue.

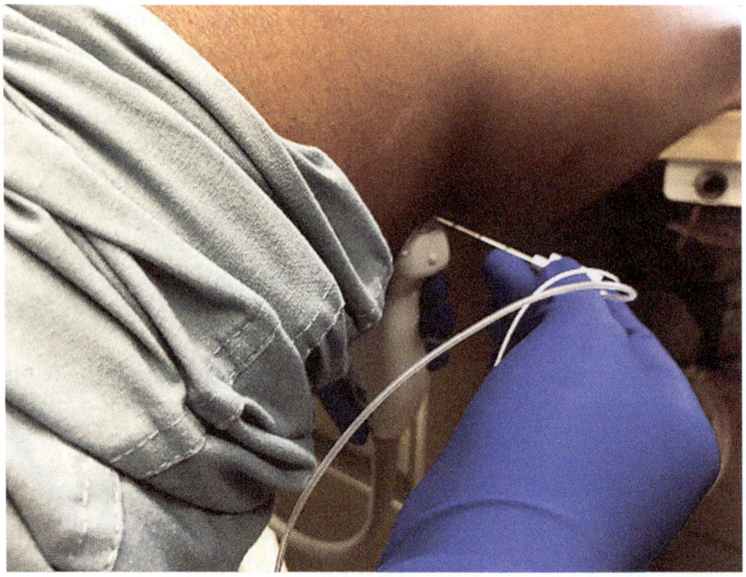

Figure 2.2. Alignment of the needle to the probe that results in maximum reflection of the needle.

effective maneuver. Tilting or toggling is not effective since it changes the angle of the incident beam.

If only the body of the needle is visible but not the tip (or vice versa), the probe needs to be rotated to align with the needle. For good needle visualization in general, it is advisable to move the transducer to the needle and not the other way around, since the needle can cause tissue injury, especially when it has not been visualized.[15]

When the target is deeper, it is especially important to make note of the depth and to start at some distance from the probe if anatomically possible. Needle insertion too close to the probe is never a good idea since it makes the needle angle too steep and prevents it from taking a more perpendicular position to the ultrasound beam. Sound waves are maximally reflected and are received by the transducer when they hit the target tissue at a perpendicular angle, resulting in the highest-quality image since the sound waves are maximally reflected at this angle.[13]

ULTRASOUND GUIDED REGIONAL ANESTHESIA (USRA) VERSUS NERVE STIMULATION

Trained hands have both advantages and disadvantages. For an experienced operator, depending upon their preference, either technique can be faster and/or more efficient. For example, in our institute we prefer to place gluteal sciatic perineural catheters guided by nerve stimulation, but prefer to use an ultrasound for popliteal sciatic block.

The ASRA, using evidence-based data, has recently created the following advisory:[16]

- USRA is comparable and equally successful when compared with traditional forms of perineural techniques.
- USRA has led to statistically, but perhaps not clinically, proven advantages in reduced onset time.
- There is no evidence that ultrasound eliminates complications; poorly performed ultrasound guidance might actually increase the risk of injury.
- USRA does not decrease the incidence of nerve injury.

ERGONOMICS

"Well begun is half done," goes the saying. The *Merriam-Webster Dictionary* defines ergonomics as an applied science concerned with designing and arranging things people use so that the people and things interact most efficiently and safely. Ergonomics plays a huge role in making any procedure successful. The location of the ultrasound and patient monitor, bed height, and hand placement are all vital in making a perineural procedure successful by preventing fatigue. The patient's bed should be elevated such that the operator does not have to bend over, and the forearm and hand holding the probe should be placed gently on the patient's body to prevent fatigue and provide stability to the probe. The ultrasound should be placed on the non-operative side of the patient's bed, aligned to the line of vision such that the operator does not have to turn their head to view it. Fifteen minutes after the block is placed, it is tested looking for at least to a decrement of sensations in the field of the block.

FAILED OR DELAYED BLOCK

In troubleshooting a delayed or potentially failed block, one has to keep the following in mind:

- The blocked nerve in question
- The properties of the local anesthetic used.

The cross-sectional area of a nerve affects the time to onset of a block, with larger nerves such as the sciatic nerve requiring more local anesthetic volume and more time to block onset.[17] As for local anesthetic properties, the pK_a of the specific local anesthetic used is one of the most crucial factors determining the block onset.

With the above factors considered, and a physical exam confirming a delayed or failed block, the next step is to administer a bolus through the perineural catheter or to reassess the block. If the additional bolus augments the block, then the patient would benefit from higher local anesthetic infusion rates. Otherwise, consider replacing the perineural catheter, paying special attention to the maximum allowable dose for the particular local anesthetic used in order to avoid local anesthetic toxicity.

PROCEDURE DOCUMENTATION

Documentation of procedures and any medical care serves the following purposes:[18,19]

- *Communication*: to the patient and among healthcare providers regarding the healthcare services administered.[20] For optimal use of documentation for communication, the notes should exhibit prioritization of information,[20] with a succinct description of the procedure, equipment used, administered medications, outcomes, and related complications if any.
- *Coding and billing*: accurate documentation facilitates billing and avoids under- or over-billing. While under-billing results in loss of revenue for the hospital, over-billing constitutes fraud!
- *A source of reference in medico-legal issues*: documenting the clinician's thought process and rationale for specific treatment choices should be conveyed as this information can be used to defend a clinician against malpractice issues.
- *Education, research, and quality improvement projects.*

AMBULATORY PERINEURAL CATHETER MANAGEMENT

Ambulatory continuous perineural infusion of local anesthetic decreases postoperative pain, opioid use, opioid-related side effects, and sleep disturbances after orthopedic surgeries.[21] When possible, certain outpatient orthopedic procedures can benefit from a continuous perineural catheter rather than a single injection nerve block. However, the patient needs a complete understanding of how the perineural infusion affects them and what precautions they need to take before going home.

Before discharging a patient with a perineural catheter, it is important that the patient is educated on the expected effects of the nerve block, how to use the ambulatory pump, and what signs/symptoms would warrant calling/returning to the hospital for help.

EFFECTS OF NERVE BLOCK

- The patient will experience muscle weakness, numbness, and altered nociception on the surgical limb. As a result, it is important that the patient does not attempt to support themselves on the affected limb. Patients are also advised to protect their surgical limb from heat and chemicals to prevent injury.[22] To this end, at our institution, we ensure that a patient has a reliable social support system in the postoperative period before discharging them with ambulatory local anesthetic infusion pumps.
- While the perineural catheter will provide analgesia, it may not alleviate all of the surgical pain, especially if the perineural catheter does not cover all the nerve distributions involved. With this in mind, the patient is advised to supplement the perineural catheter with oral analgesics as appropriate, with the goal of achieving optimal participation in physical therapy and basic functionality during the recovery period.
- Patients should also be taught to watch for signs of infection, local anesthetic toxicity, and to contact the acute pain service immediately regarding such.

HOW TO USE THE AMBULATORY PAIN PUMP

- The pump is set with a continuous basal infusion, with an option for patient bolus if needed for breakthrough pain. We teach the patient how to administer local anesthetic boluses via the pump.
- Patients are advised against showering while the perineural catheter is in place or disconnecting the catheter.
- Upon discontinuation of the local anesthetic infusion and block resolution, the perineural catheter is removed by the patient under the guidance of acute pain staff over the phone.

REFERENCES

1. Rawal N. 10 years of acute pain services: achievements and challenges. *Reg Anesth Pain Med.* 1999;24(1):68–73.
2. Fargen KM, et al. Enhanced staff communication and reduced near-miss errors with a neurointerventional procedural checklist. *J Neurointerv Surg.* 2013;5(5):497–500.
3. Neal JM, Woodward CM, Harrison TK. The American society of regional anesthesia and pain medicine checklist for managing local anesthetic systemic toxicity: 2017 Version. *Reg Anesth Pain Med.* 2018 Feb;43(2):150–153.
4. Perrenoud B, et al. The effectiveness of health literacy interventions on the informed consent process of health care users: a systematic review protocol. *JBI Database System Rev Implement Rep.* 2015;13(10):82–94.
5. Lin YK, et al. How to effectively obtain informed consent in trauma patients: a systematic review. *BMC Med Ethics.* 2019;20(1):8.
6. Singh TSS. Is it time to separate consent for anesthesia from consent for surgery? *J Anaesthesiol Clin Pharmacol.* 2017;33(1):112–113.
7. Bernards CM, et al. Regional anesthesia in anesthetized or heavily sedated patients. *Reg Anesth Pain Med.* 2008;33(5):449–460.
8. Pither CE, Ford DJ, Raj PP. The use of peripheral nerve stimulators for regional anesthesia: a review of experimental characteristics, technique, and clinical applications. *Reg Anesth Pain Med.* 1985;10(2):49–58.
9. Pinnock CA, Fischer H, Jones RP. Peripheral nerve blockade. In: Pinnock CA, Fischer HBJ, Jones RP, eds. *Peripheral Nerve Blockade.* 1st ed. Edinburgh: Churchill Livingstone; 1996:12–23.

10. Hadzic A, et al. Nerve stimulators used for peripheral nerve blocks vary in their electrical characteristics. *Anesthesiology*. 2003;98(4):969–974.
11. Ten Hoope W, Looije M, Lirk P. Regional anesthesia in diabetic peripheral neuropathy. *Curr Opin Anaesthesiol.* 2017;30(5):627–631.
12. Sites BD, et al. Artifacts and pitfall errors associated with ultrasound-guided regional anesthesia. Part I: understanding the basic principles of ultrasound physics and machine operations. *Reg Anesth Pain Med.* 2007;32(5):412–418.
13. Brull R, Perlas A, Chan VWS. Ultrasound-guided peripheral nerve blockade. *Curr Pain Headache Rep.* 2007;11;25–32. https://doi.org/10.1007/s11916-007-0018-6.
14. Abdallah FW, Brull R. Is sciatic nerve block advantageous when combined with femoral nerve block for postoperative analgesia following total knee arthroplasty? A systematic review. *Reg Anesth Pain Med.* 2011;36(5):493–498.
15. Chin KJ, et al. Needle visualization in ultrasound-guided regional anesthesia: challenges and solutions. *Reg Anesth Pain Med.* 2008;33(6):532–544.
16. Neal JM, et al. The ASRA evidence-based medicine assessment of ultrasound-guided regional anesthesia and pain medicine: executive summary. *Reg Anesth Pain Med.* 2010;35(2 Suppl):S1–S9.
17. Chen X, et al., Factors associated with minimum effective volume of lidocaine 1.5% for sciatic nerve blocks. *Clin J Pain.* 2020;36(4):296–301.
18. Davidson SJ, et al., Where's the beef? The promise and the reality of clinical documentation. *Acad Emerg Med.* 2004;11(11):1127–1134.
19. Ho YX, et al. A qualitative analysis evaluating the purposes and practices of clinical documentation. *Appl Clin Inform.* 2014;5(1):153–168.
20. Hoonpongsimanont W, et al., Assessing medical student documentation using simulated charts in emergency medicine. *BMC Med Educ.* 2018;18(1):203.
21. Ilfeld BM, et al. Popliteal sciatic perineural local anesthetic infusion: a comparison of three dosing regimens for postoperative analgesia. *Anesthesiology*. 2004;101(4):970–977.
22. Gharabawy R, Abd-Elsayed A, Elsharkawy H, Farag E, Cummings K, Eid G, Mendoza M, Mounir-Soliman L, Rosenquist R, Ali Sakr Esa W. The Cleveland Clinic experience with supraclavicular and popliteal ambulatory nerve catheters. *Sci World J.* 2014;2014:572507. doi:10.1155/2014/572507.

REVIEW QUESTIONS

(1) A 40-year-old male received an elbow replacement, and he received an infraclavicular catheter for postoperative pain relief. His arm is numb and so are all the fingers, but he complains of burning and pain on the medial side of his elbow. What is the reason for this pain?

A. Lateral cord of the brachial plexus was incompletely blocked
B. The intercostobrachial nerve block is missing
C. The posterior cord was incompletely blocked
D. None of the above

(2) During a nerve stimulation guided gluteal sciatic block, no motor response is noted at 1 mA (pulse duration 0.1 ms, frequency 2 Hz) in a patient with diabetic neuropathy. What is the next step in management?

A. Increase the current on the peripheral nerve stimulation
B. Decrease the current on peripheral nerve stimulation
C. Inject the local anesthetic
D. All the above

(3) A 32-year-old trauma patient is admitted to the hospital for repair of a tibia-fibula fracture. Per surgeon request, femoral and sciatic nerve catheters are placed and a perineural infusion of 0.2% ropivacaine is administered. Next morning, the patient starts complaining of excruciating pain at the surgical site after having a comfortable night. What is the next step in management?

A. Administer a bolus of local anesthetic to see if that will help
B. Call the orthopedic service for evaluation of compartment syndrome
C. Replace the nerve block catheters if the bolus does not help
D. All of the above

(4) A 65-year-old patient is admitted to the intensive care unit with left-sided rib fractures. Patient also has a pneumothorax on the left side. An ultrasound guided paravertebral is planned; however, on placement of the probe, the ultrasound visualization is poor even though the patient is of normal weight. What is the possible cause of this abnormality?

A. Surgical emphysema from the pneumothorax is affecting the ultrasound resolution
B. The machine is broken
C. The patient has abnormal anatomy
D. None of the above

(5) A 23-year-old patient who has a popliteal perineural catheter for a foot surgery is starting to feel pain in his sole on postoperative day 2. What is going on?

A. The tibial component of the sciatic nerve was missed during the block
B. The common peroneal component of the sciatic nerve was missed during the block
C. The saphenous nerve was missed during the block
D. None of the above

(6) A chronic pain patient receives a popliteal sciatic and saphenous nerve block for his foot surgery and is subsequently discharged with 4/10 pain. Eight hours later, his block wears off and his foot pain becomes unbearable, prompting him to go to the emergency room. What is the reason for his excruciating pain?

A. Rebound pain
B. Local anesthetic toxicity
C. Failed block
D. None of the above

(7) A patient presents for right ankle surgery and receives a single shot saphenous and a popliteal sciatic perineural catheter for postoperative pain relief with an infusion rate of 6 ml/hr. In the operating room, the surgeon calls for removal of the perineural catheters since he plans to use a sterile tourniquet. When can the block be replaced?

A. Immediately postoperatively with ultrasound guidance

B. After recovery of motor and sensory function of the leg
C. Immediately postoperatively under nerve stimulator guidance
D. After recovery of motor function only

(8) While placing an interscalene catheter, the stimulation of which muscle is considered ideal?

A. Deltoid
B. Biceps
C. Either deltoid or biceps is acceptable
D. None

ANSWERS

(1) **B.** All approaches to the brachial plexus block will miss the intercostobrachial nerve (ICBN) since ICBN arises from the collateral branch of the second intercostal nerve. Since all the fingers are numb, it's unlikely that one of the cords of the brachial plexus was missed during the infraclavicular brachial plexus block. The patient should get relief from pain once the ICBN is blocked.

Reference

Moustafa MA, Kandeel AA. Randomized comparative study between two different techniques of intercostobrachial nerve block together with brachial plexus block during superficialization of arteriovenous fistula. *J Anesth*. 2018;32(5):725–730.

(2) **A.** Patients with diabetes suffer from chronic hyperglycemia which decreases axonal conduction velocity. The electric stimulation threshold of the nerve is markedly increased whereby the risk for needle trauma in stimulator-guided nerve blocks is theoretically elevated.[2] Increasing the current from the nerve stimulation may elicit a response.

Reference

Ten Hoope W, Looije M, Lirk P. Regional anesthesia in diabetic peripheral neuropathy. *Curr Opin Anaesthesiol*. 2017;30(5):627–631.

(3) **B.** There is sparse evidence to support the claim that nerve blocks can mask the pain presentation of acute compartment syndrome (ACS). The few cases where nerve blocks were implicated in delaying/masking the diagnosis of ACS have been in the context of dense blockade. Thus, use of lower concentrations of local anesthetic for regional blocks has been advocated to prevent potential masking of ACS. If anything, nerve blocks are beneficial in patients at risk for ACS because they promote vasodilation, which in turn improves tissue perfusion. Peripheral nerve blocks are also useful in the diagnosis of ACS, with severe ischemic pain manifesting despite nerve blockade. We avoid giving boluses of local anesthetic via the nerve block if the patient is at high risk of developing ACS.

Reference

Kucera TJ, Boezaart AP. Regional anesthesia does not consistently block ischemic pain: two further cases and a review of the literature. *Pain Med*. 2014;15(2):316–319.

(4) **A.** Surgical emphysema interferes with the ultrasound image since a soft tissue air boundary reflects 99% of the beam such that none is available to reflect back to the probe, leading to poor visualization of targeted area.

Reference

Wardhan R, Kantamneni S. The challenges of ultrasound-guided thoracic paravertebral blocks in rib fracture patients. *Cureus*. 2020;12(4):e7626.

(5) **D.** Popliteal perineural catheters are continuous perineural blocks of the sciatic nerve in the popliteal region. The dorsum of the foot is innervated by the common peroneal nerve and the plantar surface by the tibial, both branches of the sciatic nerve. The nerve block catheter is usually placed above the bifurcation of the sciatic nerve before the nerve splits into common peroneal and tibial nerves. If only nerve stimulation technique was used to guide the catheter, one of the divisions of the sciatic nerve can be missed, leading to a failed block. Catheter dislodgement can also lead to displacement of the catheter away from one of the branches. An extra volume of local anesthetic can help with spread to the tibial nerve. If the bolus is not successful, either patients can be advised to take pain medications to cover the pain, or replacement of the nerve block should be considered.

References

Dufour E, et al. Combined ultrasound and neurostimulation guidance for popliteal sciatic nerve block: a prospective, randomized comparison with neurostimulation alone. *Anesth Analg*. 2008;106(5):1553–1558.
Hauritz RW, et al. Displacement of popliteal sciatic nerve catheters after major foot and ankle surgery: a randomized controlled double-blinded magnetic resonance imaging study. Br J Anaesth. 2016;117(2):220–227.

(6) **A.** Rebound pain implies the dramatic increase in pain once the regional anesthetic has dissipated. It is caused by unopposed nociceptive inputs that are brutally uncovered after peripheral nerve block resolution (PNB) resolution. In a mouse animal model, perineural dexamethasone, when added to clinical concentration of bupivacaine, prolonged sensory and motor block, along with preventing the rebound hyperalgesia.

References

Lavand'homme P. Rebound pain after regional anesthesia in the ambulatory patient. Curr *Opin Anaesthesiol*. 2018;31(6):679–684.
An K, Elkassabany NM, Liu J. Dexamethasone as adjuvant to bupivacaine prolongs the duration of thermal antinociception and prevents bupivacaine-induced rebound hyperalgesia via regional mechanism in a mouse sciatic nerve block model. *PLoS One*. 2015;10(4):e0123459.

(7) **B.** Communication is key, and not just a one-way street. At our institute we communicate with the surgeons via email or phone call daily to avoid the very situation.

Even though ultrasound guidance can be used to assist in placement of perineural catheter, especially on a blocked nerve, it is not advisable to do so for the following reasons:

(1) Intrafascicular placement of the needle can be missed because of lack of paresthesia.

(2) Any possible nerve injury from the surgery can be missed.
(3) The 24-hour maximum volume for the local anesthetic may have been attained from the initial block in the patient.

(8) **C.** Historically, biceps twitch was considered more reliable than deltoid twitch to determine the success of an interscalene block. However, new data indicate that if a clear deltoid twitch is elicited, it is as effective as a biceps twitch in determining accurate needle placement and in predicting successful motor block.

References

Urmey WF. Interscalene block: the truth about twitches. *Reg Anesth Pain Med.* 2000;25(4):340–342.

Silverstein WB, Saiyed MU, Brown AR. Interscalene block with a nerve stimulator: a deltoid motor response is a satisfactory endpoint for a successful block. *Reg Anesth Pain Med.* 2000;25(4):356–359.

3.

REGIONAL ANESTHESIA EQUIPMENT

Thomas Halaszynski

STEM CASE AND KEY QUESTIONS

A 60-year-old male was struck by a car crossing the street. In the emergency room, he complains of right upper extremity pain; he has a Glasgow Coma Score of 13 for confusion and eye opening to speech. Patient's history is remarkable for hypertension, fainting episodes, chronic obstructive pulmonary disease (COPD; 30 pack-year smoking), paroxysmal atrial fibrillation, and low back pain. Medications include dabigatran, methadone, and oxycodone. Patient's vital signs reveal atrial fibrillation and blood pressure of 130/70 mm Hg. Head computed tomography scan shows a small subdural hematoma, but neurosurgical service determined that the patient did not require interventions and will be following by observation.

(1) WHY IS IMMOBILIZATION OF THE ARM IMPORTANT FOLLOWING HUMERAL FRACTURE, AND WHAT NERVES ARE AT RISK FOR INJURY FROM HUMERAL FRACTURE?

Immobilization is important to avoid further tissue damage, brachial plexus nerve injury, and/or terminal nerve branch injury. With a midshaft humeral fracture, the radial nerve is at particular risk. With a proximal humeral fracture, the shoulder can be dislocated, causing abnormal positioning that could cause stretching, pinching, and/or pressure on the brachial plexus (axillary nerve at risk due to course around proximal humeral shaft). In a distal humeral fracture, ulnar nerve is at risk due to proximity to fracture fragments and ulnar nerve palsy can be common (up to 50%).[1] Therefore, documentation of preexisting neurologic findings should be performed; consider any regional anesthesia technique by approaching a more proximal portion of the brachial plexus in relation to site of upper extremity trauma; *ultrasound imaging* should be conducted (especially with brachial plexus blockade); maintain patient communication during regional procedure (patient acts as feedback toward reducing negative iatrogenic effects); and consider using an *insulated needle* with *nerve stimulation* (can aid in reducing negative iatrogenic effects).

(2) HOW CAN A NERVE STIMULATION TECHNIQUE WITH INSULATED PERIPHERAL NERVE BLOCK (PNB) NEEDLES REDUCE NERVE INJURY/INTRANEURAL INJECTION?

Energy density at the needle tip forms current that stimulates target nerve(s). Depolarization currents of 0.2–0.5 mA for peripheral nerve localization correspond to an appropriate needle tip-to-nerve proximity. However, with nerve stimulation and corresponding motor twitch at currents less than 0.2 mA, there is an increased risk of intraneural needle placement and possibly intrafascicular needle tip placement. Intraneural/intrafascicular needle placement will typically warrant reflexive reactions of withdraw, pain, and paresthesia (*all* possibly intense), however, this occurrence may not be 100%, as in rare situations where the needle tip is intraneural/intrafascicular without patient reaction.[2]

Individuals with glycosylation of nerves (diabetic patients), nerve trauma, nerve demyelination, and other neurologic pathology may not have a response or may reveal an atypical response to stimulation and/or may require higher currents to achieve similar degrees of motor response compared to unaffected patients.[2] In addition, biphasic behavior of cathodic nerve stimulation techniques (paradoxical decrease in nerve conduction with closer needle tip-to-nerve proximity at 2–4 cm from target nerves) could explain the incidence of intraneural injection using a nerve stimulator when compared to using an ultrasound-guided approach.[2] Another aspect influencing sensitivity/specificity of nerve stimulation techniques could be the proximity of the needle tip to nerves with a higher concentration of sensory axons that insulate motor axons at lower current densities.[3]

(3) WHAT ARE GOOD QUALITIES OF A BLOCK NEEDLE AND WHY ARE INSULATED PNB NEEDLES USED?

An appropriate motor response is achieved with a current between 0.5 and 0.2 mA (suggesting ideal needle tip to target nerve). Stimulating PNB needles should permit for nerve stimulator connection and should be insulated along the needle shaft with only the tip exposed to deliver current.[4]

Attributes of quality regional needles include: appropriate finger grips at the proximal needle end, ability to connect extension tubing (facilitate aspiration), contain centimeter markings on the shaft, and needle tips beveled at 45 degrees (versus 17 degree of infiltration needles) to enhance operator sensation as the needle passes through tissue/tissue planes and reducing trauma to sensitive structures (i.e., nerves, blood vessels, etc.).

With insulated needles (nonconductive covering of the shaft), energy density at needle tip is the current stimulating target nerve(s). Uninsulated needles experience greater current dispersion since the entire needle (portion under skin) is in contact with conductive tissues, leading to alternate electrical paths while drawing current away from the needle tip and target structures. Thus, higher currents are required to overcome the current losses through the needle shaft.[2]

There are echogenic needles with engraved needle tip patterns (dihedral/tetrahedral grooves or Xx patterns with clear coating) to enhance ultrasound wave reflections designed for optimal needle tip visibility under ultrasound.

(4) THE DECISION WAS MADE TO ADMINISTER A BRACHIAL PLEXUS BLOCK FOR POSTOPERATIVE PAIN MEDICINE. HOW CAN THE PHYSICS OF ULTRASOUND ASSIST IN THIS TECHNIQUE?

Sound is oscillating mechanical energy (ultrasound emitted at frequency above human hearing; >20 kHz) transmitted through tissue by compression/condensation and expansion/rarefaction of particles. Medical ultrasound frequencies range from 1 MHz to 20 MHz with the wavelength (λ) of a sound wave being the quotient of the speed of sound (ν) and frequency (f); $\lambda = \nu / f$. The speed of sound is defined as the square root of the quotient of elasticity/bulk modules (B) and density (ρ); therefore, related to conductive media characteristics and unrelated to amplitude or frequency.[5] Acoustic impedance (Z) is substance resistance toward sound conduction and is defined as the product of velocity of sound in and density of a substance ($Z = \nu \cdot \rho$). For example, lungs have low acoustic impedance and bone has high impedance, with differences between acoustic impedance of substances determined by how much energy is reflected/transmitted at their interfaces. As another example, tissue-bone and air-tissue interfaces reflect almost all incident sound wave.[5,6]

Piezoelectricity is the foundation of ultrasound transducer operation where *piezo* (to compress) refers to some crystals that emit electric impulse when deformed. There are 2 components to piezoelectric effects: reverse effect (deformation of a crystalline structure with input of electrical energy to the material) and direct effect (ability of crystalline structure to emit electrical impulse following deformation). Therefore, piezoelectric crystals can both emit energy (sound waves) and conduct energy (transform the energy into an image).[7]

Attenuation is loss of sound energy within tissue (absorption of energy, transmission through tissue, reflection/scattering as sound waves encounter interfaces) that cannot be processed into an image. As attenuation coefficient and length of the sound wave traveling through tissue increase, so will attenuation (source of attenuation is through absorption of sound energy by tissues). In addition, attenuation is related to the frequency of sound waves, so that as frequency of the wave increases so does attenuation; as a result, as frequency gets higher, more sound energy is lost in the tissue, which diminishes the tissue penetration at a given amplitude.[6,8]

Intensity of sound waves and power adjustments are used to overcome attenuation losses, yielding more information for ultrasound image processing. Power (P) is the rate energy is being delivered and is described as units of energy over time expressed as watts (W), and intensity is the rate energy is delivered over an area (expressed as: $I = P/4\pi r2$). Therefore, as sound waves travel through tissue, intensity decreases with the square of the distance from the source (r), and increasing power will increase intensity of the sound wave at a given distance from the source. However, increasing power comes at a cost, as heat is imparted to the tissues through attenuation (i.e., penetration at the price of resolution).

(5) WHAT IS RESPONSIBLE FOR AND WHAT ARE COMMON ULTRASOUND IMAGE ARTIFACTS: IMAGING ERRORS OR DISTORTIONS IN ECHO PROCESSING AND IMAGE DISPLAY?

False displays of structures in the incorrect anatomical location, or distorted appearance, missing, and/or nonexistent structures (artifacts) are due to ultrasound machine misconfiguration and/or operator error that can result from the following errors/distortions: acoustic shadowing, bayonet sign, refraction error, and reverberation artifact.[9]

1. Acoustic shadowing occurs at the interface between tissues of different acoustic impedance (i.e., bone and muscle). Therefore, when sound waves encounter the echo dense structure, nearly all of the sound is reflected, which results in an acoustic shadow, causing image dropout deep to the reflective surface and unresolvable objects deep to the shadow (i.e., acoustic shadowing at interface between lamina of vertebral bodies and paraspinal muscles).[6,7,10]
2. Bayonet sign is a step-off or apparent kink of the needle shaft due to needle positioning/transitioning between tissues of different propagation speeds (i.e., needle portion appearing more superficial is in tissue of faster propagation speed, such as muscle, and needle segment appearing deeper in substance with slower propagation velocity, such as fluid-filled space).[9,10]
3. Refraction error is when the reflected wave passes between tissues of different acoustic impedance, resulting in a shift in the path of sound wave from its initial axis, making the image appear to be along a deviated path rather than from its actual origin.[9]
4. Reverberation artifacts (2 acoustic interactions) occur when the sound wave strikes 2 reflectors or the transducer and a reflector (Figure 3.1). For example, sound waves

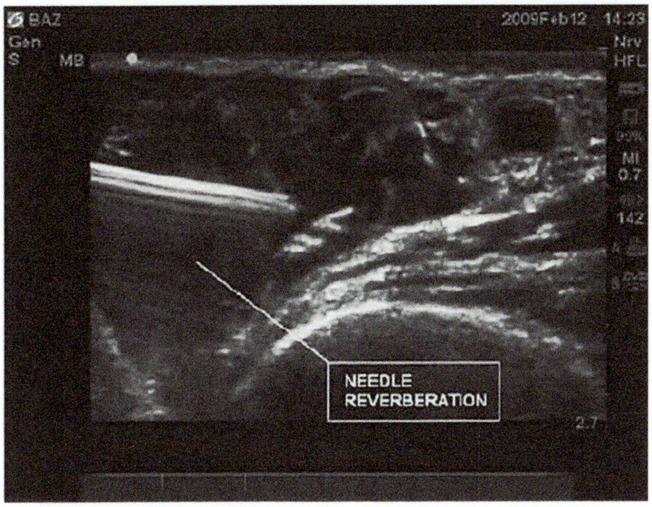

Figure 3.1. Reverberation artifact.

strike the needle, causing a reflection; the reflected beam strikes another surface with greater acoustic impedance that causes some of the energy to be transmitted to the transducer with a reflection occurring back into the tissue toward the first reflective surface (i.e., needle).[9,10]

(6) WHAT RELEVANT ANATOMIC STRUCTURES IN THE NECK AND BELOW THE NECK CAN BE INJURED OR INJECTED ACCIDENTALLY DURING BRACHIAL PLEXUS BLOCK?

Several important structures are in proximity along the brachial plexus and at risk of injury when performing regional anesthesia. These anatomical and vasculature structures include: spinal cord and/or vertebral artery, apex of the lung and subclavian artery/vein, and the axillary artery/vein.[11] Other anatomy at risk include parietal and visceral pleura, unintended neural tissues (i.e., phrenic, recurrent laryngeal, vagus, and cervical sympathetic nerve plexus). Epidural or subarachnoid spread of local anesthetic is another risk (possible during rapid and/or using high injection pressures). There is potential that aberrant needle passes can traumatize any of the above as well as neuronal components being targeted.[11,12]

(7) PERIOPERATIVELY AN ULTRASOUND AND LANDMARK PLUS NERVE STIMULATION TECHNIQUE IS PLANNED. WHAT ARE THE PHYSICS OF NERVE STIMULATION, AND HOW CAN IT BE APPLIED CLINICALLY TO REDUCE INJURY?

Nerve stimulators (electrical waveforms that trigger depolarization and are adjusted to permit detection of minimal stimulating thresholds) create a pulsed electric current causing depolarization to target nerves, resulting in muscle stimulation and/or tingling/paresthesia. Clinicians can observe motor and sensory reactions at a set current/intensity as the needle is advanced until a "brisk" response is obtained. The current is then slowly reduced until motor/sensory reaction is reduced and lost. The goal is motor/sensory loss to occur at a desired threshold current along with the optimal needle-to-target interface. If the needle is too close to the target nerve at a current lower than threshold, then the needle is too close and should be adjusted. If motor/sensory loss occurs at a higher threshold current, then additional needle adjustment is necessary to optimize needle-to-target interface.[13] Histologic features, such as nerve myelination and density of ion channels, determine the rheobase and chronaxie (waveform and current determined by physical properties of the nerve).[13]

Chronaxie is the minimum duration of current impulse to stimulate a nerve at 2 × the rheobase, and rheobase is the minimum continuous current required to depolarize a nerve.[2] The required current (I) to stimulate a nerve is related to rheobase (P), chronaxie (κ), and impulse (t) duration: $I = P \cdot (1 + \kappa/t)$. For example, each type of nerve has distinct rheobase and chronaxie that affect the current needed to cause depolarization (A-alpha motor fibers have low chronaxie [0.05–0.1ms], while smaller C-fibers have higher chronaxie [0.4ms]).[2] Therefore, clinicians can selectively stimulate motor fibers with pulse lengths of 50–100 ms and prevent stimulation-related pain since it is below the threshold (400 ms) of C-fibers. Adjustments of impulse duration permit selective nerve stimulation and stimulation of deranged nerves; for example, glycosylation of diabetic patients' nerve structures affect chronaxie by increasing pulse duration (stimulation is possible without excess current).[2,13]

(8) HOW IS THE NERVE STIMULATOR USED TO TARGET NERVE DEPOLARIZATION? WHY DOES A SUPRACLAVICULAR NERVE BLOCK HAVE A HIGH FAILURE RATE WHEN USING A LANDMARK/NERVE STIMULATOR TECHNIQUE? CAN THIS BE AVOIDED USING ULTRASOUND-GUIDED NERVE BLOCKADE?

Modern nerve stimulation models include needle- and grounding-lead, timing clock and display system with controls, along with a microprocessor controller. These stimulators can deliver a constant current by adjusting voltage to accommodate various impedances as the needle passes through different tissues. With timing inputs from the clock, the microprocessor controller creates a stimulating impulse at a desired pulse width determined by rheobase and chronaxie of the target nerve. Clinicians adjust the current delivered using an analog or digitally controlled potentiometer that allows adjustment to the pulse width to stimulate motor or sensory nerves. Operators can also set the rate at which the device produces a pulse wave with a frequency adjustment between 1 Hz and 2.5 Hz. The higher frequencies, the more pulses generated/second, and the easier to detect changes in response to needle movement. However, in those with musculoskeletal trauma, higher frequency pulses could result in patient discomfort due to more frequent contracture of traumatized tissues.[2]

Polarity of the stimulating needle tip determines how current(s) behave as needles are passed through tissue and the current/distance association with the target nerve. Nerve stimulation cathode is the negative terminal lead (electron

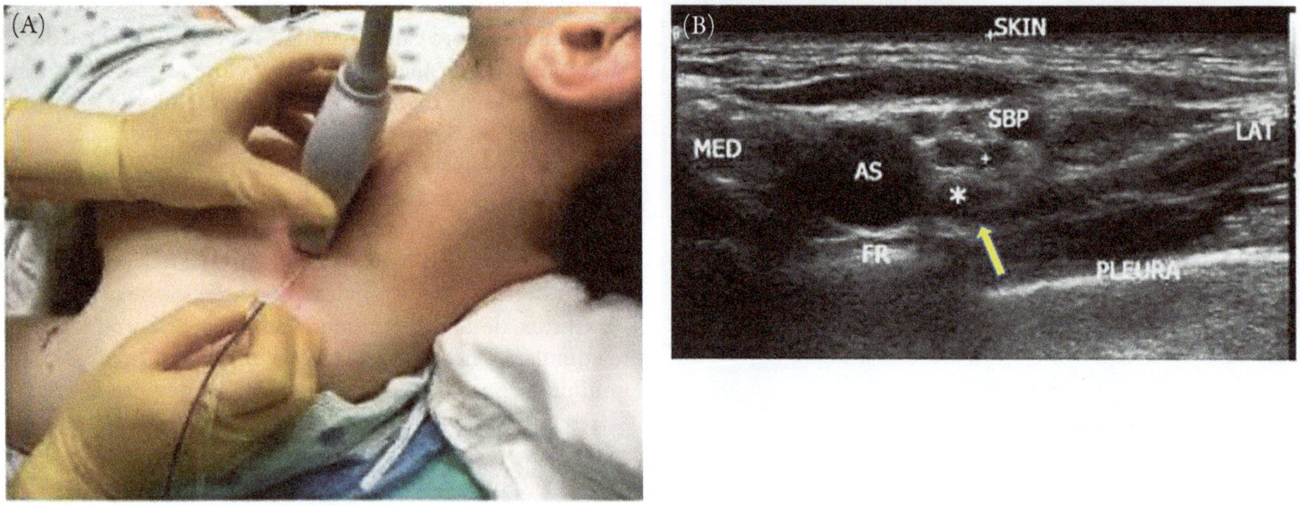

Figure 3.2. Ultrasound-guided brachial plexus block: targeting the "corner pocket." (A) Position of the ultrasound probe and the sonographer hand. (B) Ultrasound anatomy of the brachial plexus at the supraclavicular fossa.
SBP = supraclavicular brachial plexus, AS = subclavian artery, FR = rib. Yellow arrow indicates position of block needle tip, and white star identifies local being injected.

donor) and the anode or grounding lead is the positive terminal (electron acceptor). Therefore, current flows from cathode to anode, and in anode stimulation, cations are discharged from anode of the skin and flow through the body to the needle cathode where stimulation occurs. Nerve stimulators make use of cathode stimulation principles because anode stimulation results in increased cation concentration under the anode (results in hyperpolarization of nerve under the anode, placing the nerve in a refractory state; resistant to depolarization); and higher currents are required to depolarize a nerve with anode stimulation.[2]

Components of the ulnar nerve could be missed when performing a nerve stimulation or landmark ("plumb-bob") supraclavicular nerve block. This is possible as neural tissue that makes up the ulnar nerve most often lies deep to the skin and posterior, lateral, and more inferior to the subclavian artery.[14] In addition, the pulsating subclavian artery could further reduce adequate infiltration of local to the posterior and inferior divisions responsible for ulnar nerve fascicles. However, when using ultrasound, the block needle can be targeted to approach the nerve plexus posteriorly/lateral to the artery with real-time imaging.[15] By administering local anesthetics directed toward the "corner pocket," this will more successfully target local anesthetics around the brachial plexus divisions that compose the ulnar nerve (Figure 3.2A, B).

(9) DESCRIBE ULTRASOUND-GUIDED INTERSCALENE BLOCK AND EXPLAIN LANDMARK/NERVE STIMULATION TECHNIQUE WITH AN INTERSCALENE APPROACH. WHAT MOTOR RESPONSE WOULD BE ELICITED WITH A NERVE STIMULATOR AND WHAT STIMULATION LEVEL WOULD BE SAFE TO INJECT?

Three major landmarks include the clavicle, clavicular head of the sternocleidomastoid (SCM), and external jugular vein. For an interscalene block by electrical nerve stimulation, the patient's head should be turned away from the side of injection. Scalene muscles are palpated posterior/lateral to the SCM clavicular head (C6 level). The stimulating needle is advanced perpendicularly to the skin posterior to the external jugular vein above the clavicle and directed in a dorsal/medial/caudal direction until an appropriate motor response is achieved (electrical current amplitude reduction below 0.5 mAmp and pulse duration of 0.1 ms). A response from C5–C6 nerve roots (deltoid, biceps, or brachioradialis contractions) is most frequently obtained first with motor response(s) of the forearm, arm, or shoulder. The needle will have been advanced about 1–2 cm at which point local is administered.[2]

For ultrasonographic-guided interscalene blockade, a (1) in-plane or (2) out-of-plane approach is used. (1) With an in-plane approach, the needle is directed in a posterolateral to anteromedial direction along the long axis of a high-frequency linear array transducer, keeping the needle tip visualized. The middle and anterior scalene muscles are easily visualized, and nerve roots are typically stacked in a cephalo-caudad arrangement. Injection and spread of local anesthetic is visualized within the brachial plexus sheath (posterior and lateral to nerve roots).[16] (2) With an out-of-plane approach, the high-frequency linear array transducer is placed caudal to the conventional interscalene block approach above the clavicle. Transducer is oriented in a posterolateral/anteromedial direction with the center overlying the interscalene space and the nerve roots image in cross section. The needle is introduced in a dorsal/medial/caudal direction, but imaging needle tip advancement with an out-of-plane approach can be challenging.[16] Nerve stimulation can also be used to confirm position of the needle tip (Figure 3.3). Typically, a motor response should be elicited around 0.5–1 mA and ideal twitch at 0.2–0.5 mA.[17] If the motor response is observed at a higher current (>1 mA), block failure could result. Stimulation at a lower level (<0.2 mA) could be indicative of intraneural/intrafascicular needle placement and risk of neural injury.[18]

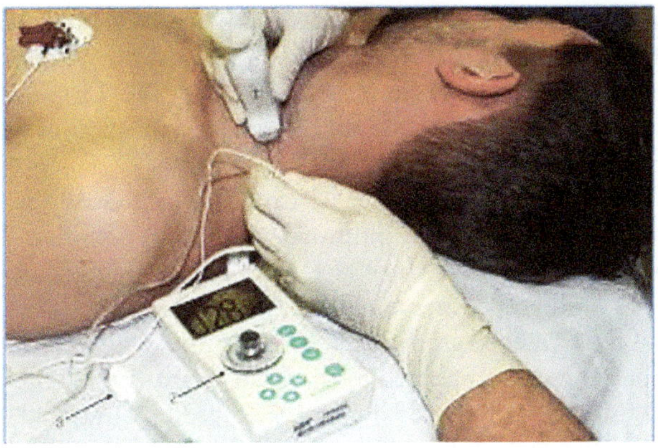

Figure 3.3. Interscalene approach to brachial plexus using a nerve stimulator.

(10) HOW CAN NERVE STIMULATION TECHNIQUE WITH INSULATED NEEDLES REDUCE INTRANEURAL INJECTION?

Energy density at the needle tip forms current that stimulates target nerve(s), and ideal depolarization currents (0.2–0.5 mA) for nerve localization will correspond to an appropriate needle tip-to-nerve placement.[17] At currents less than 0.2 mA there is an increased risk of intraneural needle tip placement (possibly intrafascicular). Intraneural/intrafassicular needle placement will typically warrant reflexive reactions of withdraw, pain, and paresthesia (*all* possibly intense); however, this occurrence may not be 100% (needle tip intraneural/intrafascicular without reaction has been reported).[17,19]

Glycosylation of nerves (i.e., diabetic patients), situations of nerve trauma and/or nerve demyelination, and other neurologic pathology may not have a response or may have an atypical response to stimulation and even require higher currents to achieve similar degrees of motor response.[17] In addition, biphasic behavior of cathodic nerve stimulation (paradoxical decrease in nerve conduction with closer needle tip-to-nerve proximity at 2–4 cm from the target nerve) could explain the incidence of intraneural injection using a nerve stimulator.[17] Another aspect influencing sensitivity/specificity of nerve stimulation could be proximity of the needle tip to nerves with a higher concentration of sensory axons insulating motor axon at lower current densities.[2]

(11) WHAT BENEFIT WOULD A PERIPHERAL NERVE CATHETER PROVIDE OVER A LONG-ACTING ANESTHETIC; ANY DOWNSIDE/CONSEQUENCES?

Peripheral nerve catheters provide continuous local infiltration that can outlast any long-acting anesthetic. Drawbacks to peripheral nerve catheters involve a more complicated placement process, catheter and insertion site infection, increased risk of bleeding, and anesthetic toxicity. Appropriately positioned catheters are a proven method for prolonging postoperative pain control with decreased reliance on intravenous and/or oral narcotic requirements.[20] Nerve plexus catheters also provide patients an ability to control their own pain medication with patient control devices.[20] Compared to single-shot injections, a catheter technique will provide analgesia beyond 24 hours (typical duration of "single-shot" block). Other limitations include malfunction/breakdown of equipment and materials, need for anesthesiologists (or other staff) to assess and manage, damage to the nerve itself (direct contact or nerve entrapment), intravascular placement and/or catheter migration, and damage to nearby anatomical structures.[21]

DISCUSSION

Regional anesthesia preparation and setup area, equipped with monitoring, should be in a quiet location, contain all necessary supplies/equipment for regional anesthesia, stocked with resuscitation drugs/equipment and supplies, and with trained personnel. Such a location could be an induction room or space for performing regional interventions (monitored, premedicated, and blocks placed before transferring patient to the operating room [OR]). Such a location may improve optimal OR efficiency. In addition, standardized documentation protocols are paramount and should include anesthesia consent, pre-block checklist (correct block/appropriate site), and anesthesia assessment (i.e., comorbidities, neurological deficits).

Regional anesthesia block and general equipment area should be stocked with a storage cart (refilled/inventoried) and contain the following:

- Sedative/hypnotic medications (midazolam, short-acting opioids along with propofol or dexmedetomidine) for blocks that may be uncomfortable/require deeper sedation
- Intravenous cannulas and solutions (intravenous line for ALL patients)
- Skin preparation solution, gauze pads, marking pen, ultrasound gel, hypodermic needles, assortment of block needles, sterile drapes (i.e., continuous catheters), and/or premade kits
- Local anesthetic options along with dextrose solutions and normal saline
- Dressings for intravenous cannulas, covering for ultrasound transducer (single shot and covers for continuous techniques), and block catheter insertion site dressing.

It is essential *to have all equipment, drugs, and monitoring readily available.*

Emergency medications/equipment should ALWAYS be readily accessible in the block area (i.e., block cart) and should include:

- Assortment of oral/nasal airways, masks, and endotracheal tubes
- Oxygen supply and bag-valve resuscitator
- Laryngoscopes along with Macintosh and Miller blades

- Suction supply/equipment
- Defibrillator and resuscitation medications (including Intralipid® 20%, succinylcholine, epinephrine, atropine, and choice of vasopressors).

PERIPHERAL NERVE BLOCK NEEDLE DESIGN(S)

There are several nerve block needle types for single-shot nerve blockade, but there are essentially insulated and non-insulated needles, with insulated needles used with nerve stimulation. Echogenic needles have been developed that can result in improved block needle-tip visualization under ultrasound.[22] Needle designs for single-shot procedures can have a pre-attached extension tubing (which facilitates aspiration and injection) along with a connection/attachment for nerve stimulation.

Needle-tip bevel design of block needles could influence the extent/degree of damage to anatomical tissues, including target nerves where injury can be caused by nerve penetration and/or forceful needle-nerve contact.[23] It is theorized that short-beveled needles (37 degrees), when compared to long-beveled (14 degrees) needles, could minimize nerve injury/damage caused by cutting or penetration of nerve structures.[24] It has been shown that long-beveled needles can more easily penetrate perineurium and possibly cause fascicular injury when compared to short-beveled needles. However, it is also theorized that short-beveled needles may result in greater damage/injury if the needle achieves penetration of nerve or nerve fascicle.[24,25] Tuohy needles and blunt/noncutting needles may provide improved operator feedback with an enhanced feel for the subtleties during needle advancement. However, a needle tip design that is too blunt may make it challenging to puncture the fascia and/or require higher insertion pressures, along with the potential of "over-penetrating" after puncturing the fascia layer(s). In addition, aberrant Tuohy needle placement may cause a greater degree of post-traumatic inflammation, myelin damage, and/or intraneural hematoma.[26,27] Block needle length should be chosen depending upon the specific block being performed. For example, deeper nerve blocks (i.e., sciatic) often require a longer length (100–120 mm) needle.[28] Ultrasound can assist in estimating the distance/trajectory of target nerve structures. Block needles that are too long may be difficult to maneuver and/or more easily bend. NOTE: The most correct needle length will permit the best needle manipulation.[28] Selection of block needle gauge/length should balance risks of the needle arching/curving as it passes through tissues along with consideration of patient comfort (22-gauge needles are most often used for single-shot nerve blocks). However, when longer needles for deeper blocks are required, they could tend to bend/arch when advancing and/or can be more challenging to "steer." Therefore, larger-gauge needles are typically used when targeting deeper nerve structures as smaller-gauge needles may lack rigidity and possibly bend/curve more easily when advancing to the needle hub. There also exists a balance between larger-gauge needles with the potential for tissue injury and/or hematoma formation during needle penetration when compared to smaller-gauge needles that may also have an increased risk of inadvertent intrafascicular needle tip placement.[24,26,29,30] NOTE: There is an increased injection resistance and slower aspiration from smaller-gauge needles.

Developing regional needles that can more easily reflect ultrasound beams may improve needle-tip visibility. This concept may also reduce the time required to complete ultrasound-guided nerve blockade. This is accomplished by: (1) placing etched grooves at the needle tip; (2) incorporating a special coating on needles that trap micro–air bubbles; or (3) integrating reflector dots on the needle's distal end that may enhance the echogenic image.[22] As an example, echogenic needles inserted at 60–70 degree angles are more easily imaged on ultrasound when compared to non-echogenic needles.[22,31]

CONTINUOUS REGIONAL ANESTHESIA/ANALGESIA

Safe and effective continuous infusion of local anesthetics is possible with specialized needle-and-catheter systems.[32] Equipment for these purposes is applicable to clinical scenarios requiring longer-term perioperative analgesia. For example, compared to traditional catheter-through-the-needle devices, catheter-over-needle assemblies have the goal of reducing catheter leakage and/or catheter migration.[33,34] Placing catheter-through-needle devices could permit gaps at the skin-catheter interface upon removal of the introducer. However, with catheter-over-needle assemblies, withdrawing the introducer doesn't alter the more secure fit of the catheter-to-skin interface (introducer housed inside the catheter).[34] Additional advantages of the catheter-over-needle design is ease of catheter insertion, confirming catheter tip placement (echogenic catheter tip), and securing of the catheter to the skin surface.

Continuous catheter-over-needle device/assemblies resemble intravenous cannulas with the distal needle end protruding through the catheter. There are other design variations of this catheter-over-needle assembly marketed by different brands, such as a catheter-within-catheter design where an inner catheter is inserted through the outer catheter. This type of catheter assembly was designed to create a unit less likely to kink the catheter.

ELECTRONIC NERVE STIMULATORS

Prior to the adoption of ultrasound-guided regional anesthesia, peripheral nerve stimulators were used for nerve target-seeking, along with confirmation of nerve and nerve plexus blockade. However, when used in combination with ultrasound, nerve stimulation can create another objective detail toward achieving a safer and more accurate/successful nerve blockade. Nerve stimulators have changed from nerve and nerve plexus target-seeking devices toward a monitoring tool for determining needle-to-nerve contact and/or proximity. Used in combination with ultrasound, nerve stimulation can be a confirmatory option that could reduce the inadvertent intraneural needle tip placement.[35]

Constant Current Output, Display Features and Variable Pulse Width

Nerve stimulators deliver a current output that can be set with variable milliamperes (mA), frequency, and pulse width. Nerve stimulators can deliver a constant and stable current, even despite varied tissue resistances. A digital display (2 decimal place accuracy) is a feature indicating the actual current being delivered and not simply a set/dialed target setting. These devices are equipped with low (6 mA) and high (80 mA) output ranges. For example, higher-output ranges are used for the epidural stimulation test, but a lower output can be used to alert for any potential intraneural needle-tip placement should muscle stimulation occur.[35]

Nerve stimulators are capable of delivering a variable pulse width (short- and long-pulse widths). When compared to long-pulse widths (1 ms) that reveal little differences in the required current to stimulate nerves (regardless of whether the needle is in direct contact with the nerve or a safe distance away), the advantages of short pulse widths (0.04 ms) serve as an indicator of the distance between needle and nerve based on changes in current. For example, there is a significant difference in the current needed, at a pulse width of 0.04 ms, to stimulate muscle tissue when comparing direct needle-tip contact with a nerve versus a needle tip 1 cm away from the target nerve.[36]

Polarity of Electrodes, Variable Pulse Frequency, and Malfunction Indicators

Polarity of block needles and grounding electrode are color-coded. The black colored lead (cathode) is more effective than the red led (anode) at depolarizing nerve membranes and is usually selected as the stimulating electrode (influence the device's ability to stimulate target nerves at a given current). The frequency of the electrical pulse being delivered can be adjusted by the device such that the optimal frequency is between 0.5 and 4 Hz, with most practitioners selecting a 2 Hz frequency (allows adjustment of frequency up to 5 Hz). NOTE: The block needle should be advanced slowly when choosing a lower frequency (i.e., 1 Hz; one stimulus/second) to avoid missing the target nerve between device stimulations. Nerve stimulators also indicate battery power, detect disconnection, and malfunction of the device. There are audible tones and/or visible light changes capable of indicating an incomplete circuit and whether the selected pulse current is being delivered or not.[37]

Electrical Impedance

Nerve stimulators can measure impedance and display the impedance between the needle tip and ground electrode.[38] Nerve stimulators use pulsating direct current (DC) (flow of electric charge in one direction). Pulsating DC has similarities to both DC and alternating current (AC) (flow of charge that can reverse direction). Capacitances of electrode-to-skin interface, the block needle tip, and tissue influence the resistance of the electrical circuit. Capacitance of the circuit varies with the frequency of the nerve stimulator current and is referred to as a *complex resistance* or *impedance* (dependent on frequency of the stimulus). Therefore, the shorter the impulse, the higher the frequency and the lower the impedance of a circuit with a given capacitance. Impedance is sensitive to the makeup of tissues (composition of water and lipid content) and since there are variations of content between intraneural and extraneural tissues (intraneural has greater nonconduction lipid amounts), a difference between intraneural and extraneural impedance exists. For example, an increase of impedance to >4.3% could identify an intraneural needle tip placement.[39] In addition, improved precision of needle tip placement may be achieved by combining impedance variables and several measurement frequencies, resulting in discrimination between nerve tissue and other types of tissue. As another example, since electrical impedance changes with injection of D5W, this may guard against injection that could cause nerve damage or other untoward results.[40]

ULTRASOUND

The clinical practice of regional anesthesia has been revolutionized and overwhelmingly accepted by anesthesia practices/practitioners with the introduction of ultrasound technology. Such technology permits real-time imaging of target nerves, block needle guidance through tissues (in-plane approach), along with imaging of other subcutaneous and surrounding anatomical structures.[41,42] Ultrasound technology advances have undergone exponential growth (i.e., improved safety and complimented performance) with several commercially available portable machines configured for regional anesthesia. However, ultrasound-guided regional anesthesia continues to be operator dependent, requires dedicated learning, practice, hand-eye coordination development, preparation for untoward clinical events, clinical and systematic development of protocols, formalized synthesis into the practice of medicine and institutional-specific culture, and consistent vigilance for safety.[43]

The ultrasound probe/transducer, along with understanding of its function, is an important component of any ultrasound machine. Transducers are configured with various footprints and beam planes that permit users to scan/image anatomical structures. Quality of ultrasound probes, machines, and images reveal evolving improvements with practitioner-friendly operation(s), easier portability, enhanced affordability of machine/transducer costs, and better image-resolution quality. Yet despite these increasing attributes of technology and enhanced ultrasound component development(s) for regional anesthesia, caution must continue to be practiced since ultrasound automation cannot completely eliminate/avoid patient harm (i.e., intraneural injection).[44,45] Therefore, the block needle tip should be always visualized to improve upon important safety measures.

Basic ultrasound physics/mechanics understanding will permit practitioners to set up and safely operate the system and select an appropriate transducer in order to obtain optimal imaging.[44] Physics of an ultrasound device (ultrasound generation, detection, propagation, and transformation) may be somewhat complex; however, clinical application of visualizing target nerves and relevant structures is simpler.[44] Ultrasound is described as high-frequency sound from piezoelectric crystals creating mechanical vibrations above 20 kHz in which the sound travels as a longitudinal wave with back-and-forth particle motion parallel to the direction of the wave.[41] As an example, humans hear with frequencies between 20 Hz and 20 kHz, whereas dolphins and bats create sounds waves in the 20–100 kHz range (for navigation).

Piezoelectric Effect

Piezoelectric concept is established by the creation of an electric charge that can lead to mechanical deformation of ceramic and quartz crystals (piezoelectric crystals) within the ultrasound probe. An electric field causing mechanical deformation to the crystals is capable of producing a sound of high frequency. These artificial and natural materials demonstrate piezoelectric properties, and lead zirconate titanate is now being used for medical imaging.[46] By stacking these elements (individual crystal components produce a small amount of energy independently) into layers, the ultrasound transducer converts the electric energy into mechanical oscillations that can in turn be converted into electric energy.[46]

Basic Terminology of Ultrasound

Ultrasound waves have a natural narrowing (self-focusing phenomenon) of the wave at a certain distance ("transition") within the ultrasound field (transition between near and far fields). The ultrasound beam width reaches the transducer diameter at a distance of 2 × the near-field length, and the beam width at this transition level equals half the diameter of the transducer. This so-called self-focusing effect will augment and intensify signals of the ultrasound by amplifying acoustic pressures.[41] The following list defines the basic terminology:

Wavelength: travel distance from beginning to end that a cycle travels (length of space of a single cycle).

Period: duration of a sound wave to complete a cycle (measured in microseconds [μs]).

Frequency: hertz (Hz) measurements representing the number of cycles repeated/second.

Speed (c): density [ρ] along with stiffness [κ] of any medium $[(\kappa/\rho)^{1/2} = c]$ determines speed (speeds within soft tissues are 1540 m/s and ultrasound for regional cannot penetrate bone).

Acoustic velocity: speed an ultrasound wave penetrates a medium and equals frequency × wavelength.

Stiffness: compression resistance of a material.

Density: concentration of a medium.

Attenuation coefficient: criterion that projects the ultrasound amplitude diminution within certain tissues as a behavior of ultrasound frequency (penetration decreases as frequency increases).

Acoustic impedance[z]: measures the obstacle/difficulty of an ultrasound wave transmitting through tissue. Increased if density of the tissue or propagation velocity is escalated (equals density[ρ] times acoustic velocity[c]; $z = \rho c$).

Two components of spatial resolution (lateral and axial resolution) exist within ultrasound imaging. Lateral is determined by ultrasound frequency and beam width describing a component of sharpness between tissue objects (i.e., side-by-side distance). Higher frequencies (narrower focus) result in improved axial and lateral resolution. Axial resolution is determined as wavelength (λ) × number of cycles per pulse (n) ÷ 2 and presented by spatial pulse length (equal to wavelength × number of cycles within a pulse).

There are three ultrasound wave interactions as it travels through tissue(s): *absorption*, *reflection*, and *scatter*.

In terms of *absorption*, ultrasound scanning can generate heat in the tissue (conversion of sound energy into heat). Tissue scanned at higher ultrasound frequencies (shorter wavelengths) absorb more heat than lower scanning frequencies (longer wavelength) and also results in improved axial resolution. However, deeper target structures cannot always be adequately visualized at higher ultrasound frequencies (i.e., poorer ultrasound penetration insufficient to visualize deeper structures). Therefore, a lower frequency would be used to improve/increase penetration, but this can result in poorer resolution since resolution of ultrasound imaging is proportional to the wavelength of the ultrasound wave. For example: 6–12 MHz provide appropriate superficial peripheral nerve resolution (less than 5 cm) and frequencies of 2–5 MHz are typically used for deeper targets and neuraxial imaging (<2 MHz or >15 MHz are rarely used due to insufficient resolution and/or penetration).

When ultrasound encounters different tissue boundaries, the ultrasound wave can be either reflected (i.e., creates an echo) or transmitted through. *Reflection* of ultrasound waves (similar to optical reflection) has a portion of the wave energy sent/reflected back into the tissue (defined by reflection and transmission angles). This reflection strength can be variable and is determined by the difference(s) of impedance between the tissue plains as well as the incident angle at their interface (i.e., equal tissue impedance results in no reflection/no echo, while significant tissue impedances can result in nearly complete reflection). As an example, a strong reflection/echo is created between soft tissue and lung/bone interfaces due to significant differences in acoustic impedance, and also depends upon the ultrasound wave angle. Therefore, to visualize intended target structure(s) more clearly, the transducer angle should also be directed as perpendicular to the target as possible. As another example of reflection, ultrasound gel is used between the transducer and skin (displaces air), but if the peripheral boundaries are irregular/curved, then the reflected waves will be diffused (i.e., no image).[41]

Scatter is caused by the redirection of ultrasound waves in several directions by the differing tissues being imaged.

Intensity of scatter is irrelevant to the direction of the ultrasound wave. Therefore, imaging of the target structure(s) is not significantly altered by nearby scattering and is irrelevant of the ultrasound wave direction.

Ultrasound echoes will have a reduced amplitude when imaging deeper structures secondary to: (a) energy is reduced with each successive reflection of the pulse wave (decreasing the formation of subsequent echoes); and (b) energy is lost as ultrasound waves travel through tissues (tissue absorbs ultrasound energy). This influence can be modified with both compression and time-gain compensation (TGC; measured in decibels; controls brightness of the image). TGC is used to improve amplitude of incoming ultrasound waves from deeper tissue depths (time-dependent amplification). However, increasing gain (i.e., brightness) also amplifies background noise as well. Ultrasound machines convert transducer echoes into visible dots, forming an anatomic image on the screen and producing a two-dimensional image or "slice" (three-dimensional imaging has recently been developed). Brightness of image dots corresponds to the echo strength and produces a gray-scale image.

During ultrasound for regional anesthesia, there are two types of probes typically used: (1) linear array and (2) curved transducer (rectangular display, and an arc-shaped image, respectively). Echoes from the transducer are converted into visible dots to form an anatomical image. NOTE: During imaging, an aqueous solution is used between the skin and transducer to eliminate air, since any such air layer could reflect the ultrasound and interfere with penetration through the tissue.

Electronic techniques of the ultrasound machine are used to optimize its focusing effects (i.e., annular and linear types of focusing, narrowing of ultrasound beam width). Adjusting the focus can result in greater resolution at the tissue plane of interest (focal zone), but this can result in poorer resolution at other tissue depths and yield less clear imaging below the focal zone. Annular focusing is achieved by directing the electronic focus in all directions of the scanning plane (concentrically arranged ring elements); and linear focusing is achieved with electronic focus applied along the lateral sides of the scanning plane.

Modes of Ultrasound Imaging

A-mode: the transducer sends an ultrasound pulse (single) into tissue, developing a one-dimensional image (A-mode not applicable to regional).

B-mode: echo from several A-mode scans together converted into dots, resulting in different brightness intensities (100–300 rather than a single A-mode), yields a two-dimensional image from a linear array of piezoelectric elements (primary mode used in regional). Varying intensities of the gray scale reveal echo strength, while horizontal and vertical imaging indicates "real" distances.

Doppler-mode: change in wavelength/frequency of the sound wave between sound source and sound receiver (sound wavelength/frequency is constant when emitted from a stationary position). As an example, a negative Doppler shift describes stretching of sound waves when the sound source is moving away from a receiver, resulting in a lower pitch sound received, compared to a positive Doppler shift describing the squeezing of sound waves as the sound source is directed toward the sound receiver, resulting in a higher-pitch sound.[47] Incident angle(s) between the ultrasound beam being emitted and the moving reflectors determine the magnitude of the Doppler shift (no Doppler shift with a 90 degree angle, and largest Doppler shift at angles of 0 degrees or 180 degrees).[47]

Color Doppler: used to image blood vessels (artery/vein) within and surrounding intended targets during ultrasound-guided regional anesthesia. Motion of blood flow toward or away from the ultrasound transducer produces a color-coded map (red/blue colors) of Doppler shifts superimposed onto a B-mode ultrasound image depicting direction and velocity of flow, with blue denoting flow away from the transducer and red indicating blood flow directed toward the transducer. As an example, depending upon tilt of the ultrasound probe/beam, the color of blood flow within the vessel(s) being imaged can switch from blue to red or red to blue (does not depict artery or vein).

Power Doppler: more sensitive compared to color Doppler in detecting blood vessels and can be used to image smaller blood vessels, but provides no information on blood flow direction or speed. Scanning with power Doppler is less dependent on transducer angle when compared to color Doppler.

M-mode: used in cardiac imaging (i.e., heart valves) with little use in regional anesthesia.

CONCLUSION

Increasing evidence and abundance of evolving literature identify how and why regional anesthesia continues to be commonplace in anesthesia practices. Much of the evidence is due to increasing patient benefits, including: reduction of opioid consumption and rescue opioid requirements; reductions in pulmonary and thromboembolic complications; pain abatement; reduced time to hospital discharge; more engaging and earlier perioperative physical therapy; and improved ultrasound equipment, along with supplies, leading to a better immediate postoperative quality of life. This interest and popularity of regional anesthesia has also resulted in improved evolving regional techniques. For example, regional anesthesia changed from paresthesia for nerve localization, then to electrical nerve stimulation, and on to ultrasound-guided nerve localization (often in conjunction with stimulators). Special equipment and specific supplies for performing regional anesthesia/analgesia are required and often are modified to ensure that techniques proceed safely and in an efficient manner. Proper equipment, surgery-specific regional protocols, practitioner skills, understanding and appropriate use of regional supplies, equipment, and medications are all necessary to ensure that regional anesthesia proceeds smoothly in a patient-safety manner throughout the perioperative period.

REFERENCES

1. Tokish JM, Alexander TC, Kissenberth MJ, Hawkins RJ. Pseudoparalysis: a systematic review of term definitions, treatment approaches, and outcomes of management techniques. *J Shoulder Elbow Surg*. 2017;26(6):177–187.
2. Klein SM, Melton MS, Warren MG, Nielsen KC. Peripheral nerve stimulation in regional anesthesia. *Reg Anesth Pain Med*. 2012;37:383–392.
3. Steinfeldt T, Schwemmer U, Volk T, et al. Nerve localization for peripheral regional anesthesia: recommendations of the German Society of Anaesthesiology and Intensive Care Medicine. *Anaesthesist*. 2014;63(7):597–602.
4. Cantrell MB, Grill WM, Klein SM. Computer-based finite element modeling of insulated Tuohy needles used in regional anesthesia. *Anesthesiology*. 2009;110(6):1229–1234.
5. Neal JM, Brull R, Horn JL, et al. The Second American Society of Regional Anesthesia and Pain Medicine evidence-based medicine assessment of ultrasound-guided regional anesthesia: executive summary. *Reg Anesth Pain Med*. 2016;41(2):181–194.
6. Neal JM. Ultrasound-guided regional anesthesia and patient safety update of an evidence-based analysis. *Reg Anesth Pain Med*. 2016;41: 195–204.
7. Shriki J. Ultrasound physics. *Crit Care Clin*. 2014;30(1):1–24.
8. Guay J, Suresh S, Kopp S. The use of ultrasound guidance for perioperative neuraxial and peripheral nerve blocks in children. *Cochrane Database Syst Rev*. 2019;2:CD011436.
9. Prabhu SJ, Kanal K, Bhargava P, Vaidya S, Dighe MK. Ultrasound artifacts: classification, applied physics with illustrations, and imaging appearances. *Ultrasound Q*. 2014;30(2):145–157.
10. Enriquez JL, Wu TS. An introduction to ultrasound equipment and knobology. *Crit Care Clin*. 2014;30(1):25–45.
11. Mian A, Chaudhry I, Huang R, et al. Brachial plexus anesthesia: a review of the relevant anatomy, complications, and anatomical variations. *Clin Anat*. 2014;27(2):210–221.
12. Tran DQ, Elgueta MF, Aliste J, Finlayson RJ. Diaphragm-sparing nerve blocks for shoulder surgery. *Reg Anesth Pain Med*. 2017;42(1):32–38.
13. Wiesmann T, Bornträger A, Vassiliou T, et al. Minimal current intensity to elicit an evoked motor response cannot discern between needle-nerve contact and intraneural needle insertion. *Anesth Analg*. 2014;118(3):681–686.
14. Guo CW, Ma JX, Ma XL, et al. Supraclavicular block versus interscalene brachial plexus block for shoulder surgery: a meta-analysis of clinical control trials. *Int J Surg*. 2017;45:85–91.
15. Tran DQ, Muñoz L, Russo G, Finlayson RJ. Ultrasonography and stimulating perineural catheters for nerve blocks: a review of the evidence. *Can J Anaesth*. 2008;55(7):447–457.
16. Koscielniak-Nielsen ZJ, Dahl JB. Ultrasound-guided peripheral nerve blockade of the upper extremity. *Curr Opin Anaesthesiol*. 2012;25(2):253–259.
17. Tsai TP, Vuckovic I, Dilberovic F, et al. Intensity of the stimulating current may not be a reliable indicator of intraneural needle placement. *Reg Anesth Pain Med*. 2008;33(3):207–210.
18. Schnabel A, Meyer-Frießem CH, Zahn PK, Pogatzki-Zahn EM. Ultrasound compared with nerve stimulation guidance for peripheral nerve catheter placement: a meta-analysis of randomized controlled trials. *Br J Anaesth*. 2013;111(4):564–572.
19. Vassiliou T, Müller HH, Limberg S, De Andres J, Steinfeldt T, Wiesmann T. Risk evaluation for needle-nerve contact related to electrical nerve stimulation in a porcine model. *Acta Anaesthesiol Scand*. 2016;60(3):400–406.
20. Ilfeld BM. Continuous peripheral nerve blocks: an update of the published evidence and comparison with novel, alternative analgesic modalities. *Anesth Analg*. 2017;124(1):308–335.
21. Merritt CK, Mariano ER, Kaye AD, et al. Peripheral nerve catheters and local anesthetic infiltration in perioperative analgesia. *Best Pract Res Clin Anaesthesiol*. 2014;28(1):41–57.
22. Abbal B, Choquet O, Gourari A, et al. Enhanced visual acuity with echogenic needles in ultrasound-guided axillary brachial plexus block: a randomized, comparative, observer-blinded study. *Minerva Anestesiol*. 2015;81:369–378.
23. Sites BD, Taenzer AH, Herrick MD, et al. Incidence of local anesthetic systemic toxicity and postoperative neurologic symptoms associated with 12,668 ultrasound-guided nerve blocks: an analysis from a prospective clinical registry. *Reg Anesth Pain Med*. 2012;37(5):478–482.
24. Franco CD, Sala-Blanch X. Functional anatomy of the nerve and optimal placement of the needle for successful (and) safe nerve blocks. *Curr Opin Anaesthesiol*. 2019;32(5):638–642.
25. Choquet O, Morau D, Biboulet P, Capdevila X. Where should the tip of the needle be located in ultrasound-guided peripheral nerve blocks? *Curr Opin Anaesthesiol*. 2012;25(5):596–602.
26. Steinfeldt T, Werner T, Nimphius W, et al. Histological analysis after peripheral nerve puncture with pencil-point or Tuohy needle tip. *Anesth Analg*. 2011;112(2):465–470.
27. Steinfeldt T, Poeschl S, Nimphius W, et al. Forced needle advancement during needle-nerve contact in a porcine model: histological outcome. *Anesth Analg*. 2011;113(2):417–420.
28. Zorrilla-Vaca A, Mathur V, Wu CL, Grant MC. The impact of spinal needle selection on postdural puncture headache: a meta-analysis and meta-regression of randomized studies. *Reg Anesth Pain Med*. 2018;43(5):502–508.
29. Selander D, Dhuner KG, Lundborg G. Peripheral nerve injury due to injection needles used for regional anesthesia: an experimental study of the acute effects of needle point trauma. *Acta Anaesthesiol Scand*. 1977;21:182–188.
30. Jeng CL, Rosenblatt MA. Intraneural injections and regional anesthesia: the known and the unknown. *Minerva Anestesiol*. 2011;77(1):54–58.
31. Uppal V, Sondekoppam RV, Ganapathy S. Effect of beam steering on the visibility of echogenic and non-echogenic needles: a laboratory study. *Can J Anaesth*. 2014;61:909–915.
32. Richman JM, Liu SS, Courpas G, et al. Does continuous peripheral nerve block provide superior pain control to opioids? A meta-analysis. *Anesth Analg*. 2006;102:248–257.
33. Ip VH, Rockley MC, Tsui BC. The catheter-over-needle assembly offers greater stability and less leakage compared with the traditional counterpart in continuous interscalene nerve blocks: a randomized patient-blinded study. *Can J Anaesth*. 2013;60:1272–1273.
34. Tsui BC, Ip VH. Catheter-over-needle method reduces risk of perineural catheter dislocation. *Br J Anaesth*. 2014;112:759–760.
35. Bigeleisen PE, Moayeri N, Groen GJ. Extraneural versus intraneural stimulation thresholds during ultrasound-guided supraclavicular block. *Anesthesiology*. 2009;110:1235–1243.
36. Robards C, Hadzic A, Somasundaram L, et al. Intraneural injection with low-current stimulation during popliteal sciatic nerve block. *Anesth Analg*. 2009;109:673–677.
37. Byrne K, Tsui BC. Practical concepts in nerve stimulation: impedance and other recent advances. *Int Anesthesiol Clin*. 2011;49:81–90.
38. Kalvoy H, Sauter AR. Detection of intraneural needle-placement with multiple frequency bioimpedance monitoring: a novel method. *J Clin Monit Comput*. 2016;30(2):185–192.
39. Vydyanathan A, Kosharskyy B, Nair S, et al. The use of electrical impedance to identify intraneural needle placement in human peripheral nerves: a study on amputated human limbs. *Anesth Analg*. 2016;123(1):228–232.
40. Bardou P, Merle JC, Woillard JB, et al. Electrical impedance to detect accidental nerve puncture during ultrasound-guided peripheral nerve blocks. *Can J Anaesth*. 2013;60:253–258.
41. Ensminger D, Bond LJ. *Ultrasonics: Fundamentals, Technologies, and Applications*. 3rd ed. Boca Raton, FL: CRC Press; 2012. doi:10.1201/b11173.
42. Vermeylen K, Engelen S, Sermeus L, Soetens F, Van de Velde M. Supraclavicular brachial plexus blocks: review and current practice. *Acta Anaesthesiol Belg*. 2012; 63(1):15–21.

43. British Medical Ultrasound Society. Guidelines for the safe use of diagnostic ultrasound equipment. *Ultrasound.* 2010;18:52–59.
44. Hara K, Sakura S, Yokokawa N, Tadenuma S. Incidence and effects of unintentional intraneural injection during ultrasound-guided subgluteal sciatic nerve block. *Reg Anesth Pain Med.* 2012;37:289–293.
45. Neal JM, Barrington MJ, Brull R, et al. The second ASRA practice advisory on neurologic complications associated with regional anesthesia and pain medicine: executive summary 2015. *Reg Anesth Pain Med.* 2015;40(5):401–430.
46. American Institute of Ultrasound in Medicine, National Electrical Manufacturers Association. *Standard for Real-Time Display of Thermal and Mechanical Acoustic Output Indices on Diagnostic Ultrasound Equipment, Revision 2.* American Institute of Ultrasound in Medicine and National Electrical Manufacturers Association; 2004.
47. White DN. Johann Christian Doppler and his effect: a brief history. *Ultrasound Med Biol.* 1982;8(6):583–591.

REVIEW QUESTIONS

(1) Which statement is correct?

A. A continuous peripheral nerve block is associated with reduced anesthetic consumption and lower opioid requirements.
B. The closer the stimulating needle or catheter to the nerve, the stronger the motor response.
C. Continuous peripheral nerve blockade (CPNB) was developed in the early 1900s and has a longer history and more clinical application than does a single-shot nerve block option.
D. When compared to insulated short bevel needles, uninsulated needles provide a more focused current and improved nerve localization.

(2) Which setting (repetition rate) of the peripheral nerve stimulator should be used to detect muscular twitches when the current is between 0.5 and 1.0 mA intensity and 0.1 ms duration?

A. 2 Hz
B. 50 Hz
C. 100 Hz
D. 200 Hz

(3) What is the most correct definition of rheobase?

A. The pulse duration at double the threshold
B. The lowest threshold current at infinitely long pulse duration
C. The pulse width at half the threshold
D. The electrical pulse that is most effective at motor stimulation

(4) Which needle localization technique requires direct contact with the nerve and/or nerve plexus?

A. Achieving a fascial click
B. Paresthesia technique
C. Under fluoroscopy
D. Ultrasound-guided technique

(5) With a nerve stimulating needle connected to the stimulator, which of the following settings is correct?

A. Select 0.1 mA as the starting current for superficial targets
B. Select 1 ms current duration for superficial blocks
C. Select 1.5 mA as the starting current for deeper targets
D. Select 1 ms current duration for deeper nerve blocks

(6) Benefits of ultrasound-guided nerve blocks include:

A. Visualization of target structures and surrounding anatomy
B. Visualization of the block needle
C. Visualization of local anesthetic spread (real-time)
D. All of the above

(7) "P" of the mnemonic PART describes what component of ultrasound imaging?

A. Placing the transducer on the body at which the underlying target is expected.
B. Reducing the distance between the nerve target and ultrasound footprint
C. "Fine-tuning" the portion of the target structure
D. Positioning the ultrasound probe perpendicular to the target nerve

(8) Nerve blocks using the short-axis, in-plane view provide all the following except:

A. Ability to visualize the entire needle
B. Increased safety
C. Improved success
D. Permits needle depth monitoring

ANSWERS

(1) **A.** Stimulating catheters for continuous techniques compared to non-stimulating catheters are associated with lower local anesthetic consumption and when compared to single-shot techniques show reduced opioid requirements. The distance between stimulating needle and target nerve/plexus is not always associated with the strength of the motor response. The CPNB needles and catheters occurred later than development of single-shot techniques, along with less clinical use. The larger uninsulated needle produces a less focused current output that can reduce nerve target accuracy.

Reference

Ilfeld BM. Continuous peripheral nerve blocks: an update of the published evidence and comparison with novel, alternative analgesic modalities. *Anesth Analg.* 2017;124(1):308–335.

(2) **A.** 2 Hz is ideal to detect motor responses.

Reference

Steinfeldt T, Schwemmer U, Volk T, et al. Nerve localization for peripheral regional anesthesia: recommendations of the German Society of Anaesthesiology and Intensive Care Medicine. *Anaesthesist.* 2014;63(7):597–602.

(3) **B.** Rheobase is the lowest threshold current at infinitely long pulse duration.

Reference

Wiesmann T, Bornträger A, Vassiliou T, et al. Minimal current intensity to elicit an evoked motor response cannot discern between needle-nerve contact and intraneural needle insertion. *Anesth Analg.* 2014;118(3):681–686.

(4) **B.** Paresthesia technique relies on the block needle advancing toward the target nerve/plexus until a sensory paresthesia is obtained. It depends upon needle tip and nerve contact. Fascial click is a "tactile pop" feeling when the needle tip pierces fascial planes. Fluoroscopy visualizes radiopaque structures (i.e., bones) in order to indirectly localize the anatomical nerve/plexus location. Nerve/plexus targets can typically be visualized using ultrasound-guided techniques and the block needle can be placed in close proximity and not requiring direct contact.

Reference

Klein SM, Melton MS, Warren MG, Nielsen KC. Peripheral nerve stimulation in regional anesthesia. *Reg Anesth Pain Med.* 2012;37:383–392.

(5) **B.** For deeper nerve/plexus targets, the operator should select 1.5 mA as the starting current intensity.

Reference

Schnabel A, Meyer-Frießem CH, Zahn PK, Pogatzki-Zahn EM. Ultrasound compared with nerve stimulation guidance for peripheral nerve catheter placement: a meta-analysis of randomized controlled trials. *Br J Anaesth.* 2013;111(4):564–572.

(6) **D.** Ultrasound permits visualization of target structures, surrounding anatomy, block needle as it is passed toward its target, and real-time spread of local.

Reference

Koscielniak-Nielsen ZJ, Dahl JB. Ultrasound-guided peripheral nerve blockade of the upper extremity. *Curr Opin Anaesthesiol.* 2012;25(2):253–259.

(7) **B.** P represents pressure (application of force on the transducer with the underlying target below the probe to improve ultrasound image), A for alignment, R for rotation, and T for tilt.

Reference

Neal JM. Ultrasound-guided regional anesthesia and patient safety update of an evidence-based analysis. *Reg Anesth Pain Med.* 2016;41: 195–204.

(8) **C.** Positioning the probe with a short-axis, in-plane approach permits A, B, and D, since there aren't any particular needle-to-probe orientations resulting in superior blockade success.

Reference

Koscielniak-Nielsen ZJ, Dahl JB. Ultrasound-guided peripheral nerve blockade of the upper extremity. *Curr Opin Anaesthesiol.* 2012;25(2):253–259.

4.

SETTING UP A MODERN ACUTE PAIN SERVICE (APS)

Jeffrey J. Mojica, Sean Washek, and Eric S. Schwenk

STEM CASE AND KEY QUESTIONS

A 45-year-old male with a history of opioid use disorder (OUD) treated with buprenorphine/naloxone 8 mg/2 mg once daily and osteoarthritis of the right knee presents for an elective total knee replacement. The patient's orthopedic team is requesting an acute pain service (APS) consult for perioperative pain management.

(1) WHAT IS THE PURPOSE OF AN ACUTE PAIN SERVICE?

The role of the APS has expanded greatly over time from purely perioperative pain control to include all hospitalized patients suffering from a variety of acute pain conditions.[1] The purpose of having an APS is for assistance and consultation in the management of complex acute pain that occurs in both surgical and nonsurgical hospitalized patients. This is usually achieved with multimodal analgesic techniques that feature regional anesthesia, opioid and non-opioid analgesic medications, and intravenous infusions, such as ketamine and lidocaine.

(2) HOW DOES UNCONTROLLED POSTOPERATIVE PAIN INFLUENCE PATIENT OUTCOMES?

Inadequately treated acute pain can increase patient morbidity, impair quality of life and physical function, delay recovery, and prolong length of stay.[2] It has been estimated that for every 10% increase in the time spent in severe postoperative pain, there is a 30% increase in chronic pain 12 months after surgery.[3]

(3) WHAT IS MULTIMODAL ANALGESIA?

The basic principle of multimodal analgesia (MMA) is using multiple groups of agents and techniques with various mechanisms of action that target different parts of the pain pathways, including pain transduction, conduction, transmission, modulation, and perception. By using agents that act on different receptors, pain can be treated more effectively, and the dosage of the medications can be decreased when used in conjunction. This can lead to fewer side effects versus exclusive use of a single agent, especially opioid-related adverse effects.

(4) WHAT ROLE DOES AN APS PLAY IN THE MANAGEMENT OF POSTOPERATIVE PAIN?

Acute pain providers work in conjunction with surgical services to treat postoperative pain. In this setting, an APS serves as a consulting service and provides recommendations to the surgical team. Commonly used techniques unique to an APS include neuraxial and peripheral nerve blocks, and ketamine and lidocaine infusions. An APS incorporates these modalities into formalized, multimodal analgesic protocols that span the entire perioperative period. MMA attenuates the stress response to surgery, decreases pain intensity, and reduces opioid-related adverse effects.[4] MMA is a core component of enhanced recovery after anesthesia and surgery (ERAS) pathways and its inclusion can facilitate postoperative recovery.[5] An APS complements the perioperative expertise of an anesthesiology department and enhances the quality of perioperative care.

(5) IS THERE A ROLE FOR A KETAMINE INFUSION IN THIS PATIENT?

In the case of the 45-year-old patient described above, a ketamine infusion that started intraoperatively and continued into the postoperative period is recommended by the APS. The postoperative continuation of ketamine requires frequent assessments by an experienced and trained team of providers that are familiar with ketamine's adverse effects.[6] With such an APS, the safety and efficacy of ketamine can be closely monitored without escalation on the level of care to telemetry or the intensive care unit.[7] It has been shown in a mixed medical-surgical patient population that the overall incidence of adverse effects is low and that almost all resolve with temporary discontinuation of the infusion.[8]

(6) IS THERE A ROLE FOR A LIDOCAINE INFUSION IN THIS PATIENT?

Lidocaine infusions have been shown to reduce the severity of postoperative pain, incidence of postoperative nausea, vomiting, and ileus duration after open and laparoscopic abdominal surgery.[9,10] It possesses potent anti-inflammatory properties that are believed to exert its analgesic effects by attenuating the stress response to surgery.[9] However, these effects are not consistent across various surgical procedures, and efficacy appears to be limited to the early postoperative period.[11] In the authors' opinion, lidocaine infusion should be reserved for patients who are contraindicated for regional anesthesia.

(7) WHY IS PAIN MANAGEMENT IN PATIENTS TAKING BUPRENORPHINE DIFFICULT? HOW SHOULD THESE PATIENTS BE MANAGED IN THE PERIOPERATIVE PERIOD?

Buprenorphine is useful in the treatment of opioid addiction and is being used with increasing frequency because, unlike methadone, it does not require frequent clinic visits and does not have the stigma that methadone carries. It is a partial agonist at μ-opioid receptors and an antagonist at κ- and ∂-opioid receptors.[12] It possesses a high receptor-binding affinity, a long half-life largely from its slow dissociation from the receptor, and a "ceiling-effect" that produces the effects of a full μ-opioid agonist but to a lesser extent.[13,14] As the daily dose of buprenorphine increases, the number of unoccupied μ-opioid receptors decreases. At a daily dose of 16 mg, the number of receptors available for interacting with another μ-opioid agonist is reduced by 85%–92% from baseline.[15] In practical terms, this means that 16 mg daily of buprenorphine will suppress opioid withdrawal symptoms and block the effects of μ-opioid agonists.

Postoperative pain management can be notoriously challenging in this population.[16,17] Non-opioid analgesics, including ketamine and local anesthetics via peripheral nerve block, peri-articular infiltration, epidural analgesia, or other vehicles, are the key to adequately managing pain when buprenorphine is involved.

As part of a MMA plan, you recommend an adductor canal catheter for postoperative analgesia. On postoperative day 1, the patient complains of severe pain located on the posterior aspect of his leg. He wants to know if something is wrong. How would you respond?

Even after a successful primary block, it is not uncommon for patients to complain of pain. The pain may represent the resolution of the primary block, equipment malfunction, catheter dislodgement, or in rare cases, an early sign of compartment syndrome.[18] In this situation, the patient is complaining of pain in a distribution not covered by an adductor canal block. Sensation to the posterior aspect of the knee is provided by the obturator, tibial, and common fibular nerve.[19] The patient should be counseled that the block is working appropriately and does not cover the posterior aspect of the knee. In many instances, posterior knee pain can be managed with opioid and non-opioid medications.

The patient is scheduled to be discharged to a rehabilitation facility on postoperative day 2. The patient's orthopedic surgeon is concerned that his pain will not be adequately controlled without the nerve block. The orthopedic surgeon asks you for analgesia recommendations for discharge.

Ambulatory pumps have been developed for the purpose of continuing local anesthetic infusions with peripheral nerve catheters after hospital discharge. In appropriate patients, ambulatory continuous peripheral nerve blocks can provide highly effective and safe analgesia.[20] Additional benefits include reduced time to discharge readiness, improved rehabilitation, range of motion, superior analgesia, and reduced opioid requirements.[21] The APS is responsible for educating patients on device management and potential adverse events to watch for, and instructing patients to call if they have any questions or concerns. We highly recommend the availability of an on-call physician to troubleshoot block-related problems over the phone or at minimum a nurse who follows a written protocol.

Oral multimodal analgesics should also be recommended at discharge for all patients without contraindications. This may include but are not limited to acetaminophen, nonsteroidal anti-inflammatory drugs (NSAIDs), gabapentinoids, tricyclic anti-depressants, N-methyl-D-aspartate (NMDA) antagonists, and opioids. We recommend prescribing all non-opioid agents around the clock and not "as needed" to establish a solid analgesic foundation, while leaving opioids for severe breakthrough pain.

DISCUSSION

The first APS was created in 1985 by the Department of Anesthesiology at the University of Washington and its purpose was to provide a 24-hour pain-management service for postoperative patients.[22] At the time, existing pain management strategies were deficient, and were limited to patient-controlled analgesia (PCA) and neuraxial techniques. In recent years, there has been a shift from opioid-based therapies to multimodal analgesia. This evolution is a result of several factors, including long-acting local anesthetics and improved delivery systems, the widespread adoption of ultrasound-guided regional anesthesia, and the need to reduce reliance on opioids in the setting of the current opioid epidemic in the United States.[23,24]

STRUCTURAL ORGANIZATION OF AN ACUTE PAIN TEAM

The majority of APS utilize an anesthesiology-led model of care.[25] Anesthesiologists are experts in perioperative medicine, pain physiology and pharmacology and are highly qualified to lead a modern APS.[1] Their skill set includes the performance of regional anesthesia techniques, and the postoperative management of these techniques reflects an extension of their duties as perioperative physicians. An APS is led by a director who is experienced in the management of pain, which may or may not include fellowship training. The director is responsible for defining the scope of practice, goals, and policies of the service. He or she is responsible for developing policies and protocols for pain assessment and treatment and regularly reviews quality assurance. The day-to-day supervision of an APS is a shared responsibility between the APS director and his or her team of attending physicians. The APS attending is typically an anesthesiologist trained in pain management and regional anesthesia techniques, although the exact skill set may vary. Fellowship training in regional anesthesia and acute pain medicine is preferable, but not mandatory. Depending on the institution or practice setting, the composition of an APS can be limited to physicians, or can include a multidisciplinary team of mid-level providers, registered nurses, residents, fellows, pharmacists, or other healthcare providers.

ACUTE PAIN NURSES AND PROTOCOL-BASED CARE

An anesthesiologist-only model may not be practical in some practice settings. A nurse-based, protocol-driven model could be a less expensive alternative.[26,27] In this model, specialty trained acute pain nurses are supervised by an anesthesiologist. The specialty trained pain nurses assist the physician in assessing pain levels and the efficacy of the prescribed pain management plan. They are knowledgeable about the adverse effects of opioids, local anesthetics, ketamine, and regional anesthesia. The acute pain nurses are in constant communication with the other members of the APS and aid in the delivery of high-quality acute pain management.

Protocol-based care allows the pain nurses to function within the scope of their practice and increases patient accessibility to specialized care. Protocols standardize clinical care and help reduce the risk of errors.[27] Protocols should define titration parameters and bolus dosing of intravenous, epidural, and peripheral nerve infusions. A summary of the roles and responsibilities of possible APS team members are summarized in Table 4.1.

THE APS IN ACADEMIC PRACTICE

An APS located within an academic hospital is more likely to have a formalized perioperative analgesic protocol compared to non-teaching institutions.[28] Its composition is also more likely to include a team of healthcare professionals in various stages of their training. The APS attending is responsible for educating and supervising the trainees. Trainees, who may include medical students, residents, and fellows, are often responsible for completing patient evaluations and developing preliminary assessments and plans for all patients on service. A finalized assessment and plan are made only after discussion with the attending physician. Resident and fellow education should also include the performance and management of regional anesthetic techniques. A typical acute pain rotation lasts for a period of 1 month, allowing trainees to become familiarized with fundamental concepts of acute pain medicine.

Nurse practitioners (NPs) and physician assistants (PAs) may also be part of the acute pain team, and their roles may vary depending on the practice and the number of residents and fellows. In practices where a resident is not consistently

Table 4.1 **ACUTE PAIN SERVICE TEAM COMPOSITION AND RESPONSIBILITIES**

ROLE	DESCRIPTION OF RESPONSIBILITIES
Director	Determines the direction of the service Defines and coordinates clinical, educational, and research goals Develops pain management policies and protocols Communicates with hospital administration, nursing management, referring physicians, and other specialists Evaluates performance of all members of the team Periodically performs quality assurance
APS Attending	Leads daily patient rounds Performs and supervises regional anesthesia procedures Performs and supervises pain consultations Participates in educational and research goals Communications any problems or issues with the director
Mid-Level Providers (Nurse Practitioner, Physician Assistant)	Functions in a similar capacity to a resident or fellow Able to titrate and administer bolus doses of medications Responds to acute pain consultation requests and formulates initial plan Frequently assesses pain and medication side effects
APS Fellow, Resident	Participates in daily rounds Responds to acute pain consultation requests Performs regional anesthesia procedures under supervision Refers complicated questions to the APS attending Supervises interns and medical students performing consults Participates in education and research goals
Clinical Nurse Specialist	Coordinates services and provides continuity of care for patients Designs and implements educational programs for the department of nursing and patients Assists the APS director in development of goals, policies, protocols, and standards
APS Nurse	Keeps service pager or phone and responds to calls Frequently assesses pain and medication side effects Adjusts pain medication regimen and frequently assesses efficacy of changes within parameters of protocols Involved in patient education for continuous infusion techniques, especially for ambulatory catheters

Modified from Schwenk ES, Baratta JL, Gandi K, Viscusi ER. Setting up an acute pain management service. *Anesthesiology Clinics*. 2014;32:893–910.

available, the role of NPs and PAs may expand and could include writing daily progress notes, providing local anesthetic bolus doses to epidural and peripheral nerve catheters, and performing regional anesthesia procedures under attending physician supervision.

THE APS IN PRIVATE PRACTICE

An APS offered in a non-teaching setting may appear quite different than one in a large academic medical center. Although some private practices may have an APS with a similar structure to that of an academic APS, it is more likely that fewer staff will cover more patients. As a result, the private practice APS may opt to manage epidural and peripheral nerve catheters only, rather than provide consultation services for complex, opioid-tolerant medical and surgical patients. In these models, efficiency is key. Epidural and peripheral nerve catheters are assessed daily for efficacy, and those that are not functioning well are usually replaced rather than troubleshooted.

Providing staff for an APS can be challenging for private practices and must be optimized to ensure sufficient coverage of all anesthesia-based services. Anesthesiologists may be asked to fulfill multiple roles and responsibilities to minimize inefficiency. For example, the performance of any regional anesthesia technique may fall on the anesthesiologist assigned to a given room. This requires all anesthesia providers to become proficient and efficient in regional anesthesia. In this scenario, those who are more adept at regional anesthesia techniques may need to cover those rooms, or alternatively the more skilled members of the group may assist the less skilled members.

If staffing permits, a dedicated regional anesthesia or APS team can help off-load perioperative regional anesthesia responsibilities. The inclusion of mid-level providers (NPs or PAs) can aid the APS team and improve the flexibility of anesthesiologists assigned to both APS and operating rooms. Mid-level providers are supervised by the APS attending and assist in rounds, coordinate patient care, troubleshoot analgesic regimens, and formulate preliminary pain plans.

In many private practices, the decision to create an APS may come down to the ability of the physicians involved to persuade leadership of the APS's value. This can be a somewhat daunting task, and a full economic analysis is beyond the scope of this chapter. However, such discussions can involve a breakdown of expected procedures to be performed each day, the number of patients being followed on average for management of an epidural or peripheral nerve catheter, and potential complications that might be prevented with regional anesthesia or multimodal analgesia, including possible decreases in length of stay.[29,30] Sometimes an illustration of the "big picture" by the APS director can reinforce its value.

MULTIMODAL ANALGESIA AND ENHANCING RECOVERY

As previously mentioned, MMA is the use of at least two analgesic medications with different pharmacologic mechanisms to achieve analgesia.[31] This strategy minimizes individual drug dosages and class-related side effects (e.g., opioid-induced respiratory depression) while also improving the quality of analgesia by targeting various receptors along the pain pathway. The route of medication delivery can be the same or via an alternative route.[31] Non-opioid agents should be considered as the first-line treatment for postoperative pain.[32,33] Though the specific agents may vary based on the patient, setting, or surgical type, evidence strongly suggests that MMA therapy can reduce perioperative surgical complications. In contrast, opioid-related adverse effects are associated with increased length of stay and healthcare costs.[34] Thus, opioid minimization and MMA have become a key element in ERAS pathways.[5] Non-opioid analgesics should be incorporated as around-the-clock therapy with or without opioids for postoperative pain relief. Many studies indicate that opioids combined with either acetaminophen or NSAIDs produced superior analgesia and decreased opioid consumption compared to opioid therapy alone.[35–37] Additionally, the combination of acetaminophen and an NSAID may offer superior analgesia compared either therapy alone.[38] Regional anesthetic techniques and continuous infusions of lidocaine and ketamine are non-opioid alternatives to pain relief and are useful adjuncts in acute pain management.

NEURAXIAL ANALGESIA

Neuraxial analgesia with local anesthetics is associated with decreased postoperative pain scores and superior analgesia when compared to systemic opioids.[39] Compared to parenteral opioids, thoracic epidural analgesia (TEA) provides superior perioperative pain relief, and decreases pulmonary complications and the duration of mechanical ventilation.[39] In upper abdominal surgery, there is a reduced incidence of postoperative ileus.[40] It attenuates the endocrine metabolic response to surgical stress and is incorporated in a variety of enhanced recovery pathways.[41]

Epidural placement is not without risk, and its complications range from minor to catastrophic. The minor complications include postdural puncture headache, postoperative back pain, and epidural failure. The more catastrophic complications, such as total spinal anesthesia, neurologic injuries, epidural hematoma, and paralysis, are fortunately very rare. The incidence of hematoma formation is approximately 1 in 150,000 for epidurals and 1 in 220,000 for spinal anesthetics.[42] Nevertheless, a surge in the literature has led to the speculation that catastrophic neuraxial complication rates are increasing.[43] This is perhaps due to a growing number of novel anticoagulants, which is a risk factor for hematoma formation. Fortunately, the American Society of Regional Anesthesia and Acute Pain Medicine (ASRA) has developed guidelines to help guide clinical management.[44] An APS can assist in the timing of anticoagulation administration for epidural placement and discontinuation.

NON-OPERATIVE APPLICATIONS OF NEURAXIAL ANALGESIA

Rib fractures are an indicator of severe trauma to the thoracic cavity. The mortality risk associated with rib fractures is directly correlated to the number of fractured ribs.[45] The pain from rib fractures can impair respiratory mechanics and may explain why pulmonary complications such as pneumothorax, aspiration pneumonia, atelectasis, empyema, hospital length of stay, and death also increase with the number of fractured ribs.[45] Thoracic epidural analgesia produces effective analgesia, allows for ambulation, and improves respiratory mechanics.[46] Retrospective analysis of the National Trauma Data Bank suggests that TEA may confer a mortality benefit,[45] leading the Eastern Association for the Surgery of Trauma and Trauma Anesthesiology Society to recommend TEA for rib fractures.[47]

MANAGEMENT OF NEURAXIAL CATHETERS

Without a structured service to monitor the safety and efficacy of neuraxial anesthesia, anesthesiologists and surgeons may be hesitant to incorporate this modality into their perioperative practices. Early identification of neuraxial candidates is essential to avoid unacceptable delays in perioperative workflows and to ensure that anticoagulants have been appropriately withheld. The APS should be proactive in identifying a patient's eligibility because this modality may be overlooked by the primary anesthesiologist.[48] When appropriate, a patient's platelet count and coagulation profile should be obtained and reviewed.

Epidurals can be administered as a continuous infusion, continuous infusions with PCA boluses, or with programmed intermittent boluses. Ropivacaine and bupivacaine are two of the most commonly administered local anesthetics. Both agents are effective in producing analgesia, but ropivacaine is associated with less motor block[49] and is less toxic to the cardiovascular and central nervous system.[50,51]

The combination of epidural opioids and local anesthetics provides a synergistic effect[52] that results in superior analgesia compared to using each class of medications alone.[39] However, this has not led to a reduction in opioid-related adverse events (i.e. respiratory depression or pruritis).[53,54] If an epidural opioid is administered, care must be taken to prevent, detect and manage respiratory depression associated with neuraxial administration.[55] Standard epidural order sets should include monitoring parameters and include reversal agents in the event of significant opioid induced respiratory depression. In this scenario, a member of the APS team should be readily available and capable in assisting with resuscitative efforts.

CONTINUOUS PERIPHERAL NERVE BLOCKS

Peripheral nerve blocks impair the transmission of nociceptive stimuli from the periphery. This effect can be prolonged when local anesthetics are administered via a continuous infusion. Continuous peripheral nerve blocks (CPNBs) are not associated with systemic hypotension, unlike neuraxial blockade.[56] Peripheral techniques have been shown to be superior to opioid-based analgesia for a variety of orthopedic surgeries involving the upper[57] and lower limb.[58] Additionally, they have been shown to enhance postoperative recovery, patient satisfaction, and reduce the incidence of postoperative nausea and vomiting.[59]

Catheter-based techniques utilize infusion delivery systems to extend the duration of analgesia. These systems can be either electronic, elastomeric, or remote controlled. Local anesthetics have historically been delivered by continuous infusion alone, continuous infusion with PCA, or by PCA alone. In recent years, automated intermittent bolus techniques have been developed.[60] The purported benefit of bolus techniques is the greater spread of local anesthetics when compared to continuous infusions, although evidence for this is lacking.[61] The optimal infusion technique has yet to be determined, but continuous infusions with or without bolus dosing are believed to be superior to bolus-only techniques.[62]

NON-OPERATIVE APPLICATIONS OF PERIPHERAL NERVE BLOCKS

CPNBs can be utilized for non-operative sources of acute pain and have been successful in providing analgesic relief for complex regional pain syndrome (CRPS),[63] phantom limb pain,[64–66] and Raynaud's syndrome,[67] among others. Occasionally, the APS may be consulted to assist in the management of these painful conditions.

ADVERSE EVENTS AND COMPLICATIONS

Nerve injury is one of the most feared complications of peripheral nerve blocks. The severity of peripheral nerve injury (PNI) can range from transient postoperative neurologic symptoms to more devastating and permanent nerve injuries. The incidence of permanent nerve injury is reported to be 2 to 4 per 10,000[43] and has remained consistent despite ultrasound-guided techniques largely replacing peripheral nerve stimulation.[68] Transient neurologic symptoms, which can persist for weeks to months, occur more frequently, with an incidence of 0%–2.2% at 3 months, and 0%–0.8% at 6 months.[43,69] Patients with preexisting peripheral neuropathies may be at a greater risk for nerve injuries.[43]

Peripheral nerve catheters are colonized by bacteria with an incidence of 7.5% to 57%, but only 0%–3% progress to an infection.[70] The microorganism most commonly associated with infectious complications is *Staphylococcus aureus*.[70] Daily inspection of catheter insertion sites is recommended because prolonged catheter use increases the risk of infection. In a recent retrospective registry analysis of 44,555 patients, the probability of infection increased starting the fourth day after catheter insertion.[71] Infected catheters should be promptly removed and monitored until resolution.

Equipment-related complications are self-limiting. Occasionally peripheral catheters can be inadvertently dislodged. The use of adhesive strips, skin sealants, transparent dressings, tunneling, and sutures have all been used to protect against premature catheter removal.[72–74] Retained catheter fragments have been reported when catheters were sutured or tunneled.[75] Surgical exploration for retained fragments is not recommended unless they are high risk for infection or producing neurological symptoms.[75,76]

NON-OPIOID INFUSIONS FOR THE MANAGEMENT OF ACUTE PAIN

The opioid crisis has led to renewed interest in non-opioid alternatives to acute pain. Lidocaine and ketamine infusions have been shown to be beneficial in several pain states and have been incorporated as part of multimodal regimens in both inpatient and outpatient settings.

INTRAVENOUS LIDOCAINE INFUSIONS

Lidocaine infusions have been used as an analgesic adjunct in numerous pain conditions, including CRPS[77] and headaches.[78] But the evidence for these conditions is limited. In contrast, the perioperative utility of lidocaine infusions has been extensively studied for a variety of surgical procedures, with the evidence strongly supporting its use for abdominal surgery.[10,79] In this patient population, lidocaine infusions have been reported to reduce postoperative pain, opioid requirements, nausea, and ileus duration.[79] Lidocaine infusions has been incorporated into numerous enhanced recovery pathways.[5]

INTRAVENOUS KETAMINE INFUSIONS

Ketamine is a phencyclidine analog and dissociative anesthetic that has been used at subanesthetic doses to treat acute and chronic pain disorders. In the era of the opioid epidemic, its usage has dramatically increased as practitioners seek effective non-opioid analgesic alternatives. This has led to the development of consensus guidelines for both acute[6] and chronic pain.[80] These guidelines established conditions for which ketamine may be beneficial, the staff qualifications, monitoring, and contraindications to ketamine. It states that ketamine administration should be limited to those trained in the "induction and maintenance of ketamine infusions" along with "appropriate credentials [that] include training in airway management."[6,80] Since ketamine is an anesthetic and most APS are anesthesiology-led, some institutions have restricted its administration to members of the APS.

Ketamine pharmacology is complex and exerts its effects via several pathways. In acute pain, the mechanism is largely from its non-competitive antagonism of the NMDA receptor.[6] The ketamine guidelines recommend a maximum dose of 0.35 mg/kg for bolus doses and up to 1 mg/kg/hour for continuous infusions.[6]

Ketamine is recommended for the most painful surgeries, including abdominal, thoracic, and orthopedic procedures, in which it has been shown to reduce opioid requirements. Opioid-tolerant or opioid-dependent patients presenting for surgery are also likely to benefit from perioperative ketamine infusions.[6] In the largest study of this patient population, infusions restricted to the intraoperative phase led to reduced opioid requirements at 48 hours and persisted until 6 weeks postoperatively.[81]

Ketamine also has utility in nonsurgical patients. For example, the use of ketamine for acute exacerbations of sickle cell disease[82,83] and chronic migraine[84] has been widely reported. The opioid-sparing properties of ketamine can assist with rapid opioid tapering in patients.[85,86]

The frequency and extent of patient monitoring are not defined in current guidelines and should be based on patient comorbidities and institutional policies. Institutional policies should be created and developed under the direction of the APS. The preemptive use of benzodiazepines and alpha-2-agonists such as clonidine is recommended in the management of adverse effects, and these medications should be incorporated in the order set for ketamine infusions.[6]

ACUTE ON CHRONIC PAIN IN THE OPIOID-TOLERANT PATIENT

Opioid-tolerant patients include patients with chronic pain, active opioid abusers, former abusers, and abusers in treatment programs with methadone, buprenorphine, or naltrexone. These patients tend to be pain-intolerant,[87] hyperalgesic,[88] and are tolerant to the anti-nociceptive effects of opioids.[89] They require larger doses of analgesics to treat the additive effects of operative pain.[90] The belief that perioperative opioids can increase the risk of drug relapse or addiction is not supported by the literature.[33] However, poorly treated pain can be a trigger for relapse.[90] Multimodal therapy with non-opioid analgesics, regional anesthesia, and ketamine is recommended in this patient population because it can reduce opioid consumption and improve pain relief.[33,81]

Prior to elective surgery, patients on chronic opioid therapy should take their regularly prescribed opioid medications. Patients on methadone maintenance therapy should have their dose verified and be given prior to surgery. There is no consensus regarding the perioperative management of patients on buprenorphine or naloxone.[91] For elective surgeries, the decision to discontinue these medications must weigh the consequences of drug relapse, overdose, and death against the benefits of improved analgesia.[92]

BARRIERS TO IMPLEMENTATION

The creation of an APS requires a significant amount of institutional commitment and planning. In the early stages of implementation, changing a hospital's culture of acute pain care is likely to be met with resistance.[93] Since the success of an APS is dependent on interdepartmental collaboration, the APS should be proactive in educating other healthcare professionals on the significance of their services.

The benefits of regional anesthesia are well documented in the literature. Yet despite its benefits, some surgical services may be hesitant to adopt the services offered by an APS.[94] In a survey of orthopedic surgeons, delay in operative time was the most common reason for forgoing regional anesthesia.[94]

Existing workflows should be modified to include the time required to perform regional anesthesia techniques. A dedicated procedure room located outside of the OR, or "block room," has been shown to improve OR efficiency.[95]

The business of healthcare requires all services to demonstrate value to the hospital enterprise. Services must be cost-efficient and operational costs must be justified in the form of revenue and/or potential cost-savings to the hospital. Unfortunately, studies have not been able to conclusively determine the cost-effectiveness of an APS.[96] Alternatively, a dedicated APS improves access to advanced analgesic therapies and can be invaluable toward a patient's perioperative experience. Adequate postoperative analgesia represents the most common preoperative concern for patients,[97] and effective strategies are tied to patient outcomes,[1] satisfaction,[98] and is a marker for healthcare quality. A satisfied customer base is linked to financial incentives, increased reimbursement, and increases the likelihood of additional referrals and profit.[99] Hospitals can also benefit from the cost-saving potential of an APS when their services are applied in the context of ERAS pathways.[99] ERAS pathways may improve perioperative outcomes, reduce complications, and decrease length of stay.[100] The sum of these benefits can result in significant cost-savings to an institution.

CONCLUSIONS

- An APS is an inpatient consultative service that uses multimodal analgesic strategies to care for the acute pain needs of surgical and nonsurgical patients.
- Anesthesiologists are experts in pharmacology, pain management, and regional anesthesia techniques, and are ideally suited to lead a modern APS.
- All members of an APS should frequently assess for treatment efficacy and adverse events.
- Regional anesthetic techniques provide superior analgesia to opioid-only therapy and require active management to optimize benefit while addressing complications, both of which may be facilitated through an APS.
- Ketamine and lidocaine are intravenous infusions that are commonly used as non-opioid adjuncts to manage acute pain conditions.
- The cost of an APS and surgical specialty acceptance of an APS are common barriers to implementing an APS.

REFERENCES

1. Werner MU, Soholm L, Rotboll-Nielsen P, Kehlet H. Does an acute pain service improve postoperative outcome? *Anesth Analg.* 2002;95(5):1361–1372.
2. Gan TJ. Poorly controlled postoperative pain: prevalence, consequences, and prevention. *J Pain Res.* 2017;10:2287–2298.
3. Fletcher D, Stamer UM, Pogatzki-Zahn E, et al. Chronic postsurgical pain in Europe: An observational study. *Eur J Anaesthesiol.* 2015;32(10):725–734.
4. Wick EC, Grant MC, Wu CL. Postoperative multimodal analgesia pain management with nonopioid analgesics and techniques: a review. *JAMA Surg.* 2017;152(7):691–697.
5. Ljungqvist O, Scott M, Fearon KC. Enhanced recovery after surgery: a review. *JAMA Surg.* 2017;152(3):292–298.
6. Schwenk ES, Viscusi ER, Buvanendran A, et al. Consensus guidelines on the use of intravenous ketamine infusions for acute pain management from the American Society of Regional Anesthesia and Pain Medicine, the American Academy of Pain Medicine, and the American Society of Anesthesiologists. *Reg Anesth Pain Med.* 2018;43(5):456–466.
7. Goldberg SF, Pozek JJ, Schwenk ES, Baratta JL, Beausang DH, Wong AK. Practical management of a regional anesthesia-driven acute pain service. *Adv Anesth.* 2017;35(1):191–211.
8. Schwenk ES, Goldberg SF, Patel RD, et al. Adverse drug effects and preoperative medication factors related to perioperative low-dose ketamine infusions. *Reg Anesth Pain Med.* 2016;41(4):482–487.
9. Dunn LK, Durieux ME. Perioperative use of intravenous lidocaine. *Anesthesiology.* 2017;126(4):729–737.
10. Kuo CP, Jao SW, Chen KM, et al. Comparison of the effects of thoracic epidural analgesia and I.V. infusion with lidocaine on cytokine response, postoperative pain and bowel function in patients undergoing colonic surgery. *Br J Anaesth.* 2006;97(5):640–646.
11. Weibel S, Jelting Y, Pace NL, et al. Continuous intravenous perioperative lidocaine infusion for postoperative pain and recovery in adults. *Cochrane Database Syst Rev.* 2018;6:CD009642.
12. Lutfy K, Cowan A. Buprenorphine: a unique drug with complex pharmacology. *Curr Neuropharmacol.* 2004;2(4):395–402.
13. Anderson TA, Quaye ANA, Ward EN, Wilens TE, Hilliard PE, Brummett CM. To stop or not, that is the question: acute pain management for the patient on chronic buprenorphine. *Anesthesiology.* 2017;126(6):1180–1186.
14. Chen KY, Chen L, Mao J. Buprenorphine-naloxone therapy in pain management. *Anesthesiology.* 2014;120(5):1262–1274.
15. Greenwald M, Johanson CE, Bueller J, et al. Buprenorphine duration of action: mu-opioid receptor availability and pharmacokinetic and behavioral indices. *Biol Psychiatry.* 2007;61(1):101–110.
16. Alford DP, Compton P, Samet JH. Acute pain management for patients receiving maintenance methadone or buprenorphine therapy. *Ann Intern Med.* 2006;144(2):127–134.
17. Roberts DM, Meyer-Witting M. High-dose buprenorphine: perioperative precautions and management strategies. *Anaesth Intensive Care.* 2005;33(1):17–25.
18. Walker BJ, Noonan KJ, Bosenberg AT. Evolving compartment syndrome not masked by a continuous peripheral nerve block: evidence-based case management. *Reg Anesth Pain Med.* 2012;37(4):393–397.
19. Tran DQ, Salinas FV, Benzon HT, Neal JM. Lower extremity regional anesthesia: essentials of our current understanding. *Reg Anesth Pain Med.* 2019 Jan 11:rapm-2018-000019.
20. Klein SM, Nielsen KC, Greengrass RA, Warner DS, Martin A, Steele SM. Ambulatory discharge after long-acting peripheral nerve blockade: 2382 blocks with ropivacaine. *Anesth Analg.* 2002;94(1):65–70.
21. Ilfeld BM, Enneking FK. Continuous peripheral nerve blocks at home: a review. *Anesth Analg.* 2005;100(6):1822–1833.
22. Ready LB, Oden R, Chadwick HS, et al. Development of an anesthesiology-based postoperative pain management service. *Anesthesiology.* 1988;68(1):100–106.
23. Schwenk ES, Mariano ER. Designing the ideal perioperative pain management plan starts with multimodal analgesia. *Korean J Anesthesiol.* 2018;71(5):345–352.
24. Wahal C, Kumar A, Pyati S. Advances in regional anaesthesia: a review of current practice, newer techniques and outcomes. *Indian J Anaesth.* 2018;62(2):94–102.
25. Ready LB. How many acute pain services are there in the United States, and who is managing patient-controlled analgesia? *Anesthesiology.* 1995;82(1):322.
26. Rawal N, Berggren L. Organization of acute pain services: a low-cost model. *Pain.* 1994;57(1):117–123.

27. Rawal N. 10 years of acute pain services: achievements and challenges. *Reg Anesth Pain Med.* 1999;24(1):68–73.
28. Nasir D, Howard JE, Joshi GP, Hill GE. A survey of acute pain service structure and function in United States hospitals. *Pain Res Treat.* 2011;2011:934932.
29. Le-Wendling L, Glick W, Tighe P. Goals and objectives to optimize the value of an acute pain service in perioperative pain management. *Tech Orthop.* 2017;32(4):200–208.
30. Said ET, Sztain JF, Abramson WB, et al. A dedicated acute pain service is associated with reduced postoperative opioid requirements in patients undergoing cytoreductive surgery with hyperthermic intraperitoneal chemotherapy. *Anesth Analg.* 2018;127(4):1044–1050.
31. American Society of Anesthesiologists Task Force on Acute Pain Management. Practice guidelines for acute pain management in the perioperative setting: an updated report by the American Society of Anesthesiologists Task Force on Acute Pain Management. *Anesthesiology.* 2012;116(2):248–273.
32. Dowell D, Haegerich TM, Chou R. CDC guideline for prescribing opioids for chronic pain: United States, 2016. *MMWR Recomm Rep.* 2016;65(1):1–49.
33. Chou R, Gordon DB, de Leon-Casasola OA, et al. Management of postoperative pain: a clinical practice guideline from the American Pain Society, the American Society of Regional Anesthesia and Pain Medicine, and the American Society of Anesthesiologists' Committee on Regional Anesthesia, Executive Committee, and Administrative Council. *J Pain.* 2016;17(2):131–157.
34. Oderda GM, Said Q, Evans RS, et al. Opioid-related adverse drug events in surgical hospitalizations: impact on costs and length of stay. *Ann Pharmacother.* 2007;41(3):400–406.
35. Aubrun F, Langeron O, Heitz D, Coriat P, Riou B. Randomised, placebo-controlled study of the postoperative analgesic effects of ketoprofen after spinal fusion surgery. *Acta Anaesthesiol Scand.* 2000;44(8):934–939.
36. Gimbel JS, Brugger A, Zhao W, Verburg KM, Geis GS. Efficacy and tolerability of celecoxib versus hydrocodone/acetaminophen in the treatment of pain after ambulatory orthopedic surgery in adults. *Clin Ther.* 2001;23(2):228–241.
37. McNicol ED, Tzortzopoulou A, Cepeda MS, Francia MB, Farhat T, Schumann R. Single-dose intravenous paracetamol or propacetamol for prevention or treatment of postoperative pain: a systematic review and meta-analysis. *Br J Anaesth.* 2011;106(6):764–775.
38. Ong CK, Seymour RA, Lirk P, Merry AF. Combining paracetamol (acetaminophen) with nonsteroidal antiinflammatory drugs: a qualitative systematic review of analgesic efficacy for acute postoperative pain. *Anesth Analg.* 2010;110(4):1170–1179.
39. Block BM, Liu SS, Rowlingson AJ, Cowan AR, Cowan JA Jr., Wu CL. Efficacy of postoperative epidural analgesia: a meta-analysis. *JAMA.* 2003;290(18):2455–2463.
40. Werawatganon T, Charuluxanun S. Patient controlled intravenous opioid analgesia versus continuous epidural analgesia for pain after intra-abdominal surgery. *Cochrane Database Syst Rev.* 2005;1:CD004088.
41. Manion SC, Brennan TJ. Thoracic epidural analgesia and acute pain management. *Anesthesiology.* 2011;115(1):181–188.
42. Horlocker TT, Wedel DJ, Rowlingson JC, et al. Regional anesthesia in the patient receiving antithrombotic or thrombolytic therapy: American Society of Regional Anesthesia and Pain Medicine Evidence-Based Guidelines (third edition). *Reg Anesth Pain Med.* 2010;35(1):64–101.
43. Neal JM, Barrington MJ, Brull R, et al. The second ASRA practice advisory on neurologic complications associated with regional anesthesia and pain medicine: executive summary 2015. *Reg Anesth Pain Med.* 2015;40(5):401–430.
44. Horlocker TT, Vandermeuelen E, Kopp SL, Gogarten W, Leffert LR, Benzon HT. Regional anesthesia in the patient receiving antithrombotic or thrombolytic therapy: American Society of Regional Anesthesia and Pain Medicine Evidence-Based Guidelines (fourth edition). *Reg Anesth Pain Med.* 2018;43(3):263–309.
45. Flagel BT, Luchette FA, Reed RL, et al. Half-a-dozen ribs: the breakpoint for mortality. *Surgery.* 2005;138(4):717–725.
46. Clemente A, Carli F. The physiological effects of thoracic epidural anesthesia and analgesia on the cardiovascular, respiratory and gastrointestinal systems. *Minerva Anestesiol.* 2008;74(10):549–563.
47. Galvagno SM Jr., Smith CE, Varon AJ, et al. Pain management for blunt thoracic trauma: a joint practice management guideline from the Eastern Association for the Surgery of Trauma and Trauma Anesthesiology Society. *J Trauma Acute Care Surg.* 2016;81(5):936–951.
48. Hanna MN, Jeffries MA, Hamzehzadeh S, et al. Survey of the utilization of regional and general anesthesia in a tertiary teaching hospital. *Reg Anesth Pain Med.* 2009;34(3):224–228.
49. Brockway MS, Bannister J, McClure JH, McKeown D, Wildsmith JA. Comparison of extradural ropivacaine and bupivacaine. *Br J Anaesth.* 1991;66(1):31–37.
50. Knudsen K, Beckman Suurkula M, Blomberg S, Sjovall J, Edvardsson N. Central nervous and cardiovascular effects of I.V. infusions of ropivacaine, bupivacaine and placebo in volunteers. *Br J Anaesth.* 1997;78(5):507–514.
51. Scott DB, Lee A, Fagan D, Bowler GM, Bloomfield P, Lundh R. Acute toxicity of ropivacaine compared with that of bupivacaine. *Anesth Analg.* 1989;69(5):563–569.
52. Kaneko M, Saito Y, Kirihara Y, Collins JG, Kosaka Y. Synergistic antinociceptive interaction after epidural coadministration of morphine and lidocaine in rats. *Anesthesiology.* 1994;80(1):137–150.
53. de Leon-Casasola OA, Parker B, Lema MJ, Harrison P, Massey J. Postoperative epidural bupivacaine-morphine therapy: experience with 4,227 surgical cancer patients. *Anesthesiology.* 1994;81(2):368–375.
54. Cullen ML, Staren ED, el-Ganzouri A, Logas WG, Ivankovich AD, Economou SG. Continuous epidural infusion for analgesia after major abdominal operations: a randomized, prospective, double-blind study. *Surgery.* 1985;98(4):718–728.
55. Practice guidelines for the prevention, detection, and management of respiratory depression associated with neuraxial opioid administration: an updated report by the American Society of Anesthesiologists Task Force on Neuraxial Opioids and the American Society of Regional Anesthesia and Pain Medicine. *Anesthesiology.* 2016;124(3):535–552.
56. Administration SAMHSA. *Key Substance Use and Mental Health Indicators in the United States: Results from the 2018 National Survey on Drug Use and Health.* Vol No. PEP19-5068. HHS Publication 2019.
57. Borgeat A, Schappi B, Biasca N, Gerber C. Patient-controlled analgesia after major shoulder surgery: patient-controlled interscalene analgesia versus patient-controlled analgesia. *Anesthesiology.* 1997;87(6):1343–1347.
58. Capdevila X, Barthelet Y, Biboulet P, Ryckwaert Y, Rubenovitch J, d'Athis F. Effects of perioperative analgesic technique on the surgical outcome and duration of rehabilitation after major knee surgery. *Anesthesiology.* 1999;91(1):8–15.
59. Hadzic A, Williams BA, Karaca PE, et al. For outpatient rotator cuff surgery, nerve block anesthesia provides superior same-day recovery over general anesthesia. *Anesthesiology.* 2005;102(5):1001–1007.
60. Taboada M, Rodriguez J, Bermudez M, et al. Comparison of continuous infusion versus automated bolus for postoperative patient-controlled analgesia with popliteal sciatic nerve catheters. *Anesthesiology.* 2009;110(1):150–154.
61. Jagannathan R, Niesen AD, D'Souza RS, Johnson RL. Intermittent bolus versus continuous infusion techniques for local anesthetic delivery in peripheral and truncal nerve analgesia: the current state of evidence. *Reg Anesth Pain Med.* 2019;44(4):447–451.
62. Singelyn FJ, Seguy S, Gouverneur JM. Interscalene brachial plexus analgesia after open shoulder surgery: continuous versus patient-controlled infusion. *Anesth Analg.* 1999;89(5):1216–1220.
63. Dadure C, Motais F, Ricard C, Raux O, Troncin R, Capdevila X. Continuous peripheral nerve blocks at home for treatment of

recurrent complex regional pain syndrome I in children. *Anesthesiology.* 2005;102(2):387–391.
64. Pisansky AJB, Brovman EY, Kuo C, Kaye AD, Urman RD. Perioperative outcomes after regional versus general anesthesia for above the knee amputations. *Ann Vasc Surg.* 2018;48:53–66.
65. Ayling OG, Montbriand J, Jiang J, et al. Continuous regional anaesthesia provides effective pain management and reduces opioid requirement following major lower limb amputation. *Eur J Vasc Endovasc Surg.* 2014;48(5):559–564.
66. Bosanquet DC, Glasbey JC, Stimpson A, Williams IM, Twine CP. Systematic review and meta-analysis of the efficacy of perineural local anaesthetic catheters after major lower limb amputation. *Eur J Vasc Endovasc Surg.* 2015;50(2):241–249.
67. Dao T, Amaro-Driedger D, Mehta J. Successful treatment of Raynaud's syndrome in a lupus patient with continuous bilateral popliteal sciatic nerve blocks: a case report. *Local Reg Anesth.* 2016;9:35–37.
68. Neal JM. Ultrasound-guided regional anesthesia and patient safety: update of an evidence-based analysis. *Reg Anesth Pain Med.* 2016;41(2):195–204.
69. Brull R, Hadzic A, Reina MA, Barrington MJ. Pathophysiology and etiology of nerve injury following peripheral nerve blockade. *Reg Anesth Pain Med.* 2015;40(5):479–490.
70. Capdevila X, Bringuier S, Borgeat A. Infectious risk of continuous peripheral nerve blocks. *Anesthesiology.* 2009;110(1):182–188.
71. Bomberg H, Bayer I, Wagenpfeil S, et al. Prolonged catheter use and infection in regional anesthesia: a retrospective registry analysis. *Anesthesiology.* 2018;128(4):764–773.
72. Cuvillon P, Ripart J, Lalourcey L, et al. The continuous femoral nerve block catheter for postoperative analgesia: bacterial colonization, infectious rate and adverse effects. *Anesth Analg.* 2001;93(4):1045–1049.
73. Compere V, Rey N, Baert O, et al. Major complications after 400 continuous popliteal sciatic nerve blocks for post-operative analgesia. *Acta Anaesthesiol Scand.* 2009;53(3):339–345.
74. Fredrickson MJ, Ball CM, Dalgleish AJ. Successful continuous interscalene analgesia for ambulatory shoulder surgery in a private practice setting. *Reg Anesth Pain Med.* 2008;33(2):122–128.
75. Despond O, Kohut GN. Broken interscalene brachial plexus catheter: surgical removal or not? *Anesth Analg.* 2010;110(2):643–644.
76. Jeng CL, Torrillo TM, Rosenblatt MA. Complications of peripheral nerve blocks. *Br J Anaesth.* 2010;105(Suppl 1):97–107.
77. Schwartzman RJ, Patel M, Grothusen JR, Alexander GM. Efficacy of 5-day continuous lidocaine infusion for the treatment of refractory complex regional pain syndrome. *Pain Med.* 2009;10(2):401–412.
78. Mooney JJ, Pagel PS, Kundu A. Safety, tolerability, and short-term efficacy of intravenous lidocaine infusions for the treatment of chronic pain in adolescents and young adults: a preliminary report. *Pain Med.* 2014;15(5):820–825.
79. Marret E, Rolin M, Beaussier M, Bonnet F. Meta-analysis of intravenous lidocaine and postoperative recovery after abdominal surgery. *Br J Surg.* 2008;95(11):1331–1338.
80. Cohen SP, Bhatia A, Buvanendran A, et al. Consensus guidelines on the use of intravenous ketamine infusions for chronic pain from the American Society of Regional Anesthesia and Pain Medicine, the American Academy of Pain Medicine, and the American Society of Anesthesiologists. *Reg Anesth Pain Med.* 2018;43(5):521–546.
81. Loftus RW, Yeager MP, Clark JA, et al. Intraoperative ketamine reduces perioperative opiate consumption in opiate-dependent patients with chronic back pain undergoing back surgery. *Anesthesiology.* 2010;113(3):639–646.
82. Hagedorn JM, Monico EC. Ketamine infusion for pain control in acute pediatric sickle cell painful crises. *Pediatr Emerg Care.* 2019;35(1):78–79.
83. Uprety D, Baber A, Foy M. Ketamine infusion for sickle cell pain crisis refractory to opioids: a case report and review of literature. *Ann Hematol.* 2014;93(5):769–771.
84. Schwenk ES, Dayan AC, Rangavajjula A, et al. Ketamine for refractory headache: a retrospective analysis. *Reg Anesth Pain Med.* 2018;43(8):875–879.
85. Strickler EM, Schwenk ES, Cohen MJ, Viscusi ER. Use of ketamine in a multimodal analgesia setting for rapid opioid tapering in a profoundly opioid-tolerant patient: a case report. *A Pract.* 2018;10(7):179–181.
86. Ocker AC, Shah NB, Schwenk ES, Witkowski TA, Cohen MJ, Viscusi ER. Ketamine and cognitive behavioral therapy for rapid opioid tapering with sustained opioid abstinence: a case report and 1-year follow-up. *Pain Pract.* 2020 Jan;20(1):95–100.
87. Compton P, Charuvastra VC, Kintaudi K, Ling W. Pain responses in methadone-maintained opioid abusers. *J Pain Symptom Manage.* 2000;20(4):237–245.
88. Angst MS, Koppert W, Pahl I, Clark DJ, Schmelz M. Short-term infusion of the mu-opioid agonist remifentanil in humans causes hyperalgesia during withdrawal. *Pain.* 2003;106(1–2):49–57.
89. Doverty M, Somogyi AA, White JM, et al. Methadone maintenance patients are cross-tolerant to the antinociceptive effects of morphine. *Pain.* 2001;93(2):155–163.
90. Huxtable CA, Roberts LJ, Somogyi AA, MacIntyre PE. Acute pain management in opioid-tolerant patients: a growing challenge. *Anaesth Intensive Care.* 2011;39(5):804–823.
91. Coluzzi F, Bifulco F, Cuomo A, et al. The challenge of perioperative pain management in opioid-tolerant patients. *Ther Clin Risk Manag.* 2017;13:1163–1173.
92. Curatolo C, Trinh M. Challenges in the perioperative management of the patient receiving extended-release naltrexone. *A A Case Rep.* 2014;3(11):142–144.
93. Powell AE, Davies HT, Bannister J, Macrae WA. Challenge of improving postoperative pain management: case studies of three acute pain services in the UK National Health Service. *Br J Anaesth.* 2009;102(6):824–831.
94. Oldman M, McCartney CJ, Leung A, et al. A survey of orthopedic surgeons' attitudes and knowledge regarding regional anesthesia. *Anesth Analg.* 2004;98(5):1486–1490.
95. Gleicher Y, Singer O, Choi S, McHardy P. Thoracic epidural catheter placement in a preoperative block area improves operating room efficiency and decreases epidural failure rate. *Reg Anesth Pain Med.* 2017;42(5):649–651.
96. Sun E, Dexter F, Macario A. Can an acute pain service be cost-effective? *Anesth Analg.* 2010;111(4):841–844.
97. Apfelbaum JL, Chen C, Mehta SS, Gan TJ. Postoperative pain experience: results from a national survey suggest postoperative pain continues to be undermanaged. *Anesth Analg.* 2003;97(2): 534–540.
98. Gupta A, Daigle S, Mojica J, Hurley RW. Patient perception of pain care in hospitals in the United States. *J Pain Res.* 2009;2:157–164.
99. Gray CF, Smith C, Zasimovich Y, Tighe PJ. Economic considerations of acute pain medicine programs. *Tech Orthop.* 2017;32(4):217–225.
100. Kehlet H, Wilmore DW. Multimodal strategies to improve surgical outcome. *Am J Surg.* 2002;183(6):630–641.

REVIEW QUESTIONS

(1) Which of the following most accurately describes an acute pain service?

A. Can be composed of a combination of physicians, nurses, pharmacists, and other clinicians who care for the acute pain needs of both surgical and nonsurgical patients.
B. Ensures the safe delivery of analgesic medications and monitors for adverse effects.

C. Incorporates regional anesthesia, ketamine or lidocaine infusions, opioid and non-opioid analgesics as part of a multimodal analgesic plan.
D. All of the above

(2) The development of pain policies, protocols, and the direction of the service is the responsibility of which member of the acute pain service (APS)?

A. Acute pain service director
B. Acute pain service attending
C. Acute pain nurse
D. Clinical nurse specialist

(3) All of the following are examples of multimodal analgesia EXCEPT:

A. Adductor canal perineural infusion and hydromorphone patient-controlled analgesia (PCA)
B. Epidural infusion of morphine alone and hydromorphone PCA
C. Intravenous ketamine infusion and oral oxycodone
D. Epidural infusion of ropivacaine and oral acetaminophen

(4) Which of the following statements about multimodal analgesia is FALSE?

A. Multimodal analgesia combines multiple analgesics of different pharmacologic classes to achieve superior analgesia while reducing the adverse effects of each individual agent.
B. Multimodal analgesia is less effective than opioid therapy alone.
C. The use of a hydromorphone PCA, around-the-clock acetaminophen and ibuprofen, and a femoral nerve block is an example of multimodal analgesia.
D. Multimodal analgesia is effective for both operative and non-operative sources of pain.

(5) A patient with a history of pancreatic cancer is scheduled for a pancreaticoduodenectomy (Whipple procedure). You would like to place an epidural for postoperative pain, but the patient's PT/INR are elevated. A colleague suggests an intravenous lidocaine infusion. What are the advantages of perioperative lidocaine infusions for abdominal surgery?

A. Decreases cardiopulmonary complications
B. Reduces mortality
C. Decreases postoperative nausea and vomiting, opioid requirements, and ileus duration
D. Decreases postoperative cognitive dysfunction

(6) Which of the following statements about ketamine is FALSE?

A. Subanesthetic doses of ketamine antagonize NMDA receptors to achieve analgesia in acute pain.
B. Ketamine antagonizes NMDA, nicotinic and muscarinic cholinergic receptors, facilitates γ-aminobutyric acid A (GABA-A) signaling, enhances the descending modulatory pain pathways, and is a μ-receptor agonist.
C. Ketamine administration requires a physician trained in airway management and ACLS.
D. None of the above statements is false.

(7) Which of the following statements about opioid-tolerant patients is FALSE?

A. Multimodal analgesic therapy is recommended for opioid tolerant patients.
B. The use of perioperative opioids does not increase the risk of relapse in patients with a history of opioid use disorder.
C. Opioid requirements are higher for patients with a history of drug abuse, but not for patients taking opioids for chronic pain.
D. Opioid-tolerant patients include those with chronic pain, and former and current illicit drug users.

ANSWERS

(1) **D.** An acute pain service is a consultative service that can be composed of a multidisciplinary team of physicians, nurses, pharmacists, and other healthcare professionals. Its purpose is to assist in the acute pain management of hospitalized surgical and nonsurgical patients. This is usually achieved with multimodal analgesia (MMA). An APS should assist in patient monitoring to optimize analgesic efficacy while reducing adverse events.

Reference

Werner MU, Soholm L, Rotboll-Nielsen P, Kehlet H. Does an acute pain service improve postoperative outcome? *Anesth Analg.* 2002;95(5):1361–1372.

(2) **A.** An APS is led by its director. The director is experienced in managing complex acute pain conditions, as well as performing regional anesthesia techniques. Their many responsibilities include: overseeing the direction of the service, developing policies and protocols, and communicating with hospital administrators.

Reference

Schwenk ES, Baratta JL, Gandhi K, Viscusi ER. Setting up an acute pain management service. *Anesthesiol Clin.* 2014;32:893–910.

(3) **B.** Both morphine and hydromorphone are opioid analgesics that target the mu receptor and have the same mechanism of action.

References

Pathan H, Williams J. Basic opioid pharmacology: an update. *Br J Pain.* 2012;6:11–16.
American Society of Anesthesiologists Task Force on Acute Pain Management. Practice guidelines for acute pain management in the perioperative setting: an updated report by the American Society of Anesthesiologists task force on acute pain management. *Anesthesiology.* 2004;100:1573–1581.

(4) **B.** Multimodal analgesia targets various nociceptive receptors along the pain pathway. Its goal is to maximize analgesia and minimize adverse effects. Multiple studies indicate that multimodal analgesia is superior to opioid therapy alone for both operative and non-operative sources of pain.

References

American Society of Anesthesiologists Task Force on Acute Pain Management. Practice guidelines for acute pain management in the perioperative setting: an updated report by the American Society of Anesthesiologists Task Force on Acute Pain Management. *Anesthesiology*. 2012;116(2):248–273.

Schwenk ES, Mariano ER. Designing the ideal perioperative pain management plan starts with multimodal analgesia. *Korean J Anesthesiol.* 2018;71(5):345–352.

(5) **C.** The analgesic mechanism of lidocaine infusions is believed to be related to its potent anti-inflammatory properties. In abdominal surgery, lidocaine infusions have been shown to reduce postoperative pain and decrease ileus duration. It also can reduce the incidence of postoperative nausea and vomiting (PONV). These benefits are not consistent across all surgical subtypes. The influence of lidocaine infusions on postoperative cognitive dysfunction has been studied in cardiothoracic surgery, not abdominal surgery. It has not been shown to decrease cardiopulmonary complications or improve patient mortality.

References

Marret E, Rolin M, Beaussier M, Bonnet F. Meta-analysis of intravenous lidocaine and postoperative recovery after abdominal surgery. *Br J Surg.* 2008;95(11):1331–1338.

Klinger RY, Cooter M, Bisanar T, et al. Intravenous lidocaine does not improve neurologic outcomes after cardiac surgery: a randomized controlled trial. *Anesthesiology.* 2019;130(6):958–970.

(6) **D.** Ketamine is an anesthetic that possesses analgesic, antidepressant, and psychomimietic effects. Subanesthetic doses are used in acute pain, while higher doses are used in chronic pain. The analgesic mechanism in acute pain is due to NMDA receptor antagonism. In high doses, ketamine can bind to mu receptors. Ketamine also antagonizes muscarinic and nicotinic cholinergic receptors, facilitates GABA signaling, and modulates descending pain pathways.

References

Schwenk ES, Viscusi ER, Buvanendran A, et al. Consensus guidelines on the use of intravenous ketamine infusions for acute pain management from the American Society of Regional Anesthesia and Pain Medicine, the American Academy of Pain Medicine, and the American Society of Anesthesiologists. *Reg Anesth Pain Med.* 2018;43(5):456–466.

Cohen SP, Bhatia A, Buvanendran A, et al. Consensus guidelines on the use of intravenous ketamine infusions for chronic pain from the American Society of Regional Anesthesia and Pain Medicine, the American Academy of Pain Medicine, and the American Society of Anesthesiologists. *Reg Anesth Pain Med.* 2018;43(5):521–546.

(7) **C.** Patients on chronic opioid therapy, former and illicit drug users, and those enrolled in medication-assisted therapy for substance abuse are considered to be opioid tolerant. These patients tend to have higher opioid requirements. Multimodal analgesia offers superior analgesia to opioid therapy alone and is recommended to avoid excessive opioid dose escalation. The use of perioperative opioids does not increase the risk of drug relapse. In contrast, poorly controlled pain can increase the risk of drug relapse.

References

Chou R, Gordon DB, de Leon-Casasola OA, et al. Management of postoperative pain: a clinical practice guideline from the American Pain Society, the American Society of Regional Anesthesia and Pain Medicine, and the American Society of Anesthesiologists' Committee on Regional Anesthesia, Executive Committee, and Administrative Council. *J Pain.* 2016;17(2):131–157.

Huxtable CA, Roberts LJ, Somogyi AA, MacIntyre PE. Acute pain management in opioid-tolerant patients: a growing challenge. *Anaesth Intensive Care.* 2011;39(5):804–823.

SECTION 2

PHARMACOLOGY

Kamen V. Vlassakov

5.

MULTIMODAL ANALGESIA

Archana O'Neill and Philipp Lirk

STEM CASE AND KEY QUESTIONS

A 54-year-old male presents with newly diagnosed colon cancer for a laparoscopic colectomy via an enhanced recovery after surgery (ERAS) pathway. He has a history of hypertension, hyperlipidemia, and lumbar radiculopathy. His past surgical history includes laparoscopic cholecystectomy and previous spine surgery. He is on lisinopril for hypertension, atorvastatin for hyperlipidemia, and gabapentin for his radiculopathy. His dose of gabapentin is 600 mg PO q8h. The patient denies taking any other medications on a regular basis.

(1) WHAT IS MULTIMODAL ANALGESIA? HOW DOES THE USE OF AN ERAS PROTOCOL AFFECT YOUR PLANS FOR ANALGESIA IN THIS CASE?

The anesthesiologist prepares to use multimodal analgesia to target multiple nociceptive pathways and receptors to facilitate postoperative pain control and reduce the chance of side effects to any of the medications chosen to achieve this goal.[1] The use of an ERAS pathway calls for standardized multimodal analgesic interventions to minimize the use of opioids in order to avoid their side effects and help speed recovery.[2]

(2) WHAT IS THE DIFFERENCE BETWEEN PREEMPTIVE ANALGESIA AND PREVENTIVE ANALGESIA? HOW DOES THIS DIFFERENCE IMPACT THE OPTIONS FOR PAIN CONTROL FOR THIS PATIENT?

Preemptive analgesia refers to the implementation of an analgesic strategy prior to the onset of a painful stimulus to minimize postoperative pain, whereas preventive analgesia aims to attenuate painful stimuli that an individual may experience in all phases of the perioperative time period (i.e., preoperative, intraoperative, and postoperative).[3] The impact of preventive interventions should extend well beyond the duration of action of the particular drugs. Preemptively, the surgical team has ordered acetaminophen 975 mg and celecoxib 200 mg to be given PO in the preoperative area. Preventively, the anesthesiologist is planning to administer intraoperatively 2 g magnesium and 8 mg dexamethasone intravenously to help with postoperative pain control.

During your preoperative interview, the patient is apprehensive about his pain control and would like to limit the use of opioids due to a history of opioid misuse in the past, so you discuss a plan for a multimodal analgesic approach combining intravenous (IV) and per os (PO) medications. Upon further questioning preoperatively, the patient reports that he did not take his morning dose of gabapentin that day.

(3) SHOULD THE PATIENT RECEIVE ANY OTHER MEDICATIONS PREOPERATIVELY TO HELP OPTIMIZE PAIN CONTROL?

Although gabapentin has recently been removed from our ERAS protocols, this patient is currently taking it on a regular basis for his history of degenerative spine issues which are an ongoing source of pain for him, so the anesthesiologist orders a dose of gabapentin to be given preoperatively in addition to the acetaminophen and celecoxib to help reduce his perioperative opioid requirements. As the patient has tolerated this medication without significant side effects, he receives 600 mg in the preoperative area. After almost 2 decades of increasing perioperative use, it has recently been questioned whether gabapentin and pregabalin should be part of the standard multimodal regimen.[4] Recent evidence suggests that the analgesic effect is less pronounced than originally anticipated, and side effects such as dizziness, sedation, and blurry vision are more common than assumed.[5] This is especially important with ERAS pathways, where excessive sedation is an obstacle to progression of care.[2]

(4) ARE THERE ANY OTHER MEDICATIONS THAT CAN BE USED INTRAOPERATIVELY TO POTENTIALLY IMPROVE PAIN CONTROL IN THIS SPECIFIC PROCEDURE?

After speaking further with the patient and understanding his concerns, the anesthesiologist decides to implement a lidocaine infusion intraoperatively in addition to the aforementioned adjuncts. A bolus dose of 1.5 mg/kg, followed by an infusion of 1 mg/kg/h, is given after the induction of general anesthesia.[6,7] These doses are calculated by ideal body weight (IBW) to avoid the chance of local anesthetic toxicity. The surgical team is made aware of the plan and the possibility that this patient may have increased pain after surgery.

During the intraoperative course after insufflation of the abdomen, the anesthesiologist notes that the patient is persistently tachycardic and hypertensive, despite being maintained on greater than 1 minimal anesthetic concentration (MAC) of sevoflurane. The anesthesiologist suspects a combination of pain and sympathetic stimulation due to laparoscopy as the likely etiology of the increased anesthetic requirements.

(5) ARE THERE ANY OTHER MEDICATIONS THAT CAN BE UTILIZED TO HELP REDUCE THE PATIENT'S ANESTHETIC REQUIREMENTS?

The anesthesiologist decides to place a bispectral index (BIS) monitor and initiate a dexmedetomidine infusion at 0.3 mg/kg/h and titrates the infusion up to 0.6 mg/kg/h over the course of the procedure, monitoring for hypotension and/or bradycardia as the dose is increased.[8] The cumulative dose of dexmedetomidine depends on its intended function. If used as a co-anesthetic, the dose depends primarily on the duration of anesthesia; if used as a co-analgesic, the dose aimed for is 0.5 mcg/kg body weight.[8,9] If used to prevent or treat shivering, the dose is 0.3 mg/kg body weight.[10] The inhaled agent dose can subsequently be decreased while ensuring that the depth of anesthesia remains appropriate. Toward the end of the procedure, after laparoscopy is complete, the dexmedetomidine infusion is stopped. Once the procedure concludes and the patient is extubated uneventfully, he is brought to the recovery room with the lidocaine infusion running.

In the recovery room, the patient continues to have pain that is difficult to control with low-dose opioids. He receives another dose of acetaminophen 1 g, now intravenously, since it has been 6 hours since his previous dose and a dose of IV ketorolac. The patient is also noted to be obstructing when he falls asleep, although he denies a history of obstructive sleep apnea. The surgical team is notified and a consult to the postoperative pain service is placed.

(6) IN LIGHT OF THE DIFFICULT TO CONTROL POSTOPERATIVE PAIN IN THIS PATIENT, ALONG WITH HIS HISTORY OF CHRONIC PAIN AS WELL AS POTENTIAL OBSTRUCTIVE SLEEP APNEA, WHAT WOULD BE THE BEST OPTION FOR POSTOPERATIVE ANALGESIA?

The postoperative pain service interviews the patient in the recovery room, and during this encounter, the patient reports that he has a history of chronic back pain. After his spine surgery, he had difficulty weaning himself off opioids, in particular oxycodone. The patient also notes persistent pain for many months after his cholecystectomy, even though his surgeon told him that "it was a piece of cake." The postoperative pain team decides on a low-dose ketamine infusion, starting at 2 mcg/kg/min to enhance analgesia and reduce opioid requirements.[11] They also recommend acetaminophen 1000 mg q6h as well as gabapentin 600 mg PO q8h and continuation of the lidocaine infusion at the previous dose of 1.5mg/kg/h IBW. As the patient has a history of oxycodone use and potential misuse, the opioid chosen for breakthrough pain is hydromorphone at the lowest effective dose. The recommendation is for hydromorphone 2–4 mg PO q4h prn.

The patient's pain is improved with this regimen, and he is transferred to the floor in stable condition on postoperative day (POD) 0 in the evening. Several hours after arriving on the floor, the patient is found to have increasing confusion and agitation. His vital signs are BP 156/84, HR 92, RR 16, and O_2 saturation 96% on room air. The responding clinician from the surgical team is called and evaluates the patient. Unable to elucidate the most likely cause of the patient's mental status changes, she notifies the postoperative pain team.

(7) WHEN THE ANESTHESIOLOGIST ARRIVES TO SEE THIS PATIENT, WHAT SHOULD BE IN HIS DIFFERENTIAL DIAGNOSIS, AND WHAT STEPS SHOULD BE TAKEN?

The anesthesiologist immediately asks the patient about hallucinations and vivid dreams as well as tinnitus. This patient is currently on multiple medications that can alter mental status, including lidocaine and ketamine. Both infusions are paused, and a stat lidocaine level is drawn to rule out symptoms of local anesthetic toxicity. The level comes back at 8.2 ng/ml, which is supratherapeutic.[12] After several hours, the patient's mental status is clearing, and he is complaining of pain again. The ketamine infusion is then restarted at a lower dose of 1.5 mcg/kg/min and the remaining postoperative course is uneventful.

DISCUSSION

Inadequate perioperative pain control delays postoperative mobilization, and may lead to development of chronic postoperative pain, amplified cardiac and pulmonary complications, and increased morbidity and mortality.[13] Pain causes enormous personal and economic problems, and in the United States, it accounts for greater healthcare expenditures than heart disease, diabetes, and cancer combined.[14] One attempt to improve awareness of the necessity of adequate pain management was the designation of pain as the "fifth vital sign."[15] Unfortunately, inadequately treated pain is still frequent even after so-called minor procedures,[13] and 30%–80% of patients continue to report moderate to severe pain immediately after surgery.[16,17]

Why is it so difficult to achieve adequate postoperative analgesia? Adequacy of pain treatment depends on multiple factors related to procedure, patient, and available (and feasible) treatment techniques. The available medications include opioids and non-opioids. Even though opioids are still widely used,[18] more information on their misuse, limitations, and side effects is becoming available, including risk of dependence and opioid-induced hyperalgesia (OIH).[15]

The goals of multimodal analgesia are to attack pain from several sides, to achieve the optimal balance between treatment effect and side effects, and to wean the patient off opioids as soon as possible. This chapter provides an introduction to the medications frequently used in multimodal analgesia, with the exception of regional anesthesia, discussed throughout this book.

MULTIMODAL ANALGESIA

Multimodal analgesia has been defined as the use of 2 or more analgesics or techniques that target different mechanisms or pathways in the nociceptive system.[19] As drugs are combined, lower doses of each class can be given, thereby lowering the side effects of each individual drug, but increasing overall efficacy.[1,20] This result may culminate in improved analgesia, enhanced functional recovery, and reduced opioid-related adverse effects.[1] The American Society of Anesthesiologists (ASA), the American Pain Society (APS), and the American Society of Regional Anesthesia and Pain Medicine (ASRA) have strongly encouraged the use of multimodal analgesia in the management of acute pain in the perioperative setting,[21,22] and it is now considered the standard of care for all postsurgical patients.[18] In addition, enhanced recovery after surgery (ERAS) protocols focus heavily on the use of multimodal analgesia with opioid-sparing techniques.[2]

Overall, however, despite the evidence, practice guidelines, and wide array of available interventions, there is still considerable heterogeneity in the practice of multimodal analgesia.[18] The following paragraphs detail the systemic analgesics available for patient- and procedure-specific pain management. They are, rather arbitrarily, grouped into classical non-opioid, opioid, and adjuvant drugs.

CLASSICAL NON-OPIOID DRUGS

Acetaminophen (Paracetamol)

Acetaminophen is one of the older and most prescribed medications in the world, with a long track record of use as an analgesic and antipyretic and a very favorable safety profile.[23] It has several routes of administration, including oral, rectal, and the recently FDA-approved intravenous formulation.[24] Interestingly, the exact mechanism of action is still unclear, but the therapeutic targets conjectured include the central cyclooxygenase (COX-3), the endogenous opioid and descending inhibitory serotoninergic system, and the nitric oxide synthase and the endocannabinoid system.[23,25] The maximum recommended adult dose of acetaminophen is 4 grams per day (or 15 mg/kg IBW four times a day), and it is considered safer than nonsteroidal anti-inflammatory drugs (NSAIDs). The major adverse effect of acetaminophen is its potential for severe hepatotoxicity, which is caused by the toxic metabolite, N-acetyl-p-benzoquinone imine (NAPQI). This toxicity is caused by absolute overdosing or failure to take into account preexisting liver damage (increased cytochrome P450 activation, decreased availability of glutathione, and chronic severe alcohol abuse).[26] Even though adequate therapeutic doses of the medication do not seem to exacerbate stable chronic liver disease, total daily dosing should be reduced, and duration of use should be minimized in these situations.[23]

Several meta-analyses have confirmed that paracetamol can reduce opioid consumption by 20%[27,28] with a very good perioperative side-effect profile. Furthermore, there is valuable evidence to support the efficacy of acetaminophen use in conjunction with another non-opioid adjunct such as an NSAID or COX-2 inhibitor to improve postoperative analgesia and reduce opioid consumption.[29,30] These studies demonstrate superior analgesia with both an NSAID or COX-2 inhibitor plus acetaminophen over either drug alone.

Acetaminophen's onset and duration of action is dependent upon its route of administration.[26] Intravenous dosing results in the fastest onset of action, about 10–20 minutes, versus oral dosing, in which the onset occurs about 35–45 minutes after administration.[23] After 45 minutes, analgesic efficacy is equivalent for both forms of administration, but pain relief lasts longer with oral dosing.[23] Intravenous administration of acetaminophen is more expensive than oral administration, while not clinically superior to the oral route.[31] This formulation may be particularly useful when a speedy onset of action is required (e.g., acute postoperative pain treatment after surgery) or when oral administration is not feasible. However, the cost of this administration route needs to be taken into account.[24]

Acetaminophen is a key component of multimodal perioperative pain management and can be used in persons with gastrointestinal disorders, renal disease, or advanced age. Except for very specific contraindications, acetaminophen and regional anesthesia should be the backbone of multimodal analgesia.

Nonsteroidal Anti-Inflammatory Drugs (NSAIDs) and COX-2 Inhibitors

Nonsteroidal anti-inflammatory drugs (NSAIDs) and COX-2 inhibitors are useful drugs with anti-inflammatory, antipyretic, and analgesic properties.[32] They act through blockade of the cyclooxygenase (COX) which is responsible for the production of prostaglandins (PGs). The two main isoforms are COX1 (expressed almost ubiquitously, especially important in the production of PG protecting the gastric mucosa and regulating renal blood flow), and COX2 (mainly involved in the inflammatory response to injury).[33] The more nonspecific the drug, the more likely, in theory, are side effects, especially gastrointestinal, renal, or hemostatic.[32,33] Another side effect observed on long-term intake is an increase in cardiovascular risk.[34] NSAIDs, both nonselective and selective, are useful analgesics as they inhibit inflammation, one of the main sources of postoperative pain. They are part of the multimodal recommendations by ASA, APS, and ASRA, and should be used whenever feasible.[21,22]

They have been shown to be as effective and, in certain cases, more effective analgesics than opioids depending on medication and dose. This is highlighted by the Oxford League Table showing NNTs between 2 and 4 for the most commonly used NSAIDs at frequently prescribed doses, including celecoxib 400 mg PO with an NNT of 2.1, ibuprofen 600 mg PO with an NNT of 2.4, and ketorolac 30 mg IM with an NNT of 3.4. Of note, the NNT for acetaminophen 1000 mg PO is 3.8.[35]

Several meta-analyses have highlighted their potential to improve analgesia and reduce opioid-induced side effects.[29,36] NSAIDs or COX-2 inhibitors were also found to have specific efficacy in total joint arthroplasty.[37]

Diclofenac

Diclofenac is the most widely used NSAID in the world, and it displays a greater selectivity for the COX-2 enzyme over COX-1.[34] The clinical efficacy is beyond doubt, and a recent Cochrane systematic review showed that diclofenac 50 mg provided effective pain relief in about 64% of patients compared to 17% with placebo (with high-quality evidence).[38] Another more recent review included 12 studies and demonstrated an opioid-sparing effect up to 50% in 6 out of the 12 trials.[39] A commonly used dose is 50 mg PO, and the total recommended daily dose is 150 mg/day.[35]

Ketorolac

This medication is one of the few NSAIDs available for intravenous use in the United States and has a rapid onset of analgesic action (approximately 10 minutes) in addition to a long duration of action (approximately 6–8 hours).[37] However, due to its increased selectivity for COX-1 over COX-2 inhibition, it has a higher chance of gastric and renal complications and should not be used for more than 5 days, or for minor pain. Several systematic reviews have supported the use of ketorolac in the perioperative period.[37,39] In terms of dosing, 15 mg is comparable to 30 mg in analgesic efficacy, so in patients with higher risk of adverse effects (e.g., the elderly with decreased baseline renal function or those with renal compromise), the lower dose should be used.[40]

Ibuprofen

Ibuprofen is another very commonly used NSAID and is available over the counter, which further expands its role in postoperative analgesia. It displays a balanced selectivity in terms of COX-1 to COX-2 inhibition, so it has a decreased potential for gastric or renal side effects compared with ketorolac and a reduced chance of cardiovascular effects in comparison to diclofenac.[41] In addition to the widely used oral formulation, it has been recently approved in intravenous form in the United States as an analgesic and anti-pyretic.[41] The vast majority of the data on oral ibuprofen also points to decreased pain scores as well as reduced opioid consumption, but a few key points are worth emphasizing. The PANSAID trial from 2019 (N = 556) investigated analgesic quality in patients undergoing total hip arthroplasty who received a combination of ibuprofen and acetaminophen. Interestingly, patients who received a combination of both drugs had a significantly greater reduction in opioid consumption than those who received acetaminophen alone, but not appreciably greater than those who received ibuprofen alone.[42] Therefore, while there is good evidence that adding an NSAID to paracetamol is beneficial, the reverse may not be as obviously true. On the other hand, a Cochrane review from 2013 including 3 studies and >1600 patients demonstrated that the combination of acetaminophen + ibuprofen provided greater analgesia than either drug alone.[43]

Celecoxib

Celecoxib is currently the only COX-2 inhibitor approved for use in the United States and is available only as an oral formulation, which may limit its utility in the postoperative setting; however, due to its greater selectivity for COX-2 inhibition, it has less effect on perioperative bleeding.[35] The COX-2 inhibitor's analgesic efficacy has been known for more than a decade[44] and was recently confirmed with the added benefit of reducing nausea and vomiting.[45] Although celecoxib has been associated with increased cardiovascular risk during long-term administration, its short-term use in the immediate perioperative period should be strongly considered for the majority of patients, wherever feasible.

In summary, the choice of NSAIDs and COX-2 inhibitor medication should be guided by surgical factors as well as patient comorbidities. Recognizing a potential for complications and in the absence of contraindications, a brief judicious perioperative course of NSAIDs or COX inhibitors should be considered safe in most settings.

ADJUVANT ANALGESICS

Glucocorticoids/Dexamethasone

Dexamethasone is routinely used by anesthesiologists to minimize postoperative nausea and vomiting (PONV),[46] and glucocorticoids are also well-known for their anti-inflammatory effects and ability to reduce tissue injury. Their analgesic properties stem from their ability to reduce prostaglandin synthesis through the inhibition of phospholipase enzyme and COX-2, thereby decreasing the proinflammatory output from the cyclooxygenase and lipoxygenase pathways.[47,48] In addition, mechanisms leading to inflammation that involve tumor necrosis factor-alpha, interleukin 1B, and C-reactive protein are modulated by these medications.[47]

Their efficacy for perioperative analgesia has been studied most notably in the context of preventive analgesia and not for established pain. In 2011, De Oliveira showed that the dose of dexamethasone needed to achieve decreased pain scores postoperatively was 0.2 mg/kg, whereas 0.1 mg/kg was not effective.[49] Another review suggested 8 mg as the commonly used dose to achieve pain reduction.[50] Another study found that intravenous dexamethasone was also effective in prolonging time to first analgesic after surgery under spinal anesthesia.[51] One surgery in which efficacy seems particularly valuable is spine surgery, where 8 mg of dexamethasone reduced postoperative pain without increasing side effects.[48]

What about side effects? A recently published retrospective study including data from 4800 orthopedic surgery patients who had received perioperative dexamethasone revealed that the small risk of elevated blood glucose levels was real but was outweighed by shorter length of stay and improved mortality, although the latter remains to be confirmed.[52] The benefit of using dexamethasone for postoperative pain control may depend on patient and procedural factors. In conclusion, dexamethasone is an inexpensive and easily administered medication frequently employed in the perioperative period for PONV prophylaxis and should be part of multimodal regimens unless contraindicated.

Gabapentinoids

Gabapentin was originally introduced as an anti-convulsant in the 1990s, followed by pregabalin, which featured improved oral pharmacokinetics and a longer half-life.[53] Both drugs were conceptualized as anticonvulsants and later were found to be useful in treating chronic pain conditions such as post-herpetic neuralgia, diabetic neuropathy, complex regional pain syndrome, and trigeminal neuralgia.[54] The main mechanism of action is through binding to $\alpha 2\delta$ subunits of presynaptic voltage-gated calcium channels in both the central and peripheral nervous system.[55] This attachment leads to the inhibition of calcium influx which, in turn, impedes the release of excitatory neurotransmitters such as glutamate, aspartate, substance P, and calcitonin gene-related peptide (CGRP) from primary afferent nerve fibers.[53] Anti-hyperalgesic and anti-allodynic properties of gabapentin are thought to rely on this reduction in neuronal hyperexcitability.[53] Over time, there was increased off-label use for perioperative analgesia, and indeed, several meta-analyses support the usefulness of gabapentinoids in reducing acute postoperative pain and opioid consumption.[53,55,56] The 2016 guidelines by the APS, ASA, and ASRA advocated for the use of gabapentinoids as a component of multimodal analgesia preoperatively as a strong recommendation with moderate quality evidence.[22] However, since then, more critical studies have emerged, highlighting the risk of respiratory depression if combined with opioids,[57] and dizziness.[5] The FDA issued a warning regarding the use of gabapentinoids with opioids in December 2019, and more recent reviews and advisories no longer advocate for the administration of gabapentinoids on a broad scale.[4] There was one more argument to use gabapentinoids perioperatively, the potential to reduce chronic pain, and the role of gabapentin in promoting opioid cessation was documented in one study from 2018 where a 24% increase in the rate of opioid cessation after surgery compared to an active placebo (lorazepam) was demonstrated.[58] It is important to note that this finding has not been replicated and may be outweighed by the risks associated with these medications noted above.

So that begs the question, does gabapentin have any role in perioperative multimodal analgesia? In our opinion, these medications should not be routinely employed as part of a multimodal analgesic plan. The caveats to that statement, though, extend to situations where patients have already been prescribed the medication prior to their surgery, especially when the surgical procedure is known to be particularly painful, e.g., thoracotomy and laparotomy, or where there will be an exacerbation of the very pain that the patient was experiencing preoperatively, e.g., spine surgery. In addition, these drugs may still be considered during the postoperative course before a patient is discharged if the individual's pain is difficult to control and/or characteristics of neuropathic pain exist. Either medication chosen in this class should be started at the lowest effective dose, and the patient should be monitored for side effects, including sedation, gait or visual disturbances, or dizziness. This pertains especially to the elderly or a patient taking opioids. As gabapentinoids are eliminated by the kidneys, caution must be exercised in patients with renal disease as well.[54]

N-methyl-D-aspartate (NMDA) Antagonists

It has been several decades since the N-methyl-D-aspartate (NMDA) receptor was implicated in nociception and characterized as an ionotropic glutaminergic receptor activated by excitatory neurotransmitters, glutamate and aspartate.[59] Importantly, these receptors have been found on primary afferents in the spinal dorsal horn.[60] Excitatory neurotransmitter stimulation of this receptor leads to persistent postoperative pain, hypersensitivity, windup, and allodynia, opioid-induced tolerance, and OIH.[60] Hence, these receptors play an important role in the genesis of "pathologic pain," which is defined as heightened pain perception resulting from sensitization.[61] NMDA receptor antagonists have been shown to prevent central sensitization caused by peripheral nociceptive stimulation in addition to mitigating its existence once established.[62]

There are several medications that have been studied for their ability to block NMDA receptors. The two that are most extensively used currently are ketamine and magnesium. We will discuss each of these medications and their roles in multimodal analgesia in the perioperative patient.

Ketamine

Ketamine was first developed in the 1960s as an anesthetic agent with analgesic properties.[60] The drug has many mechanisms of action, including effects on μ-opioid receptors, muscarinic receptors, monoaminergic receptors, γ-aminobutyric acid receptors, and multiple others.[11,60] However, its principal pharmacologic function is antagonism at NMDA receptors. Its main effects are either hypnotic/analgesic at higher doses (bolus of 0.5–1 mg/kg), or anti-hyperalgesic and preventing spinal cord sensitization at lower doses (bolus of 0.1 mg/kg followed by low-dose infusion). Ketamine use is burgeoning in the clinical area, not least as a result of the opioid crisis in parts of the Western world.[63] Consensus guidelines by ASRA, AAPM, and ASA were published in 2018, and they noted that subanesthetic doses of ketamine exhibited the most benefit in surgeries associated with significant postoperative pain such as thoracic surgery, upper and lower abdominal surgery, and orthopedic (both limb and spine) surgery.[11,64] Procedures which cause mild levels of pain, including head and neck surgery, do not seem to warrant perioperative ketamine usage in opioid-naïve patients.[64]

In addition to the type of surgery, there are some patient indications for ketamine treatment, the most compelling being an opioid-tolerant or opioid-dependent patient.[64] Although there is some conflicting evidence regarding this indication, a 2010 study by Loftus et al. (N = 102) and a more recent 2019 study by Boenigk et al. (N = 129) both demonstrated that postoperative opioid consumption was reduced in opioid-dependent and opioid-tolerant patients who received ketamine infusions perioperatively.[65,66] The consensus statement by ASRA, AAPM, and ASA mentioned above also concluded that there is at least mild benefit and more likely moderate benefit of sub-anesthetic dosing of perioperative ketamine for this particular patient population.[11]

Another potential patient indication for low-dose ketamine in the perioperative period outlined by the consensus statement is in patients at higher risk of opioid-induced respiratory depression, such as those with obstructive sleep apnea.[11] Opioids are known to increase the severity of OSA after surgery, and ketamine is recognized for its ability to preserve respiratory drive and oropharyngeal muscle tone at lower doses, as well as its utility in reducing opioid consumption.[67] Therefore, it may be beneficial in this particular patient population, although further research needs to be undertaken to verify this claim.[11]

Another topic addressed in the statement is the dose range considered sub-anesthetic but still effective for acute pain.[11] Higher doses of ketamine seem to correlate with increased adverse effects of the drug, such as hallucinations, nightmares, tachycardia, and hypertension.[68] Therefore, the consensus committee recommends limiting a bolus of ketamine to 0.35 mg/kg and infusions for acute pain to 1 mg/kg/h to provide effective analgesia while minimizing adverse reactions.[11] We suggest starting even lower, at 0.1–0.15 mg/kg as a bolus and 0.1 mg/kg/h as an infusion, and to titrate upward, with the main goal being avoidance of side effects. These thoughts help put into context the results of the 2018 PODCAST trial, a multicenter, international randomized control trial with 672 patients over 60 years old who received a single bolus dose of ketamine, either 0.5 mg/kg or 1 mg/kg, versus placebo prior to incision and demonstrated a greater incidence of hallucinations and nightmares with escalating doses of ketamine without a benefit on pain scores, opioid consumption, or reduction in postoperative delirium.[69]

It is important to also consider the contraindications to ketamine use, specifically uncontrolled cardiovascular disease, pregnancy, and psychosis.[11] In addition, ketamine should be utilized with caution in patients with moderate hepatic disease and avoided in patients with severe liver disease, i.e., cirrhosis.[11] Elevated intracranial pressure or intraocular pressure also precludes the safe use of ketamine from the available evidence.[11] One particular area of future investigation includes ketamine's utility in preventing persistent post-surgical pain (PPSP). One meta-analysis from 2014 that included 17 studies demonstrated a very small but statistically significant decrease in the risk of developing PPSP at 3 and 6 months, but the data were very heterogeneous, and no consistent regimen for timing and dosing of ketamine to achieve this goal could be extrapolated.[70]

In our experience, low-dose ketamine infusions have been particularly helpful in managing postoperative pain in the opioid-tolerant or opioid-dependent patient for reducing opioid consumption, as well as for its analgesic benefits. As a result, it has become a mainstay of our multimodal analgesia plan in these patients, especially if they are undergoing a painful surgery, as noted previously. In addition, ketamine is beneficial in patients who are on medically assisted treatment of opioid use disorder with either methadone or buprenorphine. The medication is most often initiated after induction of anesthesia with either a small bolus followed by a continuous infusion or only a continuous infusion that is maintained for 48–72 hours postoperatively and adjusted according to a patient's postoperative pain requirements and any encountered side effects. The main take-home message if ketamine is considered is "start low, go slow," meaning start with a small dose and titrate upward, rather than starting with a high dose and being forced to discontinue due to side effects.

Magnesium

Magnesium plays an important role in cellular homeostasis. It is vital for enzyme function, neurotransmission, and cell signaling, and has been touted as "nature's physiological calcium channel blocker."[71,72] This ion has been studied for decades in the context of anesthesia due to its central depressant effects, but more recently, the focus has shifted to its utility in perioperative analgesia stemming from its known antagonism of NDMA receptors and role in preventing central sensitization. Lacking any direct antinociceptive qualities, magnesium acts as a noncompetitive NMDA receptor antagonist through prevention of intracellular influx of calcium by blocking the excitatory neurotransmitters, aspartate and glutamate, from binding to these receptors.

The first trial indicating an analgesic effect of magnesium in postoperative pain, published in 1996, demonstrated that the perioperative administration of magnesium sulfate resulted in reduced opioid requirements, decreased pain, and improved sleep quality without notable side effects.[72] Since that time, one review failed to find a substantive effect of magnesium,[73] while later analyses showed a benefit.[71,74,75] The most recent meta-analysis from 2015 included 27 trials (N = 1504). Although the results from this study reinforced the notion that perioperative magnesium reduced postoperative pain scores at rest and at 24 hours with movement, the findings for opioid consumption differed in that there was a notable reduction in opioid consumption in urogenital, orthopedic, and cardiovascular surgeries, but equivocal data for gastrointestinal surgeries.[76]

To summarize, although there have been conflicting results, overall, the data demonstrate that magnesium has a favorable influence on postoperative pain by enhancing the effects of concomitantly administered opioids, as well as by preventing central sensitization stemming from peripheral tissue injury.[59,62] Dosing can be either in the form of a bolus or an infusion intraoperatively, with it typically ranging from 30 to 50 mg/kg for the bolus and infusion rates of 8–15 mg/kg/h.[77] Furthermore, magnesium has a wide therapeutic window and a good safety profile when used at therapeutic doses, although patients should be monitored closely for signs of hypermagnesemia, especially with renal insufficiency.[59] Therefore, it may be utilized safely and effectively as a component of multimodal analgesia; however, dosing parameters, time course of administration, and long-term effects on pain require additional investigation.

INTRAVENOUS LIDOCAINE

Local anesthetics have been utilized extensively for regional anesthesia both in the neuraxial space and in peripheral nerve blocks due to their ability to block voltage-gated sodium channels. However, more recently, local anesthetics, in particular lidocaine, have been studied for their analgesic, anti-hyperalgesic, and anti-inflammatory effects, which are thought to be related to a variety of other mechanisms of action.[78,79] Lidocaine, the classic amide local anesthetic, was first described as an analgesic in 1951, and this effect has been demonstrated in both the central and peripheral nervous system.[80] In addition to its effects on voltage-gated sodium channels, lidocaine has been shown to exert effects on voltage-gated calcium channels, potassium channels, glutamate receptors, G protein-coupled receptors, acetylcholine (ACh) receptors, NMDA receptors, and the glycinergic system.[7] With respect to ACh and NMDA receptors, lidocaine has been shown to display significantly heightened sensitivity for these receptors on the order of 100–1000 times, and these effects are believed to be responsible for the drug's anti-hyperalgesic properties.[79,80] Lidocaine's anti-inflammatory characteristics stem from its inhibition of leukocyte activation and release of surgical pro-inflammatory markers, such as IL-6, IL-8, and C-reactive protein.[12,80] Interestingly, the plasma concentrations of lidocaine observed when using intravenous dosing replicates plasma levels measured during epidural anesthesia, approximately 1 μMol.[81] The preventive analgesic benefit of lidocaine has been supported by the duration of the clinical effect, which can last more than 8.5 hours after termination of the infusion, or 5.5 times the half-life of the drug.[12]

These systemic effects were the reason to speculate in the early 2000s whether lidocaine could potentially play a beneficial role when administered systemically,[78] and the first prospective randomized controlled trial published in 2007 indeed showed that systemic lidocaine, compared to placebo, shortened length of hospital stay and promoted return of bowel function.[82] The gold standard for abdominal surgery had been epidural analgesia,[83] but concerns over side effects (hypotension, pruritus, urinary retention) and complications (spinal hematoma) have decreased enthusiasm for epidurals.[84,85] It is now accepted that laparoscopic visceral surgery is no longer an indication for epidural analgesia, and IV lidocaine has proven itself as a valuable analgesic adjunct in that setting. In contrast, regional anesthesia is still the gold standard for open (especially upper) abdominal surgery. There are studies which even suggest that IV lidocaine is not inferior to epidural analgesia during open abdominal surgery,[86,87] but there has been debate whether study design disfavored epidurals, and many clinicians continue to use regional, rather than intravenous, anesthesia to help with pain management after open abdominal surgery. As a side note, going beyond the scope of this chapter is the issue whether more targeted truncal blocks (paravertebral, transverse abdominis plane, rectus sheath, quadratus lumborum) combined with a good multimodal regimen can replace epidural anesthesia, and the authors do think that this approach would be more likely to succeed than intravenous lidocaine alone. Again, these blocks rely on relatively high volumes of local anesthetic; therefore systemic levels of clinical relevance are achieved, and systemic effects are a "freebie" whenever truncal nerve blocks are performed.

Intravenous lidocaine has also had positive results in breast surgery,[88] and results on the brink of clinical significance in spine [89] and thyroid [90] surgery which are still being discussed. Theoretically, large inflamed wound surfaces as noted with burns would also be an area where IV lidocaine can be used as an analgesic rescue modality.

The enthusiasm for IV lidocaine was dampened by a recently updated meta-analysis from 2018 by Weibel and colleagues who reviewed a total of 68 trials (4525 patients) spanning various types of surgeries. The authors concluded that it was unclear if IV lidocaine decreases pain in the early postoperative phase at 1–4 hours after surgery compared to placebo.[91] Furthermore, they found that there was no substantive difference in pain at 24 hours and 48 hours between patients receiving the infusion and placebo.[91] In addition, bowel function recovery, postoperative nausea, and postoperative pain were not clearly associated with the use of a lidocaine infusion.[91] Evidence was also lacking when comparing IV lidocaine and epidural anesthesia with respect to the optimal timing and dosing of these analgesic regimens.[91] The authors of this study again acknowledged that the quality of evidence on the advantage of IV lidocaine was very low due to inconsistency, imprecision, and study quality.[80,91] However, 3 more studies were still being conducted and 18 others were awaiting classification upon the completion of the updated Cochrane review, which may alter the results of this review.[91] At this time, it appears that this modality for pain control may be of most value in very specific situations such as those where regional techniques are not feasible or where other adjuncts are contraindicated based on patient specific issues. The optimal timing, dosing, and length of administration of this drug still require further investigation. Dosing in the perioperative setting is generally 1–1.5 mg/kg IBW for the bolus, followed by an infusion of 1 mg/kg/h IBW.[79] Although lidocaine is considered a very safe local anesthetic with a long history of use, when it is administered intravenously, monitoring for signs and symptoms of local anesthetic toxicity, including tinnitus, perioral numbness, and arrhythmias, must be undertaken, and plasma levels should be monitored to ensure they remain below the toxic range (<5 μg/ml).[12] Patients with significant liver dysfunction are at increased risk of local anesthetic toxicity, so further precautions should be taken when using this medication in such situations.[12]

ALPHA-2 AGONISTS

The pharmacologic attributes of α-2 agonists, including sedation, anxiolysis, hypnosis, sympathicolysis, and analgesia, all achieved without causing respiratory depression, would seem to make this class of drugs an ideal option for perioperative use.[92] There are multiple mechanisms of action that give rise to these combined effects, including the hyperpolarization of supraspinal noradrenergic neurons, which decreases neuronal firing in the locus coeruleus and leads to an inhibition of sympathetic neurotransmitter release and suppression of activity in descending sympathetic pathways and is responsible for the sedative properties of these drugs.[9,93] Further actions in the spinal cord that directly account for their analgesic effects include activation of several types of α-2 receptors in the dorsal horn, thereby decreasing the release of pro-nociceptive neurotransmitters, including substance P and glutamate, from primary afferent terminals.[9]

Dexmedetomidine and clonidine are the two α-2 agonists in which we are most interested perioperatively. These drugs have been used as additives to regional anesthesia with favorable effects, and they have also been utilized systemically. It is believed that when administered systemically, these α-2 agonists enhance the analgesic effect of opioids without augmenting their hyperalgesic qualities.[94]

Clonidine

Clonidine is best known for its anti-hypertensive effects, which it accomplishes through brain stem adrenergic receptor stimulation, leading to activation of inhibitory neurons that decrease central nervous system sympathetic outflow.[93] Due to its bioavailability, clonidine has good efficacy as an oral preparation, so it can be used preoperatively or postoperatively. It has also been used as premedication in the pediatric population with success.[93] Clonidine has multiple other routes of administration, including intravenous, perineural, neuraxial, and transdermal. When administered orally, it is rapidly and almost completely absorbed, and as a result, is effective for preoperative anxiolysis and sedation and as an adjunct to opioids in the postoperative period.[8] It is also useful as an anesthesia and analgesia adjuvant and has been shown to decrease MAC requirements, as well as a valuable additive to local anesthetics for regional techniques.[93]

In the meta-analysis by Blaudszun et al., the patients treated with clonidine had about a 25% reduction in morphine consumption in the first 24 hours postop, and pain intensity was decreased by about 0.7 cm on the 10 cm VAS scale, the latter finding being similar to what was seen with dexmedetomidine.[92] In 2014, the results of the POISE-2 study demonstrated that low-dose clonidine was associated with a greater risk of clinically significant hypotension and nonfatal cardiac arrest without improving cardiac outcomes in patients undergoing noncardiac surgery.[95] These results, coupled with the increased availability of dexmedetomidine, have led to the decreased use of clonidine in the perioperative period. The lesson for contemporary practitioners is to use good judgement on when to administer clonidine, weighing risks and benefits, and being ready to treat hypotension when it ensues. In the postoperative period, we have used it effectively as an adjunct in multimodal analgesia, especially after a patient requires transition from a dexmedetomidine infusion. If the patient receives the medication for over 1 week, it should be titrated down in order to avoid rebound hypertension, a significant side effect which can lead to a hypertensive crisis.[90] Other indications are in patients at risk of alcohol withdrawal,[96] excess anxiety,[97] or shivering.[10] Usual doses for the latter indications are 0.5 mcg/kg body weight, except for shivering, where 0.25–0.3 mcg/kg is used.

Dexmedetomidine

Dexmedetomidine was approved by the FDA in 1999 for short-term use as an analgesic and sedative medication in the intensive care setting (ICU) setting.[93] It is a much more highly selective α-2 agonist compared with clonidine, and its half-life is about 2 hours versus 9–12 hours for clonidine, and because the $\alpha\text{-}2_A$ receptor subtype is relevant for pain, it may be the better analgesic than clonidine. Several meta-analyses have examined the effectiveness of these α-2 agonists in postoperative analgesia. One such meta-analysis included 30 studies (N = 1792), with 933 receiving either clonidine or dexmedetomidine, and the authors concluded that perioperative systemic alpha-2 agonists reduced postoperative opioid consumption, pain intensity, and nausea without prolonging recovery times.[92] The reduction of morphine consumption at 24 hours was noted to be about 30% over placebo with dexmedetomidine, and the degree of analgesia was greater with dexmedetomidine compared to acetaminophen, but less than NSAIDs.[92] The most common adverse effects noted were bradycardia and arterial hypotension.[92] In contrast, the large network meta-analysis by Martinez et al. on non-opioid analgesics after major surgery found convincing evidence that α-2 agonists were similar to NSAIDs and COX-2 inhibitors in reducing opioid consumption, analgesia, and PONV, and much better than acetaminophen alone.[29] There have also been multiple other meta-analyses looking only at the perioperative administration of dexmedetomidine, with the majority demonstrating decreased postoperative pain and reduced opioid consumption, as well as other secondary outcomes such as reduced opioid-related adverse effects and PONV.[98–100] The most common adverse effects were intraoperative bradycardia and hypotension.[98]

With respect to specific types of surgery, reviews from recent years in spine surgery, intracranial neurosurgery, and bariatric surgery have all established a benefit of perioperative dexmedetomidine in reducing opioid consumption both intraoperatively and postoperatively and decreasing pain scores.[100–102] In these situations, a decreased opioid requirement is of particular value due to the need for rapid neurological assessment postoperatively with neurosurgery and spine surgery, in addition to a desire to avoid the enhanced opioid-induced respiratory depression in obese patients undergoing bariatric surgery. The reader is alerted to the fact that clonidine and dexmedetomidine have been accused of causing false-positive pathologic readings during neuromonitoring of spinal motor pathways,[103] but this finding has not been reliably replicated, and different institutions may have specific policies in place regarding dexmedetomidine and its place in neurosurgery when monitoring is used. Based on its ability to reduce both anesthetic and opioid requirements intraoperatively, dexmedetomidine appears to be a valuable tool in ERAS protocols and has significantly improved postoperative outcomes in this context.[104]

Intravenous administration of dexmedetomidine is most common, and dosing typically consists of a bolus dose between 0.25–1 mcg/kg given over 10 minutes and infusion rates of 0.2–1 mcg/kg/h. The bolus dose may be omitted in patients with tenuous hemodynamics. Due to its hemodynamic effects, dexmedetomidine should be administered in monitored settings, such as the OR, PACU, or ICU. Initial dose when used for analgesic purposes should be limited to 0.5 mcg/kg body weight.

CONCLUSION

The past decade has seen a dramatic shift from opioid-based analgesic methods to methods based primarily on non-opioids. We are now prioritizing regional anesthesia and analgesic adjuvants over opioids and have learned that judicious patient- and procedure-specific use of multimodal drug regimens can achieve equal or better pain control with less side effects compared to opioid-based analgesia. Multimodal analgesia should be standard of care and employed in all patients requiring systemic analgesia.

REFERENCES

1. Buvanendran A, Kroin JS. Multimodal analgesia for controlling acute postoperative pain. *Curr Opin Anaesthesiol.* 2009;22:588–593.
2. Joshi GP, Kehlet H. Enhanced recovery pathways: looking into the future. *Anesth Analg.* 2019;128:5–7.
3. Rosero EB, Joshi GP. Preemptive, preventive, multimodal analgesia: what do they really mean? *Plast Reconstr Surg.* 2014;134:85S–93S.
4. Kharasch ED, Clark JD, Kheterpal S. Perioperative gabapentinoids: deflating the bubble. *Anesthesiology.* 2020;133:251–254.
5. Fabritius ML, Geisler A, Petersen PL, et al. Gabapentin for postoperative pain management: a systematic review with meta-analyses and trial sequential analyses. *Acta Anaesthesiol Scand.* 2016;60: 1188–1208.
6. Lirk P, Picardi S, Hollmann MW. Local anaesthetics: 10 essentials. *Eur J Anaesthesiol.* 2014;31:575–585.
7. Lirk P, Hollmann MW, Strichartz G. The science of local anesthesia: basic research, clinical application, and future directions. *Anesth Analg.* 2018;126:1381–1392.
8. Giovannitti JA Jr, Thoms SM, Crawford JJ. Alpha-2 adrenergic receptor agonists: a review of current clinical applications. *Anesth Prog.* 2015;62:31–39.
9. Grewal A. Dexmedetomidine: new avenues. *J Anaesthesiol Clin Pharmacol.* 2011;27:297–302.
10. Lewis SR, Nicholson A, Smith AF, Alderson P. Alpha-2 adrenergic agonists for the prevention of shivering following general anaesthesia. *Cochrane Database Syst Rev.* 2015 Aug 10;2015(8):CD011107.
11. Schwenk E, Viscusi E, Buvanendran A, et al. Consensus guidelines on the use of intravenous ketamine for acute pain management, from the American Society of Regional Anesthesia and Pain Medicine (ASRA), the American Academy of Pain Medicine (AAPM), and the American Society of Anesthesiologists (ASA). *Reg Anesth Pain Med.* 2018;43:521–546.
12. Dunn LK, Durieux ME. Perioperative use of intravenous lidocaine. *Anesthesiology.* 2017;126:729–737.
13. Gerbershagen HJ, Aduckathil S, van Wijck AJ, Peelen LM, Kalkman CJ, Meissner W. Pain intensity on the first day after surgery: a prospective cohort study comparing 179 surgical procedures. *Anesthesiology.* 2013;118:934–944.
14. Kharasch ED, Avram MJ, Clark JD. Rational perioperative opioid management in the era of the opioid crisis: reply. *Anesthesiology.* 2020;133:942–943.
15. Wu CL, Raja SN. Treatment of acute postoperative pain. *Lancet.* 2011;377:2215–2225.
16. Meissner W, Zaslansky R. A survey of postoperative pain treatments and unmet needs. *Best Pract Res Clin Anaesthesiol.* 2019;33:269–286.
17. Gan TJ, Habib AS, Miller TE, White W, Apfelbaum JL. Incidence, patient satisfaction, and perceptions of post-surgical pain: results from a US national survey. *Curr Med Res Opin.* 2014;30:149–160.
18. Ladha KS, Patorno E, Huybrechts KF, Liu J, Rathmell JP, Bateman BT. Variations in the use of perioperative multimodal analgesic therapy. *Anesthesiology.* 2016;124:837–845.
19. Manworren RC. Multimodal pain management and the future of a personalized medicine approach to pain. *AORN J.* 2015;101:308–314; quiz 15–18.
20. Kehlet H, Dahl JB. The value of "multimodal" or "balanced analgesia" in postoperative pain treatment. *Anesth Analg.* 1993;77:1048–1056.
21. American Society of Anesthesiologists Task Force on Acute Pain M. Practice guidelines for acute pain management in the perioperative setting: an updated report by the American Society of Anesthesiologists Task Force on Acute Pain Management. *Anesthesiology.* 2012;116: 248–273.
22. Chou R, Gordon DB, de Leon-Casasola OA, et al. Management of postoperative pain: a clinical practice guideline from the American Pain Society, the American Society of Regional Anesthesia and Pain Medicine, and the American Society of Anesthesiologists' Committee on Regional Anesthesia, Executive Committee, and Administrative Council. *J Pain.* 2016;17:131–157.
23. Oscier CD, Milner QJ. Peri-operative use of paracetamol. *Anaesthesia.* 2009;64:65–72.
24. Gollamudi J, Marks S. Oral versus intravenous acetaminophen #302. *J Palliat Med.* 2016;19:231–232.
25. Klinger-Gratz PP, Ralvenius WT, Neumann E, et al. Acetaminophen relieves inflammatory pain through CB1 cannabinoid receptors in the rostral ventromedial medulla. *J Neurosci.* 2018;38:322–334.
26. Mattia C, Coluzzi F. What anesthesiologists should know about paracetamol (acetaminophen). *Minerva Anestesiol.* 2009;75:644–653.
27. Remy C, Marret E, Bonnet F. Effects of acetaminophen on morphine side-effects and consumption after major surgery: meta-analysis of randomized controlled trials. *Br J Anaesth.* 2005;94:505–513.
28. Toms L, McQuay HJ, Derry S, Moore RA. Single dose oral paracetamol (acetaminophen) for postoperative pain in adults. *Cochrane Database Syst Rev.* 2008 Oct 8;2008(4):CD004602.
29. Martinez V, Beloeil H, Marret E, Fletcher D, Ravaud P, Trinquart L. Non-opioid analgesics in adults after major surgery: systematic review with network meta-analysis of randomized trials. *Br J Anaesth.* 2017;118:22–31.
30. Ong CK, Seymour RA, Lirk P, Merry AF. Combining paracetamol (acetaminophen) with nonsteroidal antiinflammatory drugs: a qualitative systematic review of analgesic efficacy for acute postoperative pain. *Anesth Analg.* 2010;110:1170–1179.
31. Mallama M, Valencia A, Rijs K, Rietdijk WJR, Klimek M, Calvache JA. A systematic review and trial sequential analysis of intravenous vs. oral peri-operative paracetamol. *Anaesthesia.* 2021 Feb;76(2):270–276.
32. Candido KD, Perozo OJ, Knezevic NN. Pharmacology of acetaminophen, nonsteroidal antiinflammatory drugs, and steroid medications: implications for anesthesia or unique associated risks. *Anesthesiol Clin.* 2017;35:e145–e62.
33. Vane JR. The mechanism of action of anti-inflammatory drugs. *Ernst Schering Res Found Workshop.* 2000;(31):1–23.
34. Gupta A, Bah M. NSAIDs in the treatment of postoperative pain. *Curr Pain Headache Rep.* 2016;20:62.
35. Hurley RW, Nabil NM, Wu CL. Acute postoperative pain. In: Gropper M, Miller RD, eds. *Miller's Anesthesia.* Philadelphia: Elsevier; 2020:2614–2638.
36. Marret E, Kurdi O, Zufferey P, Bonnet F. Effects of nonsteroidal anti-inflammatory drugs on patient-controlled analgesia morphine side effects: meta-analysis of randomized controlled trials. *Anesthesiology.* 2005;102:1249–1260.
37. Fillingham YA, Hannon CP, Roberts KC, et al. The efficacy and safety of nonsteroidal anti-inflammatory drugs in total joint arthroplasty: systematic review and direct meta-analysis. *J Arthroplasty.* 2020;35:2739–2758.
38. Derry S, Wiffen PJ, Moore RA. Single dose oral diclofenac for acute postoperative pain in adults. *Cochrane Database Syst Rev.* 2015 Jul 7;2015(7):CD004768.
39. Martinez L, Ekman E, Nakhla N. Perioperative opioid-sparing strategies: utility of conventional NSAIDs in adults. *Clin Ther.* 2019;41:2612–2628.

40. Zhou TJ, Tang J, White PF. Propacetamol versus ketorolac for treatment of acute postoperative pain after total hip or knee replacement. *Anesth Analg*. 2001;92:1569–1575.
41. Southworth SR, Sellers JA. Narrative summary of recently published literature on intravenous ibuprofen. *Clin Ther*. 2020;42:1210–1221.
42. Thybo KH, Hagi-Pedersen D, Dahl JB, et al. Effect of combination of paracetamol (acetaminophen) and ibuprofen vs either alone on patient-controlled morphine consumption in the first 24 hours after total hip arthroplasty: the PANSAID randomized clinical trial. *JAMA*. 2019;321:562–571.
43. Derry CJ, Derry S, Moore RA. Single dose oral ibuprofen plus paracetamol (acetaminophen) for acute postoperative pain. *Cochrane Database Syst Rev*. 2013 Jun 24;2013(6):CD010210.
44. Straube S, Derry S, McQuay HJ, Moore RA. Effect of preoperative Cox-II-selective NSAIDs (coxibs) on postoperative outcomes: a systematic review of randomized studies. *Acta Anaesthesiol Scand*. 2005;49:601–613.
45. Khan JS, Margarido C, Devereaux PJ, Clarke H, McLellan A, Choi S. Preoperative celecoxib in noncardiac surgery: a systematic review and meta-analysis of randomized controlled trials. *Eur J Anaesthesiol*. 2016;33:204–214.
46. Gan TJ, Belani KG, Bergese S, et al. Fourth consensus guidelines for the management of postoperative nausea and vomiting. *Anesth Analg*. 2020;131:411–448.
47. Rhen T, Cidlowski JA. Antiinflammatory action of glucocorticoids: new mechanisms for old drugs. *N Engl J Med*. 2005;353:1711–1723.
48. Sharma M, Gupta S, Purohit S, Goyal AK. The effect of intravenous dexamethasone on intraoperative and early postoperative pain in lumbar spine surgery: a randomized double-blind placebo-controlled study. *Anesth Essays Res*. 2018;12:803–808.
49. De Oliveira GS Jr, Almeida MD, Benzon HT, McCarthy RJ. Perioperative single dose systemic dexamethasone for postoperative pain: a meta-analysis of randomized controlled trials. *Anesthesiology*. 2011;115:575–588.
50. Waldron NH, Jones CA, Gan TJ, Allen TK, Habib AS. Impact of perioperative dexamethasone on postoperative analgesia and side-effects: systematic review and meta-analysis. *Br J Anaesth*. 2013;110:191–200.
51. Heesen M, Rijs K, Hilber N, et al. Effect of intravenous dexamethasone on postoperative pain after spinal anaesthesia: a systematic review with meta-analysis and trial sequential analysis. *Anaesthesia*. 2019;74:1047–1056.
52. Herbst RA, Telford OT, Hunting J, et al. The effects of perioperative dexamethasone on glycemic control and postoperative outcomes. Endocr Pract. 2020;26:218–225.
53. Tiippana EM, Hamunen K, Kontinen VK, Kalso E. Do surgical patients benefit from perioperative gabapentin/pregabalin? A systematic review of efficacy and safety. *Anesth Analg*. 2007;104:1545–1556.
54. Kong VK, Irwin MG. Gabapentin: a multimodal perioperative drug? *Br J Anaesth*. 2007;99:775–786.
55. Doleman B, Heinink TP, Read DJ, Faleiro RJ, Lund JN, Williams JP. A systematic review and meta-regression analysis of prophylactic gabapentin for postoperative pain. *Anaesthesia*. 2015;70:1186–1204.
56. Arumugam S, Lau CS, Chamberlain RS. Use of preoperative gabapentin significantly reduces postoperative opioid consumption: a meta-analysis. *J Pain Res*. 2016;9:631–640.
57. Savelloni J, Gunter H, Lee KC, et al. Risk of respiratory depression with opioids and concomitant gabapentinoids. *J Pain Res*. 2017;10:2635–2641.
58. Hah J, Mackey SC, Schmidt P, et al. Effect of perioperative gabapentin on postoperative pain resolution and opioid cessation in a mixed surgical cohort: a randomized clinical trial. *JAMA Surg*. 2018;153:303–311.
59. Bujalska-Zadrozny M, Tatarkiewicz J, Kulik K, Filip M, Naruszewicz M. Magnesium enhances opioid-induced analgesia: what we have learnt in the past decades? *Eur J Pharm Sci*. 2017;99:113–127.
60. Mion G, Villevieille T. Ketamine pharmacology: an update (pharmacodynamics and molecular aspects, recent findings). *CNS Neurosci Ther*. 2013;19:370–380.
61. Himmelseher S, Durieux ME. Ketamine for perioperative pain management. *Anesthesiology*. 2005;102:211–220.
62. Woolf CJ, Thompson SW. The induction and maintenance of central sensitization is dependent on N-methyl-D-aspartic acid receptor activation; implications for the treatment of post-injury pain hypersensitivity states. *Pain*. 1991;44:293–299.
63. Zeballos JL, Lirk P, Rathmell JP. Low-dose ketamine for acute pain management: a timely nudge toward multimodal analgesia. *Reg Anesth Pain Med*. 2018;43:453–455.
64. Laskowski K, Stirling A, McKay WP, Lim HJ. A systematic review of intravenous ketamine for postoperative analgesia. *Can J Anaesth*. 2011;58:911–923.
65. Loftus RW, Yeager MP, Clark JA, et al. Intraoperative ketamine reduces perioperative opiate consumption in opiate-dependent patients with chronic back pain undergoing back surgery. *Anesthesiology*. 2010;113:639–646.
66. Boenigk K, Echevarria GC, Nisimov E, et al. Low-dose ketamine infusion reduces postoperative hydromorphone requirements in opioid-tolerant patients following spinal fusion: a randomised controlled trial. *Eur J Anaesthesiol*. 2019;36:8–15.
67. Sharma S, Balireddy RK, Vorenkamp KE, Durieux ME. Beyond opioid patient-controlled analgesia: a systematic review of analgesia after major spine surgery. *Reg Anesth Pain Med*. 2012;37:79–98.
68. Aroni F, Iacovidou N, Dontas I, Pourzitaki C, Xanthos T. Pharmacological aspects and potential new clinical applications of ketamine: reevaluation of an old drug. *J Clin Pharmacol*. 2009;49:957–964.
69. Avidan MS, Maybrier HR, Abdallah AB, et al. Intraoperative ketamine for prevention of postoperative delirium or pain after major surgery in older adults: an international, multicentre, double-blind, randomised clinical trial. *Lancet*. 2017;390:267–275.
70. McNicol ED, Schumann R, Haroutounian S. A systematic review and meta-analysis of ketamine for the prevention of persistent post-surgical pain. *Acta Anaesthesiol Scand*. 2014;58:1199–1213.
71. De Oliveira GS, Jr., Castro-Alves LJ, Khan JH, McCarthy RJ. Perioperative systemic magnesium to minimize postoperative pain: a meta-analysis of randomized controlled trials. *Anesthesiology*. 2013;119:178–190.
72. Tramer MR, Schneider J, Marti RA, Rifat K. Role of magnesium sulfate in postoperative analgesia. *Anesthesiology*. 1996;84:340–347.
73. Lysakowski C, Dumont L, Czarnetzki C, Tramer MR. Magnesium as an adjuvant to postoperative analgesia: a systematic review of randomized trials. *Anesth Analg*. 2007;104:1532–1539.
74. Albrecht E, Kirkham KR, Liu SS, Brull R. Peri-operative intravenous administration of magnesium sulphate and postoperative pain: a meta-analysis. *Anaesthesia*. 2013;68:79–90.
75. Murphy JD, Paskaradevan J, Eisler LL, et al. Analgesic efficacy of continuous intravenous magnesium infusion as an adjuvant to morphine for postoperative analgesia: a systematic review and meta-analysis. *Middle East J Anaesthesiol*. 2013;22:11–20.
76. Guo BL, Lin Y, Hu W, et al. Effects of systemic magnesium on postoperative analgesia: is the current evidence strong enough? *Pain Physician*. 2015;18:405–418.
77. Rodriguez-Rubio L, Nava E, Del Pozo JSG, Jordan J. Influence of the perioperative administration of magnesium sulfate on the total dose of anesthetics during general anesthesia: a systematic review and meta-analysis. *J Clin Anesth*. 2017;39:129–138.
78. Hollmann MW, Durieux ME. Local anesthetics and the inflammatory response: a new therapeutic indication? *Anesthesiology*. 2000;93:858–875.
79. Hermanns H, Hollmann MW, Stevens MF, et al. Molecular mechanisms of action of systemic lidocaine in acute and chronic pain: a narrative review. *Br J Anaesth*. 2019;123:335–349.
80. Beaussier M, Delbos A, Maurice-Szamburski A, Ecoffey C, Mercadal L. Perioperative use of intravenous lidocaine. *Drugs*. 2018;78:1229–1246.
81. Inoue R, Suganuma T, Echizen H, Ishizaki T, Kushida K, Tomono Y. Plasma concentrations of lidocaine and its principal metabolites during intermittent epidural anesthesia. *Anesthesiology*. 1985;63:304–310.

82. Herroeder S, Pecher S, Schonherr ME, et al. Systemic lidocaine shortens length of hospital stay after colorectal surgery: a double-blinded, randomized, placebo-controlled trial. *Ann Surg.* 2007;246:192–200.
83. Popping DM, Elia N, Van Aken HK, et al. Impact of epidural analgesia on mortality and morbidity after surgery: systematic review and meta-analysis of randomized controlled trials. *Ann Surg.* 2014;259:1056–1067.
84. Bos EME, Haumann J, de Quelerij M, et al. Haematoma and abscess after neuraxial anaesthesia: a review of 647 cases. *Br J Anaesth.* 2018;120:693–704.
85. Moen V, Dahlgren N, Irestedt L. Severe neurological complications after central neuraxial blockades in Sweden 1990–1999. *Anesthesiology.* 2004;101:950–959.
86. Swenson BR, Gottschalk A, Wells LT, et al. Intravenous lidocaine is as effective as epidural bupivacaine in reducing ileus duration, hospital stay, and pain after open colon resection: a randomized clinical trial. *Reg Anesth Pain Med.* 2010;35:370–376.
87. Terkawi AS, Tsang S, Kazemi A, et al. A clinical comparison of intravenous and epidural local anesthetic for major abdominal surgery. *Reg Anesth Pain Med.* 2016;41:28–36.
88. Lepot A, Elia N, Tramer MR, Rehberg B. Preventing pain after breast surgery: a systematic review with meta-analyses and trial-sequential analyses. *Eur J Pain.* 2020.
89. Farag E, Ghobrial M, Sessler DI, et al. Effect of perioperative intravenous lidocaine administration on pain, opioid consumption, and quality of life after complex spine surgery. *Anesthesiology.* 2013;119:932–9840.
90. Kim MH, Kim MS, Lee JH, Kim ST, Lee JR. Intravenously administered lidocaine and magnesium during thyroid surgery in female patients for better quality of recovery after anesthesia. *Anesth Analg.* 2018;127:635–641.
91. Weibel S, Jelting Y, Pace NL, et al. Continuous intravenous perioperative lidocaine infusion for postoperative pain and recovery in adults. *Cochrane Database Syst Rev.* 2018;6:CD009642.
92. Blaudszun G, Lysakowski C, Elia N, Tramer MR. Effect of perioperative systemic alpha2 agonists on postoperative morphine consumption and pain intensity: systematic review and meta-analysis of randomized controlled trials. *Anesthesiology.* 2012;116:1312–1322.
93. Nguyen V, Tiemann D, Park E, Salehi A. Alpha-2 agonists. *Anesthesiol Clin.* 2017;35:233–245.
94. Grosu I, de Kock M. New concepts in acute pain management: strategies to prevent chronic postsurgical pain, opioid-induced hyperalgesia, and outcome measures. *Anesthesiol Clin.* 2011;29:311–327.
95. Devereaux PJ, Sessler DI, Leslie K, et al. Clonidine in patients undergoing noncardiac surgery. *N Engl J Med.* 2014;370:1504–1513.
96. Ungur AL, Neumann T, Borchers F, Spies C. Perioperative management of alcohol withdrawal syndrome. *Visc Med.* 2020;36:160–166.
97. Hidalgo MP, Auzani JA, Rumpel LC, Moreira NL Jr, Cursino AW, Caumo W. The clinical effect of small oral clonidine doses on perioperative outcomes in patients undergoing abdominal hysterectomy. *Anesth Analg.* 2005;100:795–802.
98. Schnabel A, Meyer-Friessem CH, Reichl SU, Zahn PK, Pogatzki-Zahn EM. Is intraoperative dexmedetomidine a new option for postoperative pain treatment? A meta-analysis of randomized controlled trials. *Pain.* 2013;154:1140–1149.
99. Le Bot A, Michelet D, Hilly J, et al. Efficacy of intraoperative dexmedetomidine compared with placebo for surgery in adults: a meta-analysis of published studies. *Minerva Anestesiol.* 2015;81:1105–1117.
100. Liu Y, Liang F, Liu X, Shao X, Jiang N, Gan X. Dexmedetomidine reduces perioperative opioid consumption and postoperative pain intensity in neurosurgery: a meta-analysis. *J Neurosurg Anesthesiol.* 2018;30:146–155.
101. Tsaousi GG, Pourzitaki C, Aloisio S, Bilotta F. Dexmedetomidine as a sedative and analgesic adjuvant in spine surgery: a systematic review and meta-analysis of randomized controlled trials. *Eur J Clin Pharmacol.* 2018;74:1377–1389.
102. Singh PM, Panwar R, Borle A, Mulier JP, Sinha A, Goudra B. Perioperative analgesic profile of dexmedetomidine infusions in morbidly obese undergoing bariatric surgery: a meta-analysis and trial sequential analysis. *Surg Obes Relat Dis.* 2017;13:1434–1446.
103. Calderon P, Deltenre P, Stany I, et al. Clonidine administration during intraoperative monitoring for pediatric scoliosis surgery: effects on central and peripheral motor responses. *Neurophysiol Clin.* 2018;48:93–102.
104. Kaye AD, Chernobylsky DJ, Thakur P, et al. Dexmedetomidine in enhanced recovery after surgery (ERAS) protocols for postoperative pain. *Curr Pain Headache Rep.* 2020;24:21.
105. Glare P, Aubrey KR, Myles PS. Transition from acute to chronic pain after surgery. *Lancet.* 2019; 393:1537–1546.

REVIEW QUESTIONS

(1) All of the following are true statements about multimodal analgesia EXCEPT:

A. Multimodal analgesia is the use of 2 or more different classes of analgesics with different mechanisms of action and varying side effect profiles to achieve adequate pain control.
B. Multimodal analgesia is strongly supported by the ASA (American Society of Anesthesiologists), APS (American Pain Society), and ASRA (American Society of Regional Anesthesia) and is considered the standard of care for postoperative pain management.
C. Multimodal analgesia always starts prior to incision.
D. Enhanced recovery after surgery (ERAS) pathways incorporate multimodal analgesia into their protocols to help reduce the surgical stress response and improve patient outcomes.

(2) Which of the following are contributors to persistent postsurgical pain (PPSP)?

A. Patient factors including age, gender, and medical comorbidities
B. The intensity and duration of postoperative pain
C. The presence of preoperative pain
D. All of the above

(3) Acetaminophen is useful for:

A. An elderly patient with a history of renal insufficiency presenting for an ORIF of a hip fracture
B. A morbidly obese patient presenting for a laparoscopic sleeve gastrectomy with a history of obstructive sleep apnea
C. A patient with stable chronic liver disease who is scheduled for a minimally invasive esophagectomy
D. All of the above

(4) With respect to nonsteroidal anti-inflammatory drugs (NSAIDs) and cyclooxygenase (COX-2) inhibitors, which of the following statements is CORRECT?

A. They have been shown to be useful after total knee and hip replacement without an increase in adverse effects.

B. COX-2 inhibitors must be avoided in all patients with a history of cardiovascular disease perioperatively.
C. Acetaminophen used alone is comparable to NSAIDs or COX-2 inhibitors in terms of analgesic efficacy.
D. A dose of morphine 10 mg IM has better analgesic efficacy than either ibuprofen 600 mg PO or celecoxib 400 mg PO.

(5) All of the following are true regarding gabapentinoids EXCEPT:

A. They bind to pre-synaptic voltage-gated calcium channels in both the central and peripheral nervous systems.
B. Their use has been associated with increased sedation, respiratory depression, and risk of naloxone administration.
C. Due to the warning issued by the FDA regarding the concomitant use of gabapentinoids with opioids, the APS, ASA, and ASRA have discouraged the routine use of this class of medications for multimodal analgesia.
D. Gabapentin dosing should be reduced in patients with renal disease.

(6) A patient with a history of chronic opioid use for pain from a carcinoma of the head and neck presents for neck dissection. The best option for perioperative pain management would be:

A. A bolus of ketamine without an intraoperative infusion
B. A bolus of ketamine with an intraoperative infusion
C. An intraoperative remifentanil infusion
D. A preoperative dose of gabapentin and acetaminophen

ANSWERS

(1) **C.** Multimodal analgesia does not specify a time at which it is instituted in the perioperative period, and different components of this strategy may begin preoperatively, intraoperatively, or postoperatively, depending on multiple factors including patient or surgical considerations. Preemptive analgesia refers to the implementation of pain control strategies prior to incision. (A, B, D: These are all true statements regarding multimodal analgesia.)

Reference

Rosero EB, Joshi GP. Preemptive, preventive, multimodal analgesia: what do they really mean? *Plast Reconstr Surg*. 2014;134:85S–93S.

(2) **D.** Persistent post-surgical pain (PPSP) is defined as pain that continues at the surgical site for more than 3–6 months after surgery for which another explanation, such as infection, malignancy, or a preexisting pain condition, is lacking. Among the many factors that contribute to the development of PPSP are age, gender, analgesic regimen, medical comorbidities, presence of preoperative pain, and intensity and duration of postoperative pain.

Reference

Glare P, Aubrey KR, Myles PS. Transition from acute to chronic pain after surgery. *Lancet*. 2019; 393:1537–1546.

(3) **D.** Acetaminophen is a safe analgesic with a long history of use in many clinical situations and for the majority of patients, including when there is a need for minimizing opioids due to age or comorbidities such as obstructive sleep apnea. In patients with stable liver disease, it can be safely used at reduced doses for short periods of time.

References

Martinez V, Beloeil H, Marret E, Fletcher D, Ravaud P, Trinquart L. Non-opioid analgesics in adults after major surgery: systematic review with network meta-analysis of randomized trials. *Br J Anaesth*. 2017;118:22–31.
Oscier CD, Milner QJ. Peri-operative use of paracetamol. *Anaesthesia*. 2009;64:65–72.

(4) **A.** In a 2020 systematic review and meta-analysis, oral NSAIDs or COX-2 inhibitors used with intravenous (IV) ketorolac were shown to significantly reduce opioid consumption and improve postoperative analgesia without significant adverse effects in total joint arthroplasty. (B) Due to their potential for cardiovascular side effects, COX-2 inhibitors must be used cautiously in patients with cardiovascular disease, but they have been used safely in the immediate perioperative period for a short duration. (C) NSAIDs and COX-2 inhibitors have been shown to be more effective than acetaminophen in analgesic efficacy when used as the only analgesic with morphine. (D) The NNT for celecoxib 400 mg PO and ibuprofen 600 mg PO are both lower than the NNT for morphine 10 mg IM, 2.1 and 2.4 for celecoxib and ibuprofen respectively, vs. 2.9 for morphine, which translates to improved analgesic efficacy.

References

Fillingham YA, Hannon CP, Roberts KC, et al. The efficacy and safety of nonsteroidal anti-inflammatory drugs in total joint arthroplasty: systematic review and direct meta-analysis. *J Arthroplasty*. 2020;35:2739–2758.
Martinez V, Beloeil H, Marret E, Fletcher D, Ravaud P, Trinquart L. Non-opioid analgesics in adults after major surgery: systematic review with network meta-analysis of randomized trials. *Br J Anaesth*. 2017;118:22–31.
Hurley RW, Nabil NM, Wu CL. Acute postoperative pain. In: Gropper M, Miller RD, eds. *Miller's Anesthesia*. Philadelphia: Elsevier; 2020:2614–2638.

(5) **C.** Although the FDA recently issued a warning against the use of gabapentinoids together with opioids, the APS, ASA, and ASRA have not yet disavowed the routine use of these medications perioperatively, while similar professional organizations in Europe have come out against their widespread use for perioperative analgesia.[4,22] (A, B, D are all true statements about gabapentinoids.)

References

Kharasch ED, Clark JD, Kheterpal S. Perioperative gabapentinoids: deflating the bubble. *Anesthesiology*. 2020;133:251–254.

Chou R, Gordon DB, de Leon-Casasola OA, et al. Management of postoperative pain: a clinical practice guideline from the American Pain Society, the American Society of Regional Anesthesia and Pain Medicine, and the American Society of Anesthesiologists' Committee on Regional Anesthesia, Executive Committee, and Administrative Council. *J Pain*. 2016; 17:131–157.

(6) **B.** Although head and neck surgery is not considered a particularly painful surgery, the patient's history of chronic opioid use will influence the intensity of pain that the patient experiences, and a ketamine bolus with infusion has been shown to improve postoperative pain, as well as reduce opioid consumption in opioid tolerant patients. (A) A bolus of ketamine intraoperatively without a continuous infusion will not provide adequate analgesia for a significant amount of time postoperatively due to ketamine's short duration of action. (C) Remifentanil infusions have been associated with opioid-induce hyperalgesia (OIH), so it is not the best choice in an opioid-tolerant patient who may have increased pain postoperatively. (D) While preoperative acetaminophen would be useful for this patient, if the patient is not currently on gabapentin, the most recent data argue against using this medication preoperatively as there does not appear to be a clinically significant benefit to its administration and an increased chance of side effects with concurrent opioid use.

References

Schwenk E, Viscusi E, Buvanendran A, et al. Consensus guidelines on the use of intravenous ketamine for acute pain management, from the American Society of Regional Anesthesia and Pain Medicine (ASRA), the American Academy of Pain Medicine (AAPM), and the American Society of Anesthesiologists (ASA). *Reg Anesth Pain Med*. 2018;43:521–546.

Mion G, Villevieille T. Ketamine pharmacology: an update (pharmacodynamics and molecular aspects, recent findings). *CNS Neurosci Ther*. 2013;19:370–380.

Wu CL, Raja SN. Treatment of acute postoperative pain. *Lancet*. 2011;377:2215–2225.

Kharasch ED, Clark JD, Kheterpal S. Perioperative gabapentinoids: deflating the bubble. *Anesthesiology*. 2020;133:251–254.

6.

LOCAL ANESTHETIC SYSTEMIC TOXICITY

Osemeke Edobor, Veena Graff, and Taras Grosh

STEM CASE AND KEY QUESTIONS

A 63-year-old 50-kg male is scheduled to undergo a total knee arthroplasty under regional anesthesia. As part of his multimodal pain regimen, an ultrasound guided adductor canal block with indwelling perineural catheter for postoperative analgesia is performed prior to spinal anesthesia in the induction room. The patient is placed on standard American Society of Anesthesiology monitors, a block time-out is performed, and the patient is sedated with 1 mg of midazolam. Upon clear visualization of the neurovascular bundle in the adductor canal, an 18-gauge 3.5-inch Touhy needle is advanced adjacent to the saphenous nerve. After negative aspiration, a dose of 2 ml of 0.5% ropivacaine is given without complication; a total of 30 mL of 0.5% ropivacaine is injected in 5 mL increments with repeat aspiration. Ten minutes pass, the patient is repositioned, and a spinal anesthetic is performed uneventfully. The patient is transported to the operating room (OR), transferred to the OR table, and prior to initiation of propofol sedation, 80 mg of lidocaine is injected intravenously to prevent discomfort from propofol administration. The patient complains of ringing in the ears, gradually becomes irritable, and multiple premature ventricular contractions are seen on the 5-lead electrocardiogram. You attempt to recycle the blood pressure cuff, but the patient attempts to rip off the cuff. The operating room staff restrain the patient, who begins to mumble his words and then becomes unarousable.

(1) WHAT IS LOCAL ANESTHETIC SYSTEMIC TOXICITY?

Local anesthetic systemic toxicity (LAST) is a life-threatening adverse reaction resulting from local anesthetic (LA) reaching significant systemic circulating levels.[1]

The team in the operating room suspect the patient is having a seizure. The anesthesiologist in the room requests additional help from his colleagues, and then quickly draws up and administers midazolam, a short-acting benzodiazepine. The anesthesiologist asks the nurse to obtain levetiracetam from the pharmacy as well as an LA toxicity kit. The anesthesiologist begins to mask ventilate the patient with 100% FiO_2.

(2) WHAT IS THE INCIDENCE OF LAST?

Exact numbers are difficult to establish given the heterogeneous presentations, but estimates are approximately 0.03%.[1–4]

This patient has a past medical history of well-controlled insulin-dependent diabetes and nonischemic cardiomyopathy with a reduced left ventricular ejection fraction of 45%. There is no personal or family history of seizure disorder or abnormal reaction to anesthetics.

(3) WHAT ARE THE SYMPTOMS AND CLINICAL PRESENTATION OF LAST?

Symptoms are primarily central nervous system (CNS) excitation progressing to depression (seizures to coma) or cardiovascular depression.[1,2]

The pharmacy is unable to locate the LA toxicity kit. The anesthesiologist is joined by one of his colleagues, who is a cardiac anesthesiologist. She obtains additional intravenous access, is able to identify a pulse, and notifies the coordinator that a cardiopulmonary bypass machine should be primed.

(4) WHAT FACTORS INCREASE RISK OF LAST?

The total concentration of LA used, as well as absorption rate based on site of injection.[1,5]

Repeat blood pressure reading reveals significant hypotension in the setting of a ventricular arrhythmia. The nurse in the room is no longer able to feel a pulse; cardiopulmonary resuscitation (CPR) is initiated.

(5) HOW SHOULD THIS PATIENT BE TREATED? WHAT IS THE CURRENT AMERICAN SOCIETY OF REGIONAL ANESTHESIA (ASRA) GUIDELINE FOR DOSING LIPID EMULSION?

Symptom management is crucial (airway, breathing, circulation) with concomitant administration of lipid emulsion if LAST is suspected.[1,2]

Lipid emulsion is obtained from the outpatient surgical pharmacy and immediately brought to the OR, where the patient is actively being resuscitated.

(6) WHAT IS THE MECHANISM OF ACTION OF LIPID EMULSION? CAN PROPOFOL OR ANY OTHER AGENTS BE SUBSTITUTED?

Lipid emulsion therapy creates an expanded lipid phase, and the resulting equilibrium drives LA from tissue into the aqueous plasma, then to the lipid phase.[1,4,6]

The airway is secure, the lipid emulsion is administered, the patient has a return of spontaneous circulation after 5 minutes of CPR. He is transferred to the surgical intensive care unit intubated, mechanically ventilated, hemodynamically supported with pressors, sedated.

(7) SHOULD THIS PATIENT BE SENT TO THE INTENSIVE CARE UNIT, AND FOR HOW LONG BEFORE DISCHARGE?

Patient should be monitored for 6 hours in the presence of cardiovascular symptoms and 2 hours if rapidly progressing CNS symptoms. All cases should be reported to www.lipidrescue.org.[1,6]

The intensivists determine the patient is hemodynamically stable and meets extubation criteria. Once extubated, he no longer endorses signs of LA toxicity; the team readies him for the wards.

(8) WHAT OTHER SERVICES COULD BE NOTIFIED DURING A LONG DURATION OF ATTEMPTED RESUSCITATION?

The primary team as well as intensivists if the patient will remain in the hospital for additional monitoring and testing.[1,6]

The anesthesiologist has a formal meeting with the perioperative committee, including nursing, surgeons, pharmacy, and administration. Their goal is to complete a root cause analysis about why the rescue lipid emulsion was not available in the OR.

DISCUSSION

LAST is a life-threatening adverse event related to the administration of LA via a variety of routes, including regional anesthesia. Its presentation does not always follow the classic symptomatology of CNS excitatory symptoms (auditory changes, circumoral numbness, metallic taste, and agitation, leading to seizures and/or CNS depression) followed by cardiotoxicity and arrest or collapse. Although incidence is low, providers must be knowledgeable and well prepared to recognize and manage LAST in a timely manner.

INCIDENCE

The reported incidence of major LAST events in regional anesthesia (seizure and cardiac arrest) has markedly decreased due to increased awareness, routine preventive measures, and possibly ultrasound guidance.[1–4] In the past decade, the incidence of major LAST (defined as administration of lipid emulsion, seizure, or cardiac arrest) is reported in the range of 0.4 to 2 per 100,000.[3,4] Minor LAST events, such as circumoral numbness, tinnitus, and metallic taste, might occur more frequently, but likely go underreported. The push to reduce opioid prescriptions will likely increase the use of various LA-based regional techniques: large-volume fascial plane blocks, continuous perineural infusions, tumescence with LA, combination of various LAs, and new LA formulations. The dramatic increase in regional anesthetics has not resulted in an increase in LAST incidence, chiefly thanks to increased vigilance, safety guidelines, and the use of ultrasound for peripheral nerve blocks to reduce the volume of LA used and to avoid intravascular injections.[3,4]

PHARMACOLOGY

LAs are amphipathic compounds (having both a hydrophobic and hydrophilic portion). An intermediary chain has either an ester or amide linkage, which dictates the metabolism (Figure 6.1). Esters are rapidly metabolized in the plasma by plasma-, butyryl-, or pseudo-cholinesterases into inactive compounds.[7,8] Amides, on the other hand, undergo a lengthier process: hepatic oxidation.

LAs exert their effect by entering into a cell and blocking the voltage-gated sodium (Na) channels at the alpha subunit. This disrupts Na influx into the cell, resulting in a decreased amplitude of the action potential, slowed rate of depolarization, increased firing threshold, slow impulse conduction, and prolonged refractory period. Disruption of neuronal conduction ultimately results in an inability to transmit impulses from the periphery to the cortex, producing analgesia and anesthesia in a dose-dependent manner.

LAs work on various receptors, blocking not only Na channels but also potassium and calcium channels, the Na-K

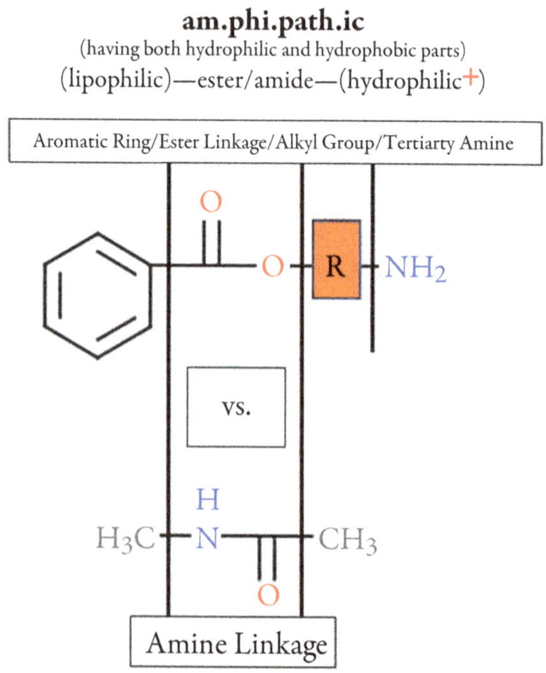

Figure 6.1. Chemical structure of ester and amide local anesthetic.

Table 6.1 PHYSICOCHEMICAL PROPERTIES OF LOCAL ANESTHETICS

FACTOR	ACTION	DESCRIPTION
pKa	Onset	LA pKa lower than tissue pH → uncharged > charged LA ⇒ faster onset LA pKa higher than tissue pH → charged > uncharged LA ⇒ slower onset
Lipid solubility	Potency	Highly soluble → high partition coefficient ⇒ more potent Able to penetrate lipid bilayer and reach target
Protein binding	Duration	More bound = longer duration of action because less effective circulating level of free/active LA Free form = actively metabolized Alpha-1-glycoprotein, albumin, tissue proteins all serves as reservoir for LA
Diffusibility	Onset	More diffusible = quicker onset
Vasodilation	Potency Duration	More blood flow = greater uptake and metabolism

ATPase channels. LAs also interact with N-methyl-D-aspartate (NMDA) receptors, and disrupt various cellular metabolic processes as well, including mitochondrial metabolism and adenosine triphosphate production, inhibiting the ryanodine receptor at the sarcoplasmic reticulum, and reducing Ca2+ sensitivity of myofilaments.[1] Being so ubiquitous, the inhibition of Na channels is responsible for variety of symptoms associated with LAST.

Most LA are achiral, but ropivacaine and levobupivacaine are S(−) enantiomers, and bupivacaine exists as a racemic mixture of R(+) and S(−) bupivacaine.[7] This chirality accounts for differences in its clinical effect and safety profiles.

The physicochemical properties of LAs are responsible for their individual pharmacokinetic differences clinically (Table 6.1).[8]

While all LAs would cause LAST once the toxic plasma level is exceeded, intrinsic and extrinsic properties contribute to the onset, severity, and differentiation between CNS versus CV toxicity. Table 6.1 lists the extrinsic and intrinsic properties contributing to LAST.

When LAs leave the initial site of injection, they enter the circulation, and redistribute to the well-perfused end organs: brain, heart, liver, and lung. Lipid-rich organs act as the greatest depot for LAs.[7,8] If the LA exceeds the capacity to be metabolized from the plasma either via cholinesterase plasma hydrolysis (esters) or hepatic oxidation (amides) and buffers (AAG, albumin, various proteins) are overwhelmed, the free fraction of the drug increases and the risks of accumulation and toxicity rise.[7,8] The underlying mechanisms of LAST are not fully understood, with diverse cellular effects in the CNS and cardiovascular system (CV) in play.[1–4]

CENTRAL NERVOUS SYSTEM

In the CNS, LAs initially compromise cortical inhibitory pathways, resulting in unopposed excitatory clinical features: circumoral numbness, tinnitus, restlessness, agitation.[7,8] As the plasma concentration of the LA rises, the excitatory pathways are interrupted, resulting in a depressive phase characterized by a loss of consciousness, coma, and finally respiratory arrest. During a seizure, increased cerebral metabolism leads to acidosis, which prolongs the seizure activity even in the presence of declining LA levels in the blood. Acidosis traps the charged/diffusible LA intracellularly, further worsening the symptoms.

CARDIOVASCULAR SYSTEM

LAs bind to Na channels in the CV system, leading to conduction and rhythm disturbances, myocardial dysfunction, and changes in vascular tone. Because LAs decrease amplitude, resting potential, and speed of conduction, a progressive prolongation in the PR, QRS, ST, and QT intervals is evident on electrocardiogram (ECG) prior to cardiovascular collapse.

PRESENTATION

Though 40% of symptoms associated with LAST are nonspecific, the majority are excitatory CNS symptoms: tinnitus, agitation, circumoral numbness, seizures (from absence to grand mal).[2,6,9] In 33% of cases, primary CNS symptoms progress to CV symptoms; 20% present primarily with isolated CV symptoms.[6] During general anesthesia, patients can also suffer from LAST, with cardiac symptoms being the initial presentation. While major symptoms are rare and usually are documented and reported, minor symptoms (tinnitus) may be underreported and even remain unnoticed.

AT RISK

The risk factors for developing LAST can be broken down into extrinsic and intrinsic events, listed in Table 6.2.

EXTRINSIC

Patient at risk for LAST include those at the extremes of age, parturients, patients with end organ dysfunction, as well as those receiving high doses of LA.[1–4] Site of injection influences significantly the peak plasma concentration and the time to reach it. Intravenous and tracheal injection result in higher plasma levels versus equal-volume subcutaneous injections. A particular area of caution is the cumulative effect of

Table 6.2 MOST COMMONLY USED LOCAL ANESTHETIC AND MAXIMUM RECOMMENDED DOSES

LOCAL ANESTHETIC	ONSET TIME	POTENCY	MAXIMUM DOSE WITHOUT EPINEPHRINE (MG/KG)	MAXIMUM DOSE WITH EPINEPHRINE (MG/KG)
Lidocaine	Fast	Moderate	5	7
Ropivacaine	Slow	Potent	3	3
Bupivacaine	Slow	Potent	2	3
Mepivacaine	Fast	Moderate	5	7

Chart adapted from data.[12]

multiple LA administrations and drugs with similar mechanism of action or competing pharmacokinetics on toxicity, e.g., the concomitant use of LA in peripheral nerve blocks, intravenous anesthesia induction, multimodal analgesia infusions, and surgical infiltration, potentially compromising clinical safety.

INTRINSIC

An important concept in the study of LAST is the ratio of the dose required to produce cardiovascular collapse (CC) to that required to induce seizures, the so-called CC/CNS ratio: the lower the number, the more likely the LA is to cause CV collapse.[7,8] A higher number indicates a higher safety margin.

Free LA plasma levels are dictated by intrinsic vasoactive properties. Generally speaking, LAs are vasodilators, with notable exceptions being cocaine and ropivacaine (at various doses).[10] The addition of epinephrine to an LA will prolong the effect of short-acting LAs (e.g., lidocaine) while also reducing systemic absorption of vasodilating agents (e.g., bupivacaine).

Lastly, the maximum safe LA dose can vary based on site of injection, absorption, speed of injection, as well as patient-specific characteristics.[7,8,10] Therefore, it is impossible to accurately determine universally applicable maximum allowable doses that predictably reflect LA plasma levels. Nevertheless, various expert references[5] describe accepted safe practices, but these must be used with vigilance and caution, taking various patient, drug, and injection-site specific characteristics into consideration. Common sense dictates that the lowest LA dose to produce a desired effect should be used.

Table 6.2 lists LAs commonly used in clinical practice, as well as their suggested maximum injected doses.

Use of liposomal formulations, such as liposomal bupivacaine, requires additional caution given the plasma concentration peaks occurring <2 hours and 36 hours after administration.[11] Additionally, other sustained-release products may soon make their way into clinical practice, requiring vigilance and acute clinical awareness.

TREATMENTS

Currently, the ASRA recommendations include symptomatic management, as well as initiating lipid rescue therapy at the first sign of LAST after securing the airway. The pharmacologic treatment of LAST differs from other cardiac arrest scenarios:[13]

- Reduce individual epinephrine boluses to ≤1 mcg/kg
- Avoid vasopressin, calcium channel blocks, beta blockers, or other local anesthetics
  - Stop injecting LA
  - Get help
    - Consider lipid emulsion therapy at the first sign of a serious LAST event
    - Call for the LAST Rescue Kit
    - Alert the nearest cardiopulmonary bypass team; resuscitation may be prolonged
  - Airway management
    - Ventilate with 100% oxygen; avoid hyperventilation; advanced airway device if necessary
  - Control seizures
    - Benzodiazepines preferred
    - Avoid large doses of propofol, especially in hemodynamically unstable patients
  - Treat hypotension and bradycardia; if pulseless, start CPR
  - Lipid emulsion 20% (precise volume and flow rate are NOT crucial)
    - Patient >70 kg
      - Bolus 100 mL lipid emulsion 20% rapidly over 2–3 minutes
      - Infuse at 200–250 mL over 15–20 minutes
    - Patient <70 kg
      - Bolus 1.5 mL/kg lipid emulsion 20% rapidly over 2–3 minutes
      - Infuse at ~0.25 mL/kg/min
    - If patient remains unstable:
      - Re-bolus once or twice at the same dose and double infusion rate; be aware of limiting dose (12 mL/kg)

- Total volume of lipid emulsion can approach 1 L in a prolonged resuscitation (e.g., >30 minutes)
- Continue monitoring
    - At least 4–6 hours after a cardiovascular event

    or

    - At least 2 hours after a limited CNS event
        - Do not exceed 12 mL/kg lipid emulsion (particularly important in the small adult or child)
    - Much smaller doses are typically needed for LAST treatment.[13]

It is important to recognize the importance of seizure management, as violent muscle contraction can result in significant injury, including fractures, dislocations, and head injury. Also, hypercontraction can exacerbate the metabolic acidosis. If the seizures are refractory, and airway is secured, consider the addition of nondepolarizing neuromuscular blockade to reduce the incidence of metabolic acidosis.

In patients experiencing nonperfusing rhythms, adequate chest compressions are paramount to ensure the distribution of the lipid emulsion. In the setting of ongoing arrhythmias or cardiac arrest, prompt advanced cardiac life support measures must be undertaken.

PREVENTION

The prevention of LAST is a multifaceted process. A thorough review of the medication administration record (MAR) is essential to identify the type, amount, and duration of present LA administration: lidocaine infusion therapy, lidocaine patches, perineural catheter infusions, etc. Determine if LA has been stopped and when it will be resumed. Drugs altering plasma cholinesterase activity (neostigmine, pyridostigmine, succinylcholine, echothiphate, phenelzine, esmolol, metocolopromaide) have the potential to decrease hydrolysis of ester-type LAs.[7,8,10] Drugs inhibiting hepatic microsomal enzymes, such as cimetidine (Tagamet), may allow the accumulation of unexpectedly high blood concentrations of amide LA.[9] Nevertheless, LAST from concomitant cimetidine use is unreported. Reduction of hepatic blood flow by drugs (propranolol) or hypotension will decrease the hepatic clearance of amide LA. Special caution must be exercised in patients taking digoxin, calcium antagonists, and/or β-blockers who receive LA with epinephrine.

Additionally, caution must be exercised at extremes of ages and in patients with significant comorbidities. Neonates and infants have reduced plasma concentration of alpha-1-glycoprotein and immature hepatic enzymes, resulting in greater free fraction of LA.[9] Dosing should be reduced by 15% in patients <4 months of age.[1]

In patients with liver disease, while LA clearance is reduced, a larger volume of distribution and maintenance of alpha-1-glycoprotein synthesis provide a safety margin; dose reductions are recommended when using repeat boluses and continuous infusions.[9]

Those with renal dysfunction may have a hyperdynamic circulation and a reduced clearance of LAs, but an increased a1-acid glycoprotein (AAG) h concentration. Therefore, unless the patient is uremic or has metabolic acidosis, dose reduction is not necessary.[9]

In the elderly a dose reduction of 10%–20% is recommended, given a reduction in skeletal muscle (which acts like a depot), as well as reduced clearance due to reduced metabolic organ perfusion and pharmacodynamic function.[9]

Parturients have increased cardiac output and reduced alpha-1-glycoprotein concentration, resulting in faster absorption and higher levels of free LA; therefore, a dose reduction is recommended.[9]

CLINICAL GUIDE TO ADMINISTERING LOCAL ANESTHETICS

When planning to initiate an intervention, calculate the maximum allowable dose of LA, and if higher volume is needed, consider reducing concentration. Ensure that adequate time has passed since prior administration, utilize the lowest volume needed to achieve the desired effect, administer slowly with frequent negative aspiration, and monitor patients. It is important to also account for the specifics of the site to which LA is being administered to best anticipate increases in plasma concentrations. Utilize ultrasound to visualize the spread of LA and reduce the risk of accidental intravascular injections, and to visualize the desired target in an effort to reduce the injectate volume. Always aspirate prior to injecting, reduce bolus aliquots to <5 mL, and consider pausing 30–45 seconds.[9] While some advocate the routine addition of epinephrine, caution must be used in anatomical areas at risk for distal ischemia and in patients with coronary artery disease or stable angina, as well as in those prone to arrhythmia.

CONCLUSIONS

- LAST is a life-threatening medical emergency that may present with a progression of CNS excitability and seizures, followed by cardiovascular collapse and cardiac arrest.
- With a high suspicion for LAST, securing the airway should be prioritized, followed by immediate initiation of intralipid therapy.
- Patients at increased risk for LAST include those at the extremes of age, patients with significant comorbidities, including organ failure, metabolic abnormalities, ischemia, etc.
- Carefully reviewing the MAR, discontinuing concomitant LA therapies, implementation of ultrasound guidance, and use of low-dose epinephrine may all lower the risk of LAST.

REFERENCES

1. El-Boghdadly K, Pawa A, Chin KJ. Local anesthetic systemic toxicity: current perspectives. *Local Reg Anesth*. 2018;11:35–44.
2. Neal JM, et al. ASRA practice advisory on local anesthetic systemic toxicity. *Reg Anesth Pain Med*. 2010;35(2):152–161.

3. Morwald EE, et al. Incidence of local anesthetic systemic toxicity in orthopedic patients receiving peripheral nerve blocks. *Reg Anesth Pain Med.* 2017;42(4):442–445.
4. Rubin DS, et al. Local anesthetic systemic toxicity in total joint arthroplasty: incidence and risk factors in the United States from the national inpatient sample 1998–2013. *Reg Anesth Pain Med.* 2018;43(2):131–137.
5. Rosenberg PH, Veering BT, Urmey WF. Maximum recommended doses of local anesthetics: a multifactorial concept. *Reg Anesth Pain Med.* 2004;29(6):564–575; discussion 524.
6. Gitman M, Barrington MJ. Local anesthetic systemic toxicity: a review of recent case reports and registries. *Reg Anesth Pain Med.* 2018;43(2):124–130.
7. Heavner JE. Local anesthetics. *Curr Opin Anaesthesiol.* 2007;20(4): 336–342.
8. Lirk P, Picardi S, Hollmann MW. Local anaesthetics: 10 essentials. *Eur J Anaesthesiol.* 2014;31(11):575–585.
9. El-Boghdadly K, Chin KJ. Local anesthetic systemic toxicity: continuing professional development. *Can J Anaesth.* 2016;63(3):330–349.
10. Liddle AM, Hall AP, Arrowsmith J, Smith G. Effect of infiltration with ropivacaine on blood loss during reduction mammoplasty. *Br J Anaesth.* 1998;81:974–975.
11. Gadsden J, Long WJ. Time to analgesia onset and pharmacokinetics after separate and combined administration of liposome bupivacaine and bupivacaine HCl: considerations for clinicians. *Open Orthop J.* 2016;10:94–104.
12. Berde CB, Strichartz GR. Local anesthetics. In: Miller RD, ed. *Miller's Anesthesia.* 8th ed. Philadelphia: Elsevier; 2015:1043.
13. Neal JM, Neal EJ, Weinberg GL. American Society of Regional Anesthesia and Pain Medicine local anesthetic systemic toxicity checklist: 2020 version. *Reg Anesth Pain Med.* 2021;46(1):81. Epub 2020 Nov 4.

REVIEW QUESTIONS

(1) A cachectic 53-year-old female with end-stage renal disease (ESRD), cirrhosis, peripheral vascular disease, and gastroesophageal reflux is scheduled for a right below-the-knee amputation. She was last dialyzed yesterday, and her INR is 1.8. The vascular surgeon asks to you consider a regional anesthetic. What is the most appropriate way to approach this patient?

A. Review the medication administration record, recent laboratory results, obtain consent, place the patient on standard ASA vital sign monitoring, and perform ultrasound guided placement of a perineural catheter with a 20% reduction in the initial bolus of LA.
B. Review the medication administration record, recent laboratory results, obtain consent, place the patient on standard ASA vital sign monitoring, and perform ultrasound guided placement of a perineural catheter without a 20% reduction in the initial bolus of LA.
C. Review the medication administration record, recent laboratory results, obtain consent, place the patient on standard ASA vital sign monitoring, and perform a high concentration and volume anatomy–based peripheral nerve block.
D. Place the patient on standard ASA vital sign monitoring without reviewing the medication administration record or recent laboratory results and perform a peripheral nerve block.

(2) In the same patient (above) a subgluteal sciatic perineural block/catheter and a single shot saphenous nerve block are completed under ultrasound guidance. In addition, at the end of the case the surgeon injects 40 mL of 0.5% bupivacaine, forgetting that the patient has a nerve block. In the post-anesthesia care unit, the patient becomes bradycardic, agitated, and starts slurring her speech. You suspect LAST; assuming the patient's weight is 40 kg, how much volume lipid emulsion should she receive in 30 minutes of resuscitation?

A. ~50 mL
B. ~330 mL
C. ~660 mL
D. ~100 mL

(3) A 21-year-old female G1P0 has been laboring for 15 hours with an L2–3 epidural that has been working well. The decision is made to proceed with an emergent cesarean section after a series of late decelerations. You decide to bolus the epidural with 20cc of 2-chloroprocaine 3%. The patient complains of heartburn and you decide to administer metoclopramide. What is the effect of metoclopramide on 2-chlorprocaine metabolism?

A. Reduced rate of ester metabolism
B. Accelerated rate of ester metabolism
C. No change in ester metabolism
D. 2-chloroprocaine is an amide

(4) All of the following statements are TRUE regarding the addition of epinephrine to local anesthetics (LA) *except*:

A. Addition of epinephrine to LA solutions can slow the rate of absorption and reduce peak plasma levels.
B. Addition of epinephrine to LA may act as a marker for intravascular injection.
C. Addition of epinephrine to LA will not speed up the onset of action.
D. Addition of epinephrine to LA increases the potency of the LA.

(5) When an LA enters a cell, it disrupts Na influx, resulting in:

A. an increased amplitude of the action potential, accelerated rate of depolarization, decreased firing threshold, fast impulse conduction, and shortened refractory period
B. a decreased amplitude of the action potential, faster rate of depolarization, increased firing threshold, fast impulse conduction, prolonged refractory period
C. a decreased amplitude of the action potential, slowed rate of depolarization, increased firing threshold, slow impulse conduction, and prolonged refractory period
D. an increased amplitude of the action potential, slowed rate of depolarization, decreased firing threshold, slow impulse conduction, and shortened refractory period

ANSWERS

(1) **A.** It is important to be systematic in your evaluation of patients prior to a procedure. Review the medication record

to identify medications that will interact with LA and potentially alter the pharmacokinetics and pharmacodynamics. Take care to understand the pathophysiologic processes of various comorbidities and their impacts on LA metabolism. In this case, the patient has ESRD, liver disease, and malnourishment; all of these comorbidities will result in a lower threshold for LA toxicity. It is imperative to reduce the concentration and volume of LA during this block utilizing the lowest effective dose. Moreover, continuous monitoring of the patient during and after the block is necessary for signs of LA toxicity.

References

El-Boghdadly K, Pawa A, Chin KJ. Local anesthetic systemic toxicity: current perspectives. *Local Reg Anesth*. 2018;11:35–44.

Neal JM, et al. ASRA practice advisory on local anesthetic systemic toxicity. *Reg Anesth Pain Med*. 2010;35(2):152–161.

Gitman M, Barrington MJ. Local anesthetic systemic toxicity: a review of recent case reports and registries. *Reg Anesth Pain Med*. 2018;43(2):124–130.

El-Boghdadly K, Chin KJ. Local anesthetic systemic toxicity: continuing professional development. *Can J Anaesth*. 2016;63(3):330–349.

(2) **B.** The patient is <70 kg and will receive a bolus of 1.5 mL/kg lipid emulsion 20% rapidly over 2–3 minutes (60mL assuming 3 min) followed by a continuous infusion at ~0.25 mL/kg/min (270mL assuming 27 min) until the signs and symptoms resolve, which is approximately 330mL. It is important to note that signs and symptoms of LAST can reoccur upon discontinuation of the infusion; therefore vigilance and a high index of suspicion are critical. Also, it is worth noting that patients who are hemodialysis dependent may become fluid overloaded, necessitating hemodialysis after administration.

References

Neal JM, Neal EJ, Weinberg GL. American Society of Regional Anesthesia and Pain Medicine local anesthetic systemic toxicity checklist: 2020 version. *Reg Anesth Pain Med*. 2021;46(1):81. Epub 2020 Nov 4.

Rubin DS, et al. Local anesthetic systemic toxicity in total joint arthroplasty: incidence and risk factors in the United States from the national inpatient sample 1998–2013. *Reg Anesth Pain Med*. 2018;43(2):131–137.

Gitman M, Barrington MJ. Local anesthetic systemic toxicity: a review of recent case reports and registries. *Reg Anesth Pain Med*. 2018;43(2):124–130.

(3) **A.** Ester LA metabolism depends on plasma esterase (pseudocholinesterase/butyryl cholinesterase) activity, which is affected by a number of medications. Metoclopramide has been shown to inhibit plasma esterase activity in vivo. When administering other medications that rely on plasma cholinesterase for metabolism, the physician must be aware that those drugs will have a reduced clearance and subsequently prolonged effect.

References

Lirk P, Picardi S, Hollmann MW. Local anaesthetics: 10 essentials. *Eur J Anaesthesiol*. 2014;31(11):575–585.

El-Boghdadly K, Chin KJ. Local anesthetic systemic toxicity: continuing professional development. *Can J Anaesth*. 2016;63(3):330–349.

(4) **D.** Epinephrine is a potent vasoconstrictor and will slow the rate of absorption and reduce peak plasma levels of LA by as much as 50% depending on the site of injection. If there is intravascular injection, tachycardia will be seen. Epinephrine prolongs but does not speed up the onset of local anesthetics; this property is attributed to concentration (greater concentration will have a quicker onset) and pKa of the LA relative to the pH of the tissue (addition of $NaHCO_3$ alkalinizes the tissue environment, creating more unionized LA molecules which can enter the cell with greater speed). Potency of an LA is related to its lipophilicity.

Reference

Bailard NS, Ortiz J, Flores RA. Additives to local anesthetics for peripheral nerve blocks: evidence, limitations, and recommendations. *Am J Health Syst Pharm*. 2014;71(5):373–385.

(5) **C.** When an LA enters the cell and binds to the Na channel, it has inhibitory effects on the cell. The best way to think about this is that LAs act to slow/numb the cell, so choose the answer which will slow the action potential the most.

References

Heavner JE. Local anesthetics. *Curr Opin Anaesthesiol*. 2007;20(4):336–342.

Lirk P, Picardi S, Hollmann MW. Local anaesthetics: 10 essentials. *Eur J Anaesthesiol*. 2014;31(11):575–585.

7.

PROLONGING NERVE BLOCKS

Brenton Alexander and Rodney Gabriel

STEM CASE AND KEY QUESTIONS

While working in a small private practice anesthesiology group, you have an otherwise healthy patient arrive following a motor vehicle accident resulting in a right lower extremity injury. Diagnostic imaging confirms a right-sided type 4 calcaneal fracture (highly comminuted), requiring surgery. Discussion with the surgical team concludes that the patient is likely to experience severe pain for at least the first 3–5 days postoperatively.

(1) WHAT OPTIONS DO YOU HAVE FOR PHARMACOLOGIC-ONLY PERIOPERATIVE PAIN CONTROL FOR THIS PATIENT?

In order to decrease preoperative, intraoperative, and postoperative pain for this patient, a well-trained anesthesia provider can offer a variety of options. Multimodal pain control is becoming increasingly popular for the perioperative period and consists of a combination of intravenous and parenteral acetaminophen/paracetamol, nonsteroidal anti-inflammatory (NSAID) (both COX-2 selective and COX-2 non-selective), gabapentin/pregabalin, topical local anesthetic (LA) patches, neuraxial opioids, regional anesthesia, and opioids. A well-organized perioperative pain strategy should be a priority for all anesthesiology departments. This can be part of an enhanced recovery after surgery (ERAS) or a perioperative surgical home (PSH) program, or can be developed independently.

(2) WHAT REGIONAL ANESTHETIC OPTIONS DO YOU HAVE TO OPTIMIZE POSTOPERATIVE PAIN MANAGEMENT FOR THIS PATIENT?

The location of this patient's injury and pain is within the distribution of the sciatic nerve, which divides into the tibial and common peroneal nerves most commonly 5–10 cm above the popliteal crease, plus a small potential area of saphenous innervation. There are many approaches to block the sciatic nerve, ranging from a single perineural injection for surgical coverage to the placement of a perineural catheter (PNC) infusing LA for up to 10 days postoperatively (or even longer depending on resources and hospital guidelines). There is a wide variety of LAs, adjuvants, and combinations that can modify the duration of clinical analgesia. At present, the only method proven to consistently provide reliable pain control beyond 48 hours after the initial injection is a continuous (or/and intermittent) LA infusion via PNC.

(3) WHAT ARE COMMON CHALLENGES PRECLUDING MORE UNIVERSAL USE OF CONTINUOUS NERVE BLOCKS? WHAT IF A PERIOPERATIVE PERINEURAL CATHETER IS NOT AN OPTION?

Unfortunately, placing a PNC requires significant attention and management effort postoperatively, which may also be insufficiently reimbursed. If one does not practice in an environment where this technique is incentivized and/or supported, it makes it quite challenging to justify the extra work and medico-legal risk of leaving a device within a patient's body with limited follow-up abilities. Until perioperative systems are adjusted to prioritize patient comfort and opioid avoidance, alternative options have to be explored. There is a wide variety of LA additives that can *potentially* increase the duration of sensory blockade and/or analgesia when PNCs are either not possible or not justified.

(4) WHEN TRYING TO INCREASE THE DURATION OF NERVE BLOCKADE VIA PERINEURAL LA ADDITIVES, WHAT ARE YOUR OPTIONS?

The most commonly investigated and clinically used additives include epinephrine, dexamethasone, buprenorphine, magnesium, clonidine, dexmedetomidine, tramadol, and most recently, liposomal bupivacaine.

(5) WHICH LA ADDITIVES HAVE PROVEN MOST CONSISTENT AND RELIABLE IN EXTENDING SENSORY BLOCKADE AND ANALGESIA DURATION?

The additives with the strongest clinical data to support their use are epinephrine, dexamethasone, and buprenorphine. The others have more limited data and require significantly more clinical research at this time to justify the risks of using a non-FDA approved substance perineurally. Ultimately, as this patient underwent surgery at a facility where PNCs were not available, a single-injection popliteal sciatic nerve block was performed using 30 cc of bupivacaine 0.5% + 5mcg/ml epinephrine + 4mg dexamethasone, resulting in 30 hours of postoperative analgesia.

(6) WHAT ARE POTENTIAL RISKS AND LIMITING FACTORS THAT NEED TO BE ADDRESSED BEFORE INSERTING AN OUTPATIENT PERIPHERAL NERVE CATHETER?

Inserting a PNC is not particularly challenging once the skill set is learned and practiced, but the difficult and time-consuming task is to ensure that these patients have appropriate follow-up. Daily communication is required to answer any questions patients may have and address any issues that have arisen, including daily checks for redness or exudate, as these are common signs of infection. A 24-hour hotline is helpful as well in order to avoid emergency room visits for small and easily addressed concerns. Patients need to be made aware of the common risks resulting from insertion of a PNC, which include infection, nerve damage, local anesthetic toxicity, displacement, and difficult removal. Removing the catheter at home is simple, and patients should be given instructions prior to discharge. Telemedicine platforms might also offer new opportunities for enhanced follow-up.

DISCUSSION

While this chapter will focus on just one feature of a multitude of relevant variables considered when choosing which LA and additives to use for extending block duration, it is important to understand that other characteristics are just as important when making this clinical decision. Time to onset, potential toxicity, and sensory versus motor blockade should be understood and considered.

PNCs constitute a well-established, well-studied, and well-understood approach for prolonging nerve blockade.[1] As PNCs are rarely used for less than 2 days, and even the most effective single shot LA +/− additive combination provides less than 30 hours of *reliable* nerve blockade, it should be noted that these two techniques are simply part of any regionalist's tool belt and can hardly compete when considering extending block duration.

When covering the topic of prolonging nerve blocks, it is important to first describe the established evidence for the expected duration of anesthesia and analgesia using the most common LAs *without* additives. The distinction between anesthesia and analgesia is significant and should be well understood by the regionalist. Surgical (regional) anesthesia typically refers to a degree of nerve blockade that allows for surgical procedures to be performed without the concurrent use of general anesthesia or any other significant doses of potent analgesics such as high-dose opioids or ketamine. Analgesia is used to describe any degree of nerve blockade that provides pain relief for the patient. The duration of analgesia is always longer than surgical anesthesia provided by equivalent nerve blockade. Table 7.1 summarizes the expected duration of anesthesia and analgesia for the most commonly used LAs in the United States.

The duration of effect of plain LAs depends on multiple pharmacologic and anatomic factors. Pharmacologically, expected average block duration depends on the LA used (Table 7.1). In the United States, most peripheral and neuraxial nerve blocks are performed using one of 4 medications: lidocaine, mepivacaine, bupivacaine, and ropivacaine. Lidocaine and mepivacaine are commonly known to have short to moderate duration of action, while bupivacaine and ropivacaine have a long duration of action. The pharmacologic characteristic that most likely affects the duration of nerve blockade to the greatest extent is the lipid solubility,[2] while concentration, vascular effects, protein binding, drug metabolism, tissue characteristics, and injection site all play important roles.[3] All of these characteristics have varying degrees of impact on duration of LA effect based on the specific clinical situation and environment, making research into the individual role of each component essential.[4]

When examining the pharmacodynamic and pharmacokinetic characteristics of the commonly used LA additives, it is apparent that their specific neural mechanisms of action in enhancing and prolonging sensory blockade and/or analgesia are insufficiently understood. It is important to also note that at the time of writing this chapter, FDA approval is lacking

Table 7.1 LOCAL ANESTHETICS COMMONLY USED IN THE UNITED STATES

LOCAL ANESTHETIC	DURATION OF ANESTHESIA* (HOURS)	DURATION OF ANALGESIA* (HOURS)	MAXIMUM DOSE* (MG/KG) WITHOUT/WITH EPI
2% lidocaine	2–5	3–7	4.5/7
1.5% mepivacaine	2–5	3–9	5/7
0.25% bupivacaine	2–5	5–24	2.5/3
0.5% bupivacaine	5–15	6–30	2.5/3
0.2% ropivacaine	Incomplete	4–14	3/3.5
0.5% ropivacaine	4–12	5–25	3/3.5

*Very dependent on the location of injection.

for all potential perineural additives (and limited approval for liposomal bupivacaine). This creates significant concerns for discussions of benefits, risk, and medico-legal issues for both patients and physicians.[5]

INDIVIDUAL ADDITIVES

EPINEPHRINE

Epinephrine was one of the first adjuvants used for nerve blocks and is thought to exert its effect by decreasing vascular absorption of LA via perineural alpha 1-mediated vasoconstriction. Multiple studies have demonstrated lower plasma concentrations of LA when co-administered with epinephrine as compared to without.[6,7] This is in addition to both its prominent function as an early warning for intravascular injection and also allowing for increases in the maximum allowable dose for commonly used LAs (Table 7.1). It is important to note that increasing the maximum allowable dose will indeed increase the duration of nerve blockade if this increase leads to additional anesthetic being injected perineurally.

It has also been demonstrated that epinephrine combined with short-acting LAs does increase the duration of nerve blockade.[8–10] The increases of anesthesia and analgesia when using epinephrine have been highly variable. One study from 1965 demonstrated that the addition of epinephrine doubles the duration of action of prilocaine and quadrupled the duration of action of lidocaine for ulnar nerve blockade.[11] Another study from 1970 found a very significant effect of epinephrine on skin wheal anesthesia using bupivacaine, although the same study found a large difference in hospital versus commercial preparations.[12] A more recent study by Dogru et al. indicates much smaller, but statistically significant, increases in axillary block duration when lidocaine 1.5% is used in combination with epinephrine.[8] That being said, there is significantly less data to support the idea that epinephrine can increase the duration of long-acting LAs with commonly used doses of epinephrine (2.5 mcg/cc–5 mcg/cc). In addition to the ropivacaine package insert denying any duration effects of epinephrine,[13] one study comparing ropivacaine with and without epinephrine (5 mcg/cc) for a femoral nerve block found no difference in duration of anesthesia between groups.[14] When examining bupivacaine, there is "inconsistent" evidence to support the use of epinephrine for increasing the duration of action, although the clinical significance may be limited.[3]

Although it has been used for over 100 years,[15] epinephrine as an LA adjuvant does not come without its own risks. An older study utilizing rat models indicated that epinephrine alone and when combined with lidocaine decreases neural blood flow more than saline or lidocaine without additives.[16] These data, combined with additional diabetic animal experimentation and the accepted susceptibility of diabetics to nerve damage, have resulted in some experts determining that avoiding epinephrine additives in diabetic patients requiring nerve blockade is justified.[17–19] Additionally, even small amounts of epinephrine injected intravascularly can have a stimulating hemodynamic effect, which may not be tolerated well by patients at risk for cardiac ischemia or arrythmias.

In summary, epinephrine is a useful addition to LA for detecting intravascular injection and increasing the maximum dose of short- to moderate-acting LAs, but shows somewhat limited evidence for significantly increasing the duration of nerve blockade, especially when combined with some long-acting LAs such as ropivacaine. Additionally, care should be taken when adding epinephrine to LAs for diabetic patients, as some evidence indicates increased potential for nerve damage.

DEXAMETHASONE

One of the promising LA additives extensively explored in the past 15 years is the glucocorticoid dexamethasone. Glucocorticoids exhibit anti-inflammatory, antiemetic, analgesic, and immunosuppressive effects systemically. The mechanism behind the dexamethasone extending nerve blockade is not completely understood but may be related to local or systemic effects.[20,21] Local action may be related to a wide variety of mechanisms, including vasoconstriction[22,23] or C-fiber nerve transmission inhibition.[24] When examining the potential for harming the peripheral nerve, there are very limited data indicating that dexamethasone (or its preservatives) and other glucocorticoids may decrease directly blood flow or cause other direct nerve injury.[23,25–28] This is in contrast with the overwhelming safety data, both clinical and basic science, indicating that perineural dexamethasone has no negative effects directly on nerves or systemically from local absorption.[29] Unfortunately, it should be mentioned that most of these studies are underpowered to detect a statistical difference in complication rate (already exceedingly rare) and most lack longer, more relevant follow-up periods.

In regard to the duration of motor, sensory, and analgesic blockade, the literature is fairly consistent. Adding a moderate dose (2–8 mg) of dexamethasone to LAs can increase nerve blockade anywhere from 5 to 8 hours (average 6.7) depending on the type of anesthetic used and location of injection.[29–31] Importantly, postoperative pain scores (12–24 hours postoperatively) and opioid requirements were also significantly lower in the perineural dexamethasone group when compared to placebo.[29] There have been some data to suggest that adding dexamethasone also decreased time to onset of peripheral nerve blockade, although the clinical significance of this is much more difficult to evaluate.[31–33] Another important caveat discovered and explored in recent years is that systemic administration (intravenous, intramuscular, or subcutaneous [IV, IM, SQ]) of dexamethasone also significantly increases the duration of nerve blockade, although possibly not to the same degree as perineural administration.[20,29,34] The most recent meta-analysis noted that duration of sensory block in the perineural dexamethasone group was significantly longer than intravenous group by 3.14 hours, although the difference in pain intensity at 12–24 hours did not reach significance.[29]

In regard to dosing of perineural dexamethasone, there have been two studies finding no difference between 4 mg and 8 mg.[29,30] One recent study did find a dose-dependent increase in efficacy of perineural dexamethasone when comparing lower doses of 1–4 mg, with 4 mg producing significantly longer duration of blockade than any lower dose.[35] Combining these two resources (although the former has much more significant data) would result in 4 mg being the logical starting dose of perineural dexamethasone.

Another important feature studied is the effect of dexamethasone on motor blockade, compared to that on sensory block and analgesia. In a meta-analysis, an approximate 5-hour increase in motor blockade with the addition of dexamethasone was demonstrated, which can significantly affect postoperative rehabilitation and potential fall risk.[31] This meta-analysis also found that adding dexamethasone to peripheral nerve blockade decreases the risk of postoperative nausea and vomiting (PONV) when compared to placebo.[31]

Lastly, caution should be exercised when choosing a preservative-free formulation of dexamethasone for perineural injection as the majority of commercially available dexamethasone vials contain preservatives with unknown potential for neurotoxicity.

Overall, perineural dexamethasone appears to be one of the promising and widely used LA adjuvants for increasing the length of nerve blockade with a relatively benign side effect profile, although safety and IV equivalency must be investigated further.

BUPRENORPHINE

Buprenorphine is classically described as a lipophilic μ-opioid receptor agonist that also has some κ-opioid receptor activity.[36] The peripheral neural activity is hypothesized to be primarily mediated by both μ-opioid receptors on C-fibers and neuronal sodium channels in a concentration-dependent manner.[37,38] This combination of opioid and LA properties has made it attractive as a perineural nerve block additive to LAs.

A recent meta-analysis on the use of buprenorphine within peripheral nerve blocks published in 2017 by Schnabel et al.[39] provides convincing evidence for the clinical effects of buprenorphine as a peripheral nerve block adjuvant. It includes 13 randomized controlled trials (RCTs) which total 685 patients. When compared with LA alone, the combination of LA and buprenorphine increased the average duration of analgesia by 8.64 hours (95% CI 6.44–10.85), while also decreasing average pain scores from 2 hours through 48 hours postoperatively.[39] Interestingly, the duration of motor blockade was only increased by 12 minutes (which is advantageous when compared to the 5-hour increase produced by dexamethasone). Importantly, PONV was increased 5-fold in the buprenorphine group, while no other side effect reached statistical significance, although pruritus trended strongly toward it.

A study by Seering et al. compared recently interscalene nerve block for shoulder surgery with either ropivacaine alone, ropivacaine with buprenorphine 300 mcg, ropivacaine with 8 mg dexamethasone, or ropivacaine with clonidine 75 mcg.[40] The results indicated a strong trend toward a significantly longer block for the dexamethasone group, although there was no statistically significant difference between the groups in median duration of analgesia.

As with dexamethasone, comparing perineural to intramuscular buprenorphine is an important experiment to establish the relative roles of systemic versus localized mechanisms of action. This approach was taken by 5 RCTs included in the 2017 meta-analysis.[39] Nerve blocks performed with LA plus (perineural) buprenorphine resulted in a 6.87-hour increase in duration of analgesia compared to plain LA blocks plus intramuscular buprenorphine. Additional studies have also concluded that perineural buprenorphine increases the time to first opioid administration and/or the time to first report of pain by a significant amount (6–10 hours).[41,42]

Overall, although it significantly increases the risk of PONV, perineural buprenorphine prolongs analgesia by a statistically significant and clinically relevant amount.

MAGNESIUM

When compared to other LA additives, magnesium has limited data supporting its modern clinical use. Known systemic mechanisms of action include N-methyl-D-aspartate (NMDA) antagonism and neuronal calcium influx modulation, while the effects on peripheral nerves is not definitively understood.[43] A recent meta-analysis on perineural magnesium demonstrates a moderate increase in duration of sensory block in combination with bupivacaine, ropivacaine, and lidocaine (108, 166, 44 minutes, respectively).[44] These increases in duration might not be judged to be clinically significant enough to justify the time spent in preparing the mixture and also the increased risk acquired by using a drug "off-label." Additionally, the studies used in this meta-analysis did have a high level of heterogeneity and likely suffer from positive reporting bias.

Importantly, no recent studies on this topic reported any clinical adverse effects of adding magnesium to perineural LA, although more studies are warranted as there are very limited basic science data on associated neurotoxicity.[45] Intravenous magnesium has been widely used and has better studied and understood mechanisms of action and side-effect profile, when compared to perineural administration. Therefore, a logical requirement for perineural administration would be to prove first that perineural administration is superior to systemic administration, especially as intravenous magnesium is known to decrease pain and analgesic requirements.[46]

Overall, magnesium may hold promise as an effective perineural adjuvant; however, comprehensive studies comparing analgesic effects between systemic and perineural routes of administration, as well as their safety profiles, are still to be conducted, published, and analyzed before widespread use can be recommended.

CLONIDINE

The mechanism of action of systemic clonidine via α-2 selective adrenergic agonism is well established and also is the proposed mechanism for epidural and intrathecal analgesia.[47,48] Clonidine is also thought to act perineurally via hyperpolarization of cation currents.[49] A meta-analysis on the effects of clonidine in peripheral nerve blockade reported that doses from 30 to 300 μg prolong nerve blockade for both intermediate and long-acting LAs by approximately 1.5 to 2 hours.[50] The same increase in duration was found for motor blockade. Importantly, when compared to LA alone, there were increases in episodes of hypotension (4.1% vs. 13.1%), bradycardia (4.1% vs. 8.5%), fainting (2.9% vs. 12.9%), and sedation (32.4% vs. 55.8%) with perineural clonidine. Among the analyzed studies, there were only two that directly compared the effects of systemic vs. perineural clonidine, yielding mixed findings.

Since this large meta-analysis, more studies with mixed results have been published. Multiple studies indicate increased peripheral nerve block duration with combined clonidine and long-acting LAs.[51–54] However, there have also been many studies of variable quality indicating no increase in nerve block duration with perineural clonidine use.[55,56] These mixed results, together with the known hemodynamic and neurologic side effects, and possible nerve block extension of only 2 hours, make it hard to justify the wide use of clonidine as an additive to LAs for peripheral nerve blockade. Future high-quality research is needed to establish a clear clinical benefit-to-risk ratio.

DEXMEDETOMIDINE

Similar to clonidine, dexmedetomidine is an α-2 selective adrenergic agonist with 7 times higher α-2/α-1 affinity.[57] As with clonidine, the presumed peripheral mechanism of action is via hyperpolarization of cation currents.[58] Two large recent meta-analyses address the efficacy of dexmedetomidine as an additive to perineural LA for prolonging nerve blockade.[59,60] The overarching conclusion among these meta-analyses is that the addition of dexmedetomidine to long-acting LAs will prolong the duration of sensory anesthesia by 230 minutes[60] and the duration of analgesia by either 264 minutes[60] or 292 minutes.[59] This result is consistent with the results in a newer volunteer study.[61]

There are important caveats that must be considered along with these positive results. Importantly, what is the systemic versus local effect of perineural dexmedetomidine? An answer to this question is offered by one of the two large recent meta-analyses by Schnabel et al.[59] They found that among all studies actually comparing the two, there was no statistical difference in peripheral nerve blockade duration between perineural versus intravenous dexmedetomidine administration. The average difference was approximately 1 hour, favoring the perineural group, but falling just short of reaching statistical significance. Although perineural dexmedetomidine has been shown to have very low risk of neural injury,[62,63] if systemic administration is as efficacious as perineural administration, it would be hard to justify wide perineural use as effects are much better known with intravenous administration.

The other major caveat to be understood before considering dexmedetomidine as a perineural adjuvant is the hemodynamic side-effect profile. Both large meta-analyses documented a statistically higher incidence in bradycardia and hypotension when compared to plain LA blocks. Bradycardia in the dexmedetomidine groups had relative risks of 2.8[59] and 3.3,[60] while hypotension had relative risks of 3.4[59] and 5.4.[60] This should be carefully weighed before deciding to administer perineural dexmedetomidine in patients with significant relevant comorbidities.

Other notable effects of perineural dexmedetomidine include a decrease in onset time for sensory (40% faster) and motor (39% faster) blockade.[60] This meta-analysis also found that perineural dexmedetomidine reduced PONV, reduced postoperative oral opioid consumption by 10.2 mg oral morphine equivalents (OME), improved pain control, and increased patient satisfaction.[60] Unfortunately, most of the included studies did not include these conclusions as primary, properly powered outcomes. The dosing of perineural dexmedetomidine is rarely standardized among different study protocols, but Vorobeichik et al. did note that a perineural dose of 50–60 μg maximized sensory blockade while minimizing hemodynamics adverse events.[60]

In summary, there exists reliable published evidence indicating that perineural dexmedetomidine significantly prolongs nerve block duration (although much less so when compared with intravenous administration) and is also associated with predictable hemodynamic side effects.

TRAMADOL

Tramadol is a centrally acting weak μ-opioid receptor analgesic that is commonly used for pain control. It is also unique in exhibiting serotonin and norepinephrine reuptake inhibition, α-2 agonism, and potassium channel blockade.[64,65] When added to LA for peripheral nerve blockade, the results have been mixed and inconsistent. A recent article on the effects of perineural tramadol on brachial plexus blockade was published in 2017 by Shin et al.[65] Although they noted high heterogeneity, it was shown that sensory blockade was prolonged by 61.5 minutes with 100 mg of perineural tramadol. Likewise, analgesia was prolonged by 125.5 minutes and motor blockade was extended by 65.6 minutes, both with high heterogeneity. Lower doses of 50 mg were ineffective, and no comparison to systemic tramadol was performed. One study has examined the effects of systemic versus perineural tramadol for supraclavicular brachial plexus block in combination with bupivacaine; both sensory block and analgesia were prolonged by approximately 60 minutes adding tramadol 100 mg perineurally.[66]

Other considerations include the side-effect profile, although no significant difference was found in key recent studies.[65,67] Unfortunately, there is minimal reliable data examining the effects of tramadol in combination with different LAs, such as short- versus long-acting. Overall, there is still a need for more basic and clinical research, before the wide clinical use of perineural tramadol can be recommended.

LIPOSOMAL BUPIVACAINE

In 2011, liposome bupivacaine was approved by the US Food and Drug Administration for use in surgical site infiltration and transversus abdominis plane blocks for the purposes of postoperative analgesia. A few years later, the drug was approved for use in interscalene blocks for major shoulder surgery. Encasing bupivacaine in liposomes allows for delivery of the medication to be prolonged over a period of multiple days with the theoretical benefit over unencapsulated bupivacaine of providing a much longer duration of analgesia with just one single injection. The advantage over continuous catheter-based perineural blocks is that it would not require *in situ* placement of a catheter or need of an external pump and medication reservoir. The first studies of liposome bupivacaine demonstrated its superiority over placebo when used in surgical-site infiltration for bunionectomy and hemorrhoidectomy.[68,69] Golf et al. conducted a randomized, double-blind phase 3 clinical trial in which patients undergoing bunionectomy received either liposome bupivacaine or placebo via wound infiltration.[68] The results demonstrated that liposome bupivacaine reduced pain scores for up to 36 hours after surgery. Gorfine et al. conducted a multicenter randomized controlled phase 3 trial comparing liposome bupivacaine versus placebo for wound infiltration following hemorrhoidectomy.[69] Their results demonstrated that when compared to placebo, liposome bupivacaine reduced opioid requirements at 72 hours postoperatively.

Following these initial placebo studies, multiple RCTs have now been published comparing liposome bupivacaine versus unencapsulated bupivacaine for surgical site infiltration. Surgical populations studied include breast surgery,[70,71] hemorrhoidectomy,[72] gynecological surgery,[73] urologic surgery,[74] plastic surgery,[75] and knee arthroplasty.[76] As demonstrated in a recent exhaustive review on the topic, there is sparse high-quality evidence from these RCTs that liposome bupivacaine when used for surgical-site infiltration is superior to standard bupivacaine.[77] More well-designed studies are needed to demonstrate liposome bupivacaine's superiority over cheaper traditional LAs, especially when LAs are mixed with commonly used additives for surgical-site infiltration analgesia.

Similar to the evidence for surgical-site infiltration, the results for liposome bupivacaine when used in peripheral nerve blocks have been mixed and inconclusive.[78–81] When mixed with standard bupivacaine for interscalene nerve blocks, liposome bupivacaine reduced worst pain scores during the first postoperative week following major shoulder surgery.[80] Two prospective RCTs reported improved pain scores and opioid requirements during the first 72 hours when used in transversus abdominis plane blocks in patients undergoing robot-assisted hysterectomy and laparoscopic hand-assisted donor nephrectomy.[78,79] More recently, a large-scale review and meta-analysis examining the evidence for the safety and effectiveness of liposomal bupivacaine in peripheral nerve blocks was completed and found that there was no benefit when compared to non-liposomal bupivacaine.[81] Once again, concrete evidence is lacking to justify the large-scale incorporation of liposomal bupivacaine into a modern regional practice. Future high-quality RCTs are needed to justify the increased cost of liposome bupivacaine when used in peripheral nerve blocks.

OTHER ADDITIVES

Historically and more recently, there has been a wide variety of other additives to LAs explored with the hope of prolonging sensory nerve blockade without adverse side effects. Some studies have yielded negative results or have raised neurotoxicity concerns, but many trials could have been better designed and conducted with more standardization, perineural safety information, and minimization of interpretation and publishing bias. Therefore, drugs such as midazolam, ketamine, fentanyl, morphine, and neostigmine cannot be recommended as perineural additives at this time. Extensive and convincing basic and clinical research is needed in order to consider incorporating the use of new LA adjuvants with clear clinical benefits and proven safety into daily practice.

PERIPHERAL NERVE CATHETERS

Although this chapter focuses on pharmacologic additives and liposomal bupivacaine for extending the duration of single-injection peripheral nerve blocks, the concept of continuous indwelling PNCs deserves a brief mention. As discussed above, the only reliable way to block a peripheral nerve beyond 24 hours is the use of repeated single injections or the insertion of a PNC attached to a continuous or intermittent bolus LA system. Appropriate safety precautions and follow-up must be a priority for any provider placing a PNC, as complications can occur with an indwelling catheter in place and after it has been removed. Appropriate sterility and strong dressings will help to decrease the risk of infection and dislodgement. Patient education and frequent contact are vital for any successful inpatient or outpatient PNC system.[1]

While traditionally placed using peripheral nerve stimulation techniques, the anesthesia community has largely transitioned to using ultrasound navigation for placement. [1] The type of LA solution used and continuous versus intermittent bolus is highly variable and an area of active research.[1] The current and future role of indwelling PNC systems is likely to change with new—potentially longer acting—pharmaceutical options, although reliable pain management beyond 24–48 hours is still only available with PNC systems.

CONCLUSIONS

- When continuous perineural catheters are not possible (for a variety of clinical, economic, and logistic reasons), certain LA additives have been used to prolong the duration of sensory blockade and/or analgesia
- To date, many of the described LA additives are not supported by well-designed basic and clinical studies, with limited proven benefit and safety to justify their use.
- Out of the many available choices, epinephrine, dexamethasone, and buprenorphine demonstrate consistent increase in analgesia duration; dexmedetomidine, clonidine, buprenorphine, and tramadol are also widely used, with their effects on block duration described as less significant.

Drug-specific side effects related to LA additives are predictable and must be reckoned with.

- Liposomal bupivacaine extends block duration further and is under continuing investigation for a variety of block techniques and surgeries, although there is very limited current evidence to justify the increased cost of this medication, with many relevant studies pending
- Most of the LA additives described in the literature require further investigations under rigorous standardized experimental and clinical trials.

REFERENCES

1. Ilfeld BM, Mariano ER. Continuous peripheral nerve blocks. *Essentials Pain Med.* Published online 2018:135–140. e2.
2. Bokesch PM, Post C, Strichartz G. Structure-activity relationship of lidocaine homologs producing tonic and frequency-dependent impulse blockade in nerve. *J Pharmacol Exp Ther.* 1986;237(3):773–781.
3. Barash PG, Cullen BF, Stoelting RK, Cahalan MK, Stock MC, Ortega R. *Clinical Anesthesia.* 7th ed. Philadelphia: Wolters Kluwer Health; 2013. Accessed September 30, 2020. https://www.scholars.northwestern.edu/en/publications/clinical-anesthesia-seventh-edition-3.
4. Miller R, Pardo M Jr. *Basics of Anesthesia.* 7th ed. Philadelphia: Elsevier; 2017.
5. Singh S, Bansal P, Dureja J. Off-label use of drugs in regional anesthesia: a need for setting up policies. *J Anaesthesiol Clin Pharmacol.* 2017;33(4):448–449.
6. Braid DP, Scott DB. Effect of adrenaline on the systemic absorption of local anaesthetic drugs. *Acta Anaesthesiol Scand.* 1966;10:334–346.
7. Schierup L, Schmidt JF, Torp Jensen A, Rye BAO. Pudendal block in vaginal deliveries mepivacaine with and without epinephrine. *Acta Obstet Gynecol Scand.* 1988;67(3):195–197.
8. Dogru K, Duygulu F, Yildiz K, Kotanoglu MS, Madenoglu H, Boyaci A. Hemodynamic and blockade effects of high/low epinephrine doses during axillary brachial plexus blockade with lidocaine 1.5%. *Reg Anesth Pain Med.* 2003;28(5):401–405.
9. Song J-H, Shim HY, Lee TJ, et al. Comparison of dexmedetomidine and epinephrine as an adjuvant to 1% mepivacaine in brachial plexus block. *Korean J Anesth.* 2014;66(4):283–289.
10. Bernards CM, Kopacz DJ. Effect of epinephrine on lidocaine clearance in vivo: a microdialysis study in humans. *Anesthesiology.* 1999;91(4):962–968.
11. Albért J, Löfström B. Bilateral ulnar nerve blocks for the evaluation of local anesthetic agents. 3. Tests with a new agent, prilocaine, and with lidocaine in solutions with and without epinephrine. *Acta Anaesthesiol Scand.* 1965;9(4):203–211.
12. Swerdlow M, Jones R. The duration of action of bupivacaine, prilocaine and lignocaine. *Br J Anaesth.* 1970;42(4):335–339.
13. Naropin® (ropivacaine HCl) package insert. Fresenius Kabi. Updated November 2018. Accessed February 19, 2021. https://www.accessdata.fda.gov/drugsatfda_docs/label/2018/020533s035lbl.pdf.
14. Weber A, Fournier R, Van Gessel E, Riand N, Gamulin Z. Epinephrine does not prolong the analgesia of 20 ml ropivacaine 0.5% or 0.2% in a femoral {three-in-one} block. *Anesth Analg.* 2001;93(5):1327–1331.
15. Nicoladoni C. Ueber die Bedeutung des Musculus Tibialis posticus und der Sohlenmuskeln für den Plattfuss. *Dtsch Zeitschrift für Chir.* 1902;67(1):348–353.
16. Myers RR, Heckman HM. Effects of local anesthesia on nerve blood flow: studies using lidocaine with and without epinephrine. *Anesthesiology.* 1989;71(5):757–762.
17. Williams BA, Murinson BB, Grable BR, Orebaugh SL. Future considerations for pharmacologic adjuvants in single-injection peripheral nerve blocks for patients with diabetes mellitus. *Reg Anesth Pain Med.* 2009;34(5):445–457.
18. Kroin JS, Buvanendran A, Williams DK, et al. Local anesthetic sciatic nerve block and nerve fiber damage in diabetic rats. *Reg Anesth Pain Med.* 2010;35(4):343–350.
19. Neal JM. Effects of epinephrine in local anesthetics on the central and peripheral nervous systems: Neurotoxicity and neural blood flow. *Reg Anesth Pain Med.* 2003;28(2):124–134.
20. Baeriswyl M, Kirkham KR, Jacot-Guillarmod A, Albrecht E. Efficacy of perineural vs systemic dexamethasone to prolong analgesia after peripheral nerve block: a systematic review and meta-analysis. *Br J Anaesth.* 2017;119(2):183–191.
21. Fanzca MJF, Fredrickson MJ, FANZCA, Danesh-Clough TK, White R. Adjuvant dexamethasone for bupivacaine sciatic and ankle blocks. *Reg Anesth Pain Med.* 2013;38(4):300–307.
22. Wang P-H, Tsai C-L, Lee J-S, Wu K-C, Cheng K-I, Jou I-M. Effects of topical corticosteroids on the sciatic nerve: an experimental study to adduce the safety in treating carpal tunnel syndrome. *J Hand Surg Eur Vol.* 2011;36(3):236–243.
23. Shishido H, Kikuchi S, Heckman H, Myers RR. Dexamethasone decreases blood flow in normal nerves and dorsal root ganglia. *Spine (Phila Pa 1976).* 2002;27(6):581–586.
24. Johansson A, Hao J, Sjölund B. Local corticosteroid application blocks transmission in normal nociceptive C-fibres. *Acta Anaesthesiol Scand.* 1990;34(5):335–338.
25. Hewson D, Bedforth N, McCartney C, Hardman J. Dexamethasone and peripheral nerve blocks: back to basic (science). *Br J Anaesth.* 2019;122(4):411–412.
26. Williams BA, Hough KA, Tsui BYK, Ibinson JW, Gold MS, Gebhart GF. Neurotoxicity of adjuvants used in perineural anesthesia and analgesia in comparison with ropivacaine. *Reg Anesth Pain Med.* 2011;36(3):225–230.
27. Ma R, Wang X, Lu C, et al. Dexamethasone attenuated bupivacaine-induced neuron injury in vitro through a threonine-serine protein kinase B-dependent mechanism. *Neuroscience.* 2010;167(2):329–342.
28. Dani C, Vestri V, Bertini G, Pratesi S, Rubaltelli FF. Toxicity of corticosteroids and catecholamines for mice neuronal cell cultures: role of preservatives. *J Matern Neonatal Med.* 2007;20(4):325–333.
29. Pehora C, Pearson AM, Kaushal A, Crawford MW, Johnston B. Dexamethasone as an adjuvant to peripheral nerve block. *Cochrane Database Syst Rev.* 2017;11:CD011770.
30. Albrecht E, Kern C, Kirkham KR. A systematic review and meta-analysis of perineural dexamethasone for peripheral nerve blocks. *Anaesthesia.* 2015;70(1):71–83.
31. Albrecht E, Reynvoet M, Fournier N, et al. Combination of dexamethasone and local anaesthetic solution in peripheral nerve blocks: a meta-analysis of randomised controlled trials. *Anesthesiology.* 2018;78(6):1001–1008.
32. Shrestha BR, Maharjan SK, Tabedar S. Supraclavicular brachial plexus block with and without dexamethasone: a comparative study. *Kathmandu Univ Med J.* 2003;1(3):158–160.
33. Yadav RK, Sah BP, Kumar P, Singh SN. Effectiveness of addition of neostigmine or dexamethasone to local anaesthetic in providing perioperative analgesia for brachial plexus block: a prospective, randomized, double blinded, controlled study. *Kathmandu Univ Med J.* 2008;6(23):302–309.
34. Desmet M, Braems H, Reynvoet M, et al. I.V. and perineural dexamethasone are equivalent in increasing the analgesic duration of a single-shot interscalene block with ropivacaine for shoulder surgery: a prospective, randomized, placebo-controlled study. *Br J Anaesth.* 2013;111(3):445–452.
35. Albrecht E, Reynvoet M, Fournier N, Desmet M. Dose–response relationship of perineural dexamethasone for interscalene brachial plexus block: a randomised, controlled, triple-blind trial. *Anaesthesia.* 2019;74(8):1001–1008. doi: 10.1111/anae.14650.
36. Kosel J, Bobik P, Tomczyk M. Buprenorphine: the unique opioid adjuvant in regional anesthesia. *Expert Rev Clin Pharmacol.* 2016;9(3):375–383.

37. Mambretti EM, Kistner K, Mayer S, et al. Functional and structural characterization of axonal opioid receptors as targets for analgesia. *Mol Pain*. 2016;12:1744806916628734.
38. Leffler A, Frank G, Kistner K, et al. Local anesthetic-like inhibition of voltage-gated Na(+) channels by the partial μ-opioid receptor agonist buprenorphine. *Anesthesiology*. 2012;116(6):1335–1346.
39. Schnabel A, Reichl SU, Zahn PK, Pogatzki-Zahn EM, Meyer-Frießem CH. Efficacy and safety of buprenorphine in peripheral nerve blocks. *Eur J Anaesthesiol*. 2017;34(9):576–586.
40. Seering MS, Bayman EO, Wong CA, Ranganath YS, Marian AA. Comparison of the effect of three different adjuvants on the analgesic duration of single injection interscalene brachial plexus block: a prospective, randomized, triple blinded clinical trial. *Reg Anesth Pain Med*. 2019 Jul 14:rapm-2018-100201.
41. Candido KD, Winnie AP, Ghaleb AH, Fattouh MW, Franco CD. Buprenorphine added to the local anesthetic for axillary brachial plexus block prolongs postoperative analgesia. *Reg Anesth Pain Med*. 2002;27(2):162–167.
42. Candido KD, Hennes J, Gonzalez S, et al. Buprenorphine enhances and prolongs the postoperative analgesic effect of bupivacaine in patients receiving infragluteal sciatic nerve block. *Anesthesiology*. 2010;113(6):1419–1426.
43. James MFM. Clinical use of magnesium infusions in anesthesia. *Anesth Analg*. 1992;74(1):129–136.
44. Li M, Jin S, Zhao X, et al. Does magnesium sulfate as an adjuvant of local anesthetics facilitate better effect of perineural nerve blocks? *Clin J Pain*. 2016;32(12):1053–1061.
45. Saeki H, Matsumoto M, Kaneko S, Tsuruta S, Cui YJ, Ohtake K, Ishida K, Sakabe T. Is intrathecal magnesium sulfate safe and protective against ischemic spinal cord injury in rabbits? *Anesth Analg*. 2004;99(6):1805–1812.
46. Koinig H, Wallner T, Marhofer P, Andel H, Hörauf K, Mayer N. Magnesium sulfate reduces intra- and postoperative analgesic requirements. *Anesth Analg*. 1998;87(1):206–210.
47. Eisenach JC, De Kock M, Klimscha W. Alpha(2)-adrenergic agonists for regional anesthesia: a clinical review of clonidine (1984–1995). *Anesthesiology*. 1996;85(3):655–674.
48. Fernandes HS, Santos SA, Ashmawi HA. Clonidine in anesthesiology: a brief review. *Biomed J Sci Tech Res*. 2018;7(2):5815–5818.
49. Kroin JS, Buvanendran A, Beck DR, Topic JE, Watts DE, Tuman KJ. Clonidine prolongation of lidocaine analgesia after sciatic nerve block in rats Is mediated via the hyperpolarization-activated cation current, not by alpha-adrenoreceptors. *Anesthesiology*. 2004;101(2):488–494.
50. Pöpping DM, Elia N, Marret E, Wenk M, Tramèr MR. Clonidine as an adjuvant to local anesthetics for peripheral nerve and plexus blocks: a meta-analysis of randomized trials. *Anesthesiology*. 2009;111(2):406–415.
51. YaDeau JT, LaSala VR, Paroli L, et al. Clonidine and analgesic duration after popliteal fossa nerve blockade: randomized, double-blind, placebo-controlled study. *Anesth Analg*. 2008;106(6):1916–1920.
52. Kohli S, Kaur M, Sahoo S, Vajifdar H, Kohli P. Brachial plexus block: comparison of two different doses of clonidine added to bupivacaine. *J Anaesthesiol Clin Pharmacol*. 2013;29(4):491–495.
53. Chakraborty S, Chakrabarti J, Mandal MC, Hazra A, Das S. Effect of clonidine as adjuvant in bupivacaine-induced supraclavicular brachial plexus block: a randomized controlled trial. *Indian J Pharmacol*. 2010 Apr;42(2):74–77.
54. Kaur G, Ahuja J, Attri J, Chatrath V, Sharan R, Kheterpal R. Comparative evaluation of 0.75% ropivacaine with clonidine and 0.5% bupivacaine with clonidine in infraclavicular brachial plexus block. *Anesth Essays Res*. 2015;9(2):189. doi: 10.4103/0259-1162.153758.
55. Andersen JH, Jaeger P, Sonne TL, Dahl JB, Mathiesen O, Grevstad U. Clonidine used as a perineural adjuvant to ropivacaine, does not prolong the duration of sensory block when controlling for systemic effects: a paired, blinded, randomized trial in healthy volunteers. Forget P, ed. *PLoS One*. 2017;12(9):e0181351. doi: 10.1371/journal.pone.0181351.
56. Fournier R, Faust A, Chassot O, Gamulin Z. Perineural clonidine does not prolong levobupivacaine 0.5% after sciatic nerve block using the Labat approach in foot and ankle surgery. *Reg Anesth Pain Med*. 2012;37(5):521–524.
57. Kamibayashi T, Maze M. Clinical uses of alpha2-adrenergic agonists. *Anesthesiology*. 2000;93(5):1345–1349.
58. Brummett CM, Hong EK, Janda AM, Amodeo FS, Lydic R. Perineural dexmedetomidine added to ropivacaine for sciatic nerve block in rats prolongs the duration of analgesia by blocking the hyperpolarization-activated cation current. *Anesthesiology*. 2011;115(4):836–843.
59. Schnabel A, Reichl SU, Weibel S, et al. Efficacy and safety of dexmedetomidine in peripheral nerve blocks: a meta-analysis and trial sequential analysis. *Eur J Anaesthesiol*. 2018;35(10):745–758.
60. Vorobeichik L, Brull R, Abdallah FW. Evidence basis for using perineural dexmedetomidine to enhance the quality of brachial plexus nerve blocks: a systematic review and meta-analysis of randomized controlled trials. *Br J Anaesth*. 2017;118(2):167–181.
61. Andersen JH, Grevstad U, Siegel H, Dahl JB, Mathiesen O, Jæger P. Does dexmedetomidine have a perineural mechanism of action when used as an adjuvant to ropivacaine? *Anesthesiology*. 2017;126(1):66–73. doi: 10.1097/ALN.0000000000001429.
62. Zhang H, Zhou F, Li C, et al. Molecular mechanisms underlying the analgesic property of intrathecal dexmedetomidine and its neurotoxicity evaluation: an in vivo and in vitro experimental study. *PLoS One*. 2013;8(2):e55556.
63. Tüfek A, Kaya S, Tokgöz O, et al. The protective effect of dexmedetomidine on bupivacaine-induced sciatic nerve inflammation is mediated by mast cells. *Clin Investig Med*. 2013;36(2):95.
64. Subedi M, Bajaj S, Kumar MS, Yc M. An overview of tramadol and its usage in pain management and future perspective. *Biomed Pharmacother*. 2019;111:443–451.
65. Shin HW, Ju BJ, Jang YK, You HS, Kang H, Park JY. Effect of tramadol as an adjuvant to local anesthetics for brachial plexus block: a systematic review and meta-analysis. *PLoS One*. 2017;12(9):e0184649.
66. Nagpal V, Rana S, Singh J, Chaudhary SK. Comparative study of systemically and perineurally administered tramadol as an adjunct for supraclavicular brachial plexus block. *J Anaesthesiol Clin Pharmacol*. 2015;31(2):191–195.
67. Soulioti E, Tsaroucha A, Makris A, Koutsaki M, Sklika E, Mela A, Megaloikonomos PD, Mavrogenis AF, Fassoulaki A. Addition of 100 mg of Tramadol to 40 mL of 0.5% Ropivacaine for Interscalene Brachial Plexus Block Improves Postoperative Analgesia in Patients Undergoing Shoulder Surgeries as Compared to Ropivacaine Alone-A Randomized Controlled Study. *Medicina (Kaunas)*. 2019 Jul 23;55(7):399.
68. Golf M, Daniels SE, Onel E. A phase 3, randomized, placebo-controlled trial of DepoFoam® bupivacaine bupivacaine (extended-release bupivacaine local analgesic) in bunionectomy. *Adv Ther*. 2011;28(9):776–788.
69. Gorfine SR, Onel E, Patou G, Krivokapic ZV. Bupivacaine extended-release liposome injection for prolonged postsurgical analgesia in patients undergoing hemorrhoidectomy: a multicenter, randomized, double-blind, placebo-controlled trial. *Dis Colon Rectum*. 2011;54(12):1552–1559.
70. Nadeau MH, Saraswat A, Vasko A, Elliott JO, Vasko SD. Bupivacaine versus liposomal bupivacaine for postoperative pain control after augmentation mammaplasty: a prospective, randomized, double-blind trial. *Aesthet Surg J*. 2016;36(2):NP47–52.
71. Smoot JD, Bergese SD, Onel E, Williams HT, Hedden W. The efficacy and safety of DepoFoam bupivacaine in patients undergoing bilateral, cosmetic, submuscular augmentation mammaplasty: a randomized, double-blind, active-control study. *Aesthet Surg J*. 2012;32(1):69–76.
72. Haas E, Onel E, Miller H, Ragupathi M, White PF. A double-blind, randomized, active-controlled study for post-hemorrhoidectomy pain management with liposome bupivacaine, a novel local analgesic formulation. *Am Surg*. 2012;78(5):574–581. doi: 10.1177/000313481207800540.

73. Yeung J, Crisp CC, Mazloomdoost D, Kleeman SD, Pauls RN. Liposomal bupivacaine during robotic colpopexy and posterior repair: a randomized controlled trial. *Obs Gynecol.* 2018;131(1):39–46.
74. Knight RB, Walker PW, Keegan KA, Overholser SM, Baumgartner TS, Ebertowski JS 2nd, Aden JK, White MA. A randomized controlled trial for pain control in laparoscopic urologic surgery: 0.25% bupivacaine versus long-acting liposomal bupivacaine. *J Endourol.* 2015;29(9):1019–1024.
75. Gatherwright J, Knackstedt RW, Ghaznavi AM, et al. Prospective, randomized, controlled comparison of bupivacaine versus liposomal bupivacaine for pain management after unilateral delayed deep inferior epigastric perforator free flap reconstruction. *Plast Reconstr Surg.* 2018;141(6):1327–1330. doi: 10.1097/PRS.0000000000004360.
76. Ilfeld BM, Gabriel RA, Eisenach JC. Liposomal bupivacaine infiltration for knee arthroplasty. *Anesthesiology.* 2018;129(4):623–626.
77. Ilfeld BM, Eisenach JC, Gabriel RA. Clinical effectiveness of liposomal bupivacaine administered by infiltration or peripheral nerve block to treat postoperative pain. *Anesthesiology.* 2021 Feb 1;134(2):283–344. doi: 10.1097/ALN.0000000000003630. PMID: 33372949.
78. Hutchins J, Delaney D, Vogel RI, et al. Ultrasound guided subcostal transversus abdominis plane (TAP) infiltration with liposomal bupivacaine for patients undergoing robotic assisted hysterectomy: a prospective randomized controlled study. *Gynecol Oncol.* 2015;138(3): 609–613.
79. Hutchins JL, Kesha R, Blanco F, Dunn T, Hochhalter R. Ultrasound-guided subcostal transversus abdominis plane blocks with liposomal bupivacaine vs. non-liposomal bupivacaine for postoperative pain control after laparoscopic hand-assisted donor nephrectomy: a prospective randomised observer-blinded study. *Anaesthesia.* 2016;71(8):930–937.
80. Vandepitte C, Kuroda M, Witvrouw R, et al. Addition of liposome bupivacaine to bupivacaine (HCl) versus bupivacaine (HCl) alone for interscalene brachial plexus block in patients having major shoulder surgery. *Reg Anesth Pain Med.* 2017;42(3):334–341.
81. Hussain N, Brull R, Sheehy B, Essandoh MK, Stahl DL, Weaver TE, Abdallah FW. Perineural liposomal bupivacaine is not superior to non liposomal bupivacaine for peripheral nerve block analgesia: a systematic review and meta-analysis. *Anesthesiology.* 2021; 134: 147–164. doi: https://doi.org/10.1097/ALN.0000000000003651.

REVIEW QUESTIONS

(1) What dose of perineural dexamethasone has been shown to provide the largest increase in duration while minimizing potential risks?

A. 1 mg
B. 2 mg
C. 4 mg
D. 8 mg

(2) What is the proposed mechanism of action of buprenorphine on local anesthetic (LA) nerve blockade in the perineural space?

A. μ-opioid receptors on C-fibers
B. κ-opioid receptor activity
C. Neuronal sodium channels
D. Both A and C

(3) What is the clinical purpose of adding epinephrine to LAs prior to perineural injection?

A. Increased duration of analgesia from long-acting LAs, such as ropivacaine
B. Increased duration of analgesia from short/moderate-acting LAs, such as lidocaine
C. Detect intravascular injection
D. Both B and C

(4) The data from multiple studies examining dexmedetomidine as a LA adjuvant for perineural injection have demonstrated an increase of approximately 250 minutes compared to LAs alone. Which of the following are known challenges to be considered with the use of perineural dexmedetomidine?

A. Hemodynamic side effects are common
B. Similar increase in analgesia duration when used systemically or perineurally
C. Neurotoxicity
D. Both A and B

(5) Which additives have been approved by the FDA for perineural injection?

A. Epinephrine
B. Dexamethasone
C. Buprenorphine
D. None of the above

(6) Which pharmacologic property of LAs likely primarily determines their duration of action?

A. Concentration
B. pK_a
C. Lipid solubility
D. Protein binding

(7) What is the proposed mechanism of action for magnesium on the peripheral nerves?

A. N-methyl-D-aspartate (NMDA) antagonism
B. Neuronal calcium influx antagonism
C. μ-opioid receptors on C-fibers
D. Unknown mechanism of action

(8) Which is not an FDA-approved site for liposomal bupivacaine injection?

A. Transversus abdominis plane block
B. Interscalene block
C. Surgical site infiltration
D. Femoral nerve block

ANSWERS

(1) **C.** While the evidence isn't extremely high quality, there are data to support a dose-dependent relationship of increased analgesia for dexamethasone doses between 1 and 4 mg. There are also data that indicate that 8 mg or higher doses do not provide any additional clinical benefit and only expose the patient to increased risk of side effects.[29–31]

References

Pehora C, Pearson AM, Kaushal A, Crawford MW, Johnston B. Dexamethasone as an adjuvant to peripheral nerve block. *Cochrane Database Syst Rev.* 2017;11:CD011770.

Albrecht E, Kern C, Kirkham KR. A systematic review and meta-analysis of perineural dexamethasone for peripheral nerve blocks. *Anaesthesia*. 2015;70(1):71–83.
Albrecht E, Reynvoet M, Fournier N, et al. Combination of dexamethasone and local anaesthetic solution in peripheral nerve blocks: a meta-analysis of randomised controlled trials. *Anesthesiology*. 2018;78(6): 1001–1008.

(2) **D.** While buprenorphine also has κ-opioid receptor activity, there has been evidence to indicate that the peripheral nerve effects are primarily due to blockade of μ-opioid receptors on C-fibers and neuronal sodium channels.

References

Desmet M, Braems H, Reynvoet M, et al. I.V. and perineural dexamethasone are equivalent in increasing the analgesic duration of a single-shot interscalene block with ropivacaine for shoulder surgery: a prospective, randomized, placebo-controlled study. *Br J Anaesth*. 2013;111(3):445–452.
Albrecht E, Reynvoet M, Fournier N, Desmet M. Dose–response relationship of perineural dexamethasone for interscalene brachial plexus block: a randomised, controlled, triple-blind trial. *Anaesthesia*. 2019;74(8):1001–1008. doi: 10.1111/anae.14650.
Kosel J, Bobik P, Tomczyk M. Buprenorphine: the unique opioid adjuvant in regional anesthesia. *Expert Rev Clin Pharmacol*. 2016;9(3):375–383.

(3) **D.** Epinephrine has been shown to modestly increase the duration of sensory blockade and analgesia from short/moderate-acting LAs such as lidocaine, but has failed to consistently increase the duration of analgesia in a clinically relevant manner for long-acting LAs, especially ropivacaine. The most common use for epinephrine as an additive to LAs is to quickly detect intravascular spread via heart rate and blood pressure changes.

Reference

Brummett CM, Williams BA. Additives to local anesthetics for peripheral nerve blockade. *Int Anesthesiol Clin*. 2011;49(4):104–116. doi: 10.1097/AIA.0b013e31820e4a49.

(4) **D.** Bradycardia and hypotension are both well-documented side effects of both systemic and perineural dexmedetomidine. Additionally, there is limited evidence suggesting that systemic dexmedetomidine provides the same increase in duration of sensory blockade. These two points complement each other as the drug is most likely exhibiting its effect via systemic endpoints versus localized nerve activity. It is important to note, however, that there has been no experimental or clinical evidence linking perineural dexmedetomidine to neurotoxicity.[59,60]

References

Schnabel A, Reichl SU, Weibel S, et al. Efficacy and safety of dexmedetomidine in peripheral nerve blocks: a meta-analysis and trial sequential analysis. *Eur J Anaesthesiol*. 2018;35(10):745–758.
Vorobeichik L, Brull R, Abdallah FW. Evidence basis for using perineural dexmedetomidine to enhance the quality of brachial plexus nerve blocks: a systematic review and meta-analysis of randomized controlled trials. *Br J Anaesth*. 2017;118(2):167–181.

(5) **A.** Unfortunately, while there has been extensive experimental and clinical evidence produced on the topic, only some LA formulations containing epinephrine have been approved by the FDA for nerve blocks.[5]

Reference

Singh S, Bansal P, Dureja J. Off-label use of drugs in regional anesthesia: a need for setting up policies. *J Anaesthesiol Clin Pharmacol*. 2017;33(4):448–449.

(6) **C.** While total dose can also significantly affect duration of sensory blockade, the other most important concept for determining duration of action is lipid solubility. Nearby vascular uptake is the most significant factor for LA removal from the peripheral nerve. Highly lipid soluble LAs are not easily dissolved in blood and therefore remain perineural longer, resulting in a longer duration of action.[2]

Reference

Bokesch PM, Post C, Strichartz G. Structure-activity relationship of lidocaine homologs producing tonic and frequency-dependent impulse blockade in nerve. *J Pharmacol Exp Ther*. 1986;237(3):773–781.

(7) **D.** As with many of the perineural additives, the exact mechanism of action on peripheral nerves is poorly understood for magnesium. This highlights the need for additional basic science research for LA adjuvants in the coming years. This also presents another significant hurdle for potential FDA approval and widespread adoption of these additives moving forward. The systemic mechanisms of action are better researched and understood, which also indicates that when systemic administration provides similar analgesia enhancement and side-effect profile, the systemic route should be favored over perineural administration.[43]

Reference

James MFM. Clinical use of magnesium infusions in anesthesia. *Anesth Analg*. 1992;74(1):129–136.

(8) **D.** At the time of writing, the only FDA-approved uses for liposomal bupivacaine are TAP block, interscalene block, and surgical-site infiltration. Although this may change with time, practitioners must be cognizant when using drugs off-label.

Reference

Ilfeld BM, Eisenach JC, Gabriel RA. Clinical effectiveness of liposomal bupivacaine administered by infiltration or peripheral nerve block to treat postoperative pain. *Anesthesiology*. 2021 Feb 1;134(2):283–344. doi: 10.1097/ALN.0000000000003630. PMID: 33372949.

SECTION 3

HEAD AND NECK

Kamen V. Vlassakov

8.

AWAKE INTUBATION AND AIRWAY BLOCKS

Choopong Luansritisakul, Kamen V. Vlassakov, and Nantthasorn Zinboonyahgoon

STEM CASE AND KEY QUESTIONS

A 50-year-old female patient diagnosed with atlantoaxial subluxation is scheduled for posterior occipito-cervical fusion. Her chief complaint is severe neck pain. The neurological examination appears normal. However, the magnetic resonance imaging (MRI) of cervical spine shows increased distance of the atlanto-dental interval. She has a history of rheumatoid arthritis, diagnosed 10 years ago, which is currently treated with methotrexate and hydroxychloroquine.

(1) HOW WOULD YOU EVALUATE THIS PATIENT PREOPERATIVELY?

At the preoperative visit, the patient can neither flex nor extend her neck. Her rheumatoid arthritis involves multiple joints, including her proximal interphalangeal joints bilaterally and both temporomandibular joints. She presents with significantly limited mouth opening and an inter-incisor distance of approximately 1 fingerbreadth. She has no symptoms of cricoarytenoid arthritis such as hoarseness, dyspnea, stridor, or tenderness over the larynx and appears otherwise unremarkable.

(2) WHAT ARE THE OPTIONS FOR MANAGING THIS PATIENT'S AIRWAY? WHAT ARE THE INDICATIONS AND CONTRAINDICATIONS FOR AWAKE FIBEROPTIC INTUBATION (AFOI)? DESCRIBE THE TECHNIQUE USED FOR FIBEROPTIC INTUBATION.

After discussion with the surgeon, the anesthesiologist decides to perform a fiberoptic intubation (a more accurate term would be *flexible endoscopic intubation*, as the majority of modern flexible bronchoscopes utilize video chips, not fiberoptic technology) in this patient in order to minimize (or completely avoid) cervical spine movement, which can lead to further neurologic damage. Due to the expected difficulty of this patient's airway, combined with her cervical spine instability, the anesthesiologist chooses to perform AFOI, as the safer method with the benefit of uninterrupted clinical monitoring and the ability to re-evaluate neurologic function after intubation. For this patient, the nasal route is preferred due to her small mouth opening.

(3) DESCRIBE THE SENSORY INNERVATION OF UPPER AIRWAY. HOW WOULD YOU PREPARE THE PATIENT'S AIRWAY FOR AN AWAKE FIBEROPTIC INTUBATION (AFOI)? WHAT LOCAL ANESTHETIC (LA) WOULD YOU CHOOSE FOR ANESTHETIZING THE PATIENT'S AIRWAY?

Prior to the AFOI, cotton pledgets soaked with 4% cocaine are inserted into the nasal cavity and left for 10 minutes. Three mL of viscous 2% lidocaine are gargled by the patient and 4 mL of 4% lidocaine are delivered via a nebulizer.

However, the patient cannot tolerate the bronchoscope being passed into the pharynx, leading to coughing, gagging, and ultimately, an unsuccessful intubation.

(4) WHAT WOULD YOU DO NEXT? WHAT ARE THE ADVANTAGES AND DISADVANTAGES OF AIRWAY BLOCKS? DESCRIBE TECHNIQUES USED TO ANESTHETIZE THE AIRWAY BY BOTH LANDMARKS AND ULTRASOUND-GUIDANCE. WHAT ARE THE BENEFITS OF ULTRASOUND-GUIDED TECHNIQUE COMPARED TO THE LANDMARK TECHNIQUE?

The anesthesiologist then decides to perform airway blocks in order to provide adequate anesthesia for awake intubation. Since this patient had limited mouth opening, the extraoral approaches are preferred. Bilateral glossopharyngeal nerve blocks (using the technique described by Azman et al.[1] Figure 8.5) and superior laryngeal nerve blocks (Figure 8.7; see figures later in the chapter) are performed under ultrasound guidance using 1% lidocaine with epinephrine 1:200,000–3 mL and 2 mL per injection, respectively. The translaryngeal block is avoided because coughing elicited by this technique could result in further displacement of the cervical spine.

Incidentally, after performing these blocks, the patient develops a sudden-onset tachyarrhythmia with heart rate 120 beats/minute, blood pressure 135/80 mmHg. She remains awake and cooperative.

(5) WHAT ARE THE POSSIBLE CAUSES OF ARRHYTHMIA IN THIS PATIENT? WHAT ARE THE COMPLICATIONS OF AIRWAY BLOCKS?

Due to the proximity of the vessels in these locations, inadvertent intravascular injection could occur.[1,2] For this reason, some recommend using intravascular markers, such as epinephrine.[3] Systemic effects from absorption of extravascular LAs and epinephrine, though typically very mild and generally well-tolerated, are also to be expected and monitored for. In addition, Doppler mode should be utilized to identify vessels in this highly vascular area. Furthermore, tachycardia could also occur from the glossopharyngeal nerve block itself via a blockade of the afferent fibers arising from the carotid sinus.[4]

Fortunately, in this patient, tachycardia is hemodynamically stable and self-limiting, not requiring pharmacologic treatment.

After the airway blocks, the patient's gag reflex is diminished to absent. Intubation is successful and tolerated well. Neurologic function is reassessed, showing no neurological damage. Then, general anesthesia is induced, and surgery is performed uneventfully.

(6) IS IT APPROPRIATE TO CONSIDER EXTUBATION AFTER THE PATIENT RECEIVES AIRWAY BLOCKS?

In general, airway blocks are not considered a contraindication to postoperative extubation. Nevertheless, they can impair some protective reflexes, such as gag reflex and cough reflex. For this reason, although not universally accepted, some advocate against airway blocks in patients at risk for aspiration.[5] Also, short-acting local anesthetics are typically used and at lower concentration, practically guaranteeing complete nerve function recovery by the end of a surgical operation of average duration.

Moreover, after cervical spine surgery, there is a significant increase in airway management difficulty as the spine is being stabilized with hardware. For this reason, the anesthesiologists must follow the criteria for extubation strictly in order to avoid challenging and dangerous reintubation. Patients at high risk for postoperative airway compromise may have to be left intubated overnight and extubated after fiberoptic evaluation.

Due to low risk for aspiration and postoperative airway compromise, this patient is extubated immediately after the operation when she meets extubation criteria. Postoperative course is uncomplicated.

DISCUSSION

Failure to intubate and/or ventilate remains a feared cause of major morbidity and mortality in anesthesia. From 1999 to 2005, difficult intubation accounted for 2.3% of 2211 anesthesia-related deaths in the United States,[6] according to US Anesthesia Closed Claims. It was reported that unsuccessful intubation with direct laryngoscopy occurred at a rate of 5 to 35 per 10,000 anesthetics.[7,8] However, with the continuing improvement in airway equipment, management techniques, and algorithms, the number of intubation-related claims have declined.[9] Over the last decade, a multitude of airway devices has been developed for difficult airway situations, including video-laryngoscopes, intubating stylets, intubating laryngeal mask airways, and flexible bronchoscopes. These devices possess specific advantages and disadvantages and thus are useful in different situations. Therefore, it is the responsibility of an anesthesiologist to choose wisely according to the patient's conditions.

Fiberoptic intubation is one of the time-tested methods for intubation in patients presenting potential risks of difficult intubation, and it is mentioned in all guidelines for difficult airway management. Despite the development of many airway devices, it is the ultimate backup nonsurgical airway technique in difficult airway patients.[10]

Compared with other methods, fiberoptic intubation has a number of advantages, as follows:

- Because of the small size and unique characteristics of flexible endoscope, it provides the highest success rate in distorted anatomy in most difficult airway patients.
- It is the most accurate method used to perform and confirm endotracheal intubation.
- This method is the least likely to cause or require cervical spine movements during intubation—an excellent option for patients with suspected unstable neck or cervical spine injury.
- Fiberoptic intubation can be used both via oral and nasal routes, and in all age groups.
- Even when performed awake, this technique produces less patient discomfort.
- It should also be the least traumatic to airway anatomy.
- With appropriate airway anesthesia and sedation, it results in less cardiovascular stress and hemodynamic changes than rigid laryngoscopy.
- Beyond intubation, it can be a useful diagnostic tool when abnormal airway is encountered perioperatively.

Fiberoptic intubation can be carried out in either awake or asleep patients, yet the awake approach is conventionally recommended when dealing with difficult airway and unpredictable ability to mask-ventilate. It allows patients to maintain airway patency and breathe spontaneously throughout the procedure. Airway anesthesia is essential to awake fiberoptic intubation. First, it helps patients better tolerate the unpleasant sensation and intense gag reflex during the procedure, the reaction of which will make intubation more challenging. Moreover, it reduces the hemodynamic response to intubation, which can be detrimental to patients with severe coexisting diseases, such as poorly controlled hypertension, coronary artery disease, and cerebrovascular disease.

SENSORY INNERVATION OF THE UPPER AIRWAY

To provide adequate anesthesia for awake fiberoptic technique, the anesthesiologist has to determine what structures need to be anesthetized along the route of intubation.

The upper airway extends from the nose to the glottis. It is divided into the nasal cavity, the oral cavity, the pharynx, and the larynx. The upper airway is mainly supplied by branches of three cranial nerves (the trigeminal nerve, the glossopharyngeal nerve, and the vagus nerve), as shown in Figure 8.1.

NASAL CAVITY

Apart from the olfaction, which is mediated via the olfactory nerve, the sensory innervation of the nasal mucosa is solely from branches of the trigeminal nerve.[11]

- The anterior ethmoidal nerve, which is a branch of the ophthalmic division, supplies the anterior third of the nasal cavity and septum. It enters the nasal cavity via the anterior ethmoidal foramen.[12,13]
- The posterior superior lateral nasal branch of maxillary nerve, posterior inferior lateral nasal branch of greater palatine nerve, and nasopalatine nerve, which are branches of the maxillary division, innervate the rest of the nasal cavity. These nerves are relayed through the sphenopalatine ganglion (pterygopalatine ganglion) found in the pterygopalatine fossa, which is located just posterior to the middle turbinate. They carry not only sensory fibers but also sympathetic and parasympathetic fibers.[13–15]

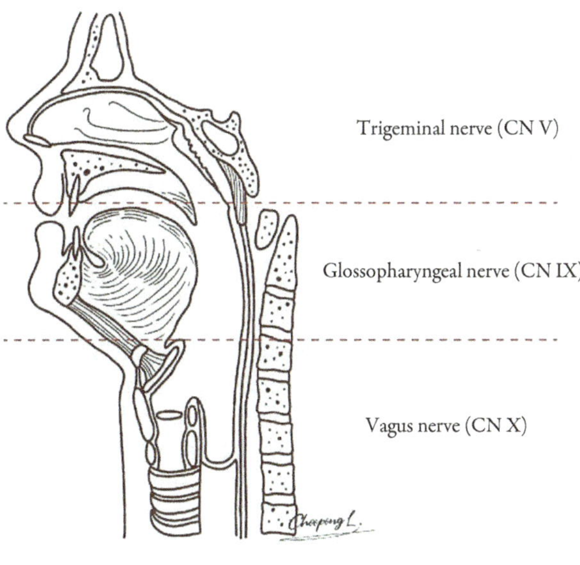

Figure 8.1. The sensory innervation of the upper airway.

ORAL CAVITY

The oral cavity receives sensory innervation from branches of the trigeminal, the facial, the glossopharyngeal, and the vagus nerves.[16–18]

- The lingual nerve of the mandibular division of the trigeminal nerve conveys general sensation from the anterior two-thirds of the tongue.
- The chorda tympani, which is a branch of the lingual branch of facial nerve, carries taste sensations from the anterior two-thirds of the tongue.
- The tonsillar branches of the glossopharyngeal nerve receive both general and taste sensation from the posterior one-third of the tongue.
- The internal branch of superior laryngeal nerve, a branch of the vagus nerve, provides only small amount of sensory supply at the base of the tongue valleculae.
- The nasopalatine and greater palatine nerves innervate the hard palate.
- The lesser palatine nerve innervates the soft palate.

Fortunately, for awake fiberoptic intubation, anesthesia for the portions of the airway anterior to the tonsillar pillars is rarely needed. In contrast, the posterior third of the tongue should be adequately anesthetized since stimulation of this area usually triggers the gag reflex and secretions, which can be problematic during awake intubation.[19,20]

PHARYNX

The pharynx is largely innervated by the pharyngeal plexus, which receives input from the glossopharyngeal and the vagus nerves.[16]

- The glossopharyngeal nerve supplies the posterior third of the tongue, vallecula, and anterior surface of the epiglottis, all parts of the pharynx. It carries visceral sensory fibers, taste sensation, sympathetic fiber, and secretomotor fibers to mucous glands in the area supplied, and motor fibers to the stylopharyngeus muscle as well. It is of note that it also innervates the carotid sinus.[13,16,18] This nerve emerges from the jugular foramen between the jugular vein and the internal carotid artery. Then, it descends anteriorly to the internal carotid artery and stays posteromedially to the styloid process, before traveling anteromedially and either piercing the lower fibers of the superior constrictor muscle or passing between the superior and middle constrictors. At the level of styloid process, it lies adjacent to the vagus nerve, the accessory nerve, and the hypoglossal nerve.[2,21]
- The vagus nerve provides extensive motor innervation to the pharynx via several branches joining the pharyngeal plexus.[16]

LARYNX

The larynx is innervated mainly by branches of the vagus nerve, which are the internal and external branches of the superior laryngeal nerve, and the recurrent laryngeal nerve.[22]

- The superior laryngeal nerve arises from the inferior ganglion of the vagus nerve and travels anteriorly to the greater cornu of the hyoid bone. It then divides into an internal and external branch. The internal branch pierces through the thyrohyoid membrane, lies in the paraglottic space, and provides both visceral sensation and secretomotor fibers to the mucosa above the vocal cords (base of tongue, posterior epiglottis, aryepiglottic folds, vestibular folds or false vocal cords, and arytenoids). The external branch supplies motor innervation to cricothyroid muscle.[21,22]
- The recurrent laryngeal nerve carries sensory input from the vocal cords and the structures below the vocal cords. It derives from the intrathoracic part of the vagus nerve. The left recurrent laryngeal nerve wraps around the aortic arch lateral to ligamentum arteriosum, while the right wraps around subclavian artery. It then ascends in the tracheoesophageal groove, passes behind the thyroid gland, and enters the larynx at the lower border of inferior constrictor muscle. It supplies motor fiber to all intrinsic muscles of the larynx except the cricothyroid muscle. Also, it provides visceral sensation, secretomotor fiber, and sympathetic fibers to the mucosa below the true vocal cords.[21,22]

TOPICAL ANESTHESIA TECHNIQUES

In most patients, effective topicalization of the upper airway is doable and critical to a successful awake intubation. Even though it is considered the safest method for anesthetizing a patient's airway, care must be taken to avoid local anesthetic systemic toxicity (LAST). Furthermore, it has been reported that topical anesthesia can result in complete airway obstruction due to loss of upper airway tone in a patient with a compromised airway.[23–25] Topical anesthesia of the upper airway can be achieved by several techniques as follows.

DIRECT APPLICATION

The simplest way to anesthetize the airway is to apply the local anesthetic (LA) directly to the mucosa. This can be accomplished by several methods, including placing of cotton-tipped swabs soaked with LA in the nasal cavity and gargling of LA solution. Occasionally, for the nasal mucosa, which is highly vascular, vasoconstrictors, such as 0.125% to 0.5% phenylephrine and 0.05% oxymetazoline, are used as adjuncts to LA such as lidocaine. This results in shrinking of the nasal mucosa, leading to less bleeding during instrumentation. In addition, it also creates more space for the fiberoptic scope and endotracheal tube. Alternatively, 4% cocaine pledgets could be used for this drug's unique combined local anesthetic and strong vasoconstricting properties.[18,19,26]

SPRAYING

Anesthesia for the upper airway could be achieved by spraying LA directly onto the mucosa via a variety of methods, such as aerosol spray and atomizer devices. A limitation of this technique results from the unpredictable distribution of the administered LA, potentially causing only a small amount of LA reaching the intended targets.[18,19]

NEBULIZATION

Nebulization can be used for topicalization of the whole airway. This method is easy, less invasive, and well tolerated. It is also beneficial for patients with limited mouth opening and patients with conditions in which coughing might be detrimental, for example, elevated intracranial pressure or open eye injury.[27] The usual dose for standard nebulizer is 4 mL of 4% lidocaine. Of note, for this technique, low oxygen flow rate of 2–4 L/min should be used in order to make the particles large enough to be accumulated in the upper airway.[28] This alludes to a limitation of this technique that often provides better coverage of the lower airway, but insufficient suppression of the gag reflex.[19,26]

"SPRAY-AS-YOU-GO" TECHNIQUE

This method can be carried out by injecting aliquots of LA through the working channel of the fiberoptic scope and onto the target area. Since the LA is applied only a short period before the intubation, this technique may be advantageous for patients at high risk for aspiration. Generally, 1–2 mL of 2% lidocaine is drawn into a 10-mL syringe. Then, the plunger is drawn back so that there is a column of air on top of the LA. When the scope is advanced to the target area, the plunger is fully depressed to disperse the LA over the mucosa.[18,19,26]

REGIONAL ANESTHESIA TECHNIQUES

In most patients, topicalization of the LA is adequate for awake fiberoptic intubation. In some, however, the gag and cough reflexes are so pronounced that airway blocks are needed. Studies have demonstrated that airway blocks provide better quality of anesthesia than nebulization in terms of patient comfort, hemodynamic stability, and ease of intubation.[29,30]

ANTERIOR ETHMOIDAL NERVE BLOCK

The anterior ethmoidal nerve can be selectively blocked when it emerges from the anterior ethmoidal foramen. This can be done by using a long cotton-tipped swab soaked in LA solution, such as 4% cocaine or 4% lidocaine with epinephrine 1:200,000. It is inserted along the dorsum of the nose, in a cephalad and slightly posterior direction, until it reaches the anterior surface of the cribriform plate, which is the location of the anterior ethmoidal foramen. The swab should be held in that position for 5 to 10 minutes[31,32] (A in Figure 8.2). As an

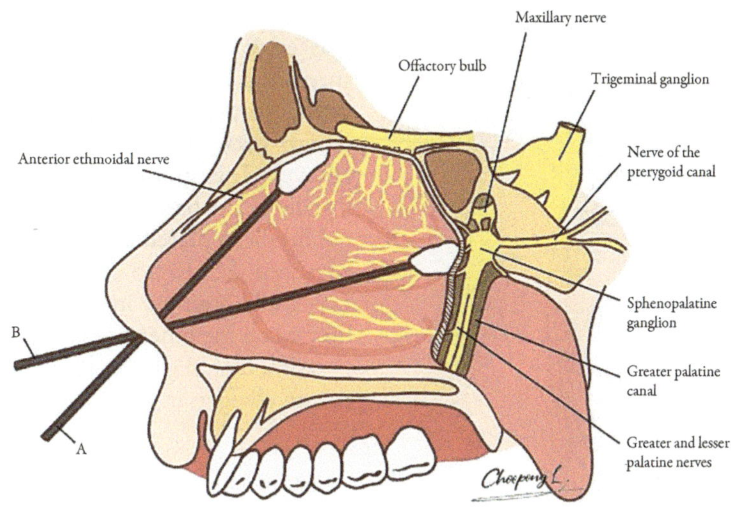

Figure 8.2. Anterior ethmoidal nerve block (A) and sphenopalatine ganglion block (B).

alternative, the cotton pledgets with bayonet forceps may be used instead of the cotton-tipped swab.[33]

SPHENOPALATINE GANGLION BLOCK

The sphenopalatine ganglion sends out multiple sensory branches, which supply the nasal cavity, the hard palate, and the soft palate.[14] Blockade of this ganglion can be useful not only for anesthetizing the airway, but also for treatment of several types of headache, including postdural puncture headache.[15,31] It can be performed by two approaches.

Nasal Approach

Due to the fact that the sphenopalatine ganglion lies beneath the nasal mucosa, it can be blocked effortlessly by applying the LA over the mucosal surface overlying the ganglion. For this approach, a long cotton-tipped swab or a cotton pledget is soaked in the LA solution, such as 4% cocaine or 4% lidocaine with epinephrine 1:200,000. After that, it is inserted posteriorly, at a 45-degree angle to the hard palate, along the upper border of the middle turbinate until the posterior wall of the nasopharynx is reached. About 5 to 10 minutes should be allowed for the anesthetic to take effect[15,19] (B in Figure 8.2).

Another technique involves the insertion of a 20-gauge angiocatheter along the path described previously. Then, anesthetic solution is rapidly injected to the mucosal surface overlying the ganglion.[20,26]

Oral Approach

The sphenopalatine ganglion can also be blocked via the greater palatine foramen. However, this technique is utilized extremely rarely for airway anesthesia, due to technical difficulty and procedural risks. The patient is placed in the supine position with the physician facing the patient on the contralateral side of the nerve to be blocked. The greater palatine foramen is palpated with the nondominant index finger. Generally, it is located near the posterior edge of the hard palate between the second and third upper molars, approximately 1 cm medial to the palatogingival margin. Before the block, a cotton soaked in LA should be applied over the foramen for 2 minutes to reduce pain on needle insertion. Then, a 25-gauge spinal needle with bending tip is inserted into the foramen in a superior and slightly posterior direction to a depth of 2–3 cm. After negative aspiration, 1–2 mL of 2% lidocaine with epinephrine 1:100,000 is injected in a slow continuous fashion. Since, in this area, the sphenopalatine artery runs together with the nerves, the epinephrine should be used to reduce the incidence of epistaxis.[15,19]

It should be noted that in approximately 15% of the population, the greater palatine foramen is closed and inaccessible to this nerve block technique.[19]

GLOSSOPHARYNGEAL NERVE BLOCK

Glossopharyngeal nerve block is highly effective in suppressing the gag reflex and minimizing hemodynamic responses to laryngoscopy. It is also useful for eliminating the gag reflex during endodontics, postoperative pain control after tonsillectomy, and the treatment of neuralgia. Several glossopharyngeal nerve block techniques have been described.

Intraoral Approach

For this approach, adequate topical anesthesia must be provided to the posterior tongue and tonsillar mucosa in order to allow manipulation of this sensitive area. Two different locations have been described for intraoral approach.

Posterior Approach

The posterior approach is a classic technique that is frequently performed by the otolaryngologist for tonsillectomy. The goal is to block the nerve more proximally than the anterior approach, at the base of the posterior tonsillar pillar

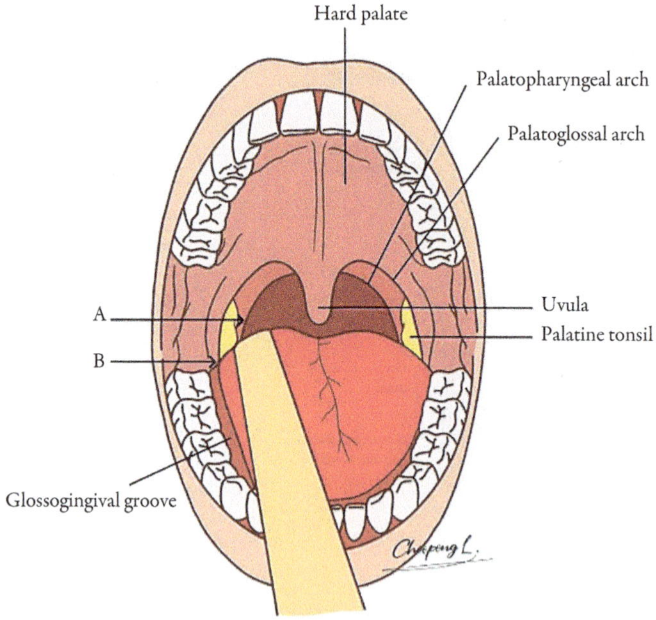

Figure 8.3. Glossopharyngeal nerve block, intraoral approach: (A) posterior approach; (B) anterior approach.

(palatopharyngeal fold). It usually blocks both sensory fibers (pharyngeal, lingual, and tonsillar branches) and the motor branch innervating the stylopharyngeus muscle.

The patient is placed in the semi-reclined position with the physician standing on the ipsilateral side of the nerve to be blocked. The patient is asked to open his/her mouth wide. Then, the tongue is displaced in an anteroinferior direction to stretch both the palatopharyngeal arch and the palatoglossal arch. This method enables the visualization of the tonsillar pillars and makes them more accessible. A size 3 Macintosh laryngoscope blade can be quite useful both for gentle retraction and additional illumination. After that, a 25-gauge sharp-bevel spinal needle bent at a right angle is inserted behind the midportion of the posterior tonsillar pillar into the submucosa. After negative aspiration, 5 mL of 0.5% to 1% lidocaine with epinephrine 1:200,000 is injected slowly. Then, the procedure is repeated on the opposite side (A in Figure 8.3).

Due to submucosal location of the nerve, LA-soaked cotton pledgets held in this area for 5 minutes can be effective as well.

Anterior Approach

This approach aims to deposit the LA at the base of the anterior tonsillar pillar (palatoglossal fold) in order to anesthetize the lingual branch of the glossopharyngeal nerve, which supplies the posterior third of the tongue and functions as the afferent limb of the gag reflex. Since it requires less exposure than the posterior approach, it is technically easier and better tolerated by patients. Some studies showed that retrograde spreading of the injectate might occur, which can lead to the blockade of more proximal branches.[34]

After sufficient topical anesthesia, the patient is placed in the sitting position with the physician facing the patient on the contralateral side of the nerve to be blocked. The patient is asked to open the mouth wide and to protrude the tongue anteriorly. The tongue is then displaced medially by using a laryngoscope blade, forming a gutter along the floor of the mouth between the tongue and the teeth (glossogingival groove). This groove is a U-shaped structure, which ends distally at the base of the palatoglossal arch. A 25-gauge spinal needle is placed at the base of the palatoglossal fold and advanced 0.25 to 0.5 cm. After negative aspiration, 2 mL of 1%–2% lidocaine is injected, and the procedure is then performed on the other side (B in Figure 8.3).

Also, this block can be achieved by using the LA-soaked cotton pledgets in the same manner as posterior approach.

Peristyloid Approach

This approach aims to infiltrate LA just posterior to the styloid process, where the glossopharyngeal nerve lies next to the internal carotid artery. This technique is highly useful for patients with limited mouth opening; however, it requires access to the lateral neck and ability to identify the bony landmark.

For the peristyloid approach, the patient should be placed supine with the head in a neutral position. In general, the styloid process lies under the midpoint of the line between the tip of the mastoid process and the mandibular angle. After the skin is infiltrated with LA, a 22-gauge needle is inserted until the styloid process is contacted, normally after less than 1–2 cm. The needle is then redirected posteriorly and walked off the styloid process. Once the contact is lost, 5–7 mL of 0.5%–1% lidocaine is injected after a negative aspiration. This is then repeated on the contralateral side. Performing bilateral glossopharyngeal block so proximally should be advised against as the vagus nerve is in immediate proximity, and bilateral vagus nerve block would predictably lead to airway compromise.

Ultrasound-Guided Technique

Two ultrasound-guided techniques have been described for the glossopharyngeal nerve block. The first method is the ultrasound-guided peristyloid approach.[35] A high-frequency linear array transducer is placed over the mastoid process in an axial plane. Then, it is moved caudally in a slight oblique direction until the styloid process is found. Subsequently, color flow Doppler is used to identify the vascular structures. A needle is then inserted in an out-of-plane approach toward the styloid process and walked off the styloid process. After a negative aspiration, LA is injected. Because of the relatively superficial location of the nerve, both echogenic needle and standard needle can be used (Figure 8.4). With this method, the chance of intravascular injection can be significantly reduced. However, the same caution against bilateral proximal blocks should be exercised.

Another method described by Azman et al. intends to block the glossopharyngeal nerve distally, at the

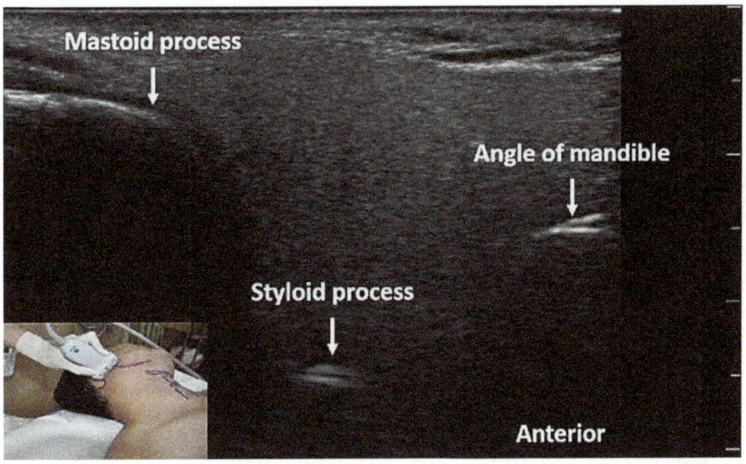

Figure 8.4. Ultrasound-guided glossopharyngeal nerve block, peristyloid approach.

parapharyngeal level, in order to reduce risk of inadvertent spread of LA to the vagus, spinal accessory, and hypoglossal nerves.[1] For this method, a high-frequency (13–6 MHz) linear probe is used. At the beginning, the probe is placed over the lateral part of hyoid bone in transverse plane. Then, the lateral tip of the probe is rotated cephalad to the mandibular angle, while the medial tip is kept on the hyoid bone. In this location, the pharyngeal wall is identified. An echogenic needle is advanced using in-plane approach, and 2–3 mL of LA is injected just superficial to the anterolateral pharyngeal wall (Figure 8.5A and B).

Complications

Apart from the general complications of nerve blockade, there are some serious specific risks associated with the glossopharyngeal nerve due to its proximity to the internal carotid artery and the internal jugular vein. Injection into the internal carotid artery could result in headache or seizure. One study using the posterior approach reported a 0.8% incidence of headache, believed to be due to an unrecognized intravascular injection, and a 0.04% incidence of seizure.[36] For this reason, incremental injection of LA, while looking for hemodynamic changes and LA toxic effects, is recommended. The potential for intra-arterial injection is greater for the peristyloid and posterior approaches because of proximity of the internal carotid artery in these regions. Additionally, puncture of these vessels can cause hematoma formation. One study reported 823 patients who had block by the posterior approach, two of whom had self-limiting hematomas.[37] Therefore, this block should be avoided in the presence of coagulopathy or anticoagulant therapy.

The peristyloid approach has also been associated with concomitant block of the hypoglossal nerve and either blockade or direct stimulation of the vagus nerve. These can result in dangerous airway obstruction, especially when occurring bilaterally. Transient hoarseness, dysphagia, and tachycardia have been reported after using this technique as well.[38,39]

Dysrhythmia can also occur from the glossopharyngeal nerve block itself, resulting from the blockade of the afferent fibers arising from the carotid sinus.[4] One study showed that, for the posterior approach, there was 1% incidence of dysrhythmia (supraventricular tachycardia and bigeminy). Of the

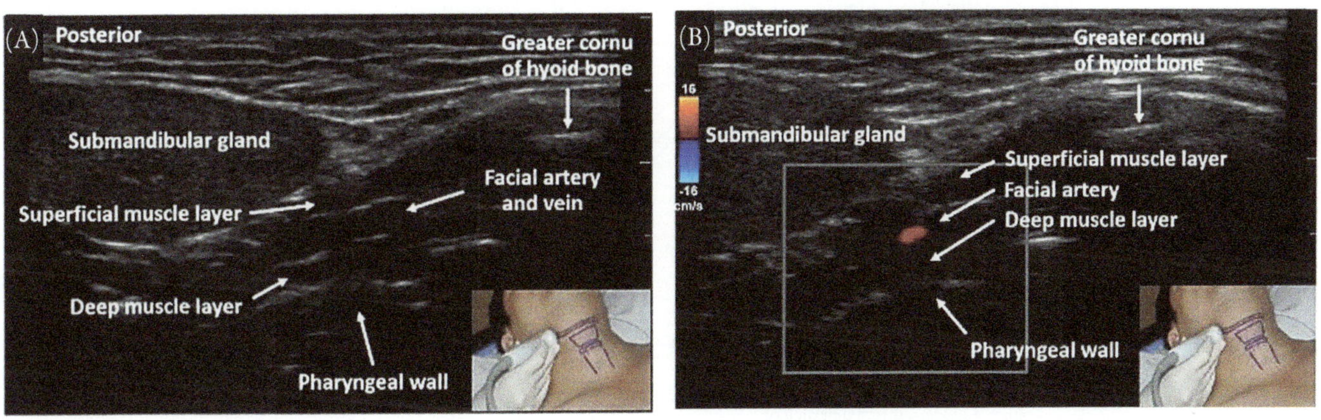

Figure 8.5. Ultrasound-guided glossopharyngeal nerve block, described by Azman et al.: (A) important structures relevant to this technique; (B) color Doppler mode used to detect facial artery.

patients with dysrhythmias, only one required treatment with propranolol.[36]

SUPERIOR LARYNGEAL NERVE BLOCK

When combined with oropharyngeal topical anesthesia, superior laryngeal nerve block can produce adequate airway anesthesia for awake intubation techniques, including AFOI. It can be performed via external or internal approaches.

External Approaches

The external approach aims to inject LA into either paraglottic space or preepiglottic space. In this approach, the patient is placed supine with the head slightly extended. This position is useful for identification of the greater cornu of the hyoid bone and the superior cornu of the thyroid cartilage, which are the key landmarks for this block. Of note, when attempting to palpate the hyoid bone, care must be taken, since it can be fractured easily if excessive force is applied.

Injection into the Paraglottic Space

The paraglottic space, containing the internal branch of the superior laryngeal nerve, is the space bound by the thyrohyoid membrane laterally and the laryngeal mucosa medially.

For this method, the greater cornu of the hyoid bone is identified by deep palpation, and the carotid artery is displaced laterally and posteriorly by the nondominant hand. A 25-gauge needle is inserted until it makes contact with the bone. After that, the needle is walked off the greater cornu in an anterior-inferior direction, and then advanced 2–3 mm more. Normally, resistance is felt as the needle is advanced through the thyrohyoid membrane. After negative aspiration, 2–3 mL of LA is injected as the needle is withdrawn. This procedure is then performed on the other side (A in Figure 8.6) The onset of this block is about 1 minute, and the success rate has been reported to be as high as 92%.[40]

As an alternative, if the greater cornu of the hyoid bone is difficult to identify, the superior cornu of the thyroid cartilage may be used as a landmark. The block needle is walked off the superior thyroid cornu in a superior-anterior direction, and the LA is injected in the same manner.

Injection into the Preepiglottic Space

The preepiglottic space usually contains the terminal branches of the internal branch of superior laryngeal nerve embedded in a fat pad. This method is very useful in morbidly obese patients, in whom the identification of anatomical landmarks might be problematic. In addition, it also decreases the likelihood of the blockade of the motor branch.

In this approach, the thyroid notch is identified, and the superior border of thyroid cartilage is traced laterally for 2 cm. A 25-gauge needle is then inserted above this point in a superior-posterior direction to a depth of 1–2 cm. After negative aspiration, 2–3 mL of LA is injected into this space. This is then repeated on the contralateral side (B in Figure 8.6).

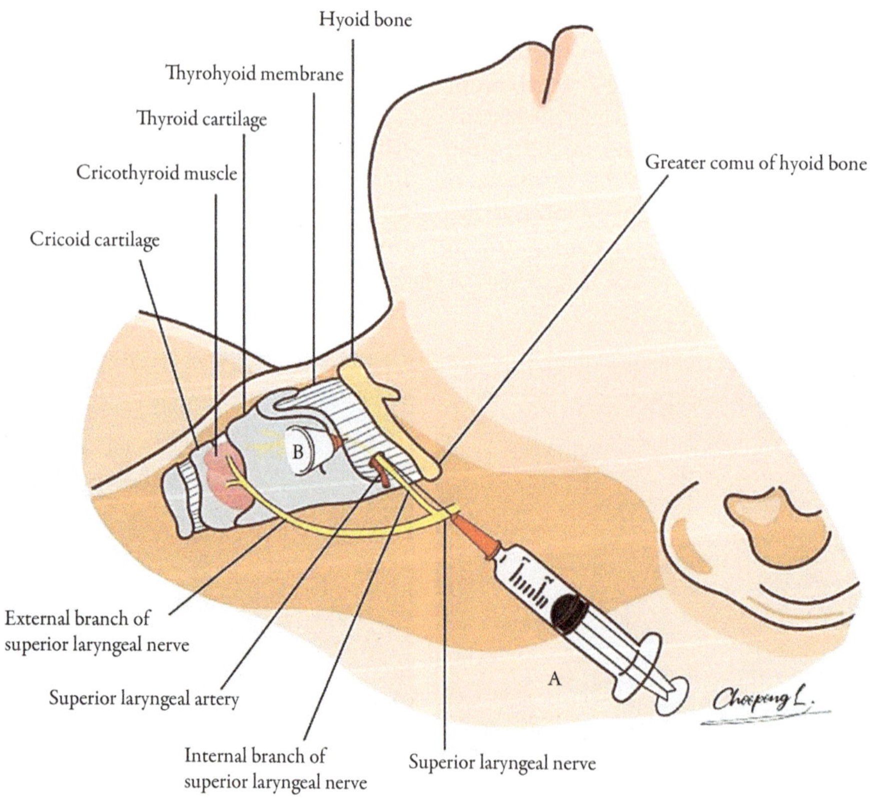

Figure 8.6. Superior laryngeal nerve block, external approach: (A) injection into the paraglottic space; (B) injection into the preepiglottic space.

Internal Approach

The superior laryngeal nerve block can also be achieved by applying LA to the pyriform fossa, where the internal branch of the superior laryngeal nerve lies just beneath the mucosa.

For this approach, after LA is applied topically to the tongue and pharynx, the patient is placed in the sitting position, and asked to open the mouth wide. The tongue is gently pulled anteriorly. A Krause forceps, armed with cottonoids soaked in 4% cocaine or 4% lidocaine, is advanced downward along the curvature of the tongue until it meets resistance. Then, the cottonoids are placed at this location for at least 5 minutes, and the procedure is performed on the other side.

Ultrasound-Guided Technique

Ultrasound guidance can be beneficial in performing the superior laryngeal nerve block, especially in patients whose anatomy is difficult to identify.[41,42] Since the hyoid bone, thyroid cartilage, and thyrohyoid membrane can be easily visualized by the ultrasound (Figure 8.7A and B), ultrasound-guided technique can improve the accuracy and reduce the risk of complications of the block.

A high-frequency linear transducer is positioned in the sagittal plane to identify the greater cornu of the hyoid bone (Figure 8.7A, B). It is then rotated 90 degrees to identify the superolateral aspect of the thyrohyoid membrane. The internal branch of the superior laryngeal nerve may be sometimes visualized with ultrasound, located near the superior laryngeal artery, just below the greater cornu of the hyoid bone and superficial to the thyrohyoid membrane.[43] Using an in-plane approach, the block needle is inserted from the lateral side, targeting slightly below the greater cornu of the hyoid bone. Then, the LA is injected after negative aspiration. In case the nerve cannot be identified, the block can also be done by injection of the LA just superficial to the thyrohyoid membrane.[44]

Complications

Several complications of the superior laryngeal nerve block have been reported. Laryngeal edema causing airway obstruction might happen due to the direct puncture of the thyroid cartilage, leading to an injection of the solution at the level of the vocal cords.[19] In addition, due to the proximity of the carotid artery, intravascular injection could occur, which might induce seizures.[45]

Furthermore, hypotension and bradycardia have also been reported.[46] These might be caused via several mechanisms, for instance, excessive pressure on the carotid sinus, vasovagal reaction, accidental intravascular injection, and direct stimulation of the vagus nerve. Other potential complications include hematoma, pharyngeal puncture, and rupture of the endotracheal tube (ET) cuff in patients already intubated.[19,20]

TRANSLARYNGEAL BLOCK

Sensory innervation of the mucosa below the vocal cords is supplied by the recurrent laryngeal nerves, but bilateral blocks of these nerves should be avoided as these would result in bilateral vocal cord paralysis, leading to airway obstruction. A safer method is topicalization of the mucosa, which can be achieved by the several techniques mentioned earlier, as well as a translaryngeal block.

Translaryngeal block is not a true peripheral nerve block technique. In fact, it is a method used for applying LA topically to the laryngeal and tracheal mucosa. A study showed that this method is favored by patients and anesthesiologists over both nebulization and "spray-as-you-go" technique.[47] The success of this method has been shown to be as high as 95% and is attributed to both topicalization of the airway and systemic absorption.[48,49]

For this technique, the patient should be placed in the supine position and ideally with neck extension (if possible and not contraindicated). The cricothyroid membrane is identified by palpating of the thyroid notch and following it caudally until a depression between the thyroid cartilage and the cricoid cartilage is found. The nondominant hand is usually used to stabilize the larynx, and mark the midline of the membrane, which is the needle-insertion point.

After skin infiltration has been made, a standard 20- or 22-gauge needle connected with 5- or 10-mL syringe containing 3–5 mL of 4% lidocaine is inserted perpendicular to the skin. This should be done with continuous aspiration of the syringe, as free aspiration of air will indicate penetration of the

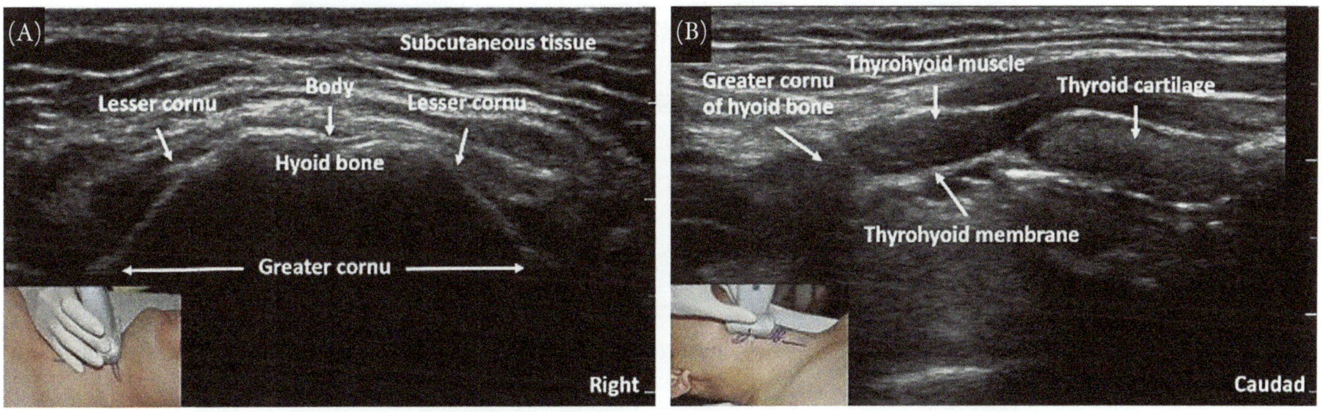

Figure 8.7. Ultrasound-guided superior laryngeal nerve block: (A) transverse scan at the level of hyoid bone; (B) parasagittal scan.

membrane and entry into the airway. Then, advancing of the needle must be stopped immediately to avoid puncturing the posterior laryngeal wall. At this point, the patient should be informed to expect coughing, and asked to exhale forcefully. The LA is then injected rapidly into the lumen. Coughing makes the patient inhale and disperse the LA, leading to adequate anesthesia of the deeper airway.

An alternative approach is to use an angiocatheter instead of the standard needle. This can minimize the risk of airway injury caused by the sharp metal bevel as the patient coughs. For this technique, the angiocatheter is connected to a 5-mL syringe containing 2–3 mL of saline. Once air is freely aspirated, the plastic sheath is advanced into the lumen, and the needle is then removed. The LA is rapidly injected through the sheath after intraluminal position is confirmed by aspiration of air. It is suggested that the catheter should be left in place until the intubation is complete to reduce the chance of subcutaneous emphysema. It can also serve as a marker to confirm entry of the bronchoscope into the trachea.

Ultrasound-Guided Technique

Ultrasound can also be used to facilitate the translaryngeal block when the patient's landmark is unidentifiable.

Using a high-frequency linear transducer, the probe is placed longitudinally in the midline of the trachea. The probe is then moved cephalad until the cricoid cartilage can be found. Normally, the cricoid cartilage is larger and more superficial than the tracheal rings. Next, the probe is further advanced until the thyroid cartilage can be seen. The cricothyroid membrane is located between the inferior border of the thyroid cartilage and the superior border of the cricoid cartilage (Figure 8.8). Finally, the midline of the membrane is marked on the patient's neck, and the translaryngeal block can be performed as described earlier. [50] The ultrasound images of thyroid cartilage, cricothyroid membrane, cricoid cartilage, and trachea are demonstrated in Figures 8.8 and 8.9. It is essential that careful scanning for adjacent vascular structures should be performed, in order to determine the safest puncture site and trajectory.

Furthermore, this block can be performed under real-time ultrasound guidance by moving the probe to a parasagittal position. Using an out-of-plane approach, the needle is then inserted just cephalad to the cricoid cartilage under ultrasound visualization and advanced until air is freely aspirated.

Complications

A serious complication of this block is bleeding and subsequent hematoma, which could cause airway compromise. Since the superior cricothyroid vessels cross this membrane horizontally in its upper third, and venous tributaries from the inferior thyroid and anterior jugular veins lie lateral to the membrane, to minimize this risk, the needle must be inserted at the lower third in the midline of the membrane.[51,52] This highlights the advantages of the ultrasound-guided and ultrasound-assisted techniques that should minimize the risks of vascular injury.

Other potential risks include injury to the vocal cords, posterior wall of the larynx, and esophagus. Therefore, it is critical that the needle should not be aimed in a cephalad direction, or advanced too far.[19]

Due to the fact that coughing is inevitable during this block, this method should be avoided when vigorous coughing is to be avoided, as in patients with increased intracranial or intraocular pressures, or unstable cervical fracture. In addition, this procedure might be considered relatively contraindicated in patients at high risk of aspiration because it significantly diminishes the cough reflex.[19,20]

Other potential complications are laryngospasm, infection, subcutaneous emphysema, pneumomediastinum, and pneumothorax.[19,49,53,54] However, these complications are rare, with an incidence of complications of less than 0.01%.[49]

CONCLUSION

There are many well-described techniques to anesthetize different parts of the airway, used in preparation for awake fiberoptic intubation. Topical anesthesia combined with minimal sedation can be effective, relatively well tolerated, and most likely to be

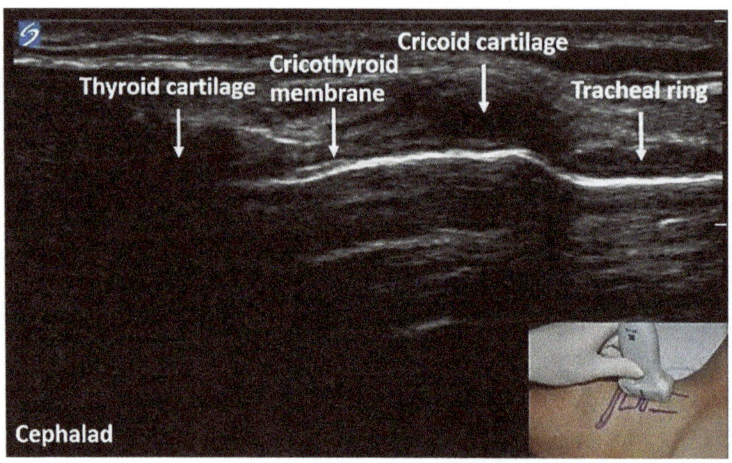

Figure 8.8. Ultrasound-guided translaryngeal block, sagittal scan.

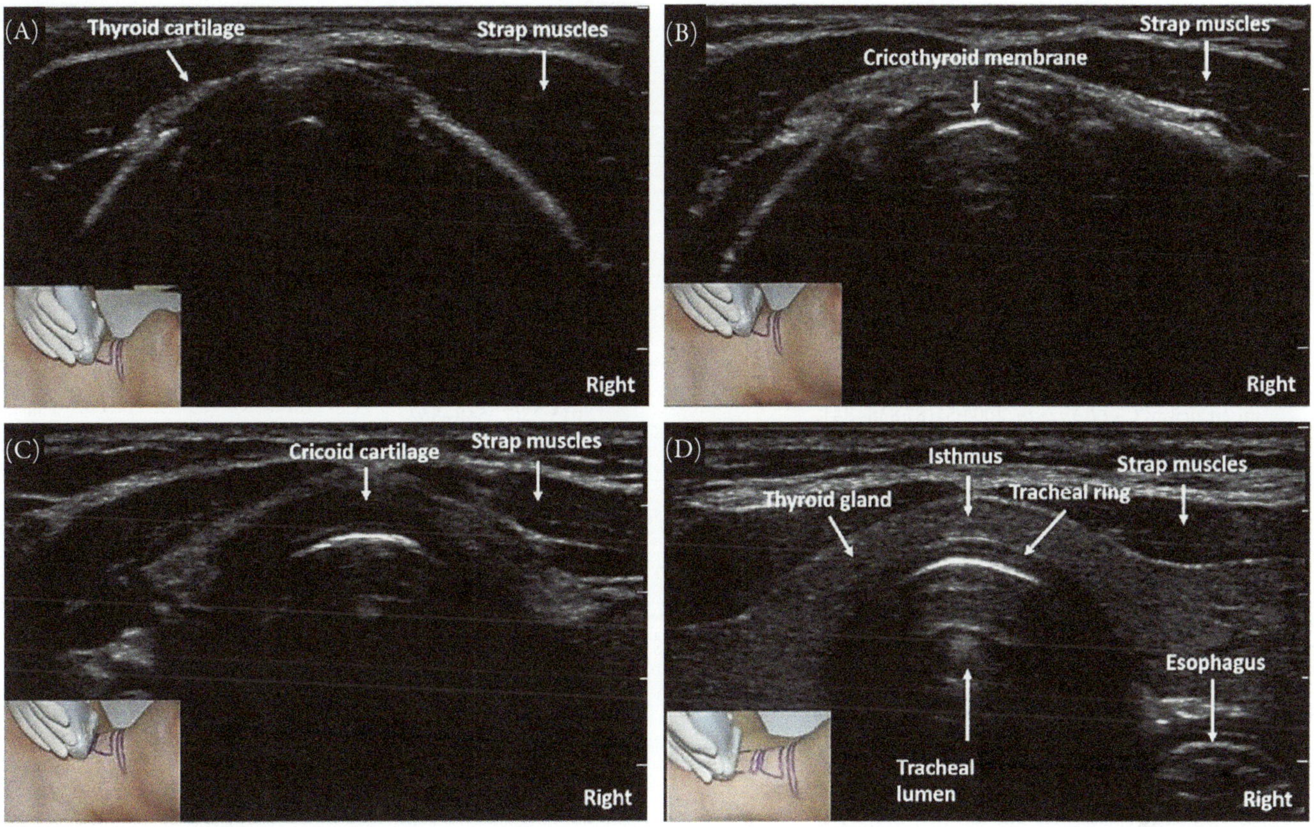

Figure 8.9. Ultrasound-guided translaryngeal block, transverse scan: (A) at the level of thyroid cartilage; (B) at the level of cricothyroid membrane; (C) at the level of cricoid cartilage; (D) at the level of the trachea.

chosen. Nevertheless, in some patients, regional anesthesia techniques are needed to provide more complete anesthesia of the airway. These typically require higher operator expertise and also carry additional risks. The anesthesiologist must weigh the risks and benefits of these methods and rationally select the safest, most effective, and best-suited approach for each patient, facilitating awake fiberoptic intubation in a difficult airway situation.

REFERENCES

1. Azman J, Stopar Pintaric T, Cvetko E, Vlassakov K. Ultrasound-guided glossopharyngeal nerve block: a cadaver and a volunteer sonoanatomy study. *Reg Anesth Pain Med.* 2017;42(2):252–258.
2. Farag E, Mounir-Soliman L, Brown DL. *Brown's Atlas of Regional Anesthesia*. Sixth ed. Philadelphia PA: Elsevier; 2021.
3. Neal JM, Barrington MJ, Fettiplace MR, et al. The Third American Society of Regional Anesthesia and Pain Medicine practice advisory on local anesthetic systemic toxicity: executive summary 2017. *Reg Anesth Pain Med.* 2018;43(2):113–123.
4. Kodama K, Seo N, Murayama T, Yoshizawa Y, Terasako K, Yaginuma T. Glossopharyngeal nerve block for carotid sinus syndrome. *Anesth Analg.* 1992;75(6):1036–1037.
5. Walts LF. Anesthesia of the larynx in the patient with a full stomach. *JAMA.* 1965;192:705–706.
6. Li G, Warner M, Lang BH, Huang L, Sun LS. Epidemiology of anesthesia-related mortality in the United States, 1999–2005. *Anesthesiology.* 2009;110(4):759–765.
7. Ramachandran SK, Klock PA. Chapter 8: Definition and incidence of the difficult airway. In: Hagberg CA, ed. *Benumof and Hagberg's Airway Management.* 3rd ed. Philadelphia: W. B. Saunders; 2013:201–208;e202.
8. Joffe AM, Aziz MF, Posner KL, Duggan LV, Mincer SL, Domino KB. Management of difficult tracheal intubation: a closed claims analysis. *Anesthesiology.* 2019;131(4):818–829.
9. Cheney FW, Posner KL, Lee LA, Caplan RA, Domino KB. Trends in anesthesia-related death and brain damage: a closed claims analysis. *Anesthesiology.* 2006;105(6):1081–1086.
10. Wong J, Lee JSE, Wong TGL, Iqbal R, Wong P. Fibreoptic intubation in airway management: a review article. *Singapore Med J.* 2019;60(3):110–118.
11. Standring S. Nose, nasal cavity and paranasal sinuses In: Strandring S, Gray H, eds. *Gray's Anatomy: The Anatomical Basis of Clinical Practice.* Philadelphia: Elsevier; 2021:686–701;e681.
12. Dalley AF, Agur AMR, Moore KL. *Moore's Clinically Oriented Anatomy.* 8th ed. Philadelphia: Wolters Kluwer; 2018.
13. Simmons ST, Schleich AR. Airway regional anesthesia for awake fiberoptic intubation. *Reg Anesth Pain Med.* 2002;27(2):180–192.
14. Srandring S. Infratemporal and pterygopalatine fossae and temporomandibular joint. In: Strandring S, Gray H, eds. *Gray's Anatomy: The Anatomical Basis of Clinical Practice.* Philadelphia: Elsevier; 2021:664–685;e662.
15. Waldman S. Sphenopalatine ganglion block: transnasal approach. In: Waldman S, ed. *Waldman: Atlas of Interventional Pain Management.* 5th ed. Philadelphia: Elsevier; 2021:13–16.
16. Standring S. Pharynx. In: Standring S, Gray H, eds. *Gray's Anatomy: The Anatomical Basis of Clinical Practice.* Philadelphia: Elsevier; 2021:702–716.
17. Standring S. Mouth In: Standring R, Gray H, eds. *Gray's Anatomy: The Anatomical Basis of Clinical Practice.* Philadelphia: Elsevier; 2021:636–663;e631.
18. Ahmad I. Regional and topical anesthesia for awake endotraceal intubation. In: Hadzic A, ed. *Hadzic's Textbook of Regional Anesthesia and Acute Pain Management.* New York: McGraw-Hill Education; 2017:289–299.

19. Artime C, Sanchez A. Preparation of the patient for awake intubation. In: Hagberg CA, Artime CA, Aziz MF, eds. *Hagberg and Benumof's Airway Management.* 4th ed. Philadelphia: Elsevier; 2018:216–234.
20. Morris I. Preparation for awake intubation. In: Hung OR, Murphy MF, eds. *Management of the Difficult and Failed Airway.* New York: McGraw-Hill Medical; 2012.
21. Standring R. Neck. In: Standring S, Gray H, eds. *Gray's Anatomy: The Anatomical Basis of Clinical Practice.* Philadelphia: Elsevier; 2021:573–606.
22. Standring R. Larynx. In: Standring R, Gray H, eds. *Gray's Anatomy: The Anatomical Basis of Clinical Practice.* Philadelphia: Elsevier; 2021:717–734;e714.
23. Ho AM, Chung DC, To EW, Karmakar MK. Total airway obstruction during local anesthesia in a non-sedated patient with a compromised airway. *Can J Anaesth.* 2004;51(8):838–841.
24. McGuire G, el-Beheiry H. Complete upper airway obstruction during awake fibreoptic intubation in patients with unstable cervical spine fractures. *Can J Anaesth.* 1999;46(2):176–178.
25. Shaw IC, Welchew EA, Harrison BJ, Michael S. Complete airway obstruction during awake fibreoptic intubation. *Anaesthesia.* 1997;52(6):582–585.
26. Gil KS, Diemunsch PA. Flexible scope intubation techniques. In: Hagberg CA, Artime CA, Aziz MF, eds. *Hagberg and Benumof's Airway Management.* 4th ed. Philadelphia: Elsevier; 2018:428–470.
27. Bourke DL, Katz J, Tonneson A. Nebulized anesthesia for awake endotracheal intubation. *Anesthesiology.* 1985;63(6):690–692.
28. Heyder J. Particle transport onto human airway surfaces. *Eur J Respir Dis Suppl.* 1982;119:29–50.
29. Kundra P, Kutralam S, Ravishankar M. Local anaesthesia for awake fibreoptic nasotracheal intubation. *Acta Anaesthesiol Scand.* 2000;44(5):511–516.
30. Gupta B, Kohli S, Farooque K, et al. Topical airway anesthesia for awake fiberoptic intubation: comparison between airway nerve blocks and nebulized lignocaine by ultrasonic nebulizer. *Saudi J Anaesth.* 2014;8(Suppl 1):S15–S19.
31. Bhatnagar N, Orebaugh S. Regional anesthesia blocks for awake intubation. In: Orebaugh S, Bigeleisen PE, eds. *Atlas of Airway Management: Techniques and Tools.* 2nd ed. Philadelphia: Lippincott, Williams & Wilkins; 2012:55–60.
32. Rosenblatt W, Abrons R, Sukhupragar W. Airway management. In: Holt NF, Ortega RA, Barash PG, et al., eds. *Clinical Anesthesia.* 8th ed. Philadelphia: Lippincott, Williams & Wilkins; 2017:767–808.
33. Hagberg. CA, Artime. CA. Airway management in the adult. In: Miller RD, ed. *Miller's Anesthesia*, Vol 1. 8th ed. Philadelphia: Saunders; 2015:1647–1683.
34. Benumof JL. Management of the difficult adult airway: with special emphasis on awake tracheal intubation. *Anesthesiology.* 1991;75(6):1087–1110.
35. Waldman S. Glosspharyngeal nerve block: extraoral approach. In: Waldman SD, ed. *Atlas of Interventional Pain Management.* Philadelphia: Elsevier; 2021:103.
36. DeMeester TR, Skinner DB, Evans RH, Benson DW. Local nerve block anesthesia for peroral endoscopy. *Ann Thorac Surg.* 1977;24(3):278–283.
37. Cooper M, Watson RL. An improved regional anesthetic technique for peroral endoscopy. *Anesthesiology.* 1975;43(3):372–374.
38. Liu Q, Zhong Q, Tang G, He G. Ultrasound-guided glossopharyngeal nerve block via the styloid process for glossopharyngeal neuralgia: a retrospective study. *J Pain Res.* 2019;12:2503–2510.
39. Singh PM, Dehran M, Mohan VK, Trikha A, Kaur M. Analgesic efficacy and safety of medical therapy alone vs combined medical therapy and extraoral glossopharyngeal nerve block in glossopharyngeal neuralgia. *Pain Med.* 2013;14(1):93–102.
40. Furlan JC. Anatomical study applied to anesthetic block technique of the superior laryngeal nerve. *Acta Anaesthesiol Scand.* 2002;46(2):199–202.
41. Ambi US, Arjun BK, Masur S, Endigeri A, Hosalli V, Hulakund SY. Comparison of ultrasound and anatomical landmark-guided technique for superior laryngeal nerve block to aid awake fibre-optic intubation: a prospective randomised clinical study. *Indian J Anaesth.* 2017;61(6):463–468.
42. Kumar A, Sinha C, Kumar A, Bhadani UK. Transverse approach for ultrasound-guided superior laryngeal nerve block for awake fiberoptic intubation. *Saudi J Anaesth.* 2017;11(3):373–374.
43. Kaur B, Tang R, Sawka A, Krebs C, Vaghadia H. A method for ultrasonographic visualization and injection of the superior laryngeal nerve: volunteer study and cadaver simulation. *Anesth Analg.* 2012;115(5):1242–1245.
44. Stopar-Pintaric T, Vlassakov K, Azman J, Cvetko E. The thyrohyoid membrane as a target for ultrasonography-guided block of the internal branch of the superior laryngeal nerve. *J Clin Anesth.* 2015;27(7):548–552.
45. Hsu CH, Lin TC, Yeh CC, Ho ST, Wong CS. Convulsions during superior laryngeal nerve block: a case report. *Acta Anaesthesiol Sinica.* 2000;38(2):93–96.
46. Wiles JR, Kelly J, Mostafa SM. Hypotension and bradycardia following superior laryngeal nerve block. *Br J Anaesth.* 1989;63(1):125–127.
47. Graham DR, Hay JG, Clague J, Nisar M, Earis JE. Comparison of three different methods used to achieve local anesthesia for fiberoptic bronchoscopy. *Chest.* 1992;102(3):704–707.
48. Boster SR, Danzl DF, Madden RJ, Jarboe CH. Translaryngeal absorption of lidocaine. *Ann Emerg Med.* 1982;11(9):461–465.
49. Gold MI, Buechel DR. Translaryngeal anesthesia: a review. *Anesthesiology.* 1959;20(2):181–185.
50. De Oliveira GS Jr., Fitzgerald P, Kendall M. Ultrasound-assisted translaryngeal block for awake fibreoptic intubation. *Can J Anaesth.* 2011;58(7):664–665.
51. Dover K, Howdieshell TR, Colborn GL. The dimensions and vascular anatomy of the cricothyroid membrane: relevance to emergent surgical airway access. *Clin Anat.* 1996;9(5):291–295.
52. Goumas P, Kokkinis K, Petrocheilos J, Naxakis S, Mochloulis G. Cricothyroidotomy and the anatomy of the cricothyroid space: an autopsy study. *J Laryngol Otol.* 1997;111(4):354–356.
53. Wong DT, McGuire GP. Subcutaneous emphysema following transcricothyroid membrane injection of local anesthetic. *Can J Anaesth.* 2000;47(2):165–168.
54. Danzl DF, Thomas DM. Nasotracheal intubations in the emergency department. *Crit Care Med.* 1980;8(11):677–682.

REVIEW QUESTIONS

(1) A 60-year-old male with squamous cell carcinoma of tongue is scheduled for glossectomy with modified radical neck dissection. The anesthesiologist plans to perform awake nasal fiberoptic intubation. Block of which nerve would provide the LEAST benefit for this patient?

A. Olfactory nerve
B. Greater palatine nerve
C. Nasopalatine nerve
D. Anterior ethmoidal nerve

(2) Regarding the innervation of larynx, which of the following is correct?

A. The superior laryngeal nerve arises from inferior ganglion of the vagus nerve and crosses anteriorly to the greater cornu of the hyoid bone.
B. Sensory innervation of the anterior surface of epiglottis is supplied by the internal branch of superior laryngeal nerve.

C. Sensory innervation of the false vocal cord is supplied by the recurrent laryngeal nerve.
D. The recurrent laryngeal nerve provides motor fibers to all intrinsic muscles of larynx.

(3) Which local anesthetic (LA) has intrinsic vasoconstrictor properties?

A. Lidocaine
B. Bupivacaine
C. Benzocaine
D. Cocaine

(4) A 20-year-old male is brought to the trauma center after a motorcycle accident. The CT scan shows a large epidural hematoma at the temporal region with cervical spine fracture at the levels of C5 and C6. He is emergently brought to the OR for craniotomy with clot removal.

Which of the following techniques for preparation of fiberoptic intubation should be avoided?

A. Bilateral superior laryngeal nerve blocks using external approach with 2 mL of 2% lidocaine each side
B. Bilateral glossopharyngeal nerve blocks using intraoral anterior approach with 2 mL of 1% lidocaine each side
C. Translaryngeal block with 3 mL of 4% lidocaine
D. Nebulization with 4 mL of 4% lidocaine

(5) Which of the following is true about sphenopalatine ganglion block?

A. The sphenopalatine ganglion lies just posterior to the inferior turbinate.
B. Epinephrine should be avoided in this block due to high absorption rate.
C. Sphenopalatine ganglion can also be blocked through the incisive foramen.
D. This block can also be useful in treatment of post-dural puncture headache.

(6) Which structures lies in close proximity to glossopharyngeal nerve at the level of styloid process?

A. Trigeminal nerve
B. Facial nerve
C. Hypoglossal nerve
D. Common carotid artery

(7) After performing superior laryngeal nerve block with 3 mL of 2% lidocaine, the patient develops sudden onset of bradycardia. Which of the following mechanisms is LEAST likely to cause bradycardia in this patient?

A. Excessive pressure on the carotid sinus
B. Blockade of the glossopharyngeal nerve
C. Accidental intravascular injection
D. Direct stimulation of the vagus nerve

(8) Which of the following statements is FALSE about translaryngeal block?

A. Ultrasound-guided technique can be useful while performing this block in obese patients.
B. The needle should be aimed in a cephalad direction in order to anesthetize the mucosa overlying the vocal cords effectively.
C. The needle should be inserted at the lower third of the membrane to avoid puncture of the superior cricothyroid vessels.
D. The success rate of this block is usually higher than 90%.

ANSWERS

(1) **A.** While the other nerves provide general sensory innervation to the septum and lateral wall of nasal cavity, the olfactory nerve carries only special sensory fibers relating to olfaction, thus its blockade is not necessary for awake intubation.

Reference

Strandring S. Nasal cavity and paranasal sinuses. In: Standring S, ed. *Gray's Anatomy*. Philadelphia: Elsevier; 2021:686–701.

(2) **A.** The superior laryngeal nerve arises from inferior ganglion of the vagus nerve and crosses anteriorly to the greater cornu of the hyoid bone. It provides sensory innervation to the mucosa above the true vocal cords, which includes the mucosa overlying false vocal cords. It also supplies motor function to cricothyroid muscle, while the other intrinsic muscles of larynx are innervated by the recurrent laryngeal nerve. However, the anterior surface of epiglottis is usually supplied by the glossopharyngeal nerve.

Reference

Standring S, Larynx. In: Standring S, ed. *Gray's Anatomy*. Philadelphia: Elsevier; 2021:717–734.

(3) **D.** The unique characteristic of cocaine is local vasoconstriction due to inhibition of local noradrenaline reuptake. This can be beneficial for the topical anesthesia as it provides both anesthesia and shrinking of the mucosa, leading to less bleeding during instrumentation.

Reference

Ahmad I. Regional and topical anesthesia for awake endotraceal intubation. In: Hadzic A, ed. *Hadzic's Textbook of Regional Anesthesia and Acute Pain Management*. New York: McGraw-Hill Education; 2017:289–99.

4. C Translaryngeal block should be avoided in a patient who has increased intracranial pressure since vigorous coughing might be detrimental. Besides, in trauma patients suspected with basilar skull fracture, direct application of LA in the nasal cavity should be avoided to prevent accidental intracranial placement.

References

Artime CA, Sanchez A. Preparation of the patient for awake intubation. In: Hagberg CA, Artime CA, Aziz MF, eds. *Hagberg and Benumof's Airway Management*. 4th ed. Philadelphia: Elsevier; 2018:216–234.
Morris IR. Preparation for awake intubation. In: Hung O, Murphy MF, eds. *Management of the Difficult and Failed Airway*. 2nd ed. China: McGraw-Hill; 2012:30–67.

(5) **D.** The sphenopalatine ganglion block is effective for anesthetizing the nasal mucosa. It can be achieved by either direct application of LA to the mucosa posterior to the middle turbinate or injection of LA via the greater palatine foramen. For this block, the epinephrine should be added to the LA to reduce the incidence of epistaxis. Apart from this indication, it is also useful for treatment of post-dural puncture headache.

Reference

Waldman SD. Sphenopalatine ganglion block: transnasal approach. In: Waldman SD, ed. *Atlas of Interventional Pain Management*. 5th ed. Philadelphia: Elsevier; 2021:13–16.

(6) **C.** At the level of styloid process, the glossopharyngeal nerve emerges from the jugular foramen and lies adjacent to the internal carotid artery, the internal jugular vein, the vagus nerve, the accessory nerve, and the hypoglossal nerve.

Reference

Farag E, Mounir-Soliman L, Brown DL. *Brown's Atlas of Regional Anesthesia*. 6th ed. Philadelphia: Elsevier; 2021.

(7) **B.** Bradycardia has been reported after the superior laryngeal nerve block. This can result from several mechanisms, including excessive pressure on the carotid sinus, accidental intravascular injection, and direct stimulation of the vagus nerve. However, blockade of the glossopharyngeal nerve is likely to cause tachycardia rather than bradycardia since it inhibits the afferent input from the carotid sinus.

Reference

Wiles JR, Kelly J, Mostafa SM. Hypotension and bradycardia following superior laryngeal nerve block. *Br J Anaesth*. 1989;63(1):125–127.

(8) **B.** Translaryngeal block is a useful and highly effective method for anesthetizing the mucosa below the vocal cords. The success rate of this technique is usually more than 90%. This can be successfully done by using either landmark or ultrasound-guided technique. For this block, the needle should be inserted at the lower third of the membrane to avoid puncture of the superior cricothyroid vessels, and advanced perpendicularly or slightly caudally to avoid laryngeal trauma.

Reference

De Oliveira GS, Jr., Fitzgerald P, Kendall M. Ultrasound-assisted translaryngeal block for awake fibreoptic intubation. *Can J Anaesth*. 2011;58(7):664–665.

9.

SCALP BLOCKS

AN OVERVIEW OF INDICATIONS, ANATOMY, AND TECHNIQUE

Arthur Formanek

STEM CASE AND KEY QUESTIONS

A 56-year-old man with chronic headaches, obstructive sleep apnea (OSA), and coronary artery disease (CAD) presents with new onset seizure. A left-sided intracranial mass is discovered on imaging and he is scheduled for craniotomy and tumor resection. Your pre-anesthesia evaluation reveals the above past medical history and no significant past surgical history. MRI T2-FLAIR reveals a mass in the left posterior portion of the superior temporal gyrus. Physical exam is notable for Mallampati 3 airway exam, blood pressure 135/85, heart rate 85, body mass index (BMI) 35 (height 5′10″, weight 245 lb.), 5/5 strength in upper and lower extremities bilaterally, no pronator drift, and fluent appropriate speech. The neurosurgeon requests the case be done "awake."

(1) WHY IS THE SURGEON REQUESTING THAT THE CASE BE DONE "AWAKE?" WHAT ARE THE INDICATIONS FOR AN AWAKE CRANIOTOMY? WHAT ARE THE CONTRAINDICATIONS?

Indications for awake craniotomy include resections in the motor strip, insula, or in eloquent brain areas such as Wernicke's or Broca's, as well as seizure surgeries to locate epileptogenic areas. Relative contraindications include patients who are unable to adequately communicate or cooperate with an intraoperative neurologic assessment, such as very young patients or those with dementia or speech deficits.[1,2]

(2) WHAT ARE THE THREE PHASES OF ANESTHETIC DEPTH IN AN AWAKE CRANIOTOMY? WHAT IS YOUR PLAN FOR ANALGESIA AND SEDATION?

Frequently, the sequence for awake craniotomy can be described as "asleep, awake, asleep"; the patient may be deeply sedated or under general anesthesia for pinning, incision, craniotomy, durotomy, and closure but must be fully interactive during mapping and resection.[3] Plan for analgesia and sedation would include a scalp block preoperatively with ropivacaine or bupivacaine, augmented with a sphenopalatine ganglion block. While not necessary, during the "asleep" portions, propofol would be administered to provide deep sedation or general anesthesia with a natural airway. During the "awake" portion, sedation and analgesia augmentation would be provided with remifentanil and dexmedetomidine.

(3) DO YOU FIND ANYTHING CONCERNING IN THE PATIENT'S PAST MEDICAL HISTORY FOR AN AWAKE CRANIOTOMY? WHAT WOULD YOU DO TO MITIGATE THESE RISKS?

The patient has a history of OSA and is obese, which could lead to obstruction during the "asleep" portions of the case. Since the patient will be in Mayfield pins, head tilt to relieve obstruction will be impossible and intubation would likely be very challenging. A nasopharyngeal airway could be useful in ameliorating airway obstruction. An Laryngeal Mask Airway could also be used for the "asleep" portions, but great care would have to be taken to avoid the occurrence of "bucking" in pins. Furthermore, the patient has CAD, and sympathetic surge from inadequate analgesia could lead to increased myocardial stress; adequate analgesia, either from the scalp block or other anesthetics, is necessary during the painful portions of the surgery.

(4) HOW WOULD YOU PERFORM A SCALP BLOCK? WOULD A UNILATERAL SCALP BLOCK BE APPROPRIATE?

A classic scalp block is performed by blocking the greater and lesser occipital nerves, the auriculotemporal nerve, the zygomaticotemporal nerve, the supraorbital nerve, and the supratrochlear nerve. Additionally, a sphenopalatine ganglion block may be performed for dural anesthesia. A unilateral scalp block is rarely performed for awake craniotomy because of the pain and sympathetic surge from Mayfield pinning. If the block is performed preoperatively for postoperative pain control, a unilateral block may be performed with the knowledge that Mayfield pinning will induce a sympathetic surge similar to an unblocked patient.

(5) WHAT ARE THE RISKS OF A SCALP BLOCK?

Risk of scalp blocks include intravascular injection or absorption of local anesthetic, as the scalp is highly vascular.

Postoperative interference with a neurological exam may also occur if the facial nerve is inadvertently blocked. Edema from large-volume injection or hematoma from vascular puncture may cause mechanical ptosis and obscure physical exam findings.

(6) THE PATIENT TOLERATES INCISION AND CRANIOTOMY WELL. DURING DUROTOMY, THAT PATENT STARTS TO COMPLAIN OF A HEADACHE. IS THERE A WAY TO AUGMENT THE SCALP BLOCK TO COVER THIS PAIN?

A sphenopalatine ganglion block will help cover dural innervation, but dural innervation is complex and the patient may still complain of headache if the dura is manipulated intraoperatively. Hence, augmentation with other analgesics is often necessary for the patient to be calmly interactive during the resection.

(7) WHILE THE SURGEON IS RESECTING THE TUMOR, THE PATIENT'S SPEECH BECOMES GARBLED. WHAT DO YOU DO?

The purpose of performing awake craniotomy is to enable real-time monitoring of physical exam changes to improve surgical resection. Such a change would warrant prompt notification of the surgeon.

(8) THE RESECTION IS PROGRESSING WELL, BUT THE PATIENT STARTS TO COMPLAIN OF A BURNING RUBBER SMELL FOLLOWED BY BILATERAL TONIC AND THEN CLONIC MUSCLE CONTRACTIONS. WHAT SHOULD BE DONE?

An interoperative seizure warrants prompt flooding of the field with cold saline and administration of a GABAergic medication such as propofol. Since the patient is in Mayfield pins, quick action is warranted to prevent cervical spine or scalp injury. Additionally, the patient's brain will likely be hyperemic postictal, worsening surgical exposure, and airway control may be needed after administration of antiepileptics.

(9) POSTOPERATIVELY, THE PATIENT IS NOTED TO HAVE A UNILATERAL PTOSIS. HOW SHOULD THE PATIENT BE EVALUATED?

A thorough neurological exam should be conducted to investigate any other focal neurological deficits or Horner's symptoms. The presence of eyelid edema or hematoma could be a cause of mechanical ptosis. Knowledge of the course of intraoperative resection would also be helpful. Blocking the auriculotemporal nerve 1 cm cranially of the tragus aids in avoiding inadvertent facial nerve blockade, which, if it occurred, should be immediately apparent after performing the block. While evolving edema may lead to mechanical ptosis, a new instance of ptosis after the patient is stable postsurgery would warrant further investigation.[4,5]

DISCUSSION

Anesthetic care of patients undergoing neurological surgery can pose unique challenges for the anesthesiologist. The anesthesiologist must have a thorough understanding of the physiology and implications of the "closed cranial box" Monro-Kellie doctrine: that the cranium is composed of a fixed-sum volume of blood, cerebral spinal fluid, and neurologic tissue.[6] In addition, the anesthesiologist must be prepared for brief painful periods during the surgery, such as Mayfield pinning and craniotomy, that produce brief but profound hemodynamic changes. Further challenges arise because of need for complete immobility while in Mayfield pins, paired with the inability to administer neuromuscular blockade given the use of neuromonitoring. Furthermore, long-acting opioids and sedatives may undesirably cloud the neurological exam in the postsurgical period. Lastly, resection in eloquent areas of brain may require "awake" surgery with the patient calm but interactive.[7]

HISTORY OF LOCAL ANESTHESIA IN NEUROSURGICAL CASES

The term "regional anesthesia" as opposed to local anesthesia infiltration was first coined by Harvey Cushing in 1902 for cocainization of major nerves for "painless operation."[8] Ironically, while he does not comment on the use of regional anesthesia for intracranial neurosurgery, he recognizes the hemodynamic benefits of regional anesthesia versus general anesthesia. In the same paper, Dr. Cushing recognized the skill and training necessary of the regional anesthetist to perform an adequate block. Published reports of subcutaneous injection of local anesthetic with vasopressors prior to surgical incision followed shortly after.[9] In 1986, Girven published the first technique describing a "scalp block" for awake craniotomy. The first double-blinded randomized study of a scalp block with bupivacaine vs. saline was not published until 1987 by Hillman et al., who recognized that despite an apparent adequate depth of anesthesia, large hemodynamic changes can still present with scalp incision.[10]

AWAKE CRANIOTOMY AND SCALP BLOCKS

INDICATIONS

Indications for awake craniotomy include resections in the motor strip, insula, or in eloquent brain areas such as Wernicke's or Broca's, as well as seizure surgeries to locate epileptogenic areas. Patients in whom awake craniotomy is contraindicated include patients who are unable to adequately communicate or cooperate with an intraoperative neurologic assessment, such as very young patients or those with dementia or speech deficits. The anesthesiologist should preoperatively perform a thorough neurologic exam to assess for preexisting neurologic deficits that may obfuscate new neurologic changes during resection.[1,2]

Brain mapping during awake craniotomy aids in maximizing the area of tumor that may be resected and limits the incidence of postoperative neurological deficits. The patient must be awake and responsive to participate in brain mapping. During brain mapping, the cortex is stimulated and the patient is conversed with and given simple commands. Any speech hesitation, aphasia, or twitches in response to stimulation are noted. Phase reversals and latency shift in somatosensory evoked potentials aid in delineating the motor cortex. Any alterations to speech are also noted during the resection.[11]

In addition to awake craniotomy, scalp blocks have been performed to augment other painful scalp and cranial surgeries, such as craniosynostosis.[12]

ANESTHETIC MANAGEMENT

The sequence for awake craniotomy frequently can be described as "asleep, awake, asleep"; the patient may be deeply sedated or under general anesthesia for pinning, incision, craniotomy, durotomy, and closure but must be fully interactive during mapping and resection.[3] Care must be taken to utilize short-acting hypnotics and analgesics to prevent oversedation during the sensitive portions of the procedure. Moreover, oversedation may lead to hypoventilation and hypercapnia with concomitant cerebral engorgement.[13] The inability to hyperventilate and control pCO_2 in such instances can make surgical exposure difficult or impossible. Reversal with naloxone or flumazenil may allow the patient to become more alert and interactive with the surgical team but may also precipitate pain and anxiety that makes the resection impossible. The anesthesiologist should note the condition of the dura as soon as craniotomy is completed; tented dura is indicative of engorged brain, while gentle pulsating dura is more suggestive of favorable exposure. Hypertonics such as mannitol or hypertonic saline may still be used to augment surgical exposure with the knowledge that no immediate improvement is possible, and the first 30 minutes may yield increased cerebral blood flow and concomitant risk of worsened exposure.[14–17] Thus, the anesthesiologist must account for time of onset of interventions before yielding to the temptation to quickly administer further hypertonic agents in hope of rapid improvement in operating conditions. As in all neurosurgical cases, reverse Trendelenburg positioning will aid in venous drainage and decrease engorgement while also increasing the risk of venous air embolism.

Short-acting opioids and sedatives that preserve the respiratory drive are optimal for awake craniotomies.[18] Remifentanil is easily and quickly titratable to optimize analgosedation, blunt coughing, and ameliorate any deficits in the scalp block.[19] In addition, opioids may relieve pain that may in turn lead to anxiety.[20] However, administering higher dose remifentanil in an awake patient may precipitate μ-related pruritis, which antihistamines are ineffective at blunting. In such cases, it would be prudent for the anesthesiologist to administer an antidopaminergic or antiserotonergic agent to combat the pruritis.[21] Dexmedetomidine also provides good sedation with preservation of spontaneous breathing, and if an adequate scalp block is performed, complete amnesia during opening and closing is not required.[22] Propofol is also a useful adjunct during the "asleep" portions of the procedure. While ketamine preserves ventilatory drive, it is a poor choice because of its potential to alter the patient's consciousness during the procedure. Insoluble volatile anesthetics such as desflurane have been described in the literature during "asleep" portions, requiring the insertion of a laryngeal mask airway.[2] Care must also be taken in patients with cardiovascular disease during craniotomy, as the drilling may precipitate intense anxiety and sympathetic stimulation if the patient is not adequately sedated.

Management of the airway during awake craniotomies can be challenging, especially in obese patients or those with obstructive sleep apnea. The head is fixed in Mayfield pins in a position to optimize surgical exposure, which frequently leads to poor neck extension. Nasopharyngeal airways, especially with lidocaine lubricant, are well tolerated in lightly sedated patients and may be of great benefit during the deeply sedated portions of the case. Great care should be exercised if an LMA or an oropharyngeal airway is used, as coughing or gagging in Mayfield pins may result in scalp laceration, or worse, cervical spine injury. If transition to general anesthesia and positive pressure ventilation is required, an LMA may be the anesthesiologist's optimal choice of airway management, as the head positioning and surgical draping will make laryngoscopy very difficult or impossible.

As the patient is awake and does not have the GABA receptor stimulation inherent to general anesthesia, the risk of intraoperative seizure exists. A discussion with the neurosurgical team regarding seizure prophylaxis should be performed. Levetiracetam is the typical first-line agent for prophylaxis because of its generally benign side-effect profile. However, the anesthesiologist should be cognizant that the addition of levetiracetam may oversedate the awake patient with an unsecured airway. If a patient suffers a seizure intraoperatively, the brain should be immediately irrigated with cold saline.[7]

SCALP BLOCK

To perform a scalp block, a total of 6 nerves bilaterally are traditionally blocked for a total of 12 injections: the greater occipital nerve, the lesser occipital nerve, the auriculotemporal nerve, the zygomaticotemporal nerve, the supraorbital nerve, and the supratrochlear nerve. As with all good regional anesthetic technique performed in a highly vascular area, negative aspiration must be confirmed before injecting local anesthetic upon needle insertion. The greater and lesser occipital nerve blocks are typically performed with the patient either sitting upright or the head turned to the opposite side to gain access to the occiput. If the anesthesiologist has better access to the occiput with the patient sitting upright, he or she may elect to perform these four injections first with the patient fully awake. Once the occipital injections are completed, the patient is allowed to lie back and be more deeply sedated for the completion of the scalp block. While unilateral scalp block is theoretically possible, it is rarely if ever performed because of the need for Mayfield pinning.

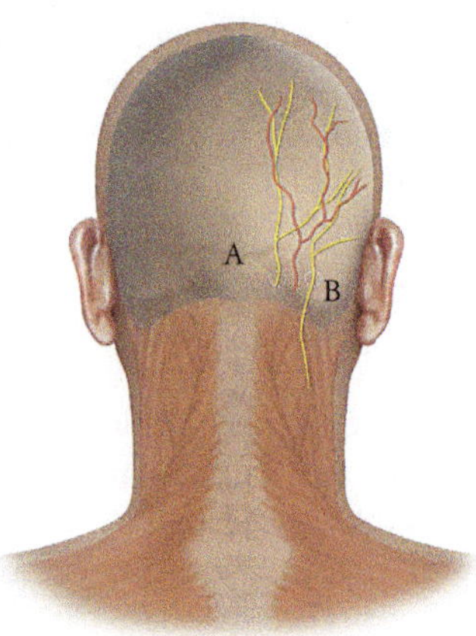

Figure 9.1. The greater occipital nerve (A) is medial to the occipital artery. The lesser occipital nerve injection site (B) should be 2.5 cm lateral to the greater occipital nerve.

Choice of Local Anesthetic

Studies describing scalp block with lidocaine, ropivacaine, bupivacaine, and levobupivacaine have been published.[23] No studies have been published investigating superiority of a specific local anesthetic, concentration, or adjuncts. This author prefers 0.5% ropivacaine for its density of blockade, duration of action, and reduced risk of cardiotoxicity given the need for injection in a highly vascular area.

Anatomy

The scalp is innervated by a mix of cranial nerves and branches of the dorsal and ventral rami. The greater and lesser occipital nerves innervate the C2 dermatome. The trigeminal nerve gives rise to the rest of the clinically relevant nerves in the classic scalp block; the supraorbital and supratrochlear nerves arise from V1, the zygomaticotemporal from V2, and the auriculotemporal from V3.[24]

The greater occipital nerve is a branch of the second cervical dorsal ramus and pierces the semispinalis capitis and trapezius muscles. It is located approximately midway between the occipital protuberance and mastoid process, where it courses medial to the occipital artery (Figure 9.1).[25,26] It innervates the posterior aspect of the head extending to the vertex.[27]

The lesser occipital nerve derives from the ventral rami of C2 and C3 and travels parallel to the posterior margin of the sternocleidomastoid. The nerve emerges from the deep fascia and courses approximately 2.5 cm lateral to the greater occipital nerve and 7 cm lateral to the greater occipital protuberance (Figure 9.1). It innervates the skin behind the ear.[24]

The auriculotemporal nerve is derived from the mandibular branch of the trigeminal nerve and innervates the anterior ear and posterior forehead. It courses from the posterior area of the temporomandibular joint to the upper preauricular area and is closely associated with the superficial temporal artery.[28]

The zygomaticotemporal nerve originates from the maxillary division of the trigeminal nerve and pierces the temporal fascia above the zygomatic arch. It innervates the posterior portion of the forehead.[24]

The supraorbital nerve is derived from the frontal nerve, which is a branch of the ophthalmic division of the trigeminal nerve. It typically courses with the supraorbital artery through the supraorbital notch at the medial third of the supraorbital margin, although variations in anatomy are not uncommon, and branches may course through accessory exits. The existence of accessory exits may lead to incomplete regional anesthesia. The supraorbital nerve innervates the scalp from the upper eyelid to the lambdoid suture.[29]

The supratrochlear nerve innervates the skin of the lower forehead and is also derived from the frontal nerve. It emerges from the cranium through the frontal notch between the trochlea of the superior oblique muscle at the superomedial corner of the orbit and the supraorbital notch. The nerve then transverses through the corrugator supercilii and the frontal belly of the occipitofrontalis muscle.[30]

Performing the Scalp Block

Locate the greater occipital nerve by palpating the occipital artery in the medial one-third to midpoint between the occipital protuberance and mastoid process. An ultrasound may be used to aid in locating the occipital artery, especially if it cannot be easily palpated. Since this location also establishes one of the landmarks for identifying the lesser occipital nerve, good localization is important. Insert the needle perpendicular to the skin and advance until cranium is contacted. After careful aspiration to ensure against intraarterial injection, inject 4–5 mL of local anesthetic medial to the artery as the needle is slowly withdrawn.[9,31]

Block the lesser occipital nerve by injecting 4–5mL of local anesthetic approximately 2.5 cm lateral to the greater occipital block along the superior nuchal line. The injection point should be approximately 1 cm superior to the mastoid tip.[24] Again, advance the needle until cranium is contacted and then inject as the needle is withdrawn.

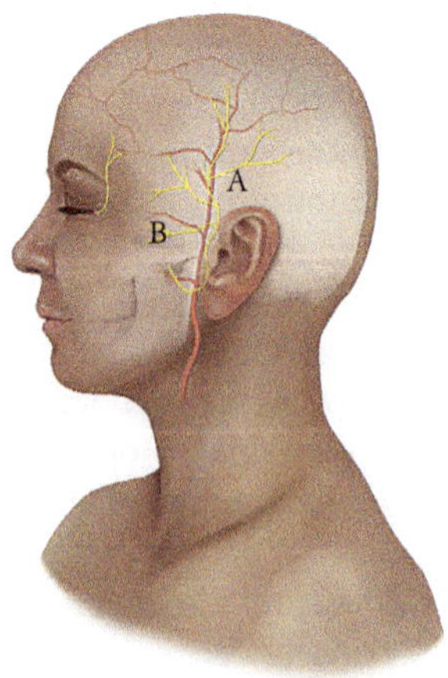

Figure 9.2. The auriculotemporal nerve injection site (A) is above the tragus and behind the superior temporal artery. Risk of inadvertent facial nerve paralysis is minimized if the injection is 1cm above the tragus. The groove along the zygomatic arch should be easily palpated for the zygomaticotemporal nerve block (B).

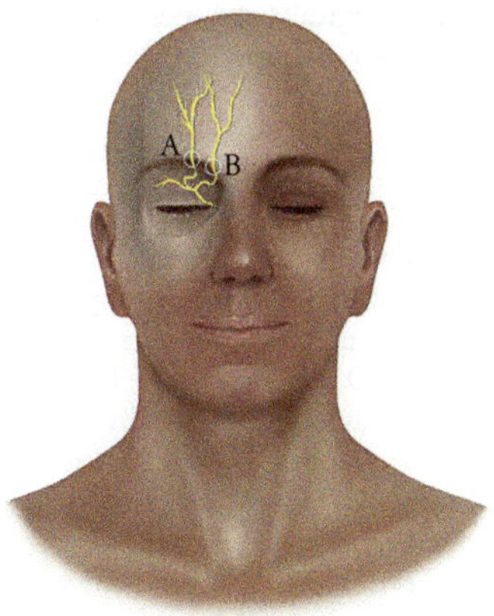

Figure 9.3. The supraorbital nerve can easily be located by palpating the supraorbital notch (A). The supratrochlear nerve (B) is blocked in the superomedial corner of the orbit.

To block the auriculotemporal nerve, insert the needle 1 cm superior to the tragus behind the superior temporal artery (Figure 9.2).[4] Advance the needle through the temporalis fascia and inject 2–3mL of local anesthetic above and below the fascia as the needle is withdrawn.[31]

For the zygomaticotemporal nerve block, find the notch along the zygomatic arch behind the lateral canthus of the eye (Figure 9.2). Advance the needle until a pop or resistance change is noted as the temporalis fascia is pierced. The zygomaticotemporal nerve ramifies as it pierces the temporalis fascia, so local anesthetic should be injected above and below the fascia. Inject 2–3 mL as you withdraw the needle through the fascia.[9,31] To ensure that local anesthetic is deposited correctly above and below the temporalis fascia, insert the needle initially fairly deep (about 1.5 cm), especially if a sharp, standard bevel injection needle is used and a fascial click is not obvious.

The supraorbital nerve traversing through the supraorbital notch may be easily located in the medial third of the supraorbital ridge (Figure 9.3). Advance the needle until it contacts bone, approximately 0.5 to 1 cm. Withdraw slightly and inject 2–3 mL of local anesthetic.[31] It may be advantageous to insert the needle next to, but not into, the supraorbital notch to avoid injecting into or causing a hematoma by piercing the supraorbital artery.

The supratrochlear nerve emerges from the superomedial angle of orbit and can be blocked by either injecting above the eyebrow 1 cm medial to the supraorbital notch or using the same injection site as the supraorbital nerve and directing the needle medially and advancing 1 cm. Inject 2–3 mL of local anesthetic.[31]

Scalp Block Efficacy

A scalp block, as opposed to surgical site infiltration of local anesthetic and vasoconstrictor, provides inhibition of nociception to both superficial and deep soft tissues.[23] Administration of a scalp block promotes hemodynamic stability after pinning, skin incision, and closure, as well as reduces pain scores and opioid consumption in the early postoperative period (up to 24–48 hours after surgery) as compared to surgical site infiltration.[32,33] Limiting opioid administration may help reduce opioid-induced hyperalgesia, especially since remifentanil is commonly used intraoperatively for craniotomies.[34]

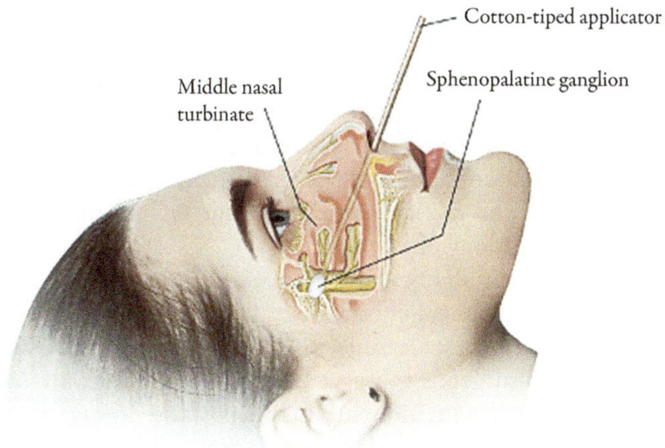

Figure 9.4. The sphenopalatine ganglion block may be performed by using a cotton-tipped applicator as a wick to guide local anesthetic past the middle turbinate.

SPHENOPALATINE GANGLION BLOCK

While scalp, pericranium, and cranium are well covered by the scalp block, the dura is not; the patient may tolerate the initial approach quite well and then complain of headache during durotomy. While opioids may be used to provide analgesia during durotomy, a sphenopalatine ganglion block may also be performed to augment the scalp block. The sphenopalatine ganglion is an attractive target to block the afferent branches of the trigeminal nerve innervating the dura mater. While only pre-ganglionic parasympathetic axons synapse in the ganglion, sensory fibers do transverse through the ganglion and hence may be blocked.[35] Additionally, activation of the trigeminal-autonomic reflex may release vasoactive peptides and present clinically as a headache.[36–38]

While most published research for sphenopalatine ganglion blocks has been in cluster migraines and post-dural puncture headaches, a large potential benefit exists for surgical patients. However, studies evaluating the perioperative utility of sphenopalatine ganglion block remain to be published.

To perform the sphenopalatine ganglion block, place a wick (a Q-tip or commercial applicator) into each nare and advance to the posterior nasopharynx (Figure 9.4). Typically, 1%–4% lidocaine is utilized, but cases with ropivacaine, bupivacaine, mepivacaine, and cocaine have been published. Drip 2–4 mL in each nare down the wick to introduce local anesthetic posterior to the middle turbinate.[35,39]

COMPLICATIONS OF THE SCALP BLOCK

It can be difficult to differentiate between symptoms of scalp block complications versus those of craniotomy. Potential complications of craniotomies include cerebral edema, cerebral hematomas, cerebral infarction, agitation, seizures, and hemodynamic instability.[2] Some of these symptoms overlap with those caused by complications of scalp blocks, such as focal deficits or seizures caused by local anesthetic toxicity. Trigeminal cardiac reflex activation and resultant bradycardia have also been observed during blockade of the supratrochlear nerve.[40] It is essential to evaluate the patient's complete neurologic exam and clinical picture to accurately diagnose and react to the etiology of a deficit.

The scalp is a highly vascular area, and risk exists for local anesthetic or block adjunct toxicity from absorption and or inadvertent intravascular injection.[5] In addition, it is quite common for surgeons to inject local anesthetic with a vasoconstrictor at the incision site for hemostasis, so care must be taken and communication made to prevent additive local anesthetic toxicity. Use of ropivacaine or levobupivacaine in lieu of bupivacaine may be considered to lessen the risk of cardiac depression. Knowledge of the surgical approach and technique is also important, as intravasation of local anesthetic neuraxially is theoretically possible in procedures that closely approximate a local anesthetic depot with the dura.

In evaluating for ptosis, the presence of Horner syndrome or other physical findings should be investigated. Mechanical ptosis caused by edema from large volumes of local anesthetic injection or hematoma has also been described.[5] Inadvertent facial nerve paralysis during auriculotemporal nerve block has also been described if the injection is made too close to the facial nerve or a large volume of anesthetic is used.[41,42] By taking care to inject not more than 1 cm cephalad to the tragus, this risk is minimized.[4]

REFERENCES

1. Bunyaratavej K, Sunisa S, Lerdsirisopon S, Tuchinda L. Continuous physical examination during subcortical resection in awake craniotomy patients: Its usefulness and surgical outcome. *Clin Neurol Neurosurg*. 2016 August;147:34–38.
2. Greenberg, MS. *Handbook of Neurosurgery*. 7th ed. New York: Thieme; 2010.
3. Barash PG, Cullen BF, Stoelting RK, Cahalan MK, Stock MC, Ortega R. *Clinical Anesthesia*. 7th ed. Philadelphia: Wolters Kluwer Lippincott Williams & Wilkins; 2013.
4. Bebawy JF, Bilotta F, Koht A. A modified technique for auriculotemporal nerve blockade when performing selective scalp nerve block for craniotomy. *J Neurosurg Anesthesiol*. 2014 Jul;26(3):271–272.
5. Hassan MH, Hassan WM, Nazaruddin Wan, Kandasamy R, Chong SE. Unilateral complete ptosis after scalp block for awake craniotomy: a rare complication. *J Neuroanaesthesiol Crit Care*. 2018;05(02):111–113.
6. Wilson MH. Monro-kellie 2.0: the dynamic vascular and venous pathophysiological components of intracranial pressure. *J Cereb Blood Flow Metab*. 2016 Aug;36(8):1338–1350.
7. Kulikov A, Lubnin A. Anesthesia for awake craniotomy. *Curr Opin Anaesthesiol*. 2018 Oct;31(5):506–510.
8. Cushing HI. on the avoidance of shock in major amputations by cocainization of large nerve-trunks preliminary to their division: with observations on blood-pressure changes in surgical cases. *Ann Surg*. 1902 Sep;36(3):321–345.
9. Osborn I, Sebeo J. "Scalp block" during craniotomy: a classic technique revisited. *J Neurosurg Anesthesiol*. 2010 Jul;22(3):187–194.
10. Hillman DR, Rung GW, Thompson WR, Davis NJ. The effect of bupivacaine scalp infiltration on the hemodynamic response to craniotomy under general anesthesia. *Anesthesiology*. 1987 Dec;67(6):1001–1003.
11. Kim SS, McCutcheon IE, Suki D, et al. Awake craniotomy for brain tumors near eloquent cortex: correlation of intraoperative cortical mapping with neurological outcomes in 309 consecutive patients. *Neurosurgery*. 2009 May;64(5):836–836.
12. Pardey Bracho GF, Pereira de Souza Neto E, Grousson S, Mottolese C, Dailler F. Opioid consumption after levobupivacaine scalp nerve block for craniosynostosis surgery. *Acta Anaesthesiol Taiwan*. 2014 Jun;52(2):64–69.
13. van Hulst RA, Hasan D, Lachmann B. Intracranial pressure, brain PCO2, PO2, and pH during hypo- and hyperventilation at constant mean airway pressure in pigs. *Intensive Care Med*. 2002 Jan;28(1):68–73.
14. Abou-Madi M, Trop D, Abou-Madi N, Ravussin P. Does a bolus of mannitol initially aggravate intracranial hypertension? A study at various PaCO2 tensions in dogs. *Br J Anaesth*. 1987 May;59(5):630–639.
15. Andrews RJ, Bringas JR, Muto RP. Effects of mannitol on cerebral blood flow, blood pressure, blood viscosity, hematocrit, sodium, and potassium. *Surg Neurol*. 1993 Mar;39(3):218–222.
16. Gu J, Huang H, Huang Y, Sun H, Xu H. Hypertonic saline or mannitol for treating elevated intracranial pressure in traumatic brain injury: a meta-analysis of randomized controlled trials. *Neurosurg Rev*. 2019 Jun;42(2):499–509.
17. Soriano SG, McManus ML, Sullivan LJ, Rockoff MA, Black PM, Burrows FA. Cerebral blood flow velocity after mannitol infusion in children. *Can J Anaesth*. 1996 May;43(5 Pt 1):461–466.
18. Goettel N, Bharadwaj S, Venkatraghavan L, Mehta J, Bernstein M, Manninen PH. Dexmedetomidine vs propofol-remifentanil conscious sedation for awake craniotomy: a prospective randomized controlled trial. *Br J Anaesth*. 2016 Jun;116(6):811–821.
19. Tung A, Fergusson NA, Ng N, Hu V, Dormuth C, Griesdale DEG. Medications to reduce emergence coughing after general anaesthesia with tracheal intubation: a systematic review and network meta-analysis. *Br J Anaesth*. 2020 Feb 22:S0007-0912(20)30012-X. doi: 10.1016/j.bja.2019.12.041. Epub ahead of print. PMID: 32098647.
20. Mirski MA, Lewin JJ. Sedation and pain management in acute neurological disease. *Semin Neurol*. 2008 Nov;28(5):611–630.
21. Kumar K, Singh SI. Neuraxial opioid-induced pruritus: an update. *J Anaesthesiol Clin Pharmacol*. 2013;29(3):303–307.
22. Garavaglia MM, Das S, Cusimano MD, et al. Anesthetic approach to high-risk patients and prolonged awake craniotomy using dexmedetomidine and scalp block. *J Neurosurg Anesthesiol*. 2014 Jul;26(3):226–233.
23. Guilfoyle MR, Helmy A, Duane D, Hutchinson PJ. Regional scalp block for postcraniotomy analgesia: a systematic review and meta-analysis. *Anesth Analg*. 2013;116(5):1093–1102.
24. Kemp WJ, 3rd, Tubbs RS, Cohen-Gadol AA. The innervation of the scalp: a comprehensive review including anatomy, pathology, and neurosurgical correlates. *Surg Neurol Int*. 2011;2:178,7806.90699. Epub 2011 Dec 13.
25. Prigge L, van Schoor AN, Bosenberg AT. Anatomy of the greater occipital nerve block in infants. *Paediatr Anaesth*. 2019;29(9):945–949.
26. Won HJ, Ji HJ, Song JK, Kim YD, Won HS. Topographical study of the trapezius muscle, greater occipital nerve, and occipital artery for facilitating blockade of the greater occipital nerve. *PLoS One*. 2018 Aug 15;13(8):e0202448.
27. Allen SM, Mookadam F, Cha SS, Freeman JA, Starling AJ, Mookadam M. Greater occipital nerve block for acute treatment of migraine headache: a large retrospective cohort study. *J Am Board Fam Med*. 2018;31(2):211–218.
28. Janis JE, Hatef DA, Ducic I, et al. Anatomy of the auriculotemporal nerve: variations in its relationship to the superficial temporal artery and implications for the treatment of migraine headaches. *Plast Reconstr Surg*. 2010;125(5):1422–1428.
29. Nanayakkara D, Manawaratne R, Sampath H, Vadysinghe A, Peiris R. Supraorbital nerve exits: positional variations and localization relative to surgical landmarks. *Anat Cell Biol*. 2018;51(1):19–24.
30. Kikuta S, Iwanaga J, Watanabe K, Kusukawa J, Tubbs RS. A relationship between the supratrochlear nerve and trochlea: anatomical study and application to migraine headaches. *J Craniofac Surg*. 2019 Nov-Dec;30(8):2497–2498.
31. Rosenblatt MA, Lai Y. *Scalp Block and Cervical Plexus Block Techniques* [Internet]. Waltham, MA: UpToDate; Jun 6, cited Oct 10, 2019]. Available from: https://www.uptodate.com

32. Akcil EF, Dilmen OK, Vehid H, Ibisoglu LS, Tunali Y. Which one is more effective for analgesia in infratentorial craniotomy? The scalp block or local anesthetic infiltration. *Clin Neurol Neurosurg.* 2017;154:98–103.
33. Yang X, Ma J, Li K, et al. A comparison of effects of scalp nerve block and local anesthetic infiltration on inflammatory response, hemodynamic response, and postoperative pain in patients undergoing craniotomy for cerebral aneurysms: a randomized controlled trial. *BMC Anesthesiol.* 2019 Jun 1;19(1):91–94.
34. Gottschalk A, Yaster M. The perioperative management of pain from intracranial surgery. *Neurocrit Care.* 2009;10(3):387–402.
35. Nair AS, Rayani BK. Sphenopalatine ganglion block for relieving postdural puncture headache: technique and mechanism of action of block with a narrative review of efficacy. *Korean J Pain.* 2017 Apr;30(2):93–97.
36. Cohen S, Levin D, Mellender S, et al. Topical sphenopalatine ganglion block compared with epidural blood patch for postdural puncture headache management in postpartum patients: a retrospective review. *Reg Anesth Pain Med.* 2018 Nov;43(8):880–884.
37. Lv X, Wu Z, Li Y. Innervation of the cerebral dura mater. *Neuroradiol J.* 2014;27(3):293–298.
38. Mojica J, Mo B, Ng A. Sphenopalatine ganglion block in the management of chronic headaches. *Curr Pain Headache Rep.* 2017;21(6):27.
39. Candido KD, Massey ST, Sauer R, Darabad RR, Knezevic NN. A novel revision to the classical transnasal topical sphenopalatine ganglion block for the treatment of headache and facial pain. *Pain Physician.* 2013;16(6):769.
40. Chowdhury T, Baron K, Cappellani RB. Severe bradycardia during scalp nerve block in patient undergoing awake craniotomy. *Saudi J Anaesth.* 2013 Jul;7(3):356–357.
41. McNicholas E, Bilotta F, Titi L, Chandler J, Rosa G, Koht A. Transient facial nerve palsy after auriculotemporal nerve block in awake craniotomy patients. *A A Case Rep.* 2014 Feb 15;2(4):40–43.
42. Sargin M, Samancioglu H, Uluer MS. Transient facial nerve palsy after the scalp block for burr hole evacuation of subdural hematoma. *Turk J Anaesthesiol Reanim.* 2018 Jun;46(3):238–240.

REVIEW QUESTIONS

(1) The patient is comfortable during craniotomy but complains of a headache during durotomy. Safe augmentation of the scalp block could prevent this by performing which of the following?

A. This pain is unavoidable.
B. Infiltrating the field with local anesthetic
C. Sphenopalatine ganglion block
D. Orbicularis oculi block

(2) A scalp block was performed, and the auriculotemporal nerve block was performed 1 cm above the level of the tragus. During follow-up the next day, the patient is noted to have unilateral ptosis. What most likely caused this?

A. Inadvertent blocking of the facial nerve
B. Surgical resection of corresponding homunculus
C. CSF drainage causing tenting of CNIII
D. Mechanical ptosis from edema

(3) A patient with moyamoya disease is scheduled to undergo encephalo-duro-arterio-myo-synangiosis (EDAMS). Would this patient be a good candidate for a scalp block?

A. Likely no, but a discussion with the surgeon would first be warranted because of risk of local anesthetic diffusion into the CSF.
B. Yes, this patient would be an ideal candidate because improved pain control postoperatively would enable reduced opioid administration and improved ability to closely follow neuro exams.
C. No, because the local anesthetic infiltration would disrupt the surgical anatomy.
D. Yes, as long as epinephrine is not administered in the local anesthetic mixture to avoid vasoconstriction in the vascular anastomosis.

(4) Your medical student states, "as long as a scalp block is performed correctly, further analgesia is never needed." You should respond that the statement is:

A. True because the scalp block will reliably cover incision and craniotomy, and the brain parenchyma is not innervated with pain receptors.
B. False because while a sphenopalatine ganglion block will provide some dural analgesia, the dura is richly innervated and the patient may complain of headache even after durotomy if the dura is touched by surgical instruments.
C. False because pericranium is not adequately covered by the scalp block and craniotomy will be intensely painful.
D. True because if the asleep-awake-asleep technique is performed, all painful portions of the surgery are completely covered while the patient is under deep sedation or general anesthesia.

(5) Which nerve innervates the posterior aspect of the scalp extending to the vertex?

A. Auriculotemporal nerve
B. Zygomaticotemporal nerve
C. Greater occipital nerve
D. Lesser occipital nerve

(6) The patient complains of pain just behind the ear. Effectively blocking which nerve would ameliorate this pain?

A. Auriculotemporal nerve
B. Zygomaticotemporal nerve
C. Greater occipital nerve
D. Lesser occipital nerve

(7) Which of the following statements is true regarding maximum safe dose of local anesthetic used in a scalp block?

A. Close communication with the surgical team is necessary because additional local anesthetic with epinephrine is routinely used for vasoconstriction at the incision site.
B. Addition of a vasopressor in the block mixture is necessary to avoid exceeding maximum safe dose of local anesthetic.
C. The highly vascular nature of the scalp makes utilization of any local anesthetic concentration greater than 0.25% unsafe.
D. Addition of adjuncts to the local anesthetic should be avoided because of the close proximity of the dura and the possibility of clouding the neurologic examination.

ANSWERS

(1) **C.** Sphenopalatine ganglion block. The patient may tolerate the initial approach quite well and then complain of headache during durotomy because the scalp, pericranium, and cranium are well covered by the conventional scalp block while the dura is not. Blocking the sensory fibers traversing through the sphenopalatine ganglion and blocking the release of vasoactive peptides from activation of the trigeminal-autonomic reflex may help relieve this pain.

References

Cohen S, Levin D, Mellender S, Zhao R, Patel P, Grubb W, Kiss G. Topical sphenopalatine ganglion block compared with epidural blood patch for postdural puncture headache management in postpartum patients: a retrospective review. *Reg Anesth Pain Med*. 2018 Nov;43(8):880–884.

Lv X, Wu Z, Li Y. Innervation of the cerebral dura mater. *Neuroradiol J*. 2014;27(3):293–298.

Mojica J, Mo B, Ng A. Sphenopalatine ganglion block in the management of chronic headaches. *Curr Pain Headache Rep*. 2017;21(6):27.

Nair AS, Rayani BK. Sphenopalatine ganglion block for relieving postdural puncture headache: technique and mechanism of action of block with a narrative review of efficacy. *Korean J Pain*. 2017 Apr;30(2):93–97.

(2) **D.** Mechanical ptosis from edema. Large volumes of local anesthetic injection and hematoma may induce eyelid edema with concomitant mechanical ptosis. If the auriculotemporal nerve injection is performed 1 cm cephalad to the tragus, the risk of inadvertent and facial nerve blockade is minimized.

References

Bebawy JF, Bilotta F, Koht A. A modified technique for auriculotemporal nerve blockade when performing selective scalp nerve block for craniotomy. *J Neurosurg Anesthesiol*. 2014 Jul;26(3):271–272.

Hassan MH, Hassan WM, Nazaruddin Wan, Kandasamy R, Chong SE. Unilateral complete ptosis after scalp block for awake craniotomy: a rare complication. *J Neuroanaesthesiol Crit Care*. 2018;05(02):111–113.

McNicholas E, Bilotta F, Titi L, Chandler J, Rosa G, Koht A. Transient facial nerve palsy after auriculotemporal nerve block in awake craniotomy patients. *A A Case Rep*. 2014 Feb 15;2(4):40–43.

Sargin M, Samancioglu H, Uluer MS. Transient facial nerve palsy after the scalp block for burr hole evacuation of subdural hematoma. *Turk J Anaesthesiol Reanim*. 2018 Jun;46(3):238–240.

(3) **A.** Likely no, but a discussion with the surgeon would first be warranted because of risk of local anesthetic diffusion into the CSF. An EDAMS operation is an indirect revascularization technique that involves draping the posterior temporalis muscle intracranially. Because of the propensity of local anesthetic to infiltrate into the soft tissue, there is a large risk of intravasation of local anesthetic into the cranial epidural space or CSF.

Reference

Ozgur BM, Aryan HE, Levy ML. Indirect revascularisation for paediatric moyamoya disease: The EDAMS technique. *J Clin Neuroscience*. 2006 Jan;13(1):105–108.

(4) **B.** False because while a sphenopalatine ganglion block will provide some dural analgesia, the dura is richly innervated, and the patient may complain of headache even after durotomy if the dura is touched by surgical instruments. While a scalp block provides excellent analgesia for the surgical approach, innervation of the dura is complex. Durotomy or touching of the dura frequently results in the patient complaining of a headache. A sphenopalatine ganglion block may be used to augment a traditional scalp block but is unlikely to reliably and completely cover dural pain.

References

Candido KD, Massey ST, Sauer R, Darabad RR, Knezevic NN. A novel revision to the classical transnasal topical sphenopalatine ganglion block for the treatment of headache and facial pain. *Pain Physician*. 2013;16(6):769.

Cohen S, Levin D, Mellender S, et al. Topical sphenopalatine ganglion block compared with epidural blood patch for postdural puncture headache management in postpartum patients: a retrospective review. *Reg Anesth Pain Med*. 2018 Nov;43(8):880–884.

Lv X, Wu Z, Li Y. Innervation of the cerebral dura mater. *Neuroradiol J*. 2014;27(3):293–298.

Mojica J, Mo B, Ng A. Sphenopalatine ganglion block in the management of chronic headaches. *Curr Pain Headache Rep*. 2017;21(6):27.

Nair AS, Rayani BK. Sphenopalatine ganglion block for relieving postdural puncture headache: technique and mechanism of action of block with a narrative review of efficacy. *Korean J Pain*. 2017 Apr;30(2):93–97.

(5) **C.** Greater occipital nerve. The greater occipital nerve courses midway between the occipital protuberance and mastoid process and innervates the posterior aspect of the head extending to the vertex.

References

Allen SM, Mookadam F, Cha SS, Freeman JA, Starling AJ, Mookadam M. Greater occipital nerve block for acute treatment of migraine headache: a large retrospective cohort study. *J Am Board Fam Med*. 2018;31(2):211–218.

Prigge L, van Schoor AN, Bosenberg AT. Anatomy of the greater occipital nerve block in infants. *Paediatr Anaesth*. 2019;29(9):945–949.

Won HJ, Ji HJ, Song JK, Kim YD, Won HS. Topographical study of the trapezius muscle, greater occipital nerve, and occipital artery for facilitating blockade of the greater occipital nerve. *PLoS One*. 2018 Aug 15;13(8):e0202448.

(6) **D.** Lesser occipital nerve. The lesser occipital nerve courses lateral to the greater occipital nerve and innervates the skin behind the ear.

Reference

Kemp WJ, 3rd, Tubbs RS, Cohen-Gadol AA. The innervation of the scalp: a comprehensive review including anatomy, pathology, and neurosurgical correlates. *Surg Neurol Int*. 2011;2:178,7806.90699. Epub 2011 Dec 13.

(7) **A.** Close communication with the surgical team is necessary because additional local anesthetic with epinephrine is routinely used for vasoconstriction at the incision site.

Reference

Greenberg, MS. *Handbook of Neurosurgery*. New York: Thieme; 2010.

10.

CERVICAL PLEXUS BLOCK FOR CAROTID ENDARTERECTOMY

Shimon Gabriel Farkas and Kamen V. Vlassakov

STEM CASE AND KEY QUESTIONS

An 81-year-old female presents to the emergency room with transient speech difficulty and left-sided weakness. Her past medical history is significant for hypertension, coronary artery disease, chronic obstructive pulmonary disease, and dyspnea on exertion. Her past surgical history includes a bare metal coronary stent placement 8 months before and a right hip replacement one year ago with no reported anesthesia-related problems. Her daily medications include aspirin 325 mg, metoprolol succinate 100 mg, and hydrochlorothiazide 25 mg. Magnetic resonance imaging (MRI) of the brain was performed and no intracranial abnormality was seen. Magnetic resonance angiography was read as without evidence of cerebral arterial occlusion, dissection, or hemorrhagic stroke. However, carotid ultrasound obtained showed a high-grade (90%) stenosis of the right internal carotid artery (ICA). The vascular surgery team has initiated a heparin infusion and scheduled her for a right-sided carotid endarterectomy (CEA) on the following day. Given her history of recent coronary stent placement and exertional dyspnea, she undergoes a preoperative echocardiogram which shows an ejection fraction of 60% with no regional wall motion abnormalities, and an electrocardiogram (EKG) showed normal sinus rhythm.

(1) WHAT ARE THE INDICATIONS FOR CAROTID ENDARTERECTOMY? WHAT PERIOPERATIVE WORKUP SHOULD BE EXPECTED FOR THIS PATIENT?

The patient is now waiting in the perioperative area and looks anxious. Her chart reveals that she weighs 90 kilograms (kg), her height is 5′7″, with a body mass index of 32.3 with no known drug allergies. She has one 20-g intravenous (IV) in the left hand and her physical exam is non-contributory, with normal heart and lung sounds, no signs of peripheral edema, and a Mallampati score of II with full dentition. The anesthesiologist explains to the patient that although general endotracheal anesthesia (GETA) is a safe and viable option, he believes that regional anesthesia combined with light sedation would be an appropriate anesthetic for this procedure and the patient is amenable to that plan. She is given 2 mg of IV midazolam and is brought into the operating room (OR) where full American Society of Anesthesiologists (ASA) monitors are applied, as well as bilateral cerebral oximetry monitors. A left-sided radial 20-g arterial line is placed using local anesthetic and a 16-g IV is placed on the same side. The patient's head is then turned to the left side and the neck is prepped and draped in the standard sterile fashion. Using real-time ultrasound guidance, the anesthesiologist scans the patient's neck from caudad to cephalad, starting with the ultrasound probe seated in the supraclavicular fossa parallel to the clavicle, working up toward the conventional brachial plexus view in the interscalene groove. The US probe is now at about the level of the cricoid cartilage in the transverse position and the US picture shows the C5 and C6 nerve roots "sandwiched" between the anterior and middle scalene muscles, with the echogenic cluster of fine cervical plexus branches sitting above the deep layer of the deep cervical fascia that encases the scalene muscles and below the sternocleidomastoid muscle (SCM), as can be seen in Figure 10.1. Then scanning continues cephalad to the C4–C5 level (thyroid cartilage level and at or close to the bifurcation of the carotid artery) and the anesthesiologist performs an intermediate cervical plexus block (CPB) by injecting local anesthetic in the plane beneath the posterior border of the SCM and beneath the superficial layer of the deep cervical fascia, observing spread of the injectate cephalad and caudad with dynamic US scanning.

(2) WHAT LANDMARKS ARE USED TO IDENTIFY THE CERVICAL PLEXUS, AND WHERE IS THE LOCAL ANESTHETIC INJECTED?

The CPB is performed without any apparent immediate complications. However, 15 minutes after its placement, the patient starts complaining of mild shortness of breath, her voice is slightly hoarse, and she feels her right eyelid drooping. Upon further questioning, she denies any ringing in her ears, numbness of the lips, or weakness in her upper extremities. The anesthesiologist comforts her by explaining that "some other nerves that control the diaphragm, vocal cords and muscles of the face, are likely anesthetized as well," a typically harmless side effect. The patient is comfortable despite these side effects and the surgeon proceeds with his incision and dissection. Moderate sedation is achieved with low-dose dexmedetomidine and propofol infusions.

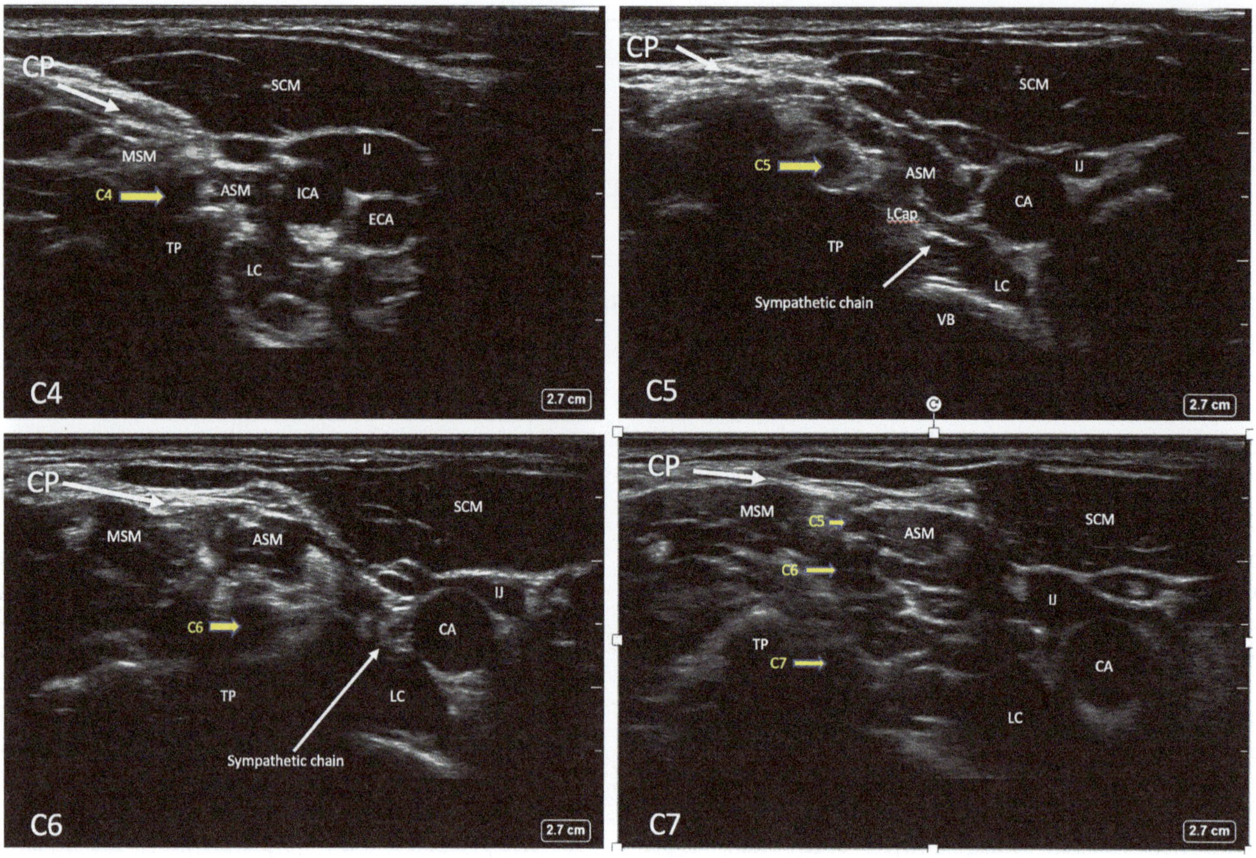

Figure 10.1. Ultrasound anatomy of the cervical plexus, scanning from C4 to C7.
CP = cervical plexus; yellow arrow = cervical nerve root; MSM = middle scalene muscle; ASM = anterior scalene muscle; LC = longus colli; TP = transverse process; ICA = internal carotid artery; LCap = longus capitis.

(3) WHAT ARE SOME POTENTIAL COMPLICATIONS AND SIDE EFFECTS ASSOCIATED WITH THE CERVICAL PLEXUS BLOCK, AND HOW CAN THEY BE AVOIDED OR MITIGATED?

After 15 minutes of meticulous dissection, the carotid artery bifurcation is clearly exposed, pulsating in the center of the surgical field. The surgeon requests that the sedation be minimized so that the patient can now perform some verbal and physical tasks. The surgeon asks the patient to squeeze the rubber toy situated in her left hand and to start counting backward from one hundred out loud. Without much delay, a high-pitched squeak echoes through the OR and the patient is heard counting, signaling to the OR staff that the patient is receiving adequate blood flow to both cerebral hemispheres. At this point in time, the patient's vital signs are stable with a heart rate of 75, arterial blood pressure of 136/80, oxygen saturation of 97%, and cerebral oxygen saturation of 70% on each side. The surgeon locates the atheromatous plaque in the internal carotid artery (ICA) and places clamps at the proximal and distal portions of the lesion in order to access it and remove it from the artery. Immediately following clamp placement, he again asks the patient to squeeze the toy in her left hand and to start counting again, but this time, there is no squeaky noise from the toy and there is a garbled verbal response coming from the patient. The carotid clamp is immediately released, and the patient is again able to squeeze her left hand and resume counting normally within the next 30 seconds. It is now clear that the patient does not have sufficient collateral circulation to support her right cerebral hemisphere. The surgeon decides to place a shunt to bypass the lesion and supply the brain with adequate cerebral blood flow. Following shunt placement and carotid cross-clamping, the patient is able to squeeze the toy and speak clearly.

(4) HOW DO WE MONITOR NEUROLOGICAL STATUS DURING CEA WHEN USING A REGIONAL ANESTHETIC APPROACH? HOW IS NEUROLOGICAL MONITORING DONE UNDER GETA?

Upon surgical manipulation of the carotid artery, the patient's heart rate precipitously drops into the 40s, but is quickly rectified with some IV glycopyrrolate. Once the plaque is removed, native blood flow through the ICA is re-established following removal of the carotid clamps and shunt. A few minutes later the patient's blood pressure starts to decline and the anesthesiologist increases the phenylephrine infusion that has been running throughout most of the case. Hemodynamic fluctuations during the case remain easy to correct with either vasopressors or vasodilators carefully titrated by the anesthesiologist.

The case concludes without any major issues and the patient is recovering in the post-anesthesia care unit (PACU).

(5) WHAT HEMODYNAMIC CHANGES SHOULD BE EXPECTED DURING A CEA AND HOW ARE THEY MANAGED?

A variety of fluctuations in heart rate and blood pressure should be expected with this surgical procedure. These are logical and somewhat predictable, considering the high concentration of critical structures affecting hemodynamics in the immediate surgical field, including arterial baroreceptors, especially in the carotid sinus, the vagus nerve, and the cervical sympathetic chain. Close monitoring, typically mandating invasive blood pressure monitoring (arterial line), immediate two-way communication with the surgeons vis-à-vis traction on sensitive structures, bleeding, patient responses, and readiness to aggressively treat hypotension and hypertension, bradycardia and tachycardia, are of paramount importance.

DISCUSSION

INDICATIONS FOR CAROTID ENDARTERECTOMY

The primary goal of CEA or carotid artery stenting (CAS) is to lower the risk of future stroke. Therefore, the decision to medically manage or surgically treat a patient is determined by the patient's neurological symptoms and degree of carotid stenosis. A carotid artery stenosis of less than 50% in a symptomatic patient, or a stenosis of less than 60% in an asymptomatic patient, should be optimized and followed with medical therapy only. Asymptomatic patients with greater than 60% carotid stenosis should be considered for CEA if their overall life expectancy is greater than 3 years and have a perioperative stroke/death rate of less than 3%. For patients who are surgical candidates, CEA is preferred over CAS for reduction of all cause stroke and peri-procedural death. CAS is preferred over CEA in symptomatic patients with >50% stenosis and a history of local tissue scarring from radiation therapy, ipsilateral neck surgery, lesions that extend proximal to the clavicle or if they have severe uncorrectable CAD, heart failure, or severe lung disease.[1,2]

PREOPERATIVE PREPARATION AND POSSIBLE COMPLICATIONS

Proper perioperative workup for patients with significant cardiac or pulmonary comorbidities (increased risk of major adverse cardiac event [MACE]) undergoing non-cardiac surgery is dependent on various factors which are explained in the most updated report of the American College of Cardiology/American Heart Association task force on practice guidelines (http://www.onlinejacc.org/content/64/22/e77). Preoperatively, an EKG is warranted in patients with history of CAD or arrhythmias, and for those with history of left ventricular dysfunction, congestive heart failure, dyspnea, or unknown exercise tolerance. An echocardiogram or cardiac stress test may be warranted, if assessment results are likely to change perioperative management. Complications associated with CEA are ipsilateral vocal cord paralysis from recurrent laryngeal nerve injury or compression, stroke, and hematoma formation at the surgical site which can compromise the airway.

CERVICAL PLEXUS BLOCK (CPB)

The patient is monitored using ASA standard monitors, a procedural consent is obtained, and a pre-block safety pause is performed; then, appropriate sedation is administered. The ultrasound-guided CPB is typically performed at the posterior border of the sternocleidomastoid muscle (SCM) at and slightly below the level of the superior border of the thyroid cartilage (which corresponds approximately to C4 level). The sonoanatomical landmarks are visualized with emphasis on identification (and counting) of the transverse processes and nerve roots in the cervical spine to visualize both the cervical plexus (target) and the beginning of the brachial plexus formation (to avoid), as well as any blood vessels in the area (Figure 10.1). To correctly establish the cervical spine level, the distinct contours of the C7 transverse process (single prominent posterior "thumb-like" process) and the C6 transverse process ("saddle-like" with a prominent anterior process—*Chassaignac tubercle, aka carotid tubercle*) are identified with their corresponding nerve "roots" (anatomically, these are the anterior primary rami of the corresponding spinal nerves, contributing to the brachial plexus). Then the probe is moved slowly cephalad and the consecutive C5, then C4 transverse processes are visualized (Figure 10.1). As the transducer travels between C6 and C4 levels, the operator focuses on identifying the interfascial plane deep to the lateral edge of the SCM and superficial to the scalene muscles and their fascia. Often a multitude of small hyperechoic structures are visualized in that area, representing the main branches of the superficial cervical plexus and *ansa cervicalis*. This plane is the target destination for the intermediate CPB, which has gained popularity with ultrasound guidance. Dynamic scanning with variable pressure, possibly utilizing color Doppler, is recommended to detect vascular structures and plan a safe block needle trajectory. Another important landmark with this block, especially when performed for CEA, is the bifurcation of the common carotid artery, which occurs with some variation between C4 and C3 level (corresponding to the upper aspect of the thyroid cartilage or hyoid bone body).

Once comfortable with the sonoanatomy, the target structures, optimal trajectory, and "danger zones," a skin wheal of local anesthetic is made and a nerve block needle is guided in-plane using a high-frequency linear ultrasound probe, placed in a transverse (axial) position/view (as depicted in Figure 10.1). The needle is advanced beneath the SCM until it pierces the superficial layer of the deep cervical fascia (as seen in Figures 10.1 and 10.2). The authors advise generous "hydrodissection" with local anesthetic to enhance the coverage of some early branches of the cervical plexus that may have already left the common space. Frequent intermittent

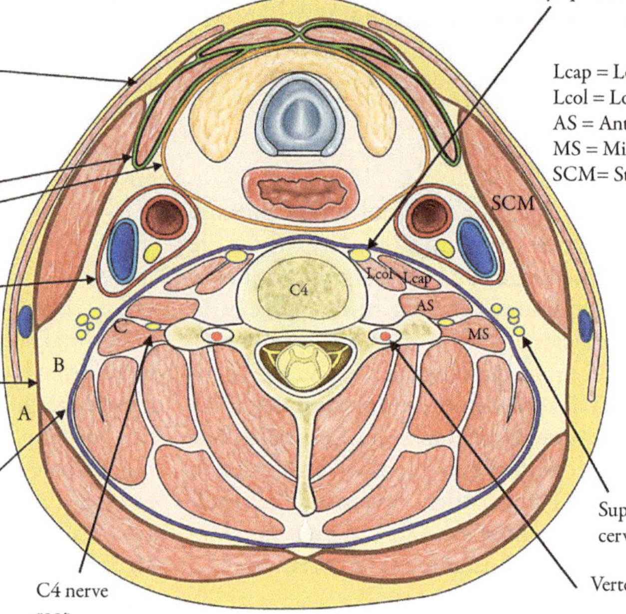

Figure 10.2. Anatomy of the cervical plexus at the level of C4.
Modified by the authors from Kim JS, Ko JS, Bang S, Kim H, Lee SY. Cervical plexus block. *Korean J Anesthesiol.* 2018 Aug;71(4):274–288. doi: 10.4097/kja.d.18.00143.

gentle aspiration, confirming extravascular needle tip position, is critical.

The cervical plexus is formed by the anterior rami (often also called "roots" of the plexus) of the first four cervical spinal nerves, C1 to C4. The superficial cutaneous branches (Figure 10.3) of the cervical plexus include the lesser occipital (C2–C3), great auricular (C2–C3), transverse cervical and supraclavicular nerves (C3–C4), all of which travel through the deep layer of the prevertebral fascia and continue to run in the interfascial plane between the prevertebral muscles and the SCM. It is within this interfascial plane that the 10–15 mL of local anesthetic is deposited. They then pierce through the superficial layer of the deep cervical fascia (also known as the investing fascia) at the middle portion of the posterior border of the SCM. The *ansa cervicalis* is a nerve loop formed from the C1 to C3 nerve roots that supplies innervation to most of the infrahyoid muscles and the SCM. It is important to note that the phrenic nerve, which innervates the diaphragm and the pericardium, arises from C3–C5.

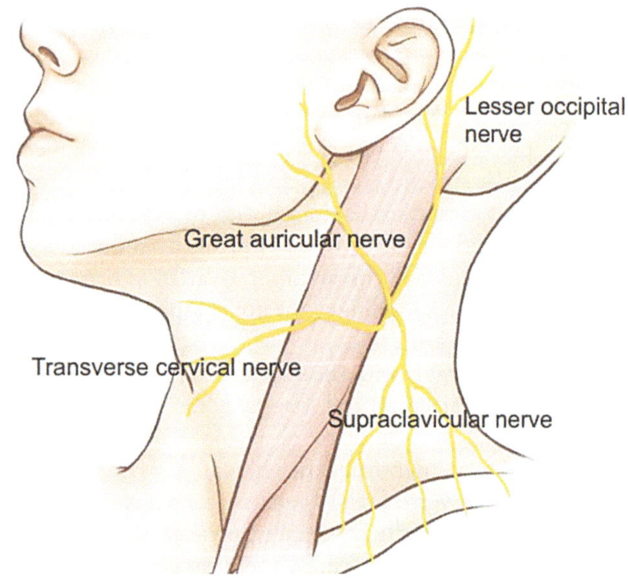

Figure 10.3. Cutaneous branches of the superficial cervical plexus. Obtained with permission from Kim JS, Ko JS, Bang S, Kim H, Lee SY. Cervical plexus block. *Korean J Anesthesiol.* 2018 Aug;71(4):274–288. doi: 10.4097/kja.d.18.00143.

A cervical plexus block provides effective anesthesia and analgesia for the head and neck region and is most commonly used for surgical anesthesia during carotid endarterectomies, but also occasionally for limited thyroid and parathyroid surgeries. The dermatomal boundaries covered by the CPB are seen in Figure 10.3. The terms that describe the various types of CPB are *superficial*, *intermediate*, and *deep*, which are loosely defined by the anatomical planes in which the injection is performed, providing a subject for academic debate within the regional anesthesiology literature. This improved working definition of functional anatomy and technique evolution from the traditional "deep" and "superficial" CPB has become possible and meaningful only with the introduction of high-resolution ultrasound imaging and needle guidance.

In the description by Kim et al.,[3] the deep cervical fascia is divided into three layers: the superficial layer, which is also called the investing fascia or submandibular fascia; the middle layer (strap muscle fascia or visceral fascia); and the deep layer, which is also known as the prevertebral fascia. This prevertebral fascia forms a tubular sheath around the vertebral column and the muscles associated with it, such as the longus colli and longus capitis anteriorly, the scalene muscles laterally, and the deep cervical muscles posteriorly (Figure 10.2). There is some disagreement as to whether or not the carotid sheath is formed by any of these layers of the deep cervical fascia or if it has its own separate fascial enclosure. The anatomical landmarks and fascial layers are depicted in Figures 10.1 and 10.2.

Before the advent of ultrasound guidance, landmark-based techniques for both the deep and superficial cervical plexus blocks were employed by experienced practitioners, but due to the complexity and frequent challenges in the landmark identification with this approach, and the associated increased risks of nerve injury, local anesthetic toxicity, and inadvertent intrathecal/intravascular (including intraarterial) injection, many clinicians have long avoided the CPB, opting for general anesthesia and electrophysiological monitoring instead. With high-resolution ultrasound imaging readily available and following recent randomized controlled trials that have demonstrated the superficial and intermediate cervical plexus blocks to be both equally efficacious and safe for carotid endarterectomy, the use of the CPB is becoming more commonplace.

COMPLICATIONS OF CERVICAL PLEXUS BLOCK

Currently, the CPB is usually performed with real-time ultrasound guidance, decreasing the risks of intrathecal or intra-vascular injection of local anesthetic. Furthermore, the landmark-based deep cervical plexus block, which was associated with most of the complications, has been largely retired since recent evidence from randomized controlled studies have shown that the "superficial" and "intermediate" cervical plexus blocks are equally efficacious at providing surgical anesthesia and are easier and safer to perform. A 2007 systematic review of complications associated with superficial and deep cervical plexus blocks was performed by Pandit et al.[4] It demonstrated that cases in which the deep CPB was utilized were more frequently associated with conversion to general anesthesia either due to block failure or patient intolerance, compared to those that utilized the superficial block technique. Furthermore, there were no reported complications from the superficial block compared to a 0.25% complication rate from the deep block, with the most common complications being either intravascular injection or respiratory distress.

Pandit et al. also performed a cadaveric study that demonstrated that injection of dye directly below the investing fascia (which by current definitions is called "intermediate CPB," coined by Telford and Stoneham[5]) had spread to the deep cervical space, staining structures such as the phrenic nerve and cervical nerve roots.[6] As with any nerve block performed under sedation and with a moderate amount of local anesthetic, there is always the risk of local anesthetic toxicity, bleeding from inadvertent puncture of nearby vessels, and respiratory distress from phrenic nerve involvement.

REGIONAL VERSUS GENERAL ANESTHESIA

Regional anesthesia allows for the patient to remain awake during the procedure, giving the surgeon and anesthesiologist the ability to continuously monitor the patient's neurological function by asking the patient to perform simple tasks with their contralateral hand (e.g., squeezing a toy that makes noise) and by monitoring their speech. Utilizing a regional anesthetic approach helps avoid some of the potential large hemodynamic shifts often seen with induction, maintenance, and emergence from general endotracheal anesthesia. This can be highly beneficial in patients who have severe comorbidities such as critical aortic stenosis, severely reduced cardiac or pulmonary function, or for those with a known difficult airway. The benefits of utilizing a general endotracheal anesthetic from the start of the procedure include complete patient immobility, decreased patient anxiety, and definitive airway protection. The GALA trial was a multicenter randomized controlled trial that compared general anesthesia to regional anesthesia for carotid surgery in 3526 patients. A primary outcome of stroke, myocardial infarction, or death within 30 days of surgery occurred in 4.8% of patients in the general anesthesia group and 4.5% in those who received regional anesthesia. There was no statistical difference in the two groups for quality of life, hospital length of stay, and the primary outcome.[7] However, the risk of stroke seemed higher during surgery under general anesthesia in patients with contralateral stenosis. A subgroup analysis from that trial has suggested that regional and local anesthesia may be associated with better neurocognitive outcomes.[8] Retrospective analyses of large databases find higher cardiovascular complication rates in patients undergoing CEA under general anesthesia; however, the conclusion has been that these differences are too small to interpret as clinically significant.[9] Ultimately, both anesthetic choices have been shown to be safe and efficacious and should be tailored to each patient's individual need.

PERIOPERATIVE MEDICAL MANAGEMENT GUIDELINES IN PATIENTS UNDERGOING CAROTID REVASCULARIZATION

Blood pressure management is crucial preoperatively for patients with asymptomatic carotid atherosclerosis, as hypertension has been directly correlated to an increased risk of stroke. Targeting a blood pressure less than 140/90 using lifestyle modifications and medical therapy is highly recommended, since each reduction of 10 mmHg in blood pressure reduces the risk of stroke by 33%.[1] Naturally, clinical judgment and adaptation of such guidelines to baseline parameters and symptoms should be considered critical. Aggressive treatment of hypertension in the setting of acute stroke is not recommended; however, treatment after the acute period is associated with reduced risk of subsequent stroke.[1]

For men aged >45 and women >55 with an anticipated cardiac risk >3%, the US Preventive Services Task Force recommends taking prophylactic daily aspirin due to its role in reducing overall cardiovascular morbidity and death, though there are no adequately powered studies that show a reduction in stroke in asymptomatic patients with carotid stenosis.[1]

Continuing beta blockade in patients already on such is very important; guiding management of beta blockade postoperatively should be based on clinical circumstances. In patients with intermediate to high risks it may be reasonable to start beta blockade. In patients with 3 or more revised cardiac risk index (RCRI) (e.g., diabetes mellitus, heart failure, CAD, renal insufficiency, cerebrovascular accident), it may be reasonable to begin beta blockers before surgery.[10]

Perioperative medical management of patients undergoing carotid revascularization should include blood pressure control (<140/90), beta blockade (heart rate 60–80 beats/min), and statin therapy (LDL <100mg/dL), and antithrombotic therapy should include aspirin (81–325 mg).[1]

ANESTHETIC GOALS

INTRAOPERATIVE ANESTHETICS GOALS FOR CEA

- Maintain blood pressure within 20% of baseline
  - o Invasive beat-to-beat blood pressure monitoring via arterial line is recommended.
  - o Be prepared to nimbly treat both hypotension and hypertension
- This includes "titration" of blood pressure to symptoms, especially during carotid cross-clamping.
- Avoid tachycardia
- Avoid permissive hypercapnia because it may cause a cerebral steal effect
  - o Hyperventilation and hypocapnia could also be detrimental via vasoconstriction.
- Quick emergence from anesthesia for an immediate postoperative neurological assessment
- Smooth emergence, avoiding coughing and bucking from the endotracheal tube which could potentially cause carotid hematoma and airway compression.

GENERAL ANESTHESIA INDUCTION

If general anesthesia is chosen, common recommendations are as follows: propofol (1–2.5 mg/kg) or etomidate (0.15–0.3 mg/kg) titrated to effect. Add a short-acting opioid like fentanyl (1–2 mcg/kg) or remifentanil (1 mcg/kg) and lidocaine (50–100 mg) or esmolol (1 mg/kg) to help blunt the sympathetic response associated with laryngoscopy and tracheal intubation. Caution is exercised to minimize or avoid, if possible, significant deviations in blood pressure during induction and endotracheal intubation.

MAINTENANCE OF ANESTHESIA

The choice between IV anesthetics and volatile agents are dependent on the type of neurological monitoring being used. Total intravenous anesthesia (TIVA) is typically employed in order to avoid interference with somatosensory evoked potential monitoring (propofol and remifentanil infusions are commonly used). If volatile anesthetics are used, they need to be delivered at a dose less than 0.5 minimum alveolar concentration (MAC) to avoid interfering with neurological monitoring. If only electroencephalography (EEG) is used for neuromonitoring, either TIVA or volatile agents may be used. The use of nitrous oxide may cause postoperative nausea and vomiting (PONV), which should be avoided because the retching could increase the risk of postoperative neck hematoma.

HEMODYNAMIC CONTROL (PERTAINS TO EITHER GETA OR REGIONAL ANESTHESIA)

- Due to the potential sudden hemodynamic fluctuations experienced throughout the case, vasopressors, beta blockers, and vasodilators should be readily available for boluses and infusions.
- Hypotension can be treated with phenylephrine (40–100 mcg boluses or an infusion 0.1 mcg–1.0 mcg/kg/min), ephedrine (5–20 mg boluses), vasopressin (0.5–2 unit boluses or an infusion of 0.02–0.1 units/kg/min), or low-dose norepinephrine (1–5 mcg/min).
- Hypertension can be treated with nitroglycerin (25–100 mcg boluses or an infusion 0.5–8 mcg/kg/min), nicardipine (100–500 mcg boluses or an infusion 2–15 mg/h), labetalol 10–20 mg boluses, or esmolol 20–50 mg boluses.

AT WHAT POINTS DURING THE PERIOPERATIVE AND POSTOPERATIVE PERIODS ARE HEMODYNAMIC FLUCTUATIONS EXPECTED?

- *Induction of anesthesia* decreases sympathetic tone and causes vasodilation, leading to abrupt decrease in preload, which may result in hypotension, myocardial depression, bradycardia, and myocardial or cerebral ischemia.
- *Intubation* of the trachea induces a sympathetic response causing tachycardia and hypertension, which can lead to myocardial demand ischemia and cerebral hyperperfusion.
- *Manipulation of the carotid body* during surgical exposure or traction can cause pronounced bradycardia due to increased parasympathetic outflow and can thus be treated with atropine, glycopyrrolate, or norepinephrine. Some surgeons infiltrate the area with local anesthetic in order to blunt the bradycardic response, but the infiltration itself may cause bradycardia and there is insufficient data to support the efficacy of this method. Hypertension and tachycardia may also occur with manipulation of the carotid sinus; therefore, clinicians must be prepared for either scenario.
- *Incision into the carotid artery* exposes the baroreceptors to atmospheric pressure, which is less than the starting intraluminal pressure, possibly leading to an increase

in sympathetic tone, resulting in hypertension and tachycardia.

- *Emergence and extubation from endotracheal anesthesia* can cause coughing and hypertension.

CONCLUSIONS

- Carotid endarterectomy surgery can be successfully performed under regional anesthesia using the ultrasound-guided superficial and intermediate cervical plexus block.
- The superficial branches of the cervical plexus are located above the investing fascia, exiting the deeper plane near the posterior border of the sternocleidomastoid muscle at the level of C4.
- The intermediate CPB is performed by depositing local anesthetic beneath the investing fascia and above the prevertebral fascia. When injected at this location, local anesthetic has been shown to reach the deep cervical plexus roots as well as consistently blocking the superficial cervical plexus.
- Complications of CPB include Horner's syndrome, temporary hemi-diaphragmatic paralysis, vocal cord paralysis, and local anesthetic toxicity.
- Hemodynamic fluctuations are common during CEA, therefore invasive blood pressure monitoring via arterial lines should be considered in higher risk patients.
- Blood pressure should be tightly maintained within 20% of baseline using both vasopressors such as phenylephrine and norepinephrine and vasodilators such as nitroglycerin or nicardipine (calcium channel blocker).

REFERENCES

1. Ricotta JJ, Aburahma A, Ascher E, Eskandari M, Faries P, Lal BK. Updated Society for Vascular Surgery guidelines for management of extracranial carotid disease: executive summary. *J Vasc Surg.* 2011;54(3):832–836. doi: 10.1016/j.jvs.2011.07.004.
2. Howell S. Carotid endarterectomy. *Br J Anaesth.* 2007;99(1):119–131. doi: 10.1201/9781315113845.
3. Kim JS, Ko JS, Bang S, Kim H, Lee SY. Cervical plexus block. *Korean J Anesthesiol.* 2018 Aug;71 (4):274–288. doi: 10.4097/kja.d.18.00143.
4. Pandit JJ, Satya-Krishna R, Gration P. Superficial or deep cervical plexus block for carotid endarterectomy: a systematic review of complications. *Br J Anaesth.* 2007;99(2):159–169. doi: 10.1093/bja/aem160.
5. Telford RJ, Stoneham MD, Pandit JJ. Correct nomenclature of superficial cervical plexus blocks (multiple letters). *Br J Anaesth.* 2004;92(5):775–776. doi: 10.1093/bja/aeh550.
6. Pandit JJ, Dutta D, Morris JF. Spread of injectate with superficial cervical plexus block in humans: an anatomical study. *Br J Anaesth.* 2003;91(5):733–735. doi: 10.1093/bja/aeg250.
7. Lewis SC, Warlow CP, Bodenham AR, et al. General anaesthesia versus local anaesthesia for carotid surgery (GALA): a multicentre, randomised controlled trial. *Lancet.* 2008;372(9656):2132–2142. doi: 10.1016/S0140-6736(08)61699-2.
8. Weber CF, Friedl H, Hueppe M, et al. Impact of general versus local anesthesia on early postoperative cognitive dysfunction following carotid endarterectomy: GALA Study Subgroup Analysis. *World J Surg.* 2009; 33:1526–1532.
9. Dakour Aridi H, Paracha N, Nejim B, et al. Anesthetic type and hospital and outcomes after carotid endarterectomy from the Vascular Quality Initiative database. *J Vasc Surg.* 2018; 67:1419–1428.
10. Fleisher LA, Fleischmann KE, Auerbach AD, et al.; American College of Cardiology; American Heart Association. 2014 ACC/AHA guideline on perioperative cardiovascular evaluation and management of patients undergoing noncardiac surgery: a report of the American College of Cardiology/American Heart Association Task Force on practice guidelines. *J Am Coll Cardiol.* 2014 Dec 9;64(22):e77–137. doi:10.1016/j.jacc.2014.07.944. Epub 2014 Aug 1. PMID: 25091544.
11. Chongruksut W, Vaniyapong T, Rerkasem K. Routine or selective carotid artery shunting for carotid endarterectomy (and different methods of monitoring in selective shunting). *Cochrane Database Syst Rev.* 2014;2014(6):CD000190. doi:10.1002/14651858.CD000190.pub3. Update in: Cochrane Database Syst Rev. 2022 Jun 22;6:CD000190. PMID: 24956204; PMCID: PMC7032624.
12. Ihnatsenka B, Boezaart AP. Applied sonoanatomy of the posterior triangle of the neck. *Int J Shoulder Surg.* 2010 Jul;4(3):63–74. doi: 10.4103/0973-6042.76963. PMID: 21472066; PMCID: PMC3063345.

REVIEW QUESTIONS

(1) Which of the following nerves are not part of the superficial cervical plexus?

A. Superior laryngeal nerve
B. Transverse cervical nerve
C. Great auricular nerve
D. Supraclavicular nerves

(2) The branches of the superficial cervical plexus can be blocked by injecting into which fascial plane?

A. Immediately superficial to the investing fascia
B. Just below the deep prevertebral fascia
C. Inside the platysma
D. Just next to the carotid sheath

(3) Local anesthetic injection into which fascial plane is considered an intermediate cervical plexus block (CPB)?

A. Above the superficial layer of the deep cervical fascia (investing fascia)
B. Above the deep layer of the deep cervical fascia (prevertebral fascia)
C. Below the prevertebral fascia
D. Above the platysma muscle

(4) Which of the following is the least likely complication associated with ultrasound-guided CPB?

A. Horner's syndrome
B. Pneumothorax
C. Dyspnea
D. Dysphonia

(5) Potential advantages of regional anesthesia versus general anesthesia for carotid endarterectomy (CEA) include all the following EXCEPT:

A. Regional anesthesia may be associated with less hemodynamic instability, perioperative morbidity, and better postoperative pain control

B. Intraoperative SSEP monitoring is highly specific in predicting perioperative neurological complications in CEA patients.
C. Regional anesthesia is associated with a higher rate of intraoperative carotid shunt placement.
D. Epidural anesthesia may be used to provide anesthesia for CEA.

(6) According to the most recent literature, all methods of cervical plexus block listed below are successfully used for carotid endarterectomies EXCEPT:

A. Combined superficial and deep CPB
B. Intermediate CPB or deep CPB
C. External CPB
D. Layer-by-layer local infiltration by the surgeon

(7) Which form of neuromonitoring is most commonly used while performing a CEA under regional anesthesia?

A. SSEPs
B. MEPs
C. Processed EEG
D. Physical and verbal responses

(8) The Chassaignac tubercle is:

A. The anterior tubercle of the C7 transverse process
B. Easily palpated in all patients
C. Often visualized with ultrasound imaging to identify the C6 nerve root
D. Situated at the level of the thyroid cartilage in adults

ANSWERS

(1) **A.** The superficial cutaneous nerves that make up the superficial cervical plexus are the lesser occipital (C2, C3), the great auricular (C2, C3), transverse cervical (C2, C3), and the supraclavicular nerves (C3, C4) as seen in Figure 10.3. They supply sensation to the skin, subcutaneous tissue, and superficial structures of the neck. CPB via the superficial or intermediate block techniques can be used to provide anesthesia and postoperative pain management for a variety of surgical procedures on the neck, such as carotid endarterectomies, internal jugular line placement, earlobe repair, clavicular surgery, and thyroid surgery.

Reference

Kim JS, Ko JS, Bang S, Kim H, Lee SY. Cervical plexus block. *Korean J Anesthesiol.* 2018 Aug;71 (4):274–288. doi: 10.4097/kja.d.18.00143.

(2) **A.** The superficial cervical plexus branches can be anesthetized by injecting local anesthetic into the subcutaneous tissue superficial to the investing fascia starting at the mid-portion of the sternocleidomastoid muscle (SCM) in a fan-like fashion, mostly along the lateral border of the SCM (superficial SCB technique). Injecting into the platysma (C) might inconsistently block some of the superficial branches; an injection below the deep prevertebral fascia (B) would produce deep cervical plexus block with some expected spread to the brachial plexus, and injecting next to the carotid sheath (D), typically performed intraoperatively by surgeons, could supplement a CPB, but would not have consistent effects on the cervical plexus nerves, while risking an immediate effect on the sympathetic chain and the vagus nerve.

References

Kim JS, Ko JS, Bang S, Kim H, Lee SY. Cervical plexus block. *Korean J Anesthesiol.* 2018 Aug;71 (4):274–288. doi: 10.4097/kja.d.18.00143.
Telford RJ, Stoneham MD, Pandit JJ. Correct nomenclature of superficial cervical plexus blocks (multiple letters). *Br J Anaesth.* 2004;92(5):775–776. doi: 10.1093/bja/aeh550.
Ihnatsenka B, Boezaart AP. Applied sonoanatomy of the posterior triangle of the neck. *Int J Shoulder Surg.* 2010 Jul;4(3):63–74. doi: 10.4103/0973-6042.76963. PMID: 21472066; PMCID: PMC3063345.

(3) **B.** The intermediate cervical plexus block is performed by injecting local anesthetic beneath the superficial layer of the deep cervical fascia (aka investing fascia), but above the prevertebral fascia, as can be seen in Figure 10.2. The superficial CPB is performed by depositing local anesthesia above the investing fascia and is essentially a subcutaneous field infiltration block.

References

Kim JS, Ko JS, Bang S, Kim H, Lee SY. Cervical plexus block. *Korean J Anesthesiol.* 2018 Aug;71 (4):274–288. doi: 10.4097/kja.d.18.00143.
Telford RJ, Stoneham MD, Pandit JJ. Correct nomenclature of superficial cervical plexus blocks (multiple letters). *Br J Anaesth.* 2004;92(5):775–776. doi: 10.1093/bja/aeh550.
Ihnatsenka B, Boezaart AP. Applied sonoanatomy of the posterior triangle of the neck. *Int J Shoulder Surg.* 2010 Jul;4(3):63–74. doi: 10.4103/0973-6042.76963. PMID: 21472066; PMCID: PMC3063345.

(4) **B.** When performed with ultrasound guidance at and above the C4–C5 levels, the block needle path should be predictably far away from the cupula of the pleura, making pneumothorax the least likely complication listed. Horner's syndrome (ptosis, miosis, anhidrosis) occurs when local anesthetic reaches the cervical sympathetic trunk which is invested by the m. longus colli layer of the deep prevertebral fascia and posterolateral to the carotid sheath (A). Dyspnea (C) that is typically mild and self-limited and can be the result of an inadvertent spread of the local anesthetic to the phrenic nerve, and dysphonia (D) may occur if the vagus nerve or its branches (superior and recurrent laryngeal nerves) are affected.

Reference

Ihnatsenka B, Boezaart AP. Applied sonoanatomy of the posterior triangle of the neck. *Int J Shoulder Surg.* 2010 Jul;4(3):63–74. doi: 10.4103/0973-6042.76963. PMID: 21472066; PMCID: PMC3063345.

(5) **C.** Regional anesthesia is a great alternative to general endotracheal anesthesia (GETA) for CEA, except for the lack of airway control. During a CEA the patient's face and airway are typically covered and far from reach, making any attempt at securing the airway mid-procedure very challenging. Cervical epidural anesthesia, while not popular likely because of its very rare potential for complications, is a validated method for anesthesia in patients undergoing CEA. GETA involves multiple points at which there can be major fluctuations in hemodynamics, including induction of anesthesia, maintenance, and emergence, all of

which may be avoided when performing the CEA under CPB and light sedation. Meta-analysis of observational studies suggests lower mortality, stroke, and myocardial infarction (MI) in patients undergoing CEA under loco-regional anesthesia. However, the analysis of the randomized-controlled trials' data did not demonstrate significant differences in mortality and morbidity rates, possibly due to a lack of pooled statistical power. Direct neurophysiological monitoring allows the surgeon and the anesthetist to be in contact with the patient at all times. SSEP and other methods of neurological monitoring are also accurate in predicting perioperative neurological complications. The rates of intraoperative shunt placement are actually lower in patients undergoing CEA under regional anesthesia

References

Macfarlane A, Vlassakov K, Elkassabany N. Regional anesthesia for vascular surgery: does the anesthetic choice influence outcome? *Curr Opin Anaesthesiol.* 2019;32(5):690–696. doi: 10.1097/ACO.0000000000000781.

Hajibandeh S, Hajibandeh S, Antoniou SA, et al. Meta-analysis and trial sequential analysis of local vs. general anaesthesia for carotid endarterectomy. *Anaesthesia.* 2018;73:1280–1289.

Nwachuku EL, Balzer JR, Yabes JG, Habeych ME, Crammond DJ, Thirumala PD. Diagnostic value of somatosensory evoked potential changes during carotid endarterectomy: a systematic review and meta-analysis. *JAMA Neurol.* 2015 Jan;72(1):73–80. doi: 10.1001/jamaneurol.2014.3071. PMID: 25383418.

(6) **C.** There is no "external" CPB method; it is called superficial CPB. Different combinations of CPB techniques and local infiltration have been used successfully to provide surgical anesthesia for CEA.

References

Kim JS, Ko JS, Bang S, Kim H, Lee SY. Cervical plexus block. *Korean J Anesthesiol.* 2018 Aug;71 (4):274–288. doi: 10.4097/kja.d.18.00143.

Telford RJ, Stoneham MD, Pandit JJ. Correct nomenclature of superficial cervical plexus blocks (multiple letters) [6]. *Br J Anaesth.* 2004;92(5):775–776. doi:10.1093/bja/aeh550

(7) **D.** One of the main advantages and cost-saving aspects of regional anesthesia is the ability to monitor brain function physiologically when performing CEA under regional anesthesia. Continual verbal interaction and intermittent motor function testing (squeezing a rubber toy with the contralateral hand) are considered sufficient in ruling out clinically relevant cerebral perfusion deficits during carotid cross-clamping and cerebral reperfusion. Of the other listed monitors, EEG and SSEP monitoring have been used extensively during CEA under general anesthesia with the latter being most common nowadays.

Reference

Lewis SC, Warlow CP, Bodenham AR, et al. General anaesthesia versus local anaesthesia for carotid surgery (GALA): a multicentre, randomised controlled trial. *Lancet.* 2008;372(9656):2132–2142. doi: 10.1016/S0140-6736(08)61699-2.

(8) **C.** The Chassaignac tubercle is the anterior tubercle of the C6 transverse process and is used to identify the origin of the C6 root of the brachial plexus. It is also known anatomically as the carotid tubercle and it is easily palpable only in young and slim patients with deep palpation that is often uncomfortable. The thyroid cartilage in adults is usually situated approximately at the C4 level, and the cricoid cartilage at the C6 level.

Reference

Ihnatsenka B, Boezaart AP. Applied sonoanatomy of the posterior triangle of the neck. *Int J Shoulder Surg.* 2010 Jul;4(3):63–74. doi: 10.4103/0973-6042.76963. PMID: 21472066; PMCID: PMC3063345.

11.

EYE BLOCKS

Gustavo A. Lozada and Alvaro Andres Macias

STEM CASE AND KEY QUESTIONS

A 67-year-old female presents to the outpatient surgery center for cataract surgery. Vision in her left eye has been worsening in the past year and a half. She has a history of hypertension, hyperlipidemia, and anxiety. Her past surgical history is limited to an appendectomy performed 40 years prior. She has no allergies. In the preop area, she appears slightly anxious. She has several questions about the type of anesthesia she is going to get. She is hoping she does not need general anesthesia. She is worried by the fact that a friend of hers has had a complication while getting an eye block in preparation for his retina surgery.

(1) WHAT ANESTHETIC OPTIONS ARE AVAILABLE FOR CATARACT SURGERY?

Anesthetic options for cataract surgery include topical anesthesia, an eye block, or, in rare cases, general anesthesia. Topical anesthesia and eye blocks are the most common modalities used for this surgical procedure. Both modalities can be combined with sedation. General anesthesia is typically limited to situations when the other modalities are not appropriate, including cases when the patients may not be cooperative or when patients with complex underlying comorbidities may not be able to undergo the procedure safely under sedation/block. Under certain circumstances, patient preference may warrant use of general anesthesia, but there should be a thorough discussion with the patient, family, and surgeon prior to following this route.

(2) WHAT ARE THE MOST FREQUENT BLOCKS PERFORMED FOR EYE PROCEDURES?

The most frequent blocks performed for eye procedures are the retrobulbar block, the peribulbar block, and the sub-Tenon's block, with the latter usually performed by the surgeon. The decision process of which block to perform should take into consideration the particular surgical procedure, the surgeon's requirements, the patient, and the proficiency of the provider performing the block.

(3) WHAT IS THE MOST LIKELY CHOICE OF ANESTHETIC FOR THIS PATIENT?

Surgery for this patient could be performed under topical anesthesia or any of the aforementioned blocks. She has an underlying history of anxiety, but with adequate sedation, this should not present as an obstacle during the surgery. If the surgeon does not require akinesia of the eye, topical anesthesia with sedation can be acceptable for her cataract surgery.

(4) WHAT MEDICATIONS CAN SHE GET FOR SEDATION?

There are multiple options for sedation. A benzodiazepine, such as midazolam, can be considered. If she is going to receive an eye block, she will require a deeper plane of sedation when the needle is introduced. This can be accomplished by combining remifentanil and midazolam, for example. Alternatively, a combination of dexmedetomidine and remifentanil can be administered. This patient has a history of anxiety. It is important to consider what anxiolytics, if any, she is taking. For instance, if she takes a benzodiazepine regularly, her response to the sedation administered might differ. She may have a higher requirement compared to a benzodiazepine-naïve patient.

(4) ARE THERE ANY CONTRAINDICATIONS FOR SEDATION IN THIS PATIENT?

This patient, based on the above history, does not have any contraindications to being sedated.

(5) WHEN OBTAINING CONSENT FROM THE PATIENT, WHAT RISKS SHOULD BE DISCUSSED?

A thorough discussion of the anesthetic risks should be an indelible part of the informed consent process. If she is going to have an eye block procedure, it is important to discuss in detail the side effects and complications that are associated with it. These include but are not limited to pain, infection, allergic reactions, bleeding, bruising, trauma to the eye, changes in the heart rate and blood pressure, nerve damage, and intravascular injection.

(6) WHAT ARE SOME POSSIBLE SIDE EFFECTS AND COMPLICATIONS FROM EYE BLOCKS? HOW ARE THESE TREATED?

Eye blocks can be associated with eliciting the oculocardiac reflex. The treatment entails stopping the stimulus that is causing the reflex, supporting the patient, and treating with glycopyrrolate or atropine if it does not subside with discontinuation of the triggering stimulus.

In the case of inadvertent intravascular injection, the patient might seize. Appropriate monitoring and basic life support measures are taken, starting with supplemental oxygen, safe positioning, airway support, and aspiration prevention. Symptomatic therapy, including benzodiazepine administrations, should be considered. Advanced airway management equipment should be readily available in the area where the block is performed in the event the airway has to be secured emergently. Administration of lipid rescue protocol should be considered in the context of evolving local anesthetic systemic toxicity and cardiotoxicity manifestations.

If an allergic reaction occurs, appropriate treatment will depend on its extent and severity. Trauma to the eye might warrant immediate surgical intervention.

DISCUSSION

Cataract surgery, the most common ophthalmic surgical procedure performed in the United States, has an increasing incidence.[1] In the United States, 30 million people were estimated to have cataracts in 2020.[2] Other common ophthalmic surgical procedures include vitreoretinal surgery, glaucoma surgery, pterygium surgery, and strabismus repair.

When providing anesthesia for any ophthalmic procedure, the goal is to ensure maximal patient comfort and safety while producing optimal conditions for a successful surgery. An understanding of relevant anatomy is essential for selecting the most appropriate technique for each patient and minimizing complications.

ANATOMY OF THE EYE

BONY STRUCTURES

Orbit

The orbit is composed of seven bones—the zygomatic, sphenoid, frontal, ethmoid, lacrimal, maxilla, and palatine.[3,4] The orbital margin is quadrilateral shaped. The frontal bone forms the *supraorbital margin*. The *supraorbital notch*, through which the supraorbital vessels and nerve pass, lies at the junction of the lateral sharp two-thirds and medial rounded third of the frontal bone. The zygomatic bone (laterally) and the maxilla (medially) form the *infraorbital margin*. The zygomatic process of the frontal bone (superiorly) and the frontal process of the zygomatic bone (inferiorly) form the *lateral margin*. The maxillary process of the frontal bone (superiorly) and the lacrimal crest of the of the frontal process of the maxilla (inferiorly) form the *medial margin* (Figure 11.1).

The orbital cavity walls, which are lined with periosteum, consist of a floor (or inferior wall), a lateral and a medial wall, and a roof (superior wall). The orbital plate of the maxilla (primarily), small orbital process of the palatine, and orbital surface of the zygomatic bone form the floor (inferior wall). The zygomatic bone forms the anterior third of the lateral wall, while the greater wing of the sphenoid bone forms its posterior two-thirds. Four bones contribute to the medial wall: the sphenoid, the ethmoid (orbital process), the lacrimal bone, and the maxilla (frontal process). The orbital plate of the frontal bone and the lesser wing of the sphenoid (small extent) form the roof.

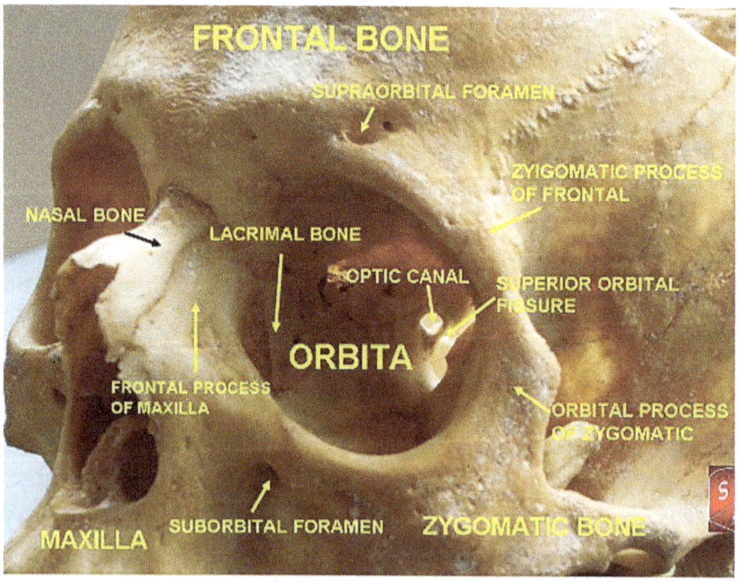

Figure 11.1. The orbital bones.
Anatomist 90 (November 21, 2011). https://commons.wikimedia.org/wiki/File:Orbital_cavity.jpg
Creative Commons Attribution-Share Alike 3.0 Unported license.

Periorbita

The walls of the orbit are lined by the periorbita or orbital periosteum. Anteriorly, it is continuous with the periosteum that lines the outer surfaces of the orbital bones. The periorbita is continuous posteriorly with the periosteal layer of the dura, which fuses with the meningeal layer of the dura at the optic canal.

FASCIAL SHEATH OF THE EYEBALL (TENON'S CAPSULE)

The facial sheath of the globe, a thin membrane that surrounds the globe, separates it from the orbital fat and forms a socket for it. It is separated from the outer surface of the sclera by the sub-Tenon space, a potential space. The fascial sheath is attached to the sclera anteriorly. It fuses with the sclera at the exit of the optic nerve and with the meninges around the optic nerve posteriorly. The fascial sheath is pierced by the tendons of all six extrinsic muscles as they pass to their insertion points on the globe.

The primary purpose of the fascial sheath is to position and support the globe within the orbit and facilitate the actions of the extrinsic muscles of the eye to cause movement of the eye.

THE GLOBE

The globe consists of three layers: an outer fibrous layer, a vascular pigmented layer, and an inner neural layer. The fibrous layer is composed anteriorly by the translucent cornea and posteriorly by the opaque sclera. Anteriorly, the sclera is lined by the conjunctiva and fascial sheath of the eyeball. It is continuous with the cornea anteriorly, joining it at the corneoscleral junction (limbus). Posteriorly, it is connected to the fascial sheath of the eyeball. At the posterior scleral foramen, the sclera fuses with the dural and arachnoid sheaths of the optic nerve. In adults, the sclera is a white structure. In children, it has a bluish tinge. In the elderly, it can have a yellowish tinge due to the deposition of fat.

The vascular pigmented layer comprises the iris and ciliary body anteriorly and the choroid peripherally and posteriorly. The inner neural layer overlying the posterior aspect of the other two layers comprises the retina.

The globe is composed of an anterior, smaller segment, which forms about one-sixth of the structure, and a posterior, larger segment, which contributes five-sixths of the structure. The convex anterior segment is composed of two chambers, anterior and posterior. The anterior chamber contains aqueous humor, produced by the ciliary body. The posterior chamber contains the lens. The iris separates the two chambers. They communicate via the pupil.

The posterior segment is composed of the vitreous humor, retina, macula, and root of the optic nerve.

The mean anteroposterior (axial) length of the globe is about 22–25 mm in adults.[5] In myopic persons, it can be significantly longer (in excess of 26 mm). The average distance from the anterior surface of the globe to the equator is 12–15 mm.

COMPARTMENTS OF THE ORBITAL CAVITY

There are three anatomical intraorbital compartments defined by the globe and muscular retrobulbar cone: intraocular, intraconal, and extraconal. The intraocular compartment comprises the globe. The intraconal compartment refers to the space within the orbital cone, which is bounded by the four rectus muscles and posterior aspect of the cone. Neural and vascular structures course within it. The cone is not a completely closed space, which has implications for procedures (e.g., local anesthetic can diffuse in or out). The extraconal compartment refers to the space outside the cone.

INNERVATION OF THE ORBIT

Sensory innervation of the globe and orbit is primarily by the frontal and nasociliary branches of the ophthalmic nerve (V1 or first branch of the trigeminal nerve). The infraorbital branch of the maxillary nerve (V2 or second branch of the trigeminal nerve) provides sensory innervation to part of the orbital floor.

THE OPTIC NERVE

The optic nerve, or cranial nerve II, is composed of approximately 1 million myelinated axons of the retinal ganglion cells.[6] It consists of four parts: intraocular, intraorbital, intracanalicular, and intracranial. The intraocular part, the only segment not enveloped by the meninges, extends from the optic disc to the posterior margins of the sclera. The intraorbital part extends from the posterior globe to the optic canal. The intracanalicular part courses inside the optic canal of the sphenoid bone. The intracranial part courses posteriorly, superior to the diaphragma sellae and cavernous sinus within the middle cranial fossa to converge with its contralateral optic nerve to form the optic chiasm.

CILIARY GANGLION

The ciliary ganglion, a 2–3-mm structure, is located approximately 2 mm posterior to the globe, between the optic nerve and lateral rectus muscle.[7] It contains preganglionic fibers, which arise from the Edinger-Westphal nucleus, and postganglionic, parasympathetic fibers which exit via the short ciliary nerves. These innervate the sphincter pupillae muscle (contracts the pupil) and the ciliary muscle (controls accommodation). Sensory fibers from the nasociliary nerve and sympathetic nerves from the internal carotid plexus also pass through the ciliary ganglion without synapsing.

Motor innervation of the extrinsic or extraocular muscles is provided by the oculomotor nerve (CN III) to the superior, inferior, and medial rectus muscles and the inferior oblique muscle, the abducens nerve (CN VI) to the lateral rectus muscle, and trochlear nerve (CN IV) to the superior oblique muscle (see Table 11.1). Of note, the trochlear nerve does not course within the muscular cone of the orbit. It is therefore an extraconal structure, which has implications for regional anesthesia procedures.

Table 11.1 SUMMARY OF THE MAIN ACTIONS ON THE EYEBALL AND INNERVATION OF THE EXTRAOCULAR MUSCLES

EXTRAOCULAR MUSCLE	ACTION ON THE EYE (ACTING ALONE)	INNERVATION
Superior rectus	Elevation, medial rotation, intorsion	Oculomotor nerve (CN III)
Inferior rectus	Depression, medial rotation, extorsion	Oculomotor nerve (CN III)
Medial rectus	Medial rotation (adduction)	Oculomotor nerve (CN III)
Lateral rectus	Lateral rotation (abduction)	Abducens nerve (CN VI)
Superior oblique	Depression, lateral rotation (abduction), medial rotation of the cornea (intorsion)	Trochlear nerve (CN IV)
Inferior oblique	Elevation, lateral rotation (abduction), extorsion	Oculomotor nerve (CN III)

THE EXTRINSIC MUSCLES OF THE EYE

There are six extrinsic muscles (extraocular muscles) which are responsible for movements of the eyeball. These consist of four rectus muscles (superior, inferior, lateral, and medial) and two oblique muscles (superior and inferior). See Table 11.1 for a summary of their action on the eyeball and innervation.

The following is a description of commonly performed eye blocks for surgical procedures. The decision process of which block or anesthetic procedure to perform is multifactorial and should include reviewing the type and complexity of the surgery, the patient, risks and benefits, the provider's level of proficiency, and the surgeon's requirements. Direct communication is critical in choosing the optimal technique.

RETROBULBAR ANESTHESIA

An intraconal procedure in essence, the retrobulbar block consists of injecting local anesthetic solution into the muscular cone. It requires a relatively smaller volume of local anesthetic solution compared to the peribulbar technique. Volumes injected can range from 3 to 5 ml.[8]

The aim of this procedure is to block the ciliary ganglia and ciliary nerves and cranial nerves II, III, IV, and VI. This technique spares the facial nerve (CN VII), which provides motor innervation to the orbicularis oculi muscle. Thus, the patient can close the eye but cannot open it (the levator palpebrae muscle receives its motor innervation from CN III). If it is desired to suppress blinking, a supplemental facial nerve block may be performed. As the trochlear nerve does not course within the muscular cone, function of the superior oblique might be spared, depending on the spread of the local anesthetic solution. This may result in incomplete akinesia of the globe.

TECHNIQUE

Assuming the patient is supine, with the eye in the neutral position (eye directed straight ahead), the retrobulbar needle (25G × 1½ inch) is inserted through the skin below the inferior lid at the junction between the medial two-thirds and lateral third of the inferior edge of the orbit (see Figure 11.2). The needle is directed slightly medially and cephalad, toward the orbital apex, and advanced to a depth of 25–35 mm; 3–5 ml of local anesthetic solution is slowly injected after negative aspiration.[8] A supplemental facial nerve block may be performed to abolish blinking.

INDICATIONS

Indications for retrobulbar anesthesia include cataract surgery, vitreoretinal procedures, glaucoma surgery, strabismus surgery, pterygium surgery, enucleation, and evisceration.

SIDE EFFECTS AND COMPLICATIONS

There is an associated increased risk of injury to the globe or the structures in the muscular cone with this block. The main

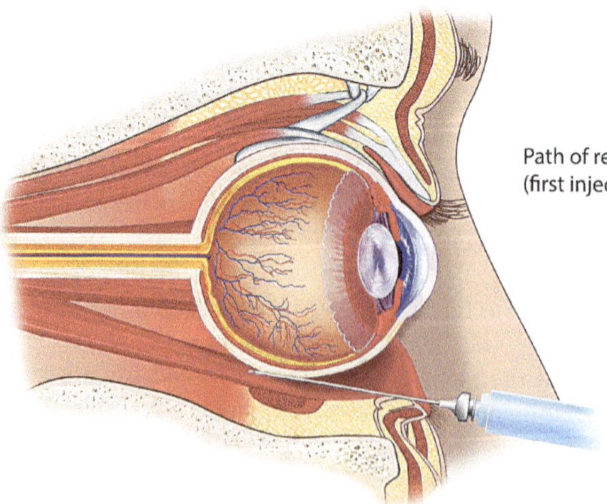

Figure 11.2. The retrobulbar block.

cause of serious side effects and complications is block needle misplacement. Possible side effects and complications include the following:

1. Chemosis (subconjunctival edema): this can usually result from injecting too rapidly or too anteriorly. Applying gentle pressure, either manually or with a pressure balloon, can reduce chemosis.
2. Pain on injection
3. Allergic reactions may happen, in particular with the use of ester local anesthetics or when hyaluronidase is used in the mix.
4. Perforation of the globe: symptoms include pain, sudden loss of vision, and a poor red reflex. The risk is increased in myopic eyes (longer eyes), eyes with scleral buckles, and when angling the needle too superficially before passing the equator of the eye.
5. Retrobulbar hemorrhage: this can manifest as motor block, a sudden rise in intraocular pressure, closing of the upper lid, and proptosis of the eye. A retrobulbar hemorrhage can induce the oculocardiac reflex. Depending on its severity, immediate surgical intervention for decompression might be required.
6. Central retinal artery occlusion: this can be caused directly by injection or can be secondary to a retrobulbar hemorrhage.
7. Brainstem anesthesia: central spread of the local anesthetic solution can result from direct injection into optic nerve sheath. This can manifest as drowsiness, contralateral blindness, agitation, confusion, convulsions, respiratory depression, and cardiac arrest. Immediate intervention is required, which includes supporting the patient and possibly securing the airway.
8. Intra-arterial injection: signs and symptoms can include cardiopulmonary arrest and convulsions from retrograde arterial spread. As above, immediate intervention is required, which includes supporting the patient and possibly securing the airway.
9. Optic nerve atrophy: injection into the optic nerve sheath or hemorrhage within the nerve sheath can cause direct damage to the optic nerve. This manifests as partial or complete loss of vision.
10. Postoperative strabismus: intramuscular injection of local anesthetic may result in myotoxicity, which can result in strabismus.
11. Oculocardiac reflex (further discussed in detail below).

THE OCULOCARDIAC REFLEX

The oculocardiac reflex is a vagally mediated reduction in heart rate of 10% or more that results from application of direct pressure to the globe, manipulation of the globe, or traction of the extraocular muscles. It most commonly manifests as sinus bradycardia but can also manifest as ectopy, atrioventricular block, junctional rhythm, ventricular tachycardia, and asystole. Its severity varies, but can result in profound bradycardia that can progress to asystole. The oculocardiac reflex can be worsened by hypercarbia, hypoxia, acidosis, concurrent administration of an opioid, and light anesthesia, if the patient is undergoing general anesthesia.

The oculocardiac reflex is a trigeminovagal reflex. It has both an afferent and efferent component. The afferent limb is the trigeminal nerve (ciliary ganglion to the ophthalmic division of the trigeminal nerve (V1) to the gasserian ganglion to the main trigeminal sensory nucleus). The efferent limb is the vagus nerve (CN X). The afferents synapse with the visceral motor nucleus of the vagus nerve in the reticular formation from where the efferents travel to the heart to have a response.[9,10]

Treatment entails stopping the stimulus (e.g., the surgery or block), supporting the patient, and administering intravenous anticholinergics such as glycopyrrolate or atropine if it does not promptly resolve after removal of the stimulus. The choice of anticholinergic to administer should be guided by the severity of the reflex. This reflex is most commonly seen in children (especially in strabismus surgery) but is also seen in adults.

PERIBULBAR ANESTHESIA

The peribulbar block is an extraconal procedure.[11–13] Local anesthetic solution is deposited outside the muscular cone. Being a volume-dependent block, it requires a larger volume of local anesthetic solution compared to the retrobulbar technique. Volumes injected can range from 6 to 12 ml.[8] The local anesthetic solution spreads into the corpus adiposum of the orbit, including within the cone. It also spreads anteriorly to the eyelids, which results in blockade of the orbicularis oculi muscle. Of note, the spread of local anesthetic solution within the orbital corpus adiposum is unpredictable, which can lead to varying results, including failed or partial blocks. In light of this, attaining full akinesia may require larger volumes of local anesthetic solution in some patients.

The aim of this technique is to block the ciliary nerves, cranial nerves III, IV, and VI. This technique does not block the optic nerve (although, if high volumes of local anesthetic solution are administered, there is potential for the injectate to diffuse intraconally, given that the cone is not a fully enclosed space).

TECHNIQUE

The eye is in the neutral position. The classical technique involves injection at two sites (see Figure 11.3). For the first injection (inferior and temporal), the peribulbar needle (25G × 7/8 inch) is introduced at the same site as for the retrobulbar block (the needle is inserted through the skin

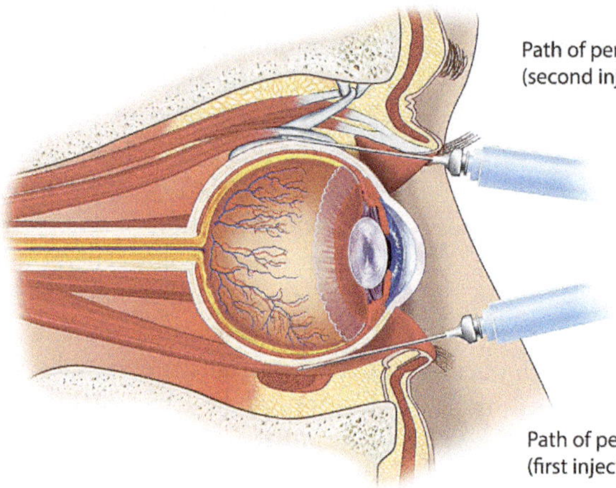

Figure 11.3. The peribulbar block, superior second injection technique.

below the inferior lid at the junction between the medial two-thirds and lateral third of the inferior edge of the orbit). However, the needle is not angled as for the retrobulbar block; it is inserted straight down, toward the floor. The needle is advanced to a maximum of 25 mm. For the second injection, which is superior and nasal, the needle is introduced between the lateral two-thirds and medial third of the superior edge of the orbit.

Although the classical technique involves two injections, a successful block can be attained with a single inferior injection with a larger volume (7–10 ml). Whittset et al.[14] and Pannu[15] advocate a single injection peribulbar technique for safety and increased patient comfort.

Should a block require subsequent supplementation, for instance, due to initial inadequate blockade, it is imperative to consider the following. The risk of complications may be increased due to anatomic distortion caused by the initial volume injected.

INDICATIONS

Indications for peribulbar anesthesia include cataract surgery, vitreoretinal procedures, glaucoma surgery, strabismus surgery, and pterygium surgery.

SIDE EFFECTS AND COMPLICATIONS

The main cause of serious side effects and complications is needle misplacement. Possible side effects and complications include the following:

1. Chemosis (subconjunctival edema); this can usually result from injecting too rapidly or too anteriorly
2. Pain on injection
3. Spread to the contralateral eye
4. Periorbital ecchymoses (periorbital hematoma)
5. Transient blindness
6. Optic nerve injury; this can result from unintentional retrobulbar injection
7. Allergic reactions
8. Oculocardiac reflex.

CONTRAINDICATIONS TO RETROBULBAR AND PERIBULBAR ANESTHESIA

1. Patient refusal
2. Uncooperative patient (including pediatric patients and underlying medical conditions)
3. Long duration of surgical procedure (in excess of 90–120 minutes). This is due to the limited duration of the block. However, this can be counteracted if the surgeon is willing to supplement the block intraoperatively if required (e.g., with a sub-Tenon's block).
4. Allergy to local anesthetic solution component(s). This should be examined on a case-by-case basis. Most allergies to local anesthetics are to the ester family of local anesthetics. Solutions can be adjusted as needed.
5. Perforated globe
6. Infection at the site
7. Coagulopathies
8. Patients on anticoagulants (e.g., warfarin—INR thresholds vary by institution. One study concluded that discontinuation of oral anticoagulants was not justified).[16]

THE SUB-TENON'S BLOCK

As previously mentioned, the sub-Tenon space is a potential space between the fascial sheath of the eyeball (Tenon's capsule) and the outer surface of the sclera. Depositing local anesthetic in this space produces analgesia of the eye via action on the short ciliary nerves as they travel to the globe. It also produces akinesia via direct blockade of anterior motor nerve fibers of the extraocular muscles. Depending on the spread of the local anesthetic, it may also affect vision as the local anesthetic diffuses along the anterior portion of the optic nerve.

TECHNIQUE

Under sterile conditions, the patient is instructed to look upward and outward (see Figure 11.4).[17–19] Surface anesthesia is first attained via the deposition of local anesthetic drops on the conjunctiva and cornea. Antiseptic eye drops are subsequently applied to the area. Surgical access of the sub-Tenon space is obtained (surgical "snip" technique): the conjunctiva and Tenon's capsule are gripped with forceps, a small incision is made through these with scissors, and a blunt cannula is inserted. Alternatively, a cannula can be introduced without a prior incision. Either a blunt cannula or sharp needle is used. The volume of local anesthetic deposited ranges from 1.5 to 5 ml (with an average of 3 ml). This procedure is primarily performed in the inferonasal quadrant of the eye.

INDICATIONS

The sub-Tenon block, used primarily for cataract surgery, can also be used for other procedures, such as vitreoretinal surgery, trabeculectomy, optic nerve fenestration, strabismus surgery, photocoagulation, and drug delivery.

SIDE EFFECTS

Common side effects/minor complications include chemosis (ranging from 23%[20] to 100%,[21] subconjunctival hemorrhage, and pain. More serious, rarer complications have been reported (in a very limited number of case reports).[22] These include brain stem anesthesia, globe perforation, orbital and/or retrobulbar hemorrhage, retinal ischemia, optic nerve damage, dysfunction of the rectus muscle, and orbital swelling.

FACIAL NERVE BLOCK

As mentioned previously, the retrobulbar block spares the facial nerve. If it is desired to prevent the patient from blinking, a supplemental partial facial nerve block could be performed. Variants of an Atkinson[23] technique are the most commonly used for this block. At the level of the lateral canthus, a skin wheel is made 2–3 cm lateral to the lateral rim of the orbit. Then 5 ml of local anesthetic are injected superiorly and inferiorly from this point to form a "V" which anesthetizes fibers of the facial nerve.

COMPARISON OF RETROBULBAR, PERIBULBAR, AND SUB-TENON'S BLOCKS

Given that an adequate volume of local anesthetic solution is injected, both the peribulbar and retrobulbar blocks accomplish the same anesthetic goals. This is due to the fact that the cone is not a completely enclosed space, which permits spread of local anesthetic (including intraconally). It has been suggested that since, theoretically, the retrobulbar block has a higher risk of complications, such as brainstem anesthesia, optic nerve injury, and retrobulbar hemorrhage, the peribulbar block is preferable.[8] Compared to both the peribulbar and retrobulbar blocks, the sub-Tenon's block, which can produce both adequate anesthesia and akinesia, has the better safety profile. The decision process of which block to perform is multifactorial and includes safety profile, provider proficiency, and depth of anesthesia and akinesia required.

LOCAL ANESTHETIC SELECTION

The local anesthetics most commonly used for performing eye blocks are bupivacaine, lidocaine, mepivacaine, and ropivacaine. These can be used either alone or as a combination of two local anesthetics. An example of a local anesthetic solution

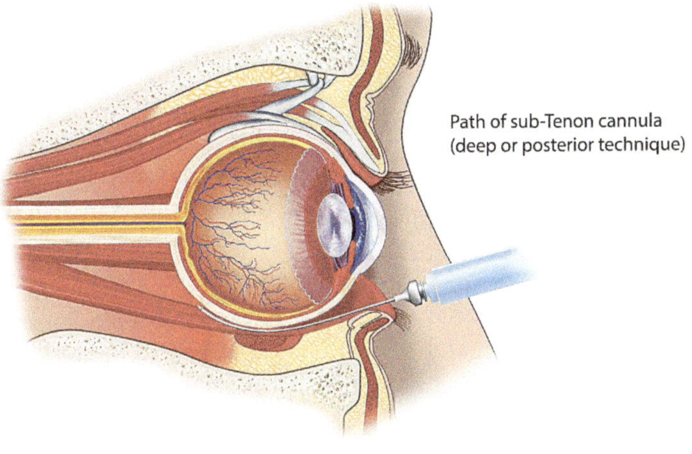

Figure 11.4. The sub-Tenon's block.

used is a combination of preservative-free lidocaine 2% with an equal volume of preservative-free bupivacaine 0.75% (e.g., 5 cc of lidocaine 2% plus 5 cc of bupivacaine 0.75 %).

ADJUVANTS

Hyaluronidase

Hyaluronidase is a proteolytic enzyme that hydrolyzes hyaluronan (hyaluronic acid), a glycosaminoglycans found in the extracellular matrix of most connective tissues. Adding it to the local anesthetic mixture facilitates the spread of the local anesthetic in the orbit. In ophthalmology, it is used for peribulbar, retrobulbar, and sub-Tenon's blocks. The rationale for its use in these procedures includes causing a quicker spread of local anesthetic solution, which limits myotoxicity, with decreased incidence of strabismus,[24,25] diminished distortion of the surgical site,[26] and decreased rise in intraocular pressure. Doses added to the local anesthetic mixture range from 1 to 150 IU/ml.[27]

α-2 Adrenergic Agonists

The use of the α-2 adrenergic agonists clonidine and dexmedetomidine for ophthalmic blocks has also been reported.[28,29]

Epinephrine

Administration of epinephrine to prolong the duration of the eye block has decreased. Vasospasm and retinal ischemia are potential side effects if it is added to the local anesthetic solution.

ALTERNATIVES TO RETROBULBAR, PERIBULBAR, AND SUB-TENON'S BLOCKS

TOPICAL ANESTHESIA

Administration of local anesthetic eye drops anesthetizes the cornea. This allows for cataract surgery to be performed. This form of anesthesia is associated with less risk than that of the needle techniques: peribulbar, retrobulbar, and sub-Tenon's blocks.[30] This method requires cooperation from the patient, as motion of the eye is fully preserved. Some surgeons, however, prefer to have full akinesia, which is not attained by this method. Nevertheless, the use of topical anesthesia for cataract surgery in the United States is increasing.

If needed, the surgeon can supplement the topical anesthetic with an intracameral injection of local anesthetic. This entails injecting a small amount of local anesthetic (0.1 ml) into the anterior chamber.

SUBCONJUNCTIVAL ANESTHESIA

Subconjunctival anesthesia, also known as perilimbal anesthesia, provides anesthesia to the anterior chamber without akinesia. It can be described as an anterior or superficial sub-Tenon's block. It can be used for pterygium, cataract, and anterior glaucoma surgery. After administering a topical anesthetic, the surgeon lifts the superotemporal or inferotemporal conjunctiva 5–8 mm from the limbus with a fine bore needle (27- to 30-gauge); 0.5–0.8 ml of local anesthetic solution is injected into the subconjunctiva.

CONCURRENT CONSIDERATION

SEDATION

There is a lot of variability on the agents used for sedation for eye procedures. Commonly used agents include a benzodiazepine, such as midazolam, an opioid such as remifentanil or fentanyl, ketamine, propofol, and dexmedetomidine.[31–34] These can be used alone or in combination. When being sedated, patients need to be properly monitored. The anesthesia provider must always be ready to treat any side effects promptly, including respiratory depression. All potentially necessary emergency equipment should be immediately available.

REVIEW OF RELEVANT POINTS

- An in-depth understanding of relevant anatomy is essential for both choosing the optimal eye block and performing it safely. This includes being familiar with the bony structures of the orbit and the structures of the globe, including its fascial sheaths, compartments, and innervation.
- There are three anatomical intraorbital compartments to consider: an intraocular, intraconal, and extraconal compartment. The globe comprises the intraocular compartment. The intraconal compartment is bound by the posterior aspect of the globe and four rectus muscles. The space outside this cone is the extraconal compartment.
- The intraconal compartment is not a completely enclosed, sealed space. This permits substances such as local anesthetic solutions to diffuse in and out of the space.
- Sensory innervation of the globe and orbit is primarily by the frontal and nasociliary branches of the ophthalmic nerve (V1 or first branch of the trigeminal nerve).
- Four extraocular muscles—the superior rectus, inferior rectus, medial rectus, and inferior oblique—receive their motor innervation from the oculomotor nerve (CN III). The motor innervation of the lateral rectus and superior oblique muscles is supplied by the abducens (CN VI) and trochlear nerves (CN IV), respectively.
- The retrobulbar block is an intraconal procedure. It provides anesthesia by blocking the ciliary ganglia and ciliary nerves and cranial nerves II, III, IV, and VI. This technique spares the facial nerve, which may warrant performing a supplemental facial nerve block. Cranial nerve IV courses outside the cone and might be spared as well.

- The retrobulbar block requires a low volume of local anesthetic solution.
- Minor complications/side effects of the retrobulbar block include chemosis and pain on injection. Major complications include globe rupture, retrobulbar hemorrhage, the oculocardiac reflex, central retinal artery occlusion, optic nerve injury, intravascular injection, and myotoxicity with possible resultant strabismus.
- The peribulbar block is an extraconal procedure. It provides anesthesia by blocking the ciliary nerves, cranial nerves III, IV, and VI. It does not block the optic nerve.
- The peribulbar block requires a higher volume of local anesthetic solution.
- The benefits of the peribulbar block, compared to the retrobulbar block, include lessened potential for intraocular, intravascular, and intradural injection, decreased risk of retrobulbar hemorrhage, and decreased risk of injury to the optic nerve.
- Minor complications/side effects of the peribulbar block include pain on injection, chemosis, and spread to the contralateral side. Major complications include periorbital ecchymoses, transient blindness, optic nerve injury, allergic reactions, and the oculocardiac reflex.
- The oculocardiac reflex is a trigeminovagal reflex with an afferent component (the trigeminal nerve) and an efferent component (the vagus nerve). Treatment includes stopping the stimulus, supporting the patient, and administering an anticholinergic as needed.
- The sub-Tenon's block produces analgesia of the eye via action on the short ciliary nerves and akinesia via blockade of the motor fibers of the extraocular muscles.
- Hyaluronidase, a proteolytic enzyme, is used as an adjuvant in the local anesthetic mixture. It facilitates the spread of the solution and is believed to limit myotoxicity and reduce rises in intraocular pressure.
- There are multiple options for patient sedation for performing eye blocks and eye surgery. Commonly used agents include midazolam, remifentanil, fentanyl, dexmedetomidine, ketamine, and propofol.

REFERENCES

1. Gollogly H, Hodge D, Sauver J, et al. Increasing incidence of cataract surgery: population-based study. *J Cataract Refract Surg.* 2013;39(9):1383–1389.
2. Congdon N, Vingerling JR, Klein BE, et al.; Eye Diseases Prevalence Research Group. Prevalence of cataract and pseudophakia/aphakia among adults in the United States. *Arch Ophthalmol.* 2004;122(4): 487–494.
3. Netter F. *Atlas of Human Anatomy*. 5th ed. Philadelphia: Saunders; 2011.
4. Snell R, Lemp M, eds. *Clinical Anatomy of the Eye*. Boston: Blackwell Scientific Publications; 1989.
5. Bhardwaj V, Rajeshbhai G. Axial length, anterior chamber depth: a study in different age groups and refractive errors. *J Clin Diagn Res.* 2013;7(10):2211–2212.
6. Rea P, ed. *Clinical Anatomy of the Cranial Nerves*. San Diego, CA: Academic Press; 2014:7–26.
7. Masland R, Albright T, Dallos P, et al., eds. *The Senses: A Comprehensive Reference*. New York: Academic Press; 2008:521–536.
8. Hadzic A, ed. *The New York School of Regional Anesthesia: Textbook of Regional Anesthesia and acute Pain Management*. New York: McGraw-Hill; 2007:362–365.
9. Schaller, B. Trigeminocardiac reflex. *J Neurol.* 2004;251(6):658–665.
10. Lord, J. Anaesthesia for eye surgery in paediatrics. *Anaesth Intensive Care Med.* 2010;11(10):429–433.
11. Bloomberg L. Administration of periocular anesthesia. *J Cataract Refract Surg.* 1986;12:677–679.
12. Davis D, Mandel M. Posterior peribulbar anesthesia: an alternative to retrobulbar anesthesia. *J Cataract Refract Surg.* 1986;12:182–184.
13. Bloomberg L. Anterior periocular anesthesia: five years' experience. *J Cataract Refract Surg.* 1991;17:508–511.
14. Whitsett J, Balyeat H, McClure B. Comparison of one-injection-site peribulbar anesthesia and retrobulbar anesthesia. *J Cataract Refract Surg.* 1990;3:71–81.
15. Pannu J. Single injection peribulbar technique for instant sight cataract surgery. In: Gills J, Sanders D, eds. *Ophthalmic Anesthesia*. Thorofare, NJ: Slack Inc; 1993:146–149.
16. Calenda E, Genevois O, et al. Peribulbar anesthesia in 750 patients treated with oral anticoagulants. *Int J Ophtalmol.* 2014;7(1): 110–113.
17. Kumar C, Williamson S, Manickam B. A review of sub-Tenon's block: current practice and recent development. *Eur J Anaesthesiol.* 2005;22:567–577.
18. Ta C. Minimizing the risk of endophthalmitis following intravitreous injections. *Retina.* 2004;24:699–705.
19. Kumar C, Dowd T, Adams W, et al. Methodology of evaluating conjunctival appearance following sub-Tenon's block for phacoemulsification cataract surgery. *Eye.* 2006;20:1110–1111.
20. Roman S, Chong D, Boureau C, et al. Sub-Tenon's anaesthesia: an efficient and safe technique. *Br J Ophthalmol.* 1997;81:673–676.
21. Kumar C, Dodds C. Evaluation of Greenbaum's sub-Tenon's block. *Br J Anaesth.* 2001;87:631–633.
22. Kumar C, Eid H, Dodds C. Sub-Tenon's anaesthesia: complications and their prevention. *Eye.* 2011;25:694–703.
23. Van Lindt M. Paralysie palpebrale transitoire provoquee dans l'operation de la cataracte. *Ann Ocul.* 1914;151:420–424.
24. Brown S, Coats D, Collins M, et al. Second cluster of strabismus cases after periocular anesthesia without hyaluronidase. *J Cataract Refract Surg.* 2001;27:1872–1875.
25. Hamada S, Devys J, Xuan T, et al. Role of hyaluronidase in diplopia after peribulbar anesthesia for cataract surgery. *Ophthalmology.* 2005;112:879–882.
26. Prosser D, Rodney G, Mian T, et al. Re-evaluation of hyaluronidase in peribulbar anaesthesia. *Br J Ophthalmol.* 1996;80:827–830.
27. Remy M, Pinter F, Nentwich M, et al. Efficacy and safety of hyaluronidase 75 IU as an adjuvant to mepivacaine for retro-bulbar anesthesia in cataract surgery. *J Cataract Refract Surg.* 2008;34: 1966–1969.
28. Bharti N, Madan R, Kaul H, et al. Effect of addition of clonidine to local anaesthetic mixture for peribulbar block. *Anaesth Intensive Care.* 2002;30:438–441.
29. Ahmed S, Elmawy M, Magdy A. Effects of the use of dexmedetomidine as an adjuvant in peribulbar anesthesia in patients presented for vitreoretinal surgeries. *Egyptian J Anaesth.* 2018;34:27–32.
30. Chuang L, Yeung L, Ku W, et al. Safety and efficacy of topical anesthesia combined with a lower concentration of intracameral lidocaine in phacoemulsification: Paired human eye study. *J Cataract Refract Surg.* 2007;33(2):293–296.
31. Yi X, Zhang Y, Jin L, et al. Anesthetic effect of propofol combined with remifentanil and propofol combined with ketamine in ophthalmic surgery. *Int J Clin Exp Med.* 2019;12(7):9387–9392.

32. Yagan O, Karakahya R, Tas N, et al. Comparison of dexmedetomidine versus ketamine-propofol combination for sedation in cataract surgery. *Turk J Anaesth Reanim*. 2015;43:84–90.
33. Yoo J, Kim S, Cho A, et al. The effect of dexmedetomidine sedation on patient and surgeon satisfaction during retinal surgery under sub-Tenon's anesthesia: a randomized controlled trial. *Korean J Anesth*. 2015;68(5):442–448.
34. Vann M, Ogunnaike B, Joshi G. Sedation and anesthesia care for ophthalmic surgery during local/regional anesthesia. *Anesthesiology*. 2007;107(3):502–508.
35. Thyssen J, Menné T, Elberling J, et al. Hypersensitivity to local anaesthetics: update and proposal of evaluation algorithm. *Contact Dermatitis*. 2008; 59:69–78.

REVIEW QUESTIONS

(1) A 59-year-old male presents for cataract surgery. He receives sedation consisting of 2 mg of midazolam and 50 mcg of remifentanil prior to getting a retrobulbar block. Ten minutes later as the eye is being prepped for surgery, it is noticed that the eye still has some movement. What nerve is most likely responsible for this movement?

A. Facial nerve
B. Oculomotor nerve
C. Trochlear nerve
D. Optic nerve

(2) A 45-year-old male presents for vitreoretinal surgery due to a retinal detachment. He receives a peribulbar block. Prior to the start of surgery, the eye is checked. It is completely akinetic and the patient reports having no sensation. The surgery is carried out successfully. Which of the following nerves is most likely **not** anesthetized with the peribulbar eye block?

A. Ciliary nerves
B. Optic nerve
C. Oculomotor nerve
D. Trochlear nerve

(3) A 79-year-old male presents for cataract surgery. A retrobulbar block is performed by the surgeon in the preop area. Two minutes after the block is performed, the patient's operative eye is noticed to be immobile, the upper lid is closing, and the eye is proptotic. The surgeon becomes concerned and checks the intraocular pressure, which she finds to be elevated. What is the most likely eye block complication in this patient?

A. Perforation of the globe
B. Central retinal artery occlusion
C. Intra-arterial injection
D. Retrobulbar hemorrhage

(4) A 38-year-old female presents for surgery for repair of a retinal detachment. She states she is allergic to benzocaine, which caused a severe rash a few years ago. She is very apprehensive about having a general anesthetic. She does not want to incur its risks. She would like to have her surgery under an eye block. Which anesthetic modality is most appropriate for this patient?

A. General anesthesia
B. Peribulbar block with a solution containing lidocaine, bupivacaine, and hyaluronidase
C. Peribulbar block with a solution containing chloroprocaine, bupivacaine, and hyaluronidase
D. Topical anesthesia

(5) A 73-year-old female presents for cataract surgery. She is sedated with 1 mg of intravenous midazolam and 50 mcg of intravenous remifentanil in preparation for peribulbar block. The needle is introduced, and injection of local anesthetic solution is begun. Suddenly, her heart rate drops from 61 to 30. What is the most likely cause for this response?

A. Intra-arterial injection
B. Brainstem anesthesia
C. Oculocardiac reflex
D. Retrobulbar hemorrhage

(6) A 12-year-old boy is undergoing strabismus repair surgery under general anesthesia. He is otherwise healthy. Shortly after the surgery begins, his heart rate decreases from 95 to 35. What anatomical structures are most likely involved in this response?

A. Vagus nerve and oculomotor nerve
B. Vagus nerve and trigeminal nerve
C. Trigeminal nerve and oculomotor nerve
D. Vagus nerve and facial nerve

(7) A 62-year-old female presents for a vitrectomy for repair of a retinal detachment. She is sedated with 2 mg of intravenous midazolam and 50 mcg of intravenous remifentanil prior to getting a retrobulbar block. A few minutes after the sedative is administered as the needle is being introduced, the patient's pulse oximetry reading is noted to drop below 90. The patient is unresponsive and apneic. What is the most likely diagnosis?

A. Oculocardiac reflex
B. Brainstem anesthesia
C. Intra-arterial injection
D. Respiratory depression

(8) An 87-year-old male presents for cataract surgery. He has a history of hypertension, non-insulin dependent diabetes, and gout. Which of the following anesthetic options has the lowest risk for his surgery?

A. Topical anesthesia
B. Peribulbar block
C. Retrobulbar block
D. Sub-Tenon's block

ANSWERS

(1) C The retrobulbar block is an intraconal procedure. The trochlear nerve does not course within the cone. Thus, it might be spared with a retrobulbar block, which results in incomplete akinesia of the eye. When is it not spared, it is most likely by diffusion of the local anesthetic solution outside the cone as it is not a completely sealed space. The facial nerve innervates the orbicularis oculi muscle, which is responsible for closing the eyelids. It has no motor function in the globe. The oculomotor nerve courses within the cone and should

not be spared with a successful block. The optic nerve has no motor function.

References

Netter F. *Atlas of Human Anatomy*. 5th ed. Philadelphia: Saunders; 2011.
Snell R, Lemp M, eds. *Clinical Anatomy of the Eye*. Boston: Blackwell Scientific Publications; 1989.
Hadzic A, ed. *The New York School of Regional Anesthesia: Textbook of Regional Anesthesia and Acute Pain Management*. New York: McGraw-Hill; 2007:362–365.

(2) **B.** The optic nerve is not anesthetized by a peribulbar block, an extraconal procedure. Hence, the patient should not lose vision. The eye in this patient is completely akinetic, which indicates successful blockade of the motor innervation of the extraocular muscles. The patient reports no sensation, which indicates blockade of the ciliary nerves, which provide sensory innervation to the globe.

References

Rea P, ed. *Clinical Anatomy of the Cranial Nerves*. San Diego, CA: Academic Press; 2014:7–26.
Bloomberg L. Administration of periocular anesthesia. *J Cataract Refract Surg*. 1986;12:677–679.
Davis D, Mandel M. Posterior peribulbar anesthesia: an alternative to retrobulbar anesthesia. *J Cataract Refract Surg*. 1986;12:182–184.
Bloomberg L. Anterior periocular anesthesia: five years' experience. *J Cataract Refract Surg*. 1991;17:508–511.
Whitsett J, Balyeat H, McClure B. Comparison of one-injection-site peribulbar anesthesia and retrobulbar anesthesia. *J Cataract Refract Surg*. 1990;3:71–81.

(3) **D.** A retrobulbar hemorrhage is the most likely complication in this case. This can manifest as motor block, a sudden rise in intraocular pressure, closing of the upper lid, and proptosis of the eye. A retrobulbar hemorrhage can also induce the oculocardiac reflex. Depending on its severity, immediate surgical intervention for decompression might be required. Central retinal artery occlusion would not manifest with the symptoms exhibited by the patient. It can result in blindness. Perforation of the eye globe symptoms include pain, sudden loss of vision, and a poor red reflex. Intra-arterial injection signs and symptoms can include cardiopulmonary arrest and convulsions from retrograde arterial spread. Immediate intervention is required, which includes supporting the patient and possibly securing the airway.

References

Hadzic A, ed. *The New York School of Regional Anesthesia: Textbook of Regional Anesthesia and Acute Pain Management*. New York: McGraw-Hill; 2007:362–365.
Bloomberg L. Administration of periocular anesthesia. *J Cataract Refract Surg*. 1986;12:677–679.
Whitsett J, Balyeat H, McClure B. Comparison of one-injection-site peribulbar anesthesia and retrobulbar anesthesia. *J Cataract Refract Surg*. 1990;3:71–81.

(4) **B.** The most appropriate anesthetic modality for this patient is a peribulbar block with a solution containing lidocaine, bupivacaine, and hyaluronidase. She is allergic to benzocaine, an ester local anesthetic. The great majority of allergies to local anesthetics are to those in the ester family due their metabolite para-aminobenzoic acid (PABA). There is no cross-reactivity between local anesthetic classes. Hence, there is no contraindication in this case to using lidocaine and bupivacaine, both amide local anesthetics. There is no need for a general anesthetic in this patient in the light of other safe options. Furthermore, the patient does not want it. Her wishes need to be considered. A peribulbar block with a solution containing chloroprocaine, bupivacaine, and hyaluronidase would not be appropriate. Chloroprocaine is an ester local anesthetic. The patient is allergic to another ester local anesthetic, benzocaine. There can be cross-reactivity within local anesthetic classes.

Reference

Thyssen J, Menné T, Elberling J, et al. Hypersensitivity to local anaesthetics: update and proposal of evaluation algorithm. *Contact Dermatitis*. 2008;59:69–78.

(5) **C.** The oculocardiac reflex is the most likely cause in this scenario. It entails a vagally mediated reduction in heart rate of 10% or more that results from application of direct pressure to the globe, manipulation of the globe, or traction of the extraocular muscles. Performing eye blocks can elicit this reflex. It most commonly manifests as sinus bradycardia but can also manifest as ectopy, atrioventricular block, junctional rhythm, ventricular tachycardia, and asystole. Its severity varies, but can result in profound bradycardia that can progress to asystole. Intra-arterial injection would manifest differently. Signs and symptoms can include cardiopulmonary arrest and convulsions from retrograde arterial spread. Brainstem anesthesia would not manifest this way. Central spread of the local anesthetic solution can result from direct injection into optic nerve sheath. This can manifest as drowsiness, contralateral blindness, agitation, confusion, convulsions, respiratory depression, and cardiac arrest. Although a retrobulbar hemorrhage can trigger the oculocardiac reflex, it would also have other manifestations. This includes motor block, a sudden rise in intraocular pressure, closing of the upper lid, and proptosis of the eye.

References

Schaller, B. Trigeminocardiac reflex. *J Neurol*. 2004;251(6):658–665.
Lord, J. Anaesthesia for eye surgery in paediatrics. *Anaesth Intensive Care Med*. 2010;11(10):429–433.

(6) **B.** The vagus and trigeminal nerves are most likely involved. The situation described with such a significant drop in heart rate most likely represents the oculocardiac reflex, which is a trigeminovagal reflex. The afferent component is provided by the trigeminal nerve. The efferent component is provided by the vagus nerve. The oculomotor and facial nerves do not play a role in this reflex or in producing any other form bradycardia.

Reference

Lord, J. Anaesthesia for eye surgery in paediatrics. *Anaesth Intensive Care Med*. 2010;11(10):429–433.

(7) **D.** Respiratory depression is the most likely diagnosis. The patient was premedicated with midazolam and remifentanil prior to performing the block. The combination of the

two agents can result in respiratory depression as seen in this case. The patient needs to be supported, including supplementing her oxygen delivery via an artificial manual ventilation with a breathing unit mask and bag as the patient is apneic. Respiratory depression resulting from this sedation is usually transient and resolves within a few minutes. As long as adequate bag/mask ventilation is attained, there is rarely a need to secure the airway more invasively in this setting. The oculocardiac reflex would manifest differently as bradycardia and possible hypotension, but not as respiratory depression as seen. Brainstem anesthesia can manifest as drowsiness, contralateral blindness, agitation, confusion, convulsions, respiratory depression, and cardiac arrest. Immediate intervention is required, which includes supporting the patient and possibly securing the airway. The patient has not exhibited most of the symptoms associated with brainstem anesthesia. Intra-arterial injection signs and symptoms can include cardiopulmonary arrest and convulsions from retrograde arterial spread. Immediate intervention is required, which includes supporting the patient and possibly securing the airway.

References

Yi X, Zhang Y, Jin L, et al. Anesthetic effect of propofol combined with remifentanil and propofol combined with ketamine in ophthalmic surgery. *Int J Clin Exp Med*. 2019;12(7):9387–9392.

Yagan O, Karakahya R, Tas N, et al. Comparison of dexmedetomidine versus ketamine-propofol combination for sedation in cataract surgery. *Turk J Anaesth Reanim*. 2015;43:84–90.

Yoo J, Kim S, Cho A, et al. The effect of dexmedetomidine sedation on patient and surgeon satisfaction during retinal surgery under sub-tenon's anesthesia: a randomized controlled trial. *Korean J Anesth*. 2015;68(5):442–448.

Vann M, Ogunnaike B, Joshi G. Sedation and anesthesia care for ophthalmic surgery during local/regional anesthesia. *Anesthesiology*. 2007;107(3):502–508.

(8) **A.** Topical anesthesia has the lowest associated risks for the patient's cataract surgery. Administration of local anesthetic eye drops anesthetizes the cornea. This allows for cataract surgery to be performed. This form of anesthesia is associated with less risk than that of the needle techniques: peribulbar, retrobulbar, and sub-Tenon's blocks. The other three choices involve needle techniques, which are associated with higher risks. These include globe rupture, optic nerve damage, brainstem anesthesia, intravascular injection, and retrobulbar hemorrhage. The use of topical anesthesia for cataract surgery is increasing in the United States.

Reference

Chuang L, Yeung L, Ku W, et al. Safety and efficacy of topical anesthesia combined with a lower concentration of intracameral lidocaine in phacoemulsification: paired human eye study. *J Cataract Refract Surg*. 2007;33(2):293–296.

SECTION 4

CARDIAC, PULMONARY AND CHEST WALL SURGERIES AND TRAUMA

Jinlei Li

12.

REGIONAL TECHNIQUES FOR CARDIOTHORACIC AND CARDIAC-RELATED PROCEDURES

Ali N. Shariat and Himani V. Bhatt

STEM CASE AND KEY QUESTIONS

A 56-year-old 75-kg male with PMHx significant for cocaine abuse, coronary artery disease (CAD), recent insertion of drug eluting stent in LAD, and ischemic cardiomyopathy with ejection fraction (EF) of 25% presented to the emergency department with shortness of breath and was found to have a non-ST segment elevation myocardial infarction (NSTEMI). Left heart catheterization showed significant new disease with in-stent stenosis of the LAD. Home medications include aspirin, clopidogrel, furosemide, metroprolol, and atorvastatin. A decision is made to schedule the patient for robotic coronary artery bypass grafting (CABG).

The robotic CABG took place in the operating room utilizing erector spinae plane (ESP) block and GETA. On the day of surgery, the patient was brought into the operating room (OR), with standard American Society of Anesthesiologists (ASA) monitors placed, and positioned sitting up. The patient was prepped and draped, a time out was performed, and the ESP block was performed on the left side under ultrasound guidance. The ultrasound was placed at the posterior midline at T4–T5 level and moved laterally until erector spinae muscle and transverse process were identified. Using an in-plane technique with a 22-ga, 2-in needle, 10 ml of 0.25% bupivacaine and 10 cc of liposomal bupivacaine were deposited between the erector spinae muscle and transverse process. The patient was then positioned supine, arterial line was placed, general anesthesia with endotracheal intubation (GETA) was initiated, and a central line was placed. Transesophageal echocardiogram (TEE) showed an EF of 25%–30% with dilated left ventricle. The robotic CABG went uneventfully, and the patient was transported to the cardiothoracic intensive care unit (CTICU). Patient was extubated the next day with 4/10 pain requiring intravenous acetaminophen.

On postoperative day 3, the patient developed episodes of ventricular tachycardia (VT) requiring resuscitation and defibrillation. After multiple episodes of VT, despite treatment with resuscitation and antiarrhythmic agents, the electrophysiology (EP) service was consulted. Repeat TEE showed an EF of 20%–25% with dilated left ventricle. After full evaluation, the EP team recommended a subcutaneous implantable cardioverter defibrillator (SICD) for secondary prevention. After full discussion with the patient and CT surgical team, the decision was made to proceed with SICD placement.

(1) WHAT ANALGESIC METHODS ARE HELPFUL IF THIS PROCEDURE WAS DONE VIA A TRADITIONAL STERNOTOMY?

Several analgesic methods are helpful in the perioperative management of cardiac surgical procedures and sternotomy pain. These techniques are the use of intrathecal opioids, epidural analgesia, bilateral paravertebral nerve block, and parasternal blocks such as pecto-intercostal fascial block (PIFB) and transversus thoracic plane block (TTP).

(2) WHAT ARE THE ACCESS POINTS FOR MINIMALLY INVASIVE CARDIAC SURGERY (MICS)?

MICS involves three 8-mm port incisions and one 3–4-cm non-rib-spreader thoracotomy incision. Postoperative pain following MICS is still substantial and is caused by rib retraction, pectoralis and intercostal muscle dissection, and intercostal nerve lesions.

(3) WHAT ARE THE APPROACHES TO TRANSAPICAL AORTIC VALVE REPLACEMENT (TAVR)?

Approaches to TAVR are subclavian, transapical, and transaortic.

(4) WOULD YOU CONSIDER ANY REGIONAL TECHNIQUES FOR SUBCUTANEOUS IMPLANTABLE CARDIOVERTER DEFIBRILLATOR (SICD) PLACEMENT? WHICH ONES AND WHY?

Implantation of the SICD involves dissection on the chest wall at the mid-axillary line, making the procedure potentially painful and requiring adequate analgesia to assure timely discharge of patients. Wound infiltration with local anesthesia has been the mainstay of analgesia for this procedure; however, this technique has a limited duration of action and achieving complete coverage is often difficult. Recently, implantation of an S-ICD under a variety of nerve blocks has been reported. A combination of thoracic paravertebral block and TTP block as the sole anesthetic has been used. A combination of the TTP block with a serratus plane block was used as well. The procedure was performed under nerve blocks alone or a combination of general anesthesia and nerve blocks.

(5) WHAT ARE THE ADVANTAGES OF DOING A REGIONAL TECHNIQUE OVER GETA IN SICD?

Deep levels of anesthesia can have deleterious effects on patients with limited left ventricular function, as well as raising the threshold for defibrillation during ICD testing. Regional anesthesia helped eliminating the risk of hemodynamic trespass inherent in the induction and maintenance of general anesthesia in patients with limited cardiovascular reserve. Even when done under general anesthesia, the truncal blocks largely reduced the need for perioperative opioids, along with the potential side effects of bradycardia, respiratory depression, and nausea/vomiting.

DISCUSSION

CARDIAC SURGERY AND POSTOPERATIVE PAIN

Acute pain following cardiac surgery, as with all postoperative pain, results from surgical manipulation and trauma initiating an inflammatory response (see Box 12.1). Inflammatory mediators, including bradykinins, serotonin, prostaglandins, histamine, leukotrienes, and cytokines are released in the process.[1] Pain intensity is usually greatest in the immediate postoperative period and improves rapidly with tissue healing. Primary risk factors for higher acute pain include younger age (<60 years old), longer duration of surgery, and location of the surgery.

Pain intensity after cardiac surgery is often severe and not adequately treated.[2,3] Following cardiac surgery, 30%–75% of patients report moderate to severe acute pain.[4] Poor pain management can have adverse physiologic effects, including atelectasis, pneumonia, increased myocardial O_2 consumption, and depression, that can lead to impaired recovery. Chronic pain following sternotomy, defined as nonanginal postoperative pain lasting more than 3 months, has an incidence ranging from 11% to 56% at 1 year after surgery.[5] Chronic poststernotomy pain most frequently affects the thorax, but may also involve the upper and lower extremities, neck, and back.[5] The variety of presentations, particularly involving pain in sites unrelated to sternal incision, is one of the main reasons that chronic poststernotomy pain is underdiagnosed.[6] Common etiologies for chronic poststernotomy pain include intercostal nerve damage, internal mammary artery harvest, brachial plexus damage, sternal retraction, and malunion.[5] One of the strongest predictors for chronic pain is severe acute postoperative pain.[7]

Box 12.1 CARDIAC SURGERY–RELATED PAIN

- Acute pain
    - Inflammatory
    - Incisional
    - Days to weeks
- Neuropathic pain
    - Nerve inflammation
    - Pressure/stretching
    - Weeks to months
- Post-Pericardiotomy Syndrome
    - Heightened inflammatory response
    - Fever, pericardial friction rub, pleuritic pain, pericardial effusion
    - Days to months

POST-PERICARDIOTOMY SYNDROME

Post-pericardiotomy syndrome (PPS) is a condition specific to cardiac surgery, with diagnosis based on 2 or more of the following criteria: (1) fever lasting beyond the first postoperative week without evidence of infection; (2) pleuritic chest pain; (3) friction rub; (4) evidence of pleural effusion; (5) evidence of new or worsening pericardial effusion.[8] Risk factors for PPS include combined cardiac surgery, pleural incision, fever, and pericardial and pleural effusions. PPS appears to have an autoimmune pathogenesis[8] with an incidence of 10%–40%, with a higher incidence seen in females and patients who had undergone pleural incision.[9] The primary medications for treating both PPS and relapses include glucocorticoids, nonsteroidal anti-inflammatory drugs (NSAIDs), and colchicine.[9]

ROLE OF REGIONAL TECHNIQUES

Effective analgesia may decrease the length of mechanical ventilation, cardiac ischemic events, and arrhythmias during the postoperative period, thereby possibly having a significant impact on hospital length of stay and overall patient satisfaction.[4] Therefore, multimodal pain management in the intraoperative and postoperative period have a high priority, and regional anesthesia has an increasingly important role. Spinal and epidural anesthesia have been extensively studied in the context of cardiac surgery. However, fear of spinal hematoma in the context of the profound anticoagulation required for cardiac procedures continues to hamper the accumulation of experience despite the lack of data supporting such a risk.[10] With the advent of truncal blocks, targeting of areas involved in cardiac surgery while avoiding the neuraxium has become possible.

NEURAXIAL TECHNIQUES

Spinal Anesthesia

Spinal anesthetic technique has been documented as early as 1980; a case series of 40 patients undergoing cardiac surgery received intrathecal morphine prior to the procedure. Thirty-six of 40 patients were extubated in the OR immediately following surgery and all patients were pain free for the first 27.5 hours postoperatively.[11] Patients undergoing coronary artery bypass graft (CABG) after receiving intrathecal morphine had decreased morphine requirements postoperatively, but the plasma norepinephrine levels were not affected, indicating that the stress response was not affected by intrathecal opioids.[12] Possible disadvantages of this technique include delay of surgery in the event of a bloody tap, postoperative urinary retention, and postoperative somnolence leading to delayed extubation. High-dose intrathecal bupivacaine combined with general anesthesia resulted in less B-receptor dysfunction and a lower stress response in patients undergoing CABG.[13]

Epidural Anesthesia

High thoracic epidural anesthesia blocks the cardiac sympathetic innervation from T1 to T5, decreases myocardial oxygen consumption, improves left ventricular function, and positively affects collateral blood flow during myocardial ischemia.[14,15] Patients who received thoracic epidural before undergoing CABG were awake sooner, resumed spontaneous ventilation sooner, and were extubated earlier.[16] Thoracic epidural blockade at T1–T2 increases myocardial oxygen supply in patients undergoing CABG with no serious hemodynamic disturbances.[17] Patients who underwent CABG and received thoracic epidural blockade had better myocardial function and perioperative hemodynamic parameters.[18]

Risk of Neuraxial Hematoma

One case report of spinal hematoma in the context of cardiac surgery occurred 57 hours postoperatively and was therefore not related to the intraoperative anticoagulation.[19]

The incidence of spinal hematoma in the context of cardiac surgery has been estimated by Ho and colleagues as being 1:150,000 to 1:1500 for epidural block and from 1:220,000 to 1:3600 for spinal anesthesia. The lower incidence is the odds of a spinal hematoma occurring in a noncardiac case, and the maximum risk was calculated using an algorithm to calculate the risk of an adverse event that has not yet occurred.[10] Although the true probability of such an event may be even lower, the possibility of a devastating complication in the context of otherwise uneventful cardiac surgery has hampered the accumulation of experience and data.

SPECIFIC USES IN CARDIOTHORACIC AND CARDIAC-RELATED PROCEDURES

Sternotomy

Due to the midline location, sternotomy requires bilateral blocks for successful analgesia. Robotic minimally mitral valve replacement (MVR) replacement will require an anterior thoracotomy at right 3rd–4th intercostal incision, while robotic minimally invasive direct coronary artery bypass (MIDCAB) requires an anterolateral thoracotomy in the 4th–5th intercostal space (Figure 12.1).

Compared to neuraxial techniques, paravertebral blocks offer the advantage of a lower risk of bleeding complications in patients undergoing cardiopulmonary bypass with full heparinization.[20] The feasibility of bilateral paravertebral catheters in patients undergoing cardiac surgery via median sternotomy was established in a study involving 111 patients. In this study, bilateral continuous paravertebral catheters provided good hemodynamic stability, analgesia, and allowed for

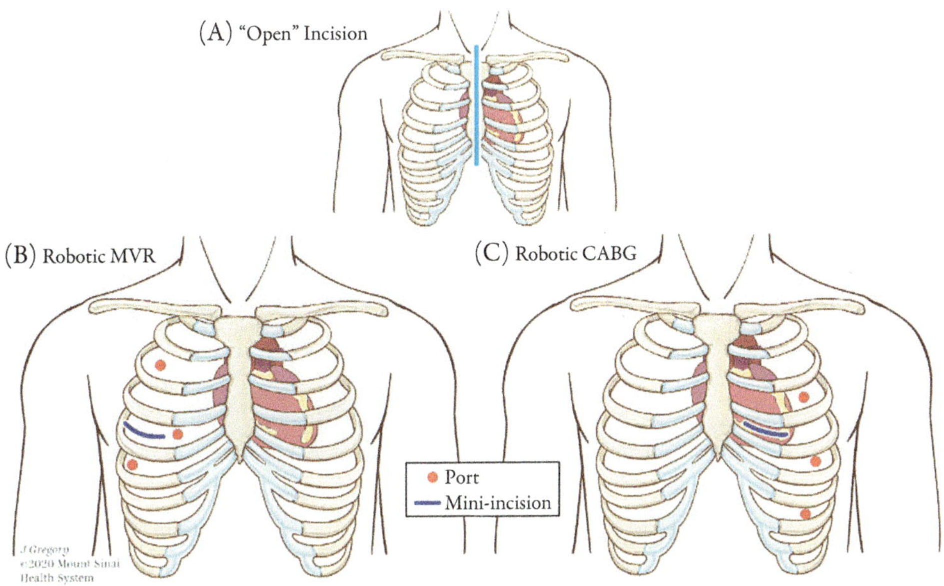

Figure 12.1. Incision sites for cardiac procedures: (A) open incision; (B) robotic MVR; (C) robotic CABG.

early extubation.[21] However, for midline sternotomy, bilateral paravertebral blocks are required, increasing the risk for local anesthetic toxicity. Concerns of possible local anesthetic toxicity using 2 paravertebral catheters for postoperative analgesia following CABG surgery were also raised by a recent study comparing this method with thoracic epidural catheters. Ho et al. inserted bilateral paravertebral blocks and administered ropivacaine boluses prior to surgery, followed by an infusion after surgery that was less than the toxic dose. All study subjects showed signs of local anesthetic toxicity, resulting in the study being terminated after only 8 patients had been enrolled.[22]

Parasternal intercostal blocks, administered by the surgeon prior to sternal closure, have been investigated in several small series. In one study, 54 mL of 0.25% levobupivacaine was injected in doses divided between multiple injections by the surgeon into the parasternal intercostal space prior to sternal closure and compared with a placebo group. Opioid use was significantly less in the block group, although pain scores and time to extubation were not reduced.[23] Several further studies have confirmed that parasternal intercostal blocks decrease opioid requirements and decrease Visual Analogue Score (VAS) pain scores, as well as shorter extubation times.[24–27] Continuous catheter-delivered bupivacaine to the sternal wound after cardiac surgery has also been shown to decrease opioid requirements and reduce pain scores.[28]

The pecto-intercostal fascial block (PIFB) (Figure 12.2A, B) was developed by de la Torre and colleagues to anesthetize the anterior cutaneous branches of the intercostal nerves that innervate the sternum. The block is performed close to the sternum, and local anesthetic is injected in the fascial plane between the pectoralis major and external intercostal muscles.[29]

The transversus thoracic plane (TTP) block (Figure 12.3A, B), first described by Ueshima and colleagues, similarly targets the anterior cutaneous branches of intercostal nerves T2–T6 by injecting local anesthetic in the fascial plane between the transversus thoracic and internal intercostal muscles at the level between the third and fourth, or fourth and fifth rib, just lateral to the sternum.[30,31] The advantages of these methods include the ability to target the multidermatomal innervation of the sternum with just one injection point on each side under ultrasound guidance, rather than multiple injections.[32] A possible risk of the TTP block is inadvertent puncture of the perforating branches of the internal thoracic artery or the anterior perforating veins that join the internal thoracic vein.[33] Ueshima et al. reported two cases using the TTP block for patients undergoing midline sternotomy.[34] Bilateral TTP blocks were performed with ultrasound guidance following anesthesia induction. Injection of 20 ml 0.375% bupivacaine on each side provided adequate incisional pain control extending into the postoperative period. Feasibility of the TTP block in the context of cardiac surgery has been demonstrated.[35]

Erector spinae plane (ESP) blocks have also been studied in the context of sternotomy. Krishna and colleagues have shown the utility of ESP blocks in cardiac surgery involving median sternotomy in reducing VAS pain scores and opioid consumption, decreasing time to extubation, and decreased intensive care unit (ICU) stay.[36] Nagaraja and colleagues compared bilateral ESP blocks to thoracic epidural analgesia in adult cardiac surgery and concluded that the ESP block was a safer alternative for optimal postoperative analgesia.[37] Another prospective study of pediatric patients undergoing cardiac surgery through a median sternotomy randomized patients to receive the ESP block at the T3 level or no block, and showed significantly lower postoperative pain scores and need for rescue opioid medication in the ESP group.[38]

Minimally Invasive Cardiac Procedures

Transapical Aortic Valve Replacement (TAVR)

Minimally invasive cardiac surgery (MICS) provides several important advantages relative to median sternotomy, including a shorter recovery period, decreased ventilator times,

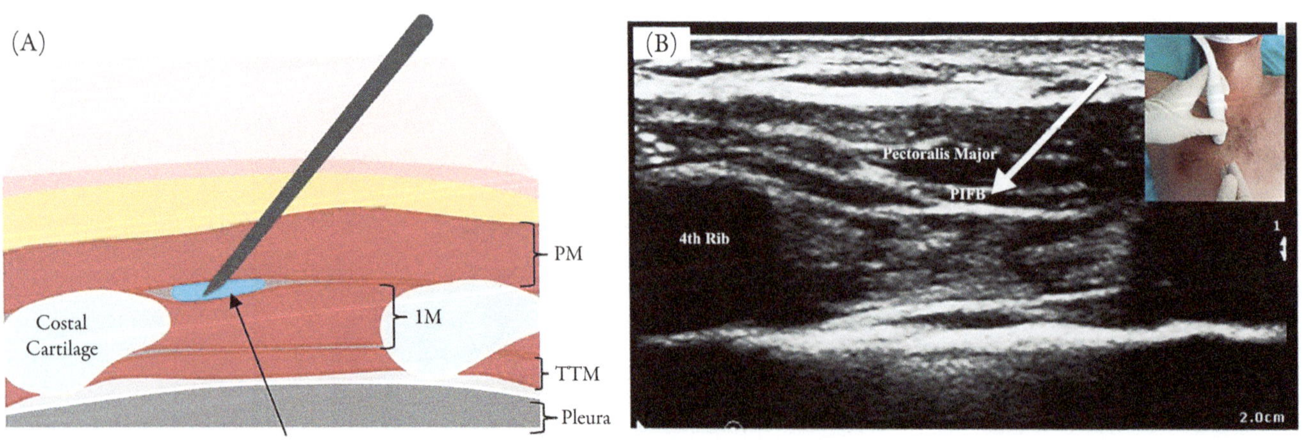

Figure 12.2. (A) The plane of injection of local anesthetics in pectointercostal fascial plane block (PIFB). (B) Pecto interfascial plane ultrasound image. PM = pectoralis major; IM = internal intercostal muscle; TTM = transversus thoracis muscle.
From: Balan C, Bubenek-Turconi SI, Tomescu DR, Valeanu L. Ultrasound-guided regional anesthesia-current strategies for enhanced recovery after cardiac surgery. *Medicina (Kaunas)*. 2021 Mar 25;57(4):312. doi: 10.3390/medicina 57040312.

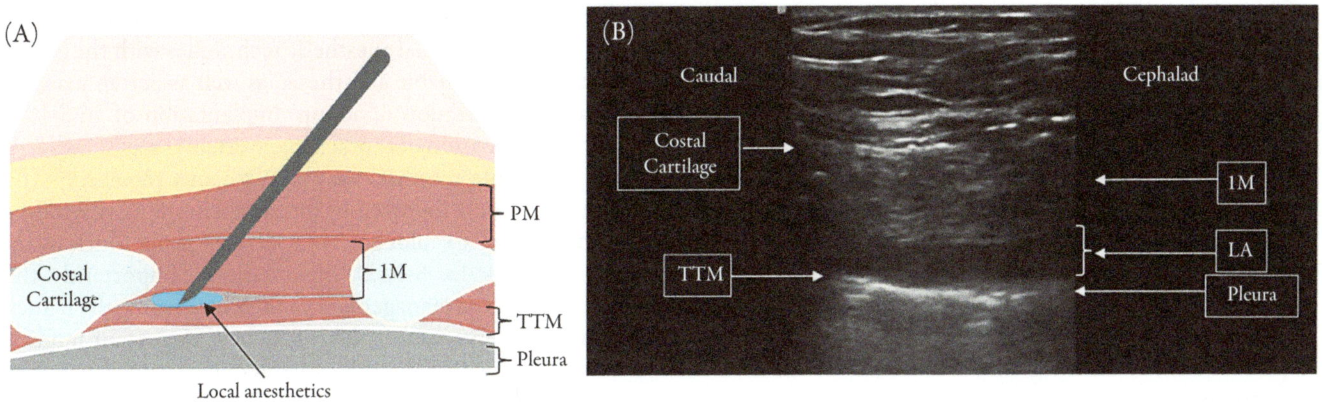

Figure 12.3. (A) The plane of injection of transversus thoracis plane (TTP) block.
PM = pectoralis major; IM = internal intercostal muscle; TTM = transversus thoracis muscle.
From: Balan C, Bubenek-Turconi SI, Tomescu DR, Valeanu L. Ultrasound-guided regional anesthesia-current strategies for enhanced recovery after cardiac surgery. *Medicina (Kaunas)*. 2021 Mar 25;57(4):312. doi: 10.3390/medicina 57040312.

(B) Ultrasound image of TTPB; note the local anesthetic (LA) above the transversus thoracis muscle (TTM).
From: Fujii S, Bairagi R, Roche M, Zhou JR. Transversus thoracis muscle plane block. *Biomed Res Int*. 2019 Jul 7; 2019:1716365. doi: 10.1155/2019/1716365.

better cosmetic results, and improved pain scores.[39] The technique involves less tissue disruption and uses three 8-mm port incisions and one 3–4-cm non-rib-spreader thoracotomy incision.[40] Nonetheless, postoperative pain following MICS is still substantial and is caused by rib retraction, pectoralis and intercostal muscle dissection, and intercostal nerve lesions.[41] Persistent pain following MICS can result in impaired respiratory mechanics and reduced mobility, resulting in hypoxemia, myocardial ischemia, and prolonged hospital length of stay.[40] Therefore, better analgesic techniques have been sought, incorporating regional anesthesia.

Since their first use, TAVRs have become a relatively common procedure. Since most patients undergoing such procedures commonly have multiple comorbidities, regional anesthesia can provide many benefits, such as superior analgesia, limiting the need for intravenous anesthesia, and reduction in the need for vasopressor support.[42]

Regional techniques are chosen according to the route of access (i.e., subclavian, transapical, transaortic) and the related nerve distribution. The use of Paravertebral Nerve Block (PVBs) for transapical TAVRs has been shown to decrease the need for high-dose remifentanil, while maintaining hemodynamic stability.[40] In a retrospective study comparing PVBs vs. no PVBs in patients receiving general anesthesia for TA-TAVR, use of paravertebral blocks resulted in lower opioid administration, earlier extubation times, and lower incidence of postoperative atrial fibrillation.[43] In a retrospective study, PVB was found to be associated with decreased opioid usage compared with serratus anterior plane (SAP) block, possibly due to better coverage of thoracostomy tube pain by the PVB. The use of SAP block as main anesthetic for TA-TAVR has been reported in a patient who was not a candidate for general anesthesia due to multiple comorbidities, including significant pulmonary hypertension and a history of laryngeal carcinoma.[44] Pectoralis Nerve Block (PECS) I block has likewise been reported for trans-subclavian TAVR with minimal intraoperative opioid use and need for vasoactive drugs.[45] PECS II block has also been reported for transapical TAVR.[41] In a retrospective study, SAP Block compared to continuous wound infiltration for MICS resulted in significantly lower morphine consumption in the first 48 hours postoperatively.[46] The parasternal pectoral block (roughly analogous to pectointerfascial plane block) has been successfully used for postoperative analgesia following a right minimally invasive thoracotomy (RMIT) for aortic valve replacement.[41]

Robotic, Endoscopic, and Thoracotomy Cardiac Surgery

Cardiac procedures are increasingly performed via small incisions in the chest wall, including robotic and minimally invasive coronary revascularization, valve repair via mini thoracotomy, and transapical valve replacement (Figure 12.3). Although coined minimally invasive, post-procedural pain is often significant, and frequently surpasses the discomfort associated with sternotomy.

Paravertebral blocks have been successfully used for minimally invasive direct coronary artery bypass (MIDCAB) surgery.[47,48] In a prospective randomized study, paravertebral catheter-delivered analgesia was as effective as Thoracic Epidural Analgesia (TEA) for pain control after MIDCAB surgery.[49] When PVB was compared to TEA in patients undergoing robotic-assisted CABG surgery, VAS pain scores and opioid consumption were shown to be similar, with fewer side effects noticed in the paravertebral group.[50] In a case series, Tahara et al. analyzed data from a variety of cardiac procedures performed via a minimally invasive surgical approach and an anesthetic technique that included continuous paravertebral catheter ropivacaine infusion. Extubation was successful in 43% of patients within 1 hour after surgery with no major complications.[48] A further review of 141 patients who underwent cardiovascular surgery with paravertebral catheter for postoperative pain control did not result in a single case of paravertebral, epidural, or spinal hematoma.[20]

Truncal plane blocks have also been successfully applied to minimally invasive cardiac surgery. PECS I and PECS II blocks were used as rescue analgesia for a patient experiencing refractory pain following minimally invasive mitral valve repair via thoracotomy.[51] Such reports may suggest a possible role for truncal blocks used preemptively as analgesic methods in cardiac procedures involving thoracotomies to improve pain scores, reduce opioid consumption, and possibly pulmonary function. Similarly, serratus anterior blocks can be used to provide additional analgesia for minimally invasive mitral valve repair.[52]

ESP continuous catheters have been successfully used for postoperative analgesia in left ventricular assist device insertions through a left anterior thoracotomy.[53] All catheters in this case series were inserted and removed in the presence of systemic anticoagulation without incidence of hematoma.

Cardiac-Related Procedures (ICD, S-ICD)

Subcutaneous implantable cardioverter-defibrillators (S-ICDs) were recently introduced as an alternative to conventional ICDs in order to circumvent the problems associated with a transvenous system due to the absence of any intravascular leads (Figure 12.4). This minimizes the risk of pneumothorax, cardiac perforation, lead dislodgement, and systemic bacteremia.[54] The maintenance of systolic blood pressure (SBP) and heart rate (HR) are of utmost concern as anesthetic goals; therefore effective analgesia that assures hemodynamic stability is of great value.[55] Implantation of the S-ICD involves dissection on the chest wall at the mid-axillary line, making the procedure potentially painful and requiring adequate analgesia to assure timely discharge of patients.[56] Wound infiltration with local anesthesia has been the mainstay of analgesia for this procedure; however, this technique has a limited duration of action and achieving complete coverage is often difficult.[56] Therefore, general anesthesia or deep sedation is often necessary to provide anesthesia for this procedure. Deep levels of anesthesia can have deleterious effects on patients with limited left ventricular function, as well as raising the threshold for defibrillation during ICD testing.[54] This has prompted investigators to seek regional anesthetic techniques with the goal of providing more reliable anesthesia, as well as better analgesia with a longer duration of action. Implantation of an S-ICD under a combination of thoracic paravertebral block and TTP block as the sole anesthetic has been recently reported.[57] This report was closely followed by another describing the combination of the TTP block with a serratus plane block as the main anesthetic for S-ICD implantation.[58] Importantly, this team reported the management of their cases using the truncal blocks as sole anesthetic, which may have important implications for eliminating the risk of hemodynamic trespass inherent in the induction and maintenance of general anesthesia in patients with limited cardiovascular reserve. These initial reports have been corroborated by a further report[59] and retrospective review[56] that established the feasibility of the routine use of TTP and serratus plane block for the analgesic management of S-ICD placement. Although these studies were performed under general anesthesia, the truncal blocks largely reduced the need for perioperative opioids, along with the potential side effects of bradycardia, respiratory depression, and nausea/vomiting.

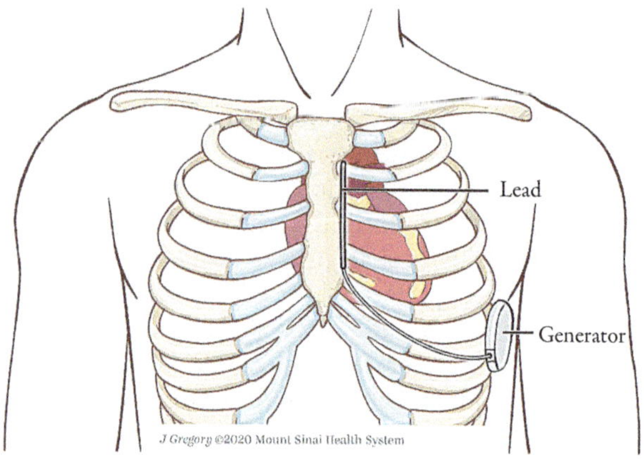

Figure 12.4. Implantable cardioverter-defibrillator lead and generator position.

REFERENCES

1. Beilin B, Bessler H, Mayburd E, et al. Effects of preemptive analgesia on pain and cytokine production in the postoperative period. *Anesthesiology*. 2003;98:151–155
2. Cogan J. Pain management after cardiac surgery. *Semin Cardiothorac Vasc Anesth*. 2010;14(3):201–204.
3. Watt-Watson J, Stevens B, Katz J, Costello J, Reid GJ, David T. Impact of preoperative education on pain outcomes after coronary artery bypass graft surgery. *Pain*. 2004;109:73–85.
4. Bigeleisen PE, Goehner N. Novel approaches in pain management in cardiac surgery. *Curr Opin Anaesthesiol*. 2015 Feb;28(1):89–94.
5. Kleiman AM, Sanders DT, Nemergut EC, et al. Chronic poststernotomy pain. *Reg Anesth Pain Med*. 2017;42:698–708.
6. van Leersum NJ, van Leersum RL, Verwey HF, Klautz RJ. Pain symptoms accompanying chronic poststernotomy pain: a pilot study. *Pain Med*. 2010 Nov;11(11):1628–1634.
7. Perkins FM, Kehlet H. Chronic pain as an outcome of surgery. *Anesthesiology*. 2000;93(4):1123–1133.
8. Imazio M, Brucato A, Rovere ME, et al. Contemporary features, risk factors, and prognosis of the postpericardiotomy syndrome. *Am J Cardiol*. 2011;108:1183–1187.
9. Lehto J, Gunn J, Karjalainen P, Airaksinen J, Kiviniemi T. Incidence and risk factors of postypericardiotomy syndrome requiring medical attention: The Finland Postpericardiotomy Syndrome Study. *J Thorac Cardiovasc Surg*. 2015;15:51–53.
10. Ho A M-H, Chung DC, Joynt GM. Neuraxial blockade and hematoma in cardiac surgery. *Chest*. 2000; 117:551–555.
11. Mathews ET, Abrams LD. Intrathecal morphine in open heart surgery. *Lancet*. 1980;2(8193):543.
12. Chaney MA, Smith KR, Barclay JC, Slogoff S. Large-dose intrathecal morphine for coronary artery bypass grafting. *Anesth Analg*. 1996;83:215–222.
13. Lee TWR, Grocott HP, Schwinn D, Jacobsohn E. High spinal anesthesia for cardiac surgery. *Anesthesiology*. 2003;98:499–510.
14. Blomberg S, Emanuelsson H, Ricksten S-E. Thoracic epidural anesthesia and central hemodynamics in patients with unstable angina pectoris. *Anesth Analg*. 1989; 69:558–562.
15. Kock M, Blomberg S, Emanuelsson H, Lomsky M, Stromberg S-O, Ricksten S-E. Thoracic epidural anesthesia improves global and

regional left ventricular function during stress-induced myocardial ischemia in patients with coronary artery disease. *Anesth Analg.* 1990;71:625–630.
16. Liem TH, Hasenbos M, Booij L, Gielen M. Coronary artery bypass grafting using two different anesthetic techniques: part 2: postoperative outcome. *J Thorac Cardiovasc Surg.* 1992;6(2):156–161.
17. Lagunilla J, García-Bengochea JB, Fernández AL, et al. High thoracic epidural blockade increases myocardial oxygen availability in coronary surgery patients. *Acta Anaesthesiol Scand.* 2006 Aug;50(7):780–786.
18. Bektas SG, Turan S, Karadeniz U, et al. Does high thoracic epidural analgesia with levobupivacaine preserve myocardium? A prospective randomized study. *Biomed Res Int.* 2015;2015:658678.
19. Rosen DA, Hawkinberry DW, Rosen KR, Gustafson RA, Hogg JP, Broadman LM. An epidural hematoma in an adolescent patient after cardiac surgery. *Anesth Analg.* 2004;98:966–969.
20. Okitsu K, Iritakenishi T, Iwasaki M, Imada T, Fujino Y. Risk of hematoma in patients with a bleeding risk undergoing cardiovascular surgery with a paravertebral catheter. *J Cardiothorac Vasc Anesth.* 2017 Apr;31(2):453–457.
21. Canto M, Sanchez, MJ, Casas MA, et al. Bilateral paravertebral blockade for conventional cardiac surgery. *Anaesthesia.* 2003;58(4):365–370.
22. Ho AM, Karmakar MK, Ng SK, et al. Local anaesthetic toxicity after bilateral thoracic paravertebral block in patients undergoing coronary artery bypass surgery. *Anaesth Intensive Care Med.* 2016;44(5):615–619.
23. McDonald SB, Jacobsohn E, Kopacz DJ, et al. Parasternal block and local anesthetic infiltration with levobupivacaine after cardiac surgery with desflurane: the effect on postoperative pain, pulmonary function, and tracheal extubation times. *Anesth Analg.* 2005;100:25–32.
24. Saini K, Chauhan S, Kiran U, Bisoi AK, Choudhury M, Hasija S. Comparison of parasternal intercostal block using ropivacaine or bupivacaine for postoperative analgesia in patients undergoing cardiac surgery. *World J Cardiovasc Surg.* 2015;5:49–57.
25. Chaudhary V, Chauhan S, Choudhury M, Kiran U, Vasdev S, Talwar S. Parasternal intercostal block with ropivacaine for postoperative analgesia in pediatric patients undergoing cardiac surgery: a double-blind, randomized, controlled study. *J Cardiothorac Vasc Anesth.* 2012 Jun;26(3):439–442.
26. Barr AM, Tutungi E, Almeida AA. Parasternal intercostal block with ropivacaine for pain management after cardiac surgery: a double-blind, randomized, controlled trial. *J Cardiothorac Vasc Anesth.* 2007;21:547–53.
27. Dowling R, Thielmeier K, Ghaly A, et al. improved pain control after cardiac surgery: results of a randomized, double-blind, clinical trial. *J Thorac Cardiovasc Surg.* 2003;126:1271–1278.
28. White PF, Rawal S, Latham P, et al. Use of a continuous local anesthetic infusion for pain management after median sternotomy. *Anesthesiology.* 2003;99:918–923.
29. De la Torre PA, Garcia PD, Alvarez SL, Miguel FJ, Perez MF. A novel ultrasound-guided block: a promising alternative for breast analgesia. *Aesthetic Surg J.* 2013;34(1):198–200.
30. Ueshima H, Otake H. Addition of transversus thoracic muscle plane block to pectoral nerves block provides more effective perioperative pain relief than pectoral nerves block alone for breast cancer surgery. *Br J Anaesth.* 2017 Mar 1;118(3):439–443.
31. Ueshima H, Kitamura A. Blocking of multiple anterior branches of intercostal nerves (Th2–6) using a transversus thoracic muscle plane block. *Reg Anesth Pain Med.* 2015;40:388.
32. Ueshima H, Takeda Y, Ishikawa S, Otake H. Ultrasound-guided transversus thoracic muscle plane block: a cadaveric study of the spread of injectate. *J Clin Anesth.* 2015;27:696.
33. Murata H, Hida K, Hara T. Transverse thoracic muscle plane block: tricks and tips to accomplish the block. *Reg Anesth Pain Med.* 2016 May–Jun;41(3):411–412.
34. Ueshima H, Hara E, Marui T, Otake H. The ultrasound-guided transversus thoracic muscle plane block is effective for the median sternotomy. *J Clin Anesth.* 2016 Mar;29:83.
35. Fujii S, Roche M, Jones PM, Vissa D, Bainbridge D, Zhou JR. Transversus thoracis muscle plane block in cardiac surgery: a pilot feasibility study. *Reg Anesth Pain Med.* 2019;44:556–560.
36. Krishna SN, Chauhan S, Bhoi D, et al. Bilateral erector spinae plane block for acute post-surgical pain in adult cardiac surgical patients: a randomized controlled trial. *J Cardiothorac Vasc Anesth.* 2019 Feb;33(2):368–375.
37. Nagaraja PS, Ragavendran S, Singh NG, Bhavya G, Manjunath N, Rajesh K. Comparison of continuous thoracic epidural analgesia with bilateral erector spinae plane block for perioperative pain management in cardiac surgery. *Ann Card Anaesth.* 2018;21:323–327.
38. Kaushal B, Chauhan S, Magoon R, et al. Efficacy of bilateral erector spinae plane block in management of acute postoperative surgical pain after cardiac surgeries through a misline sternotomy. *J Cardiothorac Vasc Anesth.* 2020;34(4):981–986.
39. Glower DD, Landolfo KP, Clements F, et al. Mitral valve operation via port access versus median sternotomy. *Eur J Cardiothorac Surg.* 1998;14 Suppl 1:S143–S147.
40. Moll V, Maffeo C, Mitchell M, et al. Association of serratus anterior plane block for minimally invasive direct coronary artery bypass surgery with higher opioid consumption: a retrospective observational study. *J Cardiothorac Vasc Anesth.* 2018;32:2570–2577.
41. Ellouze O, Missaoui A, Berthoud V, Bouhemad B, Guinot P-G. Parasternal pectoral block for right anterior minimally invasive thoracotomy in cardiac surgery. *J Cardiothorac Vasc Anesth.* 2020;34(2):450–453.
42. Dehidin B, Guinot PG, Ibrahim H, et al. Anesthesia and perioperative management of patients who undergo transfemoral transcatheter aortic valve implantation: an observational study of general versus local/regional anesthesia in 125 consecutive patients. *J Cardiothorac Vasc Anesth.* 2011 Dec;25(6):1036–1043.
43. Poltak JM, Cobey FC, Augoustides JG, Connors CW. Paravertebral analgesia in transapical transcatheter aortic valve replacement. *Heart Lung Vessel.* 2015;7(3):217–223.
44. Berthoud V, Ellouze O, Bièvre T, et al. Serratus anterior plane block for apical TAVR in an awake patient. *J Cardiothorac Vasc Anesth.* 2018;32(5):2275–2277.
45. Alexander B, Angaramo G, Walz JM, et al. A novel approach to managing trans-subclavian transcatheter aortic valve replacement with regional anesthesia. *J Cardiothorac Vasc Anesth.* 2018 Jun;32(3):1391–1393.
46. Berthoud V, Ellouze O, Nguyen M, et al. Serratus anterior plane block for minimal invasive heart surgery. *BMC Anesthesiol.* 2018 Oct 20;18(1):144.
47. Ganapathy S, Murkin JM, Boyd DW, et al. Continuous percutaneous paravertebral block for minimally invasive cardiac surgery. *J Cardiothorac Vasc Anesth.* 1999;13(5):594–596.
48. Tahara S, Inoue A, Sakamoto H, et al. A case series of continuous paravertebral block in minimally invasive cardiac surgery. *JA Clin Reports.* 2017;3(1):45.
49. Dhole S, Mehta Y, Saxena H, et al. Comparison of continuous thoracic epidural and paravertebral blocks for postoperative analgesia after minimally invasive direct coronary artery bypass surgery. *J Cardiothorac Vasc Anesth.* 2001;15(3):288–292.
50. Khalil AE, Abdallah NM, Bashandy GM, et al. Ultrasound-guided serratus anterior plane block versus thoracic epidural analgesia for thoracotomy pain. *J Cardiothorac Vasc Anesth.* 2017;31:152–158.
51. Yalamuri S, Klinger RY, Bullock WM, et al. Pectoral fascial (PECS) I and II blocks as rescue analgesia in a patient undergoing minimally invasive cardiac surgery. *Reg Anesth Pain Med.* 2017;42:764–766.
52. Costa F, Nenna A, Barbato R, Benedetto M, Del Buono R, Agrò FE. Serratus anterior plane block for right minithoracotomy revision after mitral valve repair. *Minerva Anestesiol.* 2017 Dec;83(12):1333–1334.
53. Adhikary SD, Prasad A, Soleimani B, Chin KJ. Continuous erector spinae plane block as an effective analgesic option in anticoagulated patients after left ventricular assist device implantation: a case series. *J Cardiothorac Vasc Anesth.* 2019 Apr;33(4):1063–1067.
54. Mittnacht AJC, Shariat A, Weiner MM, et al. Regional techniques for cardiac and cardiac-related procedures. *J Cardiothorac Vasc Anesth.* 2019 Feb;33(2):532–546.

55. Esandoah MK, Portillo JG, Weiss R, et al. Anesthesia care for subcutaneous implantable cardioverter/defibrillator placement: a single-center experience. *J Clin Anaesth*. 2016;31:53–59.
56. Miller MA, Bhatt HV, Weiner M, et al. Implantation of the subcutaneous implantable cardioverter-defibrillator with truncal plane blocks. *J Cardiothorac Vasc Anesth*. 2018;18:30111–30115.
57. Ueshima H, Hiroshi O. A successful case of subcutaneous implantable cardioverter-difibrillator implantation performed under the transversus thoracic muscle plane block. *J Clin Anesth*. 2016;32:253–254.
58. Ueshima H, Hara E, Otake H. Successful cases of S-ICD implantation performed under the serratus plane block. *J Clin Anesth*. 2016;33:147–148.
59. Bhatt HV, Hernandez N, Shariat A. Successful use of serratus and transversus thoracic plane blocks for subcutaneous cardioverter-defibrillator placement. *J Cardiothorac Vasc Anesth*. 2018;32(1):e22–e23.

REVIEW QUESTIONS

(1) Etiologies for pain following cardiac surgery include:

A. Internal mammary artery harvest
B. Intercostal nerve damage
C. Sternal retraction
D. All of the above

(2) Post-pericardiotomy syndrome requires which 2 of the following criteria to make the diagnosis?

A. Musculoskeletal chest pain
B. Friction rub
C. Evidence of pleural effusion
D. B and C

(3) Which of the following are regional techniques that have shown analgesic benefit in coronary artery bypass grafting (CABG) involving sternotomy?

A. Erector spinae block
B. Serratus anterior plane block
C. Transversus thoracic plane (TTP) block
D. A and C

(4) Which of the following is a possible risk of the transversus thoracic plane (TTP) block?

A. Hemidiaphragmatic paralysis
B. Puncture of a perforating branch of the internal thoracic artery
C. Brachial plexus injury
D. Recurrent laryngeal nerve palsy

(5) Which of the following blocks is **not** an analgesic method for minimally invasive cardiac surgery?

A. Intercostobrachial nerve block nerve
B. PECS I block
C. Serratus anterior block
D. PECS II block

(6) Regional blocks for subcutaneous implantable cardioverter-defibrillators (S-ICDs) must target which of the following nerve distributions?

A. Dorsal ramus and anterior cutaneous branches of the intercostal nerves
B. Anterior and lateral cutaneous branches of the intercostal nerves
C. Only lateral cutaneous branch of intercostal nerves
D. Dorsal ramus of intercostal nerves and intercostobrachial nerve

(7) Which of the following is **not** a risk factor for higher acute pain following cardiac surgery?

A. Age <60 years
B. Longer duration of surgery
C. Prior sternotomy
D. Location of surgery

(8) Which of the following is **not** a risk factor for post-pericardiotomy syndrome (PPS)?

A. Prior cardiac surgery
B. Pleural incision
C. Fever
D. Combined cardiac surgery

ANSWERS

(1) **E.** Chronic poststernotomy pain most frequently affects the thorax, but may also involve the upper and lower extremities, neck, and back. The variety of presentations, particularly involving pain in sites unrelated to sternal incision, is one of the main reasons chronic poststernotomy pain is underdiagnosed. Common etiologies for chronic poststernotomy pain include intercostal nerve damage, internal mammary artery harvest, brachial plexus damage, sternal retraction, and malunion. One of the strongest predictors for chronic pain is severe acute postoperative pain.

References

Kleiman AM, Sanders DT, Nemergut EC, et al. Chronic poststernotomy pain. *Reg Anesth Pain Med*. 2017; 42:698–708
van Leersum NJ, van Leersum RL, Verwey HF, Klautz RJ. Pain symptoms accompanying chronic poststernotomy pain: a pilot study. *Pain Med*. 2010 Nov;11(11):1628–1634.
Perkins FM, Kehlet H. Chronic pain as an outcome of surgery. *Anesthesiology*. 2000;93(4):1123–1133.

(2) **D.** Post-pericardiotomy syndrome (PPS) is a condition specific to cardiac surgery with diagnosis based on 2 or more of the following criteria: (1) fever lasting beyond the first postoperative week without evidence of infection; (2) pleuritic chest pain; (3) friction rub; (4) evidence of pleural effusion; (5) evidence of new or worsening pericardial effusion.

Reference

Imazio M, Brucato A, Rovere ME, et al. Contemporary features, risk factors, and prognosis of the postpericardiotomy syndrome. *Am J Cardiol*. 2011; 108:1183–1187.

(3) **D.** Erector spinae nerve (ESP) block and transversus thoracic nerve blocks have shown evidence of analgesic benefit in CABG procedures, while the serratus anterior plane (SAP) block did not.

References

Ueshima H, Kitamura A. Blocking of multiple anterior branches of intercostal nerves (Th2–6) using a transversus thoracic muscle plane block. *Reg Anesth Pain Med.* 2015; 40:388.

Ueshima H, Hara E, Marui T, Otake H. The ultrasound-guided transversus thoracic muscle plane block is effective for the median sternotomy. *J Clin Anesth.* 2016 Mar;29:83.

Krishna SN, Chauhan S, Bhoi D, et al. Bilateral erector spinae plane block for acute post-surgical pain in adult cardiac surgical patients: a randomized controlled trial. *Heart Rhythm.* 2018 Jul;15(7):1108–1111.

Kaushal B, Chauhan S, Magoon R, et al. Efficacy of bilateral erector spinae plane block in management of acute postoperative surgical pain after cardiac surgeries through a misline sternotomy. *J Cardiothorac Vasc Anesth.* 2019;1–9.

(4) **B.** Puncture of a perforating branch of the internal thoracic artery as it lies immediately below the thin transversus thoracic muscle.

References

Murata H, Hida K, Hara T. Transverse thoracic muscle plane block: tricks and tips to accomplish the block. *Reg Anesth Pain Med.* 2016 May–Jun;41(3):411–412.

Ellouze O, Missaoui A, Berthoud V, Bouhemad B, Guinot P-G. Parasternal pectoral block for right anterior minimally invasive thoracotomy in cardiac surgery. *J Cardiothorac Vasc Anesth.* 2019;1–4.

(5) **A.** Intercostobrachial nerve block covers the medial upper side of the arm and will not be helpful for minimally invasive cardiac surgery. PECS I, PECS II, and serratus anterior plane block were used in minimally invasive cardiac surgery procedures.

References

Samerchua A, Leurcharusmee P, Panjasawatwong K, Pansuan K, Mahakkanukrauh P. Cadaveric study identifying clinical sonoanatomy for proximal and distal approaches of ultrasound-guided intercostobrachial nerve block. *Reg Anesth Pain Med.* 2020 Nov;45(11):853–859.

Ellouze O, Missaoui A, Berthoud V, Bouhemad B, Guinot P-G. Parasternal pectoral block for right anterior minimally invasive thoracotomy in cardiac surgery. *J Cardiothorac Vasc Anesth.* 2019;1–4.

Alexander B, Angaramo G, Walz JM, et al. A novel approach to managing trans-subclavian transcatheter aortic valve replacement with regional anesthesia. *J Cardiothorac Vasc Anesth.* 2018 Jun;32(3):1391–1393.

Berthoud V, Ellouze O, Nguyen M, et al. Serratus anterior plane block for minimal invasive heart surgery. *BMC Anesthesiol.* 2018 Oct 20;18(1):144.

(6) **B.** Regional blocks for subcutaneous implantable cardioverter-defibrillators (S-ICDs) must target the anterior and lateral cutaneous branches of intercostal nerves.

References

Miller MA, Bhatt HV, Weiner M, et al. Implantation of the subcutaneous implantable cardioverter-defibrillator with truncal plane blocks. *J Cardiothorac Vasc Anesth.* 2018; 18:30111–30115.

Ueshima H, Hiroshi O. A successful case of subcutaneous implantable cardioverter-defibrillator implantation performed under the transversus thoracic muscle plane block. *J Clin Anesth.* 2016;32:253–254.

Ueshima H, Hara E, Otake H. Successful cases of S-ICD implantation performed under the serratus plane block. *J Clin Anesth.* 2016; \33:147–148.

Bhatt HV, Hernandez N, Shariat A. Successful use of serratus and transversus thoracic plane blocks for subcutaneous cardioverter-defibrillator placement. *J Cardiothorac Vasc Anesth.* 2018;32(1):e22–e23.

(7) **C.** Prior sternotomy is not a risk factor for higher postoperative pain following cardiac surgery.

References

Beilin B, Bessler H, Mayburd E, et al. Effects of preemptive analgesia on pain and cytokine production in the postoperative period. *Anesthesiology.* 2003;98(1):151–155.

Watt-Watson J, Stevens B, Katz J, Costello J, Reid GJ, David T. Impact of preoperative education on pain outcomes after coronary artery bypass graft surgery. *Pain.* 2004;109:73–85.

(8) **A.** Prior cardiac surgery is not a risk factor for post pericardiotomy syndrome (PPS).

References

Imazio M, Brucato A, Rovere ME, et al. Contemporary features, risk factors, and prognosis of the postpericardiotomy syndrome. *Am J Cardiol.* 2011;108(8):1183–1187.

Lehto J, Gunn J, Karjalainen P, Airaksinen J, Kiviniemi T. Incidence and risk factors of postypericardiotomy syndrome requiring medical attention: The Finland Postpericardiotomy Syndrome Study. *J Thorac Cardiovasc Surg.* 2015;15:51–53.

13.

VIDEO-ASSISTED THORACOSCOPY AND THORACOTOMY

Davies G. Agyekum and Taras Grosh

STEM CASE AND KEY QUESTIONS

A 65-year-old man with medical history significant for a 20-pack year of smoking and 20 years of asbestosis exposure presents with 1 year of progressive cough and dyspnea. He has been intermittently treated with a combination of antibiotics and bronchodilator therapy without improvement. In the last 3 months, the cough has increased in frequency, with an associated right-sided chest pain, chills, dyspnea on exertion, orthopnea, and poor oral intake. A subsequent chest x-ray revealed a right pleural effusion and possible right middle lobe mass of unknown etiology. He is referred to thoracic surgery by his primary physician for further evaluation. The patient is evaluated by a thoracic surgeon. A detailed physical exam revealed decreased breath sounds over the right middle and lower lung fields. A computed tomography (CT) scan to assess the lung fields confirmed a moderate-sized right pleural effusion, right pleural thickening, enlarged mediastinal lymph nodes, and a single lung nodule in the right middle lobe. An ultrasound-guided thoracentesis further characterized the effusion as an exudative effusion. A decision is made to perform a therapeutic and diagnostic video-assisted thoracoscopy surgery (VATS).

(1) IN THE PREOPERATIVE HOLDING AREA, THE PATIENT EXPRESSES CONCERN ABOUT POSTOPERATIVE PAIN. IS THERE ANY EVIDENCE TO GUIDE THE PERIOPERATIVE MANAGEMENT OF ANALGESIA?

Although no consensus exists on the optimal pain control after VATS, most physicians agree that a multimodal approach to pain management is key. A strong multimodal pain regimen consists of a combination of opioids, analgesic adjuncts (i.e., acetaminophen, NSAIDS, gabapentinoids, NMDA antagonists, Na channel antagonists, alpha-2 agonists), and regional anesthesia. Table 13.1 details frequently used medications as part of a multimodal analgesic regimen. For patients for whom regional anesthesia is not available, surgical infiltration with local anesthetic and patient-controlled analgesia (PCA) are recommended.[1]

(2) THE PATIENT IS REASSURED WHEN HE IS TOLD THAT THE TYPICAL PAIN SCORE FOR VATS IS LOW COMPARED TO OTHER OPERATIONS AND THAT SPECIAL REGIONAL TECHNIQUES CAN BE EMPLOYED TO FURTHER REDUCE THE SEVERITY OF PAIN. HE IS INTERESTED IN ANYTHING TO REDUCE THE AMOUNT OF POSTOPERATIVE PAIN AND ASKS WHAT REGIONAL ANESTHESIA TECHNIQUES ARE OFFERED FOR HIS VATS PROCEDURES.

Regional anesthesia, administered by the anesthesiologist, is a staple in every multimodal protocol. The gold standard for analgesia during major thoracic surgery has classically been the placement of a thoracic epidural analgesic (TEA) catheter.[2] With advancements in VATS techniques, strong multimodal as well as ultrasound-guided regional anesthesia, TEA is being reserved for either major open thoracic procedures or for patients with significant opioids use disorder or chronic pain pathology. Other regional anesthesia techniques include ipsilateral paravertebral block (PVB) and fascial plane blocks such as: erector spinae plane (ESP) block, serratus anterior plane block (SAPB), pectoralis I and II blocks (PECS I and II), intercostal nerve blocks (ICNB), and parasternal fascial plane blocks (PFPB). Intraoperatively, surgeons are utilizing extended-release formulations of local anesthetic for their intercostal nerve blocks placed intrathoracically. Postoperatively, surgeons can inject local anesthetic through chest tubes known as intrapleural anesthesia. Unfortunately, unless the tube can be clamped, local anesthetic will drain out of the cavity, producing only a short duration of analgesia.[3]

(3) WHAT IS THE MECHANISM OF INTERCOSTAL NERVE (ICN) BLOCKS, AND WHAT ARE THE SPECIAL CONSIDERATIONS FOR PERFORMING THEM?

Intercostal nerve carries both sensory and motor fibers as they penetrate the posterior intercostal membrane distal to the intervertebral foramen to enter the subcostal grove, where they continue to run parallel to the rib, accompanied by intercostal artery and vein. Within the thorax, the nerve

Table 13.1 FREQUENTLY USED MEDICATIONS IN A MULTIMODAL ANALGESIC REGIMEN

CLASS	MEDICATION	CONSIDERATIONS
Opioids		
Short acting	Fentanyl	100 mcg IV w/ induction, 25 mcg IV aliquots for emergence
Long acting	Tramadol	Weak opioid, suitable for elderly, caution w/ other SSRI/SNRI
	Morphine	Caution in renal disease (active metabolites), causes histamine release
	Oxycodone	1.5 × stronger than PO morphine, PO dosing 5–10 mg q 4–6 h × <5 days
	Hydromorphone	0.2 to 0.5 mg IV q 3h for breakthrough vs. PCA @ 0.2 mg q 15 min 4 × stronger than PO morphine, PO dosing 4–8 mg q 6 h × <5 days
NSAIDs	Ketorolac	30 mg IV prior to emergence after d/w surgeon (hemostasis)
NMDA antagonists	Ketamine	Administer w/ glycopyrrolate to reduce secretions or administer after bronchoscopy is completed, 0.2 mg/kg/h infusion or bolus
Na channel antagonist	Lidocaine	1–2 mg/kg/h gtt, avoid infusion if using liposomal bupivacaine
Alpha-2 agonist	Dexmedetomidine	0.2 mcg/kg/min, stop 30 minutes before emergence, hypotension in PACU
Acetaminophen	Acetaminophen	1000 mg PO preoperatively, administer prior to opioids, goal <4000 mg daily
Gabapentinoids	Gabapentin Pregabalin	300–900 mg PO preoperatively for patients already on it, on chronic opioids, or with a comorbid chronic pain condition Consider switching to 150 mg daily for those for whom gabapentin is ineffective Caution for acute fluid retention and lower extremity edema

is often found between the innermost and internal intercostal muscles. As the nerve approaches midline, it gives off the lateral cutaneous branch at the midaxillary line and subsequently turns anteriorly, piercing overlying muscles and skin to terminate as the anterior cutaneous branch. The intercostal nerves have lateral and anterior cutaneous branches. Each lateral cutaneous branch divides into anterior and posterior terminal branches, except the second intercostal nerve, which is called the intercostobrachial nerve. The anterior terminal branches run forward to the side and the forepart of the chest, supplying the skin and the breast; PECS II cannot cover this. The posterior terminal branches run backward and supply the skin over the scapula and latissimus dorsi muscle. The intercostobrachial nerve innervates the axilla and medial side of the arm (Figure 13.1).

Distal and proximal spread of local anesthetics injected into the subcostal groove blocks the ipsilateral sensory and motor fibers of the ICNs; some of the injectate may enter the paravertebral space. T1 and T2 provide nerve fibers to the upper extremities and upper thorax; T3 through T6 supply the thorax; T7 through T11 supply the lower thorax and abdomen; and T12 innervates the abdominal wall and the skin of the front section of the gluteal region.[4]

The disadvantages of intercostal block include the requirement for technical expertise, an approximately 1% risk of pneumothorax, and local anesthetic toxicity with multiple levels of blockade. Absorption of local anesthetics from the intercostal space is very rapid with peaks in plasma concentration, estimated to be around 10 minutes.[5]

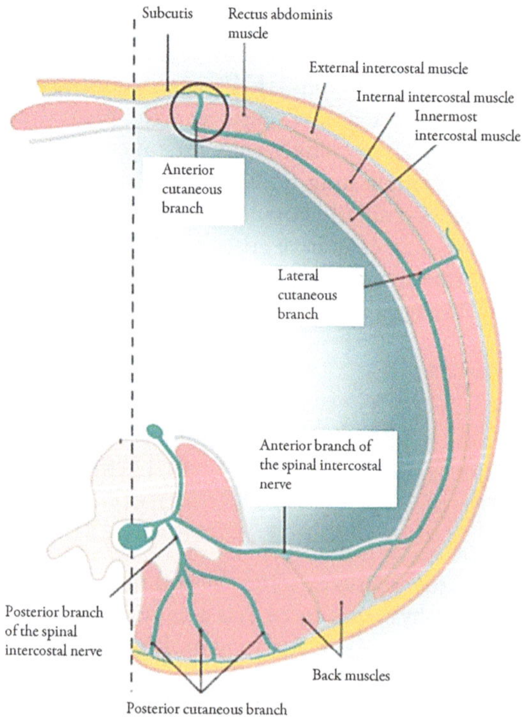

Figure 13.1. The intercostal nerve anatomy.
From: Smelt H, Pouwels S, Apers J, et al. Anterior cutaneous nerve entrapment syndrome: two case reports of the forgotten diagnosis after bariatric surgery. *Cureus*. 2020 Jun 8;12(6): e8499. doi: 10.7759/cureus.8499. License Creative Commons Attribution License CC-BY 4.0.

(4) THE PATIENT IS IMPRESSED WITH YOUR EXTENSIVE KNOWLEDGE OF THE MULTITUDE OF REGIONAL TECHNIQUES FOR THORACIC SURGERY AND ASKS HOW WELL THORACIC WALL BLOCKS WORK.

Fascial plane blocks rely on passive spread of local anesthetics, and as such, only a proportion of the total injected mass of local anesthetic will reach and act on target nerves. Factors including volume, direction of injection, speed of injection, respiratory movement, and gravity play a role in the mechanism of thoracic wall blocks. The number of factors inevitably leads to variation in the extent and intensity of sensory loss. Additional considerations include contralateral innervation across the midline and overlapping innervation between adjacent nerves. This may lead to unilateral blocks providing only partial analgesia for the medial thorax. Communications between contiguous spinal nerves may be a further reason for incomplete sensory loss. As a result, thoracic wall blocks should not be regarded as the sole anesthetic techniques, but rather as an additional component of a multimodal analgesic repertoire. Continuous local anesthetic infusion catheters have the advantage in allowing infusion or repeated boluses of local anesthetic, which can prolong and may even augment the analgesic effect.[3]

(5) ON A FOLLOW-UP APPOINTMENT WITH THE THORACIC SURGEON, IT IS REVEALED TO THE PATIENT THAT THE FLUID COLLECTION IN HIS CHEST IS EXUDATIVE AND LIKELY RELATED TO HIS YEARS OF ASBESTOS EXPOSURE. THIS IS FURTHER CONFIRMED FROM PATHOLOGICAL STUDIES, AND THE PATIENT IS DIAGNOSED WITH MALIGNANT MESOTHELIOMA. HE IS SCHEDULED TO UNDERGO A RIGHT RADICAL PLEURECTOMY VIA A POSTEROLATERAL THORACOTOMY. HOW IS THORACOTOMY PAIN DIFFERENT FROM VATS PAIN?

The thoracic cavity can be accessed via a large subcostal incision, an alternative to VATS. In this open method, an incision is made through the skin, subcutaneous fat, deep fascia, and pectoralis major muscle. The intercostal muscles are split along the superior edge of the inferior rib to avoid injury to the neurovascular bundle. The parietal pleura is visualized. Utilizing a double-lumen endotracheal tube, the anesthetist deflates the operative lung. The parietal pleura is incised or penetrated with a hemostat.[6]

The prevalence of pain before thoracotomy is generally low (12%), but persistent pain following thoracotomy is a significant problem, with estimates of pain prevalence at 1 year of 50%; for large open thoracic cases, the use of neuraxial anesthesia in the form of thoracic epidural analgesia (TEA) or thoracic paravertebral block (TPVB) is advocated. TEA and TPVB are also utilized in minimally invasive cases if opioids or adjunct agents should be avoided or minimized (i.e., patient request, NSAIDs in patients with renal insufficiency, or opioids in those with severe chronic obstructive pulmonary disease or obstructive sleep apnea). TEA and TPVB are alternatives to the thoracic wall blocks with advantages, chief of which are their ease of performance and universal familiarity.

DISCUSSION

VIDEO-ASSISTED THORACOSCOPIC SURGERY (VATS) AND THORACOTOMY

Thoracoscopic interventions were pioneered by Hans Christian Jacobeus in the early 1900s in an effort to avoid a more invasive thoracotomy. By inserting a cystoscope into the thoracic cavity, filling the cavity with air and creating an artificial pneumothorax, Jacobeus was able to inspect, visualize, and lyse multiple pleural adhesions for patients with tuberculosis.[7] In addition to a camera port, additional small incisions are made to provide access for the surgical instruments, such as staplers, dissectors, coagulators, and lasers controlled externally by either a surgeon or robot. The most common preoperative diagnosis includes pleural disease (e.g., effusions), recurrent pneumothorax, recurrent empyema, localized lung masses, pulmonary infiltrates, hyperhidrosis, and reflex sympathetic dystrophy (RSD). Advantages of VATS over open thoracotomy includes decreased postoperative pain, pulmonary impairment, and hospital stay. The relative contraindications of VATS are listed in Box 13.1.[8]

Acute postoperative pain is a combination of nociceptive, neuropathic, or inflammatory reaction, resulting from activation of peripheral pain receptors and their specific A-delta and C-sensory nerve fibers (nociceptors). Chronic pain related to ongoing tissue injury is presumably caused by persistent activation of these fibers.

During VATS, pain may be caused by the incisions, crushing of intercostal nerves during angulation of instruments through a porthole incision, rib trauma, costovertebral joint dislocation, tracheobronchial injury, pleural irritation due to

***Box 13.1* RELATIVE CONTRAINDICATIONS TO VIDEO-ASSISTED THORACOSCOPIC SURGERY**

- Inability to tolerate single-lung ventilation
- Severe pulmonary hypertension
- Severe thoracic trauma
- Hemodynamic instability
- Very dense pleural adhesions
- Superior sulcus tumor
- Extensive tumor invasion of the chest wall
- Definitive chemoradiation
- Complex esophageal surgical resection when the stomach cannot be used as a conduit

thoracostomy tubes, or visceral pain in the lung parenchyma, pericardium, or diaphragm. In addition, although more common after an open thoracotomy, ipsilateral shoulder pain can plague patients.[9]

The gold standard for analgesia during major thoracic surgery has classically been the placement of a TEA catheter. Unless the patient refuses or has a contraindication, TEA provides somatic and visceral analgesia, a sympathectomy, and is cardioprotective. With advancements in VATS techniques, and strong multimodal as well as ultrasound-guided regional anesthesia, TEA is being reserved for either major open thoracic procedures or patients with significant opioids use disorder or chronic pain pathology.

Ultrasound guided regional anesthesia techniques that the anesthesiologists can use include ipsilateral paravertebral block (PVB) and a group of blocks known as fascial plane blocks: erector spinae plane block (ESPB), serratus anterior plane (SAP) block, pectoralis I and II blocks (PECS I and II), intercostal nerve (ICN) blocks, and parasternal fascial plane blocks (PFPB). With the exception of the paravertebral block, which is considered a deep block, the other blocks can be considered in patients who are anticoagulated. Unlike PVB and TEA, though, these fascial plane blocks do not provide motor or dense blockade; therefore, a strong multimodal protocol of opioids, acetaminophen, gabapentinoids, NMDA antagonists, and NSAIDs is recommended.

Intraoperatively, surgeons are utilizing extended-release formulations of local anesthetic for their intercostal nerve blocks placed intrathoracically. Postoperatively, surgeons can inject local anesthetic through chest tubes known as intrapleural anesthesia. Unfortunately, unless the tube can be clamped, local anesthetic will drain out of the cavity, producing only a short duration of analgesia.

INTERCOSTAL NERVE BLOCK

Large parts of the skin (dermatome) and musculature (myotome) of the chest and abdominal wall are innervated by the intercostal nerves (ICN). Intercostal nerves are somatic nerves that arise from the anterior divisions of the thoracic spinal nerves from T1 to T11. Their blockade results in concomitant analgesia to their particular area. Of note, significant overlap exists among dermatomes and myotomes. In order to successfully block a particular area, multiple levels (above and below the desired segment) need to be blocked.

Although initially described in 1907, use of intercostal nerve blocks (ICNBs) did not gain prominence until the 1940s, when it was realized that they can reduce pulmonary complications and opioid requirements after upper abdominal surgery. Furthermore, the introduction of ultrasound guidance to the practice of regional anesthesia has enabled practitioners to readily offer ICNB. Continuous ICNB was introduced in the 1980s to mitigate problems associated with repeated multiple injections. Today, ICNB provides excellent analgesia in a multitude of acute and chronic pain conditions affecting the thorax and upper abdomen, including breast and chest wall surgery. Including thoracic and upper abdominal surgical procedures (e.g., thoracotomy, video-assisted thoracoscopy (VAT), chest tube placement, breast surgery, rib fractures, and upper abdominal procedures), the innervating thoracic and thoracoabdominal intercostal nerves can be blocked to provide anesthesia and/or analgesia.[10]

FASCIAL PLANE BLOCK

A variety of thoracic wall fascial plane regional anesthesia techniques have been described: pectoral nerve blocks (PECS I and II), serratus anterior plane (SAP) block, pecto-intercostal fascial block (PIFB), erector spinae plane (ESP) block, and retrolaminar blocks. Increased knowledge of the sonoanatomy in regional anesthesia has led to the identification of tissue layers and the development of newer techniques. They are nearly all fascial plane blocks, relying on the spread of local anesthetics to target nerves within the plane or in adjacent tissue compartments. Unlike a direct ultrasound-guided peripheral nerve block, fascial plane blocks can provide inconsistent analgesia since practitioners are rarely visualizing small cutaneous nerves. Before ultrasound, thoracic wall blocks were confined to TEA, TPVB, and ICNB. Here were review anterolateral, anteromedial, and posterolateral thoracic wall blocks.[3]

Our current understanding of the mechanism of thoracic fascial plane blocks indicates that they should not be expected to consistently provide the same degree of analgesia as a well-functioning epidural or TPVB. Nevertheless, the available evidence indicates that they are still highly effective in reducing opioid requirements and improving pain experience in a wide range of clinical settings. These new fascial plane blocks are therefore best employed as part of a multimodal analgesia with other systemic analgesics. Catheters or extended-release formulations of local anesthetic are beneficial in situations where moderate to severe pain is expected for more than 12 hours. It should be noted that the optimal local anesthetic dosing regimen requires further investigation. Research into these techniques is still at an early stage, and well-designed comparative trials are needed to ascertain the optimal choice of technique for specific surgical applications. Until then, they may be regarded as viable alternatives to the traditional techniques of TEA and TPVB, particularly.[3]

NEURAXIAL BLOCKS

THORACIC EPIDURAL ANALGESIA (TEA)

TEA is currently considered the gold standard in the treatment of thoracotomy pain. In many comparative studies of the use of systemic opiates, TEA was proven superior.[1]

To perform a TEA, an epidural catheter is inserted between level T3 and T8 in a midline or paramedian approach, using the "loss of resistance" or "hanging drop" technique. Typically, a combination of dilute concentration of local anesthetic (bupivacaine or ropivacaine) with a lipophilic opiate (fentanyl or sufentanil) is used pre- and intraoperatively. The local anesthetic works centrally, producing symmetric bilateral analgesia for 4–8 dermatomes and myotomes depending on the local anesthetic infusion volume. This combination allows for a reduced total local anesthetic dose and improved systemic analgesia from the opioid. Although tunneled epidural catheters have remained in place for up to 30 days, typically epidural catheters remain in situ for 3–4 days after surgery. Upon removal of thoracic drains and transition to oral pain medication, the TEA is removed.

Along with the excellent analgesic properties of TEA, the sympathetic blockade of local anesthetics has significant beneficial effects on several organ systems: increased gastrointestinal motility and perfusion and decreased myocardial ischemia and systemic stress response. However, the effective analgesia must be balanced against the possible alteration of lung function as accessory muscles of respiration can be anesthetized. Moreover, sympathectomy can result in an unopposed vagal tone with a potentially increased bronchial tone and reactivity.

THORACIC PARAVERTEBRAL BLOCK (TPVB)

The TPVB can be thought of as a unilateral TEA; both are considered neuraxial blocks requiring discontinuation of antiplatelet and anticoagulants prior to placing and provide similar analgesia.

Thoracic paravertebral space is a channel-like cavity on both sides of the thoracic spine, filled with adipose tissue, the sympathetic trunk, and small vessels. The thoracic spinal nerves run through the space as they emerge from the intervertebral foramina to become intercostal nerves. Using ultrasound guidance, TPVB can be performed using one or more injections, as well as facilitating placement of a perineural catheter for continuous analgesia. Compared to the anatomic landmark technique, the use of ultrasound guidance boosts the success rate, reduces complications, and decreases the incidence of periosteal injury.

After identification of the spinous processes from C7 to T7, injection points corresponding to the transverse process are marked 2.5 cm lateral to the midline at each desired level. Single local anesthetic injection at the T3 or T4 level or multiple injections at alternate levels are performed, depending on the required extent of the block. When TPVB is performed as the sole anesthetic for a surgical procedure, multiple injections may be more effective and preferable, while a single injection may be as effective and adequate when the block is used primarily for postoperative analgesia. Continuous catheters may be placed for continuous TPVB to provide prolonged postoperative analgesia. The technique for placing catheters is the same as for single-shot injections, using ultrasound guidance or anatomic landmarks.

The TPVB can also be completed by the surgeon intraoperatively and continued in the same fashion as a TEA.[8]

FASCIAL PLANE BLOCKS

Anterolateral Thoracic Wall Blocks (Figure 13.2)

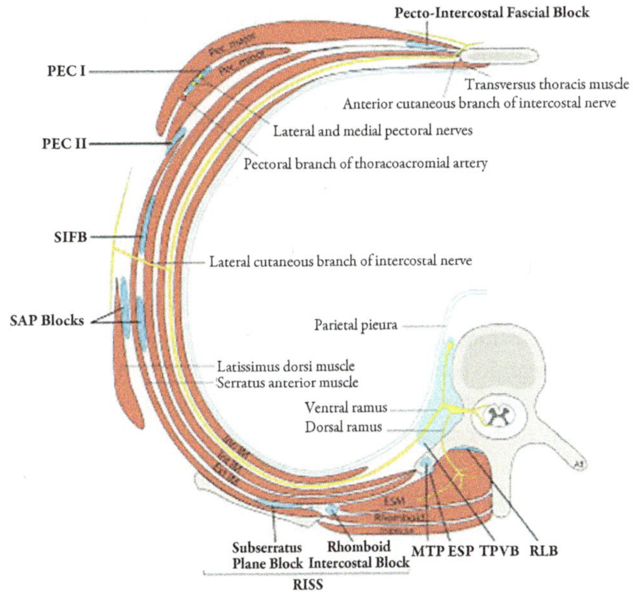

Figure 13.2. Schematic diagram of anatomy and injection sites for regional anaesthesia targets in chest wall surgery. Transverse section at the level of T3.
Ext IM = external intercostal muscle; Int IM = internal intercostal muscle; Inn IM = innermost intercostal muscle; ESM = erector spinae muscle; RLB = retrolaminar block; TPVB = thoracic paravertebral block; ESP = erector spinae plane block; MTP = mid-point transverse process to pleura block; SAP = serratus anterior plane; SIFB = serratus intercostal fascial block.
Image appears courtesy of Dr. Ann Barron.
Obtained with permission from Elsevier from: FitzGerald S, Odor PM, Barron A, Pawa A. Breast surgery and regional anaesthesia. *Best Pract Res Clin Anaesthesiol.* 2019;33(1):95–110.

Pectoral Block Type I (PECS I)

The PECS I block involves the administration of local anesthetic to block the medial (C8, T1) and lateral (C5–C7) pectoral nerves by hydro-dissecting the plane between the pectoralis major and minor muscles near the pectoral branch of the thoracoacromial artery. These nerves provide motor innervation to the pectoralis muscles and thus this block provides little to no analgesic effect in thoracic surgery.

Pectoral block type II (PECS II)

The PECS II block is a combination of local anesthetic spread between the pectoralis major and minor (PECS I) as well as infiltration deep to the pectoralis minor and superficial to the clavipectoral fascia and the superficial border of the serratus muscle. The second injection anesthetizes the lateral cutaneous branches of upper intercostal nerves (T2–T6), which will produce the dermatomal anesthesia to the chest wall (pectoral and axillary regions) and the long thoracic nerves (C5–C7), which innervate the serratus anterior muscle. The upper intercostal nerves are ventral rami of thoracic nerves. The intercostal nerves have lateral and anterior cutaneous branches. Each lateral cutaneous branch divides into anterior and posterior terminal branches, except the second intercostal nerve, which is called the intercostobrachial nerve. The anterior terminal branches run forward to the side and the forepart of the chest, supplying the skin and the breast; PECS II cannot cover this. The posterior terminal branches run backward and supply the skin over the scapula and latissimus dorsi muscle. The intercostobrachial nerve innervates the axilla and medial side of the arm (Figure 13.1).

Both blocks are completed with the patient supine, arm either at the side or abducted 90 degrees. The ultrasound probe is placed just under the coracoid process in a paramedian sagittal view to identify the pectoralis major, minor, and second rib. The goal is to identify the pectoral branch of the thoracoacromial artery while optimizing fascial plane lines. The echogenic block needle is advanced from medial to lateral, and saline should be used to create a pocket between both muscles. After completing the PECS I block, the ultrasound transducer is moved caudally and into the anterior axillary line to identify the fourth rib. The second injection is made deep to the pectoralis minor, approximately 4–6 cm from the surface. Approximately 10 cc and 20 cc are required between the first and second injection, respectively.

The PECS II block is ideal for midclavicular chest wall pain related to rib fractures or postsurgical pain.[11]

Serratus Anterior Plane Block (SAPB)

The SAPB involves injection of local anesthetics into a fascial plane either superficial to (between pectoralis minor/latissimus dorsi and serratus) or deep into the serratus anterior muscle (between the serratus and intercostal muscles/ribs). The SAPB is performed between the mid and posterior axillary lines at the level of T4–T5 ribs, at a more lateral and posterior location than the pectoral blocks. The intercostobrachialis nerve, lateral cutaneous branches of the intercostal nerves (T2–T9), long thoracic nerve, and thoracodorsal nerve are located in a compartment between the serratus anterior and the latissimus dorsi muscles, between the posterior and midaxillary lines, and are blocked with this technique. The two main anatomical landmarks are the latissimus dorsi and the serratus anterior muscles.

The block is performed with the patient positioned either lateral decubitus or supine with the arm brought forward. The two main methods exist for identifying the plane for the serratus block. The first method requires counting the ribs from the clavicle while moving the transducer laterally and distally until the fourth and fifth ribs are identified. The transducer is oriented in the coronal plane and then tilted until the latissimus dorsi is identified. The serratus muscle, a thick, hypoechoic muscle deep to the latissimus dorsi, is imaged over the ribs. Translating the transducer posteriorly enables identification of the plane between the serratus anterior and latissimus dorsi muscles. The second method is to place the transducer across the axilla, where the latissimus dorsi will appear more prominent. The location of the thoracodorsal artery is easier to identify this way. Either an in-plane and out-of-plane approach is appropriate. Following the identification of landmarks, regional anesthesia can be achieved by injecting 20–30 cc of local anesthetic.

Both superficial and deep SAP blocks primarily target the lateral cutaneous branches of the intercostal nerves. The actual nerves involved in the block are determined largely by the exact point of injection and the volume of injectate. The efficacy of the SAP block in thoracotomy and rib fractures suggests that it may also anesthetize deeper structures, although cadaveric studies have yet to demonstrate this. The long thoracic nerve and thoracodorsal nerve also run in the superficial serratus anterior muscle plane and may therefore be inadvertently or deliberately anesthetized by a superficial SAPB.[11]

The SAPB is ideal for lateral rib fractures and pain in the distribution of the axillary fossa. Depending on the volume of local anesthetic used and spread between facial planes, coverage can extend posteriorly as well as anteriorly. Dermatomal evaluation demonstrates significant cross-coverage anteriorly compared to the PECS II block, but in the axillary fossa the PECS II does not cover as well.[7]

ANTEROMEDIAL THORACIC WALL BLOCKS

Parasternal Fascial Plane Blocks

The sternum and the parasternal region are innervated by the anterior branches of the intercostal nerves. This area is not reliably covered by the PECS II and SAP blocks, both of which primarily target the lateral rather than the anterior cutaneous intercostal branches. The terminal anterior branches can be targeted in one of two fascial planes. The transversus thoracic plane block (TTPB) is an injection deep to intercostal muscles and superficial to transversus thoracis muscles. The pecto-intercostal fascial block (PIFPB) is a more superficial parasternal block requiring the deposition of local anesthetic between the pectoralis major and minor. In both cases a dilute higher volume of local anesthetic is recommended: 10–20 cc of 0.25% ropivacaine/bupivacaine. Both blocks pose the risk of cardiac and pulmonary injury, but extra care should be given for the TTPB given the proximity to the internal thoracic artery bilaterally as well as pleura.[12,13]

The parasternal blocks are ideal for the management of sternal fracture pain or costochondritis.[14]

POSTEROLATERAL THORACIC WALL BLOCKS

Erector Spinae Plane (ESP) Block

The ESP block is a technique where local anesthetic is injected into a fascial plane between the tips of the thoracic transverse processes and the overlying erector spinae muscle. It differs from the retrolaminar and the paraspinal intercostal plane blocks primarily on the bony landmark that is sought (transverse process vs. lamina vs. rib). Cadaveric and imaging studies have conflicting data whether the ESP block results in injectate spread to paravertebral and epidural spaces (3–5 segments), and intercostal nerves (6–10 levels).

Retrolaminar Block

The retrolaminar block is a recently described technique in which local anesthetics are injected into the fascial plane between the posterior surface of the thoracic lamina and the overlying transversopinalis muscles. Using ultrasound, the lamina, overlying muscle, and the local anesthetic spread between them can be directly visualized. Some cadaveric studies have confirmed that the injectate spreads anteriorly through the intertransverse ligaments into the paravertebral and epidural spaces.

Paraspinal-Intercostal Plane Blocks

The paraspinal-intercostal plane blocks consist of injecting local anesthetic into the paraspinal-intercostal plane. The injectate has been shown to spread primarily to lateral cutaneous branches of the ventral rami of spinal nerves.[3]

CONCLUSION

- Thoracic fascial plane blocks represent a significant advancement in regional anesthesia for their simplicity and safety. These blocks can be utilized for superficial and deep surgery in the chest wall and axillary regions (e.g., mastectomy, cosmetic breast surgery, chest tube placement, multiple rib fractures).
- The decision as to which block to perform is guided by factors including desired area of coverage, the available sites for ultrasound probe placement and needle insertion, patient positioning, and operator experience.
- Most single-injection techniques last 8–12 hours, while continuous catheters can be considered if a prolonged effect is desired.
- Extended-release formulations of local anesthetic are evolving; currently, the gold standard for analgesia is still neuraxial anesthesia when compared to wound infiltration with PCA vs. neuraxial.
- Thoracic fascial blocks may be considered in patients with coagulation abnormalities after careful evaluation of the potential benefit versus the risks associated with hematoma formation or vascular injury.
- Thoracic paravertebral block (TPVB) is a compartment block used most commonly to provide anesthesia and/or analgesia for mastectomy and cosmetic breast surgery, thoracic surgery, nephrectomy, and rib fractures. Compared with epidural blockade, TPVB offers the possibility of unilateral block.
- Indwelling catheters may be placed for continuous TPVB to provide prolonged postoperative analgesia.
- The use of thoracic epidural analgesia and thoracic paravertebral block or thoracic fascial blocks should always be accompanied by a systemic multimodal analgesia to maximize opioid-sparing.
- The adequate volume and dosage of local anesthetic efficacy in thoracic fascial plane blocks await further investigation. Risk of local anesthetic systemic toxicity is high, and proper precaution and monitoring must be observed.

REFERENCES

1. Marshall K, McLaughlin K. Pain management in thoracic surgery. *Thorac Surg Clin.* 2020;30(3):339–346.
2. Joshi GP, Bonnet F, Shah R, et al. A systematic review of randomized trials evaluating regional techniques for postthoracotomy analgesia. *Anesth Analg.* 2008;107(3):1026–1040.
3. Chin KJ. Thoracic wall blocks: from paravertebral to retrolaminar to serratus to erector spinae and back again—a review of evidence. *Best Pract Res Clin Anaesthesiol.* 2019;33(1):67–77.
4. Karmakar MK, Greengrass RA, Latmore M, Levin M. Thoracic and lumbar paravertebral block. In: Admir H, ed. *Hadzic's Textbook of Regional Anesthesia and Acute Pain Management.* New York: McGraw-Hill Education; 2017:721–739.
5. Behnke H, Worthmann F, Cornelissen J, Kahl M, Wulf H. Plasma concentration of ropivacaine after intercostal blocks for video-assisted thoracic surgery. *Br J Anaesth.* 2002;89(2):251–253.
6. Perkins FM, Franklin JS. 19—Prediction and prevention of persistent post-surgical pain. In: Benzon HT, Rathmell JP, Wu CL, Turk DC, Argoff CE, Hurley RW, eds. *Practical Management of Pain.* 5th ed. Philadelphia: Mosby; 2014:298–303;e292.
7. Nagy AG, Poulin EC, Girotti MJ, Litwin DE, Mamazza J. History of laparoscopic surgery. *Can J Surg.* 1992;35(3):271–274.
8. Hanna JM, Berry MF, D'Amico TA. Contraindications of video-assisted thoracoscopic surgical lobectomy and determinants of conversion to open. *J Thorac Dis.* 2013;5(Suppl 3):S182–189.
9. Hartigan P. Anesthesia for video-assisted thoracoscopic surgery (VATS) for pulmonary resection. In: Slinger PD, Nussmeier N, eds. *Anesthesia for Video-Assisted Thoracoscopic Surgery (VATS) for Pulmonary Resection.* Waltham, Ma: UptoDate; 2021.
10. Ho A, Buck R, Latmore M, Levine M, Karmakar M. Intercostal nerve block: landmarks and nerve stimulator technique. In: Hadzic A, ed. *Hadzic's Textbook of Regional Anesthesia and Acute Pain Management.* nysora.com. 2021:1376–1379.
11. Blanco R. The "pecs block": a novel technique for providing analgesia after breast surgery. *Anaesthesia.* 2011;66(9):847–848.
12. Ueshima H, Kitamura A. Blocking of multiple anterior branches of intercostal nerves (Th2–6) using a transversus thoracic muscle plane block. *Reg Anesth Pain Med.* 2015;40(4):388.
13. de la Torre PA, Garcia PD, Alvarez SL, Miguel FJ, Perez MF. A novel ultrasound-guided block: a promising alternative for breast analgesia. *Aesthet Surg J.* 2014;34(1):198–200.
14. Murata H, Hida K, Hara T. Transverse thoracic muscle plane block: tricks and tips to accomplish the block. *Reg Anesth Pain Med.* 2016;41(3):411–412.

REVIEW QUESTIONS

(1) The use of thoracic epidural analgesia (TEA) for thoracic surgery results in sympathetic blockade. Which of the following is one of the beneficial effects of this sympatholysis?

A. Increased systemic stress response
B. Increased bronchial tone and reactivity as a result of unopposed vagal tone
C. Increased gastric motility and perfusion
D. Decreased coronary blood flow and a resultant increase in myocardial ischemia

(2) The best evidence in studies supports what volume of local anesthetic to be injected for a PECS II block for optimal spread and analgesia?

A. 20 mL up to 40 mL
B. No consensus for evidence-based recommendation

C. 0.3 mL/kg
D. As much as the patient tolerates

(3) Which of the following statements is true regarding serratus plane block?

A. It is not important to visualize latissimus dorsi muscle.
B. It provides axillary region anesthesia by anesthetizing long thoracic nerve.
C. It is indicated in patients with anteriolateral rib fracture.
D. It provides axillary region anesthesia by anesthetizing the nerve to latissimus dorsi.

(4) A 60-year-old patient with COPD undergoes a thoracotomy and receives general anesthesia as well as thoracic epidural analgesia (TEA). Which of the following is true in regard to the patient's pulmonary function following surgery?

A. The patient will have an increased functional residual capacity (FRC) compared to a patient who receives general anesthesia alone.
B. The patient will have increased airway resistance compared to a patient who receives general anesthesia alone.
C. The patient will have a reduced forced expiratory volume in one second (FEV_1) compared to a patient who receives general anesthesia alone.
D. The patient will have a reduced vital capacity (VC) compared to a patient who receives general anesthesia alone.

(5) Which of the following correctly describes the anatomy of the paravertebral space?

A. The pleura forms the ventral border, the vertebrae form the medial border, and the costotransversal processes form the dorsal border.
B. As the spinal nerves travel through the paravertebral space, they are surrounded by a thick layer of fascia.
C. The paravertebral space is an isolated compartment and does not reliably communicate with the intercostal space of the epidural space.
D. The lung parenchyma forms the ventral border, the vertebrae form the medial border, and the pleura forms the dorsal border.

(6) A 65-year-old male stopped his Coumadin 3 days prior to arriving for a video-assisted thoracoscopy (VATS); his INR is 1.7. While the surgeon is comfortable with proceeding to the OR, she asks you to perform a regional technique as part of her enhanced recovery protocol. What combination of interventions and medications would be most helpful in the management of this patient?

A. Thoracic epidural analgesia, acetaminophen, gabapentin, oxycodone
B. Ipsilateral thoracic paravertebral block, ketorolac, acetaminophen, gabapentin, oxycodone
C. Ipsilateral erector spinae plane block, acetaminophen, gabapentin, oxycodone
D. Pectointercostal fascial plane block, acetaminophen, gabapentin, oxycodone

(7) A 67-year-old female presenting with right-sided anterolateral rib fractures from T3–T6; her INR is 1.9 as she receives Coumadin. You are consulted to help with the pain management. You have decided to place a single-shot serratus anterior plane block with liposomal bupivacaine. Where are the injection site and borders?

A. Third rib, mid-clavicular line, between the pectoralis major and pectoralis minor
B. Fourth rib mid-axillary, inferior to the rib, with local displacing pleura on injection
C. At the level of T4, deep to the erector spinae muscles and superficial to the T4 transverse process
D. At the level of fourth–fifth, between the serratus anterior and the latissimus dorsi muscles, between the posterior and midaxillary lines.

(8) What nerves do you hope to anesthetize with a serratus plane block?

A. Lateral and medial pectoral nerves
B. Posterior ramus of the T4 spinal nerve
C. Anterior division of the intercostal nerves
D. The intercostobrachial nerve, lateral cutaneous branches of the intercostal nerves (T3–T9), long thoracic nerve, and thoracodorsal nerve

ANSWERS

(1) **C.** The sympatholysis from the thoracic epidural analgesia (TEA) for thoracic surgery results in increased gastric motility and perfusion. It also results in decreased bronchial tone and reactivity and increased coronary blood flow and a resultant increase in myocardial ischemia because of unopposed vagal tone.

Reference

Clemente A, Carli F. The physiological effects of thoracic epidural anesthesia and analgesia on the cardiovascular, respiratory and gastrointestinal systems. *Minerva Anestesiologica*. 2008;74(10):549–563.

(2) **B.** There is no consensus for evidence-based recommendation that supports what volume of local anesthetic to be injected for a PECS II block for optimal spread and analgesia.
(3) **C.** Serratus anterior plane block (SAPB) targets the lateral cutaneous branches of the intercostal nerve from T2–T9, and that is helpful in the anterior lateral rib fractures. The block is done at the posterior to midaxillary line between ribs 4–5; the serratus anterior muscle (SAM) is clearly visible superficial to the ribs. Overlying SAM is the latissimus dorsi muscle. Anesthesia of the axilla comes from blocking the intercostobrachial nerve.

Reference

Kunhabdulla NP, Agarwal A, Gaur A, et al. Serratus anterior plane block for multiple rib fractures. *Pain Physician*. 2014;17(4):E651–E653.

(4) **A.** When compared to general anesthesia when compared with IV-PCA and general anesthesia, TEA resulted in a 27% increase in the FRC and an overall improvement in pulmonary outcome.

Reference

Wahaba WM, Don HF, Craig DB. Post-operative epidural analgesia: effects on lung volume. *Can Anaesth Soc J.* 1975; 22:519–527.

(5) **A.** The boundaries of the paravertebral space are as follows: the pleura forms the ventral border, the vertebrae form the medial border, and the costotransversal processes form the dorsal border.

Reference

Batra RK, Krishnan K, Agarwal A. Paravertebral block. *J Anaesthesiol Clin Pharmacol.* 2011;27(1): 5–11.

(6) **C.** An Ipsilateral erector spinae plane block, acetaminophen, gabapentin, oxycodone can provide acceptable postoperative pain control after a VATS procedure. Neuroaxial procedures like thoracic epidural analgesia and paravertebral blocks are contraindicated with INR above 1.4; additionally there are more conservative good alternatives. The pectointercostal fascial plane covers only the parasternal area

Reference

Salhotra R. Ultrasound-guided truncal/plane blocks: are they safe in anticoagulated patients? *J Anaesthesiol Clin Pharmacol.* 2020;36(1):118–120.

(7) **D.** The injection site for serratus anterior plane block (SAPB) is at the level of ribs 4–5, between the serratus anterior and the latissimus dorsi muscles, between the posterior and midaxillary lines; injection at the third rib, mid-clavicular line, between the pectoralis major and pectoralis minor constitutes PEC I block. Injection at the level of T4, deep to the erector spinae muscles and superficial to the T4 transverse process, constitutes the erector spinae (ESP) block.

Reference

Chin KJ. Thoracic wall blocks: from paravertebral to retrolaminar to serratus to erector spinae and back again—a review of evidence. *Best Pract Res Clin Anaesthesiol.* 2019;33(1):67–77.

(8) **D.** The nerves anesthetized in a serratus anterior plane (SAP) block are the intercostobrachial nerve, lateral cutaneous branches of the intercostal nerves (T2–T9), long thoracic nerve, and thoracodorsal nerve. The lateral and medial pectoral nerves are anesthetized in PEC block. The posterior ramus of the T4 and adjacent spinal nerve are anesthetized in erector spinae plane (ESP) block. The anterior division of the intercostal nerves are anesthetized in the parasternal blocks; i.e., the pecto-intercostal fascial block (PIFPB) and the transversus thoracic plane block (TTPB).

Reference

Chin KJ. Thoracic wall blocks: from paravertebral to retrolaminar to serratus to erector spinae and back again—a review of evidence. *Best Pract Res Clin Anaesthesiol.* 2019;33(1):67–77.

14.

THE TRAUMA PATIENT WITH FRACTURED RIBS

Dennis J. Warfield Jr. and Sanjib Das Adhikary

STEM CASE AND KEY QUESTIONS

A 70-year-old male was involved in a motor vehicle accident as a restrained driver with airbag deployment. Once extricated, he was taken to the nearest trauma center where he was confused and complaining of left-sided chest pain and difficulty breathing. Chest x-ray demonstrated multiple left-sided rib fractures. His past medical history is significant for atrial fibrillation, hypertension, and chronic obstructive pulmonary disease (COPD) with a long-standing smoking history. His medications include rivaroxaban, metoprolol, losartan, and an albuterol inhaler. After a comprehensive assessment and stabilization in the trauma bay, he was admitted to the surgical intensive care unit (SICU). A consult to the regional anesthesia and acute pain medicine team has been placed for coordination and assistance in optimizing his pain management.

(1) WHAT OTHER CONDITIONS SHOULD YOU LOOK FOR IN A PATIENT WITH MULTIPLE RIB FRACTURES? WHAT ARE THE IMPLICATIONS OF HAVING MULTIPLE RIB FRACTURES IN REGARD TO HIS PAIN MANAGEMENT?

Due to the mechanism of injury, computed tomography (CT) scans of his head, neck, chest, abdomen, and pelvis were obtained before admission to the SICU. They demonstrated no acute intracranial pathology, no acute cervical spine injury or fracture, a left-sided lung contusion, a small left-sided apical pneumothorax, multiple left-sided rib fractures involving ribs 3 through 7 anteriorly and no acute abdominal or pelvic injuries. The patient is lying in bed, moaning in pain, while he holds tight to his chest.

(2) IS THERE A ROLE FOR THE REGIONAL ANESTHESIA AND ACUTE PAIN MEDICINE SERVICE IN MANAGING THIS PATIENT'S PAIN? WHAT TYPES OF CONSERVATIVE THERAPY ARE THERE FOR PATIENTS WITH RIB FRACTURES?

As part of the trauma team's rib fracture protocol, you (as a member of the regional anesthesia and acute pain medicine service) are consulted. The patient, now located in the ICU, is noted to be flat in bed, motionless and splinting with shallow breathing. He is receiving oxygen via nasal cannula at 4 liters per minute. An intravenous patient-controlled analgesia (IVPCA) pump containing fentanyl is connected and is running at a basal rate. Nursing tasks to assist the patient to get out of bed to chair and mobilize as tolerated are in place, as well as for respiratory therapy to provide full pulmonary toilet, including aggressive chest physical therapy multiple times daily. Multimodal pain orders consisting of oral acetaminophen, ibuprofen, and oxycodone as needed are also implemented.

(3) HOW SHOULD THIS PATIENT'S PAIN BE EVALUATED? IF CONSERVATIVE THERAPY PROVIDES SUBOPTIMAL PAIN MANAGEMENT, WHAT ARE THE NEXT STEPS? WHAT OTHER FACTORS AND CONDITIONS NEED TO BE TAKEN INTO ACCOUNT BEFORE AN APPROPRIATE MODE OF ANALGESIA IS SELECTED?

By both self-assessment (pain scores) and functional assessment (incentive spirometry), you feel that this patient's pain management can be improved from his current status. You decide that the best pain relief in this situation would be provided with a continuous thoracic epidural catheter and discuss this with both the patient and his family. Owing to the anterior nature of the rib fractures, the multiple levels involved, and unilateral location, you plan for a left-sided paramedian approach to the epidural space between the fifth and sixth thoracic vertebral levels. Due to his morbid obesity, palpation of his spinous processes proves challenging. It is discovered during the safety time out that he took his metoprolol and losartan earlier today, but it is unclear when his last dose of rivaroxaban was taken. His last blood pressure in the supine position was 128/65; however, when placed in the sitting position in preparation for the procedure, it decreased to 76/54.

(4) WILL THIS NEW INFORMATION (VITAL SIGNS CHANGES AND UNCLEAR ANTICOAGULATION STATUS) CHANGE YOUR MANAGEMENT?

You decide to abort the placement of a thoracic epidural catheter due to the present hypotension. Family confirms that the patient is noncompliant with his rivaroxaban, last dose of which was said to be taken more than 3 days ago. Instead, you agree now to place a left-sided paravertebral (PVB) catheter at the fifth thoracic level. Placement of the PVB catheter took multiple attempts and a considerable amount of bleeding still is noticed at the site of needle puncture. After securing the catheter, you bolus it with 10 cc of 0.5% ropivacaine and start an infusion. Thirty minutes have passed since the bolus was administered and it appears he is breathing more comfortably with less splinting. You obtain dermatomal coverage from T3–T7 on the left as demonstrated by spot testing with ice. Both his pain score and incentive spirometry have improved from baseline. His own assessment confirms your observations and he thanks you for your efforts in caring for him.

(5) THE BLOCK IS IN PLACE AND FUNCTIONAL, WHAT ARE THE NEXT STEPS?

During acute pain management rounds the next day, the patient's nurse tells you that although his pain is better controlled, he still appears to be short of breath. As you walk into the room, you see that he is clutching his chest, is short of breath with labored breathing, tachycardic, and has an oxygen saturation in the low 90s. You auscultate the patient's chest, switch him from nasal cannula to a non-rebreather mask, obtain an arterial blood gas, order a STAT chest x-ray and immediately alert the trauma team of the patient's change in condition. The paravertebral catheter site is examined, which shows some bloody drainage around the catheter, but no erythema or tenderness to palpation. Dermatomal coverage is still adequate with ice testing. A review of his morning vital signs and labs shows him to be afebrile without an elevated white count. Both services decide that a STAT CT of his chest is warranted. This reveals a large pulmonary embolus (PE). The trauma team communicates with the acute pain management service the need for full anticoagulation with a therapeutic intravenous heparin infusion to initiate treatment for the patient's PE.

(6) WHAT ARE THE IMPLICATIONS OF THE PATIENT HAVING A PVB CATHETER IN PLACE AND NEEDING FULL ANTICOAGULATION FOR HIS PE?

Since there was profuse bleeding at the PVB catheter entrance site following the multiple attempts during placement, you decide to remove the catheter an hour before beginning heparinization in an attempt to mitigate any chance of the patient developing a neuraxial hematoma. The patient subsequently develops an intolerable increase in pain over the course of the next few hours correlating to the location of the rib fractures. Both oral and intravenous rescue analgesia with opioids proves to be both inadequate and counterproductive, now bringing you back to where you had originally started.

(7) ARE THERE ANY OTHER TREATMENT MODALITIES FOR RIB FRACTURES? WHAT ELSE DO YOU HAVE TO OFFER THE PATIENT NOW?

In consultation with the trauma team and the rest of your acute pain medicine service, you discuss analgesic options for this patient which will give him the best chance of avoiding further pulmonary compromise. The trauma team discusses bringing the patient to the operating room for rib plating while you debate other methods of pain control which are essential for his recovery. Members of your team suggest attempting additional techniques such as intrapleural analgesia, intercostal nerve and serratus anterior plane (SAP) blocks, none of which any of you feel comfortable with performing or feel would be optimal for the patient's current condition. Your team does, however, have experience in performing erector spinae plane (ESP) blocks and finally agree on this route of analgesia in an attempt to deliver better pain control for this patient. Placement of an ESP catheter at the left fifth thoracic level utilizing ultrasound was successful. A subsequent bolus of 30 mL of 0.5% ropivacaine helped achieve effective pain relief once again, which was continued by an infusion. After resolution of his PE, rib plating was ultimately performed by the trauma team. With adequate pain control in the midst of surgical correction, he was able to participate successfully with nursing care and respiratory therapy over the course of the next few days to eventually be discharged from the hospital.

DISCUSSION

Rib fractures, in particular those involving various levels, are frequent in multi-trauma patients. These injuries are typically seen after blunt thoracic trauma, most commonly involving motor vehicle accidents. Rib fractures alone are associated with significant morbidity and mortality as well as long-term disability without appropriate management.[1] In many places around the world, trauma is a significant cause of both morbidity and mortality, and is the leading the cause of death in the first four decades of life. Rib fractures, as a subset of trauma, are commonly found in at least 10% of all injured patients, most often as a consequence of blunt thoracic trauma.[2] Motor vehicle accidents are acknowledged as one of the major sources of blunt thoracic trauma with resultant rib fracture injuries.

Acute management of rib fractures, including a comprehensive analgesic plan, is critical in preventing respiratory complications while simultaneously aiding in a more rapid recovery. Rib fractures frequently require an ICU level of care for better outcomes as constant coordination of efforts between teams is essential to having superior prognoses.

PATHOGENESIS OF RIB FRACTURES

Studies have shown that rib fractures are associated with an overall mortality rate as high as 20%. Pneumonia has been recognized as the leading cause of death in the majority of these patients, with age being a strong predictor of mortality.[3] Rib

Table 14.1 **RIB FRACTURE SCORE CALCULATOR: RIB FRACTURE SCORE = (BREAKS × SIDES) + AGE FACTOR**

	CHARACTERISTICS	TOTAL
BREAKS	NUMBER (#) OF FRACTURES	TOTAL # OF FRACTURES
Sides	Unilateral	1
	Bilateral	2
Age (years) factor	<50	0
	51–60	1
	61–70	2
	71–80	3
	>80	4

Modified from Easter, A. Management of patients with multiple rib fractures. *Am J Crit Care.* 2001;10(5):320–327.

fracture scoring systems, such as *Easter's formula*,[4] as shown in Table 14.1, have been implemented as screening tools for early recognition of severity. These scoring systems attempt to identify patients at higher risk of morbidity and mortality and therefore in need of a more acute and advanced level of care. Together, they have been customized with numerous institutionally based pain management algorithms for appropriate medical and/or surgical management of rib fractures.

The number of ribs fractured correlates with the severity of injury. Four or more rib fractures are associated with higher mortality rates.[5] The location of rib fracture(s) is also a marker of severity. If a fracture of the first rib is sustained, healthcare providers should be aware of and anticipate the possibility of other major underlying injuries.[4] A flail chest in the setting of rib fractures has an incidence of 7%.[6] However, it is associated with a mortality rate as high as 33%.[7] Anatomically, a flail chest is defined by the presence of at least 3 consecutive unilateral ribs each fractured in 2 or more places. Clinically, the diagnosis is made whenever an incompetent segment of chest wall is large enough that paradoxical motion of the chest wall is visible with respiration.[8]

CLINICAL MANIFESTATIONS OF RIB FRACTURES

Rib fractures, taking into consideration number, type, and location, play a significant role in compromising both oxygenation and ventilation. The morbidity and mortality associated with rib fractures is due to a combination of three main causes:

1. Splinting or pain from rib fractures causes **hypoventilation** and an overall reduction in the total tidal volume achieved. If pain is not appropriately managed, hypoventilation can lead to the development of atelectasis, the complete or partial collapse of the entire lung, lobe, or segment, which in turn contributes to retention of secretions predisposing the patient to developing pneumonia.[4]
2. Physical damage to the lung secondary to rib fractures may result in an underlying pulmonary contusion. This causes poor lung compliance and **impaired gas exchange**, leading to intrapulmonary shunting and a decrease in P_aO_2.[2]
3. Multiple rib fractures or the presence of a flail chest may cause **altered breathing mechanics**, resulting in ventilatory insufficiency. This insufficiency is due to the disruption of normal costovertebral and diaphragmatic muscle excursion.[4] The negative intrapleural pressure generated during inhalation produces paradoxical movement of the flail section, causing it to move inward, opposite the rest of the rib cage, which moves outward. The section of lung underneath the flail chest does not expand normally. This results in a decrease in tidal volume and ultimately, inefficient breathing.[2]

TREATMENT MODALITIES FOR RIB FRACTURES

A number of *un-modifiable* risk factors affect disability, morbidity, and mortality in patients with rib fractures, including advanced age, preexisting comorbidities, and the number and location of fractures. Pain, however, is a *modifiable* risk factor of paramount importance. It is crucial that analgesia be promptly addressed to circumvent hypoventilation and the development of atelectasis and pneumonia, avoidable or prolonged endotracheal intubation, and even death. There are many approaches to effective pain management in these patients, which include both conservative management and invasive techniques. A multimodal and at times step-wise approach often gives the patient the best chance to avoid potential imminent pulmonary compromise.

CONSERVATIVE MANAGEMENT

Conservative management for rib fractures comprises individual and/or group tasks aimed at helping clear mucus and secretions from the airways, preventing atelectasis and ultimately pneumonia from occurring. They include early ambulation, chest physiotherapy (including percussion), pulmonary hygiene/toilet (including frequent suctioning and coughing), as well as deep breathing exercises by means of repeated use of incentive spirometry and vibratory positive expiratory pressure (PEP) devices. It is vital that these tasks ensue early and often to prevent the patient from decompensating.

Multimodal oral and intravenous analgesics that do not inhibit respiration (i.e., acetaminophen and nonsteroidal anti-inflammatory drugs [NSAIDs] such as ibuprofen), in addition to topical agents (i.e., lidocaine patches), are an important supplementary component to this approach. These are non-sedating and non-respiratory-drive-depressing means of pharmacotherapy that will assist in pain control, allowing the patient to participate more effusively with the above-mentioned tasks.

Intravenous patient-controlled analgesia (PCA) with opioids such as fentanyl, morphine, and hydromorphone are also commonly used for rib fracture analgesia, especially as an adjunct for breakthrough pain control. Extreme caution must be taken when this route of pharmacotherapy is utilized for pain management as unintentional over-sedation may result in hypoventilation and inhibition of coughing, the exact opposite of the goal at hand, with potential to lead the patient to respiratory failure.

Conservative therapy is commonly used for younger patients with non-severe rib fractures, often as the sole therapy.

These approaches are also generally used for older patients with more severe rib fractures as first-line therapy prior to or simultaneously with more aggressive therapy, including further invasive techniques. It is crucial to provide frequent and regular therapy with repeated assessment of patient progress to recognize when an escalation in treatment may be required.

INVASIVE TECHNIQUES

The use of invasive techniques in the treatment of rib fractures has evolved over time. To provide consistently successful analgesia for rib fractures, the practitioner must be not only skilled in performing the procedure, but knowledgeable regarding anatomy, indications, and contraindications, as well as the potential complications with an appropriate response in management if needed.

Invasive techniques range from midline neuraxial and perineuraxial procedures such as thoracic epidural and thoracic paravertebral (PVB) catheter placement, to more lateral and peripheral procedures such as the newer myofascial plane truncal nerve blocks. These innovative techniques offer an alternative when thoracic epidural or PVB catheter placement are contraindicated or not feasible. They are *less* invasive, allow for a broader application, and provide excellent analgesia with minimal side effects.

Thoracic Epidural

The use of a thoracic epidural catheter for rib fracture analgesia is both complex and conditional. The placement of a properly functional thoracic epidural catheter requires technical competence, experience, familiarity of anatomy, and discretion in choosing the appropriate patient. Thoracic epidural analgesia for rib fractures has historically been the gold standard treatment and is supported by several studies.[9,10,11] This technique is frequently applied to patients with bilateral rib fracture injuries.

The true efficacy in thoracic epidural analgesia in reducing pulmonary complications, hospital and ICU length of stay (LOS), and overall mortality, though, has been questioned.[12,13] Studies involving epidural analgesia are difficult to properly and fairly evaluate due to varying degrees and definitions of success, inconsistency in provider skill, and overall heterogeneity within the studies themselves, including the composition of the solutions infused to obtain analgesia.

The practitioner needs to be aware of both potential side effects and complications from thoracic epidural catheter placement and how to properly manage them if they occur. These include hypotension, urinary retention, pruritus, allergic reaction, motor blockade, one-sided block, patchy or no block, post-dural puncture headache (PDPH), high epidural or unintentional spinal, infection, and bleeding. It is imperative to verify the patient's **anticoagulation status** prior to attempting any neuraxial analgesic technique, inquiring about what medication and dose was taken and when it was last taken. The American Society of Regional Anesthesia (ASRA) has established evidence-based guidelines for practicing regional anesthesia in patients receiving antithrombotic or thrombolytic therapy.[14]

It is important to evaluate the clinical situation *as a whole* prior to selecting an appropriate mode of analgesia. For a patient who has sustained unilateral rib fractures, a thoracic epidural catheter for analgesia might not be the best initial choice for pain management.

Thoracic Paravertebral (PVB)

Along with continuous thoracic epidural catheter placement, thoracic paravertebral (PVB) catheter placement is one of the most widely used regional techniques for providing analgesia for rib fractures. One major advantage is that it is associated with fewer side effects. As an off-midline technique, a few differences between thoracic PVBs and epidurals are key in management. Unlike a properly placed and functional epidural, which would provide bilateral coverage, a PVB will only provide coverage to the ipsilateral side. This makes this method of analgesia more favorable for one-sided rib fractures with *less* concern over potential hypotension and coagulopathy. In comparison to an epidural injection, a PVB injection will preferentially spread caudally (i.e., with any epidural bolus, usually three-fifths of the volume spreads cephalad and two-fifths caudad, whereas with a PVB two-fifths of the volume spreads cephalad and three-fifths spread caudad).[15] This factor plays a strategic role in the optimal location(s) of catheter placement.

Both thoracic epidural and PVB catheter placement techniques provide superior analgesia while potentially saving the patient from being subject to the side effects of systemic opioids. A recent review of data from the National Trauma Data Bank (NTDB) within the United States demonstrated that there were comparable results between analgesia obtained with thoracic epidural and PVB after propensity score matching of patients in respect to development of pneumonia, length of mechanical ventilation, and overall LOS. However, in comparison to patients who did not receive any regional technique, patients who did receive either a thoracic epidural or PVB were also shown to have prolonged LOS and more frequent ICU admissions, even though this group was associated with a decrease in overall mortality.[16]

It is important to note that when thoracic epidural catheter placement is contraindicated or not feasible for patients who have sustained bilateral rib fracture injuries, PVB catheter placement or either of the following mentioned techniques can be performed in similar two-sided fashion simultaneously to obtain bilateral analgesia.

Erector Spinae Plane (ESP) Block

The increasing use of ultrasound has led to the development of several new myofascial plane nerve blocks. These novel ultrasound-guided peripheral nerve block techniques are effective alternatives to neuraxial techniques for pain management when the patient is either not amenable to or the placement of a thoracic epidural or PVB catheter is not practical. These techniques are being applied to a host of different postoperative analgesic protocols, with rib fracture analgesia now being explored as another avenue for potential use.

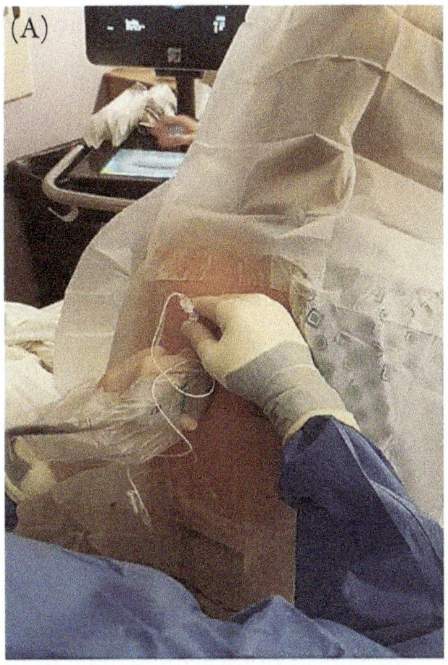

Figure 14.1A. In-plane approach to the ESP block in the sitting position. Reproduced with permission from: Thiruvenkatarajan V, Eng HC, Adhikary SD. An update on regional analgesia for rib fractures. *Curr Opin Anaesthesiol.* 2018;31(5):601–607.

The ESP block has been used for pain management after abdominal and thoracic surgery due to described extensive truncal analgesia. The presumed mechanism is thought to be attributable to coverage of both dorsal and ventral rami of the thoracic nerves with local anesthetic spread.[17] To perform this procedure the patient is placed in the sitting position. The ultrasound transducer is held sagittal, off midline to the desired side, and the block needle is introduced using an in-plane technique (Figure 14.1A).[17] Ultrasound imaging (Figure 14.1B)[17] shows the proper injection location within the erector spinae myofascial plane. This plane is located on the posterior chest wall between the anterior surface of the erector spinae muscle and the posterior surface of the spinal transverse process (TP).

The ESP block is *simpler, safer, and less invasive* than either a thoracic epidural or PVB and can be utilized in the presence of either coagulopathy or anticoagulation. As with the previously mentioned techniques, infusion catheters can also be placed within the erector spinae plane for prolonged analgesia. A limitation with this technique is the variability of the spread of local anesthetic within the myofascial plane.

Serratus Anterior Plane (SAP) Block

Another alternative myofascial plane technique in the management of rib fractures is the serratus anterior plane block. This is performed in the axillary region, above or below the serratus anterior muscle.[18] The patient is positioned either supine or lateral, with the arm placed above or across the body to allow access to the mid-axillary region (Figure 14.2A).[17] Ultrasound imaging (Figure 14.2B)[17] shows the relevant anatomy with projected needle pathways for both the superficial and deep methods of performing the SAP block.

Studies have shown, by assessing both distribution of the injection and sensory mapping, that the superficial plane technique (injection of local anesthetic within the fascial plane between the latissimus dorsi and serratus anterior muscles) provides more effective analgesia.[18] At the axillary fossa, the intercostobrachialis nerve, lateral cutaneous branches of the intercostal nerves (T3–T9), long thoracic nerve, and thoracodorsal nerve are located in a compartment between the

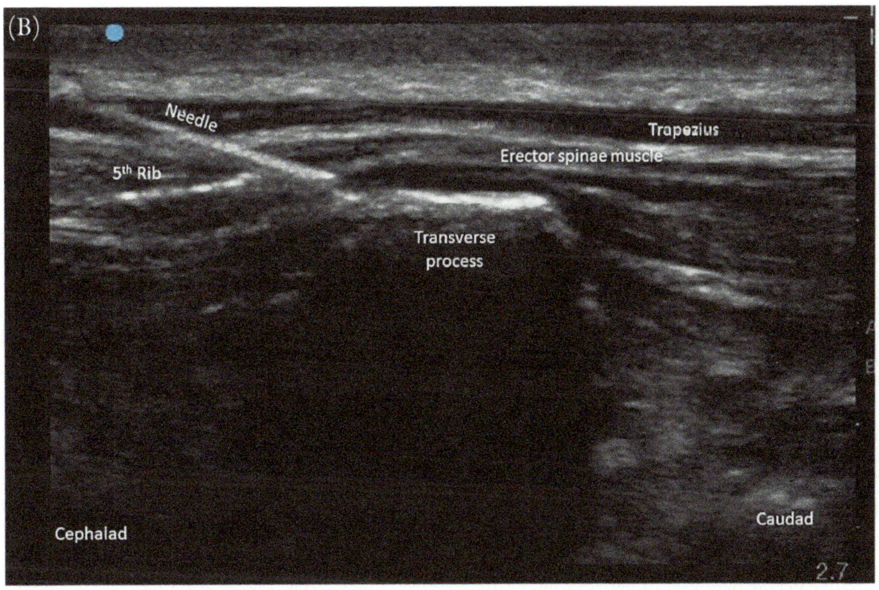

Figure 14.1B. Ultrasound image of the ESP block where transverse process is seen and the correct location of the needle tip is confirmed by injecting 0.5–1 cc of normal saline 0.9% observing linear fluid spread lifting the erector spinae muscle off the tip of the TP.
Reproduced with permission from: Thiruvenkatarajan V, Eng HC, Adhikary SD. An update on regional analgesia for rib fractures. *Curr Opin Anaesthesiol.* 2018;31(5):601–607.

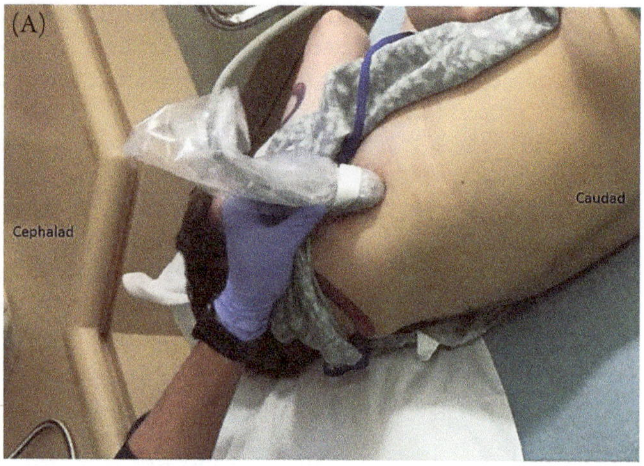

Figure 14.2A. In-plane approach to SAP block with the patient positioned laterally. Orientation of the ultrasound probe is aligned at an angle following the edge of the latissimus dorsi muscle. The arm can be placed across the body, allowing the latissimus dorsi muscle to be more lateral over the chest wall.
Reproduced with permission from: Thiruvenkatarajan V, Eng HC, Adhikary SD. An update on regional analgesia for rib fractures. *Curr Opin Anaesthesiol.* 2018;31(5):601–607.

serratus anterior and the latissimus dorsi muscles, between the posterior and midaxillary lines.[19]

These newer interfascial plane injections were originally developed as alternatives to thoracic epidural, PVB, intercostal, and intrapleural blocks, primarily for analgesia after surgery on the hemithorax.[19] Now, with advancements in practitioner skill and an increase in the utilization of ultrasound, these techniques are being applied with broader application.

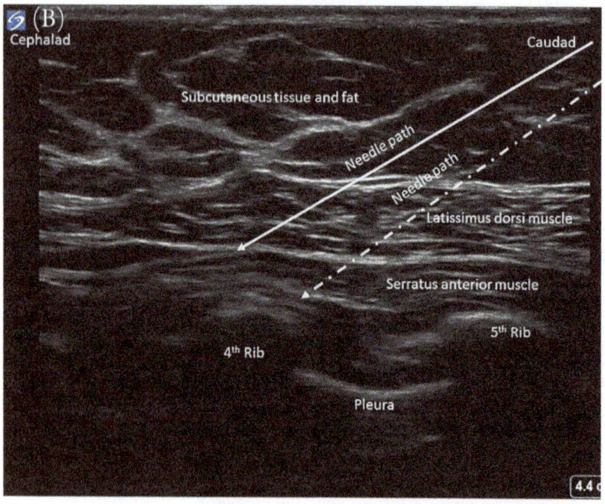

Figure 14.2B. Ultrasound image of the serratus anterior plane with surrounding anatomy and tentative needle pathways of performing both superficial (solid arrow) and deep (dashed arrow) blocks.
Reproduced with permission from: Thiruvenkatarajan V, Eng HC, Adhikary SD. An update on regional analgesia for rib fractures. *Curr Opin Anaesthesiol.* 2018;31(5):601–607.

Intercostal Nerve (ICB) Block

The intercostal nerves are the continuation of the ventral ramus. To perform an effective intercostal nerve (ICN) block), the block must be performed proximal to the midaxillary line, where the lateral cutaneous branch takes off.[19] An ICNB may need to be performed at multiple levels (for each involved level of fractured rib). This makes this block a less favorable option to perform as it requires several, often repeated, injections, each increasing the risk of complications, particularly pneumothorax due to relative location, and local anesthetic systemic toxicity (LAST) due to the highly vascularized bundle located underneath each rib.

Intrapleural Analgesia

Intrapleural analgesia consists of the injection of local anesthetic into the pleural space via a catheter. Analgesia is believed to result from the spread of local anesthetic to multiple intercostal nerves using a single interpleural injection site.[20] It is an unreliable technique that requires a large volume of local anesthetic to be infused. Its use has fallen out of favor.

Surgical Management

Rib fractures are predominantly managed nonoperatively. There is increasing evidence supporting the role of surgical management, open reduction internal fixation (ORIF) of fractured ribs, or rib plating. In 2017, clinical practice guidelines were published and intended to be an evidence-based resource for performing surgical stabilization of rib fractures (SSRF). Among these indications are flail chest, multiple severely displaced fractures, those who fail early non-operative management, and lastly, those who have symptomatic nonunion and or malunion of rib fractures.[21] Optimal timing of when surgical intervention should take place, however, has not been established, but is recommended to be performed as soon as possible after admission, preferably within 24 hours. SSRF is not recommended in the setting of hemodynamic instability, when there are higher priority injuries that need to be addressed first, or if there is an appropriate trial of non-operative management. Surgical stabilization may help improve pulmonary function, decrease mechanical ventilation time, and lower the risk of developing pneumonia and needing a tracheostomy. This may potentially avoid the need for longer hospital stays, especially within the ICU, which ultimately helps decrease costs. Large randomized controlled trials are still needed to further establish absolute indications as well as determine long-term outcomes.[21]

Rib fractures are common injuries in the setting of blunt chest trauma that without appropriate management could have severe morbidity and mortality. It is crucial to have a consistent, thorough, and effective treatment plan, implemented early, involving any and all necessary healthcare teams. Having an integrated team approach will allow for the individualized care each patient might need in order to work toward the best possible outcome.

CONCLUSIONS

- Blunt thoracic trauma is responsible for the majority of rib fractures.
- The number of ribs fractured and presence of a flail chest are associated with increased morbidity and mortality.
- Morbidity and mortality associated with rib fractures are due to hypoventilation, impaired gas exchange, altered breathing mechanics, and pneumonia.
- Conservative management of rib fractures consists of early ambulation, chest physiotherapy, pulmonary hygiene, and analgesia with oral, intravenous, and topical agents.
- The use of invasive techniques is ever-changing. The entire clinical context must be considered before choosing the most appropriate procedure.
- Thoracic epidural catheter placement has historically been the gold standard treatment for pain management in multiple rib fractures and should be considered with bilateral fractures.
- Thoracic PVBs have been shown to have comparable efficacy in pain management to thoracic epidural catheter placement.
- The ESP block is a new myofascial plane nerve block that can been used in patients with multiple rib fractures when more invasive techniques are contraindicated.
- The SAP block is more effective when the superficial plane technique is performed.
- The ICN block is not a favorable nerve block to perform with multiple rib fractures due to its high potential for complications.
- Intrapleural analgesia in an unreliable technique.
- Surgical stabilization of rib fractures is increasing in popularity for multiple rib fractures and flail chest.
- Appropriate follow-up and handling of any complication are **essential**.

REFERENCES

1. Pressley C, Fry W, Philp A, Berry S, Smith R. Predicting outcome of patients with chest wall injury. *Am J Surg.* 2012;204:910–914.
2. May L, Hillermann C, Patil S. Rib fracture management. *BJA Education.* 2016;16:26–32.
3. Brasel KJ, Guse CE. Layde P, Weigelt JA. Rib fractures: relationship with pneumonia and mortality. *Crit Care Med.* 2006;34(6):1642–1646.
4. Easter A. Management of patients with multiple rib fractures. *Am J Crit Care.* 2001;10(5):320–327.
5. Holcomb JB, Mcmullin NR, Kozar RA, Lygas MH, Moore FA. Morbidity from rib fractures increases after age 45. *J Am Coll Surg.* 2003;196(4):549–555.
6. Richardson JD, Adams L, Flint LM. Selective management of flail chest and pulmonary contusion. *Ann Surg.* 1982;196:481–487.
7. Ciraulo DL, Elliott D, Mitchell KA, Rodriguez A. Flail chest as a marker for significant injuries. *J Am Coll Surg.* 1994;178:466–470.
8. Nirula R, Diaz JJ, Trunkey DD, Mayberry JC. Rib fracture repair: indications, technical issues, and future directions. *World J Surg.* 2008;33(1):14–22.
9. Gage A, Rivara F, Wang J, Jurkovich GJ, Ababi S. The effect of epidural placement in patients after blunt thoracic trauma. *J Trauma Acute Care Surg.* 2014;76:39–45.
10. Bulger EM, Edwards T, Klotz P, Jurkovich GJ. Epidural analgesia improves outcome after multiple rib fractures. *Surgery.* 2004;136:426–430.
11. Wu CL, Jani ND, Perkins FM, Barquist E. Thoracic epidural analgesia versus intravenous patient-controlled analgesia for the treatment of rib fracture pain after motor vehicle crash. *J Trauma: Injury, Infection Crit Care.* 1999;47(3):564–567.
12. Carrier FM, Turgeon AF, Nicole PC, et al. Effect of epidural analgesia in patients with traumatic rib fractures: a systematic review and meta-analysis of randomized controlled trials. *Can J Anaesth.* 2009;56:230–442.
13. Duch P, Moller MH. Epidural analgesia in patients with traumatic rib fractures: a systematic review of randomised controlled trials. *Acta Anaesthesiol Scand.* 2015;59:698–709.
14. Horlocker TT, Vandermeuelen E, Kopp SL, Gogarten W, Leffert LR, Benzon HT. Regional anesthesia in the patient receiving antithrombotic or thrombolytic therapy: American Society of Regional Anesthesia and Pain Medicine evidence-based guidelines (fourth edition). *Reg Anesth Pain Med.* 2018;43:263–309.
15. Greengrass RA, Duclas R. Paravertebral blocks. *Int Anesthesiol Clin.* 2012;50(1):56–73.
16. Malekpour M, Hashmi A, Dove J, Torres D, Wild J. Analgesic choice in management of rib fractures: paravertebral block or epidural analgesia? *Anesth Analg.* 2017;124:1906–1911.
17. Thiruvenkatarajan V, Eng HC, Adhikary SD. An update on regional analgesia for rib fractures. *Curr Opin Anaesthesiol.* 2018;31(5):601–607.
18. Blanco R, Parras T, McDonnell JG, Prats-Galino A. Serratus plane block: a novel ultrasound-guided thoracic wall nerve block. *Anaesthesia.* 2013;68(11):1107–1113.
19. Hadžić A. *Hadzic's Textbook of Regional Anesthesia and Acute Pain Management.* New York: McGraw-Hill Education; 2017:2:650–660.
20. Dhanjal S, Shannon C. Interpleural analgesia. In: *StatPearls.* Treasure Island, FL: StatPearls; 2022. Available from: https://www.ncbi.nlm.nih.gov/books/NBK526020/.
21. McClure TT, Myers P, Triplet JJ, Johnson DB, Taylor BC. Surgical treatment of flail chest and rib fractures: a systematic review of the literature. *Int J Orth.* 2019;6(2):1039–1044.

REVIEW QUESTIONS

(1) Which rib if fractured is considered to be a hallmark of severe trauma?

A. 1st rib
B. 4th rib
C. 5th rib
D. 12th rib

(2) The erector spinae myofascial plane is found in the posterior chest wall between which corresponding anatomical structures?

A. Anterior surface of erector spinae muscle and anterior surface of spinal transverse process
B. Anterior surface of erector spinae muscle and posterior surface of spinous process
C. Anterior surface of erector spinae muscle and posterior surface of spinal transverse process

D. Posterior surface of erector spinae muscle and posterior surface of spinal transverse process

(3) A patient in the ICU with multiple bilateral rib fractures and a thoracic epidural catheter in place for analgesia had a therapeutic intravenous heparin infusion started emergently for a massive pulmonary embolus (PE). Upon resolution of the PE, how long after the discontinuation of the intravenous heparin is it recommended to wait to remove the epidural catheter?

A. 1–3 hours
B. 4–6 hours
C. 7–9 hours
D. 10–12 hours

4. A serratus anterior plane block is being planned for right-sided rib fractures. Which of the following groups of anatomical structures correspond to the superficial approach to the serratus anterior plane block?

A. Fascial plane between pectoralis major and pectoralis minor
B. Fascial plane between pectoralis minor and serratus
C. Fascial plane between latissimus dorsi and serratus
D. Fascial plane between serratus and the surface of the ribs

(5) The morbidity and mortality associated with rib fractures is due to a combination of all of the following factors EXCEPT:

A. Altered breathing mechanics
B. Hyperventilation
C. Impaired gas exchange
D. Hypoventilation

(6) Which of the following is considered a modifiable risk factor for a patient being treated for rib fractures?

A. Age
B. Preexisting comorbidities
C. Pain
D. Number and location of rib fractures

(7) You receive a consult from the trauma service for thoracic epidural catheter placement for a patient in the ICU with left-sided rib fractures from T3–T6 and right-sided rib fractures from T4–T8. When you gather a history from the patient you learn that she took her rivaroxaban this morning before arriving to the hospital. How long is it recommended to wait before attempting a neuraxial procedure from the time of last rivaroxaban administration?

A. 24 hours
B. 48 hours
C. 72 hours
D. 96 hours

(8) A patient was brought in earlier today from a motor vehicle accident with an unstable cervical spine fracture, right-sided T2–T5 and left-sided T3–T6 rib fractures, bilateral pulmonary contusions, and a pelvis fracture. Which of the following would be the best choice to provide analgesia to this patient in their present condition in addition to conservative multimodal pain management?

A. Continuous thoracic epidural
B. Bilateral paravertebral blocks
C. Bilateral erector spinae plane blocks
D. Bilateral serratus anterior plane blocks

(9) Which of the following statements is true?

A. Rib fractures alone are associated with significant morbidity and mortality as well as long-term disability with or without appropriate management.
B. Rib fractures alone are associated with significant morbidity and mortality as well as long-term disability with appropriate treatment.
C. Rib fractures alone are associated with significant morbidity and mortality as well as long-term disability without appropriate management.
D. All of the above

(10) Which of the following factors play a definitive role in choosing an effective pain management plan in patients with multiple rib fractures?

i. Body habitus
ii. Spectrum of additional injuries
iii. Coagulation status
iv. Respiratory status
v. Pain score
   A. i, ii, iii
   B. ii, iii, iv
   C. ii, iii, iv, v
   D. i, ii, iii, iv

ANSWERS

(1) **A.** A fracture of the first rib is considered a hallmark of severe trauma secondary to the amount of force required in order to break.[4] If a fracture of this rib occurs, healthcare providers should be aware of and anticipate the possibility of other major underlying injuries such as aortic and other vascular tears, cardiac injuries, brachial plexus injuries in addition to pulmonary trauma.

Reference

Easter A. Management of patients with multiple rib fractures. *Am J Crit Care.* 2001;10(5):320–327.

(2) **C.** The erector spinae plane block is directed at the erector spinae myofascial plane. This is located on the posterior chest wall between the anterior surface of the erector spinae muscle and oriented cephalocaudally to the posterior surface of the spinal transverse process.

Reference

Thiruvenkatarajan V, Eng HC, Adhikary SD. An update on regional analgesia for rib fractures. *Curr Opin Anaesthesiol.* 2018;31(5):601–607.

(3) **B.** According to ASRA guidelines, an indwelling neuraxial catheter can be removed 4–6 hours after the discontinuation of intravenous heparin (and after assessment of the patient's coagulation status).

Reference

Horlocker TT, Vandermeuelen E, Kopp SL, Gogarten W, Leffert LR, Benzon HT. Regional anesthesia in the patient receiving antithrombotic or thrombolytic therapy: American Society of Regional Anesthesia and Pain Medicine evidence-based guidelines (fourth edition). *Reg Anesth Pain Med.* 2018;43:263–309.

(4) **C.** The superficial approach to the serratus anterior plane block involves an injection technique in the fascial plane between the latissimus dorsi and serratus anterior muscles in the axillary region. In comparison to the deep method (plane between serratus anterior muscle and surface of the ribs), the superficial plane technique has been shown to provide more effective analgesia.

Reference

Blanco R, Parras T, McDonnell JG, Prats-Galino A. Serratus plane block: a novel ultrasound-guided thoracic wall nerve block. *Anaesthesia.* 2013;68(11):1107–1113.

(5) **B.** Morbidity and mortality associated with rib fractures is due to a combination of hypoventilation, impaired gas exchange, and altered breathing mechanics. Hypoventilation, secondary to splinting, leads to the development of atelectasis predisposing the patient to developing pneumonia.[8] Physical damage to the lung directly from rib fracture(s) result in pulmonary contusion. These damaged areas of lung have impaired gas exchange leading to shunting and a decrease in P_aO_2.[1] Multiple rib fractures, especially in the presence of a flail chest, may cause altered breathing mechanics, which ultimately results in inefficient breathing.

References

Nirula R, Diaz JJ, Trunkey DD, Mayberry JC. Rib fracture repair: indications, technical issues, and future directions. *World J Surg.* 2008;33(1):14–22.

Pressley C, Fry W, Philp A, Berry S, Smith R. Predicting outcome of patients with chest wall injury. *Am J Surg.* 2012;204:910–914.

(6) **C.** Pain is a modifiable risk factor that is critical to address promptly in order to avoid the development of atelectasis, pneumonia, prolonged intubation, and even death. There are various approaches to effective analgesia, including both conservative management and invasive techniques. Multimodal approaches often give the patient the best chance to avoid pulmonary compromise.

References

May L, Hillermann C, Patil S. Rib fracture management. *BJA Education.* 2016;16:26–32.

Brasel KJ, Guse CE, Layde P, Weigelt JA. Rib fractures: relationship with pneumonia and mortality. *Crit Care Med.* 2006;34(6):1642–1646.

(7) **C.** According to ASRA guidelines, rivaroxaban is recommended to be held or discontinued 72 hours prior to attempting to place a neuraxial block. Further recommendation is to consider checking rivaroxaban or anti-factor Xa activity if less than 72 hours, although no acceptable level of residual rivaroxaban activity to proceed with neuraxial block has been determined.

Reference

Horlocker TT, Vandermeuelen E, Kopp SL, Gogarten W, Leffert LR, Benzon HT. Regional anesthesia in the patient receiving antithrombotic or thrombolytic therapy: American Society of Regional Anesthesia and Pain Medicine evidence-based guidelines (fourth edition). *Reg Anesth Pain Med.* 2018;43:263–309.

(8) **D.** In the presence of an unstable cervical spine fracture, strict spinal precautions should be maintained. In this particular situation, of the listed procedures, a bilateral serratus anterior plane (SAP) block would be the only procedure that is feasible to perform with the patient remaining in the supine position. This myofascial plane block is performed in the axillary region, above or below the serratus anterior muscle, and can be implemented in a two-sided fashion for rib fracture pain management.

Reference

Blanco R, Parras T, McDonnell JG, Prats-Galino A. Serratus plane block: a novel ultrasound-guided thoracic wall nerve block. *Anaesthesia.* 2013;68(11):1107–1113.

(9) **C.** Rib fractures alone are associated with significant morbidity and mortality, as well as long-term disability without appropriate management.

Reference

Pressley C, Fry W, Philp A, Berry S, Smith R. Predicting outcome of patients with chest wall injury. *Am J Surg.* 2012;204:910–914.

(10) **A.** Patients with rib fractures require safe, effective analgesia to prevent respiratory compromise.[2] Choosing an effective pain management strategy for patients with rib fractures can prove to be challenging due to a spectrum of additional injuries, body habitus, coagulation status, and preexisting comorbidities. Many strategies have been implemented to provide pain control, ranging from opioid therapy alone to multimodal approaches, frequently including regional anesthesia.

Reference

May L, Hillermann C, Patil S. Rib fracture management. *BJA Education.* 2016;16:26–32.

15.

BREAST SURGERY

Franklin Chiao, Simon Chin, and Eman Nada

STEM CASE AND KEY QUESTIONS

A 49-year-old female presents for a left breast. Three weeks later, she is scheduled for a left mastectomy with TRAM (transversus abdominis muscle) autologous flap. Her medical history is significant for obesity, anxiety, depression, fibromyalgia, and chronic lower back pain for which she uses acupuncture and as-needed (PRN) oxycodone.

Your plan for postoperative pain management is to place a preoperative nerve block for the breast part and a postoperative abdominal block for the abdominal part.

(1) WHAT ARE NERVE BLOCK OPTIONS FOR HER LUMPECTOMY?

The options are intercostal, pectoralis (PEC), serratus anterior plane (SAP), erector spinae plane (ESP) blocks, local anesthetic infiltration with sedation, paravertebral block (PVB), and epidural blocks. However, placing an epidural or a paravertebral block for a lumpectomy is excessive.

(2) THE PATIENT COMES BACK IN A FEW WEEKS FOR A LEFT MODIFIED RADICAL MASTECTOMY (MRM) WITH A LEFT TRANSVERSE RECTUS ABDOMINIS MYOCUTANEOUS (TRAM) FLAP RECONSTRUCTION. DESCRIBE THIS PROCEDURE BRIEFLY.

In the MRM, the breast is removed along with most of the axillary lymph nodes. The borders of dissection extend superiorly to the clavicle, medially to the sternum, inferiorly to where breast tissue ends, and laterally to the border of the latissimus dorsi. The greater pectoral fascia is also removed.[1]

(3) HOW IS THE TRAM FLAP RECONSTRUCTED?

When a TRAM flap is used, the rectus abdominis muscle is used to reconstruct the breast. The rectus abdominis muscle is dissected with overlying fat and skin along with its blood supply, then it is passed subcutaneously from the upper abdomen in a tunnel to the chest. The pedicled flap is based upon the superior epigastric vessels. A free TRAM is harvested with the overlying muscle and the attached inferior epigastric vessels. This flap is completely separated from the abdomen and brought to the chest defect, where it is anastomosed to either the thoracodorsal or internal mammary vessels. The donor defect within the abdominal wall is repaired with an inlay mesh with both the pedicled and free techniques.[2]

(4) WHAT IS THE NERVE SUPPLY OF THE BREAST?

The nerve supply of the breast includes the medial and lateral pectoral nerves, thoracodorsal nerve, long thoracic nerve, anterior and lateral branches of the intercostal nerves, supraclavicular nerves, and intercostobrachial nerve[3] (Figure 15.1).

The skin overlying the axillary tail is innervated by the intercostobrachial nerve (T1–T2). The pectoralis major and minor muscles underlie the breast and are supplied by the medial (C8–T1) and lateral (C5–C7) pectoral nerves. The serratus anterior may be retracted during surgery, and this muscle is supplied by the long thoracic nerve (C5–C7).[4]

(5) WHAT NERVE BLOCK OPTIONS CAN BE USED FOR MASTECTOMY AND TRAM FLAP SURGERY?

For the breast part, options are the same as for the lumpectomy procedure in question 1; however, the literature is scarce regarding fascial plane blocks with autologous flaps. For the abdominal part: an epidural, erector spinae, transversus abdominis plane, or quadratus lumborum plane blocks can be used.

(6) WHAT ARE THE DRAWBACKS OF PECTORAL NERVE BLOCKS?

Pectoral nerve blocks do not cover the parasternal area. Adding a transversus thoracic muscle plane (TTP) block or the pecto-intercostal fascial (PIF) block can help cover the medial area

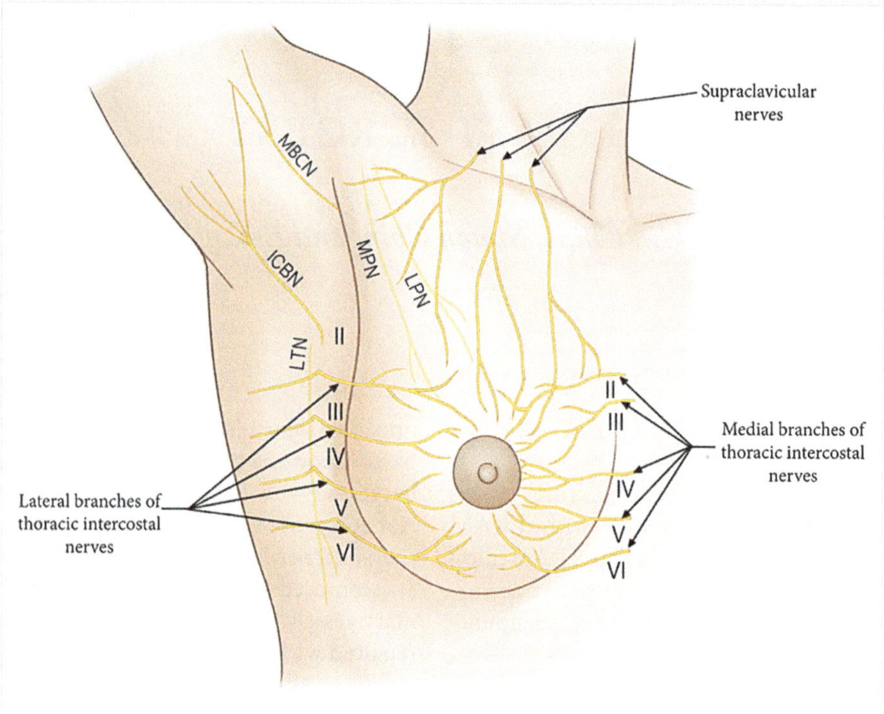

Figure 15.1. Nerve supply of the breast.
Obtained under creative common License from: Kim DH, Kim S, Kim CS, et al. Efficacy of pectoral nerve block type II for breast-conserving surgery and sentinel lymph node biopsy: a prospective randomized controlled study. *Pain Res Manag.* 2018 May 15; 2018:4315931. doi: 10.1155/2018/4315931. PMID: 29861803; PMCID: PMC5976903.

of the breast. PEC II blocks the long thoracic nerve and makes testing its integrity difficult.

(7) WHAT IS THE INCIDENCE OF PNEUMOTHORAX WITH BREAST SURGERY WITHOUT BLOCKS?

Low, but it regularly occurs.

(8) WHICH BLOCK CAUSES THE MOST HYPOTENSION? WHY IS THAT IMPORTANT?

Epidural analgesia causes more of a sympathectomy than other blocks. Hypotension can result in low perfusion and may affect flap vitality.

(9) WHICH IS MORE PAINFUL, THE BREAST COMPONENT OR THE ABDOMINAL COMPONENT?

Both components are painful, but the abdominal component is more painful.

(10) WHAT IS THE VALUE OF A PERIPHERAL NERVE BLOCK IN BREAST SURGERY?

It is effective for postoperative pain, helps early recovery, shortens the length of hospital stay, and possibly reduces the incidence of chronic post-mastectomy pain.

(11) FROM AN ANESTHESIA PERSPECTIVE, WHAT ARE SOME COMPONENTS OF ENHANCED RECOVERY AFTER SURGERY (ERAS) FOR RECONSTRUCTIVE BREAST PROCEDURES?

ERAS in breast surgery includes starting perioperative multimodal analgesia, preop carbohydrate drinks, prevention of nausea and vomiting, early ambulation, and earlier diet advancement.

DISCUSSION

Breast cancer is the second most common malignancy after lung cancer worldwide.[5] Mastectomy is a major surgical treatment, and is associated with significant pain, nausea, vomiting, and in some cases chronic pain.[1] Many women choose to undergo breast reconstruction after mastectomy to help restore their body image and psychological well-being.

Options for breast reconstruction are either using a prosthetic implant or an autologous graft.[2]

Autologous tissue reconstruction has the advantage of its soft texture with a ptotic appearance like a normal breast. It also has a long life span compared to the synesthetic graft. It has the drawback of needing a longer operating time and hospitalization, more pain and scarring, and loss of muscle function from the donor site.[6]

Common sites for autologous grafts are the abdomen, latissimus dorsi muscle, and gluteal muscles. Abdominal flaps include, from most invasive to least invasive: the free transverses abdominis muscle—TRAM-; muscle-sparing TRAM; deep and superficial inferior epigastric artery (DIEP and SIEA) flaps. When the abdominal tissue is not available or sufficient, secondary flap options from the buttock and thigh are used.[7]

NERVE BLOCK IN BREAST SURGERY

Minor surgery like breast biopsies and lumpectomies are often done under monitored anesthesia care with local anesthetic block or infiltration. Major surgeries such as mastectomies have large incisions and with TRAM flap require more analgesic supplements. Breast reconstruction is a painful surgery, it usually needs an average of 30–50 mg of morphine mg equivalents (MME)/day.[8–13] Regional anesthesia expedites and improves the quality of postoperative recovery.

THORACIC EPIDURAL ANALGESIA (TEA)

Thoracic epidural analgesia has been extensively used in breasts surgery with success. The most common levels for placement of a TEA catheter are at T3–T5 for a mastectomy to cover T2–T6 dermatomes. If used to cover the abdominal site of the graft, it is s placed at T8–T9 level. It results in good pain relief, reduced nausea, and vomiting, as well as increased patient satisfaction and earlier discharge.[14,15]

THORACIC PARAVERTEBRAL BLOCK (TPVB)

TPVB provides analgesia in a dermatomal distribution like unilateral epidural analgesia with less hypotension due to unilateral sympathectomy.[16]

The TPV space is a triangular-shaped space on both sides of the vertebrae, bounded anterolaterally by the parietal pleura, medially by the posterolateral parts of the vertebral body, and posteriorly by the transverse process, costotransverse ligament, and the endothoracic fascia. The paravertebral space contains adipose tissue within which the intercostal vessels, rami, and nerves reside. The space is continuous with the intercostal space laterally and the epidural space medially. Paravertebral injections can reach the contralateral paravertebral space through the paravertebral and epidural space.[17]

Technique

TVPB can be done in the sitting, lateral or prone position. However, the sitting position makes the procedure easier because of a better appreciation of the landmarks. It also, can be done blindly or using ultrasound guidance.

Identification of the Paravertebral Space

Blind Technique

With the patient in the sitting position, a Tuohy needle is introduced 2.5–3 cm lateral to the spinous process. It is advanced directly posteroanterior, perpendicular to the skin, until it contacts bone—pars intervertebralis, articular column, or transverse process. If bone is not contacted after 3–4 cm, withdrawal and redirection are attempted. Once bone is contacted it is then "walked off" in an inferolateral direction while a loss of resistance is continuously sought. As the costotransverse ligament is penetrated, a "pop" is usually felt, and a loss of resistance to air signifies entering the paravertebral space. The same technique can be done without loss of resistance, taking the bony contact as a landmark, then introducing the needle further no more than 1–1.5 cm.[18]

Ultrasound Guidance

Transverse Approach

The ultrasound probe is placed on the rib of the level to be blocked. The rib is identified with its hyper-echoic periosteum with its dropout effect; the probe is then moved caudally to visualize the musculature of the intercostal space with the characteristic pleura below. The paravertebral space is identified by its hypoechoic character in contrast to the hyperechoic inferior part of the transverse process medially and the pleura inferiorly (Figures 15.2A and 15.3A). The needle is passed, in-plane, to traverse the costotransverse ligament. The passage of the needle through the costotransverse ligament is heralded by a tactile "pop." After negative aspiration, a local anesthetic (LA) is injected. The anterior displacement of the pleura will aid in confirmation of needle placement within the paravertebral space.

Longitudinal or Parasagittal Approach

With the patient is in a sitting position, the ultrasound probe is placed longitudinally 2–2.5 cm lateral to the tip of the spinous processes of the desired level. Using an in-plane technique, the needle is directed toward the costotransverse ligament (Figures 15.2B and 15.3B). The passage of the needle through the costotransverse ligament is heralded by a tactile "pop." After negative aspiration, LA is injected, and the ventral movement of the pleura will signify paravertebral injection.

The clinical effect of the single-level injection is highly variable because LA spread is unpredictable. It was found that multiple small injections at different levels are preferred over one large injection because of more reliable coverage during breast surgery; however, it resulted in a more vascular puncture.[19–21] The use of the ultrasound resulted in fewer procedural complications as compared to anatomical landmarks. However, it did not change the efficacy.[22,23] The overall complications from the paravertebral block are rare and include vascular injection, pneumothorax, and hypotension.[18]

LIMITATIONS OF TEA AND TPVB

Hypotension

TEA and TPVB cause hypotension due to sympathectomy, with less hypotension with TPVB. Hypotension

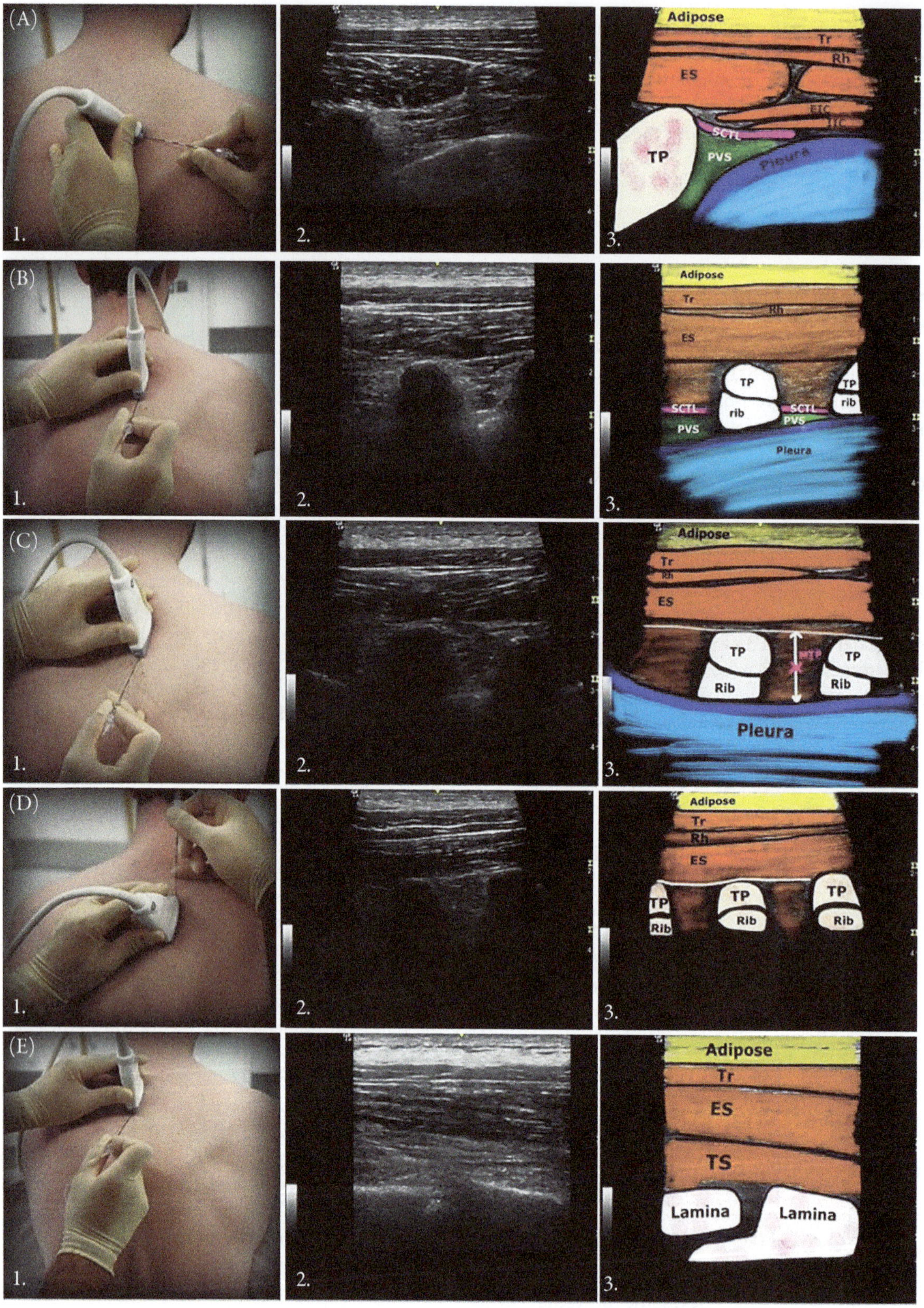

Figure 15.2. Fascial plane blocks of the chest wall. Summary of ultrasound probe position, imaging and anatomical structures for paravertebral, MTP, ESP, and retrolaminar blocks. Letters relate to block technique (A to E). 1: patient, probe, and needle position. 2: ultrasound image generated. 3: overlay of structures. A: Transverse in-plane PVB. B: Paramedian sagittal PVB. C: Mid-point transverse process to pleura (MTP) block. D: Erector spinae plane (ESP) block. E: Retrolaminar block. Tr (trapezius muscle); Rh (rhomboid muscle); ES (erector spinae muscle complex); EIC (external intercostal muscle); IIC (internal intercostal muscle); SCTL (superior costotransverse ligament); TP (transverse process); PVS (paravertebral space); TS (transversospinalis muscle). RISS, PECS, SAP, SIFB and PIFB blocks.

Letters relate to block technique (F to K). 1: patient, probe, and needle position. 2: ultrasound image generated. 3: overlay of structures. F: Rhomboid intercostal part of RISS block. G: Sub-serratus part of RISS block. H: PECS block. I: Serratus anterior plane (SAP) block. J: Serratus intercostal fascial block (SIFB). K: Pectointercostal fascial block (PIFB). Tr (trapezius muscle); Rh (rhomboid muscle); Ic (intercostal muscle); LD (lattisimus dorsi muscle); SA (serratus anterior muscle); PM (pectoralis major muscle); Pm (pectoralis minor muscle); ICM (intercostal muscles).

Obtained with permission from: FitzGerald S, Odor PM, Barron A, Pawa A. Breast surgery and regional anaesthesia. *Best Pract Res Clin Anaesthesiol.* 2019 Mar;33(1):95–110. doi: 10.1016/j.bpa.2019.03.003. PMID: 31272657.

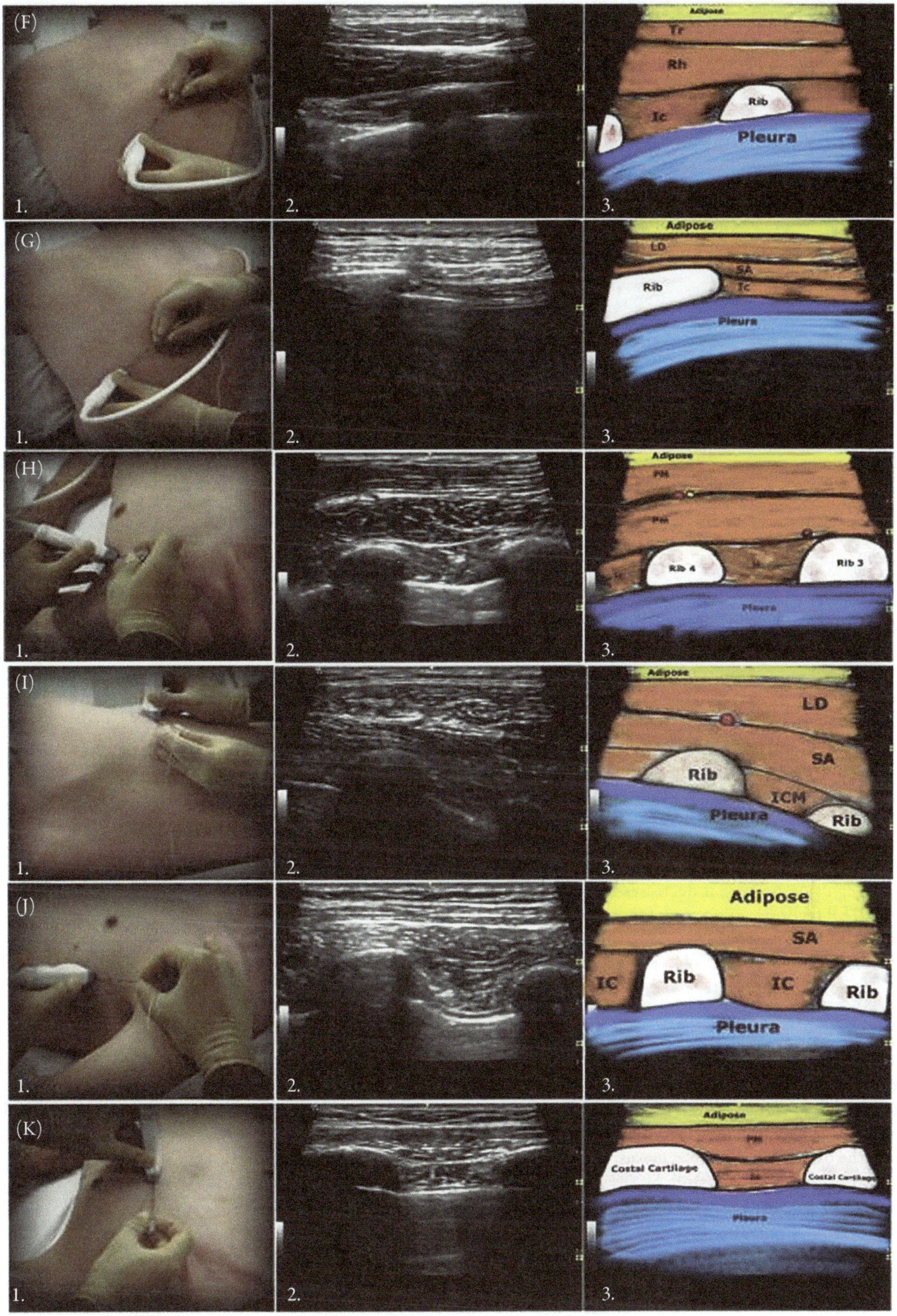

Figure 15.2. Continued

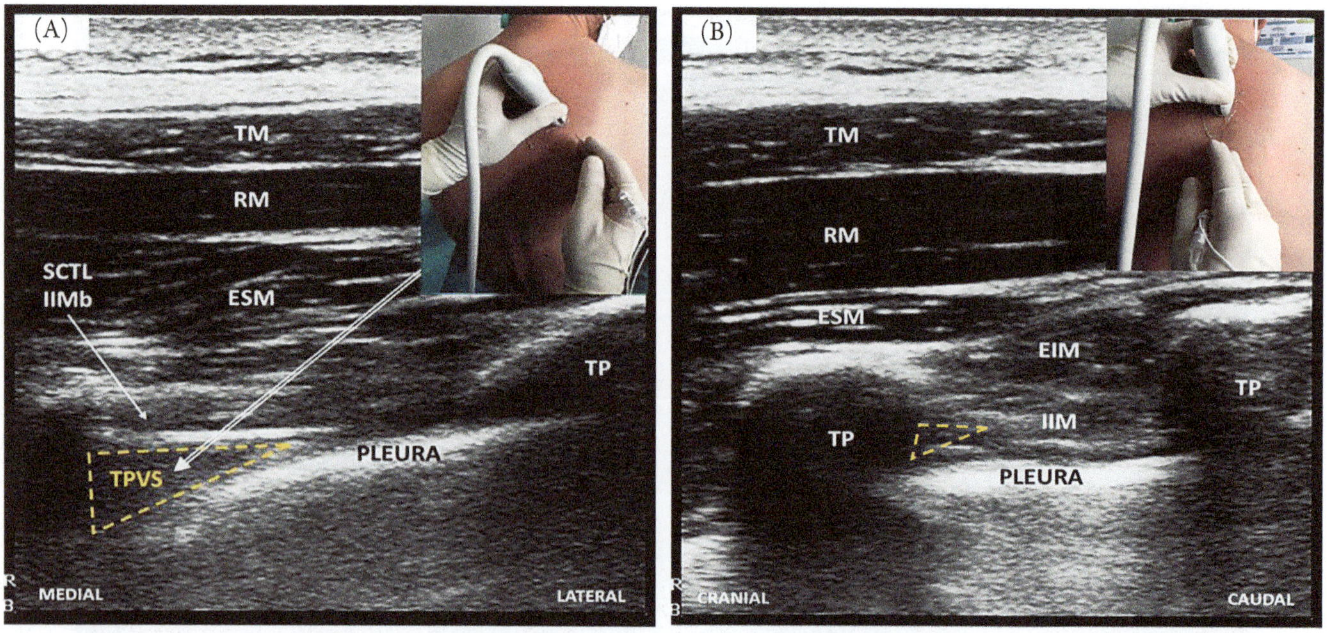

Figure 15.3. Thoracic paravertebral block: (A) parasagittal scan of thoracic paravertebral space (TPVS); (B) transverse/oblique scan of TPVS. Obtained under Creative Commons Attribution (CC BY) license from: Balan C, Bubenek-Turconi SI, Tomescu DR, Valeanu L. Ultrasound-guided regional anesthesia-current strategies for enhanced recovery after cardiac surgery. *Medicina (Kaunas)*. 2021 Mar 25;57(4):312. doi: 10.3390/medicina57040312.

can be harmful to flap viability. It can be difficult to prevent hypotension in reconstructive autologous procedures under anesthesia, as these procedures are long and involve a low degree of surgical stimulation. Treating hypertension while limiting the use of vasopressors and fluid administration may be challenging. Goal-directed fluid therapy was found to result in improved hemodynamics with less fluid administration.[24–26] Besides avoiding hypotension, it is also important to avoid hypothermia, hypo/hypervolemia, hypocapnia, and anemia during anesthesia and in the postoperative period. A target hematocrit of 30%–35% helps maintain perfusion because it decreases blood viscosity.[27] A study of DIEP reconstruction found that although epidural blocks resulted in better pain relief, a significant increase in vasopressor use was found. However, there was no difference in flap complication rate.[28]

Lack of Coverage of Certain Areas

Axillary Coverage

Due to the complex breast innervation, TEA and TPVB may not cover the axilla (T1–T2 dermatome) and the innervation from the brachial and cervical plexus. Cutaneous sensory innervation of the axilla is mainly by the intercostobrachial nerve (ICBN), while the brachial plexus contributes to the structures within the axilla. ICBN arises from the second intercostal nerve; it traverses the serratus anterior muscle and crosses the axilla toward the medial side of the arm.[4]

Adding a paravertebral block at C7–T1, placing a low cervical upper thoracic epidural block, or adding a PEC II block was used for axillary coverage.[4,29,30]

The Parasternal Area

The medial side of the breast might not be blocked due to overlapping innervation from the contralateral side. This can be treated by local infiltration or the addition of the transversus thoracic muscle plane block (TTPB) or the pecto-intercostal fascial block (PIFB).[31,32]

The Infraclavicular Area

The infraclavicular area is supplied by branches of the supraclavicular nerves C4–C5. This can be covered by blocking the ipsilateral cervical block.[33]

PERIPHERAL NERVE BLOCK

PECTORALIS (PEC) AND SERRATUS ANTERIOR PLANE (SAP) BLOCK

PEC I block targets the medial and lateral pectoral nerves in the plane between the pectoralis major and pectoralis minor muscles. PEC II block is placed in the plane between the pectoralis minor and the serratus anterior muscle over the second, third, or fourth ribs; this shares the same endpoint as the SAP block. In this plane, the anterior divisions of the lateral cutaneous branches of the second through sixth intercostal nerves are blocked, as well as the long thoracic nerve, and the thoracodorsal nerve.[34,35]

Technique

These blocks are performed with the patient supine and the back slightly inclined to 30–45 degrees. The probe is placed

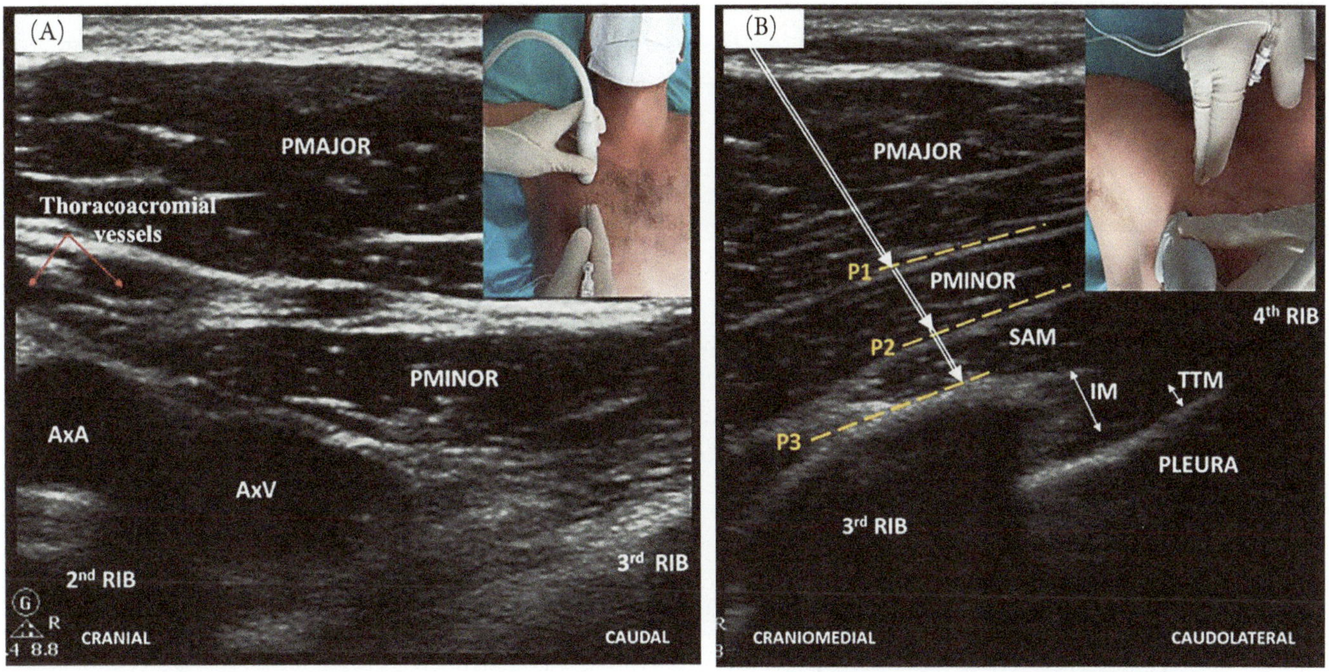

Figure 15.4. PEC and SAP blocks: (A) PEC I block parasagittal scan and sonsoanatomy. (B) PEC II / SAP block: Oblique scan after a slight medial tilt with inferolateral sliding toward the midaxillary line-4th rib level. In SAP Block, P2 or P3 need to be targeted at the 4th or 5th rib level.
Obtained under Creative Commons Attribution (CC BY) license from: Balan C, Bubenek-Turconi SI, Tomescu DR, Valeanu L. Ultrasound-guided regional anesthesia-current strategies for enhanced recovery after cardiac surgery. *Medicina (Kaunas)*. 2021 Mar 25;57(4):312. doi: 10.3390/medicina57040312.

nearly vertical and slightly lateral and distal to where the infraclavicular block is performed. The needle is usually introduced in-plane and coming from the upper part of the probe as it heads for placement at the level of the third and fourth ribs (Figures 15.2 Continuation Plate H and 15.4A.) LA is injected between the pectoralis major and minor muscles for PECI block, and between the pectoralis minor and serratus anterior muscles for the PEC II block.[35] The SAP is performed with the probe moved to a more lateral position than PEC II, overlying the fifth rib at the midaxillary line. The presence of the thoracodorsal artery can verify the plane between the latissimus dorsi and serratus anterior muscle and can help identify the plane. LA is injected between the two muscles or underneath the serratus muscle and above the rib (Figures 15.2 Continuation Plate J and 15.4B).

PEC and SAP blocks have low risk with a high analgesic profile. The area of coverage of the SAP is the anterolateral and partial posterior thoracic wall, covering dermatomes from T2 to 15.2 Continuation Plate J T9. SAP is essentially a variation of the PEC II block, affecting predominantly the lateral cutaneous branches of the thoracic intercostal nerves, along with intercostobrachial, thoracodorsal, and long thoracic nerves.[36]

A meta-analysis of 7 randomized controlled trials with 458 patients showed that pectoral nerve blocks significantly reduced postoperative opioid consumption and the pain for hours after surgery.[37] Compared to TPVB, PEC II block provided similar or better and prolonged pain relief and more reduction of opioid consumption compared to TPVB.[38–40]

Drawbacks

In PEC II blocks the long thoracic nerve is blocked; this prevents the surgeon from stimulating the nerve to test for its integrity. Attempts to inject under the serratus anterior muscle do not reliably eliminate this problem. A thorough discussion should take place with the surgeon before placing the block, so they can determine if they need to stimulate the nerve or not.[41]

PEC blocks do not cover the internal mammary region; the addition of the transversus thoracic muscle plane (TTP) block or the pecto-intercostal fascial block (PIFB) helps cover this area. The parasternal muscle layers include the pectoralis major, internal intercostal, and transversus thoracis muscle as the deepest. At the parasternal area, the intercostal nerve runs between the internal intercostal and the transversus thoracic muscle and it ends by piercing the muscles above it to end as the anterior intercostal nerve, which divides in medial and lateral branches[7] (Figure 15.5).

In the PIFB the LA is injected in the subpectoral interfascial plane between the pectoralis major and the internal intercostal muscles 2–3 cm lateral to the sternal border at the level of the fourth rib (Figure 15.2 Continuation Plate K). In the TTPB, the LA is injected between the internal intercostal and the transversus thoracis muscles. The TTPB carries the risk of pneumothorax as the transversus thoracis muscle is thin and is not easy to visualize and is close to the pleura. Moreover, it may injure the internal mammary artery which courses through the interfacial plane. For that reason, the PIFB is considered a safer block than the TTPB and will serve the same goal.[31,32]

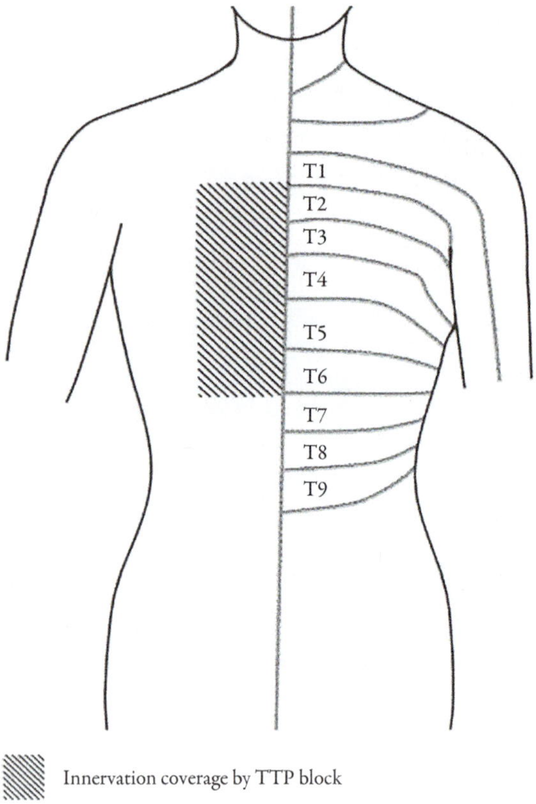

Figure 15.5. Innervation coverage by transversus thoracis plane block. Obtained under Copyright Creative Commons Attribution (CC BY) license from: Fujii S, Bairagi R, Roche M, Zhou JR, Transversus thoracis muscle plane block. *BioMed Res Int.* 2019; Article ID 1716365, https://doi.org/10.1155/2019/1716365.

POSTERIOR FASCIAL PLANE BLOCK

ERECTOR SPINAE PLANE (ESP) BLOCK

The ESP block was used successfully in breast surgery (Figure 15.2 Continuation Plate D). Two metanalyses showed improved pain relief and reduced opioid consumption by an average of 8 mg. It also decreased the need for rescue analgesia, and the incidence of postoperative nausea and vomiting.[42,43] Similarly, rhomboid intercostal nerve block also promoted enhanced recovery and decreased opioid consumption moderately after mastectomy surgery (Figure 15.2 Continuation Plate F). [44]

Complications

There are few complications from the use of regional anesthesia for mastectomy. There is no evidence basis for pneumothorax with chest wall blocks, except for rare incidence with intercostal and serratus anterior blocks. In theory, it can happen, but particularly with ultrasound, the pleura can be seen and is avoided. It can be confusing, though, as pneumothorax can occur with breast surgery.[45]

LIPOSOMAL BUPIVACAINE IN THE BREAST AREA

Strong evidence from a pooled data analysis that included 9 double-blind studies involving multiple surgery types, including breast augmentation surgery, concluded that patients injected with liposomal bupivacaine reported lower cumulative pain scores through 72 hours than those injected with plain bupivacaine.[46] However, in other randomized studies with plain bupivacaine, no significant benefit was noted, except for decreased opioid consumption through 48–60 hours.[47]

ABDOMINAL PAIN FROM TRAM FLAP SITE

The abdominal flaps—especially the non-muscle sparing—cause significant postoperative pain. Different nerve block techniques are used, such as transversus abdominis plane (TAP) block, rectus sheath block, quadratus lumborum (QL) and ESP block, thoracic epidural, and continuous local infiltration wall analgesia for the rectus site of the TRAM procedure.

TRANSVERSUS ABDOMINIS PLANE BLOCK

CONTINUOUS TAP BLOCK

Ultrasound-guided single-injection TAP block for DIEP flap surgery resulted in significantly lower morphine consumption in the first 24 hours only.[12] Surgically placed wound catheters infusing local anesthetic for abdominal donor sites or in microsurgical breast reconstruction decreased the use of narcotics and antiemetic medications and resulted in a shorter hospital stay.[48] Ropivacaine 0.2% infusion catheters, placed in both the abdominal and breast bed wound over the pectoralis major muscle under the autologous flap, resulted in better pain relief at rest and with coughing and earlier bowel movement than intravenous opioid alone.[49] A total dose of 960 mg of ropivacaine infused daily did not result in toxic plasma concentrations and did not cause a vasoconstrictive effect that affected the flap perfusion.[50] The cost of the double TAP catheters and the pump was largely returned by benefit in reduced hospital stay time and opioids and nausea medications consumption.[51]

A meta-analysis that included 10 studies of 684 patients compared the single-injection TAP block to a TAP catheter—mostly ultrasound-guided—with intermittent postoperative analgesia, and control who received systemic narcotics. Eight studies found a significant reduction in the total morphine requirements in the TAP group, and length of stay (LOS) (mean difference = −0.95 days). While TAP blocks using Liposomal Bupivacaine (LB) decreased the LOS by 0.83 days as compared with the control, which was not statistically significant.[52] Another strong evidence confirmed TAP block decreased the LOS by 1 day and opioid requirement by about 44 mg of MME.[53]

QUADRATUS LUMBORUM BLOCK

As the quadratus lumborum block was used successfully for analgesia after abdominal surgery, it can be useful for analgesia after breast reconstruction using the abdominal muscles. The literature is scarce on this topic; a case has reported the successful use of quadratus lumborum in this surgery.[54]

ENHANCED RECOVERY PROGRAM

A successful perioperative enhanced recovery protocol for breast reconstruction includes the following:[55]

Preoperative:

- Preadmission education and counseling
- Preadmission optimization; smoking cessation, weight reduction for the morbidly obese
- Preoperative flap planning, if perforators mapping is required, using computed tomographic angiography scanning
- Preoperative fasting should be minimized, and patients should be allowed to drink fluids until 2 hours before surgery. Preoperative maltodextrin-based drinks should be given until 2 hours before surgery.
- Oral premedication administered in the preoperative holding area: NSAID, acetaminophen, and gabapentin
- Thromboprophylaxis

Intraoperative:

- Maintenance of normothermia
- Goal-directed intravenous to maintain euvolemia and avoidance of fluid overload
- Multimodal, opioid-sparing pain management is recommended.
- Antiemetics

Postoperative:

- Early feeding should be encouraged within the first 24 hours.
- Multimodal analgesia
- Flap monitoring within 72 hours should occur frequently. Clinical evaluation is sufficient for monitoring with implantable buried devices recommended in the buried flaps.
- Early mobilization in the first 24 hours
- Urinary catheter removed on POD 1 in absence of surgical complications
- Post-discharge home exercise program

Afonso, et al.[56] described their specific ERAS protocol. The main elements are:

Preoperative:

- Patients avoid prolonged fasting.

Intraoperative:

- Multimodal analgesia that includes intravenous acetaminophen and/or ketorolac, TAP blocks with liposomal bupivacaine
- Antiemetic drugs (ondansetron or dexamethasone)
- Intraoperative goal-directed fluid management was guided by hemodynamic parameters, including the pulse pressure variation method.

Postoperative:

- Intravenous ketorolac (15 mg) was administered every 6 hours for the first 3 days and then was transitioned to an oral equivalent for an additional 2 days. Breakthrough pain was covered with oral or intravenous opioids. PCA was eliminated in most patients.
- All patients were instructed to ambulate and start a regular diet on the first postoperative day, with the expectation of hospital discharge on postoperative day 3.

Multiple studies have found that the ERAS protocol significantly decreased the amount of opioid consumption and LOS, with no difference in the incidence of complications.[57,58] Bedford et al.[59] found that the ERAS pathway significantly decreased LOS from 5.5 days to 3.9 days. However, the study was criticized for including more DIEP flaps rather than TRAM flaps and including more healthier patients. Cost savings is another important benefit of the ERAS protocol. ERAS protocol contributed to $279,258 savings from freeing up inpatient beds and an increase in overall contribution margins of $189,342.[60] When looking at the cost savings per patient, the adjusted mean costs of patients with ERAS were $4,576 less than those of the traditional group ($38,688 versus $43,264).[61] However, when it was calculated based on the Medicare-derived facility cost model, it resulted in only a cost savings of $732.87.[62]

PERSISTENT POSTOPERATIVE PAIN (PPP) AFTER BREAST SURGERY

Persistent postoperative pain (PPP) after mastectomy is a chronic pain that lasts at least 3 months following breast cancer therapy. The incidence is thought to be 40%–50%; however, it varies by the severity and the duration. It is moderate to severe in 25% and is still present in 25% of patients at one year.[63] The pain is neuropathic in 65% of the cases; other types include phantom pain and non-painful phantom sensations.[64]

A systematic review of 19,813 patients found that a higher prevalence of PPP was associated with axillary lymph node dissection, younger age, radiotherapy, and greater acute postoperative pain. No association was found with body mass index, type of breast surgery, chemotherapy, or endocrine therapy.[65] Association of the PPP with reconstruction is controversial; while some did not find a relationship, others reported an association with immediate reconstruction.[66,67] Regarding the type of reconstructive surgery, women undergoing immediate reconstruction reported increased pain compared to women receiving two-staged procedures in which implant placement was preceded by a temporary tissue expander.[68]

PREVENTION OF THE DEVELOPMENT OF PPP

The effect of regional anesthesia in reducing the risk of developing PPP is controversial. A metanalysis showed that a paravertebral block for breast surgery and intravenous infusion of lidocaine may reduce the risk of developing PPP 3–6 months after breast cancer surgery.[69] Small studies reported that intravenous lidocaine infusion or paravertebral blocks during breast surgery slightly decreased the incidence of PPP,[22,70,71] while a recent multicenter randomized controlled study showed no value from paravertebral nerve block.[63]

Other helpful methods include gabapentinoids, venlafaxine, intravenous lidocaine, and topical lidocaine. EMLA cream can reduce the incidence of chronic pain after mastectomy, whereas local anesthetic infiltration does not.[69,72]

REGIONAL ANESTHESIA AND BREAST CANCER RECURRENCE

Older retrospective studies suggested that a paravertebral block would reduce the incidence of recurrence after breast surgery. However, later work did not prove that. A metanalysis of 15 studies showed no difference in cancer rates between patients who had paravertebral blocks and those who did not.[73] A large randomized controlled trial looked at the incidence of local or metastatic breast cancer recurrence. The study included 2108 women with a median of 36 months as the primary outcome and incisional pain at 6 months and 12 months as the secondary outcome. Among women assigned regional anesthesia-analgesia, 10% recurrences were noted in each group; the study concluded that paravertebral block and propofol did not reduce breast cancer recurrence after potentially curative surgery compared with sevoflurane and opioids. The frequency and severity of persistent incisional breast pain were unaffected by the anesthetic technique.[63]

REFERENCES

1. Plesca M, Bordea C, El Houcheimi B, Ichim E, Blidaru A. Evolution of radical mastectomy for breast cancer. *J Med Life*. 2016;9(2):183–186.
2. Nahabedian M. Options for autologous flap-based breast reconstruction. In: Chagpar A, Butler CE, Collins KA, eds. *UpToDate*. Waltham, MA; 2021 (accessed June, 3, 2021).
3. Woodworth GE, Ivie RMJ, Nelson SM, Walker CM, Maniker RB. Perioperative breast analgesia: a qualitative review of anatomy and regional techniques. *Reg Anesth Pain Med*. 2017;42(5):609–631.
4. Pawa A, Wight J, Onwochei DN, et al. Combined thoracic paravertebral and pectoral nerve blocks for breast surgery under sedation: a prospective observational case series. *Anaesthesia*. 2018;73(4):438–443.
5. Sung H, Ferlay J, Siegel RL, et al. Global cancer statistics 2020: GLOBOCAN estimates of incidence and mortality worldwide for 36 cancers in 185 countries. *CA Cancer J Clin*. 2021;71(3):209–249.
6. Serletti JM. Breast reconstruction with the TRAM flap: pedicled and free. *J Surg Oncol*. 2006;94(6):532–537.
7. Tang A, Bordoni B. Anatomy, thorax, muscles. In: *StatPearls*. Treasure Island, FL: StatPearls; 2022. Available from: https://www.ncbi.nlm.nih.gov/books/NBK538321/
8. Heller L, Kowalski AM, Wei C, Butler CE. Prospective, randomized, double-blind trial of local anesthetic infusion and intravenous narcotic patient-controlled anesthesia pump for pain management after free TRAM flap breast reconstruction. *Plast Reconstr Surg*. 2008;122(4):1010–1018.
9. Tan KJ, Farrow H. Improving postoperative analgesia for transverse rectus abdominis myocutaneous flap breast reconstruction; the use of a local anaesthetic infusion catheter. *J Plast Reconstr Aesthet Surg*. 2009;62(2):206–210.
10. Kroll SS, Sharma S, Koutz C, et al. Postoperative morphine requirements of free TRAM and DIEP flaps. *Plast Reconstr Surg*. 2001;107(2):338–341.
11. Astanehe A, Temple-Oberle C, Nielsen M, et al. An enhanced recovery after surgery pathway for microvascular breast reconstruction is safe and effective. *Plast Reconstr Surg Glob Open*. 2018;6(1):e1634.
12. Hivelin M, Wyniecki A, Plaud B, Marty J, Lantieri L. Ultrasound-guided bilateral transversus abdominis plane block for postoperative analgesia after breast reconstruction by DIEP flap. *Plast Reconstr Surg*. 2011;128(1):44–55.
13. Jablonka EM, Lamelas AM, Kim JN, et al. Transversus abdominis plane blocks with single-dose liposomal bupivacaine in conjunction with a nonnarcotic pain regimen help reduce length of stay following abdominally based microsurgical breast reconstruction. *Plast Reconstr Surg*. 2017;140(2):240–251.
14. Woodworth GE, Ivie R, Nelson S, Walker C, Maniker R. Perioperative breast analgesia: a qualitative review of anatomy and regional techniques. *Reg Anesth Pain Med*. 2017;42(5):609–631.
15. Correll DJ, Viscusi ER, Grunwald Z, Moore JH Jr. Epidural analgesia compared with intravenous morphine patient-controlled analgesia: postoperative outcome measures after mastectomy with immediate TRAM flap breast reconstruction. *Reg Anesth Pain Med*. 2001;26(5):444–449.
16. Yeung JH, Gates S, Naidu BV, Wilson MJ, Gao Smith F. Paravertebral block versus thoracic epidural for patients undergoing thoracotomy. *Cochrane Database Syst Rev*. 2016;2:CD009121.
17. Karmakar MK. Thoracic paravertebral block. *Anesthesiology*. 2001;95(3):771–780.
18. Batra RK, Krishnan K, Agarwal A. Paravertebral block. *J Anaesthesiol Clin Pharmacol*. 2011;27(1):5–11.
19. Balan C, Bubenek-Turconi SI, Tomescu DR, Valeanu L. Ultrasound-guided regional anesthesia-current strategies for enhanced recovery after cardiac surgery. *Medicina (Kaunas)*. 2021;57(4):312.
20. FitzGerald S, Odor PM, Barron A, Pawa A. Breast surgery and regional anaesthesia. *Best Pract Res Clin Anaesthesiol*. 2019;33(1):95–110.
21. Cowie B, McGlade D, Ivanusic J, Barrington MJ. Ultrasound-guided thoracic paravertebral blockade: a cadaveric study. *Anesth Analg*. 2010;110(6):1735–1739.
22. Terkawi AS, Tsang S, Sessler DI, et al. Improving analgesic efficacy and safety of thoracic paravertebral block for breast surgery: a mixed-effects meta-analysis. *Pain p\Physician*. 2015;18(5):E757–780.
23. Tahiri Y, Tran DQ, Bouteaud J, et al. General anaesthesia versus thoracic paravertebral block for breast surgery: a meta-analysis. *J Plast Reconstr Aesthet Surg*. 2011;64(10):1261–1269.
24. Booi DI. Perioperative fluid overload increases anastomosis thrombosis in the free TRAM flap used for breast reconstruction. *Eur J Plast Surg*. 2011;34(2):81–86.
25. Zhong T, Neinstein R, Massey C, et al. Intravenous fluid infusion rate in microsurgical breast reconstruction: important lessons

learned from 354 free flaps. *Plast Reconstr Surg.* 2011;128(6): 1153–1160.
26. Funk D, Bohn J, Mutch W, Hayakawa T, Buchel EW. Goal-directed fluid therapy for microvascular free flap reconstruction following mastectomy: a pilot study. *Plast Surg (Oakv).* 2015;23(4):231–234.
27. Hagau N, Longrois D. Anesthesia for free vascularized tissue transfer. *Microsurgery.* 2009;29(2):161–167.
28. Cormier NS, Stein MJ, Zhang T, Lee H, Zhang J. Epidural nerve blocks increase intraoperative vasopressor consumption and delay surgical start time in deep inferior epigastric perforator free flap breast reconstruction. *Plast Reconstr Surg Glob Open.* 2019;7(1):e2105.
29. Wenk M, Massoth C, Popping DM, Mollmann M. Feasibility of cervical epidural anesthesia for breast cancer surgery. *Anesthesiol Res Pract.* 2017;2017:7024924.
30. Munasinghe BM, Subramaniam N, Nimalan S, Sivamayuran P. Ultrasound to the rescue: axillary clearance under complete regional blockade. *Case Rep Anesthesiol.* 2021;2021:6655930.
31. de la Torre PA, Garcia PD, Alvarez SL, Miguel FJ, Perez MF. A novel ultrasound-guided block: a promising alternative for breast analgesia. *Aesthet Surg J.* 2014;34(1):198–200.
32. Murata H, Hida K, Hara T. Transverse thoracic muscle plane block: tricks and tips to accomplish the block. *Reg Anesth Pain Med.* 2016;41(3):411–412.
33. Karmakar MK, Greengrass RA, Latmore M, Levin M. Thoracic and lumbar paravertebral block. In: Admir H, ed. *Hadzic's Textbook of Regional Anesthesia and Acute Pain Management.* New York: McGraw-Hill Education; 2017:1359–1373.
34. Blanco R. The "pecs block": a novel technique for providing analgesia after breast surgery. *Anaesthesia.* 2011;66(9):847–848.
35. Blanco R, Fajardo M, Parras Maldonado T. Ultrasound description of PECS II (modified PECS I): a novel approach to breast surgery. *Rev Esp Anestesiol Reanim.* 2012;59(9):470–475.
36. Blanco R, Parras T, McDonnell JG, Prats-Galino A. Serratus plane block: a novel ultrasound-guided thoracic wall nerve block. *Anaesthesia.* 2013;68(11):1107–1113.
37. Sercan O, Karaveli A, Ozmen S, Uslu A. Comparison of the effects of pectoral nerve block and local infiltration anesthesia on postoperative pain for breast reduction surgery: a prospective observational study. *Eurasian J Med.* 2021 Jun;53(2):102–107.
38. Kulhari S, Bharti N, Bala I, Arora S, Singh G. Efficacy of pectoral nerve block versus thoracic paravertebral block for postoperative analgesia after radical mastectomy: a randomized controlled trial. *Br J Anaesthesia.* 2016;117(3):382–386.
39. Martsiniv VV, Loskutov OA, Strokan AM, Bondar MV. Efficacy of pectoral nerve block type II versus thoracic paravertebral block for analgesia in breast cancer surgery. *Wiad Lek.* 2020;73(7):1470–1475.
40. Siddeshwara A, Singariya G, Kamal M, Kumari K, Seervi S, Kumar R. Comparison of efficacy of ultrasound-guided pectoral nerve block versus thoracic paravertebral block using levobupivacaine and dexamethasone for postoperative analgesia after modified radical mastectomy: a randomized controlled trial. *Saudi J Anaesth.* 2019;13(4):325–331.
41. Perez MF, Duany O, de la Torre PA. Redefining PECS blocks for postmastectomy analgesia. *Reg Anesth Pain Med.* 2015;40(6):729–730.
42. Zhang Y, Liu T, Zhou Y, Yu Y, Chen G. Analgesic efficacy and safety of erector spinae plane block in breast cancer surgery: a systematic review and meta-analysis. *BMC Anesthesiol.* 2021;21(1):59.
43. Huang W, Wang W, Xie W, Chen Z, Liu Y. Erector spinae plane block for postoperative analgesia in breast and thoracic surgery: a systematic review and meta-analysis. *J Clin Anesth.* 2020;66:109900.
44. Altiparmak B, Korkmaz Toker M, Uysal AI, Dere O, Ugur B. Evaluation of ultrasound-guided rhomboid intercostal nerve block for postoperative analgesia in breast cancer surgery: a prospective, randomized controlled trial. *Reg Anesth Pain Med.* 2020;45(4):277–282.
45. Schneider LF, Albornoz CR, Huang J, Cordeiro PG. Incidence of pneumothorax during tissue expander-implant reconstruction and algorithm for intraoperative management. *Ann Plast Surg.* 2014;73(3):279–281.
46. Vyas KS, Rajendran S, Morrison SD, et al. Systematic review of liposomal bupivacaine (exparel) for postoperative analgesia. *Plast Reconstr Surg.* 2016;138(4):748e–756e.
47. Ha AY, Keane G, Parikh R, et al. The analgesic effects of liposomal bupivacaine versus bupivacaine hydrochloride administered as a transversus abdominis plane block after abdominally based autologous microvascular breast reconstruction: a prospective, single-blind, randomized, controlled trial. *Plast Reconstr Surg.* 2019;144(1):35–44.
48. Raghavendra GK, Sreenivasa RH, Ashok K, et al. Surgically placed wound catheters (SPWC) and local anaesthetic infusion in breast surgery: efficacy and safety analysis. *Breast Dis.* 2011;33(1):1–8.
49. Utvoll J, Beausang-Linder M, Mesic H, Raeder J. Brief report: improved pain relief using intermittent bupivacaine injections at the donor site after breast reconstruction with deep inferior epigastric perforator flap. *Anesth Analg.* 2010;110(4):1191–1194.
50. Dagtekin O, Hotz A, Kampe S, Auweiler M, Warm M. Postoperative analgesia and flap perfusion after pedicled TRAM flap reconstruction: continuous wound instillation with ropivacaine 0.2%. A pilot study. *J Plast Reconstr Aesthet Surg.* 2009;62(5):618–625.
51. Giordano S, Verajankorva E, Koskivuo I, Suominen E. Effectiveness of local anaesthetic pain catheters for abdominal donor site analgesia in patients undergoing free lower abdominal flap breast reconstruction: a meta-analysis of comparative studies. *J Plast Surg Hand Surg.* 2013;47(6):428–433.
52. Abdou SA, Daar DA, Wilson SC, Thanik V. Transversus abdominis plane blocks in microsurgical breast reconstruction: a systematic review and meta-analysis. *J Reconstr Microsurg.* 2020;36(5):353–361.
53. Chi D, Chen AD, Ha AY, Yaeger LH, Lee BT. Comparative effectiveness of transversus abdominis plane blocks in abdominally based autologous breast reconstruction: a systematic review and meta-analysis. *Ann Plast Surg.* 2020;85(6):e76–e83.
54. Spence NZ, Olszynski P, Lehan A, Horn JL, Webb CA. Quadratus lumborum catheters for breast reconstruction requiring transverse rectus abdominis myocutaneous flaps. *J Anesth.* 2016;30(3):506–509.
55. Soteropulos CE, Tang SYQ, Poore SO. Enhanced recovery after surgery in breast reconstruction: a systematic review. *J Reconstr Microsurg.* 2019;35(9):695–704.
56. Afonso A, Oskar S, Tan KS, et al. Is enhanced recovery the new standard of care in microsurgical breast reconstruction? *Plast Reconstr Surg.* 2017;139(5):1053–1061.
57. Tan YZ, Lu X, Luo J, et al. Enhanced recovery after surgery for breast reconstruction: pooled meta-analysis of 10 observational studies involving 1,838 patients. *Front Oncol.* 2019;9:675.
58. Offodile AC, 2nd, Gu C, Boukovalas S, et al. Enhanced recovery after surgery (ERAS) pathways in breast reconstruction: systematic review and meta-analysis of the literature. *Breast Cancer Res Treat.* 2019;173(1):65–77.
59. Batdorf NJ, Lemaine V, Lovely JK, et al. Enhanced recovery after surgery in microvascular breast reconstruction. *J Plast Reconstr Aesthet Surg.* 2015;68(3):395–402.
60. Kaoutzanis C, Ganesh Kumar N, O'Neill D, et al. Enhanced recovery pathway in microvascular autologous tissue-based breast reconstruction: should it become the standard of care? *Plast Reconstr Surg.* 2018;141(4):841–851.
61. Oh C, Moriarty J, Borah BJ, et al. Cost analysis of enhanced recovery after surgery in microvascular breast reconstruction. *J Plast Reconstr Aesthet Surg.* 2018;71(6):819–826.
62. Mericli AF, McHugh T, Kruse B, DeSnyder SM, Rebello E, Offodile AC 2nd. Time-driven activity-based costing to model cost utility of enhanced recovery after surgery pathways in microvascular breast reconstruction. *J Am Coll Surg.* 2020;230(5):784–794 e783.
63. Sessler DI, Pei L, Huang Y, et al. Recurrence of breast cancer after regional or general anaesthesia: a randomised controlled trial. *Lancet.* 2019;394(10211):1807–1815.
64. Richebe P, Capdevila X, Rivat C. Persistent postsurgical pain: pathophysiology and preventative pharmacologic considerations. *Anesthesiology.* 2018;129(3):590–607.
65. Wang L, Guyatt GH, Kennedy SA, et al. Predictors of persistent pain after breast cancer surgery: a systematic review and meta-analysis of observational studies. *CMAJ.* 2016;188(14):E352–E361.
66. De Oliveira GS Jr., Bialek JM, Nicosia L, et al. Lack of association between breast reconstructive surgery and the development of

chronic pain after mastectomy: a propensity matched retrospective cohort analysis. *Breast.* 2014;23(4):329–333.
67. Wallace MS, Wallace AM, Lee J, Dobke MK. Pain after breast surgery: a survey of 282 women. *Pain.* 1996;66(2–3):195–205.
68. Roth RS, Qi J, Hamill JB, et al. Is chronic postsurgical pain surgery-induced? A study of persistent postoperative pain following breast reconstruction. *Breast.* 2018;37:119–125.
69. Levene JL, Weinstein EJ, Cohen MS, et al. Local anesthetics and regional anesthesia versus conventional analgesia for preventing persistent postoperative pain in adults and children: a Cochrane systematic review and meta-analysis update. *J Clin Anesth.* 2019;55:116–127.
70. Ibarra MM, GC SC, Vicente GU, Cuartero del Pozo A, Lopez Rincon R, Fajardo del Castillo MJ. [Chronic postoperative pain after general anesthesia with or without a single-dose preincisional paravertebral nerve block in radical breast cancer surgery]. *Rev Esp Anestesiol Reanim.* 2011;58(5):290–294.
71. Chang YC, Liu CL, Liu TP, Yang PS, Chen MJ, Cheng SP. Effect of perioperative intravenous lidocaine infusion on acute and chronic pain after breast surgery: a meta-analysis of randomized controlled trials. *Pain Pract.* 2017;17(3):336–343.
72. Fassoulaki A, Sarantopoulos C, Melemeni A, Hogan Q. EMLA reduces acute and chronic pain after breast surgery for cancer. *Reg Anesth Pain Med.* 2000;25(4):350–355.
73. Perez-Gonzalez O, Cuellar-Guzman LF, Soliz J, Cata JP. Impact of regional anesthesia on recurrence, metastasis, and immune response in breast cancer surgery: a systematic review of the literature. *Reg Anesth Pain Med.* 2017;42(6):751–756.

REVIEW QUESTIONS

(1) Which is not a donor site for autologous grafts?

A. Rectus abdominis muscles
B. Latissimus dorsi
C. Paraspinal muscles
D. Gluteus muscle

(2) Which block causes the most hypotension?

A. Thoracic paravertebral block
B. Thoracic epidural analgesia
C. Lumbar epidural analgesia
D. Erector spinae plane Block

(3) Why might a thoracic epidural or paravertebral nerve block not provide good analgesia for the axillary dissection part?

A. Missing lower cervical and upper thoracic dermatomes.
B. Missing T 4 dermatome
C. Missing the thoracodorsal nerve
D. Missing the long thoracic nerve

(4) Which one of the following is the proper place to deposit local anesthetics for a paravertebral block?

A. Between the parietal and the visceral pleura
B. Between the costotransverse membrane and the parietal pleura
C. Between the internal and the innermost intercostal muscles.
D. Above the vertebral transverse process.\

(5) Which nerve is not involved in breast innervation?

A. Supraclavicular nerve
B. Anterior intercostal nerve
C. The dorsal ramus of the intercostal nerve
D. Lateral pectoral nerve

(6) Which of the following blocks is useful to supplement an epidural or paravertebral block that is not covering the axillary tail?

A. Pectoral block I
B. Pectoral block II
C. Parasternal block
D. Cervical plexus block

(7) Which is the pectoral block unlikely to cover?

A. Lateral cutaneous branch of the intercostal nerve
B. Anterior cutaneous branch of the intercostal nerve
C. Medial pectoral nerve
D. Lateral pectoral nerve

(8) In breast cancer surgery, paravertebral nerve block has proven to:

A. Prevent cancer recurrence
B. Irrelevant to cancer recurrence
C. Be controversial
D. Slow down the progression of stage 4 breast cancer

(9) ERAS protocols in breast reconstruction have proven to:

A. Improve the outcome of the procedure
B. Reduce opioid consumption and length of hospitalization.
C. To result in higher emergency room visits after discharge.
D. Reduce the length of surgery

ANSWERS

(1) **C.** Paraspinal muscles are not a site for autologous flaps. Common sites for autologous grafts are the abdomen, latissimus dorsi muscle, and gluteal muscles. Abdominal flaps include, from most invasive to least invasive: the free transverses abdominis muscle—TRAM-, muscle-sparing deep and superficial inferior epigastric artery (TRAM, DIEP, and SIEA) flaps. When the abdominal tissue is not available or sufficient, secondary flap options from the buttock and thigh are used.[7]

Reference

Tang A, Bordoni B. Anatomy, thorax, muscles. In: *StatPearls*. Treasure Island, FL: StatPearls; 2022. Available from: https://www.ncbi.nlm.nih.gov/books/NBK538321/

(2) **B.** Thoracic epidural analgesia blocks more sympathetic nerve fibers, while a paravertebral block causes only a unilateral

sympathectomy, so it results in less hypotension. Fascial plane blocks do not cause hypotension.

Reference

Yeung JH, Gates S, Naidu BV, Wilson MJ, Gao Smith F. Paravertebral block versus thoracic epidural for patients undergoing thoracotomy. *Cochrane Database Syst Rev.* 2016;2:CD009121.

(3) **A.** Sensory innervation of the axilla is mainly by the intercostobrachial nerve, which is responsible for the major portion of the cutaneous supply. The brachial plexus also contributes to the sensory supply by innervating structures contained within the axilla, blockade of which could be required during extensive surgeries of the axilla, as a supplement to the former.

Reference

Munasinghe BM, Subramaniam N, Nimalan S, Sivamayuran P. Ultrasound to the rescue: axillary clearance under complete regional blockade. *Case Rep Anesthesiol.* 2021 Feb 11;2021:6655930.

(4) **E.** In the paravertebral block, local anesthetics are deposited between the costotransverse membrane and the parietal pleura.

Reference

Batra RK, Krishnan K, Agarwal A. Paravertebral block. *J Anaesthesiol Clin Pharmacol.* 2011;27(1):5–11.

(5) **C.** The dorsal ramus of the intercostal nerve is not involved in the breast innervation. The nerve supply of the breast includes the medial and lateral pectoral nerves, thoracodorsal nerve, long thoracic nerve, anterior and lateral branches of the intercostal nerves, supraclavicular nerves, and the intercostobrachial nerve.

Reference

Woodworth GE, Ivie RMJ, Nelson SM, Walker CM, Maniker RB. Perioperative breast analgesia: a qualitative review of anatomy and regional techniques. *Reg Anesth Pain Med.* 2017;42(5):609–631.

(6) **D.** The skin overlying the axillary tail of the breast may also have cross-innervation from the intercostobrachial nerve (T1–T2), which is not reliably blocked by TPVB. PECS II nerve block has been useful in covering this area.

Reference

Pawa A, Wight J, Onwochei DN, et al. Combined thoracic paravertebral and pectoral nerve blocks for breast surgery under sedation: prospective observational case series. *Anaesthesia.* 2018;73(4):438–443.

(7) **B.** The pectoral nerve block is unlikely to cover the anterior cutaneous branch of the intercostal branch which supplied the parasternal area medial to the breast.

Reference

Woodworth GE, Ivie RMJ, Nelson SM, Walker CM, Maniker RB. Perioperative breast analgesia: a qualitative review of anatomy and regional techniques. *Reg Anesth Pain Med.* 2017;42(5):609–631.

(8) **B.** Older retrospective studies suggested that a paravertebral block would reduce the incidence of recurrence after breast surgery. However, later work did not prove that. A large randomized controlled trial that included 2108 women who were followed for a median of 36 months found that the two groups had a 10% recurrence whether they received regional anesthesia and or not. The study concluded that paravertebral block and propofol did not reduce breast cancer recurrence after potentially curative surgery compared with sevoflurane and opioids.

References

Perez-Gonzalez O, Cuellar-Guzman LF, Soliz J, Cata JP. Impact of regional anesthesia on recurrence, metastasis, and immune response in breast cancer surgery: a systematic review of the literature. *Reg Anesth Pain Med.* 2017;42(6):751–756.

Sessler DI, Pei L, Huang Y, et al. Recurrence of breast cancer after regional or general anaesthesia: a randomized controlled trial. *Lancet.* 2019;394(10211):1807–1815.

(9) **B.** ERAS protocols in breast reconstruction have proven to reduce opioid consumption and length of hospitalization.

References

Offodile AC, 2nd, C. Gu C, S. Boukovalas S, et al. Enhanced recovery after surgery (ERAS) pathways in breast reconstruction: systematic review and meta-analysis of the literature. *Breast Cancer Res Treat.* 2019;173(1):65–77.

Batdorf NJ, Lemaine V, Lovely JK, et al. Enhanced recovery after surgery in microvascular breast reconstruction. *J Plast Reconstr Aesthet Surg.* 2015;68(3):395–402.

SECTION 5

ABDOMEN, PELVIS AND PERINEUM

Eman Nada

16.

EMERGENCY EXPLORATORY LAPAROTOMY

Francis V. Salinas

CASE STEM CASE AND KEY QUESTIONS

A 60-year-old male with a past medical history of coronary artery disease, diabetes mellitus, obesity (BMI 38), and obstructive sleep apnea (OSA) is postoperative day 1 for exploratory laparotomy and small bowel resection after presenting with an acute abdomen due to bowel obstruction in the setting of sepsis. He is currently intubated, lightly sedated, and has failed a spontaneous breathing trial. The intensivist requests a consult for postoperative pain management to facilitate extubation and to decrease his risk of pulmonary complications. The patient has a temperature of 38.0°C, with an SBP of 90 mmHg/MAP of 63 mmHg on a low-dose (0.5 mcg/kg/min) phenylephrine infusion. A review of his medications notes subcutaneous ultra-fractionated 5000 international unit (IU) twice daily, most recent dose 3 hours ago. His laboratory studies are notable for a platelet count of 75,000. On further lightening of his sedation, he is able to confirm that he has severe upper and periumbilical abdominal pain. On examination, he has a vertical midline incision extending from his xyphoid to several centimeters below the umbilicus. He has intact bilateral upper and lower extremity sensory-motor function.

(1) WHAT ARE THE PHYSIOLOGIC EFFECTS OF POSTOPERATIVE PAIN AFTER OPEN UPPER ABDOMINAL SURGERY?

Pulmonary dysfunction after major upper abdominal surgery occurs after upper abdominal surgery, because of pain and abnormal diaphragm function. Physiologically, the resultant decrease in vital capacity and functional residual capacity lead to atelectasis, hypoxemia (from ventilation-perfusion mismatch), and decreased ability to clear secretions, which increases the risk of pneumonia.

(2) HOW CAN EFFECTIVE POSTOPERATIVE ANALGESIA AID IN EXTUBATION AND DECREASING POSTOPERATIVE PULMONARY COMPLICATIONS?

Effective postoperative analgesia from regional anesthesia techniques provides superior analgesia compared to systemic opioids, decreases opioid-induced respiratory depression and sedation, and improves postoperative pulmonary function and outcomes. In addition, thoracic epidural blockade (with local anesthetic) improves postoperative diaphragm dysfunction independent of analgesic effects by blocking the reflex inhibition of the phrenic nerve associated with upper abdominal surgery.

(3) WHAT ARE THE OPTIONS FOR REGIONAL ANESTHESIA TECHNIQUES AFTER MAJOR UPPER ABDOMINAL SURGERY?

The standard for regional anesthesia technique after major upper abdominal surgery has historically been thoracic epidural analgesia (TEA). However, there are significant risks (high failure rates, nerve injury, central neuraxial hematoma, and sympathectomy-associated hypotension) and contraindications (alterations in primary and secondary hemostasis, hemodynamic instability due to sepsis or volume depletion). Other options include thoracic paravertebral block (which is associated with similar risks and contraindications to TEA). The most common ultrasound-guided peripheral nerve block techniques include transversus abdominis plane block (TAP Block) and rectus sheath block (RSB). Newer and less commonly used ultrasound-guided interfascial plane techniques include quadratus lumborum block (QL Block), and thoracic erector spinae plane block Erector Spinae block (ESP Block). In contrast to TEA, minor alterations in hemostasis, sepsis, and hemodynamic instability are considered relative contraindications for either TAPB or RSB. Additionally, ultrasound-guided TAPB and RSB may be performed safely in anesthetized patients. In addition, the blocks are performed with the patients in the supine position.

(4) WHAT ARE THE CONTRAINDICATIONS FOR THORACIC EPIDURAL ANALGESIA?

Contraindications are typically hemodynamic instability, sepsis, alterations in hemostasis that may increase the risk of neuraxial hematoma. In addition, time constraints and presence of prior spinal instrumentation may also preclude use of TEA.

(5) CAN TAPB OR RSB BE PLACED IN ANESTHETIZED PATIENTS?

In contrast to TEA, TAPB or RSB may be placed in anesthetized or sedated patients as the risk of significant nerve injury is minimal. Additional advantages of TAPB or RSB are lack of block-associated sympathectomy, which minimizes the risk of perioperative hypotension related to the block. Placement of TAPB or RSB is performed with the patient in supine position and does not require placing patients on their side or in the sitting position.

(6) CAN TAPB-RSB BE PLACED IN THE SETTING OF SUBCUTANEOUS HEPARIN OR THROMBOCYTOPENIA?

Thrombocytopenia is a relative contraindication for placement of TAPB-RSB and at a platelet count of 75,000 would have a lower risk of severe complications related to block-related bleeding (such as central neuraxial hematoma with TEA). In addition, if TEA were considered, at least 4–6 hours must have elapsed before placement. In contrast, TABP and RSB are considered superficial blocks and could be placed less than 4–6 hours after the last dose of subcutaneous heparin.

(7) WHAT IS THE SENSORY SUPPLY OF THE ANTEROLATERAL ABDOMINAL WALL?

The sensory innervation of the skin, muscles, and parietal peritoneum of the anterolateral abdominal wall is supplied by the thoracolumbar nerves which originate from the ventral rami of the lower thoracic spinal nerves (T6–T12) and a continuation of the respective intercostal nerves (T6–T11), subcostal nerve (T12), and ilioinguinal-iliohypogastric (L1) nerves. The clinically relevant nerves for abdominal surgery are T7–T12. It is important to note that only the somatic components of pain are covered when ultrasound-guided TAP Block and RS Block are utilized. Thus, a multimodal analgesic regimen is required to cover the visceral component of postoperative pain.

(8) WHAT IS THE ANATOMICAL INJECTION POINT FOR TAPB AND RSB?

The epimysium that envelops the four paired muscles of the anterolateral abdominal wall form fascial layers that are essential to the successful performance of TAP Block and RS Blocks. Along the lateral abdominal wall, the thoracolumbar nerve travel in the interfascial plane superficial to the transversus abdominis (TA) but deep to the internal oblique (IO) muscles. In the anterior upper abdomen along the subcostal margin, the thoracolumbar nerves travel superficial to the TA, but deep to the rectus abdominis (RA) muscles. The interfascial plane is termed the *transversus abdominis plane* (TAP) since the nerves course superficial to the TA muscle. Thus, the target fascial plane for TAP Block is always superficial to the TA muscle, whether along the lateral abdominal wall or along the subcostal margin.

The fascial layers of the external oblique (EO), IO, and TA converge at the lateral border of the RA to form the linea semilunaris, which subsequently continues medially to envelop the anterior and posterior borders of the rectus muscle to form the rectus sheath. The thoracolumbar nerve course from lateral to medial and within the TAP, and penetrate through the lateral edge of the rectus sheath and travel a short distance deep to the RA muscle before coursing ventrally and terminating within the anterior abdominal wall as the anterior cutaneous branches. Thus, the target fascial plane for the RSB is deep to the RA muscle, ventral to the posterior aspect of the rectus sheath.

(9) WHAT IS THE EXPECTED SENSORY DISTRIBUTION (AND INDICATION) FOR A TAPB VERSUS RSB?

Unilateral blocks are used for one-side procedures (cholecystectomy, appendectomy, renal transplantation), while bilateral blocks are used for vertical midline, and transverse abdominal incisions. Local anesthetic injection within the TAP along the lateral abdominal wall between the iliac crest and lateral costal margin (lateral TAPB) will consistently spread to the T10–T12 thoracolumbar nerve and provide sensory coverage for lower abdominal procedures such as cesarean delivery and total abdominal hysterectomy (via a low transverse incision). Local anesthetic injection between TAP just inferior to costal margin (subcostal TAP block) will consistently spread to the T7–T9 thoracolumbar nerves and provide sensory coverage for upper abdominal procedures such as hepatobiliary procedures and open gastrectomy. For extensive abdominal incisions, a bilateral dual (four-quadrant) TAP Block technique will provide coverage from the xyphoid process to the pubic symphysis from the midline to the anterior axillary line.

Injection between the RA and posterior rectus sheath (or RSB) just cephalad to the umbilicus may provide analgesia of the midline anterior abdominal wall from the xyphoid process to pubic symphysis.

(10) WHAT IS THE TYPICAL VOLUME AND CONCENTRATION OF LOCAL ANESTHETIC INJECTION FOR BILATERAL TAPB OR RSB?

The recommended volume for single-injection bilateral lateral TAP Block or subcostal TAP Blockis 15–20 mL of either bupivacaine 0.25% or ropivacaine 0.375% with 2.5 mcg of epinephrine/mL for each side. Increasing the dose beyond 20 mL for TAPB has not been shown to increase sensory block coverage as the lateral and subcostal TAP are considered functionally separate anatomical compartments. The typical dose for a four-quadrant TAPB is 15–20 mL/compartment for a total volume of 60–80 mL. The addition of epinephrine is recommended to decrease the systemic absorption and subsequent peak plasma local anesthetic concentration (Cmax).

(11) WHAT IS THE EXPECTED DURATION OF ANALGESIA FOR SINGLE INJECTION ULTRASOUND-GUIDED TAPB VS. RSB?

Based on the evidence to date, the expected duration of single-injection TAP block is 12–24 hours. In contrast, the expected duration of action a single-injection RSB is typically 8–12 hours. If prolonged analgesia (>24 hours) is desired, continuous TAPB or RSB catheters should be placed.

(12) WHAT IS THE OPTIMAL MODALITY OF LOCAL ANESTHETIC DELIVERY FOR CONTINUOUS TAPB-RSB BLOCK?

Injectate and sensory block studies indicate that intermittent bolus dosing may result in increased sensory block distribution. This may be done with automated programmed intermittent or manual intermittent bolus dosing. The alternative and technically easier modality is continuous infusion of 8–12 mL/hr per side (for bilateral catheters). There is lack of rigorous evidence for the superior analgesic efficacy of one modality versus the other. Although there is minimal risk based on clinical experience, there is a potential risk of local anesthetic systemic toxicity (LAST) given the relatively large volumes of local anesthetic per hour.

(13) WHAT ARE THE COMPLICATIONS OF TAPB OR RSB?

Although the risks for single-injection or continuous TAPB or RSB are low, risks include visceral injury, bleeding and hematoma formation, LAST, and needle site infection.

(14) WHICH BLOCK PROVIDES THE BEST CHOICE FOR MIDLINE VERTICAL INCISIONS?

To date, there has been no published randomized clinical trial directly comparing TAPB vs. RSB for emergent laparotomy with vertical midline incision. Such a trial would need to incorporate the location and extent of the incision. The choice is influenced by the experience of the anesthesiologist, the ability to visualize the target fascial plane, the location-extent of the vertical midline incision, as well as the presence of postoperative surgical drains.

DISCUSSION

Emergency laparotomy typically requires a vertical midline incision that is often accompanied by severe postoperative pain which is mainly derived from the abdominal wall incision. Thoracic epidural analgesia (TEA) has been considered the standard regional anesthetic modality for major laparotomy.[1,2] Adequate postoperative analgesia is an integral part of decreasing the stress response, enhancing earlier mobilization (decreasing risk of venous thromboembolic events), and decreasing the incidence of postoperative pulmonary dysfunction that may lead to hypoxemia and/or postoperative pneumonia.[3–5]

However, TEA is often contraindicated in emergency laparotomy due to time constraints, hemodynamic instability (due to volume depletion or sepsis), or alterations in primary or secondary hemostasis that may increase the risk for central neuraxial infection or hematoma formation.[6–8] A TPV Block may also provide effective analgesia, but is technically challenging, requires bilateral blocks, and shares similar contraindications to TEA.[9] Bilateral erector spinae plane blocks (ESP Blocks) placed at the midthoracic (T7 or T8) levels deep to the erector spinae muscle at the superficial aspect of the desired transverse process have recently been reported to provide effective analgesia for major abdominal surgery and may potentially offer a safer alternative to bilateral TPVBs.[10,11] TAP Block and RS Block are ultrasound-guided interfascial plane blocks that provide effective somatic (covering the skin, subcutaneous tissue, muscle, and fascia) analgesia for anterolateral abdominal wall incisions. They do not provide visceral analgesia; thus, a multimodal analgesic regimen is required to cover the visceral component after abdominal surgery.[12]

The key to effective use of TAPB-RSB for abdominal surgery is a thorough understanding of the applied clinical anatomy of the anterolateral abdominal wall that not only improves the technical success rate, but also determines the appropriate choice of approach (where to inject local anesthetic based on the location of the incision), technique (how the local anesthetic is delivered), and the potential risk of complications.

APPLIED CLINICAL ANATOMY

MUSCLES AND FASCIA OF THE ANTEROLATERAL ABDOMINAL WALL

The layers of the anterolateral abdominal wall from superficial to deep are skin, subcutaneous tissue, the abdominal muscles and their associated fascia and aponeuroses, transversalis fascia, extraperitoneal fat, and parietal peritoneum. There are 4 paired muscles that form the anterolateral abdominal wall: the rectus abdominis (RA), external oblique (EO), internal oblique (IO), and transversus abdominis (TA). The lateral muscles overlie one another from superficial to deep (EO, IO, and TA) and terminate medially to form an aponeurosis (linea semilunaris), which is located lateral to the paired midline RA. The linea semilunaris continues medially to encase the RA to form the anterior and posterior aspects of the rectus sheath. The rectus sheath continues medially to blend in the midline with the rectus sheath of the contralateral side to form the midline linea alba (Figures 16.1 and 16.2.1). The transition from muscle to linea semilunaris below the costal margin begins at the midclavicular line for the EO and IO. In contrast, the medial border of the TA belly courses further medially along the lower subcostal margin. Thus, in the upper abdomen, the TA runs deep to the RA before forming the linea semilunaris. Consequently, the TAP is located between the IO and TA along the lateral abdominal wall, but between the RA and TA inferior to the subcostal margin (Figures 16.2.2, 16.2.3, 16.2.4, 16.2.5). Above the level of the arcuate line (midway between the umbilicus and the pubic symphysis), the anterior rectus sheath (superficial to the RA) is formed by the aponeuroses of the EO and the anterior lamina of the IO, while the posterior rectus sheath (deep to the

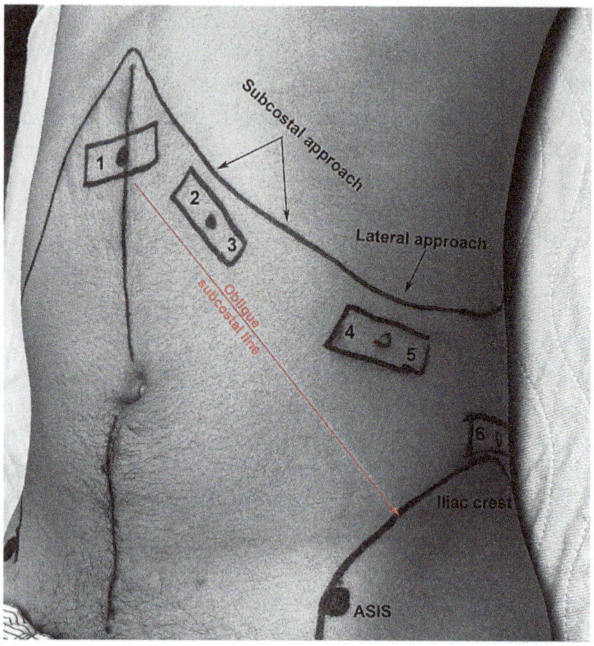

Figure 16.1. Surface anatomy of the anterolateral abdominal wall and four approaches of ultrasound-guided transversus abdominis plane (TAP) block. Red line indicates the oblique subcostal line extending from xyphoid process to anterior part of the iliac crest.

RA) is formed from the aponeuroses of the posterior lamina of the IO and TA (Figure 16.3A and B). Inferior to the arcuate line, all three aponeuroses course anterior to the RA to form the anterior layer of the rectus sheath, with the posterior layer being formed only by the epimysium of the RA and transversalis fascia. The RA is attached to the anterior aspect of the rectus sheath by 3 or 4 tendinous insertions. Thus, the anterior aspect of the rectus sheath is divided into separate sub-compartments. In contrast, the posterior aspect of the rectus sheath is unsegmented and is anatomically a continuous space along its entire course.[13–15] The transversalis fascia is a thin areolar tissue that lines the deep surface of the TA and RA and separates them from the abdominal cavity.

SENSORY INNERVATION OF THE ANTEROLATERAL ABDOMINAL WALL

The anterolateral abdominal wall is innervated by the thoracolumbar nerve, which originate from the ventral rami of the lower six thoracic spinal (T7–T12) and are a continuation of the respective intercostal (T7–T11) and subcostal (T12) nerves.[13,14] Each nerve gives rise to lateral cutaneous branches at the midaxillary line, which course superficially (through muscle, subcutaneous tissue, and skin) along the anterior axillary line to supply the sensorimotor innervation of the anterolateral abdominal wall between the midaxillary line to midclavicular line. The thoracolumbar nerves course further anteriorly and travel in the neurovascular transversus abdominis plane (TAP). The upper segmental nerves (T7–T9) enter the TAP medial to the anterior axillary line, while the lower segmental nerves (T10–T12) enter the TAP progressive more laterally. Within the TAP, the lower segmental nerves (T9–T12) give off multiple communicating branches to form a longitudinal TAP plexus, from which the terminal anterior branches arise. The terminal continuation of the thoracolumbar nerves enters the rectus sheath at its lateral margins (the linea semilunaris) (Figure 16.3A and B).[13,14] In the majority of cases, the nerves course further medially for several centimeters deep to the

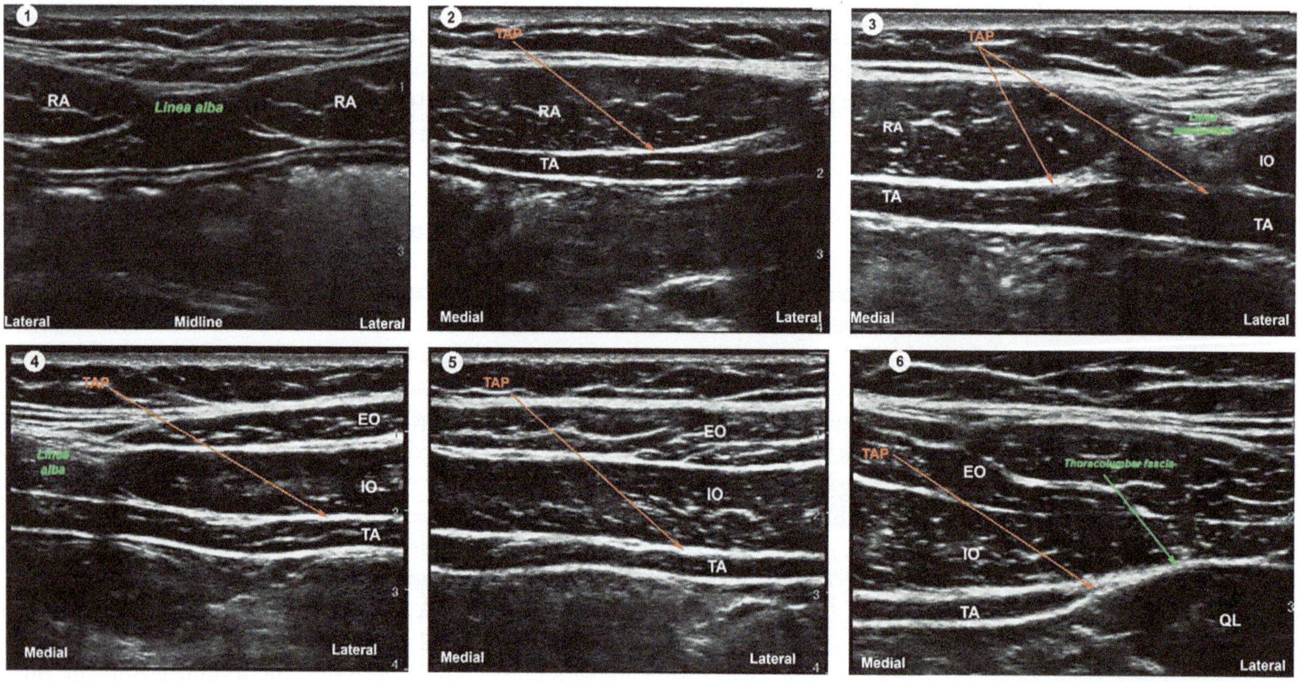

Figure 16.2. Corresponding ultrasound images of the transducer location on anterolateral abdominal wall starting in the midline below the xyphoid. The ultrasound anatomy of the muscles, aponeuroses, and transversus abdominis plane are illustrated.
RA = rectus abdominis; EO = external oblique; IO = internal oblique; TA = transversus abdominis; TAP = transversus abdominis plane.

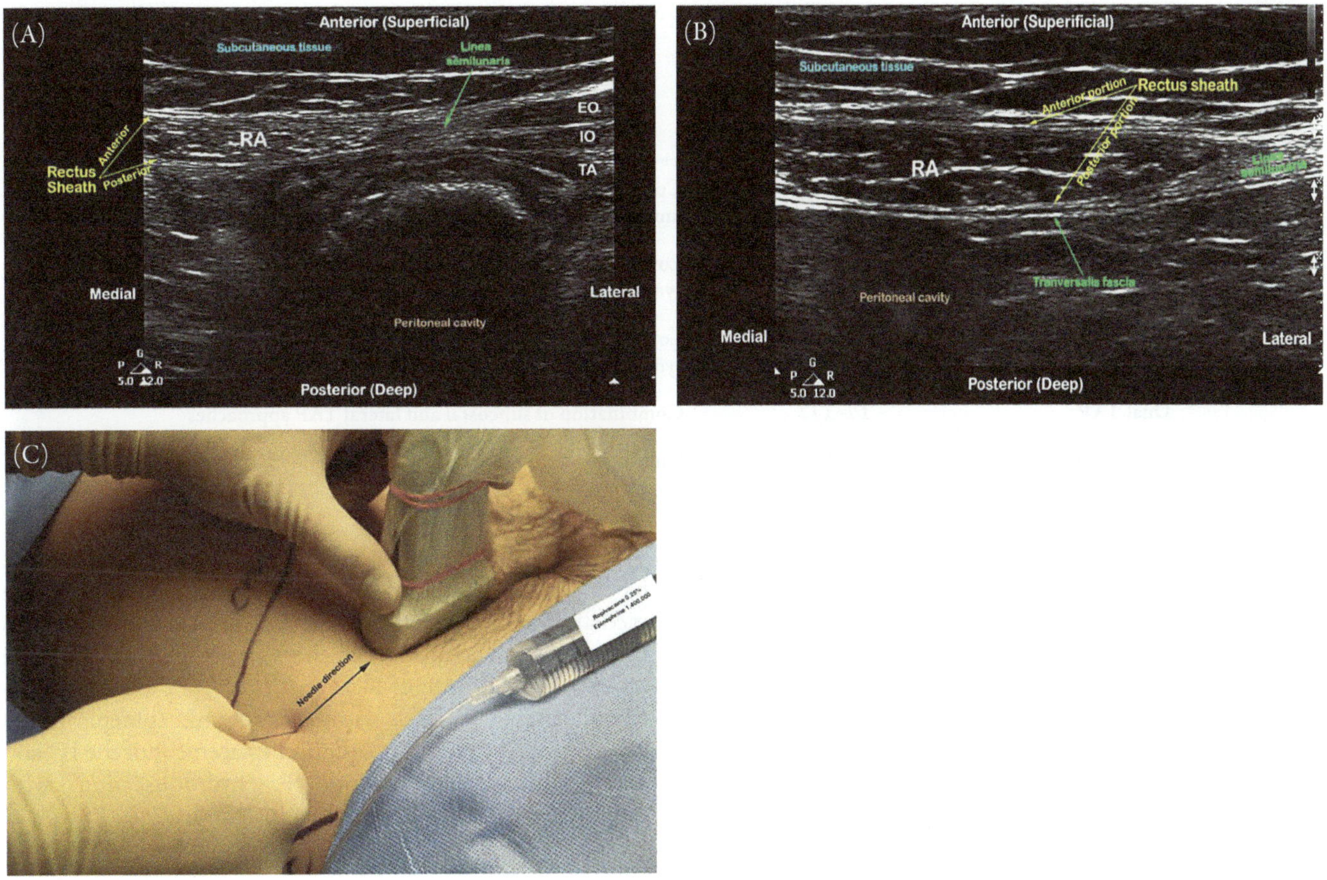

Figure 16.3. Ultrasound anatomy of rectus sheath block just above the umbilicus (T9–T10). Note the formation of the linea semilunaris from the medial continuation of the fascia of the lateral abdominal wall muscles; with the linea semilunaris giving rise to anterior and posterior sections of the rectus sheath.
RA = rectus abdominis; EO = external oblique; IO = internal oblique; TA = transversus abdominis.

RA (ventral to the posterior layer of the rectus sheath) before ascending ventrally. During their course, the nerves give rise to posterior muscular branches before terminating in the subcutaneous tissue and skin (as the anterior cutaneous branch) to provide sensory innervation to the anterior abdominal wall between the midclavicular line and midline. Once again, the nerves branch and communicate to form a longitudinal rectus sheath plexus, before entering the subcutaneous tissue of the anterior abdominal wall. In a small percentage of cases, the nerves directly pierce the lateral edge of the RA and thus may be missed with more medial injections within the posterior rectus sheath.[13,15]

Cadaveric and clinical studies have demonstrated that the TAP is not continuous within the anterolateral wall and is divided anatomically (and functionally) into lower and upper abdominal TAP compartments.[16–21] Ultrasound-guided injection of local anesthetic (or dye) between the costal margin and the iliac crest at the midaxillary line (within the lateral TAP) consistently blocks the T10–T12 thoracolumbar nerves, while the upper segmental nerves (T7–T9) are typically not blocked, as these nerves enter the TAP medial to anterior axillary line.[16,17] Ultrasound-guided injection of local anesthetic or dye just lateral to the linea semilunaris and just inferior to the lower subcostal margin consistently blocks T10–T11 but does not extend cephalad to T9.[16] If blockade of the T7–T9 nerves is desired, injection should be medial to the linea semilunaris between the RA and TA.[17,18] Thus, ultrasound-guided injections between the IO and TA (within the lateral TAP) can provide analgesia for lower abdominal surgery. Similarly, injections between the RA and TA (within the subcostal TAP) can provide analgesia for upper abdominal surgery. Although rigorous spread of RSB has not been studied as extensively as for TAPB, an injection between the RA and posterior rectus sheath at or just above the umbilicus potentially provides midline analgesia extending from the xyphoid to the pubic symphysis.[21–24]

TAPB CLASSIFICATION AND DESCRIPTION OF APPROACHES/TECHNIQUES

The nomenclature describing TAPB (Table 16.1) is confusing in light of multiple new approaches that have been recently described.[25–28] The heterogeneity of the block description nomenclature, approaches, injection techniques (medial-to-lateral vs. lateral-to-medial)[28] leads to difficulty in interpreting the true magnitude of analgesic efficacy of each approach/technique. However, the published evidence consistently demonstrates the analgesic efficacy of TAPB and RSB when

Table 16.1 **CLASSIFICATION OF ULTRASOUND-GUIDED TAP BLOCK AND CORRESPONDING SUPPLIED AREAS**

APPROACH	SEGMENTAL THORACOLUMBAR NERVES BLOCKED	SUPPLIED AREA OF ANTEROLATERAL ABDOMINAL WALL
Subcostal TAPB	T7–T9	Upper abdomen below xyphoid to just above the umbilicus and parallel to costal margin
Lateral TAPB	T10–T12	Lower abdomen from umbilicus to just above pubic symphysis from midline to midclavicular line
Posterior TAPB	T10–T12	Lower abdomen from umbilicus to just above pubic symphysis from midline to posterior axillary line
Dual TAP	T7–T12	Combination of subcostal and lateral TAP approaches
Oblique subcostal	T7–T12	Combination of subcostal and lateral TAP approaches

compared to either traditional systemic opioid-based and/or TEA.[29–34] In addition, the additional descriptions of the TAPB were based on landmark-based loss-of-resistance (LOR) technique targeting the posteriorly located triangle of Petit.[35] Controversy exists whether this LOR technique and approach (injection site along the iliac crest at the posterior axillary line) acts by blocking both the thoracolumbar nerves within the TAP, as well as possible retrograde to the thoracic paravertebral spaces.[21,35–38] The vast majority of published studies, as well as in daily clinical practice, utilize ultrasound guidance to increase the success rate of local anesthetic placement, as well as to avoid potential complications associated with blind needle placement.[39]

The most commonly used ultrasound-guided approaches (based on where the local anesthetic is injected) include: (1) lateral (midaxillary) TAPB; (2) posterior (posterior axillary) TAPB; (3) subcostal TAPB; (4) dual (four-quadrant) TAPB; and (5) oblique subcostal TAPB. The ultrasound-guided posterior TAPB approach has also been described but is not as extensively studied as the subcostal and lateral approaches.[21] The transducer locations for the lateral and posterior TAPB are both along the lateral abdominal wall. However, the injection target for the lateral TAPB is along the midaxillary line, and in contrast, the injection point for the posterior TAPB is at the posterior midaxillary line. The posterior TAPB approach provides better local anesthetic spread to the lateral cutaneous branches and may provide better analgesia of the lateral abdominal wall.[20,21,28,40] Clinical evidence indicates that posterior TAPB provides a longer duration of analgesia compared to lateral TAPB.[41]

LATERAL TAP BLOCK

The lateral TAP Block (Figures 16.1, 16.2.4, 16.2.5) targets the T10–T12 thoracolumbar nerves and is indicated for lower abdominal (infraumbilcal) surgery. It is performed by placement of the transducer in an axial orientation at the anterior-to-midaxillary line between the costal margin and iliac crest. The three layers of the lateral abdominal wall (from superficial to deep), EO, IO, and TA, their accompanying fascia, and the peritoneal cavity are easily visualized. The fascial planes appear hyperechoic relative to the hypoechoic muscles. The block needle is inserted several centimeters away from the medial edge of the transducer and is advanced in plane into the interfascial layer between the IO and TA. After negative aspiration, 15–20 mL of local anesthetic (bupivacaine 0.25% or ropivacaine 0.375%, with 2.5 mcg/mL epinephrine) is injected, observing for superficial displacement of the IO and downward displacement of the TA ("hydrodissection") with an elliptical hypoechoic spread within the TAP.

POSTERIOR TAPB

The posterior approach (Figures 16.1, 16.2.6) is similar to the lateral approach, but the ultrasound transducer is moved more posteriorly in order to view where the IO and TA taper off into a common aponeurosis (thoracolumbar fascia), which is connected to the lateral border of the quadratus lumborum muscle (QL). The TAP is between the IO and TA and is continuous with the thoracolumbar fascia. The injection site is along the posterior axillary line and is superficial to thoracolumbar fascia near the lateral border of the QL. After negative aspiration, 15–20 mL of local anesthetic (bupivacaine 0.25% or ropivacaine 0.375%, with 2.5 mcg/mL epinephrine) is injected, observing for superficial displacement of the IO and downward displacement of the TA ("hydrodissection") with an elliptical hypoechoic spread within the TAP and posterior spread anterior to the thoracolumbar fascia.

SUBCOSTAL TAPB

The subcostal TAPB (Figures 16.1, 16.2.2, 16.2.3, 16.2.4) targets the T7–T9 thoracolumbar nerves and is indicated for upper abdominal (supraumbilical) surgery. It is performed by placement of the transducer in an oblique orientation along the costal margin, starting with the medial edge of the transducer at the xyphoid process. The transducer is systematically moved along the costal margin to initially visualize the RA and posterior rectus sheath. As the transducer is moved further lateral, the interfascial TAP between the RA and TA is visualized. With further lateral scanning along the costal margin, the linea semilunaris is visualized, and followed by the transition to the three lateral abdominal wall muscle layers (EO, IO, TA). The fascial planes appear hyperechoic relative to the hypoechoic muscles. The block needle is inserted from the medial edge of the transducer and advanced in plane into the interfascial layer between the RA and TA. After negative aspiration, 15–20 mL of local anesthetic (bupivacaine 0.25% or ropivacaine 0.375%, with 2.5 mcg/mL epinephrine) is injected, observing for hydrodissection, with an elliptical hypoechoic spread within the TAP.

OBLIQUE SUBCOSTAL TAP BLOCK

The oblique subcostal TAPB (Figures 16.1, 16.2) is a technical modification of the subcostal TAPB and targets both the upper (T7–T9) and lower (T10–12) thoracolumbar nerves.[13,14,42] The oblique subcostal line extends from the xyphoid to the anterior aspect of the iliac crest. The technique is initially the same as for the subcostal TAP. After initial hydrodissection between the RA and TA, the interfascial plane is opened anterior to the block needle tip, and the needle is subsequently advanced toward the lateral inferior end of the dilating plane (with simultaneous manipulation of transducer movement, needle advancement, and hydrodissection. The sequence is repeated until the lateral edge of the transducer reaches the anterior aspect of the iliac crest.[42] With a combination of hydrodissection, and needle and transducer advancement (starting from the xyphoid process along the costal), the needle is passed between the RA and TA, then deep to the linea semilunaris, and subsequently between the IO and TA toward the anterior aspect of the iliac crest. The initial description of this technique used a single needle insertion site and required a long block needle (15–20 cm) and a large volume (40 mL) of local anesthetic to hydrodissection the entire TAP.[42] Despite the initial description, it is often technically difficult to advance the needle along the hydrodissection plane with a single needle insertion point and requires a large volume of local anesthetic (80 mL) for a bilateral block. A technically easier modification involves withdrawing and reinserting (then advancing) the block needle repeatedly as a multi-injection technique.[43,44] Although this requires several needle insertions, it is technically easier and requires lower volumes (20 mL of either bupivacaine 0.25% or ropivacaine 0.375%, with 2.5 mcg/mL epinephrine) of local anesthetic to fill the entire TAP from the xyphoid to the anterior aspect of the iliac crest. Using this technique results in 100% successful block of the T7–T12, as well as 50% successful block of the T6 and L1 thoracolumbar nerves.[32,42,43]

DUAL TAPB

An alternative to the oblique subcostal TAPB approach is simply combining the subcostal TAPB and lateral TAPB, which is described as a dual TAPB. It is described as a "four-point" or "four-quadrant" approach since it involves four separate injections to perform bilateral lateral and subcostal TAP blocks.[19,27]

RS BLOCK APPROACH

The RSB approach (Figure 16.3A and B) provides analgesia of the midline anterior abdominal wall from the xiphoid process to the pubic symphysis. It is performed by placement of the transducer in an axial orientation over the lateral edge of the RA, typically at or just cephalad to the umbilicus.[22] With the linea semilunaris, lateral portion of the RA, and posterior rectus sheath in view, a block needle is inserted several centimeters lateral to the lateral edge of the transducer. The needle is advanced in plane in a lateral-to-medial direction, entering the RA at its lateral border. The linea semilunaris and posterior rectus sheath both appear hyperechoic relative to the hypoechoic RA. The needle tip is placed between the posterior aspect of the RA and the posterior rectus sheath. After negative aspiration, 20–25 mL of local anesthetic (bupivacaine 0.25% or ropivacaine 0.25 to 0.375%, with 2.5 mcg/mL epinephrine) is injected, observing for hydrodissection with an elliptical hypoechoic spread within the lateral aspect of the posterior "rectus sheath compartment." For upper midline incision, place an RSB halfway between the umbilicus and xyphoid (targeting T7–T10). For vertical lower abdominal incision below the umbilicus, place halfway between the umbilicus and pubic symphysis (targeting T9–12). For extensive incision that extends from xyphoid to below umbilicus, place at or just above level of the umbilicus (targeting T7–T12). Recently published clinical trials support the clinical efficacy of RSB for postoperative analgesia for major surgical procedures for vertical midline incisions.[44–46]

CONTINUOUS TAPB-RSB

The analgesic duration of a single injection TAPB (10–12 hours) and RSB (6–8 hours) may be extended by placement catheters for extended continuous postoperative analgesia.[47–50] The technique for placement of catheters is the same as for single-injection techniques.[22] Either continuous low-dose infusion (typically 8–10 mL/hr) or repeated intermittent bolus dosing (10–15 mL every 8–12 hours for TAPB and every 6–8 hours for RSB) provide effective analgesia. The current evidence demonstrates perhaps increased spread with intermittent bolus dosing, but no evidence of increased analgesic efficacy.[47–50] Thus, the choice will be determined by availability of equipment (infusion pumps), institutional manpower, and protocols. Typical local anesthetics used are either ropivacaine 0.2% or bupivacaine 0.125%.

PHARMACOKINETICS

Single-injection bilateral TABP or RSB typically requires high volumes (30–40 mL for TABP or RSB and 60–80 mL for dual-TAPB) of local anesthetics. Thus, knowledge of the mean maximum plasma concentration (Cmax) and mean time to reach Cmax (Tmax) can provide guidelines for dosing as well as duration of observation after placement of single injection techniques. As would be expected, there are dose-dependent increases in Cmax with either approach. There is no significant difference in Cmax when comparing TABP versus RSB when utilizing comparable doses.[51] In contrast, Tmax is significantly longer with RSB (40–60 minutes) compared to TABP (18–30 minutes).[51–54] Epinephrine added to local anesthetic dosing consistently decreases Cmax by approximately 40%–50% for both TAPB and RSB, thus potentially decreasing the risk for LAST.[52,55] In a systematic review of 15 studies with 381 total patients, the predefined threshold for LAST was exceeded in 8.7% of patients. However, only 0.8% patients exhibited clinical symptoms of mild central nervous system (CNS) toxicity and no symptoms or electrocardiogram (ECG) findings of cardiac toxicity.[51] Continuous peripheral nerve blocks and specifically continuous TABP have not demonstrated clinically relevant episodes of LAST. The apparent lack of LAST with continuous infusions is likely due to a postoperative increase in alpha-acid glycoprotein, and consequently, an increase in protein-binding capacity for local anesthetics.[56–58]

COMPLICATIONS

Potential complications for TAP-RSB include vascular injury with resulting bleeding and hematoma formation, visceral damage, and LAST.[59–62] Blind loss of resistance techniques should not be used, as they are associated a significant incidence of incorrect needle placement.[46,63,64] The ascending branch of the deep circumflex artery is located within the lateral TAP, while the superior and inferior and epigastric arteries are located deep to the RAM and should be avoided during performance of the block.[13,14,65] Both TAPB and RSB require relatively higher volumes of local anesthetic, especially with bilateral blocks/catheters. Although the risk of LAST is low, studies have shown that TAPB and RSB may result in systemic local anesthetic concentrations that exceed the threshold for LAST.[51] Epinephrine should be used both as a marker for intravascular injection and to decrease the systemic absorption of local anesthetics, thus decreasing the risk for LAST.[51,52,55]

LIPOSOMAL BUPIVACAINE

The current evidence does not support the use liposomal bupivacaine compared to single-injection conventional bupivacaine in terms of clinically relevant postoperative opioid-sparing nor pain scores.[66–68]

REFERENCES

1. Popping DM, Elia N, Van Aken KH, et al. Impact of epidural analgesia on mortality and morbidity after surgery: systematic review and meta-analysis of randomized controlled trials. *Ann Surg.* 2014;259(6):1056–1067.
2. Vester-Andersen M, Lundstrøm LH, Møller MH, et al. The associate between epidural analgesia and mortality in emergency abdominal surgery: a population-based cohort study. *Acta Anaesthesiol Scand.* 2020;64(1):104–111.
3. Liu S, Carpenter RL, Neal JM. Epidural anesthesia and analgesia: their role in postoperative outcome. *Anesthesiology.* 1995;82(6):1474–1506.
4. Manikian B, Cantineau JP, Betrand M, et al. Improvement in diaphragmatic function by a thoracic extradural block after upper abdominal surgery. *Anesthesiology.* 1988;68(3):379–386.
5. Pansard JL, Manikian B, Bertrand M, et al. Effects of thoracic extradural block in diaphragmatic electrical activity and contractility after upper abdominal surgery. *Anesthesiology.* 1993;78(1):63–71.
6. Bos EME, Haumann J, de Quelerj M, et al. Haematoma and abscess after neuraxial anaesthesia: a review of 647 cases. *Br J Anaesth.* 2018;120(4):693–704.
7. Horlocker TT, Vandermeuelen E, Kopp SL, et al. Regional anesthesia in the patient receiving antithrombotic or thrombolytic therapy: American Society of Regional Anesthesia and Pain Medicine evidence-based guidelines (fourth edition). *Reg Anesth Pain Med.* 2018;43(3):263–309.
8. Lee O, Bateman BT, Kheterpal S, et al. Risk of epidural hematoma after neuraxial techniques in thrombocytopenic parturients: a report from the multicenter perioperative outcomes group. *Anesthesiology.* 2017;126(6):1053–1063.
9. Sondekaoppam RV, Uppal V, Brookes J, Ganapathy S. Bilateral thoracic paravertebral blocks compared to thoracic epidural analgesia after midline laparotomy: a pragmatic non inferiority clinical trial. *Anesth Analg.* 2019;129(34):855–863.
10. Abu Elyazed MM, Mostafa SF, Abdelghany MS, Eid GM. Ultrasound-guided erector spinae plane blocks in patients undergoing open epigastric hernia repair: a prospective randomized controlled study. *Anesth Analg.* 2109;129(1):235–240.
11. Erector spinae plane block for multimodal analgesia after wide midline laparotomy. *Medicine.* 2019;98(20):e15654.
12. Hemmerling TM. Pain management after abdominal surgery. *Lagenbecks Arch Surg.* 2018;403(78):791–803.
13. Rozen W, Tran TMN, Ashton MW, et al. Refining the course of the thoracolumbar nerves: a new understanding of the innervation of the abdominal wall. *Clin Anat.* 2008;21:325–333.
14. Chin KJ, McDonnell JG, Carvahalo B, et al. Essentials of our current understanding: abdominal wall blocks. *Reg Anesth Pain Med.* 2017;42(2):133–183.
15. Seidel R, Wree A, Schulze M. Does the approach influence the success rate of ultrasound-guided rectus sheath blocks? An anatomical case series. *Local Reg Anesth.* 2017;July 5;10:61–65. doi: 10.2147/LRA.S133500. eCollection.
16. Tran TMN, Ivanusic JJ, Hebbard P, et al. Determination of spread of injectate after ultrasound-guided transversus abdominis plane bock: a cadaveric study. *Br J Anaesth.* 2009;102 (1):123–127.
17. Barrington MJ, Ivanusic JJ, Rozen WM, Hebbard P. Spread of injectate after ultrasound-guided subcostal transversus abdominis plane block. *Anaesthesia.* 2009;64(7):745–750.
18. Lee THW, Barrington MJ, Tran TMN, et al. Comparison of extent of sensory block following posterior and subcostal approaches to ultrasound-guided transversus abdominis plane block. *Anaesth Intensive Care.* 2010;38(3):452–460.
19. Børglum J, Jensen K, Christensen AF, et al. Distribution patterns, dermatomal anesthesia, and ropivacaine serum concentrations after bilateral dual transversus abdominis plane block. *Reg Anesth Pain Med.* 2012;37(3):294–301.
20. Støving K, Rothe C, Rosenstock CV, et al. Cutaneous sensory block area, muscle-relaxing effect, and block duration of the transversus abdominis plane block: a randomized, blinded, and placebo-controlled study in healthy volunteers. *Reg Anesth Pain Med.* 2015;40(4):355–362.
21. Carney J, Finnerty O, Rauf J, et al. Studies on the spread of local anaesthetic solution in transversus abdominis plane block. *Anaesthesia.* 2011;68(11):1023–1030.
22. Salinas FV. How I do it; ultrasound-guided rectus sheath blocks. *Am Soc Reg Anesth Pain Med Newsl.* 2014:5–8.
23. Cornish P, Deacon A. Rectus sheath catheters for continuous analgesia after upper abdominal surgery. *ANZ J. Surg* 2007;77(1–2):84.
24. Visou M, Hauber J, Scholz S. Single-injection ultrasound-guided rectus sheath blocks for children: distribution of injected anesthetic. *Paediatr Anaesth.* 2019;29(3):280–285.
25. Hebbard P. TAP block nomenclature. *Anaesthesia.* 2015:70(1):112–113.
26. Mokini Z, Vitale G. Yet more on TAP block nomenclature. *Anaesthesia.* 2015;70(3):369–370.
27. Børglum J, Maschmann C, Belhage B, Jensen K. Ultrasound-guided bilateral dual transversus abdominis plane block: a new four-point approach. *Acta Anaesthesiol Scand.* 2011;55:658–663.
28. Sondekoppam RV, Brookes J, Morris L, et al. Injectate spread following ultrasound-guided lateral to medial approach for dual transversus abdominis plane blocks. *Acta Anaesthesiol Scand.* 2015;59:369–376.

29. Brogi E, Kazan R, Cyr S, et al. Transversus abdominis plane block for postoperative analgesia: a systematic review and meta-analysis of randomized controlled trials. *Can J Anaesth* 2016;63(10):1184–1196.
30. Baerswyl M, Zeiter F, Piubellini D, et al. The analgesic efficacy of transversus abdominis plane block versus epidural analgesia: a systematic review and with metanalysis. *Medicine*. 2018;97(26):e11261.
31. Qin C, Liu Y, Xiong J, et al. The analgesic efficacy compared ultrasound-guided transverse abdominis plane block with epidural analgesia following abdominal surgery: a systematic review and meta-analysis of randomized controlled trials. *BMC Anesthesiol.* 2020;28(20):52.
32. Yoshida T, Furutani K, Watanabe Y, et al. Analgesic efficacy of bilateral continuous transversus abdominis plane blocks using an oblique subcostal approach in patients undergoing laparotomy for gynaecological cancer: a prospective randomized, triple-blinded, placebo-controlled study. *Br J Anaesth*. 2016;117(6):812–820.
33. Guo J, Li H, Pei Q, Feng Z. The analgesic efficacy of subcostal transversus abdominis plane block with Mercedes incision. *BMC Anesthesiol.* 2018;18(1):36.
34. Ganapathy S, Sondekoppam RV, Terlecki M, et al. Comparison of efficacy of and safety of lateral-to-medial continuous transversus abdominis plane block with thoracic epidural analgesia in patients undergoing abdominal surgery. *Eur J Anaesthesiol.* 2015;32:797–804.
35. McDonnell JG, O'Donnell B, Curley G, et al. The analgesic efficacy of transversus abdominis plane block after abdominal surgery. *Anesth Analg.* 2007;104(1):L193–197.
36. McDonnell JG, O'Donnell B, Farrell T, et al. Transversus abdominis plane block: a cadaveric and radiological evaluation. *Reg Anesth Pain Med.* 2007;32(5):399–404.
37. Jankovic ZB, du Feu FM, McConnell P. An anatomical study of the transversus abdominis plane block: location of the triangle of Petit and adjacent nerves. *Anesth Analg.* 2009;109(3):981–985.
38. Nteli Chatzioglou G, Bagheri H, Pinar Y, Govsa F. Anatomical topography of the inferior lumbar triangle for transversus abdominis plane block. *Surg Radiol Anat.* 2018;40(1):99–107.
39. Abrahams M, Derby R, Horn JL. Update on ultrasound for truncal blocks: a review of the evidence. *Reg Anesth Pain Med.* 2016;41(2):275–288.
40. Desmet M, Helsoot D, Vereecke E, et al. Pneumoperitoneum does not influence the spread of local anesthetics in midaxillary approach transversus abdominis plane block. *Reg Anesth Pain Med.* 2015;40(4):349–354.
41. Abdallah F, Laffey JG, Halpern SH, Brull R. Duration of analgesic effectiveness after the posterior and lateral transversus abdominis plane techniques for transverse lower abdominal incisions: a meta-analysis. *Br J Anaesth.* 2013;111(5):721–735.
42. Hebbard PD, Barrington MJ, Vasey C. Ultrasound-guided continuous oblique transversus abdominis plane block. description of a new anatomy and technique. *Regional Anesth Pain Med.* 2011;35(5):436–441.
43. Chen YC, Shi K, Xia Y, et al. Sensory assessment and regression of bilateral oblique subcostal transversus abdominis plane block in volunteers. *Reg Anesth Pain Med.* 2018;43(2):174–179.
44. Yassin HM, Abd Elmoneim AT, El Moutaz H. The analgesic efficacy of ultrasound-guided rectus sheath analgesia compared with low thoracic analgesia after elective abdominal surgery with midline incision: a prospective randomized controlled trial. *Anesth Pain Med.* 2017;7(3): e14244.
45. Elbarhawy K, El-Deeb A. Rectus sheath block for postoperative analgesia in patients with mesenteric vascular occlusion undergoing laparotomy: a randomized single-blinded study. *Anesth Essay Res.* 2016;10(3):5216–520.
46. Bakshi SG, Mapari A, Shylasree TS, et al. Rectus sheath block for postoperative analgesia in gynecological oncology surgery (RESONS): a randomized-control trial. *Can J Anesth.* 2012;63(12):1335–1344.
47. Rao Kadam V, Van Wijk RM, Moran JL, et al. Continuous transversus abdominis plane block vs intermittent bolus for analgesia after abdominal surgery: a randomized controlled trial. *J Pain Res.* 2017;10:1705–1712.
48. Khatibi B, Said ET, Sztain JF, et al. Continuous transversus abdominis plane nerve blocks: does varying local anesthetic delivery method-automatic bolus versus continuous basal infusion-influence the extent of sensation to cold? A randomized, triple-masked, cross-over study in volunteers. *Anesth Analg.* 2017;124(4):1298–1303.
49. Bojaxhi E, Clendenen SR. A comparative study of automated pulsed bolus versus continuous basal infusion on distribution of contrast in the transversus abdominis fascial plane in a cadaver: a technical report. *Cureus.* 2019 Sep 16;11(9):e5664. doi: 10.7759/cureus.5664.
50. Purdy M, Kinnunen M, Kokki M, et al. A prospective, randomized, open label, controlled study investigating the efficiency and safety of 3 analgesia methods of rectus sheath block analgesia following midline laparotomy. *Medicine.* 2018 Feb;97(7):e996.
51. Rahiri J, Tuhoe J, Svirskis, et al. Systematic review of systemic concentrations of local anaesthetic after transversus abdominis plane block and rectus sheath block. *Br J Anaesth.* 2017;118(4):517–526.
52. Kitayama M, Wada M, Hashimoto H, et al. Effects of adding epinephrine on early systemic absorption of local anesthetics in abdominal truncal blocks. *J Anesth.* 2014;28(4):631–634.
53. Murouci T, Isakawa S, Yamakage M. Chronological changes in ropivacaine concentration and analgesic effects between transversus abdominis plane block and rectus sheath block. *Reg Anesth Pain Med.* 2015;40(5):568–571.
54. Yasumura R, Kobayashi Y, Ochia R. A comparison of plasma levobupivacaine concentrations following transversus abdominis plane block and rectus sheath block. *Anaesthesia.* 2016;71(5):544–549
55. Miranda P, Corvetto MA, Altermatt FR, et al. Levobupivacaine absorption pharmacokinetics with and without epinephrine during TAP block: analysis of doses based on associated risks of local anesthetic toxicity. *Eur J Clin Pharmacol.* 2016;72(10):1221–1227.
56. Bleckner LL, Bina KH, McKnight G, et al. Serum ropivacaine concentrations and systemic local anesthetic concentrations in trauma patients receiving long-term continuous peripheral nerve catheters. *Anesth Analg.* 2010;110(2):630–634.
57. Bleckner LL, Solia C, Fileta BB, et al. Serum free ropivacaine concentrations among patients receiving continuous peripheral catheters: is it safe for long term infusions? *Anesth Analg.* 2014;118(1):225–229.
58. Hessian EC, Evans BE, Woods JA, et al. Plasma ropivacaine concentrations during bilateral transversus abdominis plane infusions. *Br J Anaesth.* 2013;111(3):488–495.
59. Farooq M, Carey M. A case of liver trauma with blunt regional anesthesia needle while performing transversus abdominis plane block. *Reg Anesth Pain Med.* 2008;33(3):274–275.
60. Lancaster P, Chadwick M. Liver trauma secondary to ultrasound-guided transversus abdominis plane block. *Br J Anaesth.* 2010;104(4): 509–510.
61. Griffiths JD, Le NV, Grant S, et al. Symptomatic local anaesthetic toxicity and plasma ropivacaine concentrations after transversus abdominis plane block for cesarean section. *Br J Anaesth.* 2013;110(6):996–1000.
62. Weiss E, Jolly C, Dumoulin JL, et al. Convulsions in two patients after bilateral ultrasound-guided transversus abdominis plane block for cesarean analgesia. *Reg Anesth Pain Med.* 2014;39(3): 248–251.
63. Dolan J, Ludie P, Geary T, et al. The rectus sheath block: accuracy of local anesthetic placement by trainee anesthesiologists using a loss of resistance approach. *Reg Anesth Pain Med.* 2009;34(3): 247–250.
64. McDermott G, Korba E, Mata U, et al. Should we stop doing blind transversus abdominis plane block? *Br J Anaesth.* 2012;108(4): 499–502.
65. Le Saint-Grant A, Taylor A, Varsou O, Grant C, Cezayirli E, Bowness J. Arterial anatomy of the anterior abdominal wall: ultrasound evaluation as a real-time guide to percutaneous instrumentation. *Clin Anat.* 2021;34(1):5–10.
66. Ha AY, Keane G, Parikh R, et al. The analgesic effects of liposomal bupivacaine versus bupivacaine hydrochloride administered as tranversus abdominis plane block after abdominally based microvascular

breast reconstruction: a prospective single-blind, randomized, controlled trial. *Plast Reconstr Surg*. 2019;144:35–44.
67. Nedeljikovic AA, Kett A, Vallejo MC, et al. Transversus abdominis plane block with liposomal bupivacaine for pain after cesarean delivery in a multicenter, randomized, double-blind, controlled trial. *Anesth Analg*. 2020;131:1830–1839.
68. Hussain N, Brull R, Sheehy B, et al. Perineural liposomal bupivacaine is not superior to nonliposomal bupivacaine for peripheral nerve block analgesia a systematic review and meta-analysis. *Anesthesiology*. 2021;134:147–164.

QUESTIONS

(1) All of the following may provide effective analgesia after upper abdominal midline laparotomy except:

A. Thoracic epidural analgesia
B. Thoracic paravertebral block
C. Lateral TAPB
D. Subcostal TAPB

(2) Which of the following are contraindication to thoracic epidural analgesia?

A. Last dose of enoxaparin 1 mg/kg every 12 hours prior to surgery
B. Last dose of clopidogrel 7 days prior to surgery
C. Last dose of apixaban 4 days prior to surgery
D. Prior lumbar fusion from L1–L5

(3) Which of the following is true?

A. TAPB and RSB provide somatic and visceral analgesia
B. Epidural analgesia blocks the somatic pain fibers only
C. Paravertebral nerve block visceral analgesia only
D. TAPB and RSB provide somatic analgesia only

(4) All of the following are muscles of the anterolateral abdominal wall except:

A. External oblique
B. Internal oblique
C. Transversus abdominis
D. Quadratus lumborum

(5) The transversus abdominis plane is located deep all of the structures except:

A. Rectus abdominis muscle
B. Linea semilunaris
C. Internal oblique
D. Quadratus lumborum

(6) Which of the following regarding the rectus sheath is true?

A. It is located anterior (superficial) and posterior (deep) to rectus abdominis muscle.
B. It is it is located deep to the transversalis fascia.
C. It is located deep to the internal oblique muscle.
D. It is located lateral to the linea semilunaris.

(7) All of the following blocks provide analgesia for lower abdominal surgery except:

A. Lateral TAPB
B. Oblique subcostal TAPB
C. Dual TAPB
D. Subcostal TAPB

(8) Which of the following is not a potential complication of TAPB or RSB?

a. Vascular injury
b. Visceral injury
c. Urinary retention
d. Local anesthetic toxicity

ANSWERS

(1) **C.** Studies found that ultrasound-guided injection of local anesthetic (or dye) between the costal margin and the iliac crest at the midaxillary line (within the lateral TAP) consistently blocks the T10–T12 thoracolumbar nerves, while the upper segmental nerves (T7–T9) are typically not blocked, as these nerves enter the TAP medial to anterior axillary line.

References

Tran TMN, Ivanusic JJ, Hebbard P, et al. Determination of spread of injectate after ultrasound-guided transversus abdominis plane bock: a cadaveric study. *Br J Anaesth*. 2009;102(1):123–127.
Barrington MJ, Ivanusic JJ, Rozen WM, Hebbard P. Spread of injectate after ultrasound-guided subcostal transversus abdominis plane block. *Anaesthesia*. 2009;64(7):745–750.

(2) **A.** The ASRA guidelines recommend stopping clopidogrel 5–7 days prior to placing a neuraxial block. The ASRA guidelines recommend stopping enoxaparin at least 24 hours for treatment doses (1 mg/kg q 12 hours or 1.5 mg/kg daily). The ASRA guidelines recommend stopping apixaban at least 72 hours (3 days) prior to surgery. A lumbar spinal fusion should not be contraindication to mid-thoracic (T7–T10) epidural analgesia that is commonly used for abdominal incisions.

Reference

Horlocker TT, Vandermeulen E, Kopp SL, et al. Regional anesthesia in the patient receiving antithrombotic or thrombolytic therapy: American Society of Regional Anesthesia and Pain Medicine evidence-based guidelines (fourth edition). *Reg Anesth Pain Med*. 2018;43(3):263–309

(3) **D.** TAP Block and RS Block cover only the somatic components of pain are covered. Thus, a multimodal analgesic regimen is required to cover the visceral component of postoperative pain. In contrast, both TEA and TPVB provide both somatic and visceral analgesia.

Reference

Hemmerling TM. Pain management after abdominal surgery. *Lagenbecks Arch Surg*. 2018;403(78):791–803.

(4) **D.** Quadratus lumborum is a posterior abdominal wall muscle that originates from the posteromedial iliac crest and inserts into the medial border of the twelfth rib and the transverse processes of the first to fourth lumbar vertebrae. There are 4 paired muscles that form the anterolateral abdominal wall: the rectus abdominis (RA), external oblique (EO), internal oblique (IO), and transversus abdominis (TA). The lateral muscles overlie one another from superficial to deep (EO, IO, and TA) and terminate medially to form an aponeurosis (linea semilunaris), which is located lateral to the paired midline RA.

Reference

Chin KJ, McDonnell JG, Carvalho B, et al. Essentials of our current understanding: abdominal wall blocks. *Reg Anesth Pain Med.* 2017;42:133–183.

(5) **D.** The quadtraus lumborum muscle is a posterior muscle and does not participate in the TAP plane.

Reference

Chin KJ, McDonnell JG, Carvalho B, et al. Essentials of our current understanding: abdominal wall blocks. *Reg Anesth Pain Med.* 2017;42:133–183.

(6) **A.** The anterior rectus sheath (superficial to the RA) is formed by the aponeuroses of the external oblique (EO) and the anterior lamina of the internal oblique (IO), while the posterior rectus sheath (deep to the RA) is formed from the aponeuroses of the posterior lamina of the IO and TA Inferior to the arcuate line, all three aponeuroses course anterior to the RA to form the anterior layer of the rectus sheath with the posterior layer being formed only by the epimysium of the RA and transversalis fascia. The RA is attached to the anterior aspect of the rectus sheath by 3 or 4 tendinous insertions. Thus, the anterior aspect of the rectus sheath is divided into separate sub-compartments. In contrast, the posterior aspect of the rectus sheath is unsegmented and is anatomically a continuous space along its entire course. The transversalis fascia is a thin areolar tissue that lines the deep surface of the TA and RA and separates them from the abdominal cavity.

References

Chin KJ, McDonnell JG, Carvahalo B, et al. Essentials of our current understanding: abdominal wall blocks. *Reg Anesth Pain Med.* 2017;42(2):133–183.

Seidel R, Wree A, Schulze M. Does the approach influence the success rate of ultrasound-guided rectus sheath blocks? An anatomical case series. *Local Reg Anesth.* 2017 July 5;10:61–65. doi: 10.2147/LRA.S133500. eCollection.

(7) **D.** The subcostal TAPB targets the T7–T9 thoracolumbar nerves and is indicated for upper abdominal (supraumbilical) surgery. The oblique subcostal TAP Block and the four quadrant TAPB target both the upper (T7–T9) and lower (T10–12) thoracolumbar nerves. The lateral TAP Block targets the T10–T12 thoracolumbar nerves and is indicated for lower abdominal (infraumbilcal) surgery.

References

Chin KJ, McDonnell JG, Carvahalo B, et al. Essentials of our current understanding: abdominal wall blocks. *Reg Anesth Pain Med.* 2017;42(2):133–183.

Hebbard PD, Barrington MJ, Vasey C. Ultrasound-guided continuous oblique transversus abdominis plane block: description of a new anatomy and technique. *Reg Anesth Pain Med.* 2011;35(5):436–441.

(8) **C.** Potential complications for TAP Block -RS Block include vascular injury with resulting bleeding and hematoma formation, visceral damage, and local anesthetic systemic toxicity (LAST). The ascending branch of the deep circumflex artery is located within the lateral TAP, while the superior and inferior and epigastric arteries are located deep to the rectus abdominis muscle and should be avoided during performance of the block. Although the risk of LAST is low, studies have shown that TAP Block -RS Block may result in systemic local anesthetic concentrations that exceed the threshold for LAST.

References

Chin KJ, McDonnell JG, Carvahalo B, et al. Essentials of our current understanding: abdominal wall blocks. *Reg Anesth Pain Med.* 2017;42(2):133–183.

Rahiri J, Tuhoe J, Svirskis, et al. Systematic review of systemic concentrations of local anaesthetic after transversus abdominis plane block and rectus sheath block. *Br J Anaesth.* 2017;118(4):517–526.

17.

POSTOPERATIVE PAIN MANAGEMENT FOR LIVING LIVER DONOR

Victor Polshin and Engy T. Said

STEM CASE AND KEY QUESTIONS

A 35-year-old healthy male is scheduled for right lobe donor hepatectomy (RLDH) to serve as donor graft for his mother's living liver donor transplant (LLDT) surgery. He has no prior medical or surgical history. He is active and exercises 3–4 times per week.

His preoperative workup includes a normal electrocardiogram, negative hepatitis serology, and normal range complete blood count, metabolic panel, liver function tests, and coagulation profile.

Preoperatively, he was given acetaminophen 975 mg and gabapentin 300 mg orally. He was offered thoracic epidural analgesia (TEA) and consented to the procedure after extensive counseling of risks and benefits. A TEA catheter was placed at T6–T7 interspace, and an epidural infusion with 0.0625% bupivacaine and 8 mcg/mL hydromorphone was started at 6 mL/hr.

He received general anesthesia, which was uneventful. Throughout the surgical procedure, central venous pressure (CVP) was maintained around 0–4 mmHg. Operative time was 6 hours, total estimated blood loss was 2 liters, and urine output was 450 mL. In total, the patient received 4 liters of crystalloid in addition to 550 mL of autologous salvaged blood.

On emergence, he was extubated and transferred to the intensive care unit. Once he was awake, he reported 8/10 abdominal pain, and was started by the surgical resident on an intravenous hydromorphone patient-controlled analgesia (PCA) to supplement TEA and other medications in the pain regimen. His pain improved, and he was able to rest at night.

On postoperative day (POD) 1, he was evaluated by the Acute Pain Service and reported pain scores in the moderate to severe range 5–7/10; however, he is somnolent at rest but complains that pain limits his movement, deep breathing, and cough. On exam, there is no sensory deficit to alcohol swab or ice throughout his chest or abdomen. He has 5/5 strength throughout his lower extremities, though the exam is limited by pain and guarding.

(1) IN THE SETTING OF POORLY CONTROLLED ACUTE POSTOPERATIVE PAIN, SOMNOLENCE, AND DECREASED SENSORY EXAM TO ICE, HOW WOULD YOU PROCEED WITH EPIDURAL INFUSION MANAGEMENT?

Assuming normal hemodynamics, the increase in local anesthetic concentration would yield a decrease in somatic pain and a change in sensory exam to ice. With 0.0625% bupivacaine concentration, a sensory deficit to alcohol swab or ice is difficult to elicit. The concentration can be increased to 0.1%, 0.125%, or 0.15% bupivacaine as blood pressure tolerates. The increase in hydromorphone in the epidural infusion can alleviate visceral pain but can have systemic effects, adding to worsening somnolence.

In this case, the epidural infusion was increased to 0.125% bupivacaine with 16 mcg/mL hydromorphone. The patient was given 8 mL loading dose and started on 8mL/hr infusion. Within 30 minutes, the patient reports feeling more comfortable and has a sensory deficit to alcohol swab from T4 level to T10.

(2) ON THE EVENING OF POD 1, HE CONTINUES TO REPORT LOWER PAIN SCORES, THOUGH HE COMPLAINS OF MODERATE TO SEVERE PAIN WITH MOVEMENT. HIS NURSE INQUIRES ABOUT ADDING KETOROLAC TO HIS PAIN REGIMEN. IN REVIEW OF HIS LABORATORY RESULTS, YOU NOTE THAT HIS LIVER FUNCTION TESTS ARE TRENDING UP, AND ARE MODERATELY ELEVATED. HOW DO YOU PROCEED? DOES KETOROLAC PROVIDE AN OPIOID-SPARING EFFECT POST–LIVER RESECTION?

A study showed that ketorolac in combination with IV-PCA is non-inferior to TEA for patients undergoing open liver resection and has shown to have an opioid-sparing effect. The American Society of Regional Anesthesia's (ASRA's) recommendation for management of nonsteroidal anti-inflammatory drugs (NSAIDs) in the setting of TEA is that they do not appear to present significant risk for epidural hematomas when used alone. However, in the setting of liver resection and acutely abnormal coagulation profile, it is not advisable to proceed with NSAID therapy in the setting of an epidural.

The patient continues to meet his postoperative milestones, his diet is advanced to clears on POD 2, and full liquid diet on POD 3. He is then transitioned from hydromorphone IV PCA to oral oxycodone. Evening of POD 3, he is transferred to the floor, and transitioned to a full diet.

(3) WHAT TYPICAL ALTERATIONS IN COAGULATION PROFILE ARE TO BE EXPECTED IN THE POSTOPERATIVE PERIOD?

Several studies have evaluated the coagulopathic effects of liver resection, all of which agree on its transient nature. The coagulation profile is altered with maximal increase in prothrombin time (PT) around POD 2, a nadir in platelets around POD 3, and a maximal increase in liver function test (LFTs) on POD 1 and a downward trend thereafter.

(4) IN ANTICIPATION OF UPCOMING HOSPITAL DISCHARGE, WHEN IS THE BEST TIME TO REMOVE THE EPIDURAL CATHETER?

A major concern for patients with TEA after RLDH is an increased risk of epidural hematoma postoperatively. The recommendation is to normalize the coagulation status at the time of removal of the epidural catheter. It is suggested that optimal time for epidural catheter removal is between POD 4 and POD 5. However, there has been no reported epidural hematomas in the literature in this surgical population.

(5) WHAT ARE SOME OF THE DRAWBACKS OF EPIDURAL ANALGESIA IN RLDH?

Several studies have described other possible side effects of postoperative epidural analgesia. These include increased intravenous resuscitation and possibly even higher transfusion rates. This is possibly due to hypotension that can be associated with employing TEA, associated with higher amounts of resuscitation with crystalloids, resulting in higher degrees of anemia due to hemodilution. On the other hand, TEA plays an important role in lowering of CVP and decreasing surgical blood loss.

(6) WHAT ARE THE RISKS AND BENEFITS OF STARTING NEURAXIAL ANALGESIA INFUSION PREOPERATIVELY VS. POSTOPERATIVELY?

Several studies have shown that in patients undergoing RLDH there is a benefit to starting neuraxial analgesia preoperatively when compared to postoperatively or even intraoperatively, either with spinal or TEA. However, there is no complete agreement on this point. This leads to a conclusion that if TEA is employed, it should be started prior to incision and continued throughout the surgery.

Pre-incisional neuraxial analgesia can provide a challenge for the anesthesiologist, as this is a major surgery with potential for very significant blood loss. However, in the case of liver resection, a lower CVP is beneficial, and has been shown by some studies to decrease intraoperative blood loss when maintained below 4 mmHg. Utilizing neuraxial anesthesia can therefore make it easier to maintain the CVP at the desired level. Of course, the amounts of other anesthetic agents, such as opioids and inhaled anesthetics, will need to be decreased, and vasopressors need to be readily available to manage any resulting intraoperative hypotension.

(7) IS SINGLE-SHOT SPINAL A GOOD ALTERNATIVE TO TEA FOR POSTOPERATIVE ANALGESIA FOR RLDH?

Despite the limitations of TEA, TEA is still the best-studied modality for intraoperative and postoperative analgesia after RLDH. A preoperative spinal using bupivacaine and long-acting opioid such as preservative-free morphine has shown to be of great analgesic benefit.

(8) WHAT ARE SOME PERIPHERAL NERVE BLOCK ALTERNATIVES TO TEA FOR A RIGHT SUBCOSTAL INCISION AND FOR A MIDLINE INCISION? ARE TRANSVERSUS ABDOMINIS PLANE (TAP) BLOCKS HELPFUL HERE?

TAP blocks have proven to be beneficial in liver resection surgery. Some studies have been done employing a combination of multiple bilateral subcostal TAP blocks and a right lateral TAP block with some efficacy. Paravertebral block (PVB) provides visceral and incisional pain coverage and has been studied in patients' status post-RLDH with good outcomes. It also provides the benefits of sympathectomy associated with epidurals, while decreasing the risk of hypotension and concern for lower extremity motor blockade. There are case reports of favorable pain control with erector spinae nerve (ESP) catheter blocks in the setting of liver resection.

(9) WHAT ARE SOME OPIOID-SPARING ANALGESICS THAT CAN BE USED POST-RLDH?

Multimodal pain management is a beneficial component of postoperative pain in RLDH. However, caution is advised in using nonsteroidal anti-inflammatory drugs (NSAIDs) in the setting of postoperative coagulopathy, especially for patients with TEA. Administration of acetaminophen for patients after liver resection should be carefully considered, and underlying liver function and risk-factor profile should be thoroughly considered.

(10) WHAT ARE SOME SURGICAL TECHNIQUES FOR DECREASING POSTOPERATIVE PAIN AFTER LIVING LIVER DONATION?

Most commonly RLDH is carried out with a right subcostal incision, and an epigastric midline incision (which may need to be extended to the umbilicus). These incisions have been shown to increase splinting in patients, resulting in shallow breathing and increasing morbidity by increasing atelectasis and risk of pulmonary infections.

Even so, some surgeons have attempted to use minimally invasive techniques to decrease morbidity associated with large incisions in order to improve recovery. Minimally invasive techniques are challenging for this surgery, due to the complexity of the surgery and also because the specimen that is resected tends to be large. RLDH is a complex procedure and often lengthy, as the entire left lobe requires meticulous care in resection while preserving vascular supply; for this reason, laparoscopic or a minimally invasive approach can be particularly challenging. Infiltration of local anesthetics at the incision sites can also be employed as one technique in a multimodal analgesia plan.

DISCUSSION

LIVING DONOR LIVER TRANSPLANT SURGICAL CONSIDERATIONS

Liver transplant is the treatment of choice for end-stage liver disease. However, the need for liver transplants has far outpaced the supply of available cadaveric livers. Unlike many organs, the liver is an organ that is capable of regeneration and adaptation. Taking advantage of these properties, partial living donor liver transplant has been employed as an alternative. Functionally, the liver is divided into two lobes and 8 segments: the smaller left lobe, comprising segments I, II, III, and IV, and the larger right lobe comprised of segments V, VI, VII, and VIII (see Figure 17.1). It is innervated by a sympathetic neuron derived from the spinal cord (T7–T12), and a parasympathetic neuron from the vagus nerve.

Partial living liver donation was initially employed for pediatric liver transplants. Typically, parents or adult relatives would donate the smaller left liver lobe, or even a portion of the left liver lobe with left lateral segmentectomy, which would provide an adequate graft for the recipients. However, for adult recipients the smaller left liver lobe is often insufficient and results in higher rates of graft failure. Over time, it became apparent that the smaller left liver lobe or a left liver segmentectomy for living liver donation in the adult population led to small-for-size syndrome, and that a larger volume of liver graft was often required. For this reason, in many centers, right liver donor hepatectomy (RLDH) has become the standard surgery for living liver donor transplant in adults.[1]

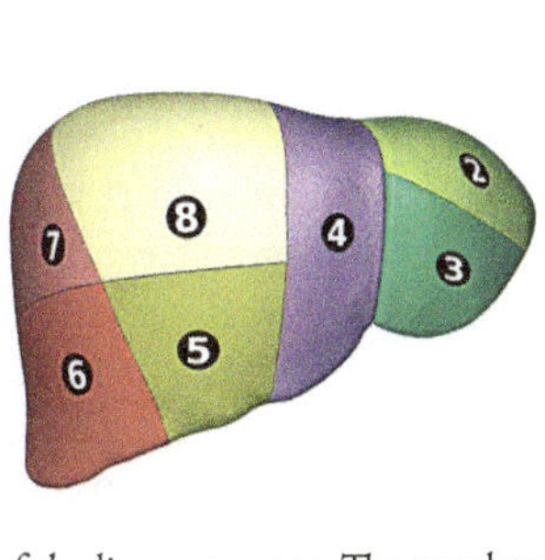

Figure 17.1. Anatomy of the liver segments. The numbered segments are the segments of the liver in anterior view. Segment 2, 3, and 4 form the left lobe of the liver. Segments 5 through 8 make up the right lobe of the liver.

Surgical approach for RLDH commonly includes a bilateral subcostal incision (chevron incision) with or without vertical extension, or a right subcostal incision with a midline sub-xyphoid extension (reserve L incision), a J-shaped incision, or an upper midline incision. (Figure 17.2). The type of incision often depends on the circumstance and surgeon preference. There have been some centers reporting results of fully laparoscopic, or minimally invasive hand-assisted techniques.[2–4] These approaches may help reduce the postoperative morbidity from pain; however, it is unclear if other surgical morbidity is reduced, and many centers have yet to adopt this approach as standard.[5] The vascular complexity, risk of major bleeding, and biliary variations make a technically challenging laparoscopic approach to liver resection, with an average learning curve of 30–60 laparoscopic hepatectomies before blood loss and surgical time can be optimized.[6]

Donor hepatectomy patients are generally healthy; therefore minimizing post-RLDH complications, with minimal impact on the donor's future quality of life, is important.[7] In general, while donor hepatectomy procedure complications are rare, there is an associated 0.1%–0.2% mortality and 25%–35% morbidity.[8,9] Up to 10% of patients develop biliary complications and will have decreased liver function for days or week postoperatively.[10] Likewise, Pomfret et al.[11] examined the morbidity after RLDH and found that despite the regeneration capacity of the liver, a donor's liver regenerated only to about 85.6% ± 8.2% of their original size, even after 1 year.

POSTOPERATIVE PAIN AFTER RLDH

Acute postoperative pain management for patients undergoing RLDH for altruistic reasons is often challenging. Most commonly, the surgical approach requires bilateral subcostal ("chevron") incisions, or right subcostal incision and a midline xyphoid to umbilicus incision. In either case, these are some of the most painful incisions, and can impact postoperative pulmonary function due to guarding and splinting with breathing. In comparison to patients who undergo liver resection for tumors, RLDH patients with similar incisions experience more significant postoperative pain.[12] In this retrospective analysis, Cywinski et al.[12] compared patients undergoing RLDH with patients undergoing major hepatic resection for tumors, both groups with patient-controlled TEA infusion and similar incision, and found that despite no difference between groups in the amount of bupivacaine used via TEA, RLDH patients had higher postoperative pain scores. Barring major surgical complications, this moderate to severe range of poorly controlled postoperative pain can become a limiting factor for recovery. There are several theories to explain

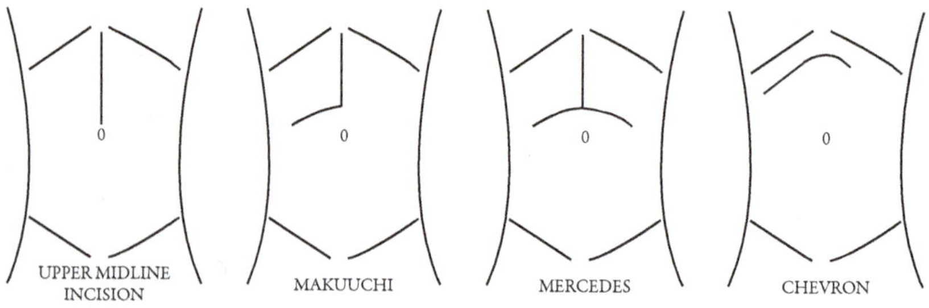

Figure 17.2. Incisions for liver surgery.

this phenomenon. One explanation is that living liver resection for donation is more complicated—the blood supply must be preserved both to the remaining left lobe, and to the right liver lobe that is being resected in order to preserve the viability of the tissues. Furthermore, the amount of the liver tissue being resected is often far larger for living liver donors than for patients undergoing liver resection due to primary or metastatic tumors of the liver. This results in increased surgical time; Cywinski et al.[12] found the surgical time for RLDH to be 707 ± 79.3 minutes, while patients undergoing major hepatic resection had an average surgical time of 255 ± 65 minutes. The extended surgical stimulation can produce more pronounced central sensitization, resulting in postoperative hyperalgesia. Another explanation is that healthy patients are selected for liver donation; thus the majority do not have experience with abdominal pain or discomfort preoperatively. This can make new onset acute pain more noticeable.[7] Conversely, patients undergoing major liver resection, or other major thoracic, abdominal, and orthopedic surgeries, commonly have pain for weeks, if not months and years, prior to their surgery. Therefore, treatment of postoperative pain can sometimes represent an improvement, or at least not a significantly higher amount of pain than usual for this patient population. Likewise, there are significant psychosocial variables that can play an important role in the perception and management of pain.[13] This is a particularly important consideration in the setting of organ donation, where the patient is temporarily debilitated for altruistic reasons. In fact, pain was reported to being more than anticipated in 44% of liver donor patients, even with the use of TEA and IV-PCA.[14]

OPIOIDS AND OPIOID-SPARING ANALGESIC OPTIONS

Opioid metabolism can be affected by liver function impairment. Some animal models have demonstrated increased plasma levels of systemic opioids in the setting of acute hepatic failure.[15] Morphine is metabolized primarily by the liver, and may be significantly affected by a liver impairment.[16] Fentanyl PCA was thought to have a favorable pharmacokinetics profile compared to morphine in liver patients. Nada et al.[17] compared fentanyl PCA to morphine PCA in donor hepatectomy. They found that although both groups had adequate pain control, the morphine group reached faster pain control with less morphine equivalent dose with less PCA demands in liver resection patients; both groups had similar side effect profile as regards respiratory depression episodes; however, the morphine was more sedating in the first 12 hours. Studies show that liver function impairment has to be severe to affect the metabolism of morphine. In chronic liver disease or in the freshly transplanted liver, there was minimal effect on the metabolites. During the anhepatic phase of liver transplantation, morphine was metabolized by extrahepatic sites such as the kidneys or intestines.[18-20]

In addition to traditional opioid-based pain management regimen, the use of other agents can reduce the amount of opioid-related side effects. The idea of multimodal analgesia is the use of a combination of drugs with different mechanisms of action, thus potentially reducing the undesirable side effects of one single drug at higher doses.

NSAIDs are included in the list of adjuvant drugs with opioid-sparing effects and have been shown to successfully decrease opioid-related side effects; however, their use is often limited by risk of bleeding, damage to gastrointestinal mucosa, and renal complications.[21] Caution is advised in the setting of postoperative coagulopathy, especially for patients with TEA. Data from the OSLO-COMET trial showed that ketorolac in combination with IV-PCA is non-inferior to TEA for patients undergoing open liver resection and that it may have an opioid-sparing effect. [22] Cyclooxygenase-2 selective NSAIDs, such as celecoxib, have demonstrated their safety profile for management of postoperative pain after hepatectomy in the setting of liver dysfunction studies.[23]

Low-dose ketamine, defined as less than 1mg/kg when administered as intravenous bolus and ≤20 μg/kg/min as an infusion, has been associated with superior pain control and opioid-sparing effects.[24] Similarly, a retrospective study of perioperative ketamine for donor hepatectomy has been found to have improved analgesia and opioid-sparing effects when compared to IV-PCA opioids alone, without ketamine-related adverse events.[25]

Postoperative liver dysfunction often limits the use of acetaminophen as the effect of the acute reduced liver volume on metabolism is not clear. Galinski et al.[26] demonstrated an increase of plasma acetaminophen level after liver resection compared with non-liver resection patients, while Hughes et al.[27] demonstrated that the greatest increase in level correlated with largest liver resections, suggesting a volume-related component. Acetaminophen is also metabolized via the cytochrome P450 pathway in liver, producing the toxic metabolite N-acetyl-p-benzoquinone imine (NAPQI) in the healthy liver.[28] Administration of acetaminophen after liver resection should be carefully considered, and underlying liver function and risk factor profile should be thoroughly considered.

POSTOPERATIVE ACUTE PAIN MANAGEMENT: NEURAXIAL ANALGESIA

Thoracic Epidural Analgesia

Thoracic epidural analgesia (TEA) is the best-studied neuraxial or regional modality for postoperative pain relief after RLDH. A study of patients undergoing liver resection for demonstrated no difference between TEA IV-PCA group, has no difference in pain score, and but a significantly lower use of additional pain medication, with an overall no difference in fluid requirement or complications.[29] Likewise, recent studies have demonstrated the use of TEA as part of fast-track protocols or enhanced recovery pathways for liver resection patients with a reduced hospital stay.[30,31] A 2014 Nationwide Inpatient Sample review of patients undergoing major liver resection showed that TEA is low in prevalence, and does not seem to influence postoperative complications, though it is associated with increased use of blood transfusions.[32] The concerns about the risks of developing an epidural hematoma given the postoperative coagulation profile changes led some transplant centers to abandon the use of TEA, despite its established advantages.[33–35] While there have been no published case reports or incidents in the published studies of epidural hematomas in patients receiving TEA and undergoing RLDH, all studied epidurals were removed only once, when coagulation profiles had normalized. Generally, given the low incidence of epidural hematomas in healthy subjects, the published studies do not provide a large enough sample to accurately calculate the incidence of epidural hematomas in this patient population. Therefore, some centers still utilize TEA after discussing with the patients at length the benefits and the possible risks.

Postoperative disturbances in coagulation profile after RLDH is a major concern given the devastating risk of epidural hematoma. Typically, these healthy patients receive their TEA preoperatively, when their coagulation profile is normal. The concern is during the postoperative period, and the timing of epidural catheter removal. Liver function tests, and blood clotting in particular, are often abnormal for several days postoperatively. A more recent study analyzing coagulation profile via Thromboelastography (TEG) after major liver resection, suggests that although the prothrombin time (PT) and partial prothrombin time (PTT) are prolonged postoperatively in patients undergoing RLDH, the actual coagulation is not altered.[36] Likewise, Barton et al.[37] found no statistically significant differences in clot formation and breakdown in patients undergoing liver resection despite an elevation in PT-INR. But rather, they suggest a brief hypercoagulable state, give the decreased time to onset (R-value) postoperatively; this may be explained by the fact that although pro-coagulant factors and platelets are decreased, anticoagulant factors are decreased as well. Furthermore, the changes in PT and PTT can be more dependent on the size of the graft relative to the donor and amount of resuscitation and transfusion during surgery.[11] Borromeo[38] reported decreasing liver function, including increased PT and PTT, in patients undergoing RLDH; this was later confirmed by Siniscalchi and Schumann.[39,40] Another study, by Choi et al.,[41] evaluated outcomes of 360 liver donations, and found that INR was highest on POD 1—with a mean of 1.53 with values ranging from 1.07 to 2.38; the Activate Partial thrombin time (aPTT) was highest on POD 0 with a mean of 66.1 with values ranging from 27.2–300. Several studies have evaluated the coagulopathic effects of liver resection, all of which agree on its transient nature.[38,39,41] The coagulation profile is altered with maximal increase in PT around POD 2, a nadir in platelets around POD 3, and a maximal increase in LFTs on POD 1and a downward trend thereafter.[38,42]

Several studies have shown that in patients undergoing RLDH there is a benefit to starting neuraxial analgesia preoperatively when compared to postoperatively or even intraoperatively, either with spinal or TEA. Other studies have shown that there is no benefit to starting postoperative TEA when compared to IV medications alone when looking at pain scores and morphine consumption. This leads to a conclusion that if TEA is employed, it may to be started prior to incision and continued throughout the surgery. [30,43] Typically, during operations like these, anesthesiologists employ short-acting, potent opioids such as fentanyl or remifentanil, and may even add hydromorphone or morphine at the end of the case. As demonstrated by Katz et al.,[38] pre-incisional administration of local anesthetic with fentanyl into the epidural space was associated with decreased postoperative hyperalgesia and decreased postoperative morphine IV-PCA requirement. It also has been well documented that any opioid exposure, even as a single dose, not only increases the tolerance of the subjects but also can exaggerate responses to noxious stimuli. Therefore, by employing pre-incisional neuraxial analgesia, and decreasing intraoperative opioid utilization, postoperative pain and opioid consumption would be decreased.

Pre-incisional TEA activation can also cause a decrease in mean arterial pressure (MAP) and CVP. For liver resection surgery, this can be advantageous intraoperatively, as a decreased CVP can result in a decrease in surgical blood loss, and many centers target a CVP <5 intraoperatively.[44,45] Conversely, postoperatively this can result in a higher requirement for vasopressors and fluid resuscitation. These include increased intravenous resuscitation and possibly even higher transfusion rates, resulting in higher degrees of anemia due to hemodilution. [46] TEA, in combination with balanced fluid management, can enable maintenance of low CVP and decrease risk of hepatic congestion secondary to fluid overload. [43]

Su et al.[47] searched retrospectively their cases of hepatic resections who received epidural analgesia over 9 years (1644) cases. They found the incidence of postoperative coagulopathy was 47.0%, similar Jacquenod et al.'s[48] report of 50% incidence. However, no epidural hematomas were discovered; meanwhile, they noted a higher incidence of plasma transfusion during epidural catheter removal after hepatic resection. There are also cases where platelets and vitamin K were administered as well. Tzimas et al.[49] reviewed papers published about epidural analgesia in liver resection surgery and looked for four areas of controversy, including the safety of epidural catheters with postoperative coagulopathy; analgesic efficacy; associated perioperative fluid administration; and the role of epidural analgesia in enhanced recovery protocols. They found that the evidence available is insufficient to provide definitive answers and called for more studies to answer these questions. Su et al.[47] believe the increased availability of alternative techniques to epidural analgesia may limit the future study of epidural analgesia for hepatic resection cases.

Despite the limitations of TEA listed above, and the concerns about increased risk of epidural hematoma in patients undergoing right liver lobe hepatectomy, TEA is still the best studied modality for intraoperative and postoperative analgesia after RLDH. [10] If TEA is employed, patients need to be counseled extensively about the risks and benefits of TEA, including a possibly increased risk of epidural hematoma. Furthermore, the catheter should be removed on POD 4 or 5 when the coagulation profile is starting to return to normal. Elterman et al.[42] suggest that optimal time for epidural catheter removal is between POD 4 and POD 5, without evidence of epidural hematoma. Similarly, other studies agree that POD 4 is optimal for removal,[41,43] while others suggest POD 5[50,51] However, there has been no reported epidural hematomas in the literature in this surgical population.

Spinal Analgesia

Preoperative intrathecal analgesia with long-acting opioids and local anesthetic has many of the same advantages as epidural analgesia.[52,53] Additionally, it avoids the risk of epidural hematoma as there is no catheter removal postoperatively.[54]

Regional Anesthesia Techniques: Peripheral Nerve Blocks

Transversus abdominal plane (TAP) blocks have been studied for lower abdominal surgeries, with a classic lateral approach covering T10–L1 sensory dermatomes, which would be inadequate for covering a right subcostal incision or a midline incision starting below the xyphoid process.[55] Therefore, some studies have been done employing a combination of multiple bilateral subcostal TAP blocks and a right lateral TAP block with some efficacy.[56] Subcostal approach to a TAP block covers T6–T9 of the thoracolaumbar nerves and provides analgesia below the xiphoid and parallel to the costal margin. Kitlik et al.[57] report a reduced 24-hour postoperative morphine consumption in living donor patients with right subcostal incision who received bilateral subcostal TAP blocks. TAP blocks have not been shown to improve other morbidity or mortality like neuraxial anesthesia.[57,58]

One of the limitations to single-shot block is the limited duration. A few studies have looked at employing a mixture of liposomal bupivacaine and bupivacaine for TAP blocks; although this was shown to be superior to no regional analgesia, it did not seem to be superior to TAP blocks with bupivacaine alone.[58]

Paravertebral block (PVB) provides visceral and incisional pain coverage and has been studied in patients' status post-RLDH with good outcomes.[59] One of the advantages over TEA is that while it provides the benefits of sympathectomy associated with epidurals, there is smaller risk of hypotension and concern for lower extremity motor blockade. Possible side effects are the risk of pneumothorax, and likewise the need for two catheters would be required instead of one, increasing the complexity and time of placement and management. Furthermore, the same anticoagulation guidelines are recommended for catheter removal. Chen et al.[60] demonstrated that continuous right thoracic paravertebral catheter, following bolus initial, can have opioid-sparing effect compared with sufentanil IV-PCA in patients undergoing right lobe hepatectomy, as well as lower pain scores at rest and with coughing. However, Schreiber et al.[61] demonstrated that PVBs are less effective than thoracic epidurals in the setting of liver resection and have similar risks to epidurals such as potential for hypotension and hematoma formation.

Erector spinae nerve (ESP) block is an interfascial plane block, superficial to a PVB, and thus offers the advantage of lesser risk of pneumothorax and is a technically less challenging procedure.[62]

CONCLUSION

Postoperative physiologic changes including coagulopathy and transient hepatitis can present challenges for acute postoperative pain management of patients undergoing RLDH. Multimodal analgesic regimen, including thoracic epidural analgesia or peripheral nerve block, with close monitoring can be effective.

REFERENCES

1. Roll GR, Parekh JR, Parker WF, et al. Left hepatectomy versus right hepatectomy for living donor liver transplantation: shifting the risk from the donor to the recipient. *Liver Transpl.* 2013;19(5):472–481.
2. Kurosaki I, Yamamoto S, Kitami C, et al. Video-assisted living donor hemihepatectomy through a 12-cm incision for adult-to-adult liver transplantation. *Surgery.* 2006;139(5):695–703.
3. Koffron AJ, Kung R, Baker T, Fryer J, Clark L, Abecassis M. Laparoscopic-assisted right lobe donor hepatectomy. *Am J Transplant.* 2006;6(10):2522–2525.
4. Nitta H, Sasaki A, Fujita T, et al. Laparoscopy-assisted major liver resections employing a hanging technique: the original procedure. *Ann Surg.* 2010;251(3):450–453.
5. Zhang B, Pan Y, Chen K, et al. Laparoscopy-assisted versus open hepatectomy for live liver donor: systematic review and meta-analysis. *Can J Gastroenterol Hepatol.* 2017;2017:2956749.
6. Cai X, Li Z, Zhang Y, et al. Laparoscopic liver resection and the learning curve: a 14-year, single-center experience. *Surg Endosc.* 2014;28(4):1334–1341.
7. Trotter JF, Talamantes M, McClure M, et al. Right hepatic lobe donation for living donor liver transplantation: impact on donor quality of life. *Liver Transpl.* 2001;7(6):485–493.
8. Cheah YL, Simpson MA, Pomposelli JJ, Pomfret EA. Incidence of death and potentially life-threatening near-miss events in living donor hepatic lobectomy: a world-wide survey. *Liver Transpl.* 2013;19(5):499–506.
9. Abecassis MM, Fisher RA, Olthoff KM, et al. Complications of living donor hepatic lobectomy—a comprehensive report. *Am J Transplant.* 2012;12(5):1208–1217.

10. Ghobrial RM, Freise CE, Trotter JF, et al. Donor morbidity after living donation for liver transplantation. *Gastroenterology.* 2008;135(2):468–476.
11. Pomfret EA, Pomposelli JJ, Gordon FD, et al. Liver regeneration and surgical outcome in donors of right-lobe liver grafts. *Transplantation.* 2003;76(1):5–10.
12. Cywinski JB, Parker BM, Xu M, Irefin SA. A comparison of postoperative pain control in patients after right lobe donor hepatectomy and major hepatic resection for tumor. *Anesth Analg.* 2004;99(6):1747–1752, table of contents.
13. Katz J, Cohen L, Schmid R, Chan VW, Wowk A. Postoperative morphine use and hyperalgesia are reduced by preoperative but not intraoperative epidural analgesia: implications for preemptive analgesia and the prevention of central sensitization. *Anesthesiology.* 2003;98(6):1449–1460.
14. Diaz GC, Renz JF, Mudge C, et al. Donor health assessment after living-donor liver transplantation. *Ann Surg.* 2002;236(1):120–126.
15. Kostopanagiotou G, Markantonis SL, Arkadopoulos N, et al. The effect of acutely induced hepatic failure on remifentanil and fentanyl blood levels in a pig model. *Eur J Anaesthesiol.* 2006;23(7):598–604.
16. Bosilkovska M, Walder B, Besson M, Daali Y, Desmeules J. Analgesics in patients with hepatic impairment: pharmacology and clinical implications. *Drugs.* 2012;72(12):1645–1669.
17. Nada EM, Alabdulkareem A. Morphine versus fentanyl patient-controlled analgesia for postoperative pain control in major hepatic resection surgeries including living liver donors: a retrospective study. *Saudi J Anaesth.* 2018;12(2):250–255.
18. Bodenham A, Quinn K, Park GR. Extrahepatic morphine metabolism in man during the anhepatic phase of orthotopic liver transplantation. *Br J Anaesthes.* 1989;63(4):380–384.
19. Mazoit JX, Sandouk P, Zetlaoui P, Scherrmann JM. Pharmacokinetics of unchanged morphine in normal and cirrhotic subjects. *Anesth Analg.* 1987;66(4):293–298.
20. Shelly MP, Quinn KG, Park GR. Pharmacokinetics of morphine in patients following orthotopic liver transplantation. *Br J Anaesthes.* 1989;63(4):375–379.
21. Marret E, Kurdi O, Zufferey P, Bonnet F. Effects of nonsteroidal anti-inflammatory drugs on patient-controlled analgesia morphine side effects: meta-analysis of randomized controlled trials. *Anesthesiology.* 2005;102(6):1249–1260.
22. Fretland AA, Hausken J, Edwin B, et al. Does ketorolac have an opioid sparing effect after open liver resection? data from the OSLO-COMET trial. Paper presented at International Hepato-Pancreato-Biliary Association, 2018.
23. Hokuto D, Nomi T, Kawaguchi C, et al. The administration of celecoxib as an analgesic after liver resection is safe. *Dig Surg.* 2017;34(2):108–113.
24. Schmid RL, Sandler AN, Katz J. Use and efficacy of low-dose ketamine in the management of acute postoperative pain: a review of current techniques and outcomes. *Pain.* 1999;82(2):111–125.
25. Halaszynski TM, Dai F, Huang Y. Donor hepatectomy surgery using ketamine to compliment analgesia and reduce morbidity: a retrospective chart review investigation. *Turk J Anaesthesiol Reanim.* 2018;46(1):28–37.
26. Galinski M, Delhotal-Landes B, Lockey DJ, et al. Reduction of paracetamol metabolism after hepatic resection. *Pharmacology.* 2006;77(4):161–165.
27. Hughes MJ, Harrison EM, Jin Y, Homer N, Wigmore SJ. Acetaminophen metabolism after liver resection: a prospective case-control study. *Dig Liver Dis.* 2015;47(12):1039–1046.
28. McGill MR, Jaeschke H. Metabolism and disposition of acetaminophen: recent advances in relation to hepatotoxicity and diagnosis. *Pharm Res.* 2013;30(9):2174–2187.
29. Allen S, DeRoche A, Adams L, et al. Effect of epidural compared to patient-controlled intravenous analgesia on outcomes for patients undergoing liver resection for neoplastic disease. *J Surg Oncol.* 2017;115(4):402–406.
30. Lin DX, Li X, Ye QW, Lin F, Li LL, Zhang QY. Implementation of a fast-track clinical pathway decreases postoperative length of stay and hospital charges for liver resection. *Cell Biochem Biophysics.* 2011;61(2):413–419.
31. van Dam RM, Hendry PO, Coolsen MM, et al. Initial experience with a multimodal enhanced recovery programme in patients undergoing liver resection. *Br J Surg.* 2008;95(8):969–975.
32. Rosero EB, Cheng GS, Khatri KP, Joshi GP. Evaluation of epidural analgesia for open major liver resection surgery from a US inpatient sample. *Proc (Bayl Univ Med Cent).* 2014;27(4):305–312.
33. Hase T, Takita K, Hashimoto T, Morimoto Y. [Coagulation profiles following donor hepatectomy and implications for the risk of epidural hematoma associated with epidural anesthesia]. *Masui.* 2011;60(7):840–845.
34. Cammu G, Troisi R, Cuomo O, de Hemptinne B, Di Florio E, Mortier E. Anaesthetic management and outcome in right-lobe living liver-donor surgery. *Eur J Anaesthesiol.* 2002;19(2):93–98.
35. Akpek EA, Arslan G, Erkaya C, et al. Anesthetic risks for donors in living-related liver transplantation: analysis of 30 cases. *Transpl Int.* 2003;16(8):486–490.
36. Cerutti E, Stratta C, Romagnoli R, et al. Thromboelastogram monitoring in the perioperative period of hepatectomy for adult living liver donation. *Liver Transpl.* 2004;10(2):289–294.
37. Barton JS, Riha GM, Differding JA, et al. Coagulopathy after a liver resection: is it over diagnosed and over treated? *HPB (Oxford).* 2013;15(11):865–871.
38. Borromeo CJ, Stix MS, Lally A, Pomfret EA. Epidural catheter and increased prothrombin time after right lobe hepatectomy for living donor transplantation. *Anesth Analg.* 2000;91(5):1139–1141.
39. Siniscalchi A, Begliomini B, De Pietri L, et al. Increased prothrombin time and platelet counts in living donor right hepatectomy: implications for epidural anesthesia. *Liver Transpl.* 2004;10(9):1144–1149.
40. Schumann R, Zabala L, Angelis M, Bonney I, Tighiouart H, Carr DB. Altered hematologic profiles following donor right hepatectomy and implications for perioperative analgesic management. *Liver Transpl.* 2004;10(3):363–368.
41. Choi SJ, Gwak MS, Ko JS, et al. The changes in coagulation profile and epidural catheter safety for living liver donors: a report on 6 years of our experience. *Liver Transpl.* 2007;13(1):62–70.
42. Elterman KG, Xiong Z. Coagulation profile changes and safety of epidural analgesia after hepatectomy: a retrospective study. *J Anesth.* 2015;29(3):367–372.
43. Koul A, Pant D, Rudravaram S, Sood J. Thoracic epidural analgesia in donor hepatectomy: an analysis. *Liver Transpl.* 2018;24(2):214–221.
44. Feltracco P, Brezzi ML, Barbieri S, Serra E, Milevoj M, Ori C. Epidural anesthesia and analgesia in liver resection and living donor hepatectomy. *Transplant Proc.* 2008;40(4):1165–1168.
45. Jones RM, Moulton CE, Hardy KJ. Central venous pressure and its effect on blood loss during liver resection. *Br J Surg.* 1998;85(8):1058–1060.
46. Page A, Rostad B, Staley CA, et al. Epidural analgesia in hepatic resection. *J Am Coll Surg.* 2008;206(6):1184–1192.
47. Su J, Soliz JM, Popat KU, Gebhardt R. Incidence of epidural hematoma from use of epidural analgesia for hepatic resection surgery: a retrospective study. *J Clin Anesth.* 2020;62:109719.
48. Jacquenod P, Wallon G, Gazon M, et al. Incidence and risk factors of coagulation profile derangement after liver surgery: implications for the use of epidural analgesia: a retrospective cohort study. *Anesth Analg.* 2018;126(4):1142–1147.
49. Tzimas P, Prout J, Papadopoulos G, Mallett SV. Epidural anaesthesia and analgesia for liver resection. *Anaesthesia.* 2013;68(6):628–635.
50. Stamenkovic DM, Jankovic ZB, Toogood GJ, Lodge JP, Bellamy MC. Epidural analgesia and liver resection: postoperative coagulation disorders and epidural catheter removal. *Minerva Anestesiol.* 2011;77(7):671–679.
51. Karna ST, Pandey CK, Sharma S, Singh A, Tandon M, Pandey VK. Postoperative coagulopathy after live related donor hepatectomy: incidence, predictors and implications for safety of thoracic epidural catheter. *J Postgrad Med.* 2015;61(3):176–180.

52. Tang JZJ, Weinberg L. A literature review of intrathecal morphine analgesia in patients undergoing major open hepato-pancreatic-biliary (HPB) surgery. *Anesth Pain Med.* 2019;9(6):e94441.
53. Lee SH, Gwak MS, Choi SJ, et al. Prospective, randomized study of ropivacaine wound infusion versus intrathecal morphine with intravenous fentanyl for analgesia in living donors for liver transplantation. *Liver Transpl.* 2013;19(9):1036–1045.
54. Nguyen M, Vandenbroucke F, Roy JD, et al. Evaluation of the addition of bupivacaine to intrathecal morphine and fentanyl for postoperative pain management in laparascopic liver resection. *Reg Anesth Pain Med.* 2010;35(3):261–266.
55. Tsai HC, Yoshida T, Chuang TY, et al. Transversus abdominis plane block: an updated review of anatomy and techniques. *Biomed Res Int.* 2017;2017:8284363.
56. Milan ZB, Duncan B, Rewari V, Kocarev M, Collin R. Subcostal transversus abdominis plane block for postoperative analgesia in liver transplant recipients. *Transplant Proc.* 2011;43(7):2687–2690.
57. Kitlik A, Erdogan MA, Ozgul U, et al. Ultrasound-guided transversus abdominis plane block for postoperative analgesia in living liver donors: a prospective, randomized, double-blinded clinical trial. *J Clin Anesth.* 2017;37:103–107.
58. Amundson AW, Olsen DA, Smith HM, et al. Acute benefits after liposomal bupivacaine abdominal wall blockade for living liver donation: a retrospective review. *Mayo Clin Proc Innov Qual Outcomes.* 2018;2(2):186–193.
59. Mistry K, Hutchins J, Leiting J, Mangalick K, Pruett T, Chinnakotla S. Continuous paravertebral infusions as an effective adjunct for postoperative pain management in living liver donors: a retrospective observational study. *Transplant Proc.* 2017;49(2):309–315.
60. Chen H, Liao Z, Fang Y, et al. Continuous right thoracic paravertebral block following bolus initiation reduced postoperative pain after right-lobe hepatectomy: a randomized, double-blind, placebo-controlled trial. *Reg Anesth Pain Med.* 2014;39(6):506–512.
61. Schreiber KL, Chelly JE, Lang RS, et al. Epidural versus paravertebral nerve block for postoperative analgesia in patients undergoing open liver resection: a randomized clinical trial. *Reg Anesth Pain Med.* 2016;41(4):460–468.
62. Tulgar S, Ahiskalioglu A, De Cassai A, Gurkan Y. Efficacy of bilateral erector spinae plane block in the management of pain: current insights. *J Pain Res.* 2019;12:2597–2613.

REVIEW QUESTIONS

(1) A 37-year-old female presents for open right liver donor hepatectomy (RLDH). What is the most effective technique for pain management?

A. Bilateral lateral tranversus abdominis plane (TAP) block
B. Thoracic epidural analgesia at the mid thoracic level (T5–T8)
C. Lumbar epidural analgesia
D. Bilateral erector spinae blocks

(2) A major concern for patients with thoracic epidurals after RLDH is an increased risk of epidural hematoma postoperatively. Liver function tests, and blood clotting in particular, are often abnormal for several days postoperatively for living liver donors. When is typically the best day to remove the thoracic epidural catheter?

A. POD 1–2
B. POD 3–4
C. POD 4–5
D. POD 5–6

(3) A 33-year-old healthy patient underwent RLDH. The patient received preoperative T6–T7 thoracic epidural, and an infusion of 0.125% bupivacaine and 4 mcg/mL fentanyl was started prior to incision. The surgery proceeded without a complication, and the patient was extubated and brought to the surgical intensive care unit (SICU). On POD 1 you find the patient to be tachypneic and complaining of 10/10 upper abdominal pain. The SICU nurse tells you that the patient has been in severe pain despite many boluses of IV fentanyl. On exam there is no sensory deficit, and boluses through the epidural with increasing concentrations of local anesthetics do not provide relief. What is the most appropriate management?

A. Remove the epidural catheter and replace a thoracic epidural catheter at T7–T8 or T8–T9 level.
B. Remove the epidural catheter and perform bilateral transversus abdominis plane (TAP) blocks.
C. Start patient on IV hydromorphone patient-controlled analgesia (PCA); stop the epidural infusion. Check the coagulation profile and platelet count and remove the catheter once the coagulation profile normalizes.
D. Perform bilateral TAP blocks, start patient on IV hydromorphone PCA; stop epidural infusion and remove the catheter on POD 4 once coagulation profile normalizes.

(4) Your medical center has a high volume of liver transplants. You are developing an enhanced recovery after surgery (ERAS) protocol to improve outcomes for patients undergoing open RLDH via a right subcostal and a midline incision extending from xyphoid process to umbilicus. What levels need to be covered by regional or neuraxial technique to decrease incisional pain?

A. Right T6–T12 levels
B. Right T6–T10 levels
C. Right T6–T 12 levels, left T6–T10 levels
D. Bilateral T6–T10 levels

(5) A healthy 35-year-old gravida 2 para 2 female is scheduled for right liver donor hepatectomy (RLDH). She had lumbar epidural analgesia catheters for her 2 normal spontaneous deliveries NSVD and has not had any other surgeries or procedures requiring anesthesia. You are seeing her 2 weeks prior to her surgery in order to perform a pre-anesthesia evaluation as well as consent her for anesthesia. What is the most appropriate approach for discussing options for postoperative analgesia?

A. Let her know that thoracic epidural analgesia (TEA) is the best and most studied option for postoperative analgesia. Mention higher risk of hematomas but reassure her that it is still very low and there are no known incidents of this.
B. Your institution does not normally perform TEA due to a higher possibility of epidural hematomas but performs bilateral subcostal TAP blocks. Discuss TAP blocks with the patient, and mention that this is a very safe, effective technique.
C. All of the above
D. None of the above

(6) Which of the following is NOT a good regional anesthesia alternative to TEA in terms of postoperative coagulopathy concerns?

A. Preoperative spinal morphine
B. Bilateral erector spinae catheters
C. Bilateral paravertebral block catheters
D. Bilateral subcostal TAP blocks

(7) A 39-year-old male, with no significant past medical or surgical history, undergoes RLDH, with a T6–T7 TEA catheter placed preoperatively. Postoperatively, he is in severe pain, despite receiving preoperative and postoperative intravenous acetaminophen, gabapentin, TEA with 0.125% bupivacaine, and 16 mcg/mL hydromorphone, with an adequate sensory level and being started on a hydromorphone IV PCA. On the night of POD 0, the epidural solution is switched to 0.2% bupivacaine with 16 mcg/mL of hydromorphone at rate of 10 mL/hr. When you see him at 11 a.m. on POD 1, his pain control is improved, 4–5/10. However, on motor exam he cannot move his lower extremities and has bilateral foot drop. What is the most appropriate action?

A. Let the primary team know that this is an expected finding, as the patient is receiving a higher dose of epidural bupivacaine. Continue with current pain management.
B. Obtain a STAT magnetic resonance imaging (MRI) of thoracic and lumbar spine to look for infection or hematoma.
C. Let the primary team and the patient know that you are concerned for a possibility of epidural hematoma. Stop the epidural infusion and remove the catheter. Obtain STAT CT of the spine. Consent the patient for bilateral TAP, paravertebral, or ESP block catheters.
D. Let the primary team and the patient know that you are concerned for a possibility of epidural hematoma. Turn off epidural infusion immediately, obtain CBC, PT, and PTT. If motor function does not return promptly, STAT CT and MRI of the spine.

ANSWERS

(1) **B.** Thoracic epidural analgesia (TEA) at the mid thoracic level (T5–T8) is the best-studied neuraxial or regional modality for postoperative pain relief after RLDH and has been associated with decreased use of opioids as well as a reduction in morbidity and mortality, including deep venous thrombosis (DVT), PE, and odds of pneumonia. Likewise, recent studies have demonstrated the use of TEA as part of fast-track protocols or enhanced recovery pathways for liver resection patients with a reduced hospital stay.

References

Lin DX, Li X, Ye QW, Lin F, Li LL, Zhang QY. Implementation of a fast-track clinical pathway decreases postoperative length of stay and hospital charges for liver resection. *Cell Biochem Biophys.* 2011;61(2):413–419.

Koul A, Pant D, Rudravaram S, Sood J. Thoracic epidural analgesia in donor hepatectomy: An analysis. *Liver Transpl.* 2018 Feb;24(2):214–221. doi: 10.1002/lt.24989. PMID: 29205784.

(2) **C.** Optimal time for epidural catheter removal after liver resection is postoperative day (POD) 4 or POD 5. The coagulation profile is altered with maximal increase in prothrombin time (PT) around POD 2, a nadir in platelets around POD 3, and a maximal increase in liver function tests on POD 1 and a downward trend thereafter. Some studies suggest that while PT and PTT may be prolonged postoperatively in patients undergoing major liver resection surgery, analysis via TEG shows that actual coagulation is not altered. If removal is needed before that, a coagulation profile and platelet count can be checked, as it may come back within normal.

References

Borromeo CJ, Stix MS, Lally A, Pomfret EA. Epidural catheter and increased prothrombin time after right lobe hepatectomy for living donor transplantation. *Anesth Analg.* 2000;91(5):1139–1141.

Cerutti E, Stratta C, Romagnoli R, et al. Thromboelastogram monitoring in the perioperative period of hepatectomy for adult living liver donation. *Liver Transpl.* 2004;10(2):289–294.

Elterman KG, Xiong Z. Coagulation profile changes and safety of epidural analgesia after hepatectomy: a retrospective study. *J Anesth.* 2015;29(3):367–372.

(3) **C.** Start patient on intravenous hydromorphone patient-controlled analgesia; stop the epidural infusion and remove the catheter once coagulation profile normalizes, usually around the fourth postoperative day. Given that there is no evidence of sensory blockade on exam and no pain relief with a bolus, most likely this epidural catheter is misplaced. Intravenous opioids should be started to alleviate the acute pain. In light of postoperative coagulopathy, removal of epidural catheter is not recommended until the coagulation profile and plate count normalize given the risk of epidural hematoma. TAP blocks are not recommended since they provide sensory block T10 and below. Subcostal TAP block can be an option.

References

Stamenkovic DM, Jankovic ZB, Toogood GJ, Lodge JP, Bellamy MC. Epidural analgesia and liver resection: postoperative coagulation disorders and epidural catheter removal. *Minerva Anestesiol.* 2011;77(7):671–679.

Karna ST, Pandey CK, Sharma S, Singh A, Tandon M, Pandey VK. Postoperative coagulopathy after live related donor hepatectomy: incidence, predictors and implications for safety of thoracic epidural catheter. *J Postgrad Med.* 2015;61(3):176–180.

(4) **D.** Surgical approach for RLDH commonly include a bilateral subcostal incision (chevron incision) with or without vertical extension, or a right subcostal incision with a midline sub-xyphoid extension (reserve L incision), a J-shaped incision, or an upper midline incision. Most commonly RLDH is carried out with a right subcostal incision, and an epigastric midline incision, which may need to be extended to the umbilicus. Thus bilateral T6–T10 blocks are often required.

Reference

Roll GR, Parekh JR, Parker WF, et al. Left hepatectomy versus right hepatectomy for living donor liver transplantation: shifting the risk from the donor to the recipient. *Liver Transpl.* 2013;19(5):472–481.

(5) **C.** Thoracic epidural analgesia (TEA) is still the best-studied modality for intraoperative and postoperative analgesia after RLDH. Despite the low incidence, some centers opt to avoid TEA, while others still utilize it after discussing with the patient at length the benefits and potential rare risks. Subcostal approach to a TAP block covers T6–T9 of the thoracolaumbar nerves and provides analgesia below the xiphoid and parallel to the costal margin. Studies have shown a decreased 24-hour postoperative morphine consumption in living donor patients with right subcostal incision who received bilateral subcostal TAP blocks.

References

Koul A, Pant D, Rudravaram S, Sood J. Thoracic epidural analgesia in donor hepatectomy: an analysis. *Liver Transpl.* 2018;24(2):214–221.

Kitlik A, Erdogan MA, Ozgul U, et al. Ultrasound-guided transversus abdominis plane block for postoperative analgesia in living liver donors: a prospective, randomized, double-blinded clinical trial. *J Clin Anesth.* 2017;37:103–107.

(6) **C.** Bilateral paravertebral block (PVB) is not a good alternative to epidural catheters in cases of coagulopathy. PVBs provide visceral and incisional pain coverage and have been studied in patients' status post-RLDH with good outcomes. PVBs provide the benefits of sympathectomy associated with epidurals, while decreasing the risk of hypotension and concern for lower extremity motor blockade. However, the same anticoagulation guidelines are recommended for catheter removal to avoid the development of a hematoma.

Reference

Mistry K, Hutchins J, Leiting J, Mangalick K, Pruett T, Chinnakotla S. Continuous paravertebral infusions as an effective adjunct for postoperative pain management in living liver donors: a retrospective observational study. *Transplant Proc.* 2017;49(2):309–315.

(7) **D.** Epidural hematoma, while rare, is considered a medical emergency. Typically, it presents with back pain, progressive sensory and/or motor deficit, and can lead to complete or partial paraplegia. For this reason, early detection and immediate surgical decompression are key to prevent further deterioration of neurologic deficits. The clinical factors that affect neurologic prognosis are progression of clinical signs, grade of neurologic deficits, and duration and location of spinal cord compression. MRI is considered the gold standard for imaging; make sure to verify that your epidural catheter is MRI compatible.

Reference

Horlocker TT, Wedel DJ, Rowlingson JC, Enneking FK, Kopp SL, Benzon HT, Brown DL, Heit JA, Mulroy MF, Rosenquist RW, Tryba M, Yuan CS. Regional anesthesia in the patient receiving antithrombotic or thrombolytic therapy: American Society of Regional Anesthesia and Pain Medicine Evidence-Based Guidelines (Third Edition). *Reg Anesth Pain Med.* 2010;35(1):64–101.

18.

POSTOPERATIVE PAIN MANAGEMENT OF OPEN NEPHRECTOMY

Stanislav Sidash and Yatish Ranganath

STEM CASE AND KEY QUESTIONS

A 57-year-old obese female is scheduled for open left nephrectomy for renal cell carcinoma. The procedure is going to be done through a left subcostal incision. The patient's past medical history is significant for sleep apnea, hypertension, and coronary heart disease. The patient had a thoracic epidural placed preoperatively at T7–T8. One hour before the end of the procedure you start the epidural infusion, and the patient seems to be comfortable; however, in the middle of the night you are called because of uncontrolled pain.

(1) WHAT ARE THE SURGICAL IMPLICATIONS OF SUBCOSTAL INCISION?

A flank-subcostal incision has the advantage of direct access to the kidney and the ability to avoid entry into the peritoneal cavity. This is especially advantageous in obese patients. Therefore, surgical complications are minimized as the approach remains extra-peritoneal and extra-pleural.

(2) DESCRIBE THE SEVERITY OF POSTOPERATIVE PAIN, IMPORTANCE OF THE SITE, AND THE RELATIONSHIP TO THE DIAPHRAGM AND THE RESPIRATORY MUSCLES.

Open nephrectomy is associated with a significant degree of acute pain. The pain has two nociceptive components: somatic and visceral pain. Somatic pain arising from the anterior abdominal wall, usually in the distribution of (T9–T11) for flank incisions, represents 70%–75% of the pain and is mainly significant for 72 hours following open surgery. Visceral pain is intense but short-lived, diffuse, and usually is significant for 24–36 hours.

The incidence of significant respiratory muscle dysfunction after upper abdominal surgery has been shown to approach 20%–40%.[1,2] Furthermore, postoperative respiratory failure after abdominal surgery has a 10-fold increase of 30-day mortality.[3]

(3) LIST THE COMMON REGIONAL ANALGESIA TECHNIQUES FOR OPEN NEPHRECTOMY. DISCUSS THE ADVANTAGES AND DISADVANTAGES OF THORACIC EPIDURAL ANALGESIA FOR ABDOMINAL SURGERY.

There are many ways to treat postoperative pain in this patient. Medical treatment alone is always a choice. Thoracic epidural analgesia (TEA) has been the standard practice. Other regional anesthesia options include the use of intrathecal opioids, paravertebral, transversus abdominis plane (TAP block), quadratus lumborum block (QLB block), and erector spinae block (ESPB) (Table 18.1).

(4) AFTER THE PATIENT'S AGREEMENT, YOU DECIDE TO PLACE A TEA. WHAT IS THE BEST SITE FOR PLACING A THORACIC EPIDURAL FOR NEPHRECTOMY?

The epidural blockade is most effective when the site of catheter insertion is in a location that corresponds to the dermatomes covered by the surgical incision. The most rapid onset and the densest block occur at the site of injection. By inserting the catheter closer to the dermatomal distribution of the surgical site, a lower dose of drug can be given, thereby reducing side effects. A mid-thoracic epidural (T6–T8) with a T5–T10 sensory level is appropriate for most open nephrectomies and upper abdominal surgeries.

(5) ONE HOUR BEFORE THE END OF THE PROCEDURE, AN EPIDURAL BOLUS OF 5 ML OF MIXTURE OF BUPIVACAINE 0.125% AND FENTANYL 2 MCG/ML WAS ADMINISTERED, THEN 6 ML/H CONTINUOUS INFUSION WAS STARTED. THE PATIENT WAKES UP COMFORTABLE; HOWEVER, IN THE MIDDLE OF THE NIGHT, YOU ARE CALLED BECAUSE OF UNCONTROLLED PAIN AT THE INCISION SITE. WHAT TO DO?

To evaluate whether an epidural is functioning appropriately (correct placement with the catheter tip in the epidural space), perform the following steps:

Table 18.1 COMMON REGIONAL ANESTHESIA TECHNIQUES FOR OPEN NEPHRECTOMY

REGIONAL TECHNIQUE	EFFECT ON PAIN	ADVANTAGES	DISADVANTAGES	CATHETER PLACEMENT
Thoracic epidural analgesia (TEA)	Somatic and visceral analgesia	Strong evidence Earlier recovery of bowel function Improved pulmonary outcomes Attenuation of the stress response Improved failure rate with fluoroscopic guidance	Not shown to decrease length of stay Complicates thromboprophylaxis	Convenient
Paravertebral blocks (PVBs)	Somatic and visceral analgesia	Analgesia like neuraxial anesthesia Fewer side effects Improved safety profile with ultrasound guidance	Technically difficult Highly operator dependent Risk of pneumothorax Increased catheter displacement	Convenient
TAP blocks	Somatic analgesia only	Opioid sparing Less complicated thromboprophylaxis Fewer side effects	No visceral analgesia Short duration of effect with single injection	Convenient but needs to be placed postop
Quadratus lumborum blocks (QLBs)	Somatic and possible visceral analgesia	Potentially opioid sparing Longer duration of action compared to TAP block Fewer side effects	Effectiveness not well studied	Convenient but needs to be placed postop
Erector spinae blocks (ESPBs)	Somatic and possible visceral analgesia	Potentially opioid sparing Less invasive compared to TEA and PVB Less complicated thromboprophylaxis Fewer side effects	Effectiveness not well studied	Convenient

- Inspect the epidural catheter and the dressing.
- Assess whether the patient has a "sensory level"; temperature discrimination (ice) and response to pinprick should be diminished or absent in the dermatomes that correspond to the level of sensory blockade.
- Feel the area expected to be blocked by the epidural and determine if it is warm to touch.
- If the above steps yield equivocal or negative results, consider testing the epidural with a 5 mL of 1%–2% lidocaine with or without epinephrine. This test dose should be administered in a monitored setting with resuscitation medications and drugs available. Evaluate the dermatomes expected to be blocked for temperature discrimination and pain perception at regular intervals for up to 20–30 minutes following a test dose. Ask the patient to rate their pain scores before and after the test dose. Monitor vital signs for any indication of sympathectomy-induced hypotension. Improvement in analgesia, hypotension, and presence of a sensory level after a test dose are indicative of a working epidural. If negative or equivocal, repeat the testing with 5 mL of 2% lidocaine. In cases of unilateral blockade despite appropriate depth of insertion, consider pulling the catheter back by 1–2 cm, leaving 3–4 cm of the catheter inside prior to testing.
- It is advisable not to administer more than 100 mg lidocaine at a time while testing for a thoracic epidural. If the catheter remains equivocal, the catheter should be removed and replaced at this stage.

(6) YOU HAVE DONE ALL THE ABOVE TESTING AND YOU FOUND THAT THE EPIDURAL IS FUNCTIONING, BUT THE PATIENT IS STILL COMPLAINING OF SIGNIFICANT PAIN. WHAT SHOULD YOU DO?

Persistent pain despite a functioning epidural may occur on several occasions and the following things need to be reviewed:

- Check the epidural pump for proper functionality and programming. Make sure all the catheter and tubing connections are adequate.
- Appropriate selection of agents to be used in the epidural infusion and adequate dosing of the epidural are key factors to be considered. Common drugs used in a thoracic epidural infusion include bupivacaine (0.05%–0.25%), fentanyl (2–5 mcg/mL) and hydromorphone (5–15 mcg/mL). For the opioids, the higher end of the dose range is used for opioid-tolerant patients and the lower end for older patients. In a hypotensive patient, running the epidural infusion at the desired rate may not be feasible.
- If the blockade is unilateral and the operative side is less blocked, placing the patient operative side down may be helpful. This issue can sometimes be corrected by withdrawing the catheter 1–2 centimeters. Replacement of the catheter may be required in other cases to achieve optimal pain control.
- Patchy block is treated with a bolus dose of local anesthetic (LA), or addition of opioids may be helpful in such a

scenario, with catheter replacement being the ultimate management. Patchy block may also be indicative of subdural catheter.

- Larger incisions, multiple incisions, and incisions farther away from the area covered by the epidural may require higher doses, frequent top-ups, and adjunctive measures for pain control.
- Site of pain needs to be examined. A patient may not have much pain at the incision site but may complain of referred pain in the shoulder due to the phrenic nerve neuropraxia (with nephrectomy or thoracotomy). Nonsteroidal anti-inflammatory drugs (NSAIDs) and other adjuncts may be helpful in such cases, as any type of surgery causes both inflammation and pain.

(7) YOU GAVE A 5 ML BOLUS OF BUPIVACAINE 0.125% WITH 2 MCG/ML OF FENTANYL, AND THE INFUSION WAS INCREASED AT 8 ML/H. THE PATIENT REPORTS SOME IMPROVEMENT, BUT THE PAIN IS STILL SO SIGNIFICANT THAT SHE CANNOT USE THE INCENTIVE SPIROMETRY. WHAT ARE THE NEXT STEPS?

In case of inadequate analgesia with TEA, a reasonable strategy would be increasing the total amount of medication the patient receives per hour. This can be done either by increasing solution concentration, rate of infusion, or both. If the patient has a functioning epidural, the rate of bupivacaine 0.125% can be safely increased to 10 mL/hr depending on the level of epidural catheter insertion and patient's body habitus. Curatolo et al.[4] applied an optimization model in 190 patients to find the best dosage combination and infusion rates of bupivacaine and fentanyl for TEA in major abdominal surgery. The two optimal regimens were: (1) 13 mg/h bupivacaine with 25 mcg/h fentanyl, and (2) 8 mg/h bupivacaine with 30 mcg/h fentanyl.

(8) YOU DISCUSS THE NEED TO PROVIDE SOME OPIOIDS AND NSAIDS WITH YOUR SURGICAL COLLEAGUES. THEY TELL YOU THAT SHE WILL DEVELOP RESPIRATORY DEPRESSION BECAUSE SHE HAS OPIOIDS IN THE EPIDURAL SOLUTION AND NSAIDS ARE NOT SAFE IN NEPHRECTOMY. HOW DO YOU RESPOND?

Although epidural analgesia forms the mainstay for postoperative pain management, supplementation with other measures is frequently necessary for reasons discussed earlier (see questions 4 and 5). Use of parenteral opioids as the second line for pain management is often required for patients with poor pain control. Parenteral opioids can be used safely when administered with neuraxial opioids in the presence of adequate monitoring. The use of NSAIDs should be considered on a case-by-case basis.

(9) THE NEXT DAY, THE FLOOR NURSE ASKS YOU IF IT IS OKAY TO AMBULATE THE PATIENT. HOW DO YOU RESPOND?

TEA covering just the surgical dermatomes has a low incidence of sympathetic and motor blockade of the lower limbs. The choice of appropriate level for the epidural placement is critical.[5] However, the proximity of the epidural catheter to lumbar levels seems to increase the risk of lower extremity motor block.[6] Usually, the spread of LA to the lower lumbar levels to affect the lower extremities would not be expected. Unreasonably high levels of TEA would be limited by other side effects, such as hemodynamics changes, prior to causing lower extremity motor blockade.

(10) WILL THE TEA RESULT IN URINARY RETENTION? WHAT IS THE INCIDENCE USING THE MIXTURE OF 0.125% BUPIVACAINE AND 2 MCG/ML FENTANYL?

Urinary retention is a common problem, with an overall incidence of 5% to 70%, depending on a multitude of factors.[7] With mixture of bupivacaine and fentanyl in a thoracic epidural for abdominal surgery, the incidence is 5.5%–13%.[8,9]

(11) BRIEFLY REVIEW THE OTHER REGIONAL ANESTHESIA TECHNIQUES THAT CAN BE USED FOR OPEN NEPHRECTOMY.

A variety of regional anesthesia techniques other than TEA can be used to provide analgesia for abdominal surgeries. Paravertebral block has been used for analgesia of unilateral procedures of the abdomen and thorax. Several studies have looked at the efficacy of TAP block for renal surgery. In addition, multiple case reports involving QLBs and a case series utilizing a modified QLB technique with subcostal approach to the anterior QLB have been described. The modified subcostal anterior QLB approach provides appropriate thoracic dermatome level (T6–L 2) needed for analgesia following open urological surgical procedures. Multiple case reports describe the usefulness of erector spinae plane block (ESPB) for nephrectomies. Intrathecal morphine (ITM) is associated with great analgesia for up to 24 hours without serious complications. However, side effects such as pruritus, urinary retention, nausea, and vomiting remain common, with respiratory depression being uncommon.

Surgical site infiltration is another available mode of analgesia as part of multimodal approach and advanced recovery protocols. Continuous LA infusions have been shown to be effective for pain control after abdominal surgeries.

DISCUSSION

Renal cell carcinoma (RCC) accounts for 2%–3% of all cancers and is the third most common malignancy of the genitourinary tract.[10,11] Open nephrectomy is still a common surgical procedure used in the management of resectable renal masses.

With advances in minimally invasive surgery, laparoscopic nephrectomy is now a widely performed feasible treatment alternative.[12,13] The surgical approach is individualized and largely determined by surgeon preference, disease process, the patient's body habitus and comorbidities, known anatomic anomalies, prior surgical history, and renal function. Partial nephrectomy or nephron-sparing surgery is performed in patients with small tumors (<7 cm in diameter, tumors at poles and not extending to renal hilum), polycystic kidney disease, and in those at risk of significant renal impairment or disease recurrence.[3]

The indications for radical surgical excision are: stage I–II RCC confined to the kidneys; stage III RCC with involvement of major vessels/extra-renal tissues or retroperitoneal lymph nodes; RCC with involvement of cardiac muscle/inferior vena cava or adrenal gland. Patients with radical nephrectomy for RCC confined to the kidney have a 5-year survival rate of 80%–90%, but these patients are at a high risk for further renal function impairment.[14]

In many institutions across the United States, open procedures have been replaced by laparoscopic techniques (especially with tumor size < 10 cm) because they offer similar RCC outcomes, decrease analgesic requirements, reduce length of stay, reduce intraoperative blood loss, and enable faster patient recuperation after surgery. Open techniques are preferable when warm ischemia times matter, such as in cases of solitary kidney, as laparoscopic techniques require a great deal of technical skill and may take longer times. Therefore, in the new era of minimally invasive surgery, highly complex renal tumors in the setting of patient comorbidity may still be better managed with open nephrectomy.[15,16]

SURGICAL INCISIONS

The most commonly used surgical approaches for open nephrectomy are flank, trans-abdominal (anterior subcostal, chevron, or midline trans-peritoneal), and thoraco-abdominal (Figure 18.1). A *flank incision* has the advantage of direct access to the kidney and the ability to avoid entry into the peritoneal cavity. This is especially advantageous in the growing obese population of patients with increased intra-abdominal adipose deposition and patients with "non-virgin" abdomens. Therefore, surgical complications are minimized as the approach remains extra-peritoneal and extra-pleural. However, lateral incisions necessitate division of large muscles, risk peripheral nerve injury, and may result in postoperative flank bulge or hernia, as well as significant pain and increased postoperative opioid requirement. It is more appropriate for partial nephrectomies. A standard *anterior subcostal incision* gives very limited visibility, so it is best reserved for small renal tumors or benign conditions. *Bilateral subcostal (Chevron)* or *extended subcostal* incision may be required to obtain better anterior access for large complex kidney tumors, bilateral renal tumors, inferior vena cava (IVC) thrombus, and polycystic bilateral nephrectomies. An *anterior trans-peritoneal incision* (laparotomy) is a popular approach for major procedures of the kidney, ureter, and adrenal gland. It provides an opportunity to evaluate other intra-abdominal organs, allows rapid access to the renal hilum and excellent exposure of bladder and retroperitoneal lymph nodes, and affords good control of the great vessels if they are injured. Pain is also minimized by avoiding muscle division. However, a midline laparotomy provides relatively poor access to the kidney because the renal hilum is at the upper limit of the incision and the overlying colon, liver, and spleen must be mobilized widely. There is risk of late bowel obstruction and incisional hernia.[17,18] Dermatomes requiring regional anesthesia blockade vary depending upon the surgical incision used: flank (T9–T11); trans-abdominal subcostal (T6–T9); trans-abdominal midline (T6–T10); thoraco-abdominal (T5–T12) (Figure 18.1–18.2).

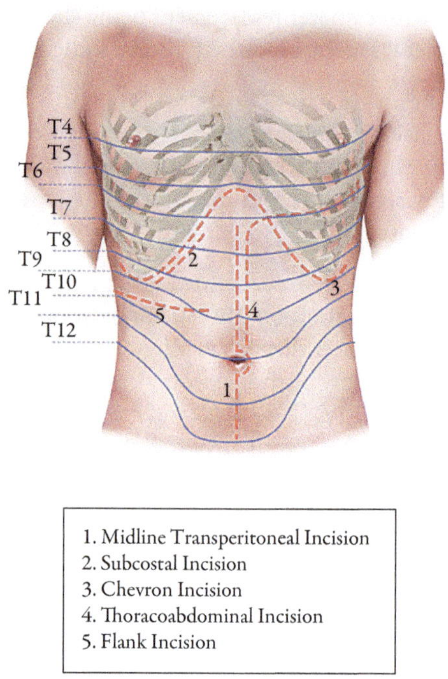

Figure 18.1. Open nephrectomy incisions and dermatomes.

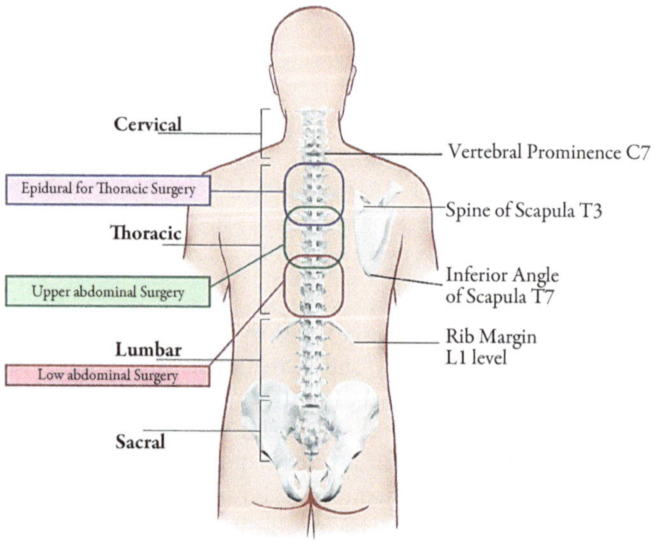

Figure 18.2. Thoracic epidural surface landmarks and areas of the thoracic spine for epidural catheter insertion for various surgeries.

THE SEVERITY OF PAIN AND EFFECT ON RESPIRATION

Open nephrectomy is associated with a significant degree of acute pain. It is well reported that the function of the respiratory muscles is affected during and after abdominal surgery. The site of the operation, as well as the type, are the most important factors affecting the respiratory muscles.[1] Indeed, it has been shown that the incidence of significant respiratory muscle dysfunction after lower abdominal surgery is very low (2%–5%) while that of upper abdominal surgery may approach 20%–40%.[2] The diaphragm covers the upper third of the kidneys posteriorly and is the predominant respiratory muscle to be affected during upper abdominal surgery. However, intercostal muscles can also be affected, depending on the surgical approach and due to positioning. The mechanism that underlies the reduction in diaphragmatic strength and the shift to predominantly rib cage breathing is not fully understood. Diaphragmatic muscle contractility does not seem to be directly affected by upper abdominal surgery. Pain afferents and inhibitory reflex generated due to manipulation of the diaphragm and the surrounding intra-abdominal organs during the surgical procedure are believed to be the main factors responsible for reflex inhibition of the phrenic nerve output following surgery.[2,19] Besides, there have been reports of decrease in maximum inspiratory, transdiaphragmatic, and expiratory muscle pressures observed after upper abdominal surgery in several studies.[2,20] This decrease is sustained for 48 hours after surgery and may persist for a week, gradually returning to normal.[21] Besides, a shift to predominantly rib cage breathing indicates that the intercostal inspiratory muscles are more active.[27]

Dysfunction of the respiratory muscles is greatly reduced when upper abdominal surgery is performed with laparoscopy rather than open laparotomy.[19,21,23] TEA has also been shown to attenuate inhibition of phrenic motor output following upper abdominal incision in animal studies.[24] In another human study, TEA has also shown to improve post–abdominal surgery diaphragmatic dysfunction in humans, as measured by abdominal contribution to tidal volume.[25] Several physical maneuvers have been tested in order to reverse this inhibition of the respiratory muscles. Inspiratory muscle training including maneuvers such as intermittent positive pressure breathing, incentive spirometry, and deep breathing exercises have been shown to significantly reduce pulmonary complications and length of hospital stay after abdominal surgery.[26–28]

ADVANTAGES OF REGIONAL ANESTHESIA

When no regional anesthesia was used, the cumulative intravenous (IV) morphine consumption median for open nephrectomy with patient-controlled analgesia (PCA) was 32.5 mg, 44 mg, and 55.5 mg at 24, 48, and 72, hours respectively. This was reduced by over 50% to 10 mg, 20.5 mg, and 28.5 mg in the study group with TEA.[29] Common regional techniques employed for open nephrectomy are listed in Table 18.1. TEA has been the most common regional anesthesia technique employed during any major abdominal surgery, including open nephrectomy. To this day it remains the gold standard for postoperative pain control and overall complication risk reduction. TEA provides optimal analgesia, decreases persistent postoperative pain, minimizes opioid consumption, ensures earlier weaning from mechanical ventilation, and decreases pulmonary complications, attenuates stress response from surgery, reduces perioperative cardiac stress and morbidity, improves gastrointestinal motility, and lowers all-cause mortality.[30,31] However, the role of TEA has been questioned recently with the implementation of enhanced recovery after surgery (ERAS) protocols, as there are some undesirable effects related to epidural that may hinder recovery.[32] These include hypotension, excessive fluid administration, difficulty in early mobilization, and need for intensive nursing care. Further, TEA placement can present challenges related to technical difficulties (traditional TEA techniques have failure rates of 12%–40%, depending on study design and definition of "failure" used) and management of postoperative thromboprophylaxis. [33] Patients undergoing radical nephrectomy are at a higher risk of thromboembolic phenomena due to malignancy. They often undergo IVC thrombectomy and may need full therapeutic anticoagulation postoperatively.

CHOOSING THE SITE FOR EPIDURAL PLACEMENT

A midthoracic epidural (T6–T8) with a T5–T10 sensory level is appropriate for most open nephrectomies and upper abdominal surgeries. Epidural catheter placement between T8 and T10 is usually appropriate for lower abdominal procedures. For thoracotomies, epidural catheters may be placed slightly higher, between T5 and T7, to obtain segmental level of T4–T8 to cover thoracotomy incision as well as the chest tube insertion site (Figure 18.1).

TROUBLESHOOTING NONWORKING EPIDURAL ANALGESIA

The epidural space is a nonuniform space, and distribution of the LA can vary widely among patients due to anatomical variations, leading to high, low, one-sided, or patchy dermatomal blocks. The eventual location of the catheter tip within the space can also be a major factor in infusion distribution and effectiveness of therapy. To trouble-shoot an epidural, a systematic approach is strongly advised. (For more details, please refer to questions 5 and 6 above.)

THE CONCENTRATION VERSUS VOLUME OF LA

There are inconsistencies in the evidence regarding this topic. Type of local anesthetic and type of surgery were suggested as being responsible for some of the irregularities in data, but this has not been supported.[34] In general, several principles regarding TEA infusion solutions apply. When infusing plain local anesthetic with or without opioid through thoracic epidural, the total dose of medication is more important

Table 18.2 INFUSIONS COMMONLY USED FOR THORACIC EPIDURAL ANALGESIA

LOCAL ANESTHETIC	OPIOID	ADVANTAGES	DISADVANTAGES
Bupivacaine 0.0625% or 0.125% Ropivacaine 0.1% or 0.2%	None	Less nausea/vomiting Less itching Less sedation Less respiratory depression	More hypotension More motor blockade May need higher concentration
Bupivacaine, 0.05% or 0.1% Ropivacaine 0.1% or 0.2%	Fentanyl 2–5 mcg/mL or Hydromorphone 5–15 mcg/mL	Less hemodynamic or opioid-related side effects	More itching More nausea/vomiting compared to plain LA
None	Fentanyl 5–10 mcg/ mL or Hydromorphone 20–40 mcg/mL	Less hypotension Less motor blockade	More nausea/vomiting More itching More sedation More respiratory depression

than solely concentration.[35] Indeed, multiples studies have shown that TEAs with high concentration/low volume vs. low concentration/high volume provide comparable levels of analgesia postoperatively.[36,37] In case of inadequate analgesia with TEA, a reasonable strategy would be increasing the total amount of medication the patient receives per hour. With functioning epidural, the rate of bupivacaine 0.125% can be safely increased to 8mL/h to 10 mL/h depending on the level of epidural and patient body habitus. Either way, adding an opioid such as hydromorphone or fentanyl to the LA solution usually is a good strategy to improve quality of analgesia as well.

The American Society of anesthesiologists (ASA) task force on neuraxial opioids recommends for all patients with continuous infusion of neuraxial opioids[38] continual monitoring for the first 20 minutes after initiation; followed by monitoring at least once per hour for the first 12 hours; at least once every 2 hours from 12 to 24 hours; and after 24 hours, at least once every 4 hours until discontinuation of infusion. Further monitoring schedule should be dictated by the clinical scenario. There is no evidence of increased incidence of respiratory depression or hypoxemia when parenteral opioids are used cautiously in the presence of neuraxial opioids (Table 18.2).

Multiple studies have shown the safe use of NSAIDs in patients undergoing nephrectomy.[39–42] However, a retrospective study found that the use of NSAIDs increased the risk for renal dysfunction in the long term after laparoscopic donor nephrectomy. In general, NSAIDs should be used for a short period of time in patients with preserved renal function (GFR > 45 mL/min).[43]

POSTOPERATIVE URINARY RETENTION (POUR)

Multiple studies link TEA to increased risk of POUR. However, several factors can lead to POUR, which is a common problem with a reported incidence of 5% to 70%.[7] Most frequent factors include duration and type of surgery, previous pelvic surgery, preexisting neurologic disease, increased age (risk increases by 2.4 times over the age of 50), gender (twice as prevalent in men due to prostate-related issues), increased intravenous fluid administration and bladder overdistention (bladder volume >270 mL), postoperative pain, and use of opioids and other medications and neuraxial anesthesia.[44] While neuroaxial blockade resulted in overall significantly greater rates of POUR compared to general anesthesia in a comprehensive meta-analysis, POUR related to epidural analgesia did not significantly differ from systemic analgesia.[7]

With lumbar epidurals, local anesthetics act on the sacral and lumbar nerve fibers (S2–S4), directly blocking the transmission of afferent and efferent nervous impulses from and to the bladder. In contrast, detrusor activity is significantly impaired with TEA, resulting in clinically relevant urinary retention.[45] The incidence of urinary retention in patients with lumbar epidurals *may be as high as* 53% (orthopedic surgery)[46] and 80% (labor analgesia).[47] Torda et al.[48] reported higher incidence of POUR with lumbar vs. thoracic administration of opioids. Naloxone (0.8 mg IV), having no innate influence on bladder function, has been shown to reverse POUR associated with epidural opioids.[49] The incidence of POUR in patients receiving TEA for intra-abdominal surgery ranges between 9% and 43%. High-dose TEA infusions using bupivacaine 0.25% have been associated with POUR rates as high as 33%,[50] while rates of less than 5% have been reported with lower doses (0.1% bupivacaine).[8] Use of hydrophilic opioids in TEA is associated with higher incidence of POUR. In a study by Kim et al.,[51] patients undergoing gastric bypass surgery receiving TEA using ropivacaine and sufentanil (S) or ropivacaine and morphine (M) in equipotent doses, resulted in S: 10% vs. M: 66% on postoperative day 2. In a recent study, POUR was significantly lower using 0.2% ropivacaine compared to 0.12% bupivacaine for TEA, reflecting less impairment of detrusor function with ropivacaine[52] (Box 18.1).

Early removal of urinary catheters with thoracic epidurals in place is associated with a high incidence of urinary retention (26.7% vs 12.4%, $p = 0.003$).[53] Despite this, an early catheter removal protocol may play a role in a multifaceted approach to reducing the incidence of catheter-associated urinary tract infections.[53]

Box 18.1 **EPIDURAL ANALGESIA AND URINARY RETENTION: RISK FACTORS**

Site of insertion: Lumbar epidural > thoracic epidural
Higher dose of local anesthetics
Hydrophilic opioids (morphine)
Type of agent: bupivacaine > ropivacaine
Epinephrine

OTHER REGIONAL ANESTHESIA TECHNIQUES

A variety of regional anesthesia techniques other than TEA can be used to provide anesthesia and/or analgesia for abdominal surgeries (Figure 18.3).

THORACIC PARAVERTEBRAL BLOCK (TPVB)

Baik et al.[54] compared TPVB with systemic analgesia in patients having elective open nephrectomy under general anesthesia. Pain scores and opioid requirements were significantly lower in the TPVB group for up to 24 hours. Mishra et al.[55] also compared TPV Block with IV PCA to IV PCA alone for nephrectomies and found that TPVB provided excellent postoperative analgesia and significantly reduced consumption of opioids. When TPV Block was compared to single-shot TEA for open renal surgery, analgesic requirements and pain scores were reported to be similar between both groups for the first 24 hours.[56] A systematic review of TPVB for abdominal surgeries found that single-shot TPVB provides postoperative analgesia in the first 12 to 24 hours, reducing pain scores, opioid consumption, and postoperative nausea and vomiting (PONV) compared with patients who receive no block. The reported block failure rate was less than 3% and complications were uncommon. [57]

TAP BLOCK

Several recent studies looked at the efficacy of TAP block for renal surgery.[58–60] Niraj et al.[59] looked at the efficacy of subcostal TAP blocks versus epidural analgesia for upper abdominal surgery. They found that continuous subcostal TAP block and epidural groups had comparable VAS scores at 8 and 75 hours after surgery with increased tramadol consumption in TAP group. In another study, Aditianingsih et al.[58] reported three-quadrant TAP block (bilateral posterior and subcostal at the side of the surgery) with addition of dexamethasone provided comparable analgesia to continuous epidural analgesia in the first 24 hours after transperitoneal laparoscopic donor nephrectomy.

QUADRATUS LUMBORUM BLOCK (QLB)

Several case reports demonstrate the utility of QLBs for nephrectomy, but randomized controlled trials (RCTs) comparing QLBs to other modalities for open nephrectomy patients are lacking.[61–64]

Longer duration of analgesia has been reported with QLBs as compared with more conventional TAP blocks.[65] A modified subcostal approach to the anterior QLB has been described for pain control following open urological procedures. It provides appropriate dermatome coverage for open urological surgical procedures between T6 and L2.[66]

Technique of the Subcostal Approach

Patients are positioned in lateral decubitus with the spine flexed. A curvilinear transducer is placed posteriorly below the 12th rib approximately 6–8 cm from the spinous process in a parasagittal oblique plane tilted medially at L1–L2 level. The QL muscle is visualized at its point of insertion on the lower border of the 12th rib, and the latissimus dorsi (LD) muscle is posterior (superficial) to it, while the diaphragmatic zone of apposition, the kidney, and perinephric fat and fascia are anterior (deep) to the QL muscle and transversalis fascia. When the ultrasound transducer is moved further medially, the LD muscle becomes thinner and disappears. At this location, the erector spinae (ES) muscle can be visualized posteriorly, and the psoas major (PM) muscle anterior to the QL muscle. The block can be performed at either of those ultrasound probe locations (Figure 18.4).

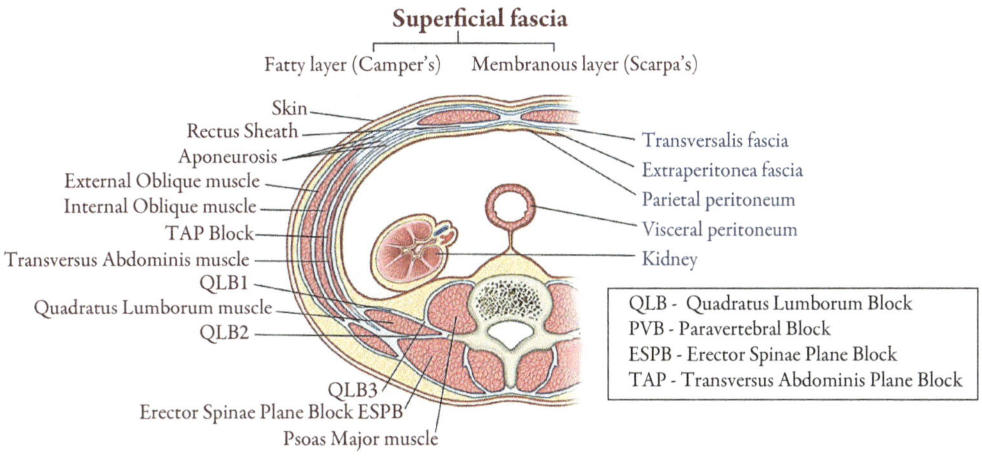

Figure 18.3. Transverse section of the abdomen: regional anesthesia techniques for abdominal surgery.

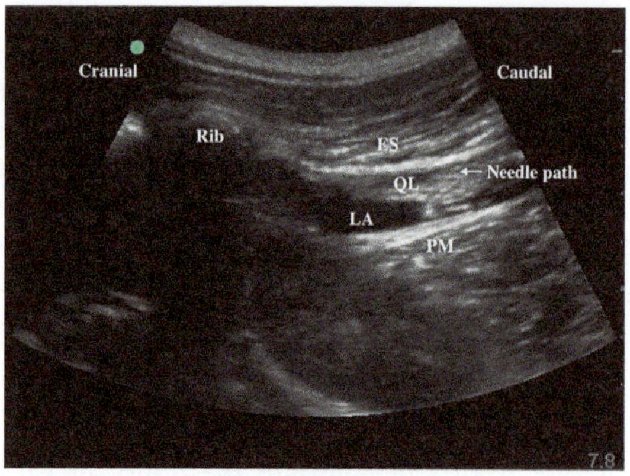

Figure 18.4. Ultrasound image of the subcostal approach to transmuscular QLB. LA spread between QL and PM muscle.
LA = local anesthetic; QL = quadratus lumborum muscle; ES = erector spinae muscle; arrow shows the needle path.
From: Zhu M, Qi Y, He H, et al. Analgesic effect of the ultrasound-guided subcostal approach to transmuscular quadratus lumborum block in patients undergoing laparoscopic nephrectomy: a randomized controlled trial. *BMC Anesthesiol.* 2019;19:154. https://doi.org/10.1186/s12871-019-0825-4.
License: Creative Commons Attribution License 4.0.

ERECTOR SPINAE BLOCK (ESP BLOCK)

Multiple case reports describe the usefulness of ESPB for nephrectomies, but RCTS are lacking.[67–69] In a recently published pooled review of 242 cases of ESPB, the block was reported as part of multimodal approach to perioperative pain management with overall reduction of opioids consumption in 34.7% of cases and 1 adverse event reported (pneumothorax).[70] More quality research is needed to evaluate the efficacy of this block for abdominal and thoracic surgery.

INTRATHECAL ADMINISTRATION OF OPIOIDS

Intrathecal morphine (ITM) was associated with great analgesia for up to 24 hours without serious complications in patients undergoing open nephrectomy.[71,72] A side effects include pruritus (30%–100% depending on the opioid used), urinary retention (35% with morphine), nausea and vomiting (30%).[73] The true incidence of clinically significant respiratory depression (the most feared complication) is not known, but evidence from smaller controlled trials and large observational studies confirm that it is infrequent.[74–76]

Lastly, bilateral *rectus sheath blocks* may be used when a midline incision is used for open nephrectomy. Although there are no specific studies looking at their usefulness for nephrectomy, there are several studies which show their benefits in terms of better analgesia and reduced opioid consumption for laparotomies involving other surgical procedures.[77–79]

LIPOSOMAL BUPIVACAINE

Only one study, by Hutchins et al., investigated liposomal bupivacaine (LB) vs. 0.25% non-liposomal bupivacaine with epinephrine in subcostal TAP block for donor nephrectomy.[80] This study found a decrease in maximum pain scores 24–48 and 48–72 hours after surgery with use of LB vs. 0.25% non-liposomal bupivacaine as part of multimodal approach. Limitations include comparing different bupivacaine concentrations, TAP technique, incomplete blinding, and small sample size. A recent metanalysis comparing perineural LB with plain bupivacaine showed a small insignificant improvement of pain scores, with no significant difference in the opioid consumption, hospital discharge, first analgesic request, opioid-related side effects, patient satisfaction length of hospital stay, and functional recovery.[81]

CONCLUSION

Regional analgesia techniques firmly remain the mainstay of the multimodal approach to postoperative analgesia and ERAS protocols after abdominal surgery. Continuous epidural blockade has been definitively demonstrated to improve pain scores, decrease opioid consumption and deleterious side effects associated with narcotic use, decrease inflammatory response, improve cardiovascular outcomes, morbidity, and mortality. Various single injection and continuous truncal blocks and surgical wound infiltration improve pain scores and rehabilitation, and decrease opioid consumption. Further insights and techniques will be developed in this area of medical knowledge with regional anesthesia at its core.

REFERENCES

1. Sasaki N, Meyer MJ, Eikermann M. Postoperative respiratory muscle dysfunction: pathophysiology and preventive strategies. *Anesthesiology.* 2013;118(4):961–978.
2. Ford GT, Rosenal TW, Clergue F, Whitelaw WA. Respiratory physiology in upper abdominal surgery. *Clin Chest Med.* 1993;14(2):237–252.
3. Kim M, Brady JE, Li G. Interaction effects of acute kidney injury, acute respiratory failure, and sepsis on 30-day postoperative mortality in patients undergoing high-risk intraabdominal general surgical procedures. *Anesth Analg.* 2015;121(6):1536–1546.
4. Curatolo M, Schnider TW, Petersen-Felix S, et al. A direct search procedure to optimize combinations of epidural bupivacaine, fentanyl, and clonidine for postoperative analgesia. *Anesthesiology.* 2000;92(2):325–337.
5. Wheatley RG, Schug SA, Watson D. Safety and efficacy of postoperative epidural analgesia. *Br J Anaesth.* 2001;87(1):47–61.
6. Kaneko T, Iwama H. The association between injected volume of local anesthetic and spread of epidural anesthesia: a hypothesis. *Reg Anesth Pain Med.* 1999;24(2):153–157.
7. Baldini G, Bagry H, Aprikian A, Carli F. Postoperative urinary retention: anesthetic and perioperative considerations. *Anesthesiology.* 2009;110(5):1139–1157.
8. Senagore AJ, Delaney CP, Mekhail N, Dugan A, Fazio VW. Randomized clinical trial comparing epidural anaesthesia and patient-controlled analgesia after laparoscopic segmental colectomy. *Br J Surg.* 2003;90(10):1195–1199.
9. Paulsen EK, Porter MG, Helmer SD, Linhardt PW, Kliewer ML. Thoracic epidural versus patient-controlled analgesia in elective bowel resections. *Am J Surg.* 2001;182(6):570–577.
10. Siegel RL, Miller KD, Jemal A. Cancer statistics, 2019. *CA Cancer J Clin.* 2019;69(1):7–34.

11. Cohen HT, McGovern FJ. Renal-cell carcinoma. *N Engl J Med.* 2005;353(23):2477–2490.
12. Zhao PT, Richstone L, Kavoussi LR. Laparoscopic partial nephrectomy. *Int J Surg (London, England).* 2016;36(Pt C):548–553.
13. Ng AM, Shah PH, Kavoussi LR. Laparoscopic partial nephrectomy: a narrative review and comparison with open and robotic partial nephrectomy. *J Endourol.* 2017;31(10):976–984.
14. Jonasch E, Gao J, Rathmell WK. Renal cell carcinoma. *BMJ (Clin Res Ed).* 2014;349:g4797.
15. Anastasiadis E, O'Brien T, Fernando A. Open partial nephrectomy in renal cell cancer: essential or obsolete? *Int J Surg (London, England).* 2016;36(Pt C):541–547.
16. Sharma V, Margreiter M. Partial nephrectomy: is there still a need for open surgery? *Curr Urol Reports.* 2013;14(1):1–4.
17. Barmparas G, Branco BC, Schnüriger B, Lam L, Inaba K, Demetriades D. The incidence and risk factors of post-laparotomy adhesive small bowel obstruction. *J Gastrointest Surg.* 2010;14(10):1619–1628.
18. Kaneko T, Funahashi K, Ushigome M, et al. Incidence of and risk factors for incisional hernia after closure of temporary ileostomy for colorectal malignancy. *Hernia.* 2019;23(4):743–748.
19. Rovina N, Bouros D, Tzanakis N, et al. Effects of laparoscopic cholecystectomy on global respiratory muscle strength. *Am J Respir Crit Care Med.* 1996;153(1):458–461.
20. Watters JM, Clancey SM, Moulton SB, Briere KM, Zhu JM. Impaired recovery of strength in older patients after major abdominal surgery. *Ann Surg.* 1993;218(3):380–390; discussion 390–383.
21. Putensen-Himmer G, Putensen C, Lammer H, Lingnau W, Aigner F, Benzer H. Comparison of postoperative respiratory function after laparoscopy or open laparotomy for cholecystectomy. *Anesthesiology.* 1992;77(4):675–680.
22. Wu A, Drummond GB. Respiratory muscle activity and respiratory obstruction after abdominal surgery. *Br J Anaesth.* 2006;96(4):510–515.
23. Bablekos GD, Michaelides SA, Analitis A, Charalabopoulos KA. Effects of laparoscopic cholecystectomy on lung function: a systematic review. *World J Gastroenterol.* 2014;20(46):17603–17617.
24. Chae WS, Choi S, Sugiyama D, Richerson GB, Brennan TJ, Kang S. Effect of thoracic epidural anesthesia in a rat model of phrenic motor inhibition after upper abdominal surgery. *Anesthesiology.* 2018;129(4):791–807.
25. Manikian B, Cantineau JP, Bertrand M, Kieffer E, Sartene R, Viars P. Improvement of diaphragmatic function by a thoracic extradural block after upper abdominal surgery. *Anesthesiology.* 1988;68(3):379–386.
26. Celli BR. Perioperative respiratory care of the patient undergoing upper abdominal surgery. *Clin Chest Med.* 1993;14(2):253–261.
27. Chuter TA, Weissman C, Starker PM, Gump FE. Effect of incentive spirometry on diaphragmatic function after surgery. *Surgery.* 1989;105(4):488–493.
28. do Nascimento Junior P, Modolo NS, Andrade S, Guimaraes MM, Braz LG, El Dib R. Incentive spirometry for prevention of postoperative pulmonary complications in upper abdominal surgery. *Cochrane Database Syst Rev.* 2014(2):Cd006058.
29. Capdevila X, Moulard S, Plasse C, et al. Effectiveness of epidural analgesia, continuous surgical site analgesia, and patient-controlled analgesic morphine for postoperative pain management and hyperalgesia, rehabilitation, and health-related quality of life after open nephrectomy: a prospective, randomized, controlled study. *Anesth Analg.* 2017;124(1):336–345.
30. Guay J, Nishimori M, Kopp SL. Epidural local anesthetics versus opioid-based analgesic regimens for postoperative gastrointestinal paralysis, vomiting, and pain after abdominal surgery: a Cochrane review. *Anesth Analg.* 2016;123(6):1591–1602.
31. Popping DM, Elia N, Van Aken HK, et al. Impact of epidural analgesia on mortality and morbidity after surgery: systematic review and meta-analysis of randomized controlled trials. *Ann Surg.* 2014;259(6):1056–1067.
32. Hughes MJ, Ventham NT, McNally S, Harrison E, Wigmore S. Analgesia after open abdominal surgery in the setting of enhanced recovery surgery: a systematic review and meta-analysis. *JAMA Surg.* 2014;149(12):1224–1230.
33. Hermanides J, Hollmann MW, Stevens MF, Lirk P. Failed epidural: causes and management. *Br J Anaesth.* 2012;109(2):144–154.
34. Liu SS, Moore JM, Luo AM, Trautman WJ, Carpenter RL. Comparison of three solutions of ropivacaine/fentanyl for postoperative patient-controlled epidural analgesia. *Anesthesiology.* 1999;90(3):727–733.
35. Laveaux MM, Hasenbos MA, Harbers JB, Liem T. Thoracic epidural bupivacaine plus sufentanil: high concentration/low volume versus low concentration/high volume. *Reg Anesth.* 1993;18(1):39–43.
36. Dernedde M, Stadler M, Bardiau F, Seidel L, Boogaerts JG. Low vs. high concentration of levobupivacaine for post-operative epidural analgesia: influence of mode of delivery. *Acta Anaesthesiol Scand.* 2006;50(5):613–621.
37. Dernedde M, Stadler M, Taviaux N, Boogaerts JG. Postoperative patient-controlled thoracic epidural analgesia: importance of dose compared to volume or concentration. *Anaesth Intensive Care.* 2008;36(6):814–821.
38. Practice guidelines for the prevention, detection, and management of respiratory depression associated with neuraxial opioid administration: an updated report by the American Society of Anesthesiologists Task Force on Neuraxial Opioids and the American Society of Regional Anesthesia and Pain Medicine. *Anesthesiology.* 2016;124(3):535–552.
39. Diblasio CJ, Snyder ME, Kattan MW, Russo P. Ketorolac: safe and effective analgesia for the management of renal cortical tumors with partial nephrectomy. *J Urol.* 2004;171(3):1062–1065.
40. Freedland SJ, Blanco-Yarosh M, Sun JC, et al. Ketorolac-based analgesia improves outcomes for living kidney donors. *Transplantation.* 2002;73(5):741–745.
41. Freedland SJ, Blanco-Yarosh M, Sun JC, et al. Effect of ketorolac on renal function after donor nephrectomy. *Urology.* 2002;59(6):826–830.
42. Varela-Santoyo E, Escamilla-Lopez MI, Izquierdo-Tolosa CD, et al. Impact of the type of analgesic therapy on postsurgical complications of patients with kidney cancer undergoing nephrectomy. *Oncology.* 2020;98(2):117–122.
43. Takahashi K, Patel AK, Nagai S, et al. Perioperative ketorolac use: a potential risk factor for renal dysfunction after live-donor nephrectomy. *Ann Transplant.* 2017;22:563–569.
44. Choi S, Mahon P, Awad IT. Neuraxial anesthesia and bladder dysfunction in the perioperative period: a systematic review. *Can J Anaesth.* 2012;59(7):681–703.
45. Wuethrich PY, Kessler TM, Panicker JN, Curatolo M, Burkhard FC. Detrusor activity is impaired during thoracic epidural analgesia after open renal surgery. *Anesthesiology.* 2010;112(6):1345–1349.
46. Capdevila X, Barthelet Y, Biboulet P, Ryckwaert Y, Rubenovitch J, d'Athis F. Effects of perioperative analgesic technique on the surgical outcome and duration of rehabilitation after major knee surgery. *Anesthesiology.* 1999;91(1):8–15.
47. Weiniger CF, Wand S, Nadjari M, et al. Post-void residual volume in labor: a prospective study comparing parturients with and without epidural analgesia. *Acta Anaesthesiol Scand.* 2006;50(10):1297–1303.
48. Torda TA, Pybus DA. Comparison of four narcotic analgesics for extradural analgesia. *Br J Anaesth.* 1982;54(3):291–295.
49. Rawal N, Mollefors K, Axelsson K, Lingardh G, Widman B. Naloxone reversal of urinary retention after epidural morphine. *Lancet.* 1981;2:1411.
50. Conacher ID, Paes ML, Jacobson L, Phillips PD, Heaviside DW. Epidural analgesia following thoracic surgery: a review of two years' experience. *Anaesthesia.* 1983;38(6):546–551.
51. Kim JY, Lee SJ, Koo BN, et al. The effect of epidural sufentanil in ropivacaine on urinary retention in patients undergoing gastrectomy. *Br J Anaesth.* 2006;97(3):414–418.
52. Girsberger SA, Schneider MP, Loffel LM, Burkhard FC, Wuethrich PY. Effect of thoracic epidural ropivacaine versus bupivacaine on lower urinary tract function: a randomized clinical trial. *Anesthesiology.* 2018;128(3):511–519.

53. Hu Y, Craig SJ, Rowlingson JC, et al. Early removal of urinary catheter after surgery requiring thoracic epidural: a prospective trial. *J Cardiothorac Vasc Anesth.* 2014;28(5):1302–1306.
54. Baik JS, Oh AY, Cho CW, Shin HJ, Han SH, Ryu JH. Thoracic paravertebral block for nephrectomy: a randomized, controlled, observer-blinded study. *Pain Med (Malden, Mass).* 2014;15(5):850–856.
55. Mishra A, Verma R, Bhatia V, Chandra G, Gupta R, Chaudhary A. Thoracic paravertebral block for postoperative pain management in patients undergoing for nephrectomy: a randomised clinical trial. *J Clin Diagn Res.* 2018;12(10):UC05–UC08.
56. Moawad HE, Mousa SA, El-Hefnawy AS. Single-dose paravertebral blockade versus epidural blockade for pain relief after open renal surgery: a prospective randomized study. *Saudi J Anaesth.* 2013;7(1):61–67.
57. El-Boghdadly K, Madjdpour C, Chin KJ. Thoracic paravertebral blocks in abdominal surgery: a systematic review of randomized controlled trials. *Br J Anaesth.* 2016;117(3):297–308.
58. Aditianingsih D, Mochtar CA, Chandra S, Sukmono RB, Soamole IW. Comparison of three-quadrant transversus abdominis plane block and continuous epidural block for postoperative analgesia after transperitoneal laparoscopic nephrectomy. *Anesth Pain Med.* 2018;8(5):e80024.
59. Niraj G, Kelkar A, Jeyapalan I, et al. Comparison of analgesic efficacy of subcostal transversus abdominis plane blocks with epidural analgesia following upper abdominal surgery. *Anaesthesia.* 2011;66(6):465–471.
60. Qu G, Cui XL, Liu HJ, Ji ZG, Huang YG. Ultrasound-guided transversus abdominis plane block improves postoperative analgesia and early recovery in patients undergoing retroperitoneoscopic urologic surgeries: a randomized controlled double-blinded trial. *Chin Med Sci J.* 2016;31(3):137–141.
61. Corso RM, Piraccini E, Sorbello M, Bellantonio D, Tedesco M. Ultrasound-guided transmuscular quadratus lumborum block for perioperative analgesia in open nephrectomy. *Minerva Anestesiol.* 2017;83:1334–1335.
62. Graca R, Miguelez P, Cardoso JM, et al. [Continuous quadratus lumborum type II block in partial nephrectomy]. *Revista Brasileira Anestesiol.* 2018;68(6):653–656.
63. Sindwani G, Sahu S, Suri A, Saeed Z. Bilateral quadratus lumborum block for postoperative analgesia in a Von Hippel-Lindau syndrome patient undergoing laparoscopic radical nephrectomy. *Saudi J Anaesth.* 2017;11(4):513–514.
64. Warusawitharana C, Basar S, Jackson BL, Niraj G. Ultrasound guided continuous transmuscular quadratus lumborum analgesia for open renal surgery: a case series. *J Clin Anesth.* 2017;42:100–101.
65. Blanco R, Ansari T, Riad W, Shetty N. Quadratus lumborum block versus transversus abdominis plane block for postoperative pain after cesarean delivery: a randomized controlled trial. *Reg Anesth Pain Med.* 2016;41(6):757–762.
66. Elsharkawy H, Ahuja S, DeGrande S, Maheshwari K, Chan V. Subcostal approach to anterior quadratus lumborum block for pain control following open urological procedures. *J Anesth.* 2019;33(1):148–154.
67. Aksu C, Gurkan Y. Ultrasound guided erector spinae block for postoperative analgesia in pediatric nephrectomy surgeries. *J Clin Anesth.* 2018;45:35–36.
68. Kim S, Bang S, Kwon W. Intermittent erector spinae plane block as a part of multimodal analgesia after open nephrectomy. *Chin Med J (Engl).* 2019;132:1507–1508.
69. Luis-Navarro JC, Seda-Guzmán M, Luis-Moreno C, Chin KJ. Erector spinae plane block in abdominal surgery: case series. *Indian J Anaesth.* 2018;62:549–554.
70. Tsui BCH, Fonseca A, Munshey F, McFadyen G, Caruso TJ. The erector spinae plane (ESP) block: a pooled review of 242 cases. *J Clin Anesth.* 2019;53:29–34.
71. Kim HC, Bae JY, Kim TK, et al. Efficacy of intrathecal morphine for postoperative pain management following open nephrectomy. *J Int Med Res.* 2016;44:42–53.
72. Yoon S, Min JJ, Kim H-C, Hong DM. The efficacy of intrathecal morphine for the postoperative pain management in open nephrectomy: 14AP8–3. *Eur J Anaesthesiol. (EJA).* 2014;31:235.
73. Rathmell JP, Lair TR, Nauman B. The role of intrathecal drugs in the treatment of acute pain. *Anesth Analg.* 2005;101(5 Suppl):S30–S43.
74. Etches RC, Sandler AN, Daley MD. Respiratory depression and spinal opioids. *Can J Anaesth.* 1989;36(2):165–185.
75. Gwirtz KH, Young JV, Byers RS, et al. The safety and efficacy of intrathecal opioid analgesia for acute postoperative pain: seven years' experience with 5969 surgical patients at Indiana University Hospital. *Anesth Analg.* 1999;88(3):599–604.
76. Ko S, Goldstein DH, VanDenKerkhof EG. Definitions of "respiratory depression" with intrathecal morphine postoperative analgesia: a review of the literature. *Can J Anaesth.* 2003;50(7):679–688.
77. Bakshi SG, Mapari A, Shylasree TS. REctus Sheath block for postoperative analgesia in gynecological ONcology Surgery (RESONS): a randomized-controlled trial. *Can J Anaesth.* 2016;63(12):1335–1344.
78. Elbahrawy K, El-Deeb A. Rectus sheath block for postoperative analgesia in patients with mesenteric vascular occlusion undergoing laparotomy: a randomized single-blinded study. *Anesth Essays Res.* 2016;10(3):516–520.
79. Tudor EC, Yang W, Brown R, Mackey PM. Rectus sheath catheters provide equivalent analgesia to epidurals following laparotomy for colorectal surgery. *Ann R Coll Surg Engl.* 2015;97(7):530–533.
80. Hutchins JL, Kesha R, Blanco F, Dunn T, Hochhalter R. Ultrasound-guided subcostal transversus abdominis plane blocks with liposomal bupivacaine vs. non-liposomal bupivacaine for postoperative pain control after laparoscopic hand-assisted donor nephrectomy: a prospective randomised observer-blinded study. *Anaesthesia.* 2016;71(8):930–937.
81. Hussain N, Brull R, Sheehy B, et al. Perineural liposomal bupivacaine is not superior to nonliposomal bupivacaine for peripheral nerve block analgesia. *Anesthesiology.* 2021;134(2):147–164.

REVIEW QUESTIONS

(1) Regarding abdominal surgery and involvement of respiratory muscles, each of the following statements are true EXCEPT:

A. The site of the operation and the type of surgery are the most important factors affecting the respiratory muscles.
B. Diaphragm is the predominant muscle affected during upper abdominal surgery.
C. There is reflex stimulation of the phrenic nerve output following upper abdominal incision and surgery.
D. Incidence of significant respiratory muscle dysfunction after abdominal surgery is much higher with upper abdominal surgery when compared to lower abdominal surgery.

(2) Which of the following statements regarding the use of thoracic epidural analgesia (TEA) for major abdominal surgery is NOT true?

A. It provides good pain control and minimizes opioid consumption.
B. It decreases the length of stay and promotes early discharge from the hospital.
C. It promotes early recovery of bowel function.
D. Management may be complicated due to the use of anticoagulants/antithrombotic agents.

(3) All the following factors regarding trouble shooting an epidural are true EXCEPT:

A. Unilateral blockade can sometimes be corrected by withdrawing the catheter 1–2 centimeters.
B. Testing of the thoracic epidural catheter with 5 mL of 1% lidocaine should be considered in a patient with uncontrolled pain.
C. Uncontrolled postoperative pain is rare in patients in the presence of a definitive functioning epidural.
D. A sensory level with diminished temperature sense and response to pinprick in bilateral dermatomes is indicative of a functioning epidural.

(4) Compared to TEA, the newer fascial plane blocks used for major abdominal surgery are likely to offer all the following advantages EXCEPT:

A. Less opioid consumption and better control of visceral pain
B. Lower incidence of hypotension and need for fluid resuscitation
C. Less complicated management of perioperative thromboprophylaxis
D. Lower incidence of neurological complications after regional anesthesia

(5) Which of the following patients is most likely to have urinary retention following placement of TEA for management of postoperative pain?

A. 27-year-old male receiving an infusion of 0.15% bupivacaine in his epidural for management of pain after gastrectomy
B. 45-year-old female receiving an infusion of 0.125% bupivacaine with 4 mcg/mL of fentanyl in her epidural for management of pain after open cholecystectomy
C. 72-year-old male receiving an infusion of 0.125% bupivacaine with 30 mcg/mL of morphine in his epidural for management of pain after open nephrectomy
D. 72-year-old female receiving an infusion of 0.2% ropivacaine with 3 mcg/mL of fentanyl in her epidural for management of pain after partial hepatectomy

(6) Each of the following is correctly matched for site of insertion of thoracic epidural and type of surgery EXCEPT:

A. Thoracotomy with lower lobe resection: T6–T7
B. Open nephrectomy with subcostal incision: T7–T8
C. Exploratory laparotomy with colectomy: T8–T9
D. Total abdominal hysterectomy: T6–T7

(7) Which of the following statements regarding common regional anesthesia techniques employed for major abdominal surgery is NOT true?

A. Quadratus lumborum blocks reduce opioid requirement when used for abdominal surgery and provide a duration of analgesia longer than TAP blocks with single injections.
B. Proposed mechanism of action of erector spinae block is via blockade of the dorsal and occasionally ventral rami of the thoracic spinal nerves and sympathetic fibers.
C. Use of ultrasound has not changed the risk of pneumothorax associated with placement of thoracic paravertebral blocks.
D. TAP blocks do not provide visceral analgesia and have a short duration of action following single injections.

(8) Each of the following is true regarding renal cell carcinoma (RCC) EXCEPT:

A. Epidural blockade for thoraco-abdominal surgical approach requires coverage of T5–T12 dermatomes.
B. Open surgical technique is preferable in solitary kidney patients due to shorter warm ischemia times.
C. RCC with involvement of cardiac muscle/IVC or adrenal gland is an absolute contraindication for surgical tumor resection.
D. A flank incision is optimal surgical approach in obese patients but has increased risk of peripheral nerve injury and escalating postoperative opioid requirement.

(9) Which of the following is true regarding TEA and TAP block commonly employed for nephrectomy?

A. TEA minimizes total opioid consumption, decreases pulmonary complications, and attenuates stress response from surgery, but does not decrease all-cause mortality.
B. Thoracic epidural placement via traditional landmark-based techniques has negligible failure rates of less than 3%.
C. TEAs with high-concentration/low-volume infusions provide more effective analgesia compared to low-concentration/high-volume infusions.
D. Some studies report three-quadrant TAP block plus dexamethasone provide similar analgesia as TEA in the first 24 hours after transperitoneal laparoscopic donor nephrectomy.

ANSWERS

(1) **C.** Diaphragmatic dysfunction is common after upper abdominal surgery. Injury-induced reflex inhibition not stimulation of phrenic motor neuron drive is one of the main factors responsible for diaphragmatic dysfunction

Reference

Chae WS, Choi S, Sugiyama D, Richerson GB, Brennan TJ, Kang S. Effect of thoracic epidural anesthesia in a rat model of phrenic motor inhibition after upper abdominal surgery. *Anesthesiology*. 2018; 129:791–807.

(2) **B.** In a systemic review and meta-analysis, epidural analgesia was associated with faster return of gut function and

reduced pain scores and superior pain control; however, no difference was observed in length of stay.

Reference

Hughes MJ, Ventham NT, McNally S, Harrison E, Wigmore S. Analgesia after open abdominal surgery in the setting of enhanced recovery surgery: a systematic review and meta-analysis. *JAMA Surg* 2014; 149:1224–1230

(3) **C.** Suboptimal dosing, inappropriate site of epidural insertion, large incisions, multiple incisions, referred pain can all lead to uncontrolled pain even in the presence of a functioning epidural. Although incorrect primary placement is one of the major causes for failed epidural, uncontrolled pain is not uncommon even in the presence of a functioning epidural. With continuous infusion, dose is the primary determinant of epidural anesthesia quality, with volume and concentration playing a lesser role. Addition of adjuvants, especially opioids and epinephrine, may substantially increase the success rate of epidural analgesia. The use of patient-controlled epidural analgesia with background infusion appears to be the best method for postoperative analgesia. Multimodal analgesia techniques need to be employed to optimize pain not covered by the epidural in case of large incisions, multiple incisions, and referred pain.

Reference

Hermanides J, Hollmann MW, Stevens MF, Lirk P. Failed epidural: causes and management. *Br J Anaesth*2012; 109:144–154.

(4) **A.** Afferent fibers innervating abdominal viscera mostly project to the CNS through autonomic sympathetic nerves. Sympathetic afferents are more likely to be blocked by the traditional blocks (epidural and paravertebral blocks) than the fascial plane blocks.

Reference

Borglum J, Gogenur I, Bendtsen TF. Abdominal wall blocks in adults. *Curr Opin Anaesth*. 2016;29:638–643.

(5) **C.** Use of hydrophilic opioid and higher dose of local anesthetics in thoracic epidurals is more likely to cause urinary retention. The potency/dose of local anesthetic and the presence of opioids affect detrusor dysfunction and the time to return micturition. With long-acting epidural opioids, the reported incidence of urinary retention is as high as 60%–70%.

Reference

Choi S, Mahon P, Awad IT. Neuraxial anesthesia and bladder dysfunction in the perioperative period: a systematic review. *Can J Anaesth*. 2012;59:681–703.

(6) **D.** Key point: Epidural catheter placement between T8 and T10 is usually appropriate for lower abdominal procedures such as hysterectomy. Beneficial effects of TEA require that catheter placement and the infusate be targeted at the thoracic segments innervating injured skin, muscle, and viscera from which the nociceptive input originates.

Reference

Manion SC, Brennan TJ. Thoracic epidural analgesia and acute pain management. *Anesthesiology*. 2011;115:181–188.

(7) **C.** Paravertebral block is a deep block, and ultrasound guided PVBs may be technically challenging due to poor needle visualization at steep angles, especially in patients with high BMI. The risk of pneumothorax with PVBs has been reported to be about 0.8% using a landmark technique with nerve stimulation. However, use of ultrasound has certainly reduced the risk of complications associated with paravertebral block.

Reference

Pace MM, Sharma B, Anderson-Dam J, Fleischmann K, Warren L, Stefanovich P. Ultrasound-guided thoracic paravertebral blockade: a retrospective study of the incidence of complications. *Anesth Analg*. 2016;122:1186–1191.

(8) **C.** Stage I–II RCC confined to the kidneys, stage III RCC with involvement of major vessels/extra-renal tissues or retroperitoneal lymph nodes, and RCC with involvement of cardiac muscle/IVC or adrenal gland are the indications for radical surgical excision. Laparoscopic techniques may require longer operative time, and open approach is preferred in solitary kidney patients to shorten warm ischemia.

Reference

Cohen HT, McGovern FJ. Renal-cell carcinoma. *N Engl J Med* 2005;353:2477–2490.

(9) **D.** TEA is a gold standard for providing optimal postoperative analgesia. Some studies have shown comparable quality of analgesia with three-point TAP blocks with addition of adjunct medications in select patients in the first 24 hours postoperatively; specifically, in laparoscopic nephrectomy. However, in patients undergoing open nephrectomy, TEA is still the most effective modality

Reference

Aditianingsih D, Mochtar CA, Chandra S, Sukmono RB, Soamole IW. Comparison of three-quadrant transversus abdominis plane block and continuous epidural block for postoperative analgesia after transperitoneal laparoscopic nephrectomy. *Anesth Pain Med*. 2018 Oct 8;5:e80024.

19.

REGIONAL ANESTHESIA FOR ABDOMINOPLASTY

Sanchit Ahuja and Sree Kolli

STEM CASE AND KEY QUESTIONS

A 46-year-old female actress underwent an uncomplicated bariatric surgery the previous year, after which she lost 60 kg of weight. Her total body weight remained unchanged thereafter. Her past medical history includes rheumatoid arthritis with mild ventilatory restrictive defect. Given her significant surgery-related weight loss, she expressed concern over the abdominal skin laxity and drooping of dermo-adipose tissue. She read about "tummy tuck" surgery on the internet and wanted to know if she can be a possible candidate. The patient was presented with the options with associated risks, and the decision was made to proceed for combined abdominoplasty and liposuction. The plan for general anesthesia with oral endotracheal tube was made, and the team proactively contacted the regional anesthesia team for managing acute postoperative pain control.

(1) WHAT ARE THE IMPLICATIONS FOR COMBINING LIPOSUCTION WITH ABDOMINOPLASTY?

Conventional abdominoplasty is done to tighten the underlying muscle fascia in a vertical line by incising hip to hip while freeing the surrounding skin, whereas liposuction dissects between neurovascular mesenteries through small incisions that are usually <1 cm in length and sucks fat cells. Since the advent of abdominoplasty, many advances, such as the combined lipoabdominoplasty procedure, have revolutionized abdominal aesthetic surgery. Lipoabdominoplasty (also known as suction-assisted abdominoplasty or abdominolipoplasty) is referred to as extensive liposuction in conjunction with abdominoplasty.

(2) WHAT ARE THE SURGICAL INCISIONS OF DIFFERENT TYPES OF ABDOMINOPLASTY/ LIPOABDOMINOPLASTY?

Most commonly, lipoabdominoplasty includes two processes: (1) contouring procedure, done via liposuction throughout the abdomen (including epigastric and mesogastric areas), followed by (2) inverted v-pattern surgical dissection laterally limited to 7.5 cm from the midline.

(3) WHAT IS TUMESCENT ANESTHESIA?

Tumescent anesthesia involves large volumes of subcutaneous injections of dilute concentrations of lidocaine-epinephrine solution into the adipose tissue to achieve widespread local anesthesia. The local anesthesia is subsequently removed/aspirated, termed as *detumescence*, which usually takes place after approximately half an hour. The maximum recommended lidocaine dose ranges from 35 to 55 mg/kg, and 0.055 mg/kg for epinephrine. It depends mainly on the maximum dose, and the vascularity of surrounding tissue of surgical excision. Overall, for a given local anesthetic (LA) dose, tumescent absorption continues beyond 24 hours. This slow absorption is presumed to be the reason for the extended drug dosage safety profile.

(4) WHAT IS THE RELATIONSHIP BETWEEN THE USE OF LOCAL ANESTHETICS AND SKIN GRAFT FAILURE?

Laboratory data suggest delayed wound healing related to myotoxic, chondrotoxic, and vasculotoxic effects of LAs. These untoward effects may be relevant especially to aesthetic surgeries; however, to date this has not been shown in human studies.

(5) WHAT IS THE BEST TIME TO PLACE THE BLOCKS FOR ABDOMINOLIPOPLASTY?

Regarding the timing, preoperative blocks are much more sonographically convenient because of related postoperative muscle plane distortion, peri-suture line edema, and associated expected hematomas. Additionally, extensive dissection may lead to significant muscle plane distortion and may therefore interfere with the spread of LAs postoperatively. Although research is scarce in terms of "when to perform" a block, the plausible effects of preemptive infiltrative blocks are thought to reduce intraoperative and immediate postoperative analgesic requirements.

(6) DISCUSS THE VARIOUS REGIONAL BLOCKS THAT CAN BE OFFERED TO THIS PATIENT FOR POSTOPERATIVE PAIN CONTROL RELATED TO ABDOMINOPLASTY, LIPOSUCTION, OR COMBINED LIPOABDOMINOPLASTY.

As a part of multimodal analgesia, regional blocks for lipoabdominoplasty are broadly divided into neuraxial and muscle plane fascial blocks. Neuraxial blocks relevant to lipoabdominoplasty include thoracic epidural analgesia (TEA) and paravertebral block (PVB). More peripheral blocks include intercostal and or interfascial plane block (intercostal, pararectus, and ilioinguinal-iliohypogastric and quadratus lumborum block [QLB]).

(7) WHAT ARE THE CHALLENGES OF PERFORMING TRANSVERSE ABDOMINIS PLANE (TAP) BLOCK IN ABDOMINOPLASTY PATIENTS? AND HOW CAN YOU WORK AROUND THESE CHALLENGES?

Morbidly obese patients or patients with multiple previous abdominal surgeries pose certain recognizable challenges in determining the muscle layers. In such difficult scenarios, (1) identify the muscle layer by first determining transversus abdominis muscle, which can be located just above the peritoneal cavity (identified by peristalsis); (2) probe scanning from medial and lateral while confirming the continuity of muscle planes is also helpful.

(8) WHAT ARE THE TYPES OF QUADRATUS LUMBORUM BLOCKS (QLBS)?

Types of QLB depend on the site of injection relative to the QL muscle; various approaches to QLB were identified, most commonly, lateral, posterior, and anterior, with subcostal transmuscular as a modification of the anterior approach.

(9) DESCRIBE BRIEFLY HOW TO PERFORM A QLB.

The procedure is done in the lateral position. A curvilinear (low frequency) ultrasound probe is placed in transverse orientation at the posterior mid axillary line (at level L2–L4). The QL muscle is identified as a quadrangular structure, hypoechoic (in relation to surrounding muscle). At this level, lumbar transverse process and vertebral body may be identified. According to the planned approach, the LA is deposited in relation to QL muscle (see Figure 19.3A, B later in the chapter).

(10) OUT OF THE DISCUSSED REGIONAL INTERVENTIONS, WHICH BLOCK MOST IMPROVES PULMONARY FUNCTION FOLLOWING SURGERIES ON ABDOMINAL MUSCULATURE SUCH AS LIPOABDOMINOPLASTY?

With background of mild restrictive ventilatory defect in our patient, the incisional postoperative pain may encumber the overall lung volumes, leading to postoperative pulmonary complications. The exquisite pain control provided by TEA serves to improve postoperative pulmonary function and decrease postoperative pulmonary complications following major upper abdominal surgery by allowing deep breathing. This is one of the few reasons why thoracic epidural is considered protective in open abdomen surgeries. Four-quadrants TAP block has been shown to not affect pulmonary function. Paravertebral blocks (PVBs) and other fascial plane blocks, on the other hand, may have some plausible effects; however, the comparative research is scarce.

DISCUSSION

ABDOMINOPLASTY

Abdominoplasty is the most commonly performed aesthetic reconstructive procedure.[1] Traditionally, abdominoplasty and liposuction were separate procedures; the earlier data, however, suggest increased risk of associated complications when both are combined.[2] The reported complications, including hematoma, wound dehiscence, seroma, and skin necrosis, ranged from 30% to 50%, primarily attributed to traumatic forces of liposuction leading to restricted vascularity of the abdominal flap. This combined surgery is known to improve outcomes and simultaneously reduced risk and associated complications.[3,4]

Lipoabdominoplasty includes two processes: (1) contouring procedure, done via liposuction throughout the abdomen (including epigastric and mesogastric areas), followed by (2) abdominoplasty, which is done through inverted v-pattern surgical dissection laterally limited to 7.5 cm from the midline.[5,6] However, there are multiple variations of abdominoplasty (Table 19.1).

TUMESCENT ANESTHESIA

Tumescent anesthesia involves large volumes of subcutaneous injections of dilute concentrations of lidocaine-epinephrine solution into the adipose tissue to achieve widespread local anesthesia. The LA is subsequently removed/aspirated, termed as *detumescence*, which usually takes place after approximately half an hour. This method assumes that less than 3–4 L of aspirate is performed and is strictly local, without any sedation or general anesthesia. The commonly utilized diluent solutions are normal saline or lactated Ringers.[7] Typically, the amount of infiltration solution used is 1–2 mL per 1 cm^3 of adipose tissue. Fluid overload is more likely to occur when higher volumes of tumescent solution are being utilized. The American Society of Plastic Surgeons recommended that physicians who are planning to perform tumescent anesthetics with volumes greater then 5 liters should be trained in comprehensive fluid resuscitation. The maximum recommended lidocaine dose ranges from 35 to 55 mg/kg, and 0.055 mg/kg for epinephrine.[8] The maximum dose, however, may also depend on the difference in vascularity of surrounding tissue of surgical excision. Overall, for a given LA dose, tumescent absorption continues beyond 24 hours. This slow absorption is presumed

Table 19.1 VARIOUS TYPES OF ABDOMINOPLASTY

	TYPES OF ABDOMINOPLASTY	COMMONLY UTILIZED SURGICAL INCISIONS
1.	Extended abdominoplasty/Complete abdominoplasty with lateral thigh lift	Lower transverse abdominal incision—undermining the skin flap—resection of excessive skin—suturing of musculofascial layers and finally closure of flap.
2.	High lateral tension abdominoplasty[59]/modified lower body lifting procedure	Involves low transverse abdominal extended scar—while vertical-vector muscles tightening, as well horizontal vector tightening. Undermining only to central skin flap and resection of lateral excess skin with controlled high-tension closure. Better aesthetic results
3.	Floating abdominoplasty or FAB technique[60]	Tightening and shaping of abdominal muscles from sternum to pubic area via small incisions while temporarily detaching (floating) the umbilicus.
4.	Circumferential abdominoplasty[61]	Extended abdominoplasty with buttock lift. Circumferential contouring procedure involving anterior and posterior belt incisions addressing buttocks, flanks, and thigh. Positioning usually involves prone first, followed by the supine position.
5.	Partial/mini abdominoplasty[62]	Relatively small single incision above pubic area; midline tightening followed by resection of excess skin.

to be the reason for the extended drug dosage safety profile. Other attributable reasons include poor vascularity of adipose tissue, and decreased uptake due to epinephrine-induced localized vasoconstriction. A study comparing concentration profile in equidosage of tumescent lidocaine in patients with liposuction and without liposuction concluded that 28% reduced plasma concentration occurred in patients with liposuction—possibly due to removal of lidocaine-impregnated adipose tissue.[9] Laboratory data suggest delayed wound healing related to myotoxic, chondrotoxic, and vasculotoxic effects of LAs.[10] These untoward effects may be relevant especially to aesthetic surgeries; however, to date this has not been shown in human studies.

Several concerns exist with tumescent anesthesia. Early postoperative complications include surgical site infections, deep venous thromboembolism (DVT), and pulmonary embolism. The risk of DVT is low, but is significantly increased when liposuction is combined with other surgical procedures. Importantly, the signs and/or symptoms of LA toxicity may be masked by sedation or general anesthesia, although complications due to LA toxicity during tumescent liposuction are relatively uncommon. However, the high dosage of tumescent lidocaine increases the risk of LA toxicity.

ABDOMINAL INCISION

A high incidence of pulmonary complications is noted after upper abdominal incisions, primarily due to alterations in pulmonary function tests.[11] Extensive upper abdominal surgery leads to a functional restrictive lung disease state, with apparent decrease in inspiratory reserve volume (IRV), functional residual capacity (FVC), and forced expiratory volume 1 (FEV1)—presumably due to decreased inspiratory effort, secondary to increased pain with respiration.[12,13] Previous work suggests that epidural anesthesia affects negatively the intercostal muscles' function; however, this has minimal effect on actual respiratory function.[14,15] The exquisite pain control provided by TEA serves to improve postoperative pulmonary function following major upper abdominal surgery by allowing deep breathing unaffected by severe pain. A study found that bilateral dual TAP blocks do not result in clinically significant changes in the pulmonary function in healthy subjects.[16] Paravertebral blocks (PVBs) and other fascial plane blocks, on the other hand, may have some plausible effects; however, the comparative research is scarce. Advancements in abdominoplasty surgery have allowed for a paradigm shift in the demographic risk profile of patients, which frequently includes elderly and advanced disease individuals for complex surgeries. For example, restrictive lung disease, itself a significant risk factor for postoperative pulmonary complications, predisposes our patient to extended length of stay and increased morbidity. "Splinting," or rapid shallow breathing in the setting of incisional pain, can create a functional restrictive disease in an already diseased lung and most commonly presents following upper abdominal surgeries. In such scenarios, there is an extremely high risk of developing postoperative pneumonia, primarily due to decreased inspiratory effort due to their surgical discomfort. TEA provides excellent analgesia but also affects multiple muscles of respiration. While a reduction of vital capacity and FEV1 due to motor blockade of the intercostal muscles is observed, however, these effects are negated in the face of the functional restrictive lung disease that occurs with splinting, and the benefits from the analgesia generally outweigh the minimally decreased pulmonary function.[17,18]

THORACIC EPIDURAL ANALGESIA (TEA)

Epidural placement at the level of thoracic spine is considered challenging due to relatively narrow intervertebral foramen. Additionally, lack of palpable landmarks, increased skin to epidural space distance, and "false" loss of resistance in fatty tissues are important determinants of difficult placement, presumably common in lipoabdominoplasty patients with higher body mass index (BMI).[19]

PARAVERTEBRAL BLOCKS

This space exists on either side of T1 to L1 vertebra, bounded by parietal pleura anterolaterally, transverse process of vertebral body laterally, superior costotransverse ligament superiorly, with apex communicating with potential intercostal space.[20]

PARAVERTEBRAL BY PROXY OR PARAVERTEBRAL VARIANT OR PARASPINAL BLOCKS

Relatively newer blocks (such as erector spinae, retrolaminar, mid-point transverse process to pleura block, and intercostal paraspinal blocks) achieve thoracic nerve blockade—without actually entering paravertebral space.[21,22] Recent identification of communicating pathways in muscle plane blocks (such as paravertebral, subcostal QL) address the visceral component and broader sensory dermatomal coverage in preliminary studies.

TAP BLOCK

For midline incisions, bilateral catheters with appropriate tunneling can be performed with continuous infusion of LAs. Importantly, this block provides somatic analgesia (not visceral) related to midline abdominal incision. Theoretical risks include needle injury to superior epigastric vessels and visceral organ puncture. These risks can be significantly minimized by ultrasound-guided technique.

Combination of blocks such as intercostal, ilioinguinal, iliohypogastric, and pararectus is also another consideration.[5] While the literature about PVBs in abdominoplasty is scares, they were generally superior when compared to fascial plane blocks for other abdominal surgeries.[23,24] A meta-analysis—limited by high risks of bias and heterogeneity—suggests improved analgesia in most abdominal procedures when compared with systemic opioids.[25] Importantly, the plausible analgesic effects of PVB suggest anterior to posterior extension with additional visceral coverage, whereas muscle plane blocks, such as TAP, provide somatic effects that are potentially limited to anterior midaxillary line. Due to these communicating pathways, more medial injections are reported to have bilateral spread, with a reported incidence of 10%, although unpredictable. An imaging study described 20 cc LA in paravertebral space to cover approximately 4 vertebrae levels; however, the craniocaudal spread was noted to be variable.[26] In summary, the limited current evidence appears to support the use of PVBs in abdomen surgeries with seemingly low side-effects profile.[20]

The advent of ultrasound allows precise and accurate deposition of LA between internal oblique and transversus abdominis muscle, targeting the neurovascular plane where anterior branches of terminal rami T7–L1 are situated. Limited primarily to somatic anesthesia of the anterior abdominal wall, the effective spread relies on volume and spread of LA injected. A few reports suggested 15 cc as an optimal volume for an adult unilateral TAP block.[27,28] The reported sensory dermatomal spread with classical TAP block is T10 to L1. The ability of classic/lateral TAP block to anesthetize sensory dermatome is limited and rarely extends beyond T10. Similarly, an imaging study also revealed no communication whatsoever between anterior and lateral compartments.[29] Therefore, a variation of TAP block, subcostal TAP block, was developed, which aimed to deposit LA injection between rectus abdominis and posterior rectus sheath or transversus abdominis. In combination with bilateral classical TAP, this is referred to as 4-point TAP block. Subcostal TAP blocks have shown extended and more cranial coverage until the sensory dermatome of T7, while posterior TAP provides blockade from T10 to L1.[30]

RECTUS SHEATH BLOCK (RS)

The block aims to anesthetize the terminal branches of the intercostal nerves between the internal oblique and transverse abdominis muscles. These nerve branches penetrate the posterior wall of rectus muscle and end in an anterior cutaneous branch supplying the skin of the umbilical area; studies showed good pain scores and no complications.[31–33] Generally, for lipoabdominoplasty, bilateral indwelling catheters are recommended. Securing the catheter to prevent inadvertent dislodgment and avoiding surgical field interference with techniques (such as subcutaneous tunneling, suture catheters) are desirable. Regardless of that, catheter displacement remains a significant concern.[34] The next important concern is catheter-related infections. Liposomal bupivacaine appears to offer reduced risks of catheter-related infections, decreased follow-up, and at least comparable efficacy. Extensive ongoing research focusing on comparing long-acting LA formulations and continuous catheters for extensive open abdomen surgeries is still in the recruitment phase.

TAP block has been used extensively in abdominoplasty. It was found to reduced pain scores and analgesic requirements and earlier ambulation also.[35,36] However, patients with increased BMI and large flap resected are more likely to fail the anesthetic block and require more postoperative analgesia.[36] When TAP block was compared to RSB Block, and subcutaneous infiltrations (SCI), a significantly longer analgesia was recorded in the TAP group compared with both the RSB and SCI groups. A significantly higher pain and morphine consumption was noted in the SCI group was compared with the other two groups.[37] TAP block was compared to a combination of pararectus injections and ilioinguinal/iliohypogastric nerve blocks for abdominoplasty in addition to bupivacaine injection in the rectus plication in both groups. It was found that patients in the TAP block group required significantly less hydromorphone postoperatively (TAP block group: 2.63 mg; standard treatment group: 4.31 mg) and had a significantly longer time to first request of pain medications (3 hours 11 minutes; standard treatment group: 1 hour 27 minutes).[38] Salama et al.[39] compared bilateral continuous TAP block to wound infiltration with LA, or a continuous wound infusion with saline. Morphine requirements in the first 48 hours were significantly higher in the saline wound infiltration compared to LA wound infiltration and TAP group (61.9 ± 12.8, 21.5 ± 9.5, and 18.9 ± 8.1 mg) but the wound infiltration and TAP group were comparable.

QUADRATUS LUMBORUM BLOCK (QL) BLOCK

Quadratus lumborum (QL) muscle originates from posteromedial iliac crest and inserts into the medial border of the 12th rib and the transverse process of L1–L4. An important landmark, thoracolumbar fascia, is a complex tubular fibrous aponeurotic sheath that encases back muscles, including QL muscle.

It extends from thoracic to lumbar spine and connects the anterolateral abdominal wall with lumbar paravertebral. Two models were described in literature with respect to splitting of thoracolumbar fascia, i.e., two-layered and three-layered models. The two-layered model comprises anterior layer (between erector spinae and QL muscle) and posterior layer (surrounding erector spinae muscle). The three-layered model incorporates three layers: anterior (anterior to QL muscle), middle (layer between erector spinae and QL), and posterior (posterior to erector spinae) (Figures 19.1 and 19.2).

Lateral Quadratus Lumborum Block (QL1)

QL Block 1 involves LA deposition at the lateral border of the QL muscle (transversalis fascia junction) (Figures 19.2, 19.3A, B).

Posterior Quadratus Lumborum Block (QL 2)

QLB 2 is defined as LA deposition posterior to QL muscle, between the junction of erector spinae and latissimus dorsi muscles.

Anterior Quadratus Lumborum Block (QL 3)

In QLB 3, LA deposition is in the fascial plane between the QL, psoas major muscles fascia, and thoracolumbar fascia[40,41] (Figure 19.4A, B).

The point of injection is demonstrated to have an impact on the dermatome spread. For example, previous cadaveric and clinical studies noted an extended dermatomal spread to even T5, by injecting LA with different approaches.[41–43]

Procedure

The procedure can be done with the patient supine, especially the QLB 1, or best in the lateral position. For anterior approach the patient is positioned in lateral decubitus position, slightly flexed hip and knee joint, with the desired block site to face toward the ceiling. A towel roll may be placed below the lower flank to facilitate the sonographic visualization of QL muscle. A curvilinear (low-frequency) ultrasound probe is placed in transverse orientation at the posterior or mid-axillary line (at level L2–L4) and QL muscle is identified as a quadrangular structure, hypoechoic (in relation to surrounding muscle). At this level, lumbar transverse process and vertebral body may be identified (Figure 19.4A, B).

Subcostal Anterior Approach

The curvilinear ultrasound probe is placed in a parasagittal oblique plane, at the level of the 12th rib (approximately 6–8 cm from the spinous process). The transducer is tilted medially, producing an oblique sagittal view at QL muscle (identified as the point of its insertion from lower border of last rib), latissimus dorsi muscle, diaphragmatic zone of apposition, perinephric fat, and fascia and the kidney are identified. If ultrasound probe is tilted more medially toward neuroaxis and the cranial side of the transducer moved lateral with the caudal side moved medially, the long axis of the psoas major

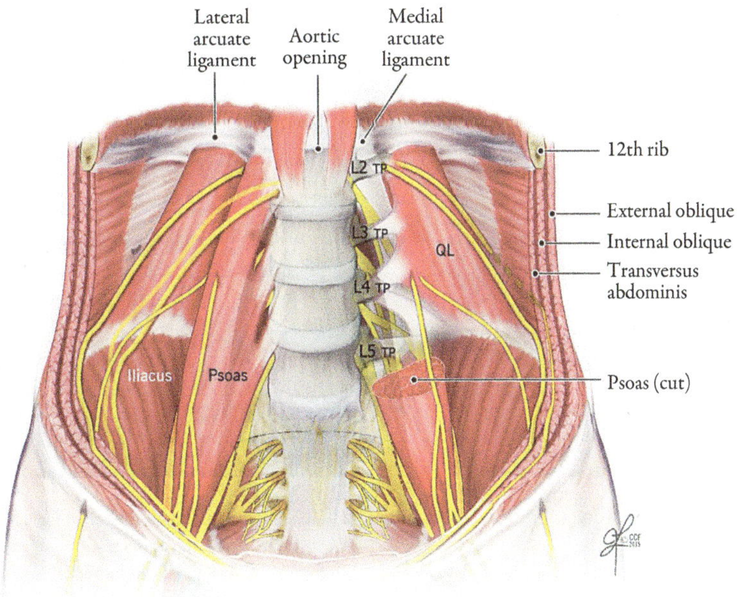

Figure 19.1. Anatomy of the quadratus lumborum and the nerves related to it.

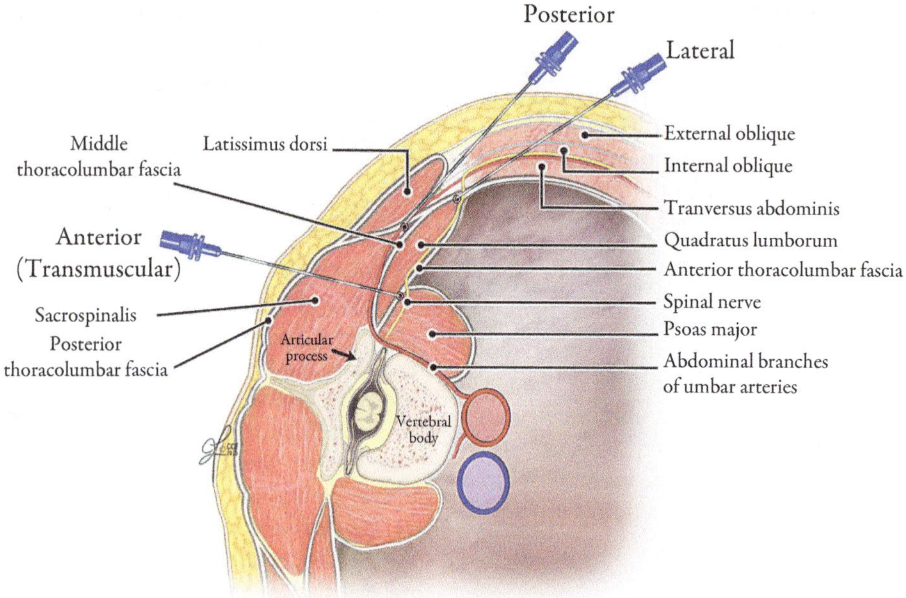

Figure 19.2. Types of quadratus lumborum block; note the tip of the needle insertion.

muscle can be seen anterior to the QL muscle. According to the planned approach, the LA is deposited in relation to QL muscle. Several approaches to QLBs have been defined in the literature and are currently under investigation; insufficient evidence exists to recommend one approach over the another. In addition, there is no consensus on type, volume, and concentration of LAs utilized to perform QLBs. Nonetheless, ongoing clinical trials are still in the recruitment phase, and prior studies remain inconclusive to determine the hypothesized clinical effect. In the interim, the author's experience suggests that QLBs are a reasonable option for lipoabdominoplasty.

Reports of spread of the LAs in the QLB differ from study to study. A small volunteer study of QLB 2 that used the response to pin prick and MRI to track the LA spread showed spreads into the paravertebral space from T10–T12, resulting in lower and lateral abdominal sensory loss. In contrast, LA administered in the QL muscle does not spread into

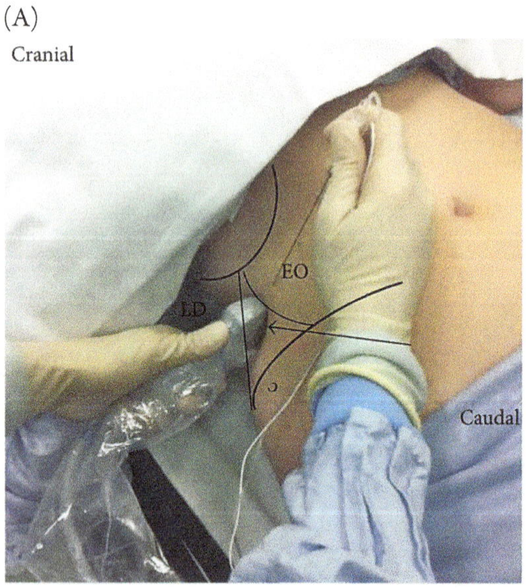

Figure 19.3A. Lateral QL block. A high-frequency linear probe was attached in the area of the triangle of Petit.
EO = external abdominal oblique; LD = latissimus dorsi; black arrow = the triangle of Petit.
From: Ueshima H, Otake H, Lin JA. Ultrasound-guided quadratus lumborum block: an updated review of anatomy and techniques. *Biomed Res Int*. 2017;2017:2752876. doi: 10.1155/2017/2752876.

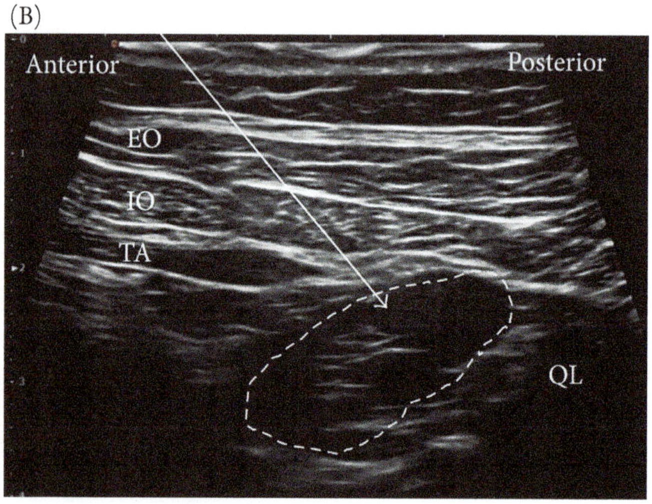

Figure 19.3B. Ultrasound images of lateral QLB.
EO = external oblique muscle; IO = internal oblique muscle; TA = transversus abdominis; QL = quadratus lumborum; white arrow = needle trajectory; white dotted line = spread of local anesthetic.
From: Ueshima H, Otake H, Lin JA. Ultrasound-guided quadratus lumborum block: an updated review of anatomy and techniques. *Biomed Res Int*. 2017;2017:2752876. doi: 10.1155/2017/2752876.

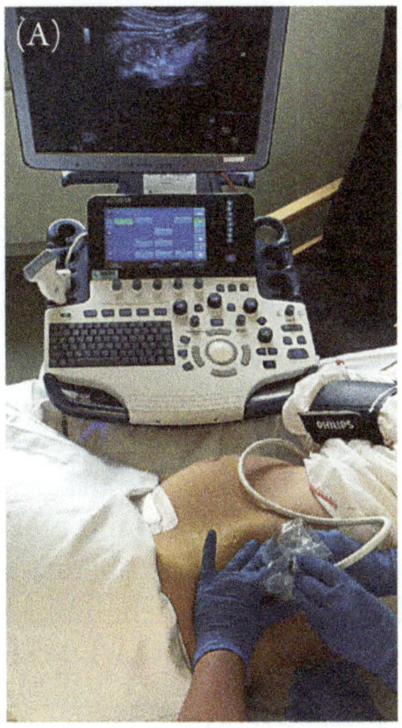

Figure 19.4A. The patient is in the right lateral position and the transducer is positioned in the transverse position in the posterior axillary line above the iliac crest.
From: Mænchen N, Hansen CK, Dam M, Børglum J. Ultrasound-guided transmuscular quadratus lumborum (TQL) block for pain management after caesarean section. *Int J Anesthetic Anesthesiol.* 2016;3:048. 10.23937/2377-4630/3/2/1048. Creative Commons Attribution License,

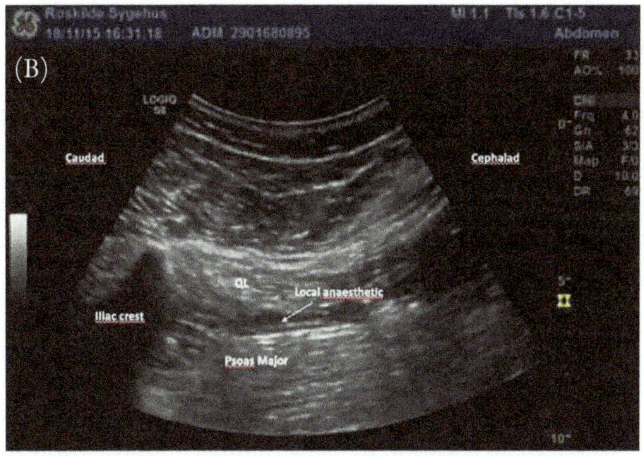

Figure 19.4B. Confirming correct spread of the injectate. After injection of the local anesthetic the transducer is rotated 90 degrees in the longitudinal plane. The correct spread of local anesthetic is confirmed by the clear visualization of injectate advancing along the interfascial compartment from the iliac crest (caudad) toward the diaphragm (cranial) separating the two muscles of quadratus lumborum (QL) and psoas major (PM).
From: Mænchen N, Hansen CK, Dam M, Børglum J. Ultrasound-guided transmuscular quadratus lumborum (TQL) block for pain management after caesarean section. *Int J Anesthetic Anesthesiol.* 2016;3:048. 10.23937/2377-4630/3/2/1048. Creative Commons Attribution License.

the PVS and results in only lateral abdominal sensory loss.[44] Another cadaver study showed that QLB 2 consistently stained the iliohypogastric, ilioinguinal, subcostal nerve, T11 to T12 and L1 nerve roots. Meanwhile, the anterior subcostal approach demonstrated predictable deep staining of the same nerves and in addition traversing the arcuate ligaments to involve T9 to T12 nerve roots with variable staining of higher thoracic nerve roots.[42] A cadaver study of QLB 3 demonstrated lumbar paravertebral space in 63% of specimens, laterally in the TAP in 50% and caudally to the anterior superior iliac spine in 63% of specimens. There was no radiographic evidence of spread to the thoracic paravertebral space. Anatomical dissection revealed dye staining of the upper branches of the lumbar plexus and the psoas major muscle in 70% of specimens.[45]

Another cadaver study showed that in QLB 3 the dye was seen to spread into the thoracic paravertebral space and the intercostal spaces to surround the somatic nerves and the thoracic sympathetic trunk. The injectate took a pathway posterior to the medial and lateral arcuate ligaments. Caudad to the diaphragm, the injected dye surrounded the subcostal, iliohypogastric, and ilioinguinal nerves in all cases, whereas the genitofemoral and lateral femoral cutaneous nerves were dyed in a varying degree. No dye was seen to surround the lumbar plexus, femoral nerve, or lumbar sympathetic trunk.[43] In a recent study the QLB was done on 34 patients using LA with radiopaque contrast, followed by tracing the injectate spread using three-dimensional computed tomography (3D-CT) images. The QLB 3 was done at the level of L2 transverse process and was called TOP QLB 3. The study found that QLB 1 spread in the TAP, QLB 2 in the TAP *and* posterior aspect of the QL muscle, whereas TOP QLB 3 spread consistently in the anterior aspect of the QL muscle *with* occasional spread to the lumbar and thoracic paravertebral areas. Of the three studied techniques, only TOP QLB 3 injections reached the paravertebral space, lumbar nerve roots, and sympathetic chain, although not in a consistent pattern. QLB 1 and QLB 2 injections reached the intercostal plane more frequently than the TOP QLB 3. In these cases, the spread reached the lateral side of the intercostal planes of the 10th and 11th ribs in more than half of the cases. Finally, the spread of the QLB 2 and TOP QLB 3 injections to the thoracic paravertebral space occurred only in one block (5%). In these two cases, the most cranial extent of the spread reached the T12 transverse process after a QLB 2 injection and the T11 transverse process after a TOP QLB 3 injection. The maximum craniocaudal extension of the paravertebral spread occurred at the L1 and L4 vertebrae. Only three TOP QLB 3 injections (15%) reached the lateral side of the vertebral body (sympathetic chain), mainly at the L2 level. This spread did not demonstrate a wide craniocaudal extension.[46] Advantages of extended dermatomal sensory coverage and possible additional visceral coverage may be provided by utilizing previously identified muscle plane communications. For example, more dorsal injections, such as subcostal transmuscular QLB, are known to cover a broader range (T6–L1) of dermatomes.[41,42,47]

Patients with BMI >30 pose technical challenges when performing deeper fascial plane blocks. So far, complications associated with QLBs have not been well described in the literature; however, risks of quadriceps weakness, visceral organ injury, infections, and muscle hematoma exist. At authors' institutions, we did not encounter any visceral organ injury (unpublished data), but the possibility of potential injury to visceral organs cannot be denied with inexperienced hands.[41,48]

QLB is not adequately studied in abdominoplasty surgery in particular. However, there are studies that examined its effect in lower abdominal surgeries. The results of the studies are conflicting and further research is needed. A randomized controlled study (RCT) of posterior bilateral QLB in abdominoplasty using either ropivacaine or placebo using saline did not find a difference in morphine consumption in the first 24 hours. The morphine consumption during the first 24 hours was 26 ± 25 mg vs. 33 ± 33 mg in the ropivacaine and placebo group, respectively.[40] The morphine consumption seems high in spite of administering perioperative paracetamol, in addition to using tumescent liposuction and injection of 20 mL bupivacaine 2.5 mg/mL with epinephrine in the rectus sheet along the suture line. Comparative studies have shown that the QLB covered more dermatomes (T7–T12) and provided more prolonged pain-free condition compared to the TAP block (24–48 h QLB versus 8–12 h TAP block).[49–52]

A meta-analysis tried to examine the effect of nerve blocks in abdominoplasty. The nerve blocks represented included TAP, rectus sheath, pararectus in addition to ilioinguinal/iliohypogastric, intercostal, and quadratus lumborum. The meta-analysis found that all modalities were effective in reducing opioid consumption except quadratus lumborum. They also concluded that TAP was more efficacious than rectus sheath and pararectus + ilioinguinal/iliohypogastrice blocks. However, the study suffered many limitations; it only included 8 studies, some of them were prospective while the others were retrospective, with high heterogeneity in terms of the type of the blocks. The QLB was represented by only one study that used the QLB 2 approach.[53]

COMBINED INTERCOSTAL AND PARARECTUS BLOCKS

A combination of interfascial (intercostal, pararectus, and ilioinguinal-iliohypogastric) blocks to possibly cover the upper and lower abdomen quadrants also has shown to provide improved pain scores and reduced recovery time.

A study compared intercostal nerve block only to general anesthesia (GA) for abdominoplasty. The blocks were placed by the surgeon and supplemented by intravenous sedation. The intercostal nerve blocks were performed blindly by the surgeon from the 4th–12th ribs. The study did not find a reduction of intraoperative opioids use in the intercostal block group compared to GA group (17 mg versus 20 mg). Some of the patients needed to be converted to GA or given more sedation or LA infiltration as they did have the procedure done under the block and sedation. The reasons for that may be because the block was done blindly, and some the procedures were combined with some other plastic procedures remote from abdominoplasty. However, they found significant decreases in the recovery room time, postoperative narcotics, postoperative nausea and vomiting, and better pain control in the intercostal block group.[54] Another study tested what is called "painless" abdominoplasty. They used a combination of intercostal and pararectus blocks for postoperative pain control. They looked into the data over 10 years retrospectively over a 10-year period and found 77 received the block and 20 worked as controls. All intercostal blocks were performed from T7 to T12 at the posterior axillary line before incision; the blocks were extended superiorly from T6 to T2 in the midaxillary line. Before plication, the iliohypogastric and ilioinguinal nerves were blocked, the pararectus block was injected above and below this point, on either side of the rectus muscle from the costal margin to the groin, in the plane of the internal oblique muscle and from the costal margin to the groin, in the plane of the internal oblique muscle. Skin incisions were anesthetized by tumescent infiltration and received a combination of nerve blocks, using bupivacaine, tetracaine, and Depo-Medrol. The study found that the treatment group had significantly less pain and required significantly less narcotics and less time in the recovery room. Patients had significantly less nausea, took less pain medication, and resumed normal activities significantly sooner than the control group. Pain scores continued to be significantly lower at home.[5]

LIPOSOMAL BUPIVACAINE

TAP block with liposome bupivacaine in open abdominal wall reconstruction demonstrated significant reductions in narcotic consumption and improved pain control. It allowed for earlier discontinuation of intravenous narcotics and shorter length of stay.[55] However, another study in ventral hernia repairs with mesh placed showed no apparent clinical benefits compared to plain bupivacaine and placebo when used in TAP block for open abdominal wall reconstruction.[56]

THE USE OF KETOROLAC

Ketorolac has important opioid-sparing effect; however, it is known to increase the bleeding rates due to its antiplatelets effect. A study that examined 106,279 patients who underwent breast and body contouring procedures found that 4924 (4.6%) received postoperative ketorolac. The study revealed that ketorolac was not associated with hematoma formation, while absolute differences in reoperation rates were low. Ketorolac was also associated with fewer readmissions, with an estimated savings of $157 per patient.[57] Firriolo et al.[58] studied the use of perioperative ketorolac in 500 reduction mammaplasty procedures. They found that Ketorolac use was largely associated with decreased perioperative opioid use, without increasing the risk of hematoma formation.

CONCLUSIONS

The decision to perform a regional block or a combination of blocks should be assessed on a case-by-case basis. The clinical profile of the patient must be the primary focus for any such decision-making. Obvious contraindications to neuraxial blocks necessitate other modalities such as truncal blocks. Research is scarce and ongoing regarding which regional block is better for lipoabdominoplasty and similar surgeries. TAP block and RSB seem to provide good analgesia for lipoabdominoplasty. Ongoing research focusing on head-to-head randomized trials comparing epidural and newer muscle plane blocks is still in the recruitment phase.

REFERENCES

1. Richter D, Stoff A Abdominoplasty procedures. In: Song DH Neligan PC. *Plastic Surgery*. Vol. 4: Trunk and Lower Extremity. Philadelphia: Elsevier Saunders; 2012:530–558.
2. Hensel JM, Lehman JA Jr, Tantri MP, Parker MG, Wagner DS, Topham NS. An outcomes analysis and satisfaction survey of 199 consecutive abdominoplasties. *Ann Plast Surg.* 2001;46(4):357–363.
3. Rangaswamy M. Lipoabdominoplasty: a versatile and safe technique for abdominal contouring. *Indian J Plast Surg.* 2008;41(Suppl):S48–S55.
4. Heller JB, Teng E, Knoll BI, Persing J. Outcome analysis of combined lipoabdominoplasty versus conventional abdominoplasty. *Plast Reconstr Surg.* 2008;121(5):1821–1829.
5. Feng LJ. Painless abdominoplasty: the efficacy of combined intercostal and pararectus blocks in reducing postoperative pain and recovery time. *Plast Reconstr Surg.* 2010;126(5):1723–1732.
6. Abdallah FW, Chan VW, Brull R. Transversus abdominis plane block: a systematic review. *Reg Anesth Pain Med.* 2012;37(2):193.
7. Sood J, Jayaraman L, Sethi N. Liposuction: anaesthesia challenges. *Indian J Anaesth.* 2011;55(3):220–227.
8. Svedman KJ, Coldiron B, Coleman WP 3rd, et al. ASDS guidelines of care for tumescent liposuction. *Dermatol Surg.* 2006;32(5):709–716.
9. Klein JA, Jeske DR. Estimated maximal safe dosages of tumescent lidocaine. *Anesth Analg.* 2016;122(5):1350–1359.
10. Hanci V, Hakimoglu S, Ozacmak H, et al. Comparison of the effects of bupivacaine, lidocaine, and tramadol infiltration on wound healing in rats. *Rev Bras Anestesiol.* 2012;62(6):799–810.
11. Miskovic A, Lumb AB. Postoperative pulmonary complications. *Br J Anaesth.* 2017;118(3):317–334.
12. Bulger EM, Edwards T, Klotz P, Jurkovich GJ. Epidural analgesia improves outcome after multiple rib fractures. *Surgery.* 2004;136(2):426–430.
13. Manion SC, Brennan TJ. Thoracic epidural analgesia and acute pain management. *Anesthesiology.* 2011;115(1):181–188.
14. Groeben H. Epidural anesthesia and pulmonary function. *J Anesth.* 2006;20(4):290–299.
15. Clemente A, Carli F. The physiological effects of thoracic epidural anesthesia and analgesia on the cardiovascular, respiratory and gastrointestinal systems. *Minerva Anestesiol.* 2008;74(10):549–563.
16. Petersen M, Elers J, Borglum J, Belhage B, Mortensen J, Maschmann C. Is pulmonary function affected by bilateral dual transversus abdominis plane block? A randomized, placebo-controlled, double-blind, crossover pilot study in healthy male volunteers. *Reg Anesth Pain Med.* 2011;36(6):568–571.
17. Xu J, Zhou J, Xiao H, et al. A systematic review and meta-analysis comparing programmed intermittent bolus and continuous infusion as the background infusion for parturient-controlled epidural analgesia. *Sci Rep.* 2019;9(1):2583–2583.
18. Bullingham A, Liang S, Edmonds E, Mathur S, Sharma S. Continuous epidural infusion vs programmed intermittent epidural bolus for labour analgesia: a prospective, controlled, before-and-after cohort study of labour outcomes. *Br J Anaesth.* 2018;121(2):432–437.
19. Lotia S, Bellamy MC. Anaesthesia and morbid obesity. *Cont Educ Anaesth Crit Care Pain.* 2008;8(5):151–156.
20. Rudkin GE, Gardiner SE, Cooter RD. Bilateral thoracic paravertebral block for abdominoplasty. *J Clin Anesth.* 2008;20(1):54–56.
21. Costache I, Pawa A, Abdallah FW. Paravertebral by proxy: time to redefine the paravertebral block. *Anaesthesia.* 2018;73(10):1185–1188.
22. Pawa A, Wojcikiewicz T, Barron A, El-Boghdadly K. Paravertebral blocks: anatomical, practical, and future concepts. *Curr Anesthesiol Rep.* 2019;9(3):263–270.
23. Melnikov AL, Bjoergo S, Kongsgaard UE. Thoracic paravertebral block versus transversus abdominis plane block in major gynecological surgery: a prospective, randomized, controlled, observer-blinded study. *Local Reg Anesth.* 2012;5:55–61.
24. Law LS, Tan M, Bai Y, Miller TE, Li YJ, Gan TJ. Paravertebral block for inguinal herniorrhaphy: a systematic review and meta-analysis of randomized controlled trials. *Anesth Analg.* 2015;121(2):556–569.
25. El-Boghdadly K, Madjdpour C, Chin KJ. Thoracic paravertebral blocks in abdominal surgery: a systematic review of randomized controlled trials. *Br J Anaesth.* 2016;117(3):297–308.
26. Marhofer D, Marhofer P, Kettner SC, et al. Magnetic resonance imaging analysis of the spread of local anesthetic solution after ultrasound-guided lateral thoracic paravertebral blockade: a volunteer study. *Anesthesiology.* 2013;118(5):1106–1112.
27. Abdallah FW, Chan VW, Brull R. Transversus abdominis plane block: a systematic review. *Reg Anesth Pain Med.* 2012;37(2):193–209.
28. Moeschler SM, Murthy NS, Hoelzer BC, Gazelka HM, Rho RH, Pingree MJ. Ultrasound-guided transversus abdominis plane injection with computed tomography correlation: a cadaveric study. *J Pain Res.* 2013;6:493–496.
29. Borglum J, Jensen K, Christensen AF, et al. Distribution patterns, dermatomal anesthesia, and ropivacaine serum concentrations after bilateral dual transversus abdominis plane block. *Reg Anesth Pain Med.* 2012;37(3):294–301.
30. Soliz JM, Lipski I, Hancher-Hodges S, Speer BB, Popat K. Subcostal transverse abdominis plane block for acute pain management: a review. *Anesthesiol Pain Med.* 2017;7(5):e12923–e12923.
31. Dutton TJ, McGrath JS, Daugherty MO. Use of rectus sheath catheters for pain relief in patients undergoing major pelvic urological surgery. *BJU Int.* 2014;113(2):246–253.
32. Tudor ECG, Yang W, Brown R, Mackey PM. Rectus sheath catheters provide equivalent analgesia to epidurals following laparotomy for colorectal surgery. *Ann R Coll Surg England.* 2015;97(7):530–533.
33. Yassin HM, Abd Elmoneim AT, El Moutaz H. The analgesic efficiency of ultrasound-guided rectus sheath analgesia compared with low thoracic epidural analgesia after elective abdominal surgery with a midline incision: a prospective randomized controlled trial. *Anesth Pain Med.* 2017;7(3):e14244.
34. Capdevila X, Pirat P, Bringuier S, et al. Continuous peripheral nerve blocks in hospital wards after orthopedic surgery: a multicenter prospective analysis of the quality of postoperative analgesia and complications in 1,416 patients. *Anesthesiology.* 2005;103(5):1035–1045.
35. Sforza M, Andjelkov K, Zaccheddu R, Nagi H, Colic M. Transversus abdominis plane block anesthesia in abdominoplasties. *Plast Reconstr Surg.* 2011;128(2):529–535.
36. Araco A, Pooney J, Araco F, Gravante G. Transversus abdominis plane block reduces the analgesic requirements after abdominoplasty with flank liposuction. *Ann Plast Surg.* 2010;65(4):385–388.
37. Abo-Zeid MA, Al-Refaey AK, Zeina AM. Surgically-assisted abdominal wall blocks for analgesia after abdominoplasty: a prospective randomized trial. *Saudi J Anaesth.* 2018;12(4):593–598.
38. Fiala T. Tranversus abdominis plane block during abdominoplasty to improve postoperative patient comfort. *Aesthet Surg J.* 2015;35(1):72–80.
39. Salama ER. Post-operative bilateral continuous ultrasound-guided transversus abdominis plane block versus continuous local anaesthetic wound infusion in patients undergoing abdominoplasty. *Indian J Anaesth.* 2018;62(6):449–454.

40. Bjelland TW, Yates TGR, Fagerland MW, Froyen JK, Lysebraten KR, Spreng UJ. Quadratus lumborum block for postoperative analgesia after full abdominoplasty: a randomized controlled trial. *Scand J Pain.* 2019 May 21;19(4):671–678.
41. Elsharkawy H, Ahuja S, DeGrande S, Maheshwari K, Chan V. Subcostal approach to anterior quadratus lumborum block for pain control following open urological procedures. *J Anesth.* 2019;33(1):148–154.
42. Elsharkawy H, El-Boghdadly K, Kolli S, et al. Injectate spread following anterior sub-costal and posterior approaches to the quadratus lumborum block: a comparative cadaveric study. *Eur J Anaesthesiol.* 2017;34(9):587–595.
43. Dam M, Moriggl B, Hansen CK, Hoermann R, Bendtsen TF, Borglum J. The pathway of injectate spread with the transmuscular quadratus lumborum block: a cadaver study. *Anesth Analg.* 2017;125(1):303–312.
44. Tamura T, Yokota S, Ito S, Shibata Y, Nishiwaki K. Local anesthetic spread into the paravertebral space with two types of quadratus lumborum blocks: a crossover volunteer study. *J Anesth.* 2019;33(1):26–32.
45. Adhikary SD, El-Boghdadly K, Nasralah Z, Sarwani N, Nixon AM, Chin KJ. A radiologic and anatomic assessment of injectate spread following transmuscular quadratus lumborum block in cadavers. *Anaesthesia.* 2017;72(1):73–79.
46. Balocco AL, Lopez AM, Kesteloot C, et al. Quadratus lumborum block: an imaging study of three approaches. *Reg Anesth Pain Med.* 2021;46(1):35–40.
47. Elsharkawy H, El-Boghdadly K, Barrington M. Quadratus lumborum block: anatomical concepts, mechanisms, and techniques. *Anesthesiology.* 2019;130(2):322–335.
48. Elsharkawy H, Bajracharya GR, El-Boghdadly K, Drake RL, Mariano ER. Comparing two posterior quadratus lumborum block approaches with low thoracic erector spinae plane block: an anatomic study. *Reg Anesth Pain Med.* 2019;44(5):549.
49. Blanco R, Ansari T, Riad W, Shetty N. Quadratus lumborum block versus transversus abdominis plane block for postoperative pain after cesarean delivery: a randomized controlled trial. *Reg Anesth Pain Med.* 2016;41(6):757–762.
50. Murouchi T, Iwasaki S, Yamakage M. Quadratus lumborum block: analgesic effects and chronological ropivacaine concentrations after laparoscopic surgery. *Reg Anesth Pain Med.* 2016;41(2):146–150.
51. Oksuz G, Bilal B, Gurkan Y, et al. Quadratus lumborum block versus transversus abdominis plane block in children undergoing low abdominal surgery: a randomized controlled trial. *Reg Anesth Pain Med.* 2017;42(5):674–679.
52. Kumar GD, Gnanasekar N, Kurhekar P, Prasad TK. A comparative study of transversus abdominis plane block versus quadratus lumborum block for postoperative analgesia following lower abdominal surgeries: a prospective double-blinded study. *Anesth Essays Res.* 2018;12(4):919–923.
53. Vonu PM, Campbell P, Prince N, Mast BA. Analgesic efficacy of nerve blocks after abdominoplasty: a systematic review. *Aesthet Surg J.* 2020;40(11):1208–1215.
54. Michaels BM, Eko FN. Outpatient abdominoplasty facilitated by rib blocks. *Plast Reconstr Surg.* 2009;124(2):635–642.
55. Fayezizadeh M, Majumder A, Neupane R, Elliott HL, Novitsky YW. Efficacy of transversus abdominis plane block with liposomal bupivacaine during open abdominal wall reconstruction. *Am J Surg.* 2016;212(3):399–405.
56. Fafaj A, Krpata DM, Petro CC, et al. The efficacy of liposomal bupivacaine on postoperative pain following abdominal wall reconstruction: a randomized, double-blind, placebo-controlled trial. *Ann Surg.* 2022;276(2):224–232.
57. Kelley BP, Chung KC, Chung TT, et al. Postoperative ketorolac in breast and body contouring procedures: a nationwide claims analysis. *Plast Reconstr Surg.* 2018;142(4):472e–480e.
58. Firriolo JM, Nuzzi LC, Schmidtberg LC, Labow BI. Perioperative ketorolac use and postoperative hematoma formation in reduction mammaplasty: a single-surgeon experience of 500 consecutive cases. *Plast Reconstr Surg.* 2018;142(5):632e–638e.
59. Teitelbaum S. Demystifying high-lateral-tension abdominoplasty. *Aesthet Surg J.* 2006;26(3):325–329.
60. Wan D, Hubbard BA, Byrd HS. Achieving aesthetic results in the umbilical float mini-abdominoplasty: patient selection and surgical technique. *Plast Reconstr Surg.* 2019;143(3):722–732.
61. Carloni R, De Runz A, Chaput B, et al. Circumferential contouring of the lower trunk: indications, operative techniques, and outcomes: a systematic review. *Aesthetic Plast Surg.* 2016;40(5):652–668.
62. Lee ET, Park HM, Lee DG, et al. Application of mini-abdominoplasty after conservative excision of extensive cesarean scar endometriosis. *Arch Plast Surg.* 2012;39(5):551–555.

REVIEW QUESTIONS

(1) The following statements are true EXCEPT:

A. Strong evidence suggests an association between local anesthetic use and skin graft failure.
B. Abdominoplasty is the most commonly performed aesthetic reconstructive procedure.
C. Combining abdominoplasty and lipoplasty is known to improve outcomes and simultaneously reduce the risk of associated complications.
D. None of the above are true.

(2) The following are effects of low thoracic epidural analgesia EXCEPT:

A. Increased functional expiratory volume first second (FEV1)
B. Decreased vital capacity
C. Improved diaphragm function
D. Improved cough

(3) Two days after an abdominoplasty, the patient started complaining of pain and numbness in the anterolateral border of the thigh. Which of the following nerves is most commonly injured during this operation?

A. Lateral cutaneous nerve of thigh
B. Sciatic nerve
C. Gluteal nerve
D. Ilioinguinal nerve

(4) Post-abdominoplasty, the patient is about to be discharged, and the anesthesia resident was called to remove an epidural catheter. However, the patient complains of backache following an epidural analgesia. This is most likely the result of:

A. Traumatic nerve injury from the needle
B. Disruption of the ligaments from the epidural needle
C. Hematoma formation
D. Prolonged immobilization

(5) Which of the following is true regarding paravertebral block?

A. Useful for thoracic surgeries only
B. Loss of resistance is due to penetration of the costovertebral membrane.

C. Mostly done in higher thoracic space
D. "Lung sliding sign" is indicative of pneumothorax.

(6) The following statements regarding transversus abdominis plane (TAP) block are true EXCEPT:

A. Visceral puncture may go unnoticed even with ultrasound guided blocks.
B. Sensory dermatomal coverage extends from T10 to L1.
C. It covers visceral pain.
D. Subcostal approach provides adequate analgesia for upper quadrants of the abdomen.

(7) The followings statements regarding quadratus lumborum block (QLB) are true EXCEPT:

A. The QLB 1 is done at the lateral edge of the QL muscle.
B. The QLB 2 is done between the QL and latissimus dorsi.
C. The QLB 3 is done between the QL muscle and erector spinae.
D. The QLB may cover visceral pain.

ANSWERS

(1) **A.** Currently, laboratory data suggest a possible delayed wound healing related to myotoxic, chondrotoxic, and vasculotoxic effects of local anesthetics. To date, no human studies have shown any association of LA use and skin graft failure.

Reference

Hanci V, Hakimoglu S, Ozacmak H, et al. Comparison of the effects of bupivacaine, lidocaine, and tramadol infiltration on wound healing in rats. *Rev Bras Anestesiol.* 2012;62(6):799–810.

(2) **A.** Gold standard for analgesia in major upper abdominal surgery is epidural anesthesia. *Low thoracic* epidural analgesia may produce small changes in pulmonary function parameters such as decrease in vital capacity and FEV1 from the baseline, possibly due to motor blockade of the inspiratory muscles. However, the beneficial effects, such as improved diaphragm function, decreased pain, and earlier extubation, greatly outweigh the drawbacks of minimally decreased pulmonary function.

References

Groeben H. Epidural anesthesia and pulmonary function. *J Anesth.* 2006;20(4):290–299.
Clemente A, Carli F. The physiological effects of thoracic epidural anesthesia and analgesia on the cardiovascular, respiratory and gastrointestinal systems. *Minerva Anestesiol.* 2008;74(10):549–563.

(3) **A.** The lateral femoral cutaneous nerve is the most commonly injured nerve after abdominoplasty. The incidence ranges from 0.36% to 10%.

Reference

Ducic I, Zakaria HM, Felder JM, 3rd, Arnspiger S. Abdominoplasty-related nerve injuries: systematic review and treatment options. *Aesthet Surg J.* 2014;34(2):284–297.

(4) **B.** The incidence of new-onset backache after epidural analgesia ranges from 2% to 31%. The most likely causes of back pain after epidural analgesia include ligamentous trauma or strain due to epidural needle or paraspinous muscle spasm. Other listed options may be possible but rare in occurrence.

Reference

Munnur U, Suresh MS. Backache, headache, and neurologic deficit after regional anesthesia. *Anesthesiol Clin North Am.* 2003 Mar;21(1):71–86.

(5) **B.** This space exists on either side of T1 to L1 vertebra bounded by parietal pleura anterolaterally, transverse process of vertebral body laterally, superior costotransverse ligament posteriorly, with apex communicating with potential intercostal space. It is useful for thoracic and abdominal pain as well. Lack of lung sliding is a sign of pneumothorax.

Reference

El-Boghdadly K, Madjdpour C, Chin KJ. Thoracic paravertebral blocks in abdominal surgery: a systematic review of randomized controlled trials. *Br J Anaesth.* 2016;117(3):297–308.

(6) **C.** TAP block covers only somatic nerves; classic TAP block usually covers sensory dermatomal spread from T10 to L1. The subcostal TAP block was developed in combination with bilateral classical TAP; this is referred to as 4-point TAP block. With this variation, the spread extends from T7 to L1.

Reference

Chakraborty A, Khemka R, Datta T. Ultrasound-guided truncal blocks: A new frontier in regional anaesthesia. *Indian J Anaesth.* 2016;60(10):703–711.

(7) **C.** QLB 1 is done at the lateral edge of the QL muscle; QLB 2 is done posterior to QLB and the latismus dorsi; and QLB 3 is done anterior to the QL muscle and posterior to the psoas major. The QLB may cover visceral pain because of possible spread to the paraveretebral space.

Reference

Tamura T, Yokota S, Ito S, Shibata Y, Nishiwaki K. Local anesthetic spread into the paravertebral space with two types of quadratus lumborum blocks: a crossover volunteer study. *J Anesth.* 2019 Feb;33(1):26–32.

20.

INGUINAL HERNIA REPAIR

Derek Blankenship, Mitchell Cahan, and Gustavo Angaramo

STEM CASE AND KEY QUESTIONS

A 78-year-old male patient is having a repeat open left inguinal hernia repair. The patient recounts the nature of the uncontrolled postoperative pain and urinary retention he had in his first surgery. Also, the pain had persisted in the same location for the past year. He uses gabapentin and oxycodone as needed to help manage his pain.

(1) HOW ARE INGUINAL HERNIAS CLASSIFIED?

Inguinal hernias are classified as direct, indirect, or femoral based upon the site of herniation. Indirect hernias protrude lateral to the inferior epigastric vessels, through the deep inguinal ring. Direct hernias are medial to the inferior epigastric vessels, within Hesselbach's triangle. The borders of the triangle are the inguinal ligament inferiorly, the lateral edge of rectus sheath medially, and the inferior epigastric vessels superolateral. Femoral hernias protrude through the femoral ring. They traverse the space between the femoral vein and the lymphatic channels. The femoral ring borders include Cooper's ligament posteriorly, the inguinal ligament anteriorly, the lacunar ligament medially, and the femoral vein laterally.

(2) WHAT IS THE NERVE SUPPLY OF THE INGUINAL HERNIA SURGERY AREA?

The inguinal region is customarily innervated within the inguinal canal by the iliohypogastric (IHN) and ilioinguinal (IIN) nerves and the genital branch of the genitofemoral nerve (GFN).

(3) WHAT TYPES OF ANESTHESIA ARE APPROPRIATE FOR INGUINAL SURGERY?

General anesthesia is used for laparoscopic and open procedures; however, regional (spinal, epidural, nerve blocks) and local infiltration have been used in open inguinal hernia repairs as the sole anesthetic. Regional anesthesia techniques have the advantage of preemptive and postoperative analgesia.

(4) WHAT IS THE NERVE BLOCK OPTIONS FOR INGUINAL HERNIA SURGERY?

Different regional techniques can be used for anesthesia and analgesia for an inguinal hernia repair. These include the IIN and IHN nerve blocks, transversalis fascia plane block (TFP) Block, transversus abdominis plane (TAP) block, quadratus lumborum (QL) block, paravertebral nerve block (PVB), local anesthesia infiltration, and caudal block.

(5) HOW CAN YOU BLOCK THE IIN AND IHN NERVES?

The IIN and IHN are blocked blindly 2 cm medial and 2 cm superior to the iliac crest, and injection is done after feeling 1 or 2 fascial pops. Using ultrasound guidance, the local anesthetic is injected in the fascial plane between the internal oblique muscle (IOM) and transversus abdominis muscle (TAM).

(6) WHAT ARE THE PROS AND CONS OF A PARAVERTEBRAL BLOCK (PVB) FOR INGUINAL HERNIA SURGERY?

It is performed at the level of T10–L2. It provides unilateral motor, sympathetic, and prolonged sensory blockade that usually lasts for 13–15 hours. Being segmental, it can be expected to have some advantages regarding hemodynamic stability and early ambulation when compared with other neuroaxial techniques; however, epidural extension of anesthesia can cause lower limb numbness and delay the discharge of patients. The PVB has become less popular after the development of the fascial plane block.

(7) DESCRIBE THE ANATOMY AND INNERVATION IN RELATIONSHIP TO THE TRANSVERSALIS FASCIAL PLANE BLOCK (TFPB).

The TFP Block is a truncal block that targets the L1 nerve branches, namely the IIN and IHN. The fascia of the TAM is also called the thoracolumbar fascia. This is formed when the TAM and IOM muscles taper off posteriorly into a common aponeurosis. This transversalis fascia is a thin aponeurotic membrane that lies between the TAM and the extraperitoneal fascia. It is part of the general layer of fascia lining the abdominal cavity.

(8) DESCRIBE THE DIFFERENCES BETWEEN THE TFPB AND THE TAP BLOCK.

The TFPB blocks T12–L1 nerve branches, especially L1 nerve branches which the TAP block does not reliably cover. The TFPB does not include the dermatomes above L1 and T12, while the TAP block does. Local anesthetic is injected deep to the TAM for the TFPB, compared to staying superficial to the muscle for the TAP block (see Figures 20.3 and 20.4 later in the chapter).

DISCUSSION

Around 75% of abdominal wall hernias occur in the groin region. Groin hernias are inguinal or femoral hernias. Inguinal hernia constitutes 90% of the cases, while femoral hernias constitute 10% of the cases. Surgical hernia repair is a common procedure with approximately 20 million inguinal hernia repairs performed worldwide every year, and in the Unites States alone the number reaches 800,000.[1]

Of inguinal hernia repairs, 90% are performed in men, and 10% in women. The median age at presentation is 60–79 years of age for women compared with 50–69 years of age for men.[2,3] Femoral hernias usually present with complications (incarceration, strangulation). Seventy percent of femoral hernia repairs are performed in women; however, the most common subtype of groin hernia in men and women is still the indirect inguinal hernia.[8]

Risk factors for hernia development include history of hernia or prior hernia repair, older age, male sex, Caucasian race, chronic cough, chronic constipation, abdominal wall injury, smoking and family history of hernia.[4] Low body mass index (BMI) <20 is independently associated with a higher incidence of acquired femoral hernia in women; also obesity is a negative risk factor for groin hernia in males and females.[5]

Inguinal hernia repair is a routine procedure in general surgery. Several repair techniques have been reported to date; despite that, tension-free mesh repairs are commonly used due to the low recurrence rates.[6]

Pain after inguinal hernia repair is classified into acute or chronic. Pain after hernia is sharp, burning, or tearing sensation. It has three mechanisms: nociceptive (somatic), neuropathic, and visceral pain. Nociceptive pain is the most common and is due to ligamentous or muscular trauma and inflammation. Neuropathic pain occurs because of direct nerve damage or entrapment. Visceral pain is transmitted through afferent autonomic pain fibers.[7]

Since the progression of a hernia by time is natural, most surgeons recommend repairing them promptly. Conversely, a small number of recent articles have reported that watchful waiting is a safe and acceptable choice with mildly symptomatic or asymptomatic cases since delay in treatment does not increase complication rates. Nonetheless, when hernia complications like incarceration or strangulation occur sporadically, they can be treated uneventfully.[8,9]

TYPES OF HERNIA REPAIR TECHNIQUES

Over the last decades the operative repair techniques have been refined and have resulted in open and laparoscopic tension-free approaches utilizing advanced prosthetic mesh-material as the gold standard. Therefore, hernia recurrence incidence rates have dropped significantly (1%–5%), to the point that today chronic pain is rather recognized as the most significant complication.[10]

Current repair options for inguinal hernias are presented in the following.

TENSION-FREE PROSTHETIC REPAIRS

1. Anterior repairs
2. Posterior (preperitoneal) repairs
3. Open techniques via inguinal incision.

TISSUE-SUTURE REPAIRS

A metanalysis has revealed that Shouldice four-layer inguinal hernia repair is the preferred non-mesh technique in terms of recurrence. However, it is more time-consuming and needs a slightly longer postoperative hospital stay.[11] During the repair, the transversalis fascia is incised from the internal ring laterally to the pubic tubercle medially, and upper and lower flaps are created. These flaps are then overlapped (double-breasted) with two layers of sutures. The conjoined tendon is then sutured to the inguinal ligament, again in two overlapping layers. This reinforces the posterior wall and narrows the deep inguinal ring. A mesh is placed while performing a total extraperitoneal technique (TEP) or a transabdominal preperitoneal approach (TAPP). A totally TEP repair is preferred to a TAPP since complications like bowel injury are a concern in TAPP. In practice, TAPP makes more sense in terms of the surgical anatomy when compared to TEP and is also easily taught in an academic setting.[12]

OPEN VERSUS LAPAROSCOPIC INGUINAL HERNIA REPAIR

Endoscopic and laparoscopic repairs result in low postoperative pain, less wound infection, and a prompt return to daily activity and working.[13] Open and laparoscopic/endoscopic techniques have been compared in several studies, demonstrating that the latter are more expensive than open repairs; however, the reimbursement is remarkably higher since the procedure is performed in ambulatory surgery centers, making laparoscopic hernia repair far more cost-effective.[14] A multicenter study revealed that recurrences and complications were more common in the laparoscopic group (this was no longer the case when the analysis factored in laparoscopic cases done by fellowship-trained surgeons); however, they had less immediate postoperative pain at 2 weeks, along with a faster return to daily activities.[15]

Globally, the most used types of mesh-based repairs are the Lichtenstein open repair and one of the variations of the laparoscopic repair. The Lichtenstein repair is a tension-free technique known to cause discomfort and debilitating pain in some patients. [15] However, the laparoscopic procedures generally have decreased the development of chronic pain after inguinal hernia repair.[16]

NERVE SUPPLY OF THE INGUINAL AREA

The IIN and IHN originate from the anterior ramus of the lumbar plexus and emerge from the lateral border of psoas major muscle, inferior to the 12th rib, and course over the anterior surface of the quadratus lumborum muscle (QLM). Lateral to the QLM, they initially run deep to TAM for a variable distance before piercing it to enter the TAP between the IOM and TAM muscles with free communications between their branches. In the preperitoneal space, innervation is provided by the genital branch of the GFN within the inguinal canal and the GFN trunk and its femoral branch, the lateral cutaneous (LFC) nerve, and the femoral nerve (FN). There is a significant variation during the course of these nerves, and aberrant anatomy with shared, duplicated, or absent nerves is common.[17]

NERVE BLOCKS FOR INGUINAL HERNIA REPAIR

Local and regional anesthesia have been demonstrated to shorten time spent in the operating room, to decrease the incidence of nausea and urinary retention, and to bring higher patient satisfaction. The use of regional anesthesia has been also associated with less postoperative analgesic requirements, shorten length of stay, and decreased costs when compared with general anesthesia. In fact, local infiltration and regional anesthesia are the preferred methods for open repair.[18,19]

PARAVERTEBRAL NERVE BLOCK (PVB)

PVB is a regional technique involving the injection of local anesthesia immediately lateral to the vertebral column into the paravertebral space. In the paravertebral space, the nerves emerge from the spinal cord through the intervertebral foramina and bifurcate into the dorsal and ventral rami. This technique provides unilateral motor, sympathetic, and prolonged sensory blockade that usually lasts for 13–15 hours. It provides more hemodynamic stability and early ambulation compared to other neuraxial techniques; however, epidural extension of anesthesia can cause lower limb numbness and motor weakness and delay the discharge of patients.[20] A systematic review of PVB reduced postoperative nausea and vomiting (PONV) compared with general anesthesia/systematic analgesia. When compared with neuraxial blocks, PVB resulted in less postoperative nausea and urinary retention. However, more time was needed to perform PVB than neuraxial blocks. It also showed decreased postoperative pain scores and analgesic requirement as compared with ilioinguinal block and TAP block.[21]

PVB has become less popular today, especially after the development of fascial plane blocks. It is performed at the level of T10–L2 and can be executed with the patient in the sitting, lateral, or prone position. The midline is represented by the spinous process of the vertebral column. The iliac crest represents the L3–L4 interspace, and the tip of the scapula corresponds to the T7 spinous process. Traditionally, skin markings can also be made 2.5 cm lateral to the midline at the levels that are to be blocked. The block needle is then inserted perpendicular to the skin until the transverse process is contacted. Once identified, the depth marker is adjusted so that it is 1.0 cm beyond the skin–transverse process depth.[18] The needle is withdrawn to the subcutaneous tissue and reinserted at a 10- to 15-degree superior or inferior angle so that it slides off the superior or inferior edge of the transverse process. The needle is advanced 1.0 cm beyond the contact with the transverse process. After negative aspiration for blood or cerebrospinal fluid, the local anesthetic is injected. Since the spread of local anesthetic after a single large-volume lumbar paravertebral injection is uncertain, a multiple-injection technique in which 4–5 mL of local anesthetic is injected at each level is more frequently used.

IIN AND IHN BLOCKS

Nerve blocks of the IIN, IHN, and GFN have been used for postoperative pain management and in diagnostic and therapeutic purposes in the treatment of chronic post-herniorrhaphy inguinal pain (CPIP). In several trials, these nerve blocks have been used preoperatively to determine which patients could respond to surgical neurectomy.

Conventionally, these blocks were performed by using anatomic landmarks. Currently they are done under ultrasound guidance under direct visualization, reducing the risk of intraperitoneal needle placement and improved accuracy.[7,22] The landmark technique involves inserting the needle 2 cm medial and 2 cm superior to the anterior superior iliac spine. As the needle penetrates the external oblique muscle (EOM) aponeurosis, an initial pop sensation will be felt, and then a local anesthetic is injected. The needle is then advanced deeper to puncture the aponeurosis of the internal oblique muscle (IOM). The bevel of the needle lies in the fascial plane between the IOM and transversus abdominis muscle (TAM). This technique is a TAP block in the region where the IIN and IHN nerves are located. However, this technique might not be always successful given the anatomical location variability of the II and IH nerves with regard to the ASIS.[23,24]

The ultrasound-guided technique involves identifying the IIN and IHN between the TAM and IOM. The ultrasound probe should be placed parallel to the line connecting the umbilicus and anterior superior iliac spine (ASIS), and three muscles should be identified: EOM, IOM, and the TAM. The hypoechoic IIN is then identified within this fascial plane

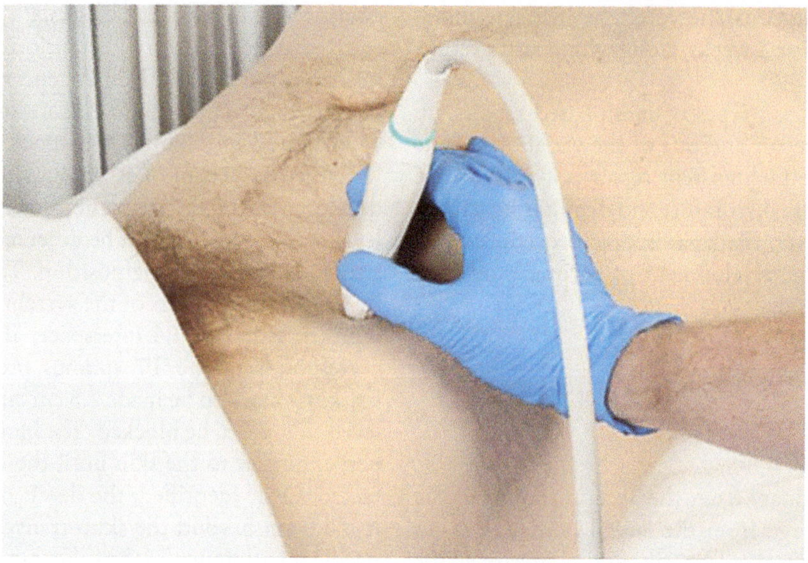

Figure 20.1. Ilioinguinal nerve block: ultrasound positioning. The transducer is placed between the anterior superior iliac spine and the umbilicus. Reproduced with permission from: Waldman RA, Willis S. A simplified approach to ultrasound guided ilioinguinal nerve block. *Phys Med Rehabil Res.* 2016;1: doi: 10.15761/PMRR.1000104.

(Figures 20.1 and 20.2A and B). The local anesthetic should be deployed between the TAM and IOM. The IHN may also be seen to be lying medial to the IIN within this fascial plane. Color Doppler image is then utilized to identify the deep circumflex iliac artery, which also lies within this fascial plane near the IIN, so it can be avoided.[25]

Conflicting results have emerged from some studies that have evaluated the efficacy of ultrasound-guided IIN/IHN blocks in the treatment of CPIP. Thomassen et al.[26] found out that ultrasound- or nerve stimulator–guided IIN/IHN blocks were equally effective in treating CPIP with successful prolonged pain relief after a median follow-up time of 20 months. However, a randomized, double-blind, placebo-controlled study failed to provide substantial evidence to support the use of ultrasound-guided IIN/IHN blocks in the diagnosis and treatment of CPIP. A viable explanation for this result is that nerve branches are divided from the IIN and IHN nerves more proximally than the anterior superior iliac spine, where blocks were performed, and a possible central sensitization where the short interruption of peripheral sensory nerve

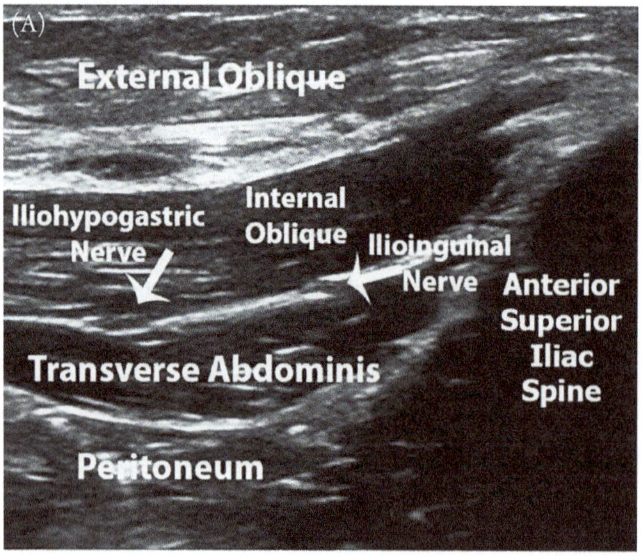

Figure 20.2A. Oblique ultrasound image demonstrating the acoustic shadow of the anterior superior iliac spine and the muscles layers and facial plane containing the ilioinginal and iliohypogastric nerves.

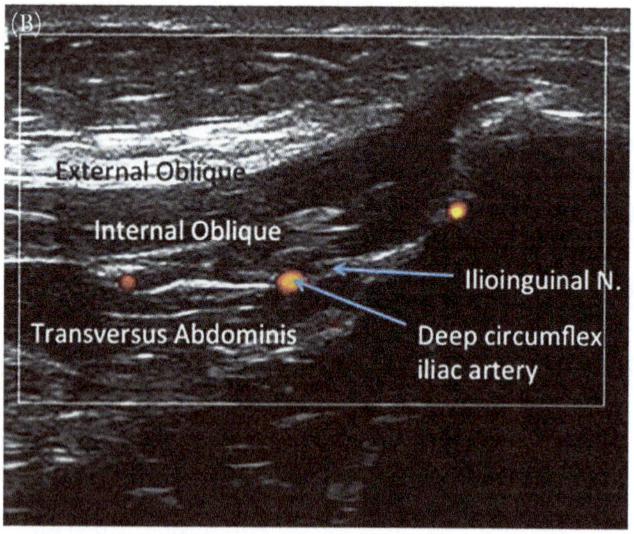

Figure 20.2B. Ilioinguinal nerve block: deep circumflex location. Color Doppler demonstrating the relationship between the deep circumflex iliac artery and ilioinguinal nerve.

Reproduced with permission from: Waldman RA, Willis S. A simplified approach to ultrasound guided ilioinguinal nerve block. *Phys Med Rehabil Res.* 2016;1: doi: 10.15761/PMRR.1000104.

transmission by the lidocaine block may not be sufficient to mitigate these changes in central pain processing.[27]

TRANSVERSUS ABDOMINIS PLANE (TAP) BLOCK AND TRANSVERSALIS FASCIA PLANE BLOCK (TFPB)

A retrospective observational study that compared TAP and TFP Blocks with a multimodal approach for postoperative inguinal herniorrhaphy pain found that they are easy to perform and have fewer complications. TFPB reaches the highest sensory level, but there were no differences in the requirements for additional analgesia.[28]

The ultrasound-guided TFPB was first described as a novel technique that may have a role for postoperative analgesia after surgical procedures that involve the area of T12–L1 dermatomes primarily. Chin et al.[29] reported the similarity of the ultrasound-guided TFPB and the QLB in terms of approach and anesthetic effectiveness. However, in the ultrasound-guided TFPB, the point of injection is more caudal and more anterior. This results in a more localized spread, explicitly targeting the IIN and IHN, where they run deep to the transversus abdominis muscle (TAM) before ascending into the transversus abdominis plane.[28] These anatomical landmarks have suggested that there is a possible relationship between the lumbar plexus and the fascia transversalis which has been corroborated by recent studies demonstrating the unanticipated finding of quadriceps and hip flexor weakness after a ultrasouns-guided TFPB.[30]

Transversalis Fascia Plane Block Technique

This nerve block can be used in inguinal hernia repair, appendectomies, cecostomies, and iliac crest bone harvest. With the patient in a supine position, an ultrasound high-frequency linear probe is placed in transversely over the lateral abdomen between the iliac crest and the costal margin. The needle is advanced in an in-plane technique once the EOM, IOM, and TAM are recognized, and the more posterior transversus aponeurosis is distinguished. The perinephric fat is generally more prominent closer to the iliac crest. The quadratus lumborum muscle is identified medial to the aponeurosis of the TAM. The endpoint is more visible if the needle is passed through the posterior quadrant of the TAM. It is then advanced into the triangular area surrounded by the posterior edge of the TAM, the QLM, and the fascia transversalis.[29] Twenty to 30 mL of bupivacaine 0.5% are injected, observing the downward displacement of the retroperitoneal fat (perinephric) into the transversalis fascia and the spread of the local anesthetic over the surface of the QLM (Figure 20.3). Hebbard[31] described in his original study that local anesthetics can be injected into the TAP upon the needle's withdrawal to achieve a more extensive block of the anterior branches of nerves above T12 (Figure 20.4).

As demonstrated by Scimia et al.[32] in their work, the ultrasound-guided TFPB provides a solid block of the nerves T12–L1 by deploying the local anesthesia in the anatomical triangular plane between the TAM and the transversalis fascia

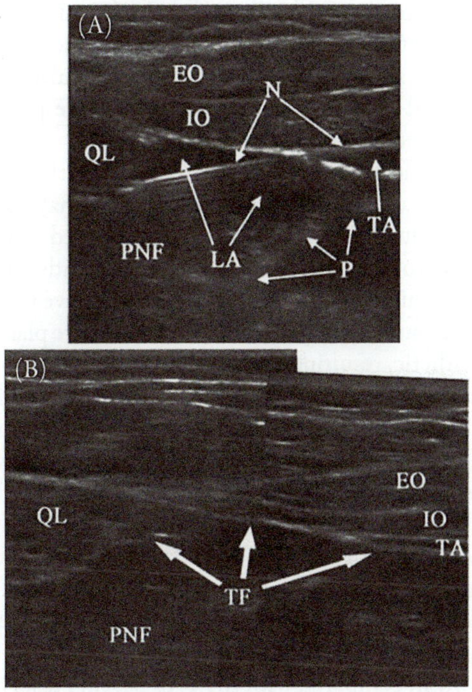

Figure 20.3A and B. Transversalis fascia plane block.

(A): The US image of a completed block. The needle (N) was advanced into the hydro-dissected space anterior to the quadratus lumborum (QL). Local anesthetic (LA), peritoneum (P), and external oblique (EO), internal oblique (IO), and transversus (TA) muscles are also shown.

(B): A sonogram of the lateral abdominal wall, including the perinephric fat (PNF) and the transversalis fascia (TF).

Reproduced with permission from: Hebbard PD. Transversalis fascia plane block, a novel ultrasound-guided abdominal wall nerve block. *Can J Anesth*. 2009;56:619.

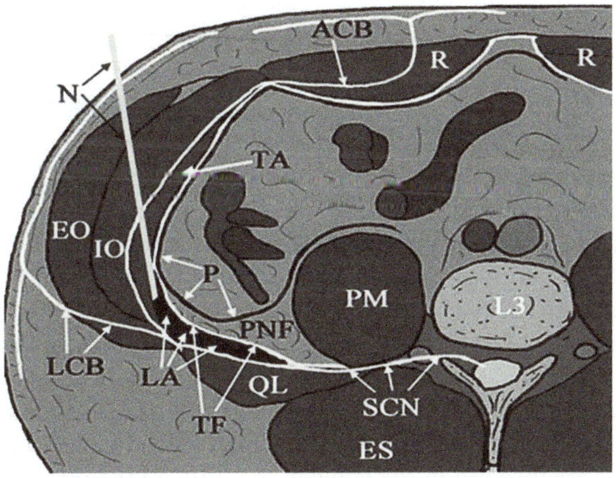

Figure 20.4. Transversalis fascia plane block. Transverse diagram through the abdomen above the iliac crest. The course of the subcostal nerve (SCN) is indicated, including the lateral cutaneous branch (LCB) and the anterior cutaneous branch (ACB). The location of the local anesthetic (LA) across the anterior surface of the quadratus lumborum (QL) and behind the transversalis fascia (TF) is shown, and the needle position (N), perinephric fat (PNF), peritoneum (P), and transversalis fascia (TF) are indicated. The following muscles are involved: rectus abdominis (R), erector spinae (ES), psoas (PM), transversus abdominis (TA), internal oblique (IO), and external oblique (EO).

Reproduced with permission from Hebbard PD. Transversalis fascia plane block, a novel ultrasound-guided abdominal wall nerve block. *Can J Anesth*. 2009;56:619.

anterolateral to the QLM. A multimodal analgesic regimen technique that includes this regional technique may provide good-quality analgesia, reducing opioid requirements and opioid-related side effects in the postoperative period, with excellent patient satisfaction.

Because the IIN and IHN course within the TAP for a short and variable length, the L1 dermatomes may not reliably be blocked during standard ultrasound-guided TAP block. Various anatomical landmark and ultrasound-based techniques for achieving IIN and IHN blockade have been widely performed, but they may often lead to inaccurate placement of local anesthetic, resulting in block failure.[29]

It has been proposed that insufficient analgesia could happen because of possible GFN nociceptive afferent inputs during inguinal hernia repair. Previous studies suggested that the benefit of adding a GFN block to IIN and IHN blocks is limited.[29]

A metanalysis of 6 studies with 632 patients found no statistically significant difference between the II/IH and TAP groups in postoperative opioid use. The II/IH block provides excellent analgesic effects at 6 and 8 hours after inguinal herniorrhaphy in compared with the TAP block. However, more high-quality randomized controlled trials with long-term follow-up are still required to make the conclusion.[33]

CHRONIC POST-HERNIORRHAPHY INGUINAL PAIN (CPIP)

Chronic postsurgical pain has been defined as pain that develops after a surgical intervention and lasts for at least 2 months when other causes of pain have been excluded.[7] For CPIP, 6 months is usually used because the inflammation around the mesh is usually still ongoing after 3 months, and there is a chance that some patients will improve substantially from 3 to 6 months postoperatively.[34,35]

The estimated frequency of moderate to severe chronic pain after hernia repair is 10%–12% and the incidence of chronic pain affecting daily activities or employment is agreed to be 0.5%–6.0%, translating to 4,000–48,000 new cases only in the United States annually, making it a serious health concern.[7]

The accurate cause of CPIP is complex and fluctuating, although it can be described by separating it into the different categories of pain encountered in CPIP: neuropathic, somatic, and or visceral pain. Neuropathic pain arises from damage or trauma to the inguinal nerves and usually develops in the sensory distribution of the affected nerves.[36] The inguinal nerves that are involved in the etiology of CPIP are the IHN, IIN, the genital branch of the GFN, and infrequently the femoral branch of the GFN or the LFC nerve. Intraoperatively, nerves can be damaged by stretching, crushing, electrical/thermal damage, partial or complete transection, becoming entrapped in suture during an open repair, or entrapment in tacks, suture, or fixation used during laparoscopic repair. Postoperatively, nerves can become damaged or entrapped in a meshoma, irritation secondary to an excessive fibrotic reaction, or inflammatory processes such as granuloma or neuroma formation.[7] Non-neuropathic causes of pain include hernia recurrence, excessive scar tissue formation, pain from the bulk of the mesh, mesh-related excess, or periosteal anchoring of the mesh near the pubic tubercle, a condition termed *periostitis pubis*.[37]

Eventually visceral pain arises from intestinal involvement with recurrence, incarceration, or mesh adherence, spermatic cord compromise, or other periurethral structures.

Interventions that can be used to treat or manage the chronic pain include watchful waiting, pharmacological treatments, local anesthetic blocks, nerve stimulation or ablation, and surgery (mesh removal, reoperation for recurrence, and neurectomy).[16]

NERVE BLOCKS AS PREDICTORS OF NEURO-ABLATIVE TECHNIQUES FOR TREATMENT OF CPIP

Once nerve blocks have shown significant pain relief, neuro-ablative techniques such as cryoablation, chemical neurolysis, and pulsed radiofrequency ablation may be considered for longer-lasting effect.[7]

Patients with risk factors for developing CPIP should be identified preoperatively, and precautionary multimodal analgesia and anesthesia should be prioritized. Preemptive measures such as peri- and postoperative gabapentinoids (the routine use of pregabalin and/or gabapentin for the management of acute postoperative pain has been recently challenged by a systematic review and meta-analysis),[38] ketamine treatment, infiltration with local anesthetics, and therapeutic ultrasound-guided nerve blocks should minimize the inflammatory cascade, reduce central sensitization, and prevent the development of severe chronic pain.

CONCLUSION

Inguinal hernia surgery is a common procedure; laparoscopic hernia repair is more common than open procedures. General anesthesia is used for laparoscopic procedure with hernial site infiltration with local anesthetics. Chronic pain after inguinal hernia repair is the most common complication after surgery. Nerve blocks like IHN, IIN, TAP and TFPB are options for postoperative pain, especially after complicated, open, or recurrent procedures. They are also useful for the diagnosis and treatment of chronic pain from inguinal hernia repair.

REFERENCES

1. Fitzgibbons RJ, Richards AT, Quinn TH. Open hernia repair. In: Souba WS, Mitchell P, Fink MP, et al., eds. *ACS Surgery: Principles and Practice.* Philadelphia: Decker; 2002:828–849.
2. Abramson JH, Gofin J, Hopp C, Makler A, Epstein LM. The epidemiology of inguinal hernia: a survey in western Jerusalem. *J Epidemiol Community Health.* 1978;32(1):59–67.
3. Kark AE, Kurzer M. Groin hernias in women. *Hernia.* 2008;12(3): 267–270.
4. Ruhl CE, Everhart JE. Risk factors for inguinal hernia among adults in the US population. *Am J Epidemiol.* 2007;165(10):1154–1161.

5. Rutkow IM. Epidemiologic, economic, and sociologic aspects of hernia surgery in the United States in the 1990s. *Surg Clin North Am.* 1998;78(6):941–951, v–vi.
6. Kulacoglu H. Current options in inguinal hernia repair in adult patients. *Hippokratia.* 2011;15(3):223–231.
7. Bjurstrom MF, Nicol AL, Amid PK, Chen DC. Pain control following inguinal herniorrhaphy: current perspectives. *J Pain Res.* 2014;7:277–290.
8. Turaga K, Fitzgibbons RJ Jr, Puri V. Inguinal hernias: should we repair? *Surg Clin North Am.* 2008;88(1):127–138, ix.
9. Fitzgibbons RJ Jr, Giobbie-Hurder A, Gibbs JO, et al. Watchful waiting vs repair of inguinal hernia in minimally symptomatic men: a randomized clinical trial. *JAMA.* 2006;295(3):285–292.
10. Bittner R, Schwarz J. Inguinal hernia repair: current surgical techniques. *Langenbecks Arch Surg.* 2012;397(2):271–282.
11. Amato B, Moja L, Panico S, et al. Shouldice technique versus other open techniques for inguinal hernia repair. *Cochrane Database Syst Rev.* 2012;4:CD001543.
12. Kapoor VK. Open inguinal hernia repair medication. *Medescape.* 2020. Updated Sep 14, 2020. Accessed Jan 19, 2021.
13. Karthikesalingam A, Markar SR, Holt PJ, Praseedom RK. Meta-analysis of randomized controlled trials comparing laparoscopic with open mesh repair of recurrent inguinal hernia. *Br J Surg.* 2010;97(1):4–11.
14. Jacobs VR, Morrison JE, Jr. Comparison of institutional costs for laparoscopic preperitoneal inguinal hernia versus open repair and its reimbursement in an ambulatory surgery center. *Surg Laparosc Endosc Percutan Tech.* 2008;18(1):70–74.
15. Neumayer L, Giobbie-Hurder A, Jonasson O, et al. Open mesh versus laparoscopic mesh repair of inguinal hernia. *N Engl J Med.* 2004;350(18):1819–1827.
16. Andresen K, Rosenberg J. Management of chronic pain after hernia repair. *J Pain Res.* 2018;11:675–681.
17. Graham D, MacQueen I, Chen D. Inguinal neuroanatomy: implications for prevention of chronic postinguinal hernia pain. *Int J Abdom Wall Hernia Surg.* 2018;1(1):1–8.
18. Hadzic A, Kerimoglu B, Loreio D, et al. Paravertebral blocks provide superior same-day recovery over general anesthesia for patients undergoing inguinal hernia repair. *Anesth Analg.* 2006;102(4):1076–1081.
19. Ozgun H, Kurt MN, Kurt I, Cevikel MH. Comparison of local, spinal, and general anaesthesia for inguinal herniorrhaphy. *Eur J Surg.* 2002;168(8–9):455–459.
20. Weltz CR, Klein SM, Arbo JE, Greengrass RA. Paravertebral block anesthesia for inguinal hernia repair. *World J Surg.* 2003;27(4):425–429.
21. Law LS, Tan M, Bai Y, Miller TE, Li YJ, Gan TJ. Paravertebral block for inguinal herniorrhaphy: a systematic review and meta-analysis of randomized controlled trials. *Anesth Analg.* 2015;121(2):556–569.
22. Hu QL, Chen DC. Approach to the patient with chronic groin pain. *Surg Clin North Am.* 2018;98(3):651–665.
23. Ndiaye A, Diop M, Ndoye JM, et al. Emergence and distribution of the ilioinguinal nerve in the inguinal region: applications to the ilioinguinal anaesthetic block (about 100 dissections). *Surg Radiol Anat.* 2010;32(1):55–62.
24. Klaassen Z, Marshall E, Tubbs RS, Louis RG Jr, Wartmann CT, Loukas M. Anatomy of the ilioinguinal and iliohypogastric nerves with observations of their spinal nerve contributions. *Clin Anat.* 2011;24(4):454–461.
25. Waldman RA, Willis S. A simplified approach to ultrasound guided ilioinguinal nerve block. *Phys Med Rehabil Res 1.* 2016. doi:10.15761/PMRR.1000104
26. Thomassen I, van Suijlekom JA, van de Gaag A, Ponten JE, Nienhuijs SW. Ultrasound-guided ilioinguinal/iliohypogastric nerve blocks for chronic pain after inguinal hernia repair. *Hernia.* 2013;17(3):329–332.
27. Bischoff JM, Koscielniak-Nielsen ZJ, Kehlet H, Werner MU. Ultrasound-guided ilioinguinal/iliohypogastric nerve blocks for persistent inguinal postherniorrhaphy pain: a randomized, double-blind, placebo-controlled, crossover trial. *Anesth Analg.* 2012;114(6):1323–1329.
28. Lopez-Gonzalez JM, Lopez-Alvarez S, Jimenez Gomez BM, Arean Gonzalez I, Illodo Miramontes G, Padin Barreiro L. Ultrasound-guided transversalis fascia plane block versus anterior transversus abdominis plane block in outpatient inguinal hernia repair. *Rev Esp Anestesiol Reanim.* 2016;63(9):498–504.
29. Chin KJ, McDonnell JG, Carvalho B, Sharkey A, Pawa A, Gadsden J. Essentials of our current understanding: abdominal wall blocks. *Reg Anesth Pain Med.* 2017;42(2):133–183.
30. Lee S, Goetz T, Gharapetian A. Unanticipated motor weakness with ultrasound-guided transversalis fascia plane block. *A A Case Rep.* 2015;5(7):124–125.
31. Hebbard PD. Transversalis fascia plane block, a novel ultrasound-guided abdominal wall nerve block. *Can J Anaesth.* 2009;56(8):618–620.
32. Scimia P, Basso Ricci E, Petrucci E, Behr AU, Marinangeli F, Fusco P. Ultrasound-guided transversalis fascia plane block: an alternative approach for anesthesia in inguinal herniorrhaphy: a case report. *A A Pract.* 2018;10(8):209–211.
33. Zhou Y, Chen M, Zhang Y, Zhou H, Yu X, Chen G. Ilioinguinal/iliohypogastric nerve block versus transversus abdominis plane block for pain management following inguinal hernia repair surgery: a systematic review and meta-analysis of randomized controlled trials. *Medicine (Baltimore).* 2019;98(42):e17545.
34. Kehlet H, Jensen TS, Woolf CJ. Persistent postsurgical pain: risk factors and prevention. *Lancet.* 2006;367(9522):1618–1625.
35. Alfieri S, Amid PK, Campanelli G, et al. International guidelines for prevention and management of post-operative chronic pain following inguinal hernia surgery. *Hernia.* 2011;15(3):239–249.
36. Loos MJ, Roumen RM, Scheltinga MR. Classifying post-herniorrhaphy pain syndromes following elective inguinal hernia repair. *World J Surg.* 2007;31(9):1760–1765; discussion 1766–1767.
37. Rivat C, Bollag L, Richebe P. Mechanisms of regional anaesthesia protection against hyperalgesia and pain chronicization. *Curr Opin Anaesthesiol.* 2013;26(5):621–625.
38. Verret M, Lauzier F, Zarychanski R, et al. Perioperative use of gabapentinoids for the management of postoperative acute pain: a systematic review and meta-analysis. *Anesthesiology.* 2020;133(2):265–279.

REVIEW QUESTIONS

(1) From all abdominal wall hernias, what percentage happen in the groin?

A. 25%
B. 50%
C. 60%
D. 75%

(2) Since hernia recurrence rates have decreased significantly, what is the most significant late complication observed after surgery?

A. Testicular complication
B. Mesh infection
C. Recurrence
D. Persistent groin pain and post-herniorrhaphy neuralgia

(3) From all the types of anesthesia for inguinal hernia repair, which one remains as the most used?

A. Regional
B. General

C. Neuraxial
D. Local infiltration

(4) Which are the nerves involved in the development of neuropathic pain as part of the chronic post-herniorrhaphy inguinal pain syndrome (CPIP)?

A. Ilioinguinal (IIN) and greater saphenous
B. Iliohypogastric (IHN), obturator, femoral
C. IHN, IIN, and GFN (genitofemoral)
D. Femoral lateral cutaneous, ilio-hypogastric

(5) The paravertebral block, being segmental in nature, can be expected to produce some advantages regarding hemodynamic stability and early ambulation, and may be a viable alternative in inguinal hernia repairs when compared with other regional techniques, except for:

A. Unilateral sympathetic block
B. Urinary retention
C. Prolonged sensory blockade
D. Lower limb numbness and motor weakness

(6) When the transversus abdominis plane (TAP) block is compared with transversalis fascia plane block (TFPB) for pain after inguinal hernia repair, the insufficient analgesia effect provided by TAP is due to lack of coverage of:

A. L1
B. T12
C. Genitofemoral nerve (GFN)
D. Ilioinguinal nerve (IIN)

(7) In the TFPB the local anesthetic is injected:

A. Between the external oblique (EO) and transversus abdominis muscle (TAM)
B. Between the external oblique (EO) and internal oblique (IO) muscles
C. Between the TAM and thoracolumbar fascia
D. Between the IO and the QL muscles

ANSWERS

(1) **D.** Approximately 75% of all abdominal wall hernias are seen in the groin. An inguinal hernia is much more common in men than women. Age is a factor for incidence and type of inguinal hernia; incidence increases by age. Indirect hernias are more common in young adults and direct ones in the elderly.

Reference

Ruhl CE, Everhart JE. Risk factors for inguinal hernia among adults in the US population. *Am J Epidemiol.* 2007;165:1154–1161.

(2) **D.** Complications that occur in the perioperative period include wound seroma/hematoma, urinary retention, bladder injury, and superficial incisional surgical site infection, while complications that occur later following hernia repair involve persistent groin pain, post-herniorrhaphy neuralgia, testicular complications, deep incisional/mesh infection, recurrent hernia, mesh migration, and erosion.

Reference

Abi-Haidar Y, Sanchez V, Itani KM. Risk factors and outcomes of acute versus elective groin hernia surgery. *J Am Coll Surg.* 2011;213(3):363–369.

(3) **B.** General, regional (spinal-epidural-nerve block) and local infiltration have been used in inguinal hernia repairs; however, general anesthesia remains the most used everywhere because of the widespread use of laparascopy.

Reference

Falk SA, Fleisher LA. Overview of anesthesia and anesthetic choices. In: Post TW, ed. Waltham, MA: UpToDate.

(4) **C.** Neuropathic pain in CPIP is thought to arise from damage or trauma to the inguinal nerves. The resultant pain usually develops in the sensory distribution of the affected nerves. The inguinal nerves that are involved in causing chronic post-herniorrhaphy inguinal pain (CPIP) are the IHN, IIN, the genital branch of the GFN, and more rarely, the femoral branch of the GFN or the LFC nerve.

Reference

Bjurstrom M, Nicol A, Amid P, Chen D. Pain control following inguinal herniorrhaphy: current perspectives. *J Pain Res.* 2014;7: 277–290.

(5) **D.** The paravertebral block, being segmental in nature, can be expected to produce some advantages regarding hemodynamic stability and early ambulation and may be a viable alternative in inguinal hernia repairs when compared with other regional techniques. However, epidural extension of anesthesia, resulting in lower limb numbness and motor weakness, has caused delays in the discharge of patients.

Reference

Mandal MC, Das S, Gupta S, Ghosh TR, Basu SR. Paravertebral block can be an alternative to unilateral spinal anesthesia for inguinal hernia repair. *Indian J Anaesth.* 2011;55(6):584–589.

(6) **A.** The inguinal area receives highly variable sensory innervation from IIN, IHN, and GFN. The IIN and IHN originate from the lumbar plexus and travel across the lower abdominal wall with free communications between their branches before piercing the TAM to course within the TAP Because the IIN and IHN course within the TAP for a short and variable length, the L1 dermatomes may not reliably be blocked during standard ultrasound-guided TAP block. Various anatomical landmarks and ultrasound-based techniques for achieving IIN and IHN blockade have been widely performed, but they may often lead to inaccurate placement of local anesthetic, resulting in block failure.

Reference

Konschake M, Zwierzina M, Moriggl B, et al. The inguinal region revisited: the surgical point of view: An anatomical-surgical mapping and sonographic approach regarding postoperative chronic groin pain following open hernia repair. *Hernia*. 2020;24(4): 883–894.

(7) **C.** The TFPB is a truncal block that targets the L1 nerve branches, namely the IIN and IHN nerves that emerge from the lateral border of psoas major muscle, inferior to the 12th rib, and course over the anterior surface of the QLM. Lateral to the QLM, they initially run deep to TAM for a variable distance before piercing it to enter the TAM plane between the IO and TAM.

Reference

Hammi C, Ahn K. Transversus abdominis plane block. [Updated 2020 Jul 31]. In: *StatPearls* [Internet]. Treasure Island, FL: StatPearls; 2020 Jan.

21.

ANESTHESIA FOR ANORECTAL SURGERY

Luiz Eduardo Imbelloni, José Eduardo De Aguilar-Nascimento, Iris Chu,

Engy T. Said, and Eman Nada

STEM CASE AND KEY QUESTIONS

A 25-year-old patient with Crohn's disease comes for a perianal fistulotomy. His past medical history includes chronic abdominal pain and bronchial asthma. He receives an average of 60 mg of oxycodone daily. Aside from his chronic treatment of asthma, he requires the use of multiple doses of bronchodilators every day. His past surgical history is significant, and includes a perianal abscess drained under general anesthesia, and two fistulectomies—one under local anesthetic infiltration with sedation and the other under spinal anesthesia. He recalls that his previous anesthetics were complicated by inadequate pain relief. The procedure performed under spinal anesthesia provided adequate pain relief, but he had to be catheterized for urinary retention.

(1) WHAT ARE THE ANESTHESIA OPTIONS FOR ANORECTAL SURGERY?

Local anesthetics (LAs) infiltration and sedation

Regional anesthesia

(a) Spinal anesthesia or saddle block

(b) Caudal anesthesia

(c) Pudendal nerve block

General anesthesia

(2) WHAT ARE THE ADVANTAGES AND DISADVANTAGES OF EACH TECHNIQUE?

Local infiltration with local anesthetic (LA) and sedation

Advantage: lower cost, limiting the degree of sedation, expedient with quick operating room turnover.

Disadvantage: inadequate analgesia that can result in patient movement during surgery and the necessity for deeper sedation in the prone position.

Regional anesthesia

(a) Spinal anesthesia

Advantage: Predictable efficacy, complete analgesia, and reduction in the amount of systemic sedation with adequate relaxation of the sphincter and surgical ease.

Disadvantage: prolonged post-anesthesia care unit (PACU) stay secondary to urinary retention and motor block. The risk of post-spinal headache, transient neurologic syndrome.

(b) Saddle block

Advantages: adequate anesthesia and analgesia, early discharge from PACU due to lack or minimal motor block.

Disadvantages: The time needed to place the block and set in.

(c) Caudal anesthesia

Advantages: prolonged postoperative analgesia without delaying discharge (spontaneous micturition).

Disadvantages: technically challenging: patient needs to be in the lateral or the prone position.

(d) Pudendal nerve block

Advantages: good postoperative analgesia, no urinary retention, quick recovery.

Disadvantages: requires a specific skill set.

General anesthesia

Advantages: considered the gold standard of anesthesia; no patient movement with a protected airway.

Disadvantages: airway manipulation, can result in varying hemodynamic changes, time-consuming, and delayed PACU discharge.

(3) HOW CAN REGIONAL ANESTHESIA BE USED AS THE SOLE ANESTHETIC?

Local anesthetic (LA) infiltration

LA infiltration of 10–30 mL is used; epinephrine is used to prolong the duration. This type of LA is especially helpful in fissure cases in which one must overcome the extreme internal sphincter spasm. Usually, patient requires some degree of sedation with local infiltration.

Spinal anesthesia

Lidocaine and bupivacaine have been used successfully. Recently, chloropropane and prilocaine are used as well. The use of hypobaric LAs is beneficial in the jackknife position, as it produces the least motor block compared to the hyperbaric form in the sitting position to produce saddle anesthesia.

Saddle block

The use of small amount of hyperbaric LA intrathecally and keeping the patient sitting for few minutes result in adequate operating conditions with no or minimal motor block.

Caudal block

The use of a 15–20 mL of LA in a caudal epidural block provides the added benefit of prolonged postoperative analgesia and better patient satisfaction.

(4) WHAT IS THE ROLE OF PUDENDAL NERVE BLOCK IN ANORECTAL SURGERY?

Pudendal nerve is derived from sacral nerves S2, S3, and S4 and has been used with success in anorectal surgery, as it provides prolonged pain relief after surgery.

(5) WHAT IS THE INNERVATION OF THE ANAL CANAL?

The internal anal sphincter is supplied by sympathetic (L5) and parasympathetic nerve (S2–S4) fibers. Sensation of the anal canal comes from the inferior rectal nerve, which is a branch of the pudendal nerve.

(6) YOU DISCUSS WITH THE PATIENT THE OPTIONS AND HE AGREES TO A SADDLE BLOCK FOR THE PROCEDURE. WHAT ARE THE OPTIONS FOR POSTOPERATIVE PAIN MANAGEMENT?

This patient's pain treatment is complicated by his tolerance to opioids, his chronic pain state, and the area of surgery. Postoperative pain after anal surgery is usually severe since the area is very sensitive and rich with somatic nerve endings. Pain during defecation is problematic. The options include intrathecal morphine, bilateral pudendal blockade, wound infiltration with LAs. Liposomal bupivacaine was successful in hemorrhoidectomies.

(7) IS IT SAFE TO USE NONSTEROIDAL ANTI-INFLAMMATORY DRUGS (NSAIDS) IN PATIENTS WITH CROHN'S DISEASE?

There is some evidence that the use of NSAIDs and acetaminophen in patients with Crohn's disease can activate the disease and result in exacerbation.

DISCUSSION

ANATOMY AND NERVE SUPPLY OF THE ANORECTAL AREA

Anatomically, the anal canal extends from the level of the upper aspect of the pelvic diaphragm to the anus. Surgically, it is usually defined as the part below the pectinate line; this part differs from the part above the pectinate line in several respects, including innervation, venous and lymphatic drainage, and possibly lining epithelium. The external sphincter ani consists of three parts: the subcutaneous, the superficial, and the deep.[1]

The anal canal receives innervation from both sympathetic and parasympathetic fibers. Sympathetic nerves arise from the first L1–L3, then fibers travel down in the pelvis and join the parasympathetic nerves to form the sacral plexus. The parasympathetic nerve supply originates from S2–S4 nerve roots.

The pudendal nerves arise from the S2, S3, and S4 nerve roots. They pass through the greater sciatic foramen, where it transverses through the sacrospinous and sacrotuberous ligaments. It then re-enters the perineum through the lesser sciatic foramen and accompanies the internal pudendal artery and vein. The pudendal nerve courses through the ischiorectal fossa and then through Alcock's canal, also known as the pudendal canal. Inside the pudendal canal, the nerve gives off the inferior rectal nerve and then the perineal nerve. Then it continues as the dorsal nerve innervating penis and clitoris. Branches of the pudendal nerve are the perineal nerve, inferior rectal nerve (also called the inferior anal or the inferior hemorrhoidal nerve) and dorsal nerve of the penis or clitoris (Figure 21.1).

The internal anal sphincter is supplied by sympathetic nerve L5, which initiates the tonic contractions, while parasympathetic nerve (S2–S4) fibers mediate anorectal relaxation. The external sphincter is supplied by the inferior rectal branch of the internal pudendal nerve, and the perineal branch of the S4 is under voluntary control.[2]

Crohn's disease is a relapsing systemic inflammatory disease of unknown etiology which primarily affects the gastrointestinal tract. Perianal fistulizing Crohn's disease affects one-quarter of the global Crohn's disease population, with 18% of cases presenting as penetrating lesions. It is commonly associated with the presence of perianal abscesses. Surgical drainage of these abscesses should be complimentary to medical therapy.[3]

COMMON ANORECTAL PROCEDURES

PERIANAL FISTULA

A perianal fistula is a tunnel with an internal opening, usually at the dentate line of the anal canal, and an external opening in the skin around the anal verge. It happens when an abscess

Nerve roots	Branchings			Sensory innervation	Motor innervation	Autonomic
Pudendal nerve (Pn) S1 S2–S4 S5 Anatomic presentation 30% autonomic and 70% somatic: 50% sensory and 20% motor	Dorsal branch of the penis/clitoris S2 (DBp/c)		Clitorid branch	Erectile tissue of the corpus cavernosum and crus of the penis/clitoris and the skin over the dorsolateral aspect of the foreskin, glans and penis/clitoris	Muscles involved in erection	Erection initiation and maintenance (parasympathetic)
			Pubic Branch			
	Perineal branch (Pb)	Deep/muscular (d)		Lower third of the vagina and urethra	Superficial and deep transverse perineal muscle, bulbospongiosus, ischiocarvernous, urethral sphincter, ant. portion of the ext. anal sphincter and variable areas of the levator ani	Conscious sensation of the need to urinate
		Superficial:	Medial Branch	Posterior portion of the perineal skin and scrotum/labia majora and labia minora	To the external sphincter and variable innervation of the levator ani	
			Posterolateral Branch			
	Inferior rectal branch S3 (Irb)			Sensory innervation of the anal circumference skin, the caudal third of the rectum and posterior vulvar	Levator ani muscle and external anal sphincter	Conscious awareness of the need to defecate

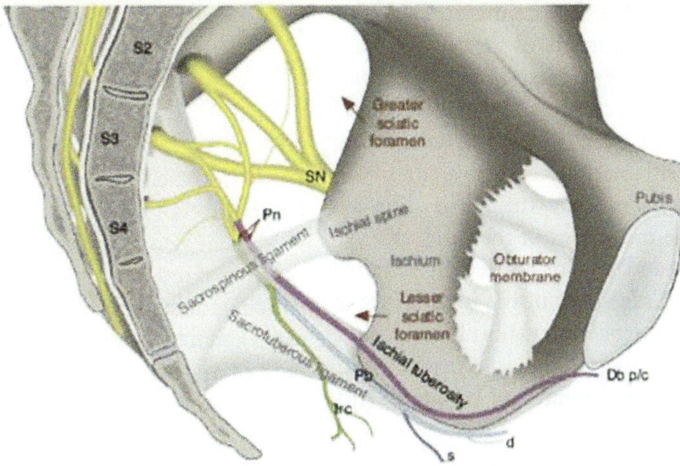

Figure 21.1. Anatomy and function of the pudendal nerve (Pn), formed by the roots of S2–S4. Its branches include the dorsal branch of the penis/clitoris DBp/c; the perineal branch (Pb) with its deep (d) and superficial (s) branches, as well as the inferior rectal branch (Irb) in its relation with the sacrospinous and sacrotuberous ligaments; the greater and lesser sciatic foramen; the ischial spine and the sciatic nerve (SN).
Obtained with permission from: Rojas-Gómez MF, Blanco-Dávila R, Tobar-Roa V, Gómez-González AM, Ortiz-Zableh AM, Ortiz-Azuero A. Regional anesthesia guided by ultrasound in the pudendal nerve territory. *Colombian J Anestesiology*. 2017;45(3):200–209. Retrieved February 20, 2021, from http://www.scielo.org.co/scielo.php?script=sci_arttext&pid=S0120-33472017000300200&lng=en&tlng=en.

ruptures or is drained, an epithelialized track forms. The chief complaint is daily soiling of purulent discharge in the perianal region. Pain is frequently associated and related to periods of reduced discharge of the pus.[4]

Anal fistula typically is treated by a single or multiple surgical procedure. The aim of the procedure is to promote the healing of the tract and preserve the sphincters. Perianal fistulas are divided into two categories: simple and complex. Simple fistulas are low, below the dentate line, with a single external opening without other complications. Complex fistulas are high, arising above the dentate line, and may have multiple external openings. They may be associated with perianal abscesses, rectal stricture, proctitis, or connections with the bladder or vagina. Treatment includes placement of noncutting setons in combination with medical and surgical treatment. Surgical treatment includes drainage of perianal abscesses, fistulotomy, or advancement of rectal flaps.[4]

Drainage of Perianal Abscesses

Surgical drainage, as opposed to spontaneous drainage, minimizes the risk of further septic complications.

Fistulotomy

The fistulous tract and is laid open and is scraped of its contents, then its sides are stitched to the sides of the incision.

Advancement of Rectal Flap

A surgeon may core out the tract, then close off the internal opening of the fistula by a mobilized flap of mucosa and submucosa to cover the tract internal opening, allowing the tract to heal and close. This is often done to reduce the amount of sphincter muscle to be cut.

Seton Placement

A seton (silk string or rubber band) is used to create scar tissue around part of the sphincter muscle before cutting it with a knife or allowing the seton to slowly cut all the way through the muscle over the course of several weeks.

The choice for a single operation (fistulotomy or fistulectomy) or placement of a seton and the scheduling of a second procedure is dependent on the trajectory of the fistula. High fistulas may require multiple procedures, which usually require the seton to slowly cut the muscle in order to prevent new abscesses, or to be used as a bridge to definitive surgery, or to control the fistula over the long term. New sphincter-preserving procedures have been introduced and they include video-assisted anal fistula treatment, insertion of anal plug, the ligation of the intersphincteric fistula tract, placement of fibrin glue, and injection of adipose mesenchymal adult stem cells into the tract and into the walls of the fistula.[4]

HEMORRHOIDAL DISEASE

Hemorrhoids are vascular cushions that help closure of the anal canal and provide sensory information that help differentiate between stool, liquid, and gas. Hemorrhoids become a disease when these veins become enlarged or inflamed. It affects up to one-quarter of all adults. Hemorrhoidal veins above the dentate line are called internal hemorrhoids and are tributaries of the portal vein. Those below the dentate line are external hemorrhoids and are tributaries of the inferior vena cava via the pudendal veins and are innervated by cutaneous sensitive nerves. As the enlargement of the internal veins progress, the patient can experience nonpainful prolapsing and occasional bleeding. Depending on the degree of internal hemorrhoids prolapse, they can be classified as 1st degree (no prolapsing), 2nd degree (prolapsing with spontaneous reduction), 3rd degree (prolapsing necessitating odd digital help to reduce), and 4th degree (irreducible prolapsing).

The chief complaint of patients suffering from internal hemorrhoid is bleeding with or without prolapsing. Bleeding usually appears during bowel movements. Advanced degrees can produce anal soiling, pruritus, and sensation of incomplete defecation, which also decrease quality of life of the patients. Inflammation and edema due to strangulation of the prolapsing can produce important pain and can lead to necrosis of the exteriorized rectal mucosa. External hemorrhoid manifests by acute inflammation which produces edema and pain. After the edema reduction, the nonretractable skin can become a plicoma, which causes soiling, pruritus, and difficulty cleaning the anal region after a bowel movement, thus decreasing quality of life.

First- and second-degree internal hemorrhoids can be treated medically or by in-office procedure. Popular in-office procedures are the rubber-band ligation and injection sclerotherapy. However, 3rd- and 4th-degree hemorrhoids necessitate surgical treatment. Surgical interventions include mucopexy, stapled hemorrhoidopexy, Doppler-guided hemorrhoidal artery ligation, and the traditional hemorrhoidectomy. The less-invasive procedures result in less anal discomfort and an earlier return to normal activities when compared with the conventional surgical hemorrhoidectomy. However, advanced disease may need traditional hemorrhoidectomy. Surgical excisions of hemorrhoids include a variety of surgical techniques. Open excision (Milligan-Morgan procedure) and closed hemorrhoidectomy (Ferguson procedure) are the most performed operations.[5]

A hemorrhoidectomy is performed in the following settings.

CLOSED HEMORRHOIDECTOMY

The most commonly performed procedure for hemorrhoids, this consists of the excision of hemorrhoidal bundles, followed by complete wound closure with absorbable suture. Postoperative care includes frequent sits baths, mild analgesics, and avoidance of constipation.

OPEN HEMORRHOIDECTOMY

The same is done as the closed hemorrhoidectomy, but the incision is left open. It is done when the location or amount of disease makes wound closure difficult or the likelihood of postoperative infection high.

STAPLED HEMORRHOIDECTOMY FOR PROLAPSING HEMORRHOIDS

Done in patients with 3rd- and 4th-degree hemorrhoids and those who fail prior minimally invasive treatments. The technique uses a circular stapling device to excise a circumferential column of mucosa and submucosa from the upper anal canal, which reduces the hemorrhoidal tissues back into the anal canal and fixates them into position. The device also interrupts part of the hemorrhoidal blood supply, thereby decreasing vascularity. Stapled hemorrhoidectomy results in less postoperative pain and shorter recovery compared with conventional surgery.

RUBBER BAND LIGATION

A rubber band is placed around the base of the hemorrhoid inside the rectum. The band cuts off circulation, and the hemorrhoid withers away within a few days.

LATERAL INTERNAL SPHINCTEROTOMY

Lateral internal sphincterotomy is sometimes performed during hemorrhoidectomy in patients with high resting sphincter pressures. It also reduces postoperative pain.[5]

ANAL FISSURE

Anal fissure is a linear ulcer in the squamous epithelium of the anus, distal to the dentate line. It is one of the most common and painful anorectal conditions encountered in surgical practice. Lateral anal sphincterotomy remains the gold standard of treatment for chronic anal fissures.[6]

ANESTHETIC CONSIDERATIONS AND TECHNIQUES

Anorectal surgical procedures are among the most common surgical operations, often performed as outpatient surgery. Minor anorectal diseases constitute 4%–5% of the adult Western population. Operations are performed on an ambulatory basis. Ambulatory anesthesia requires using medications and techniques that result in rapid onset and recovery while remaining cost-effective. However, anorectal surgery requires deep levels of anesthesia. To achieve these goal, regional blocks alone or in combination with monitored anesthesia care, or deep general anesthesia usually with tracheal intubation, are usually used.

LOCAL ANESTHETIC INFILTRATION

This is usually done using 10–30 mL of LA. Several mixtures and techniques were used with success. There are also various techniques for LA infiltration in the anorectal zone. The topical application of 5% lidocaine cream, or eutectic mixture of local anesthetics (EMLA) cream, 1 hour before surgery increases patient tolerability for injection of LA.[7,8] Subcutaneous, subendodermal, and submucosal injection of low-volume LA followed by further infiltration is another technique.[9] The posterior perineal block entails infiltration of 40–50 mL of LA in the deep plane to block the inferior rectal nerves, the posterior branch of the internal pudendal nerves, and the anococcygeal nerves. Infiltration of the superficial plains blocks the inferior gluteal nerves and perineal branches of minor nerves from the sacral plexus.[10] It is performed with a finger in the rectum, as a needle is introduced at 2 cm behind the anal verge in posterior commissure. It is introduced further until 5 cm into the presacral compartment and 10 mL of LA is injected to block the anococcygeal nerves. The needle is then redirected laterally and forward, into each ischiorectal fossa to block the branches of the pudendal nerve; 10 mL of LA is injected in both the right and left fossa. Finally, 5 mL of LA is injected fanwise in both the right and left perianal skin to anesthetize the branches of the superficial perineal nerves.[11]

Different sedation methods have been used, and the combination of propofol-ketamine has been advocated for anorectal surgery in the jackknife position.[12]

A few studies have compared general, neuraxial, and LA infiltration with sedation for outpatient rectal surgery, the latter being described as safe and effective, with the advantage of decreasing the PACU and hospital stay with substantial cost savings.[12–15] However, sedation in the prone position can result in respiratory problems that can be unmanageable. It should be considered on an individual basis and after taking all the safety precautions. Additional studies are needed to confirm the safety and efficacy of this technique, especially with the use of sedation in the prone position.[16]

When LA infiltration was compared to spinal anesthesia, no difference in the frequency of side effects, pain scores, and in-patient satisfaction was noted.[14,17,18] Moreover, the LA group incurred lower cost, reduced hospital stays, and reduced risk of anesthesia.[17,18] Cost-benefit analysis was performed in a study by Li, Coloma, et al. where 93 patients undergoing anorectal surgery were randomly assigned to 1 of 3 anesthetic treatments. LA with propofol sedation, compared to spinal and general anesthesia, provided the fastest time to oral intake, home readiness, less need for pain medications, no complaints of nausea, and high satisfaction, with the lowest cost of anesthesia.[19]

SPINAL

Spinal anesthesia is another effective and safe way of anesthetizing these patients. However, using conventional doses of LA for spinal blocks results in longer recovery time than those who received general anesthesia.[20] On the other hand, by modifying the dose, concentration, and position at the time of injection, an effective anesthesia with rapid recovery can be reached. Dr. Imbelloni, one of this chapter's authors, has published extensively on this topic with good recovery times, no post-spinal headache or hemodynamic changes.[21–25]

Spinal lidocaine has been used successfully with rapid onset, predictable efficacy, and prompt regression. However, its use is limited by the possible development of transient neurologic symptoms (TNS). TNS is characterized by pain in the buttocks and legs that develops within days after spinal. A metanalysis that included 4733 patients found that the incidence of TNS was 10.8% in the lidocaine group, compared to 2.2% when the other LAs are used intrathecally (bupivacaine, levobupivacaine, prilocaine, chloroprocaine, procaine, and articaine). TNS was also higher in the hyperbaric or isobaric lidocaine compared with the hypobaric lidocaine group.[26,27] However, the use of 2-chloroprocaine and mepivacaine had a similar risk to lidocaine.[26,28]

A large study of 1045 screened specifically for the incidence of TNS in anorectal surgery. Patients received 1–1.5 mL of 3% hyperbaric lidocaine intrathecally under in the jackknife position. Only 4 patients (0.4%) reported TNS on postoperative day (POD) 3. Three of them resolved without any treatment by POD 5, whereas in one patient, numbness of the lower extremities lasted until POD 7. The study concluded that the incidence is very low with intrathecal lidocaine 3% in the jackknife position, as compared to the previously higher reports of the lithotomy position with the higher concentrations.[28,29]

However, spinal lidocaine was used in anorectal surgery successfully with no incidence of TNS. When a small dose of 18 mg of hypobaric lidocaine 0.5%–0.6% was administered intrathecally in jackknife position, it predominantly provided a sensory block.[25] When comparing spinal 30 mg of 1.5% to the same dose of 2% hyperbaric lidocaine in the lithotomy position in anorectal patients, both concentrations resulted in adequate surgical conditions and rapid recovery from sensory and motor blockade.[21] A study looked into 150 anorectal surgery patients who received 3 mL (4.5 mg) of hypobaric 0.15% bupivacaine or 3 mL (18 mg) of hypobaric 0.6% lidocaine in the jackknife position. Adequate surgical blockade was achieved when the mean level of cephalad dispersion was L1 for both medications, grade 1 motor blockade of 7% in the lidocaine and 12% in bupivacaine group that was no longer present at 60 minutes. The sensory blockade lasted 99.1 ± 11.0 minutes with bupivacaine, and 64.1 ± 7.6 minutes with lidocaine.[22]

Low-dose bupivacaine was also effective in anorectal surgery. A comparison was done using 6 mg of 0.15% hypobaric bupivacaine in a jackknife position, to 6 mg of hyperbaric 0.5% bupivacaine in the sitting position for 5 minutes, after which they were placed in a jackknife position. Every patient in the spinal hypobaric bupivacaine in the jackknife position had selective blockade of the posterior sacral nerve roots, while patients in the spinal hyperbaric bupivacaine in the sitting position experienced blockade of the anterior and posterior nerve roots. Sensory blockade was significantly higher and motor blockade was significantly less severe in hypobaric groups. Eighty% in hyperbaric bupivacaine while only 98% of the patients in the hypobaric bupivacaine group self-transferred to the stretcher unassisted. However, recovery time, prevalence of hemodynamic changes, nausea or vomiting, urine retention, or post-spinal headache were similar between the two groups.[24] A similar study administered spinal hypobaric bupivacaine 0.15% (6 mg) in the prone position, found that the block spread spanned from T10 to L2 with only three patients suffering from motor block. The blockade lasted 122.17 ± 15.35 minutes. No hemodynamic changes were observed in all patients.[23]

The baricity of a solution is determined by the relationship between its density and the density of the CSF. The mean density of the CSF is 1.00059 ± 0.00020 g·ml−1. Local anesthetics can be made hypobaric by dilution in distilled water or made hyperbaric by adding 8% dextrose in water. For example, hypobaric 0.6% lidocaine can be obtained using isobaric 2% lidocaine (1.5 mL or 30 mg) + distilled water (3.5 mL) to make a total of 30 mg in 5 cc. Likewise, hypobaric 0.15% bupivacaine can be obtained by mixing 1.5 mL of isobaric 0.5% bupivacaine (7.5 mg) with 3.5 mL of distilled water.[30]

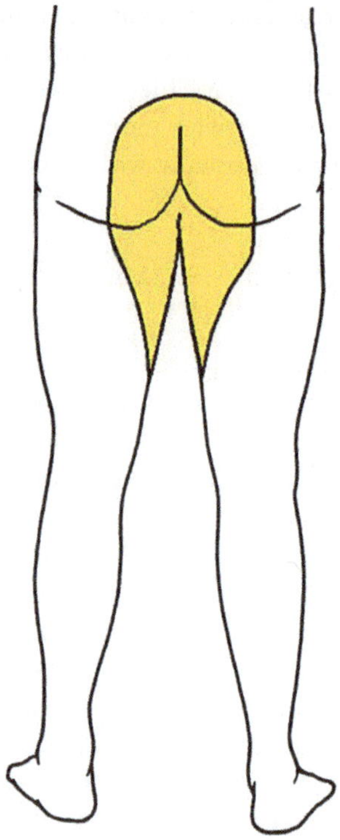

Figure 21.2. Saddle anesthesia.
From: https://en.wikipedia.org/wiki/Saddle_anesthesia.

SADDLE BLOCK

The saddle block (SB) is a segmental block for the area of perineum and inner sides of thigh that would touch a saddle when riding a horse, and this corresponds to the area innervated by sacral component of spinal roots (S2–S5) (Figure 21.2).

Benefits of SB are namely preservation of motor strength and lack of hemodynamic changes over traditional spinal and even superior to total intravenous anesthesia and general anesthesia in terms of postoperative recovery and of analgesic consumption after surgery.[31,32] The duration of the sitting position after spinal anesthesia is more important than the baricity of bupivacaine in determining the cephalad spread of spinal anesthesia. Maximum cephalad spread levels of T5, T9, and T11 were reached at 2, 5, and 10 minutes, respectively, after the patients assumed the jackknife position. However, the sensory block levels progressively increased until 15 or 20 minutes in all groups.[33]

Gudaityte et al.[34] compared 4 mg to 5 mg of hyperbaric bupivacaine for an SD in anorectal surgery. They resulted in similar block, but the 4 mg resulted in shorter duration and faster recovery. Yung et al.[32] describe their clinical experience at the University of Toronto of using 3 mg hyperbaric bupivacaine 0.75% successfully in SB. SB was also reported to be successful with 2.5 mg hyperbaric levobupivacaine with 12.5 μg or 25 μg fentanyl added. Patients were kept sitting for 5 minutes after the block with resultant sensory block of S1–S2 with no motor block.[35] Adjuvants, such as fentanyl and sufentanil, potentiate the afferent sensory blockade and facilitate reductions in the dose of local anesthetics.[36] Wassef et al.[37] went further and reduced the dose to 1.5 mg and compared it to 6 mg of the hyperbaric bupivacaine. They found that 1.5 mg produced a more limited block, earlier time to ambulation (98 vs. 147 minutes), and earlier hospital discharge (126 vs. 249 minutes) with satisfactory anesthetic conditions. Similar results were also reported when 1.5 mg was compared to 6 mg of hyperbaric levobupivacaine.[38] However, Carron et al.[39] warn that lower dose spinal may not be successful in every patient, and the block is dose dependent. They report low rates at 2 mg (20%), near maximal (90%) at 3 mg, and maximal (100%) at the highest doses.[39]

Short-acting local anesthetics like chlorprocaine, prilocaine, lidocaine, and mepivacaine are beneficial as they provide adequate anesthesia for short perianal surgery. The new preparation of chloroprocaine is devoid of neurotoxicity, with negligible incidence of TNS. Plain chloroprcaine 2% shows hyperbaric effects without dextrose being added.[40] SB using a dose of 20 mg of 1% chloroprocaine was deemed to be the optimal dose for short perianal surgery given the avoidance of prolonged motor blockade with the 30 mg dose, while 10 mg may result in block failure.[41] Hyperbaric 2% prilocaine can used successfully for spinal anesthesia in perianal surgery. A dose-finding study concluded that 10 mg provide sufficient analgesia, without motor block and shorter recovery times. Higher doses tend to cause motor block and prolonged PACU stay.[42]

Yung et al.[32] conducted a systematic review on SB in anorectal surgery. Eleven randomized controlled studies of 1063 patients were included. They investigated several outcomes based on the types of the LAs used. Longer-acting local anesthetics included bupivacaine, levobupivacaine, and ropivacaine; a dose of ≤5 mg distinguished LA-LD (long acting–low dose) from LA-HD (long acting–high dose) groups. Shorter acting agents included chloroprocaine, lidocaine, mepivacaine, and prilocaine; similarly, a dose of ≤20 mg distinguished SA-LD (short acting–low dose) from SA-HD (short acting–high dose) groups (Table 21.1). Interestingly, the SA-LD regimen reported the most prolonged times to sensory block regression (SBR) (median of 210 min), while the LA-LD regimen reported the fastest times to SBR (median 136 min). The fastest time to SBR was 76 minutes, reported in patients receiving 1.5 mg of hyperbaric bupivacaine 0.75%, while the most prolonged sensory block of 312 minutes was reported in patients receiving 5 mg of hyperbaric chloroprocaine 0.5%. Likewise, 5 mg of 0.5% hyperbaric chloroprocaine resulted in prolonged motor blockade of 240 min. The block success rate was 98.9% across all trials.[32]

Table 21.1 **COMPARISON OF OUTCOMES OF LONGER ACTING AND SHORTER ACTING LOCAL ANESTHETICS, HIGH AND LOW DOSE, USED IN SADDLE BLOCK**[32]

		MEDIAN IQR (MIN)
Time to discharge	Overall	182 ± 102
	Longer acting, higher dose	182 (70)
	Longer acting, lower dose	119 (7)
	Shorter acting, higher dose	182 (48)
	Shorter acting, lower dose	196 (78)
Time to sensory block regression	Overall	145± 35
	Longer acting, higher dose	149 (28)
	Longer acting, lower dose	136 (30)
	Shorter acting, higher dose	–
	Shorter acting, lower dose	210 (93)
Time to motor block regression	Overall	60 (100)
	Longer acting, higher dose	100 (12)
	Longer acting, lower dose	0 (0)
	Shorter acting, higher dose	72 (N/A)
	Shorter acting, lower dose	60 (119)
Time to first urine voiding	Overall	202 (68)
	Longer acting, higher dose	236 (76)
	Longer acting, lower dose	205 (142)
	Shorter acting, higher dose	211 (N/A)
	Shorter acting, lower dose	186 (17)
Time to first ambulation	Overall	116 (46)
	Longer acting, higher dose	146 (1)
	Longer acting, lower dose	100 (2)
	Shorter acting, higher dose	116 (N/A)
	Shorter acting, lower dose	135 (74)

CAUDAL EPIDURAL

The use of a caudal epidural block for anorectal surgery provides the added benefit of prolonged postoperative analgesia. Caudal epidural block with 15–20 mL 2% lidocaine with epinephrine or bupivacaine 0.25% with epinephrine provides higher patient satisfaction and longer-lasting analgesia than local anesthetic infiltration without delaying discharge.[43,44]

PUDENDAL NERVE BLOCK (PNB)

Pudendal nerve block (PNB) is effective as an anesthetic technique or as a postoperative pain-control method.[45–48] It can be done either by landmark, nerve stimulator, or under ultrasound guidance.

PNB using bupivacaine after spinal anesthesia provided analgesia for 23.8 hours and all of the patients had spontaneous micturition.[45] When it was added to general anesthesia, it resulted in better pain relief and reduced postoperative morphine consumption.[46–48] It was used as the sole anesthetic with an 80% success rate, despite good nerve stimulator response.[48] The PB group reported higher patient satisfaction, faster return-to-normal activities including better walking, sitting, and defecation, and shorter hospital stays compared to general anesthesia.[47–52] Two important systematic reviews have confirmed the results of these individual studies on the benefits of using PNB in anorectal surgery.[53,54] On the other hand, drawbacks of PB are the need for multiple needle injections, special equipment, skill, and time needed to place and establish the block.

Ultrasound-guided blockade of the PB assists in finding landmarks. It is performed at the level of the ischial spine and transperineally. PNB done inside Alcock canal with small local anesthetic volume minimizes the risk of sacral plexus blockade and would anesthetize all three branches of the pudendal nerve before they ramify in the ischioanal fossa.[55,56]

Technique

Using nerve stimulator: a 100 mm insulated needle is introduced medial to the ischial tuberosity in each side, transperineally perpendicular to the skin in a sagittal plan. The proximity of the nerve is indicated by the anal sphincter contraction. Then, 20 mL of local anesthetics is injected on each side.[45,57]

Using ultrasound: with the patient lying prone, the ultrasound probe is placed at the level of the ischial tuberosity to capture the transverse view of the ischial spine, the sacrospinous and sacrotuberous ligaments, the internal pudendal artery, and the pudendal nerve. A 22-gauge needle is advanced

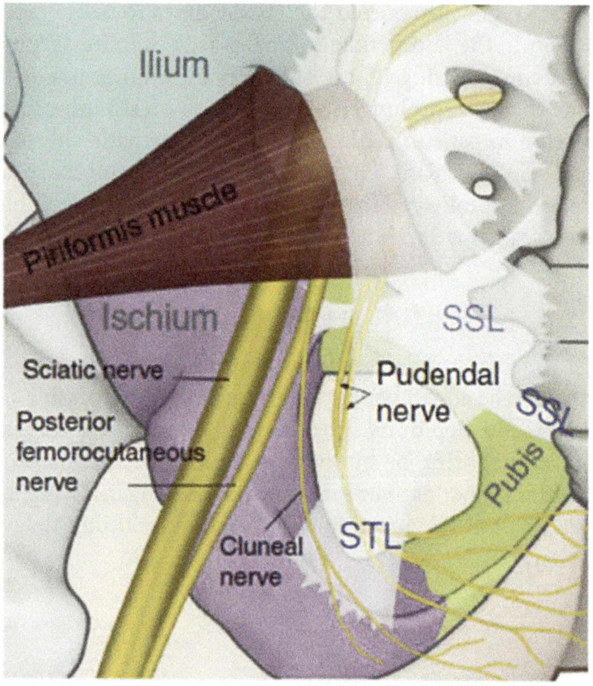

Figure 21.3. Relationship of the sacrospinous (SSL) and sacrotuberous (STL) ligaments (made transparent in order to show the deep structures), and the course of the pudendal, sciatic and posterior femorocutaneous nerves. Obtained with permission from: Rojas-Gómez MF, Blanco-Dávila R, Tobar-Roa V, Gómez-González AM, Ortiz-Zableh AM, Ortiz-Azuero A. Regional anesthesia guided by ultrasound in the pudendal nerve territory. *Colombian J Anestesiology*. 2017;45(3):200–209. Retrieved February 20, 2021, from http://www.scielo.org.co/scielo.php?script=sci_arttext&pid=S0120-33472017000300200&lng=en&tlng=en.

under real-time ultrasound guidance to reach the pudendal nerve in the plane between both ligaments. Then local anesthetic is injected and is visualized around the nerve and expanding between the sacrospinous and sacrotuberous ligaments[56] (Figures 21.3 and 21.4A, B).

EFFECT OF NERVE BLOCK ON ANAL SPHINCTER TONE

When comparing epidural, caudal, and SB for the degree of inhibition of the anal sphincter tone, SB produced the highest inhibition of maximal squeezing pressure, although it was inhibited by the other two as well. PNB results in incomplete puborectalis muscle relaxation.[52] Relaxation of the anal sphincter tone is related to the sympathetic blockade.[2]

POSTOPERATIVE PAIN AFTER ANORECTAL SURGERY

The anal canal is extremely sensitive, especially below the pectinate line, and thus external hemorrhoids may be very painful. Anorectal surgery requires deep anesthesia as the area is rich with somatic nerve endings and is reflexogenic. Operations under light planes of anesthesia cause intense pain and reflex body movements. Dilation of the anus has been well known to trigger laryngospasm under lighter planes of anesthesia.

Postoperative pain is one of the greatest problems in ambulatory patients after anal surgery. A retrospective study of 1100 patients submitted to the ambulatory hemorrhoidectomy showed that 35% experienced moderate to severe pain at home, even on analgesic therapy.[58] Pain during defecation is problematic and finding a solution for it remains challenging.[59] Several methods help in the early postoperative period. Intrathecal morphine of <0.3 mg after spinal anesthesia is effective in reducing pain; however, it results in increased incidence of nausea, vomiting, and pruritus and a slightly increased risk of respiratory depression. Doses higher than ≥0.3 mg result in an increased risk of pruritus and more episodes of respiratory depression compared to the lower dose.[60] Bilateral pudendal blockade is associated with prolonged postoperative analgesia.[45] Wound infiltration with liposomal bupivacaine in

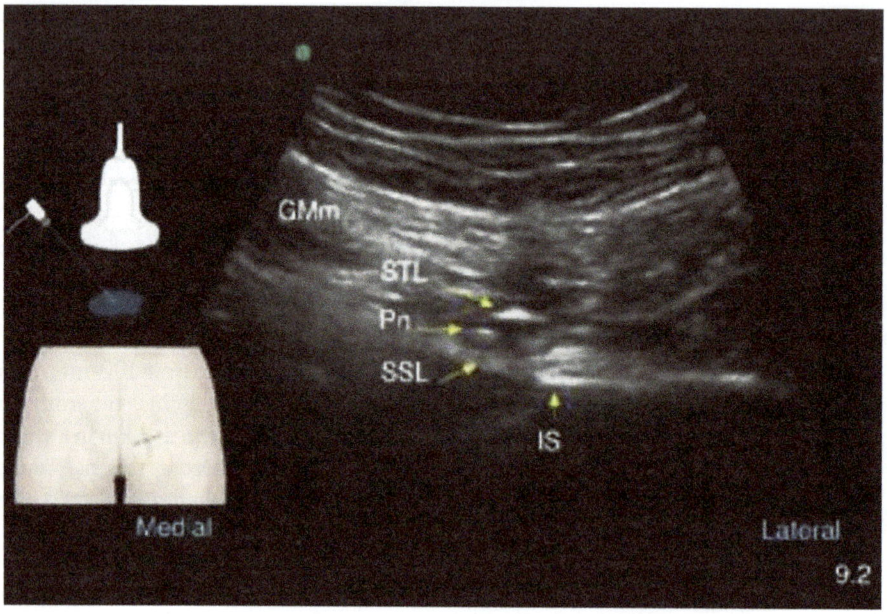

Figure 21.4A. Gluteal ultrasound during pudendal nerve (Pn) recognition. The nerve is deep to the gluteus maximus muscle (GMm), the sacrotuberous ligament (STL), and superficial to the sacrospinous ligament (SSL). The ischial spine (IS) is found lateral to those structures.

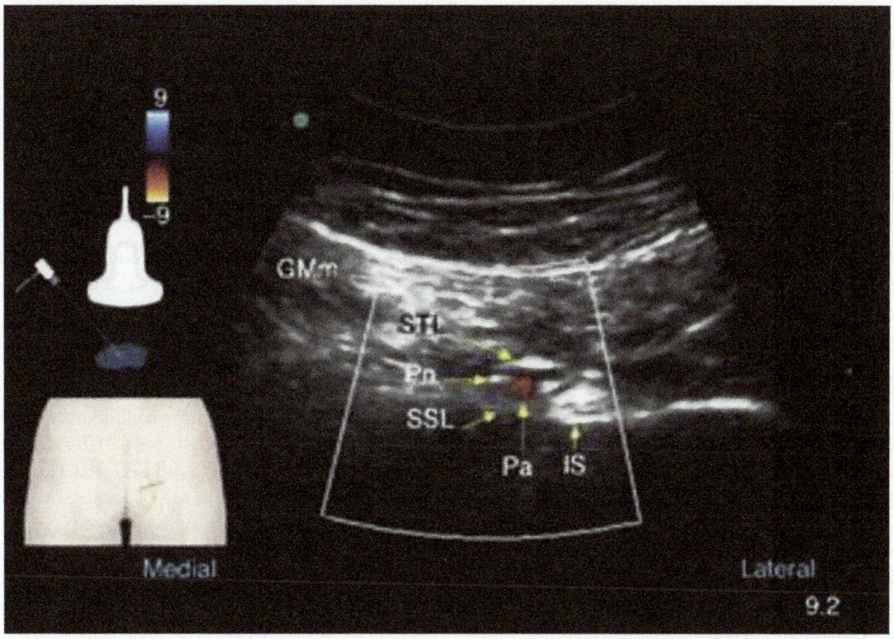

Figure 21.4B. Color Doppler ultrasound at the gluteal level: pudendal nerve (Pn), gluteus maximus muscle (GMm), deep to the sacrotuberous ligament (STL) and superficial to the sacrospinous ligament (SSL); the internal pudendal artery (Pa) and the ischial spine are found lateral to these structures. Obtained with permission from: Rojas-Gómez MF, Blanco-Dávila R, Tobar-Roa V, Gómez-González AM, Ortiz-Zableh AM, Ortiz-Azuero A. Regional anesthesia guided by ultrasound in the pudendal nerve territory. *Colombian J Anestesiology*. 2017;45(3):200–209. Retrieved February 20, 2021, from http://www.scielo.org.co/scielo.php?script=sci_arttext&pid=S0120-33472017000300200&lng=en&tlng=en.

hemorrhoidectomy has demonstrated significant reduction in pain scores through 72 hours, opioid requirements, delayed time to first opioid use, and improved patient satisfaction. [61]

The PROSPECT (procedure specific postoperative pain management) systematic review rigorously analyzed 74 studies related to postoperative pain in hemorroidectomy. The review recommended the use of PNB, with or without general anesthesia, for all patients undergoing hemorrhoidal surgery, in addition to multimodal pain management, glyceryl trinitrate, laxatives, and oral metronidazole after hemorrhoidectomy. [54]

THE USE OF NSAIDS AND ACETAMINOPHEN IN INFLAMMATORY BOWEL DISEASE

A study has shown that using NSAIDs and acetaminophen more than 5 times per month was associated with activation of Crohn's disease, but not ulcerative colitis.[62] Clinical relapse was noted in 20% of patients with quiescent inflammatory bowel disease, which may be due to dual inhibition of the COX enzymes. However, some COX-2-selective NSAIDs appear to be safe.[63]

CONCLUSION

Anorectal surgery is a commonly performed procedure that is done on an ambulatory basis. Although it is considered a minor procedure, anesthesia for these procedures needs careful planning. General anesthesia, spinal, caudal epidural, pudendal nerve block, and local anesthetic infiltration are all options. In order to balance good anesthesia, good postoperative analgesia, resources, costs, early recovery, and return to normal daily activities, a thorough understanding of the pros and cons of each technique is needed.

REFERENCES

1. Jorge JMN, Habr-Gama A. Anatomy and embryology. In: Beck DE, Roberts PL, Saclarides TJ, Senagore AJ, Stamos MJ, Wexner SD, eds. *The ASCRS Textbook of Colon and Rectal Surgery*. New York: Springer; 2011:1–22.
2. Shon YJ, Huh J, Kang SS, Bae SK, Kang RA, Kim DK. Comparison of saddle, lumbar epidural and caudal blocks on anal sphincter tone: a prospective, randomized study. *J Int Med Res*. 2016;44(5):1061–1071.
3. Panes J, Rimola J. Perianal fistulizing Crohn's disease: pathogenesis, diagnosis and therapy. *Nat Rev Gastroenterol Hepatol*. 2017;14(11):652–664.
4. Lachance S, Boutros M. Anal conditions: fistula-in-ano. In: Steele S, Maykel J, Wexner SD, eds. *Clinical Decision Making in Colorectal Surgery*. Cham: Springer; 2020:101–109.
5. Rubbini M, Ascanelli S. Classification and guidelines of hemorrhoidal disease: Present and future. *World J Gastrointest Surg*. 2019;11(3):117–121.
6. Wiley M, Day P, Rieger N, Stephens J, Moore J. Open vs. closed lateral internal sphincterotomy for idiopathic fissure-in-ano: a prospective, randomized, controlled trial. *Dis Colon Rectum*. 2004;47(6):847–852.
7. Anannamcharoen S, Cheeranont P, Boonya-usadon C. Local perianal nerve block versus spinal block for closed hemorrhoidectomy: a ramdomized controlled trial. *J Med Assoc Thai*. 2008;91(12):1862–1866.
8. Schwartz DA, Loftus EV Jr, Tremaine WJ, et al. The natural history of fistulizing Crohn's disease in Olmsted County, Minnesota. *Gastroenterology*. 2002;122(4):875–880.
9. Argov S, Levandovsky O. Local anesthesia in anal surgery: a simple, safe procedure. *Am J Surg*. 2006;191(1):111–113.

10. Gabrielli F, Cioffi U, Chiarelli M, Guttadauro A, De Simone M. Hemorrhoidectomy with posterior perineal block: experience with 400 cases. *Dis Colon Rectum.* 2000;43(6):809–812.
11. Brunat G, Pouzeratte Y, Mann C, Didelot JM, Rochon JC, Eledjam JJ. Posterior perineal block with ropivacaine 0.75% for pain control during and after hemorrhoidectomy. *Reg Anesth Pain Med.* 2003;28(3):228–232.
12. Kelley KA, Kaur T, Tsikitis VL. Perianal Crohn's disease: challenges and solutions. *Clin Exp Gastroenterol.* 2017;10:39–46.
13. Sandborn WJ, Fazio VW, Feagan BG, Hanauer SB, American Gastroenterological Association Clinical Practice C. AGA technical review on perianal Crohn's disease. *Gastroenterology.* 2003;125(5):1508–1530.
14. Sungurtekin H, Sungurtekin U, Erdem E. Local anesthesia and midazolam versus spinal anesthesia in ambulatory pilonidal surgery. *J Clin Anesth.* 2003;15(3):201–205.
15. Macario A, Weinger M, Carney S, Kim A. Which clinical anesthesia outcomes are important to avoid? The perspective of patients. *Anesth Analg.* 1999;89(3):652–658.
16. Smith ZL, Das KK, Kushnir VM. Anesthesia-administered sedation for endoscopic retrograde cholangiopancreatography: monitored anesthesia care or general endotracheal anesthesia? *Curr Opin Anaesthesiol.* 2019;32(4):531–537.
17. Manoharan R, Jacob T, Benjamin S, Kirishnan S. Lateral anal sphincterotomy for chronic anal fissures: a comparison of outcomes and complications under local anaesthesia versus spinal anaesthesia. *J Clin Diagn Res.* 2017;11(1):PC08–PC12.
18. Jinjil K, Dwivedi D, Bhatnagar V, Ray RK, Tara S. Perianal block: is it as good as spinal anesthesia for closed hemorrhoidectomies? *Anesth Essays Res.* 2018;12(1):36–41.
19. Gebhardt V, Kiefer K, Bussen D, Weiss C, Schmittner MD. Retrospective analysis of mepivacaine, prilocaine and chloroprocaine for low-dose spinal anaesthesia in outpatient perianal procedures. *Int J Colorectal Dis.* 2018;33(10):1469–1477.
20. Pavlin DJ, Rapp SE, Polissar NL, Malmgren JA, Koerschgen M, Keyes H. Factors affecting discharge time in adult outpatients. *Anesth Analg.* 1998;87(4):816–826.
21. Imbelloni LE, Gouveia MA, Cordeiro JA. Low dose of lidocaine: comparison of 15 with 20 mg/ml with dextrose for spinal anesthesia in lithotomy position and ambulatory surgery. *Acta Anaesthesiol Scand.* 2008;52(6):856–861.
22. Imbelloni LE, Gouveia MA, Cordeiro JA. Hypobaric 0.15% bupivacaine versus hypobaric 0.6% lidocaine for posterior spinal anesthesia in outpatient anorectal surgery. *Rev Bras Anestesiol.* 2010;60(2):113–120, 164–118.
23. Imbelloni LE, Vieira EM, Gouveia MA, Cordeiro JA. [Restricted dorsal spinal anesthesia for ambulatory anorectal surgery: a pilot study.]. *Rev Bras Anestesiol.* 2004;54(6):774–780.
24. Imbelloni LE, Vieira EM, Gouveia MA, Netinho JG, Cordeiro JA. [Hypobaric 0.15% bupivacaine versus hyperbaric 0.5% bupivacaine for posterior (dorsal) spinal block in outpatient anorectal surgery.]. *Rev Bras Anestesiol.* 2006;56(6):571–582.
25. Imbelloni LE, Gouveia MA, Vieira EM, Cordeiro JA. Selective sensory spinal anaesthesia with hypobaric lidocaine for anorectal surgery. *Acta Anaesthesiol Scand.* 2008;52(10):1327–1330.
26. Koo CH, Shin HJ, Han SH, Ryu JH. Lidocaine vs. other local anesthetics in the development of transient neurologic symptoms (TNS) following spinal anesthesia: a meta-analysis of randomized controlled trials. *J Clin Med.* 2020;9(2):493.
27. Zaric D, Pace NL. Transient neurologic symptoms (TNS) following spinal anaesthesia with lidocaine versus other local anaesthetics. *Cochrane Database Syst Rev.* 2009;2:CD003006.
28. Forget P, Borovac JA, Thackeray EM, Pace NL. Transient neurological symptoms (TNS) following spinal anaesthesia with lidocaine versus other local anaesthetics in adult surgical patients: a network meta-analysis. *Cochrane Database Syst Rev.* 2019;12:CD003006.
29. Morisaki H, Masuda J, Kaneko S, Matsushima M, Takeda J. Transient neurologic syndrome in one thousand forty-five patients after 3% lidocaine spinal anesthesia. *Anesth Analg.* 1998;86(5):1023–1026.
30. Imbelloni LE. Spinal hemianesthesia: unilateral and posterior. *Anesth Essays Res.* 2014;8(3):270–276.
31. Schmittner MD, Schreiber H, Janke A, et al. Randomized clinical trial of perianal surgery performed under spinal saddle block versus total intravenous anaesthesia. *Br J Surg.* 2010;97(1):12–20.
32. Yung EM, Abdallah FW, Todaro C, Spence E, Grant A, Brull R. Optimal local anesthetic regimen for saddle block in ambulatory anorectal surgery: an evidence-based systematic review. *Reg Anesth Pain Med.* 2020;45(9):733–739.
33. Ariyama J, Hayashida M, Sugimoto Y, Imanishi H, To-Oyma Y, Kitamura A. Spread of spinal anesthesia in patients having perianal surgery in the jackknife position: effects of baricity of 0.5% bupivacaine and positioning during and after induction of spinal anesthesia. *J Clin Anesth.* 2009;21(6):408–413.
34. Gudaityte J, Marchertiene I, Karbonskiene A, et al. Low-dose spinal hyperbaric bupivacaine for adult anorectal surgery: a double-blinded, randomized, controlled study. *J Clin Anesth.* 2009;21(7):474–481.
35. Honca M, Dereli N, Kose EA, et al. [Low-dose levobupivacaine plus fentanyl combination for spinal anesthesia in anorectal surgery]. *Rev Bras Anestesiol.* 2015;65(6):461–465.
36. Shim SM, Park JH, Hyun DM, Jeong EK, Kim SS, Lee HM. The effects of adjuvant intrathecal fentanyl on postoperative pain and rebound pain for anorectal surgery under saddle anesthesia. *Korean J Anesthesiol.* 2018;71(3):213–219.
37. Wassef MR, Michaels EI, Rangel JM, Tsyrlin AT. Spinal perianal block: a prospective, randomized, double-blind comparison with spinal saddle block. *Anesth Analg.* 2007;104(6):1594–1596, table of contents.
38. Kazak Z, Ekmekci P, Kazbek K. Hyperbaric levobupivacaine in anal surgery: spinal perianal and spinal saddle blocks. *Der Anaesthesist.* 2010;59(8):709–713.
39. Carron M, Freo U, Veronese S, Innocente F, Ori C. Spinal block with 1.5 mg hyperbaric bupivacaine: not successful for everyone. *Anesth Analg.* 2007;105(5):1515–1516; author reply 1516.
40. Kopacz DJ. Spinal 2-chloroprocaine: minimum effective dose. *Reg Anesth Pain Med.* 2005;30(1):36–42.
41. Gebhardt V, Mueller-Hansen L, Schwarz A, Bussen D, Weiss C, Schmittner MD. Chloroprocaine 10 mg/ml for low-dose spinal anaesthesia in perianal surgery: a randomised dose finding study. *Acta Anaesthesiol Scand.* 2017;61(2):241–249.
42. Gebhardt V, Herold A, Weiss C, Samakas A, Schmittner MD. Dosage finding for low-dose spinal anaesthesia using hyperbaric prilocaine in patients undergoing perianal outpatient surgery. *Acta Anaesthesiol Scand.* 2013;57(2):249–256.
43. Van Elstraete AC, Pastureau F, Lebrun T, Mehdaoui H. Caudal clonidine for postoperative analgesia in adults. *Br J Anaesth.* 2000;84(3):401–402.
44. Siddiqui ZI, Denman WT, Schumann R, Hackford A, Cepeda MS, Carr DB. Local anesthetic infiltration versus caudal epidural block for anorectal surgery: a randomized controlled trial. *J Clin Anesthes.* 2007;19(4):269–273.
45. Imbelloni LE, Vieira EM, Gouveia MA, Netinho JG, Spirandelli LD, Cordeiro JA. Pudendal block with bupivacaine for postoperative pain relief. *Dis Colon Rectum.* 2007;50(10):1656–1661.
46. Wey PF, Lions C, Rimmele T, Ould-Ahmed M, Escarment J. [Nerve stimulator guided pudendal nerve block for postoperative analgesia. An evaluation of professional practice]. *Ann Fr Anesth Reanim.* 2007;26(12):1087–1088.
47. Naja Z, Ziade MF, Lonnqvist PA. Nerve stimulator guided pudendal nerve block decreases posthemorrhoidectomy pain. *Can J Anaesth.* 2005;52(1):62–68.
48. Naja Z, El-Rajab M, Al-Tannir M, et al. Nerve stimulator guided pudendal nerve block versus general anesthesia for hemorrhoidectomy. *Can J Anaesth.* 2006;53(6):579–585.
49. Alkhaldi HM, Salaita WM, Shabaneh MA, Al-Horut MI, Aldabbas RM, Uraiqat AA. Postoperative outcome comparison between pudendal nerve block and caudal block after lateral open internal sphincterotomy. *Med Arch.* 2015;69(3):187–189.
50. Kim SH, Song SG, Paek OJ, Lee HJ, Park DH, Lee JK. Nerve-stimulator-guided pudendal nerve block by pararectal approach. *Colorectal Dis.* 2012;14(5):611–615.

51. Di Giuseppe M, Saporito A, La Regina D, et al. Ultrasound-guided pudendal nerve block in patients undergoing open hemorrhoidectomy: a double-blind randomized controlled trial. *Int J Colorectal Dis.* 2020;35(9):1741–1747.
52. Kim J, Lee DS, Jang SM, Shim MC, Jee DL. The effect of pudendal block on voiding after hemorrhoidectomy. *Dis Colon Rectum.* 2005;48(3):518–523.
53. Fadel MG, Peltola L, Pellino G, Frunza G, Kontovounisios C. The role of pudendal nerve block in colorectal surgery: a systematic review. *J Invest Surg.* 2021:34(11):1238–1245.
54. Sammour T, Barazanchi AW, Hill AG, Group P. Evidence-based management of pain after excisional haemorrhoidectomy surgery: a PROSPECT review update. *World J Surg.* 2017;41(2):603–614.
55. Bendtsen TF, Parras T, Moriggl B, et al. Ultrasound-guided pudendal nerve block at the entrance of the pudendal (Alcock) Canal: description of anatomy and clinical technique. *Reg Anesth Pain Med.* 2016;41(2):140–145.
56. Rofaeel A, Peng P, Louis I, Chan V. Feasibility of real-time ultrasound for pudendal nerve block in patients with chronic perineal pain. *Reg Anesth Pain Med.* 2008;33(2):139–145.
57. Imbelloni LE, Beato L, Beato C, Cordeiro JA, de Souza DD. Bilateral pudendal nerves block for postoperative analgesia with 0.25% S75:R25 bupivacaine: pilot study on outpatient hemorrhoidectomy. *Rev Bras Anestesiol.* 2005;55(6):614–621.
58. Rawal N, Hylander J, Nydahl PA, Olofsson I, Gupta A. Survey of postoperative analgesia following ambulatory surgery. *Acta Anaesthesiol Scand.* 1997;41(8):1017–1022.
59. Ceulemans A, De Looze D, Van de Putte D, Stiers E, Coppens M. High post-operative pain scores despite multimodal analgesia in ambulatory anorectal surgery: a prospective cohort study. *Acta Chir Belg.* 2019;119(4):224–230.
60. Li S, Coloma M, White PF, et al. Comparison of the costs and recovery profiles of three anesthetic techniques for ambulatory anorectal surgery. *Anesthesiology.* 2000;93(5):1225–1230.
61. Haas E, Onel E, Miller H, Ragupathi M, White PF. A double-blind, randomized, active-controlled study for post-hemorrhoidectomy pain management with liposome bupivacaine, a novel local analgesic formulation. *Am Surg.* 2012;78(5):574–581.
62. Long MD, Kappelman MD, Martin CF, Chen W, Anton K, Sandler RS. Role of nonsteroidal anti-inflammatory drugs in exacerbations of inflammatory bowel disease. *J Clin Gastroenterol.* 2016;50(2):152–156.
63. Kvasnovsky CL, Aujla U, Bjarnason I. Nonsteroidal anti-inflammatory drugs and exacerbations of inflammatory bowel disease. *Scand J Gastroenterol.* 2015;50(3):255–263.

REVIEW QUESTIONS

(1) All the following are true regarding the incidence of transient neurologic syndrome (TNS) EXCEPT:

A. Higher in hyperbaric, isobaric compared to hypobaric lidocaine
B. Higher in 2-chlorprocaine compared to bupivacaine
C. Higher in mepivacaine compared to ropivacaine
D. Higher in the jackknife than the lithotomy position

(2) Which of the following is NOT a treatment for anal fistula?

A. Mucopexy
B. Seton placement
C. Fistulotomy
D. Advancement rectal flap

(3) Which of these doses/concentrations of local anesthetic is most appropriate for a patient getting a spinal with the least amount of motor blockade in the jackknife position for surgery?

A. Hyperbaric: 20 mg of lidocaine 5%
B. Hypobaric: 6 mg bupivacaine 0.15%
C. Hyperbaric: 6 mg bupivacaine 0.2%
D. Hypobaric: 40 mg of lidocaine 5%

(4) Which of the anesthetic techniques results in the lowest maximal squeezing pressure (MSP) of the anal sphincter?

A. Local anesthetic infiltration
B. Caudal
C. Lumbar epidural
D. Saddle block

(5) Which of the following is more important in limiting the cephalad spread of local anesthetics (LAs)?

A. Higher baricity of LA
B. Sitting position
C. Jackknife position
D. The type of the spinal needle

(6) All of the following are branches of the pudendal nerve EXCEPT:

A. Perineal nerve
B. Inferior rectal nerve
c. Dorsal nerve of the penis or clitoris
d. Inferior hypogastric nerve

(7) Which of these degrees of hemorrhoid prolapsing is true?

A. 1st degree: slight prolapse
B. 2nd degree: prolapse necessitating odd digital help to reduce
C. 3rd degree: prolapsing with spontaneous reduction
D. 4th degree: irreducible prolapse

(8) Which ligament needs to be surpassed to reach the sacral hiatus?

A. Superior costotransverse ligament
B. Ligamentum flavum
C. Sacrococcygeal ligament
D. Fascia lata

(9) Dilation of the anus can result in a reflex stimulated by:

A. Parasympathetic nerves
B. Pudendal nerves
C. Inferior hypogastric nerves
D. Sacral plexus—sympathetic nerves

ANSWERS

(1) **D.** The risk of TNS after spinal anesthesia is found to be higher when the hyperbaric or isobaric lidocaine is used, compared to when hypobaric lidocaine is used. This is also true when lidocaine was used compared to bupivacaine, levobupivacaine, prilocaine, procaine, and ropivacaine. Mepivacaine and 2-chloroprocaine had a similar risk to lidocaine in terms

of TNS development after spinal anesthesia. A large study concluded that the incidence is very low when intrathecal lidocaine 3% was used and surgery was done in the jackknife position, compared to the lithotomy position with the higher concentrations.

References

Forget P, Borovac JA, Thackeray EM, Pace NL. Transient neurological symptoms (TNS) following spinal anaesthesia with lidocaine versus other local anaesthetics in adult surgicalpatients: a network meta-analysis. *Cochrane Database Syst Rev.* 2019;12(12):CD003006.

Morisaki H, Masuda J, Kaneko S, Matsushima M, Takeda J. Transient neurologic syndrome in one thousand forty-five patients after 3% lidocaine spinal anesthesia. *Anesth Analg.* 1998;86(5):1023–1026.

(2) **A.** All the answers aside from mucopexy are treatments for anal fistula. Fistulotomy is where a fistula is cut open over a probe and scraped of its contents and its sides are stitched to the sides of the incision. Advancement of rectal flap is when the tract is opened and the mucosa and submucosa are moved to cover the internal opening. Seton placement is where a seton (silk string or rubber band) is used to create scar tissue around part of the sphincter muscle before cutting it with a knife or allowing the seton to slowly cut all the way through the muscle over the course of several weeks.

Reference

Vasilevsky CA. Anorectal abscess and fistula. In: Beck DE, Roberts PL, Saclarides TJ, Senagore AJ, Stamos MJ, Wexner SD, eds. *The ASCRS Textbook of Colon and Rectal Surgery*. New York: Springer; 2011:219–243. https://doi.org/10.1007/978-1-4419-1584-9_13.

(3) **B.** Low-dose bupivacaine is effective in anorectal surgery. When 6 mg of 0.15% hypobaric bupivacaine in a jackknife position was compared with 6 mg of hyperbaric 0.5% bupivacaine in the sitting position for 5 minutes, patients with the hypobaric bupivacaine in the jackknife position had selective blockade of the posterior sacral nerve roots, while patients with the spinal hyperbaric bupivacaine in the sitting position experienced blockade of the anterior and posterior nerve roots. Sensory blockade was significantly higher and motor blockade was significantly less severe in hypobaric groups.

The low dose of 6 mg is more ideal than 40 mg of lidocaine to prevent motor blockade.

Reference

Imbelloni LE, Vieira EM, Gouveia MA, Netinho JG, Cordeiro JA. [Hypobaric 0.15% bupivacaine versus hyperbaric 0.5% bupivacaine for posterior (dorsal) spinal block in outpatient anorectal surgery.]. *Rev Bras Anestesiol.* 2006;56(6):571–582.

(4) **D.** Saddle block compared to the lumbar epidural and caudal block produced the maximum squeezing inhibition of the anal sphincter. No differences were detected between epidural lumbar and caudal blocks.

Reference

Shon YJ, Huh J, Kang SS, Bae SK, Kang RA, Kim DK. Comparison of saddle, lumbar epidural and caudal blocks on anal sphincter tone: a prospective, randomized study. *J Int Med Res.* 2016;44(5): 1061–1071.

(5) **B.** The patient position after the spinal anesthesia is more important than the baricity of bupivacaine in determining the cephalad spread of spinal anesthesia. In the jackknife position, however, the sensory block levels progressively increased until 15 or 20 minutes in all groups.

Reference

Ariyama J, Hayashida M, Sugimoto Y, Imanishi H, To-Oyma Y, Kitamura A. Spread of spinal anesthesia in patients having perianal surgery in the jackknife position: effects of baricity of 0.5% bupivacaine and positioning during and after induction of spinal anesthesia. *J Clin Anesth.* 2009;21(6):408–413.

(6) **D.** The pudendal nerve arises from the S2, S3, and S4 nerve roots. Branches of the pudendal nerve are the perineal nerve, inferior rectal nerve (also called the inferior anal or inferior hemorrhoidal nerve), and dorsal nerve of the penis or clitoris. The inferior hypogastric nerve is not a branch of the pudendal nerve.

Reference

Barleben A, Mills S. Anorectal anatomy and physiology. *Surg Clin North Am.* 2010;90(1):1–15.

(7) **D.** Depending on the degree of internal hemorrhoids prolaps,e they can be classified as 1st degree (no prolapsing), 2nd degree (prolapsing with spontaneous reduction), 3rd degree (prolapsing necessitating odd digital help to reduce, and 4th degree (irreducible prolapsing).

Reference

Rubbini M, Ascanelli S. Classification and guidelines of hemorrhoidal disease: present and future. *World J Gastrointest Surg.* 2019;11(3):117–121.

(8) **C.** The sacrococcygeal ligament is the ligament that needs to be surpassed to enter the caudal space. The superior costotransverse ligament is a fibrous band that arises from the neck of a rib to the transverse process of the vertebra above; it needs to be surpassed to place a paravertebral nerve block. Surpassing the ligamentum flavum heralds the entry into the epidural space. Fascia lata needs to be surpassed in a femoral/fascia iliaca block.

References

Kao SC, Lin CS. Caudal epidural block: an updated review of anatomy and techniques. *Biomed Res Int.* 2017;2017:9217145.

Ardon AE, Lee J, Franco CD, Riutort KT, Greengrass RA. Paravertebral block: anatomy and relevant safety issues. *Korean J Anesthesiol.* 2020 Oct;73(5):394–400.

(9) **D.** The sacral splanchnic nerves come from the sacral sympathetic ganglia which innervate the vascular smooth muscle of the pelvic viscera and conduct pain fibers from the pelvic viscera. Somatic motor fibers supply the external sphincter. Sensory fibers are concerned with the reflex control of the sphincters and with pain. The anal canal is very sensitive below the pectinate line, so that external hemorrhoids may be very painful. In fact, dilation of the anus has been well known to trigger laryngospasm under lighter planes of anesthesia.

Reference

Gudaityte J, Marchertiene I, Pavalkis D. Anesthesia for ambulatory anorectal surgery. *Medicina (Kaunas).* 2004;40(2):101–111.

SECTION 6

UPPER EXTREMITY

Linda Thi Le-Wendling

22.

SHOULDER ARTHROSCOPY

Alberto E. Ardon, Steven B. Porter, and Robert L. McClain

STEM CASE AND KEY QUESTIONS

A 63-year-old man with a long-standing history of left shoulder pain is scheduled for a left arthroscopic, possibly open, subacromial decompression. He has a history of non-insulin-dependent diabetes mellitus and lung cancer, for which he has had a right upper lobe resection. His medications include metformin daily. He has regular follow-ups with his primary care provider, and his most recent glycosylated hemoglobin value was 7.5%. He is also prescribed 10 mg of oxycodone by mouth 4 times per day as needed for his chronic left shoulder and lower back pain. The patient is concerned about postoperative pain. He elaborates that his friend had an arthroscopic rotator cuff repair and was in "excruciating pain" for 24 hours after the procedure. The surgeon states, "This procedure is typically not very painful. We have ways to make sure you do not hurt."

During his preoperative visit, the patient tells the nurse that he knows an arthroscopic technique can help decrease postoperative pain compared to an open incision. However, he is fearful of having significant pain after his surgery. Additionally, he has been told to avoid certain pain medications because of his kidneys. The patient's preoperative laboratory values reveal a serum creatinine of 2.0 mg/dL, consistent with values over the past year. A previous nephrology consultation recommended avoiding nephrotoxic medications and better diabetic management.

On the morning of surgery, the patient arrives at the hospital, still apprehensive about pain control. The anesthesiologist discusses the different systemic multimodal analgesics available to the patient for his procedure. The anesthesiologist also explains that peripheral nerve blocks (PNBs), either as a single injection or continuous infusion, can help decrease postoperative pain.

The patient states that he is interested in "getting a nerve block" but does not know if he wants nerve catheter placement because he has been told that this procedure will not be very painful.

The patient is interested in receiving a nerve block; however, he remarks that "someone told me I could not get a block because I had part of my lung removed."

The patient wants a single-injection block for the procedure. The anesthesiologist performs an ultrasound-guided interscalene block with 10 mL of 0.5% ropivacaine. Twenty minutes after the block, the patient cannot abduct his left arm and reports numbness in his left thumb. While his breathing has become shallower, he denies dyspnea, and his pulse oximetry reading is 93%. The patient then undergoes arthroscopic subacromial decompression. His recovery is uneventful, and he is discharged home that afternoon with no discomfort in his shoulder. Early the next morning, the patient is awakened by severe pain in his left shoulder. He receives no relief from his prescribed analgesics. The patient calls his surgeon and says that he is in agony. Per the surgeon's advice, the patient visits the emergency department. The consulting anesthesiologist suspects the patient has had an episode of rebound pain and recommends peripheral nerve catheter placement.

The patient requests an interscalene catheter because he wants "all of my pain to go away." The regional anesthesia team explains to the patient that although the nerve catheter may eliminate much of the pain, it may not prevent all discomfort.

The patient understands and wishes to proceed. The nerve catheter is placed uneventfully, and the patient obtains significant pain relief. The regional anesthesia team connects the infusion pump and verifies the correct settings and function. The patient's wife arrives at his bedside and asks the anesthesiologist how to care for the catheter.

(1) WHAT IS THE SENSORY DISTRIBUTION OF THE SHOULDER?

Most of the dermatomes, myotomes, and osteotomes of the shoulder are covered by the brachial plexus, generally arising from C5 to T1. The two terminal branches of the brachial plexus that innervate the shoulder are the suprascapular nerve and the axillary nerve. In addition, cutaneous innervation is from the superficial cervical plexus (C1–C4), and the axilla derives sensory innervation from T2.

(2) WHAT ARE SOME OF THE CONSIDERATIONS WHEN ASSESSING A PATIENT FOR REGIONAL ANESTHESIA FOR SHOULDER SURGERY?

Considerations for regional anesthesia include a discussion of whether the patient can tolerate any expected physiological consequence from the nerve block, such as the high potential for phrenic nerve blockade and subsequent hemidiaphragmatic paralysis in a patient with poor pulmonary function, the benefits and concerns between the use of single injection versus continuous techniques of the brachial plexus, and setting the expectations for postoperative pain control.

(3) WHAT ARE THE ADVANTAGES AND DISADVANTAGES OF SINGLE-INJECTION NERVE BLOCKS AND NERVE CATHETERS?

Single-injection techniques require less time and resources, result in less mechanical trauma and bleeding, and do not require aggressive needle tip placement within brachial plexus sheath for efficacy. However, the duration of analgesia is short. Continuous techniques allow longer duration but require more technical skills from the proceduralist, as well as a dedicated and available anesthesiology team for catheter management.

(4) WHAT ARE THE REGIONAL ANESTHETIC OPTIONS WHEN A PATIENT FOR SHOULDER ARTHROSCOPY HAS POOR PULMONARY FUNCTION?

Options include a superior trunk block (although phrenic nerve block can still occur with this technique), a suprascapular block (with or without the addition of an axillary nerve block), or local anesthetic infiltration by surgeons (if the other options are not feasible).

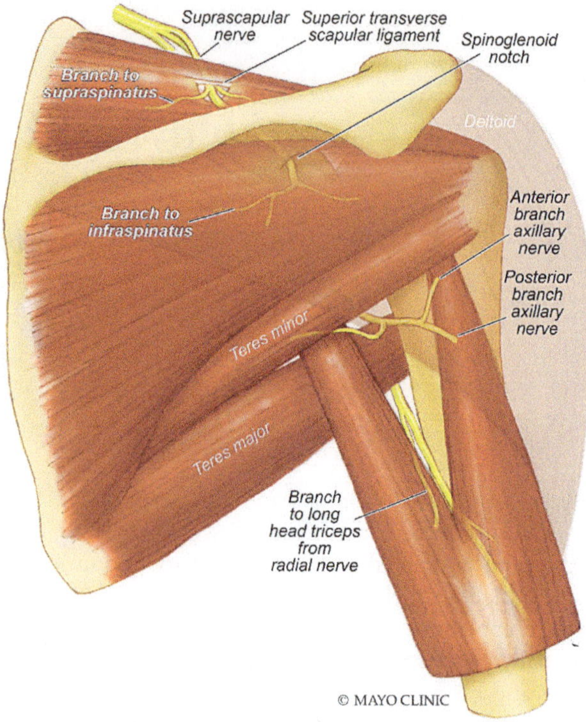

Figure 22.1. Innervation of the shoulder, posterior view.
Used with permission from Mayo Foundation for Medical Education and Research.

(5) WHAT IS REBOUND PAIN?

Rebound pain is the quantifiable difference in pain scores when a PNB is working versus the increase in acute pain that is encountered as the effects of PNB resolve. It occurs approximately 16–24 hours after an interscalene block, has been described more commonly in younger patients (ages <60), lasts about 2–6 hours, can be resistant to opioids despite other multimodal analgesics, and is independent of the type of local anesthetic used for the PNB.

DISCUSSION

SENSORY DISTRIBUTION OF THE SHOULDER AND ARTHROSCOPIC SURGERY

Most of the dermatomes, myotomes, and osteotomes of the shoulder are covered by the brachial plexus, generally arising from C5 to T1. Contributions from C4, also referred to as a prefixed brachial plexus, appear in approximately 30%–60% of cases,[1] and contributions from T2, also referred to as a postfixed brachial plexus, appear in approximately 15%–70%.[2] The two terminal branches of the brachial plexus that innervate the shoulder are the suprascapular nerve (from C5–C6) and the axillary nerve (from the posterior cord). Innervation of the shoulder is demonstrated in Figures 22.1 and 22.2. Blockade of the suprascapular nerve with or without the axillary nerve can be performed for analgesia when interscalene or upper trunk blockades are contraindicated. It is possible for certain areas of the shoulder to be sensate even after successful interscalene brachial plexus block. These would include cutaneous areas innervated by the superficial cervical plexus (C1–C4) as well as the axilla (T2), which can be anesthetized by infiltrating a local anesthetic along the posterior border of the sternocleidomastoid muscle or by performing a selective T2 thoracic paravertebral block, respectively.

Although arthroscopic shoulder procedures involve only small incisions for surgical access, pain after surgery can be significant. In addition to patient-associated risk factors such as a history of chronic pain and preoperative opioid use, the type of arthroscopic surgery may also influence the level of postoperative pain. Some authors have suggested that rotator cuff repair[3,4] may be associated with greater degrees of postoperative pain compared to other arthroscopic shoulder surgeries. Compared to open techniques, shoulder arthroscopy overall is generally associated with less postoperative pain and a decreased risk of damage to the deltoid muscle.[5] Patient positioning during surgery can influence the type of anesthetic used. For example, the beach chair position does not necessarily require general anesthesia if an interscalene nerve block is performed. Additionally, it is considered easier to convert to open surgery from the beach chair position if the need arises. Most often, fluid extravasation from arthroscopy occurs in the chest and upper arm and does not cause edema in the neck or airway, which can occur in the lateral position. The beach chair position, however, carries a rare but catastrophic risk of cerebral ischemia if cerebrovascular parameters are not maintained.[6] Conversely, the lateral position simplifies hemodynamic management and allows for easier access to the most

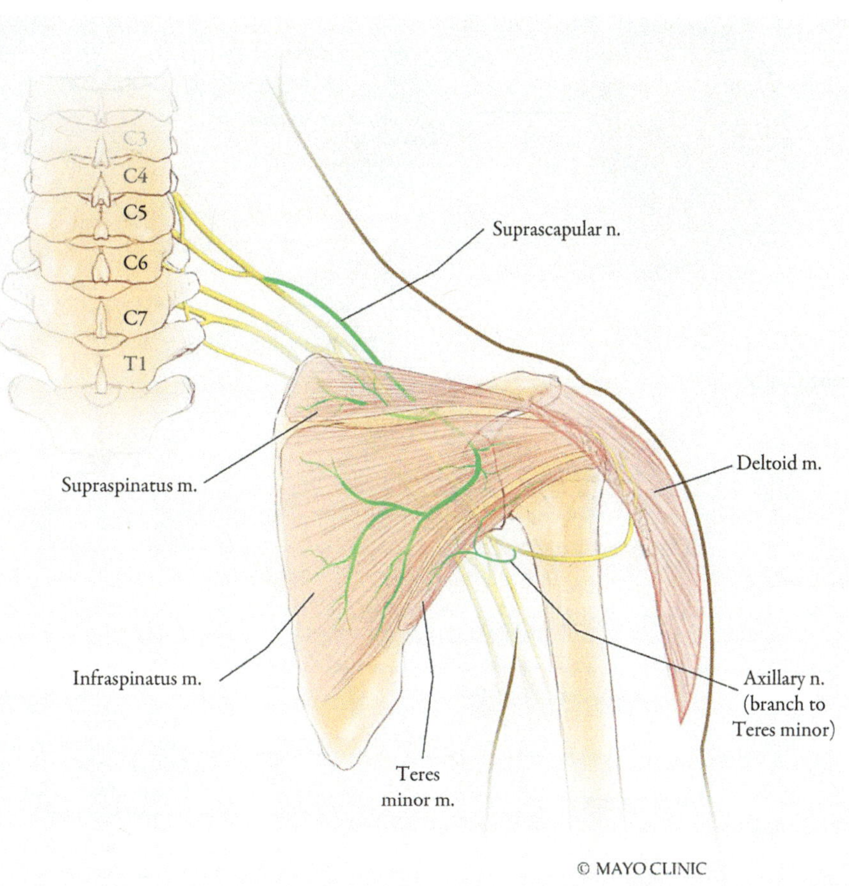

Figure 22.2. Innervation of the shoulder, posterior view
Used with permission from Mayo Foundation for Medical Education and Research.

inferior portion of the glenoid, which may be necessary in some instability operations.

MULTIMODAL ANALGESIA AND SHOULDER ARTHROSCOPY

Opioid use in the United States has reached crisis proportions. According to the Centers for Disease Control and Prevention, over 47,000 Americans die annually from opioid-related overdoses, and over 28,000 of those deaths are attributed to overdosing on synthetic opioids.[7] Recent data analyses suggest that the use of perioperative opioids to treat acute pain can be associated with increased risk of chronic opioid use.[8] Patients receiving opioids within 7 days of outpatient surgery are 44% more likely to continue to be on opioids a year later, compared to patients who were not given opioids for postoperative analgesia.[8] In 2017, the US Department of Health and Human Services issued a statement declaring a public health emergency related to opioid use.[9] Despite these developments, opioids continue to be a common choice for analgesia after shoulder surgery, even with evidence that opioid use after orthopedic surgery is associated with worse patient outcomes and more intense postoperative pain management requirements.[10–12]

Recent data on the use of enhanced recovery after surgery protocols indicate that multimodal analgesia is effective at reducing or eliminating the use of opioids in the perioperative period for shoulder arthroscopy.[13–17] These medications frequently include local anesthetics, nonsteroidal anti-inflammatory drugs (NSAIDs), acetaminophen, corticosteroids, gabapentinoids, alpha-2 receptor agonists, N-methyl-D-aspartate receptor antagonists, and opioids when appropriate. Nonpharmacological methods such as transcutaneous electrical nerve stimulation[18] and cryotherapy[19] have also been shown to be useful for ameliorating pain after shoulder arthroscopy.

Various analgesic medications have different targets to interrupt nociception (Figure 22.3). These synergistic interruptions in nociception can decrease the need for opioids and thus decrease the risk of μ-receptor-associated side effects. NSAIDs have long been used for analgesia after surgery. Their benefits are derived from the inhibition of cyclooxygenase, and they help to decrease the formation of proinflammatory eicosanoids.[20] NSAIDs, although generally safe, should be used with caution in some patient populations. For example, patients with kidney disease may be at risk of developing worsened renal function when given NSAIDs. Prostaglandins are involved in the regulation of blood flow in the afferent arterioles of nephrons; inhibition of their function can decrease renal blood flow and consequently glomerular filtration rate.[20] Gabapentinoids act centrally and peripherally to block a specific subset of voltage-gated calcium channels. These agents have been found

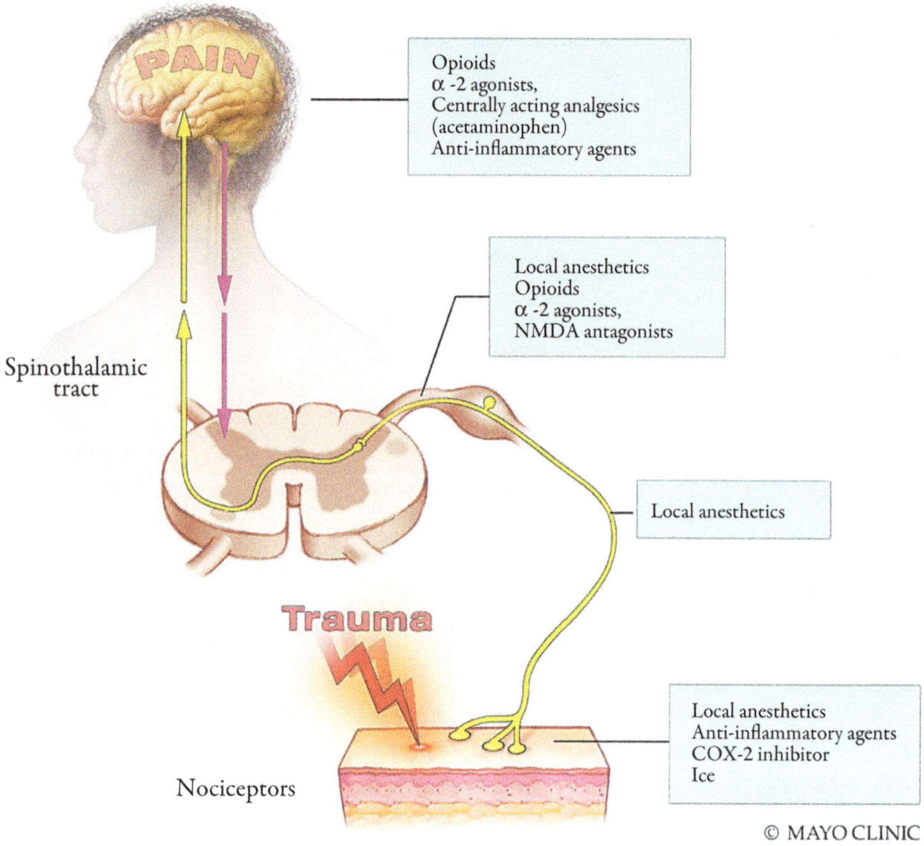

Figure 22.3. Targets for interruption of nociceptive signals.
Used with permission from Mayo Foundation for Medical Education and Research.

to be effective analgesics for post-herpetic neuralgia and diabetes-associated neuropathic pain.[21] The efficacy of gabapentinoids for postoperative analgesia, on the other hand, is controversial. Some reports show a modest opioid-sparing effect from these medications,[22,23] whereas others suggest that gabapentin provides little benefit but can be associated with significant postoperative respiratory depression.[24]

Ketamine is unique among non-opioid analgesics. It is an anesthetic agent that produces a dissociative hypnotic state when given in high doses, but it can reduce perioperative opioid consumption and improve pain scores when administered in lower doses.[25,26] Over the last decade, there has been a resurgence of low-dose ketamine use for acute postoperative pain control with minimal side effects.

REGIONAL ANESTHESIA AND SHOULDER ARTHROSCOPY

Proper assessment of whether a patient is a candidate for a regional anesthetic technique is important,[27] but particularly for a technique such as the interscalene PNB, which has the potential to alter respiratory dynamics and has a higher risk of serious complications if bleeding occurs. Anesthesiologists who plan to perform a PNB should ensure that the patient can tolerate any expected physiological consequence from the nerve block. For example, a deconditioned patient with a history of significant obstructive pulmonary disease may not be eligible for an interscalene PNB. Patient participation during medical decision-making should be encouraged; most patients prefer to be active participants in the process, and their involvement can increase satisfaction with clinical care.[28,29]

After the decision has been made to proceed with a regional anesthetic technique, informed consent should be obtained. The informed consent process should be a discussion of the most significant effects, side effects, and risks involved. Informed consent is not a one-way conversation, nor a rushed patient signature on a document, but rather a dialogue between a patient and a physician.[30] Because of the detail-oriented nature of this dialogue, the informed consent process can require a significant amount of time; anesthesiologists should budget for this time in the preoperative period, in addition to the time required to perform the block. Although some medical centers have moved the process of discussing informed consent to the preoperative clinic arena with a resulting decrease in surgical delays,[31] some studies suggest that information recall by the patient may be limited even when benefits and risks are discussed in this clinical setting.[32]

SINGLE-INJECTION NERVE BLOCKS AND NERVE CATHETERS

Interscalene PNB has been used for analgesia after shoulder surgery since the 1990s. Although nerve stimulator-guided techniques achieved satisfactory analgesia, significant concern regarding events such as inadvertent neuraxial spread hindered widespread popularity of the technique. With the wide adoption of ultrasound-guided regional anesthesia over the past 15 years, brachial plexus PNBs for analgesia of the upper extremity have become the norm for anesthesiologists.[33–37] Ultrasound-guided interscalene PNBs have been shown to effectively and reliably provide analgesia after shoulder surgery with a minimal risk of complications.[38] An interscalene PNB can dramatically reduce the need for opioids in the first 6–8 hours after surgery and improve patient satisfaction with anesthetic care.[39–41] The decision to proceed with a single-injection or continuous perineural catheter should be based on the potential advantages and disadvantages of each technique.

SINGLE-INJECTION BLOCKADE

Compared to an indwelling catheter, a single-injection brachial plexus PNB may offer some advantages regarding logistics and risk.

Single-Injection Advantage: Logistics

(1) Placing a single-injection PNB requires fewer resources and is faster. Typically, all that is required is an ultrasound with a sterile probe cover, a skin disinfectant, a 21- or 22-gauge blunt-tip needle, and local anesthetic. In contrast, interscalene catheter placement requires a sterile drape, a 17- or 18-gauge needle and appropriate catheter, and multiple sterile dressing supplies.

(2) A single-injection PNB can be placed more easily by one provider. In an effort to facilitate efficiency, the presence of an assistant is typically very helpful when placing a catheter. Reliable availability of this additional help, however, may be challenging in a fast-paced practice environment.

(3) A single interscalene PNB injection does not require an anesthesiologist to have 24-hour availability to address issues related to an inpatient or ambulatory continuous local anesthetic infusion.

Single-Injection Advantage: Lower Risk

In addition, a single-injection interscalene block may have less risk compared to a catheter. First, given the smaller caliber of needle required, the risk of bleeding may be reduced. This decreased risk of bleeding can be particularly important for patients who are anticoagulated. These patients may not be eligible for catheter placement or maintenance. Second, advancing the needle into the brachial plexus sheath is not required for an effective single-injection block,[42] and this more conservative needle placement may decrease the risk of respiratory side effects.[43,44] Although somewhat controversial,[45] classic teaching suggests that optimal interscalene catheter placement involves insertion into the interscalene space proper, rather than into the middle scalene muscle.[46–48]

Alternatively, single-injection blockade for shoulder arthroscopy presents some significant disadvantages compared to a catheter technique.

Single-Injection Disadvantages

(1) Relatively short duration: a typical single-injection brachial plexus PNB lasts 8–12 hours, which may not be adequate to address the duration of pain after an arthroscopic shoulder procedure.

(2) Although the minimum effective dose of 0.75% ropivacaine for interscalene PNB may be as little as 7 mL,[49] such a reduction in dosage will decrease the duration of analgesia.

(3) Significant shoulder swelling can occur during extended arthroscopy. This saline-induced swelling can lead to discomfort, as well as decrease the efficacy of the nerve block. Similar to the process of local anesthetic "washout," which has been reported in the literature regarding reversal of local anesthetic-induced side effects,[50,51] the excessive use of arthroscopic fluid may lead to a decrement in PNB. Establishing nerve blockade prior to incision decreases the need for systemic opioids and prevents large sympathetic responses to surgical stimuli.[52]

INDWELLING CATHETER

Compared to a single-injection PNB, an indwelling continuous perineural catheter can offer distinct advantages for arthroscopic shoulder surgery. Continuous interscalene blockade use in particular can be so effective that it has become the analgesic technique of choice for same-day shoulder surgery in some hospitals and ambulatory surgical centers.

Catheter Advantage: Longer Analgesia

The most significant advantage of a perineural catheter is the duration of analgesia. Continuous perineural catheters typically deliver 48–72 hours of local anesthetic and can infuse for longer periods if needed.

Catheter Advantage: Greater Flexibility with Initial Dosing

Although dosages of local anesthetic can be decreased with a single-injection block if desired, the duration of the blockade will be proportionately shortened. In the case of ambulatory surgery, this may present a situation in which the nerve block wears off shortly after the patient arrives at home. In contrast, perineural catheters allow for some adjustment in initial dosage without jeopardizing the duration of pain control.

Catheter Advantage: Individualization

A perineural catheter, when used with a digital pump, provides a greater opportunity to deliver local anesthetic in a personalized form, via changes in infusion rate, bolus volumes, and intervals between boluses. Such individualization can be very useful in patients whose requirements may differ from those of a standard patient, such as those with chronic pain.

Alternatively, nerve catheters placed for shoulder arthroscopy can present some significant challenges compared to a single-injection technique.

Nerve Catheter Disadvantages

(1) Follow-up for continuous catheters is labor intensive. An anesthesiologist must be available in real time to provide appropriate follow-up for the patient's care (whether hospitalized or ambulatory) and to address any issues that may arise.[53] From our experience, it is not uncommon for patients with an interscalene catheter to call the regional anesthesia team with questions regarding the extent of arm numbness, subjective changes in respiration, and leakage of local anesthetic from the catheter site. Similarly, a nonfunctioning catheter should be rapidly assessed and replaced if needed. An anesthesiologist versed in addressing these concerns would ideally be available at all times; this may not be feasible in some centers.

(2) Patients may be dissatisfied with a prolonged blockade. Despite appropriate preoperative education, some patients may find the sensation of upper extremity numbness distressing, particularly aft(er the first 24 hours of infusion.

(3) If postoperative use of anticoagulants is required when an interscalene nerve catheter is in place, another mechanism of analgesia may be needed.

REGIONAL ANESTHESIA FOR THE PATIENT WITH POOR PULMONARY FUNCTION

Patients with compromised pulmonary function who present for shoulder arthroscopy are a challenge for anesthesiologists because they are at increased risk of developing perioperative pulmonary complications, including respiratory failure.[54] In addition, these patients are at increased risk of opioid-induced respiratory depression[55] and may be at risk of developing respiratory failure after a regional anesthetic technique that could anesthetize the ipsilateral phrenic nerve. Likewise, any patient with a contralateral phrenic nerve palsy or nonfunctioning contralateral diaphragm has an absolute contraindication to interscalene PNB.[56] Although rare, changes in diaphragmatic excursion and relative decreases in lung function can also occur with a more distal brachial plexus block such as an infraclavicular approach.[57] A problem arises as to how to provide adequate analgesia to fragile patients while minimizing opioids and avoiding regional techniques that would put them at risk of any perioperative pulmonary complications.

Alternatives and modifications to the interscalene brachial plexus block allow clinicians to provide excellent analgesia to the shoulder while avoiding the complications and side effects of phrenic nerve blockade. Originally described in 2014,[58] the superior trunk block has been shown to be associated with a significantly lower incidence of phrenic nerve palsy compared to the traditional interscalene approach. A randomized controlled trial of 126 patients for shoulder arthroscopy found that with comparable pain scores, the incidence of hemidiaphragmatic paralysis was recorded as only 4.8% in patients who received a superior trunk block, compared to 71% of those who received an interscalene block.[59] In another study, 80 patients were randomized to receive an interscalene PNB or superior trunk block for shoulder arthroscopy; complete hemidiaphragmatic paresis was seen in 72% of those receiving an interscalene block versus 5% in those with a superior trunk block.[60] Superior trunk block also provided non-inferior pain control compared to an interscalene block.

The suprascapular nerve provides approximately 70% of the sensory innervation to the glenohumeral joint and also innervates the supra- and infraspinatus muscles (Figures 22.1 and 22.2). Selective blockade of the suprascapular nerve has been shown to provide adequate analgesia after arthroscopic shoulder surgery, while also sparing the phrenic nerve.[61–63] Although it is slightly less effective than the interscalene block for pain control, it can be used for patients when an interscalene block is contraindicated. One meta-analysis reviewed 1382 patients across 14 randomized trials comparing suprascapular nerve block (SSNB) to interscalene PNB.[64] This study concluded that although the SSNB proved effective for postoperative analgesia, it did not reduce opioid consumption or pain scores compared to interscalene PNB. However, major complications such as pneumothorax, Horner's syndrome, and recurrent laryngeal nerve paresis were less common with SSNB compared to interscalene PNB.

Adding an axillary nerve block to a SSNB can provide improved analgesia over the SSNB alone and could be considered for patients who have inadequate pain control in the recovery room.[65]

One other technique to consider in this patient population is local anesthetic infiltration (LAI) for postoperative analgesia. LAI is placed by the orthopedic surgeon at the conclusion of surgery. Although LAI can be helpful for pain control and avoiding respiratory compromise, this technique has been shown to be inferior to an interscalene PNB or an SSNB.[63,66] Furthermore, it is most commonly used in open-surgical procedures. We recommend it only when other techniques are contraindicated or unavailable.

REBOUND PAIN

Rebound pain is defined as the quantifiable difference in pain scores when a PNB is working versus the increase in acute pain that is encountered as the effects of PNB resolve.[67] It has been described more commonly in younger patients (ages <60), lasts about 2–6 hours, and is generally independent of the type of local anesthetic used for the PNB.[68,69] During those hours, pain can be severe (visual analog scale >7) and resistant to opioids, even in patients receiving scheduled multimodal analgesia. It is commonly reported as a burning pain. Rebound pain may be more severe after shoulder surgery compared to other orthopedic surgeries.[67]

Rebound pain has been demonstrated in animal models, although the clinical relevance of the *thermal* hypersensitivity noted at block resolution remains controversial. Kolarczyk and Williams noted a transient increase in thermal sensitivity in rats who received sciatic nerve blocks in the absence of surgery.[70] Janda and colleagues also found thermal sensitivity in a similar rat model following sciatic PNB but concluded that this was short-lived and clinically insignificant.[71] These animal studies are limited by the fact that the sciatic nerve blocks were performed in the absence of surgical trauma. Both studies point away from mechanical hypersensitivity, however, which suggests that the untreated surgical pain being felt for the first time is not the primary source of rebound pain.

Rebound pain is clinically relevant, in our opinion, when it changes a patient's recovery trajectory. For example, Sunderland and colleagues documented an increase in the incidence of unplanned physician visits within 48 hours after surgery for wrist fracture in patients who received a PNB compared to those who did not.[72] Additionally, more patients who received a PNB sought some form of medical attention for pain and more often reported severe postoperative pain compared to patients who received general anesthesia only. Along the same line, a small randomized trial of patients undergoing distal radius fixation found that patients who received a PNB had better pain scores and a shorter length of stay in the recovery room compared to patients who received general anesthesia only; however, 12 hours after surgery, the PNB patients had significantly worse pain scores compared to the general anesthesia–only patients.[73]

Specifically regarding interscalene PNB, one study found that although single-injection interscalene PNB can provide effective postoperative analgesia for 6–8 hours after shoulder surgery, these patients can suffer rebound pain (described as a visual analog scale score approximately 1 cm higher than those who did not receive a PNB) between 16 and 24 hours after their block.[74]

In general, single-injection PNBs will wear off the evening of postoperative day 0, when the ambulatory patient is already at home, with few resources to avoid a trip to the emergency room if the pain is intolerable. If a perineural adjuvant can provide a clinically significant increase in postoperative analgesia that preempts a patient from being awakened by severe pain, there may be a role for it in the perioperative period. (For more information on adjuvants to PNBs, see Chapter 7.) There is a role for a continuous PNB any time a surgery can be associated with moderate to severe postoperative pain; data have shown that the duration of a PNB may influence rebound pain scores.[67]

As regional anesthesiologists, we need to do a better job of discussing rebound pain and how to manage it effectively. Work is ongoing to gain a better understanding of the impact of rebound pain on a patient's quality of recovery.[75]

EXPECTATION SETTING REGARDING PAIN CONTROL

Expectations regarding appropriate analgesic techniques for shoulder surgery are best set in the preoperative period. Patients who understand the expected distribution of analgesia, duration of PNB, and anticipated postoperative discomfort (even after a successful technique) may be better equipped to tolerate the incidence of postoperative pain or the expected effects of the analgesic technique.

During the expectation-setting process, the role of any regional anesthetic technique should be clarified in the context of the overall postoperative analgesic plan. Although an ambulatory interscalene catheter may negate the need for any opioid analgesic in some patients, the patient and family should be informed that multiple analgesic methods can and may need to be used for postoperative pain after shoulder arthroscopy. In collaboration with the surgeon, information regarding analgesics and instructions for their use should be provided to patients. Likewise, the overall analgesic plan should be discussed with the surgeon so that a coordinated effort is in place and analgesic expectations are set for the patient, surgeon, and anesthesiologist.

AMBULATORY NERVE CATHETER CARE AND EDUCATION

The patient and family should be adequately educated regarding ambulatory catheter care. This can typically be accomplished preoperatively or in the postoperative bay if the patient is lucid and family/companions are also available. In general, education consists of:[27,53,76]

- Infusion pump user interface and bolus function
- Water precautions
- How to manage breakthrough pain
- How to address infusion leaks
- Safety concerns
    - Signs and symptoms of local anesthetic toxicity
    - Signs of bleeding or hematoma
    - How to turn off the infusion pump
    - Contact information for the acute pain service or anesthesiologist.

This information can be presented to the patient in a concise document given at discharge. Examples of content to include in a patient handout can be seen in Box 22.1. Common logistical problems that anesthesiologists can anticipate include accidental dislodgement, local anesthetic leakage from the catheter site, and an inability to directly troubleshoot the catheter via telephone.[27] Notably, however, the incidence of problems that require physician intervention can be as low as 4%.[76] During the education process, the educator should clarify situations that require an immediate phone call to the anesthesiology team or emergent medical care, such as dyspnea, changes in mental status, or intolerable pain. Patient understanding and contact information for both the patient and provider should be confirmed prior to patient discharge.

Box 22.1 EXAMPLE OF INFORMATION TO INCLUDE IN PERIPHERAL NERVE CATHETER HOME INSTRUCTIONS LISTED BY CATEGORY

Setting expectations regarding function

A peripheral nerve catheter was placed by your anesthesiologist to help with pain control after your surgery. It is not in a vein or an artery. You received a very strong surgical block that will wear off sometime during the night of surgery or the next morning.

Someone from the Acute Pain Service will call you each day that your peripheral nerve catheter is in place.

Contact information

Call the Acute Pain Service if you have any questions or concerns regarding your peripheral nerve catheter or pain control while the peripheral nerve catheter is in place.

We are available at XXX-XXX-XXXX, 24 hours a day, 7 days a week. If no answer, call the hospital operator and ask for the Acute Pain Service.

Call the Acute Pain Service immediately if you have:

- Pain that is not controlled
- A temperature greater than 101° Fahrenheit
- Pain at the catheter insertion site
- Bleeding, swelling, skin redness, or tenderness at the catheter insertion site

Medication facts and warnings

You are being administered a 0.2% ropivacaine infusion via a ________ nerve catheter. Bag volume is 600 mL.

The infusion device delivers medication continuously.

To help reduce pain, you may have a dose button that you can press every 1 hour as needed.

Stop the infusion and call the Acute Pain Service immediately if you experience:

- Numbness or tingling around your mouth or tongue
- A new instance of ringing in your ears
- Shortness of breath

Daily use information

Do not place the infusion in water.

Do not shower.

Leakage around the nerve catheter dressing frequently occurs. Do not change the peripheral nerve catheter dressing. You may reinforce the top of the dressing as needed by applying gauze and tape as provided.

Keep your extremity protected as it may be weak and numb.

CONCLUSIONS

- Most of the innervation of the shoulder arises from C5 to T1, with occasional contributions from C4 or T2. Assessment of a patient's pulmonary status and ability to tolerate a change in diaphragmatic function should be assessed prior to an interscalene block.
- Regional anesthetic options for a patient with compromised pulmonary function include a more distal brachial plexus block, superior trunk block, and suprascapular nerve block.
- Expectations regarding the regional anesthetic technique should be set with the patient. The role of the block in the context of the overall pain-control plan and other analgesic agents should be explained.
- Rebound pain is significant when it alters the recovery trajectory of a patient. A single-injection interscalene block may not be sufficient to properly address pain after shoulder surgery.
- Anesthesiologists should properly educate patients about peripheral nerve blockade, including expected pain control, possible side effects, and ambulatory nerve catheter care, if applicable.

REFERENCES

1. Bonnel F. Microscopic anatomy of the adult human brachial plexus: an anatomical and histological basis for microsurgery. *Microsurgery*. 1984;5:107–118.
2. Shin AY, Spinner RJ, Steinmann SP, Bishop AT. Adult traumatic brachial plexus injuries. *J Am Acad Orthop Surg*. 2005;13:382–396.
3. de Boer FA, Schouten TTJ, Boekestein EP, et al. Risk factors for postoperative pain in the first three weeks after arthroscopic or open shoulder surgery. *Orthop Traumatol Surg Res*. 2019;105:241–244.
4. Calvo E, Torres MD, Morcillo D, Leal V. Rotator cuff repair is more painful than other arthroscopic shoulder procedures. *Arch Orthop Trauma Surg*. 2019;139:669–674.
5. Yamaguchi K, Levine WN, Marra G, Galatz LM, Klepps S, Flatow EL. Transitioning to arthroscopic rotator cuff repair: the pros and cons. *Instr Course Lect*. 2003;52:81–92.
6. Li X, Eichinger JK, Hartshorn T, Zhou H, Matzkin EG, Warner JP. A comparison of the lateral decubitus and beach-chair positions for shoulder surgery: advantages and complications. *J Am Acad Orthop Surg*. 2015;23:18–28.
7. Rudd RA, Aleshire N, Zibbell JE, Gladden RM. Increases in drug and opioid overdose deaths: United States, 2000–2014. *MMWR*. 2016;64:1378–1382.
8. Alam A, Gomes T, Zheng H, Mamdani MM, Juurlink DN, Bell CM. Long-term analgesic use after low-risk surgery: a retrospective cohort study. *Arch Intern Med*. 2012;172:425–430.
9. US Department of Health & Human Services. *HHS Acting Secretary Declares Public Health Emergency to Address National Opioid Crisis*. 2017. Available at: https://www.hhs.gov/about/news/2017/10/26/hhs-acting-secretary-declares-public-health-emergency-address-national-opioid-crisis.html.
10. Franklin PD, Karbassi JA, Li W, Yang W, Ayers DC. Reduction in narcotic use after primary total knee arthroplasty and association with patient pain relief and satisfaction. *J Arthroplasty*. 2010;25:12–16.
11. Morris BJ, Laughlin MS, Elkousy HA, Gartsman GM, Edwards TB. Preoperative opioid use and outcomes after reverse shoulder arthroplasty. *J Shoulder Elbow Surg*. 2015;24:11–16.
12. Morris BJ, Sciascia AD, Jacobs CA, Edwards TB. Preoperative opioid use associated with worse outcomes after anatomic shoulder arthroplasty. *J Shoulder Elbow Surg*. 2016;25:619–623.
13. Jo CH, Shin JS, Huh J. Multimodal analgesia for arthroscopic rotator cuff repair: a randomized, placebo-controlled, double-blind trial. *Eur J Orthop Surg Traumatol*. 2014;24:315–322.
14. Cho CH, Song KS, Min BW, et al. Multimodal approach to postoperative pain control in patients undergoing rotator cuff repair. *Knee Surg Sports Traumatol Arthrosc*. 2011;19:1744–1748.
15. Han SS, Lee YH, Oh JH, Aminzai S, Kim SH. Randomized, controlled trial of multimodal shoulder injection or intravenous

patient-controlled analgesia after arthroscopic rotator cuff repair. *Knee Surg Sports Traumatol Arthrosc*. 2013;21:2877–2883.
16. Uquillas CA, Capogna BM, Rossy WH, Mahure SA, Rokito AS. Postoperative pain control after arthroscopic rotator cuff repair. *J Shoulder Elbow Surg*. 2016;25:1204–1213.
17. Elkassabany NM, Wang A, Ochroch J, Mattera M, Liu J, Kuntz A. Improved quality of recovery from ambulatory shoulder surgery after implementation of a multimodal perioperative pain management protocol. *Pain Med*. 2019;20:1012–1019.
18. Mahure SA, Rokito AS, Kwon YW. Transcutaneous electrical nerve stimulation for postoperative pain relief after arthroscopic rotator cuff repair: a prospective double-blinded randomized trial. *J Shoulder Elbow Surg*. 2017;26:1508–1513.
19. Speer KP, Warren RF, Horowitz L. The efficacy of cryotherapy in the postoperative shoulder. *J Shoulder Elbow Surg*. 1996;5:62–68.
20. Chou R, Gordon DB, de Leon-Casasola OA, et al. Management of postoperative pain: a clinical practice guideline from the American Pain Society, the American Society of Regional Anesthesia and Pain Medicine, and the American Society of Anesthesiologists' Committee on Regional Anesthesia, Executive Committee, and Administrative Council. *J Pain*. 2016;17:131–157.
21. Nicol AL, Hurley RW, Benzon HT. Alternatives to opioids in the pharmacologic management of chronic pain syndromes: a narrative review of randomized, controlled, and blinded clinical trials. *Anesth Analg*. 2017;125:1682–1703.
22. Dauri M, Faria S, Gatti A, Celidonio L, Carpenedo R, Sabato AF. Gabapentin and pregabalin for the acute post-operative pain management: a systematic-narrative review of the recent clinical evidences. *Curr Drug Targets*. 2009;10:716–733.
23. Fabritius ML, Wetterslev J, Mathiesen O, Dahl JB. Dose-related beneficial and harmful effects of gabapentin in postoperative pain management: post hoc analyses from a systematic review with meta-analyses and trial sequential analyses. *J Pain Res*. 2017;10:2547–2563.
24. Adam F, Ménigaux C, Sessler DI, Chauvin M. A single preoperative dose of gabapentin (800 milligrams) does not augment postoperative analgesia in patients given interscalene brachial plexus blocks for arthroscopic shoulder surgery. *Anesth Analg*. 2006;103:1278–1282.
25. Cengiz P, Gokcinar D, Karabeyoglu I, Topcu H, Cicek GS, Gogus N. Intraoperative low-dose ketamine infusion reduces acute postoperative pain following total knee replacement surgery: a prospective, randomized double-blind placebo-controlled trial. *J Coll Physicians Surg Pak*. 2014;24:299–303.
26. Brinck EC, Tiippana E, Heesen M, et al. Perioperative intravenous ketamine for acute postoperative pain in adults. *Cochrane Database Syst Rev*. 2018;12:CD012033.
27. Greengrass RA, Nielsen KC. Management of peripheral nerve block catheters at home. *Int Anesthesiol Clin*. 2005;43:79–87.
28. Huang J, Chagpar A. Active participation in decision-making in contralateral prophylactic mastectomy for patients with breast cancer. *J Surg Res*. 2019;242:129–135.
29. Babac A, von Friedrichs V, Litzkendorf S, Zeidler J, Damm K, Graf von der Schulenburg JM. Integrating patient perspectives in medical decision-making: a qualitative interview study examining potentials within the rare disease information exchange process in practice. *BMC Med Inform Decis Mak*. 2019;19:188.
30. Lin CJ, Luke C, Sullivan D, Kidwell R. Development of specific peripheral nerve block consent form. *J Clin Anesth*. 2019;54:33–36.
31. Brooks BS, Barman J, Ponce BA, Sides A, Vetter TR. An electronic surgical order, undertaking patient education, and obtaining informed consent for regional analgesia before the day of surgery reduce block-related delays. *Local Reg Anesth*. 2016;9:59–64.
32. Bai JW, Abdallah FWW, Cohn M, Ladowski S, Madhusudan P, Brull R. Say what? Patients have poor immediate memory of major risks of interscalene block disclosed during the informed consent discussion. *Reg Anesth Pain Med*. 2019;pii: rapm-2019-100858.
33. Alfred VM, Srinivasan G, Zachariah M. Comparison of ultrasound with peripheral nerve stimulator-guided technique for supraclavicular block in upper limb surgeries: a randomized controlled trial. *Anesth Essays Res*. 2018;12:50–54.
34. Kolny M, Stasiowski MJ, Zuber M, et al. Randomized, comparative study of the effectiveness of three different techniques of interscalene brachial plexus block using 0.5% ropivacaine for shoulder arthroscopy. *Anaesthesiol Intensive Ther*. 2017;49:47–52.
35. Singh S, Goyal R, Upadhyay KK, Sethi N, Sharma RM, Sharma A. An evaluation of brachial plexus block using a nerve stimulator versus ultrasound guidance: a randomized controlled trial. *J Anaesthesiol Clin Pharmacol*. 2015;31:370–374.
36. Girdler-Hardy TP, Webb C, Menon G. Improved safety and efficacy of ultrasound-guided interscalene nerve block vs a nerve-stimulator guided technique. *Br J Anaesth*. 2015;115:474–475.
37. Orebaugh SL, Kentor ML, Williams BA. Adverse outcomes associated with nerve stimulator-guided and ultrasound-guided peripheral nerve blocks by supervised trainees: update of a single-site database. *Reg Anesth Pain Med*. 2012;37:577–582.
38. Singh A, Kelly C, O'Brien T, Wilson J, Warner JJ. Ultrasound-guided interscalene block anesthesia for shoulder arthroscopy: a prospective study of 1319 patients. *J Bone Joint Surg Am*. 2012;94:2040–2046.
39. Trompeter A, Camilleri G, Narang K, Hauf W, Venn R. Analgesia requirements after interscalene block for shoulder arthroscopy: the 5 days following surgery. *Arch Orthop Trauma Surg*. 2010;130:417–421.
40. Kim JH, Koh HJ, Kim DK, et al. Interscalene brachial plexus bolus block versus patient-controlled interscalene indwelling catheter analgesia for the first 48 hours after arthroscopic rotator cuff repair. *J Shoulder Elbow Surg*. 2018;27:1243–1250.
41. Hughes MS, Matava MJ, Wright RW, Brophy RH, Smith MV. Interscalene brachial plexus block for arthroscopic shoulder surgery: a systematic review. *J Bone Joint Surg Am*. 2013;95:1318–1324.
42. Maga J, Missair A, Visan A, et al. Comparison of outside versus inside brachial plexus sheath injection for ultrasound-guided interscalene nerve blocks. *J Ultrasound Med*. 2016;35:279–285.
43. Ayyanagouda B, Hosalli V, Kaur P, Ambi U, Hulkund SY. Hemidiaphragmatic paresis following extrafascial versus conventional intrafascial approach for interscalene brachial plexus block: a double-blind randomised, controlled trial. *Indian J Anaesth*. 2019;63:375–381.
44. Palhais N, Brull R, Kern C, et al. Extrafascial injection for interscalene brachial plexus block reduces respiratory complications compared with a conventional intrafascial injection: a randomized, controlled, double-blind trial. *Br J Anaesth*. 2016;116:531–537.
45. Albrecht E, Bathory I, Fournier N, Jacot-Guillarmod A, Farron A, Brull R. Reduced hemidiaphragmatic paresis with extrafascial compared with conventional intrafascial tip placement for continuous interscalene brachial plexus block: a randomized, controlled, double-blind trial. *Br J Anaesth*. 2017;118:586–592.
46. Swenson JD, Davis JJ, DeCou JA. A novel approach for assessing catheter position after ultrasound-guided placement of continuous interscalene block. *Anesth Analg*. 2008;106:1015–1016.
47. Mariano ER, Loland VJ, Ilfeld BM. Interscalene perineural catheter placement using an ultrasound-guided posterior approach. *Reg Anesth Pain Med*. 2009;34:60–63.
48. Mariano ER, Loland VJ, Sandhu NS, et al. A trainee-based randomized comparison of stimulating interscalene perineural catheters with a new technique using ultrasound guidance alone. *J Ultrasound Med*. 2010;29:329–336.
49. Vandepitte C, Gautier P, Xu D, Salviz EA, Hadzic A. Effective volume of ropivacaine 0.75% through a catheter required for interscalene brachial plexus blockade. *Anesthesiology*. 2013;118:863–867.
50. Smith LM, Barrington MJ. A novel approach to reversal of respiratory distress following insertion of an interscalene nerve catheter. *J Clin Anesth*. 2018;47:43–44.
51. Ngai LK, Ma W, Costouros JG, Cheung EV, Horn JL, Tsui BCH. Successful reversal of phrenic nerve blockade following washout of interscalene nerve block as demonstrated by ultrasonographic diaphragmatic excursion. *J Clin Anesth*. 2019;59:46–48.
52. Lavand'homme P, De Kock M, Waterloos H. Intraoperative epidural analgesia combined with ketamine provides effective preventive analgesia in patients undergoing major digestive surgery. *Anesthesiology*. 2005;103:813–820.

53. Ilfeld BM, Enneking FK. Continuous peripheral nerve blocks at home: a review. *Anesth Analg*. 2005;100:1822–1833.
54. Licker M, Schweizer A, Ellenberger C, Tschopp JM, Diaper J, Clergue F. Perioperative medical management of patients with COPD. *Int J Chron Obstruct Pulmon Dis*. 2007;2:493–515.
55. Gupta K, Prasad A, Nagappa M, Wong J, Abrahamyan L, Chung FF. Risk factors for opioid-induced respiratory depression and failure to rescue: a review. *Curr Opin Anaesthesiol*. 2018;31:110–119.
56. Urmey WF, Gloeggler PJ. Pulmonary function changes during interscalene brachial plexus block: effects of decreasing local anesthetic injection volume. *Reg Anesth*. 1993;18:244–249.
57. Rettig HC, Gielen MJ, Boersma E, Klein J, Groen GJ. Vertical infraclavicular block of the brachial plexus: effects on hemidiaphragmatic movement and ventilatory function. *Reg Anesth Pain Med*. 2005;30:529–535.
58. Burckett-St Laurent D, Chan V, Chin KJ. Refining the ultrasound-guided interscalene brachial plexus block: the superior trunk approach. *Can J Anaesth*. 2014;61:1098–1102.
59. Kim DH, Lin Y, Beathe JC, et al. Superior trunk block: a phrenic-sparing alternative to the interscalene block: a randomized controlled trial. *Anesthesiology*. 2019;131:521–533.
60. Kang R, Jeong JS, Chin KJ, et al. Superior trunk block provides noninferior analgesia compared with interscalene brachial plexus block in arthroscopic shoulder surgery. *Anesthesiology*. 2019;131:1316–1326.
61. Wiegel M, Moriggl B, Schwarzkopf P, Petroff D, Reske AW. Anterior suprascapular nerve block versus interscalene brachial plexus block for shoulder surgery in the outpatient setting: a randomized controlled patient- and assessor-blinded trial. *Reg Anesth Pain Med*. 2017;42:310–318.
62. Desroches A, Klouche S, Schlur C, Bauer T, Waitzenegger T, Hardy P. Suprascapular nerve block versus interscalene block as analgesia after arthroscopic rotator cuff repair: a randomized controlled noninferiority trial. *Arthroscopy*. 2016;32:2203–2209.
63. Singelyn FJ, Lhotel L, Fabre B. Pain relief after arthroscopic shoulder surgery: a comparison of intraarticular analgesia, suprascapular nerve block, and interscalene brachial plexus block. *Anesth Analg*. 2004;99:589–592.
64. Kay J, Memon M, Hu T, et al. Suprascapular nerve blockade for postoperative pain control after arthroscopic shoulder surgery: a systematic review and meta-analysis. *Orthop J Sports Med*. 2018;6(12):2325967118815859.
65. Lee JJ, Kim DY, Hwang JT, et al. Effect of ultrasonographically guided axillary nerve block combined with suprascapular nerve block in arthroscopic rotator cuff repair: a randomized controlled trial. *Arthroscopy*. 2014;30:906–914.
66. Fontana C, Di Donato A, Di Giocomo G, et al. Postoperative analgesia for arthroscopic shoulder surgery: a prospective randomized controlled study of intraarticular, subacromial injection, interscalenic brachial plexus block and intraarticular plus subacromial injection efficacy. *Eur J Anaesthesiol*. 2009;26:689–693.
67. Williams BA, Bottegal MT, Kentor ML, Irrgang JJ, Williams JP. Rebound pain scores as a function of femoral nerve block duration after anterior cruciate ligament reconstruction: retrospective analysis of a prospective, randomized clinical trial. *Reg Anesth Pain Med*. 2007;32:186–192.
68. Henningsen MJ, Sort R, Møller AM, Herling SF. Peripheral nerve block in ankle fracture surgery: a qualitative study of patients' experiences. *Anaesthesia*. 2018;73:49–58.
69. Sort R, Brorson S, Gögenur I, Nielsen JK, Møller AM. Rebound pain following peripheral nerve block anaesthesia in acute ankle fracture surgery: an exploratory pilot study. *Acta Anaesthesiol Scand*. 2019;63:396–402.
70. Kolarczyk LM, Williams BA. Transient heat hyperalgesia during resolution of ropivacaine sciatic nerve block in the rat. *Reg Anesth Pain Med*. 2011;36:220–224.
71. Janda A, Lydic R, Welch KB, Brummett CM. Thermal hyperalgesia after sciatic nerve block in rat is transient and clinically insignificant. *Reg Anesth Pain Med*. 2013;3:151–154.
72. Sunderland S, Yarnold CH, Head SJ, et al. Regional versus general anesthesia and the incidence of unplanned health care resource utilization for postoperative pain after wrist fracture surgery: results from a retrospective quality improvement project. *Reg Anesth Pain Med*. 2016;41:22–27.
73. Galos DK, Taormina DP, Crespo A, et al. Does brachial plexus blockade result in improved pain scores after distal radius fracture fixation? a randomized trial. *Clin Orthop Relat Res*. 2016;474:1247–1254.
74. Abdallah FW, Halpern SH, Aoyama K, Brull R. Will the real benefits of single-shot interscalene block please stand up? a systematic review and meta-analysis. *Anesth Analg*. 2015;120:1114–1129.
75. Sort R, Brorson S, Gögenur I, Møller AM. An Ankle Trial study protocol: a randomised trial comparing pain profiles after peripheral nerve block or spinal anaesthesia for ankle fracture surgery. *BMJ Open*. 2017;7:e016001.
76. Swenson JD, Cheng GS, Axelrod DA, Davis JJ. Ambulatory anesthesia and regional catheters: when and how. *Anesthesiol Clin*. 2010;28:267–280.

REVIEW QUESTIONS

(1) Regarding shoulder arthroscopy, which of the following statements is TRUE?

A. The lateral position is associated with an increased risk of cerebral ischemia.
B. The interscalene block provides surgical anesthesia to the anterior and posterior shoulder and axilla.
C. Contributions from C4 and T2 to the brachial plexus are rare.
D. The beach chair position carries a low risk of fluid extravasation to the neck and airway.

(2) Which of the following regional anesthetic techniques can be considered best for patients with poor pulmonary function after shoulder arthroscopy?

A. Supraclavicular brachial plexus block
B. Infraclavicular brachial plexus block
C. Suprascapular nerve block
D. Ulnar nerve block

(3) A 54-year-old woman with chronic renal insufficiency (glomerular filtration rate <30 mL/min/BSA) is scheduled for shoulder arthroscopy. Which of the following should NOT be considered part of her multimodal analgesic plan?

A. Acetaminophen
B. Dexmedetomidine
C. Ketamine
D. Ketorolac

4. Which of the following is TRUE of rebound pain after PNB resolution?

A. It is associated with patients who are >60 years old.
B. It occurs after PNB with bupivacaine rather than ropivacaine.
C. It is associated with complex knee surgery rather than shoulder surgery.
D. It generally lasts 2–6 hours.

(5) Regarding rebound pain, which of the following statements is TRUE?

A. Following distal radius repair, patients with PNB had better pain scores than patients with general anesthesia only, 12 hours after surgery.
B. Following wrist fracture surgery, patients with PNB had fewer unplanned physician visits compared to patients with general anesthesia only.
C. The longer the duration of a PNB, the lower the rebound pain score.
D. Patients generally comprehend the preoperative oral and written instructions about what to expect regarding the duration of PNB, when it will wear off, and how they will feel after the PNB resolves.

(6) Patient participation during medical decision-making:

A. Can lead to increased satisfaction with patient care
B. Is detrimental to quality of care
C. Takes patient preferences into consideration
D. Both A and C

(7) Regarding use of an ambulatory nerve catheter:

A. Patients with cognitive dysfunction, unreliability, or lacking a social support system may not be appropriate candidates.
B. Real-time availability of an anesthesiologist is required for appropriate follow-up.
C. The nerve catheter's role in the complete analgesic plan should be explained.
D. All of the above.

(8) All of the following should be included in ambulatory nerve catheter patient education EXCEPT:

A. How to manage breakthrough pain
B. Signs and symptoms of local anesthetic toxicity
C. How to reinsert the catheter
D. Contact information for the acute pain service

ANSWERS

(1) **D.** Shoulder arthroscopy can be performed in the lateral or beach chair position. The beach chair position allows for transitioning to an open repair if the need arises and has a low risk of irrigation solution extravasation to the neck or airway compared to the lateral position. A brachial plexus with contributions from C4 (a *prefixed* brachial plexus) occurs in approximately 30%–60% of patients, and a brachial plexus with contributions from T2 (a *postfixed* brachial plexus) occurs in approximately 15%–70% of patients. The sensory distribution of the superficial cervical plexus and T2 nerve root are not anesthetized with an interscalene block and may require supplementation following major shoulder surgery.

Reference

Shin AY, Spinner RJ, Steinmann SP, Bishop AT. Adult traumatic brachial plexus injuries. *J Am Acad Orthop Surg.* 2005;13:382–396.

(2) **C.** Of the choices listed, the isolated the suprascapular nerve block (SSNB) is the most appropriate regional anesthetic choice for a patient with poor pulmonary reserve. The suprascapular nerve provides most of the sensory innervation to the glenohumeral joint, and SSNB has been shown to spare the phrenic nerve and therefore preserve diaphragmatic function. The ulnar nerve provides little innervation to the shoulder.

Reference

Wiegel M, Moriggl B, Schwarzkopf P, Petroff D, Reske AW. Anterior suprascapular nerve block versus interscalene brachial plexus block for shoulder surgery in the outpatient setting: a randomized controlled patient- and assessor-blinded trial. *Reg Anesth Pain Med.* 2017;42:310–318.

(3) **D.** Multimodal analgesia should be a part of any perioperative acute pain management plan. Ketorolac is a nonsteroidal anti-inflammatory drug and an effective analgesic for most patients. However, it is associated with acute renal failure in patients with severe renal insufficiency and thus should be avoided in patients with low glomerular filtration rates.

Reference

Chou R, Gordon DB, de Leon-Casasola OA, et al. Management of postoperative pain: a clinical practice guideline from the American Pain Society, the American Society of Regional Anesthesia and Pain Medicine, and the American Society of Anesthesiologists' Committee on Regional Anesthesia, Executive Committee, and Administrative Council. *J Pain.* 2016;17:131–157.

(4) **D.** Rebound pain has been associated with younger patients (ages <60) and shoulder surgery more than knee surgery, and it appears to be independent of the type of long-acting local anesthetic used. It is generally described as lasting 2–6 hours and is resistant to opioid analgesics. Older patients presenting for surgery with a PNB appear to be at lower risk for rebound pain than younger patients.

References

Williams BA, Bottegal MT, Kentor ML, Irrgang JJ, Williams JP. Rebound pain scores as a function of femoral nerve block duration after anterior cruciate ligament reconstruction: retrospective analysis of a prospective, randomized clinical trial. *Reg Anesth Pain Med.* 2007;32:186–192.

Henningsen MJ, Sort R, Møller AM, Herling SF. Peripheral nerve block in ankle fracture surgery: a qualitative study of patients' experiences. *Anaesthesia.* 2018;73:49–58.

Sort R, Brorson S, Gögenur I, Nielsen JK, Møller AM. Rebound pain following peripheral nerve block anaesthesia in acute ankle fracture surgery: an exploratory pilot study. *Acta Anaesthesiol Scand.* 2019;63:396–402.

(5) **C.** Unfortunately, published data suggest increased healthcare use following wrist fracture surgery with PNB compared to patients with general anesthesia only. Additionally, 12 hours after surgery, patients with single-injection PNB had worse pain scores compared to patients who received general anesthesia only. Data suggest that for every additional hour of PNB, a patient's pain score is reduced by 0.03 units. Patients may not fully comprehend how long a PNB is expected to last or what to expect as it resolves.

References

Williams BA, Bottegal MT, Kentor ML, Irrgang JJ, Williams JP. Rebound pain scores as a function of femoral nerve block duration after anterior cruciate ligament reconstruction: retrospective analysis of a prospective, randomized clinical trial. *Reg Anesth Pain Med.* 2007;32:186–192.

Henningsen MJ, Sort R, Møller AM, Herling SF. Peripheral nerve block in ankle fracture surgery: a qualitative study of patients' experiences. *Anaesthesia.* 2018;73:49–58.

Sunderland S, Yarnold CH, Head SJ, et al. Regional versus general anesthesia and the incidence of unplanned health care resource utilization for postoperative pain after wrist fracture surgery: results from a retrospective quality improvement project. *Reg Anesth Pain Med.* 2016;41:22–27.

Galos DK, Taormina DP, Crespo A, et al. Does brachial plexus blockade result in improved pain scores after distal radius fracture fixation? A randomized trial. *Clin Orthop Relat Res.* 2016;474:1247–1254.

(6) **D.** Most patients prefer to be active participants in the medical decision-making process. Patient involvement in decision-making can increase satisfaction with clinical care.[28,29] There is no evidence that involving patients in this process negatively affects quality of care.

References

Huang J, Chagpar A. Active participation in decision-making in contralateral prophylactic mastectomy for patients with breast cancer. *J Surg Res.* 2019;242:129–135.

Babac A, von Friedrichs V, Litzkendorf S, Zeidler J, Damm K, Graf von der Schulenburg JM. Integrating patient perspectives in medical decision-making: a qualitative interview study examining potentials within the rare disease information exchange process in practice. *BMC Med Inform Decis Mak.* 2019;19:188.

(7) **D.** Patients with cognitive dysfunction, unreliability, or lacking a social support system may not be able to appropriately care for a nerve catheter or identify signs of complications. Appropriate home care assumes that an anesthesiologist is available via telephone to address any concerns or complications that may arise with an ambulatory nerve catheter. Anesthesiologists should communicate to the patient the expected analgesic effect of the nerve block and catheter to appropriately set expectations regarding pain control.

References

Greengrass RA, Nielsen KC. Management of peripheral nerve block catheters at home. *Int Anesthesiol Clin.* 2005;43:79–87.

Ilfeld BM, Enneking FK. Continuous peripheral nerve blocks at home: a review. *Anesth Analg.* 2005;100:1822–1833.

(8) **C.** Overall pain management strategy, signs of local anesthetic toxicity, and contact information should all be part of patient education regarding ambulatory nerve catheter use. A patient should not be instructed to reinsert a catheter. Instead, the patient should be evaluated for catheter replacement in the event of potential catheter failure.

References

Greengrass RA, Nielsen KC. Management of peripheral nerve block catheters at home. *Int Anesthesiol Clin.* 2005;43:79–87.

Ilfeld BM, Enneking FK. Continuous peripheral nerve blocks at home: a review. *Anesth Analg.* 2005;100:1822–1833.

Swenson JD, Cheng GS, Axelrod DA, Davis JJ. Ambulatory anesthesia and regional catheters: when and how. *Anesthesiol Clin.* 2010;28:267–280.

23.

SHOULDER ARTHROPLASTY ANALGESIC STRATEGIES

Olga "Kiki" Nin and Taras Grosh

STEM CASE AND KEY QUESTIONS

A 25-year-old man is admitted by the trauma service after a backcountry skiing injury. The patient undergoes a magnetic resonance imaging scan of his shoulder, which reveals multiple rotator cuff tears and a small fracture in the humeral head. His past medical history is significant for previous opioid use disorder; he reports his last dose of Suboxone (8 mg of buprenorphine/2 mg of naloxone) was 24 hours ago. He is otherwise healthy and actively attempting to taper his Suboxone. The patient is scheduled to go to the operating room the next day for shoulder arthroplasty. His family is concerned about the patient's history of opioid use disorder.

The patient's sister, a fourth-year medical student working with an orthopedic surgeon at her community hospital, is curious about the methods of anesthetizing the shoulder. More specifically, she wants to learn about the differences between local infiltration compared to continuous interscalene blocks (ISBs) and nerve blocks using liposomal bupivacaine.

Because the patient is at a level 1 trauma center hospital with a robust regional anesthesia and acute pain service, you decide to perform a continuous block.

The patient's family researched his condition and learned that there are different types of shoulder arthroplasties, including anatomical versus reverse shoulder arthroplasty. They want to know what type of shoulder replacement he will have and how it will impact his pain.

The patient undergoes a hemiarthroplasty under general anesthesia, with a superior trunk peripheral nerve catheter for continuous postoperative analgesia. The patient's sister is impressed with how her brother's care is managed. As part of her Quality Initiative, she would like to be an advocate for enhanced recovery after surgery (ERAS) protocols at her community hospital.

KEY QUESTIONS

(1) WHICH NERVES INNERVATE THE SHOULDER? WHICH NERVES NEED TO BE ANESTHETIZED FOR SHOULDER ARTHROPLASTY FOR PATIENT COMFORT?

The nerve roots of the brachial plexus combine to form trunks (superior [C5, C6], middle [C7], and inferior [C8, T1]) that pass between the anterior and middle scalene muscles. The innervation to the glenohumeral joint is complicated and overlapping: the axillary, suprascapular, supraclavicular, and lateral pectoral nerves are chiefly responsible for sensation in the joint. The skin over the medial parts of the shoulder receives nerves from the cervical plexus.

(2) WHAT DISTRIBUTION DOES THE INTERSCALENE BLOCK (ISB) TARGET? WHAT ARE THE RISKS AND SIDE EFFECTS OF AN ISB?

An ISB targets the superior trunk (derived from the nerve roots of C5, C6), and often the middle trunk (nerve root of C7), between the anterior and middle scalene muscles. Side effects include ipsilateral phrenic nerve blockade resulting in hemidiaphragmatic paralysis, Horner's syndrome from blockade of the stellate ganglion, and hoarseness from recurrent laryngeal nerve block. More devastating complications include epidural or subarachnoid injection, vertebral artery injury, carotid injury, or pneumothorax.

(3) HOW DOES THE EFFICACY OF LOCAL ANESTHETIC INFILTRATION IN THE SURGICAL FIELD COMPARE TO A PERIPHERAL NERVE BLOCK?

Compared to a peripheral nerve block, local anesthetic infiltration on the surgical field by the surgical team requires high local anesthetic volumes, provides about 4–12 hours of analgesia, and is unable to be prolonged with a continuous infusion. The goal is in situ diffusion of local anesthetics blocking the nociceptive nerve message at the nerve endings, thereby avoiding paresthesia or muscle weakness of the surgical limb. Some studies list this modality as comparable to ISB in analgesia.[6] Local infiltration is an option in facilities where anesthesiologists are unfamiliar with regional anesthesia, when patients cannot tolerate phrenic nerve palsy and concomitant hemidiaphragmatic paralysis, or when a patient refuses a regional technique. Providers must carefully monitor the total local anesthetic dose because local infiltration of an anesthetic is frequently a high-volume intervention.

(4) WHAT ARE THE DIFFERENT TYPES OF SHOULDER ARTHROPLASTIES? ARE THERE DIFFERENCES IN PAIN OR MOBILITY?

There are three main categories of shoulder replacement: hemiarthroplasty (humerus replacement only), anatomic total shoulder replacement (humerus and glenoid replacement), and reverse shoulder arthroplasty (anatomy is reversed). Hemiarthroplasty procedures are usually the most painful due to the subscapularis being cut and the repair being metal against bone. Anatomic total shoulder arthroplasty is less painful than hemiarthroplasty, but it still has repairing of the subscapularis. This surgical approach is the one that provides the best motion. Reverse shoulder arthroplasty has the least amount of pain postoperatively if the subscapularis is not repaired, but has limited internal rotation compared to the other approaches.

(5) ASIDE FROM REGIONAL ANESTHESIA, WHAT ARE THE PHARMACOLOGIC OPTIONS FOR POSTOPERATIVE PAIN CONTROL AFTER TOTAL SHOULDER ARTHROPLASTY?

The goal of a multimodal pain protocol is to improve postoperative analgesia and decrease opioid use and its side effects, while facilitating discharge and improving patient satisfaction. Multimodal pain medications include acetaminophen, nonsteroidal anti-inflammatory drugs (NSAIDs), gabapentin, ketamine, alpha-2 agonists (e.g., dexmedetomidine and clonidine) and/or systemic local anesthetic infusions (e.g., lidocaine infusion).

DISCUSSION

Postoperative pain control after shoulder arthroplasty is best accomplished with multimodal analgesia. A combination of an NSAID, acetaminophen, a gabapentinoid, an N-methyl-D-aspartate (NMDA) antagonist, an opioid, and a local anesthetic has consistently proved to be superior to a single modality.[1] How the local anesthetic is applied (local infiltration versus peripheral nerve block) depends on the facility, patient comorbidities, and user experience.

Cutaneous, bony, and muscular innervation of the shoulder is derived from the brachial plexus, which itself is formed by the ventral rami of the lower cervical and upper thoracic nerve roots. The nerve roots emerge from the neck adjacent to the transverse processes of the cervical vertebrae and posterior to the vertebral artery. The nerve roots of the brachial plexus combine to form trunks (superior [C5, C6], middle [C7], and inferior [C8, T1]) that pass between the anterior and middle scalene muscles. The innervation to the glenohumeral joint is complicated and overlapping: the axillary, suprascapular, supraclavicular, and lateral pectoral nerves are chiefly responsible for sensation in the joint. The skin over the medial parts of the shoulder receives nerves from the cervical plexus. Table 23.1 lists the nerves involved in innervating the shoulder joint.

Traditionally known as the ISB, placing local anesthetic into the brachial plexus sheath between the anterior and middle scalene muscles results in successful blockade of the superior (C5, C6) and, often, middle (C7) trunks. Anatomic variations exist, such as a C6 split (Figure 23.1); therefore, careful understanding of the sonoanatomy is crucial. For more complete analgesia, injecting local anesthetic posterior to the sternocleidomastoid along the superficial cervical plexus (C3, C4) results in analgesia over the clavicle (the cape of the shoulder) and the first two anterior intercostal spaces.

Practitioners should be aware that blockade of the ipsilateral phrenic nerve is common. The phrenic nerve receives a branch from the C5 nerve root (Figure 23.1) and travels along the anterior scalene muscle. Blocking the brachial plexus more proximally at the level of the C5 nerve root will always result in ipsilateral phrenic blockade, especially with high-volume injections (> 10 mL) of local anesthetic. Phrenic block is associated with an approximately 20%–30% reduction in forced expiratory volume in 1 second and forced vital capacity (and possibly greater reductions in obese patients) and may not be tolerated by patients with limited pulmonary reserve.[2] In patients with oxygen-dependent chronic obstructive pulmonary disease, morbid obesity with obstructive sleep apnea, and contralateral hemidiaphragmatic paralysis, the practitioner should consider a suprascapular nerve block. Additional common side effects include Horner's syndrome from blockade of the stellate ganglion and hoarseness from recurrent laryngeal nerve block; while short-lived, these side effects can provoke anxiety and should be discussed with patients prior to blockade. More devastating complications include epidural or subarachnoid injection, vertebral artery injury, carotid injury, or pneumothorax.

In patients unable to tolerate ipsilateral phrenic paralysis (poorly controlled chronic obstructive pulmonary disease, contralateral hemidiaphragmatic paralysis), there are alternatives to the traditional interscalene approach to brachial plexus blockade. The suprascapular nerve provides 70% of the sensory input to the glenohumeral joint and innervates the infraspinatus and supraspinatus muscles.[3] Although small randomized controlled trials have shown mixed results regarding its efficacy, a recent meta-analysis found that the two approaches provided similar analgesia. Compared to patients who received the interscalene approach, patients who received suprascapular nerve blocks had similar 24-hour morphine consumption and pain scores with fewer pulmonary complications.[4] The ISB provided superior analgesia compared to the suprascapular nerve block only in the first hour after surgery, allowing for shorter post-anesthesia care unit (PACU) stays. Beyond that, outcomes such as opioid-related side effects, analgesic duration, PACU opioid consumption, and procedural discomfort were not significantly different between the groups.

Alternatively, a more distal approach to the ISB using ultrasound guidance and targeting the superior trunk (distal to the roots) of the brachial plexus using a low volume of local anesthetic can reduce inadvertent spread to the phrenic nerve and provide comparable analgesia to a more proximal ISB.[5] The superior trunk can be seen distal to the convergence

Table 23.1 NERVES RELATED TO THE SHOULDER WITH MUSCLES INNERVATED AND GENERAL FUNCTION

NERVE	ORIGIN	INNERVATION	FUNCTION
Supraclavicular nerve	C3–4	Cutaneous	Sensation over the clavicle
Dorsal scapular nerve	C5	Levator scapula muscle, rhomboid major muscle, rhomboid minor muscle	Elevates and adducts the scapula toward the spinal column
Long thoracic nerve	C5–C7	Serratus anterior muscle	Pulls the scapula forward around the thorax, allowing for anteversion of the arm
Suprascapular nerve	Upper trunk: C5–C6	Supraspinatus muscle, infraspinatus muscle, glenohumeral joint, capsule of shoulder	Supraspinatus m: Abducts humerus 0–10 degrees Infraspinatus m: externally rotates humerus
Subclavian nerve	Upper trunk: C5–C6	Subclavius muscle	Depresses the shoulder
Lateral and medial pectoral nerve	Lateral and medial cords	Pectoralis major muscle, pectoralis minor muscle	Depresses the shoulder, adducts and medially rotates the arm
Upper and lower subscapular nerve	Posterior cord	Subscapularis muscle, teres major muscle	Internally rotates arm
Thoracodorsal nerve	Posterior cord: C6–C8	Levator scapulae muscle, latissimus dorsi muscle	Extends, rotates, and adducts the arm
Medial cutaneous nerves of the arm and forearm	Medial cord	Cutaneous	Sensation to medial arm and forearm
Musculocutaneous	C5–C6	Brachialis muscle, brachioradialis muscle, coracobrachialis muscle, biceps brachii long head	Flexes the shoulder, humeroulnar joint
Axillary	C5–C6	Deltoid, teres minor, cutaneous	Deltoid m: abducts, flexes, and extends the shoulder Teres minor m: laterally rotates the shoulder, stabilizes glenohumeral joint Superior lateral brachial cutaneous nerve: sensation to posterior arm and shoulder; Articular branches: acromioclavicular joint and anterior aspect of glenohumeral joint
Radial	C5–T1	Triceps brachii brachioradialis	Extends the arm and forearm, supinates the forearm, sensation to posterior and posterolateral arm

of the C5 and C6 nerve roots but proximal to the takeoff of the suprascapular nerve (Figure 23.1). Avoiding needle advancement through the middle scalene muscle mitigates the risk of nerve injury to the long thoracic nerve and dorsal scapular. Nevertheless, practitioners must be aware that the transverse cervical artery and dorsal scapular artery cross over and through the brachial plexus at this level. These vessels can be in proximity to the superior trunk. Careful evaluation and identification of pulsatile structures on ultrasound are needed to avoid vascular injury.

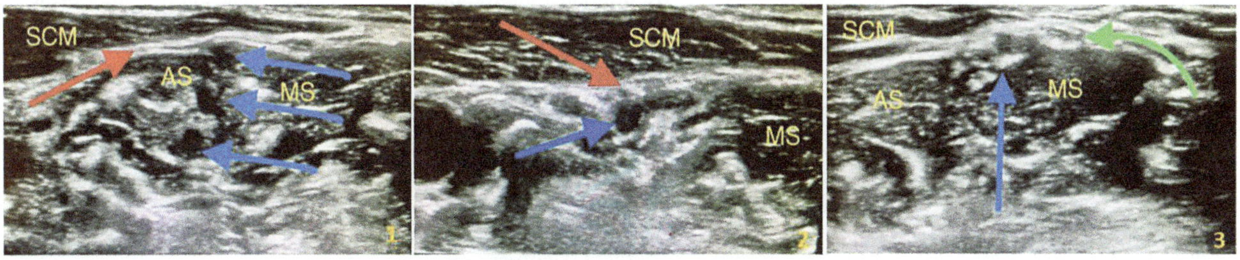

Figure 23.1. The brachial plexus for interscalene block depicting a C5 and split C6 (blue arrows) in the interscalene groove flanked by the anterior scalene (AS) and middle scalene (MS) muscles in image 1. Note the phrenic nerve (red arrow) between the sternocleidomastoid (SCM) and the AS muscles. Ultrasound image 2 is at the level of C5 nerve root (blue arrow) with the phrenic nerve (red arrow) at the 12 o'clock position. Image 3: The superior trunk (blue arrow) with the suprascapular nerve (green arrow) above the middle scalene (MS). The phrenic nerve is not visible.
Image obtained from Taras Grosh, MD, personal neck anatomy.

In facilities where peripheral nerve blocks were not performed, surgical infiltration with local anesthetic was found to have comparable results to ISB for postoperative pain control and opioid consumption in the first 48 hours, as well as after 1 month.[6] Opioids have an important role in managing acute postoperative pain, especially as part of a multimodal protocol. Scheduled oral opioid and as-needed intravenous (IV) breakthrough dosing can be sufficient for opioid-naïve patients. In the small number of patients who cannot receive a nerve block or for whom surgical infiltration is insufficient, patient-controlled analgesia with a short-acting opioid (e.g., hydromorphone/morphine) for 24 hours is a reasonable alternative, during which time continuous pulse oximetry, and possibly capnography, should be available to detect apnea. Nevertheless, sole opioid use for postoperative analgesia is not as effective as a multimodal approach to treat pain.[7] Even low doses of opioids predispose patients to more frequent complications than NSAIDs, namely constipation, nausea, vomiting, lethargy, somnolence, and hyperalgesia.

Patients with opioid use disorder or on an opioid-deterrent therapy such as Suboxone or methadone should be encouraged to receive a continuous perineural infusion of local anesthetic.

MODALITIES OF REGIONAL ANESTHESIA

Total shoulder arthroplasty is a painful surgery that requires a carefully thought-out multimodal pain regimen. For shoulder arthroplasties, a continuous catheter-based infusion of local anesthetic in the interscalene groove provides continuous analgesia until the catheter is removed. An overview of modalities is shown in Table 23.2.

SURGICAL INFILTRATION

Local infiltration by the surgeon has become an increasingly popular technique for analgesia after shoulder arthroplasty. Ultimately, the goal is in situ diffusion of local anesthetics blocking the nociceptive nerve message at the nerve endings, thereby avoiding paresthesia or muscle weakness of the surgical limb. Some studies list this modality as comparable to ISB in analgesia.[6] Local infiltration is an option in facilities where anesthesiologists are unfamiliar with regional anesthesia, when patients cannot tolerate phrenic nerve palsy and concomitant hemidiaphragmatic paralysis, or when a patient refuses a regional technique. Providers must carefully monitor the total local anesthetic dose because local infiltration of an anesthetic is frequently a high-volume intervention. Additionally, surgeons can place a catheter into the glenohumeral joint and administer a constant infusion of local anesthetic after surgery to provide continuous analgesia. The downside of intra-articular injections of local anesthetics is postoperative chondrolysis, a condition in which patients present with a stiff, painful shoulder and a decreased range of motion.[8]

Table 23.2 MODALITIES OF REGIONAL ANALGESIA

ACTIONS/ CHARACTERISTICS	LOCAL INFILTRATION	INTERSCALENE CATHETER	LIPOSOMAL BUPIVACAINE
Placed by	Surgeon	Anesthesiologist	Surgeon/anesthesiologist
Location	Intracapsular, pericapsular, intramuscular	At upper and middle trunk of the brachial plexus	Incisional, intracapsular pericapsular, interscalene nerve block
Volume of local anesthetic injected	~110 mL (0.2%)	~20 mL initial dose (0.2%–0.5%) and 6 mL/hour for 48 to 72 hours (0.1%–0.2%)	266 mg (20-mL vial)
Duration of analgesia	4 to 12 hours	Continuous until catheter removed or migrated	12 to 36 hours
Adjuncts required	Yes	No	Yes
Injectate (typical)	Ropivacaine/ bupivacaine ± epinephrine, nonsteroidal anti-inflammatory drugs, dexamethasone, epinephrine, clonidine	Ropivacaine/ bupivacaine ± dexamethasone	Liposomal bupivacaine ± plain bupivacaine
Complications	Failure to provide analgesia Nerve injury Infection Local anesthetic toxicity	Failure to provide analgesia Nerve injury Infection Local anesthetic toxicity Phrenic nerve palsy Horner's syndrome Dorsal scapular and long thoracic nerve injury	Failure to provide analgesia Nerve injury Infection Local anesthetic toxicity
Challenges	Experienced surgeon needed for successful block	Experience with regional anesthesia Follow-up service	Experience with regional anesthesia

CONTINUOUS ISB

Use of an interscalene catheter is the preferred method of analgesia for shoulder arthroplasty. By providing a catheter through which local anesthetic can be continuously infused and additional doses of local anesthetics (at varying concentrations) can be delivered, the density and spread of the nerve block can be altered. Unfortunately, at concentrations greater than 0.2% ropivacaine or bupivacaine, patients may experience altered motor function in addition to the desired sensory block. ISB catheters are preferred in patients for whom opioids should be avoided or are ineffective, such as patients with opioid use disorder, those on an opioid-deterrent therapy (e.g., Suboxone), those refusing opioids, or those who have an opioid intolerance. ISB catheter management can be challenging for multiple reasons, including:

1. They can dislodge or migrate.
2. They are a nidus for infection.
3. Placement can be time-consuming
4. A follow-up support service is needed.

Nevertheless, ISB catheters continue to be a popular option given the significant benefits of the sensory block.

LIPOSOMAL BUPIVACAINE

Liposomal bupivacaine, trademarked as Exparel by Pacira Pharmaceuticals, comprises free bupivacaine molecules encapsulated in a liposome. Over 72 hours, the bupivacaine is released from the liposome and acts as free bupivacaine on surrounding tissue and nerves. In multiple randomized control trials and in vivo studies, the duration of analgesia has not been consistent with the manufacturer's claims. The duration of action has varied from 12 to 36 hours; analgesia, side effects, and opioid-sparing claims have not differed significantly or have been demonstrated to be worse compared to nonliposomal local anesthetics.[9,10] Compared to placebo, liposomal bupivacaine has been shown to reduce opioid consumption and pain scores.[11] Compared to an ISB catheter, analgesia in the group that received liposomal bupivacaine was inferior, and opioid consumption was higher.[12]

Table 23.3 INDICATIONS FOR VARIOUS SURGERIES[13]

TYPE OF SURGERY	INDICATIONS
Total shoulder arthroplasty	Primary osteoarthritis Inflammatory arthroplasties Post-traumatic osteoarthritis Osteonecrosis with an affected glenoid
Hemiarthroplasty	Proximal fracture of the humerus Cuff-tear arthroplasty Inflammatory arthroplasty with massive cuff tear or insufficient glenoid bone stock Osteonecrosis with a preserved glenoid
Resurfacing hemiarthroplasty	Healthy intact glenoid No fractures Healthy humeral bone
Reverse total shoulder	Complete rotator cuff tear (not repairable) with or without arthritis. Previous shoulder replacement. Proximal humerus fracture or non-unions Reimplantation for deep periprosthetic infection Reconstruction after tumor resection

TYPES OF SHOULDER ARTHROPLASTIES

Total shoulder arthroplasty surgery is needed in patients who have severe osteoarthritis, rheumatoid arthritis ("inflammatory arthritis"), rotator cuff tear arthropathy, post-traumatic arthritis, severe fractures, avascular necrosis, or failed previous shoulder replacement surgery. The surgeon will determine the type of total shoulder arthroplasty that will relieve pain and improve function. There are three main categories of shoulder replacement (Table 23.3): hemiarthroplasty (humerus replacement only); anatomic total shoulder replacement (humerus and glenoid replacement); and reverse shoulder arthroplasty (anatomy is reversed). The type of shoulder arthroplasty varies depending on patient anatomy and diagnosis, which includes humeral-sided hemiarthroplasty alone, resurfacing, or replacement, and/or with a stemless, short stem, or standard stem. Anatomic shoulder replacements indicated for arthritis and a good rotator cuff include a glenoid replacement with a stemless, short stem, or standard stem replacement on the humerus side. Finally, the most common replacement in 2019 was reverse shoulder arthroplasty, which is indicated for a wide variety of pathologies and consists of a metal ball connected to the native glenoid and a cup connected to the humerus with a short or standard stem.

Hemiarthroplasties are used sparingly because long-term pain relief has been shown to be less predictable compared to an anatomic shoulder replacement. However, they are still used to treat severe fractures in young patients, avascular necrosis without glenoid arthritis, and osteoarthritis and cuff tear arthropathy in the very young. The trend is to use stemless or short-stem implants without cement (Figure 23.2). Hemiarthroplasties are also used in salvage situations in which no viable glenoid can be reconstructed.

Resurfacing hemiarthroplasty replaces the joint surface of the humeral head with a cap prosthesis without a stem. This is usually done if the glenoid has an intact cartilage surface and no fractures and there is a desire to preserve humeral bone. This procedure is frequently done in young, active patients.

An anatomic total shoulder replacement uses a metal ball attached to a stem and a plastic glenoid socket (Figure 23.2B). Glenoid sockets can be completely polyethylene and are mostly cemented. There are also metal composite engrossed options, as well as metal-backed engrossed glenoid socket options. Patients with bone-on-bone osteoarthritis, mild glenoid erosion, and an intact rotator cuff are good candidates for this type of surgical implant. Patients with osteoarthritis,

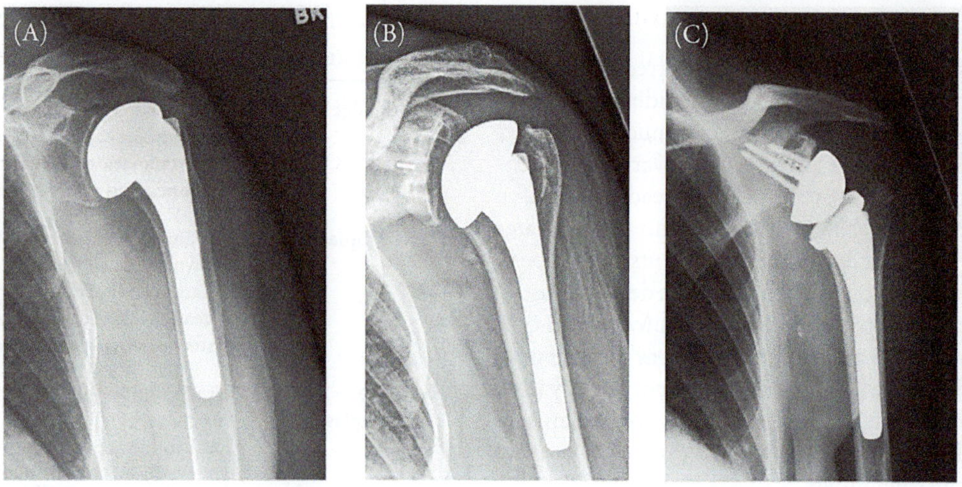

Figure 23.2 (A) A standard-stem hemiarthroplasty; (B) standard-stem anatomic total shoulder arthroplasty; (C) standard reverse total shoulder arthroplasty. Images courtesy of Thomas W. Wright, MD.

inflammatory disease, and glenoid disease benefit more from total shoulder replacement than hemiarthroplasty.

In reverse total shoulder arthroplasty, the socket and metal ball are switched. The metal ball is attached to the native glenoid bone, and the plastic socket is attached to the upper humerus with a standard or short stem (Figure 23.2C). As a highly versatile procedure, reverse shoulder arthroplasty has many indications, including cuff tear arthropathy, failed cuff syndrome (irreparable rotator cuff tear), fractures, osteoarthritis in the elderly, inflammatory arthritis, and revision shoulder arthroplasty. It is also indicated for arthroplasty in patients with severe glenoid erosion, patients older than 80 years, patients with tumors, patients with neuromuscular conditions, and patients requiring a weight-bearing shoulder. Reverse total shoulder arthroplasty provides a fixed fulcrum for an intact deltoid to raise the arm in the absence of a rotator cuff. The procedure leaves open the option for surgery if the rotator cuff is torn or malfunctioning by reversing the ball and socket and using the deltoid muscle for shoulder mobility. An anatomical total shoulder requires that the muscles and tendons (rotator cuff) around the shoulder joint be intact.

IMPLICATIONS FOR POSTOPERATIVE PAIN MANAGEMENT

Pain after shoulder arthroplasty can vary depending on the patient and surgical technique. Patients on chronic opioid management are a challenge. However, for most patients, significant pain abates in 48–72 hours. Not all shoulder arthroplasty procedures are the same regarding pain. Patients who have a major motor tendon unit violated and repaired (subscapularis) will experience more pain. When performing a reverse shoulder arthroplasty, some surgeons will opt not to repair the subscapularis, which leads to significantly less pain because no major motor tendon unit has been repaired or under tension.

MULTIMODAL ANALGESIA IN SHOULDER ARTHROPLASTY

Most anesthetic protocols for total shoulder arthroplasty are designed to deliver quality care to patients by improving pain control, reducing length of stay, and decreasing postoperative complications and readmission rates. Postoperative pain control protocols usually include a combination of regional anesthesia and multimodal analgesia.[14] The goal of a multimodal pain protocol is to improve postoperative analgesia and decrease opioid use and its side effects, while facilitating discharge and improving patient satisfaction. Patients should achieve a tolerable and functional pain score before discharge so that they can continue daily activities at home.

All patients should have a focused preoperative examination, including pain history, and a pain control plan should be discussed before surgery. Preoperative patient education and preparation are essential for a good outcome.[15] Preoperative patient preparation should include discussion of any current pain medication regimen and its continuation to treat preexisting pain, premedication before surgery, and a discussion with the patient of a multimodal pain plan, as well as family education of a surgical pain management plan. The American Society of Anesthesiologists Task Force provides clinical guidelines for the use of acetaminophen, NSAIDs, gabapentin, and ketamine as part of multimodal analgesia.[1,15,16] Table 23.4 presents an overview of doses and properties of various multimodal analgesics.

ACETAMINOPHEN

Acetaminophen is a commonly used non-opioid analgesic medication. It has a well-established efficacy profile, minimal adverse effects, and a low potential to cause drug–drug interaction.[17] Its formulations include oral, rectal, and, since 2010, IV routes. Since 2010, the price of IV acetaminophen has increased more than 400-fold ($10.36–$40.39). The IV formulation has advantages when a patient is strictly NPO,

Table 23.4 **MULTIMODAL ANALGESIA MEDICATIONS**

NAME	DOSE	INDICATIONS AND PROPERTIES
Acetaminophen	Recommended dosage: 1000 mg every 6 hours or 650 mg every 4 hours Maximum single dose: 1000 mg Maximum daily dose: 4000 mg, 3000 mg in elderly 2000 mg with chronic alcohol use	Use with caution in patients with liver disease No antiplatelet properties like NSAIDs. Oral acetaminophen when possible should be used 45–60 min before surgery for gastric absorption (less expensive than IV acetaminophen)
NSAIDs	Propionic acid: 400 to 800 mg of ibuprofen every 4 to 8 hours (maximum dose: 2400 mg) 220 mg of naproxen every 8 hours (maximum dose: 660 mg) Coxib: 200 mg of celecoxib every 12 hours (maximum dose: 400 mg)	Concerns regarding cardiovascular events in high-risk patients, bleeding, renal dysfunction, gastric ulceration, and bone healing
Gabapentinoid	Pregabalin: 75 mg daily, up to 600 mg daily Gabapentin: 300 mg three times a day, up to 3600 mg daily	Pregabalin: higher bioavailability but higher cost Gabapentinoids: anxiolytics, reduce perioperative delirium, and improve sleep Careful in the elderly and with sedation
Ketamine	IV bolus: 0.5 mg/kg followed by infusion: 0.15 to 0.25 mg/kg/hour	Side effects: sympathomimetic, hallucinations, salivation, and nystagmus

NSAIDs = nonsteroidal anti-inflammatory drugs; IV = intravenous

when actively vomiting, or when unable to tolerate oral intake (developmental delay). It provides a faster onset of analgesia relative to the other modes of administration. If the oral route is available, oral acetaminophen should be given 45–60 minutes prior to surgery to allow adequate time for gastric absorption. Acetaminophen should be given on a schedule, instead of as needed, when used as part of a multimodal plan. Precautions should be taken in patients with preexisting severe liver dysfunction.

GABAPENTINOIDS

The gabapentinoids, gabapentin and pregabalin, bind to voltage-gated calcium channels and promote antinociceptive actions by inhibiting the release of excitatory neurotransmitters. Initially used to treat chronic neuropathic pain, they may also work to prevent and reduce acute pain and opioid consumption and to reduce the incidence of chronic post-surgical pain.[18]

Eskander and colleagues showed that 300 mg of pregabalin at 12 hours and 1 hour preoperatively decreased pain scores (Visual Analog Scale scores) at 1 to 8 hours after surgery. Their study demonstrated lower opioid consumption, higher satisfaction scores, and no statistically significant increase in somnolence or dizziness.[19] Bang et al. showed that 300 mg of pregabalin 2 hours before surgery decreased pain scores (Visual Analog Scale) 2 to 12 hours post-surgery but did not decrease opioid use 24 hours after surgery.[20] Adam et al. showed that 100 mg of gabapentin 2 hours before surgery did not significantly lower pain scores, oral opioid consumption, or first analgesic request compared to the control group.[21] Common side effects of these medications are dizziness, somnolence, and drowsiness, which can be undesirable in the elderly and have a cumulative effect with narcotics.[20] The first dose should be given at night due to the sedating effects. Other common side effects of gabapentin include peripheral extremity swelling and weight gain. Dose reductions should be considered for the elderly and in patients with chronic kidney disease.

NSAIDS

NSAIDs interrupt the cyclooxygenase (COX) pathway and its subsequent potent inflammatory end products. Nonsteroidal medications can reduce perioperative pain and opioid use.[22] Toivonen et al. reported lower postoperative pain scores from 30 to 180 minutes after surgery when using a COX-2 inhibitor and longer time lapses to the first analgesic. Patients on the COX 2 inhibitor consumed fewer narcotics, were discharged home faster, and continued to have lower pain scores up to 7 days post-surgery.[23] Potential side effects of COX-1 inhibitors are platelet dysfunction, peptic ulcer disease, fluid retention, hypertension, renal impairment, and delayed bone-tendon healing.[24,25] COX-modulated prostaglandins E2 and F2a promote active bone formation. Early studies in rats have found impaired bone healing with indomethacin,[26–28] but subsequent systematic reviews of studies have found significant variability in study design, yielding inconsistent results.[29] COX-2 selective inhibitors showed fewer side effects than the COX-1 inhibitors.[30] Precautions should also be taken with COX-2 inhibitors and high-risk cardiovascular patients.[31]

Combined with NSAIDs, acetaminophen reduces the dose and possibly the need for opioids to treat moderate pain.[32,33] This oral combination is recommended 30 minutes prior to administration of an opioid; frequently, the opioid dose can be reduced.

KETAMINE

Ketamine is a non-barbiturate with amnestic, analgesic, and hypnotic effects. It provides analgesia through the inhibition of NMDA-gated calcium channels. Ketamine can prevent hyperalgesic effects through its mechanism of action.[33] Subanesthetic doses can help treat acute, neuropathic, and chronic pain.[34] Precautions should be taken if patients suffer from coronary artery disease, increased intracranial pressures, or psychiatric conditions. Side effects include hallucinations, nystagmus, and increases in salivation, sympathetic tone, and intracranial pressure.

Other multimodal pain medications to consider in patients with chronic pain or those who have uncontrolled pain are alpha-2 agonists and systemic local anesthetic infusions. Alpha-2 agonists act directly on the alpha-2-adrenoreceptors in the central nervous system and the spinal cord.[35] The two most commonly used medications in this class are dexmedetomidine and clonidine. These agents can reduce opioid consumption, anxiety, postoperative nausea and vomiting, shivering, and the stress response.[36] These medications can cause severe bradycardia and hypotension, and their use for perioperative pain control has not been officially approved. The loading dose for dexmedetomidine is 0.5–1 mcg/kg over 10 minutes, followed by an infusion of 0.2–1.7 mcg/kg/hour. Clonidine can also cause severe hypotension and lead to withdrawal if stopped abruptly. Dosing is usually 0.2 mg orally twice per day.

IV lidocaine infusions have been shown to decrease opioid use, pruritus, postoperative nausea and vomiting, urinary retention, and inflammatory cytokines, as well as modulate NMDA, which can help prevent chronic pain. Contraindications to a lidocaine infusion include an allergy to lidocaine, heart disease (heart block, dysrhythmias, severe heart failure), severe hepatic or renal disease, uncontrolled seizures, or acute porphyria. Some acute pain departments and physicians have developed protocols for lidocaine infusion. These protocols usually involve a bolus of 1–1.5 mg/kg (ideal body weight), followed by an infusion of 1–2 mg/kg/hour (ideal body weight). To improve efficacy, the infusion should be continued for 48 hours at the lowest dose of 1 mg/hg/hour. For safety, the patient should be followed by the hospital's acute pain service, and local anesthetic toxicity guidelines need to be in place.[37]

ERAS FOR SHOULDER ARTHROPLASTY

Establishing an ERAS protocol requires a multidisciplinary team involving surgeons, anesthesiologists, physical therapists, nurses, discharge planners, social workers, and, most importantly, patients and their families. This collaboration will help patient recovery and discharge planning, depending on patient selection. An effective ERAS protocol has four critical phases: preadmission, preoperative, intraoperative, and postoperative.[1] Appropriate patient screening and optimization during the preadmission stage is important for a successful surgery and recovery. Patient and family education is a key component of an ERAS protocol, and needs to start at the surgical clinic appointment. At this appointment, expectations should be clearly discussed. The surgical coordinator and discharge planners need to ensure that all necessary equipment is available to the patient before the day of surgery.

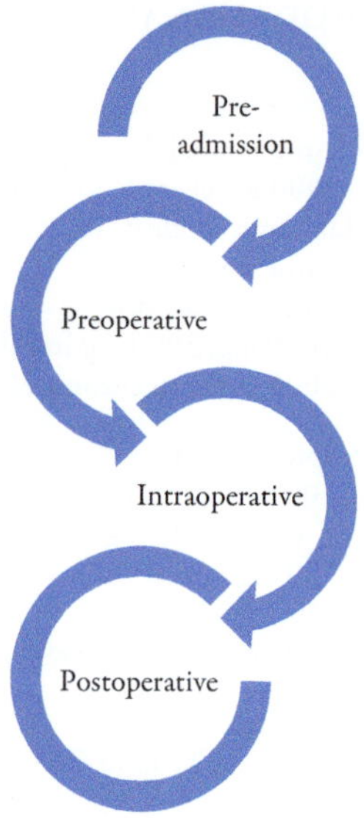

Figure 23.3. Enhanced recovery after surgery protocol phases. Image created by Olga C. Nin, MD.

Physical therapy before and after surgery is a key component of patient recovery. The better the physical condition of the shoulder before surgery, the easier the recovery will be. A physical therapy appointment before the surgery can help explain the exercises the patient will do after surgery, as well as set expectations for recovery. Physical therapists will be able to show the patient range-of-motion exercises, strengthening exercises, and functional training, as well as job- or sport-specific training.

ERAS protocols have helped reduce complications and increase patient satisfaction. Research has shown a reduction of up to 35% in healthcare costs with the implementation of an ERAS protocol.[38] ERAS protocols have been shown to help standardize patient care, reduce medical errors, decrease length of stay, and help increase the number of patients a hospital treats, among other benefits.[39] While multimodal pain control or patient education may differ, a good guideline to follow is shown in Table 23.5.

CONCLUSIONS

- Cutaneous, bony, and muscular innervation of the shoulder is derived from the brachial plexus, which itself is formed by the ventral rami of the lower cervical and upper thoracic nerve roots (superior [C5, C6], middle [C7], and inferior [C8, T1].
- The innervation to the glenohumeral joint is complicated and overlapping: the axillary, suprascapular, supraclavicular, and lateral pectoral nerves are chiefly responsible for

Table 23.5 ENHANCED RECOVERY AFTER SURGERY PROTOCOL GUIDELINES

PREADMISSION	PREOPERATIVE	INTRAOPERATIVE	POSTOPERATIVE
Patient and family education	Pre-medication	Postoperative nausea and vomiting prophylaxis	Education on continuing multimodal pain management
Physical therapy and preconditioning	Multimodal pain control	Multimodal pain control	Physical therapy
Social worker support	Regional nerve block	Fluid management	Functional pain control
Home supplies	Anxiety management	Normothermia	
Medical optimization	Patient expectation setting	Blood conservation	
	Active prewarming		
	Optimize preoperative fasting		

sensation in the joint. The skin over the medial parts of the shoulder receives nerves from the cervical plexus.

- Regional anesthesia modalities include an interscalene block (ISB), whose duration can be extended with a continuous infusion. However, an ISB can result in hemidiaphragmatic paralysis from phrenic nerve blockade.
- Alternatives to ISB include the more distal superior trunk block (lower incidence of phrenic nerve blockade), suprascapular nerve block combined with axillary nerve block, and surgical local anesthetic infiltration.
- The goal of a multimodal pain protocol is to improve postoperative analgesia and decrease opioid use and its side effects, while facilitating discharge and improving patient satisfaction.
- Patients should achieve a tolerable and functional pain score before discharge so that they can continue daily activities at home.
- Establishing an ERAS protocol requires a multidisciplinary team involving surgeons, anesthesiologists, physical therapists, nurses, discharge planners, social workers, and, most importantly, patients and their families.
- ERAS protocols have helped reduce complications and increase patient satisfaction.
- The surgeon will determine the type of total shoulder arthroplasty that will relieve pain and improve function. There are three main categories of shoulder replacement: hemiarthroplasty (humerus replacement only); anatomic total shoulder replacement (humerus and glenoid replacement); and reverse shoulder arthroplasty (anatomy is reversed).

REFERENCES

1. Grosh T, Elkassabany NM. Enhanced recovery after shoulder arthroplasty. *Anesthesiol Clin*. 2018;36:417–430.
2. Caleffi-Pereira M, Pletsch-Assunção R, Cardenas LZ, et al. Unilateral diaphragm paralysis: a dysfunction restricted not just to one hemidiaphragm. *BMC Pulm Med*. 2018;18:126.
3. Burckett-St Laurent D, Chan V, Chin KJ. Refining the ultrasound-guided interscalene brachial plexus block: the superior trunk approach. *Can J Anaesth*. 2014;61:1098–1102.
4. Cros Campoy J, Domingo Bosch O, Pomés J, Lee J, Fox B, Sala-Blanch X. Upper trunk block for shoulder analgesia with potential phrenic nerve sparing: a preliminary anatomical report. *Reg Anesth Pain Med*. 2019. pii:rapm-2019-100404. doi:10.1136/rapm-2019-100404.
5. Kang R, Jeong JS, Chin KJ, et al. Superior trunk block provides noninferior analgesia compared with interscalene brachial plexus block in arthroscopic shoulder surgery. *Anesthesiology*. 2019;131:1316–1326.
6. Sicard J, Klouche S, Conso C, et al. Local infiltration analgesia versus interscalene nerve block for postoperative pain control after shoulder arthroplasty: a prospective, randomized, comparative noninferiority study involving 99 patients. *J Shoulder Elbow Surg*. 2019;28:212–219.
7. Bhatia A, Buvanendran A. Anesthesia and postoperative pain control-multimodal anesthesia protocol. *J Spine Surg*. 2019;5:S160–S165.
8. Anderson SL, Buchko JZ, Taillon MR, Ernst MA. Chondrolysis of the glenohumeral joint after infusion of bupivacaine through an intra-articular pain pump catheter: a report of 18 cases. *Arthroscopy*. 2010;26:451–461.
9. Kolade O, Patel K, Ihejirika R, et al. Efficacy of liposomal bupivacaine in shoulder surgery: a systematic review and meta-analysis. *J Shoulder Elbow Surg*. 2019;28:1824–1834.
10. Namdari S, Nicholson T, Abboud J, Lazarus M, Steinberg D, Williams G. Interscalene block with and without intraoperative local infiltration with liposomal bupivacaine in shoulder arthroplasty: a randomized controlled trial. *J Bone Joint Surg Am*. 2018;100:1373–1378.
11. Patel MA, Gadsden JC, Nedeljkovic SS, et al. Brachial plexus block with liposomal bupivacaine for shoulder surgery improves analgesia and reduces opioid consumption: results from a multicenter, randomized, double-blind, controlled trial. *Pain Med*. 2020;21:387–400.
12. Abildgaard JT, Lonergan KT, Tolan SJ, et al. Liposomal bupivacaine versus indwelling interscalene nerve block for postoperative pain control in shoulder arthroplasty: a prospective randomized controlled trial. *J Shoulder Elbow Surg*. 2017;26:1175–1181.
13. Sanchez-Sotelo J. Total shoulder arthroplasty. *Open Orthop J*. 2011;5:106–114.
14. Niesen AD, Hebl JR. Multimodal clinical pathways, perineural catheters, and ultrasound-guided regional anesthesia: the anesthesiologist's repertoire for the 21st century. *Minn Med*. 2011;94:31–34.
15. American Society of Anesthesiologists Task Force on Acute Pain Management. Practice guidelines for acute pain management in the perioperative setting: an updated report by the American Society of Anesthesiologists Task Force on Acute Pain Management. *Anesthesiology*. 2012;116:248–273.
16. Memtsoudis SG, Poeran J, Zubizarreta N, et al. Association of multimodal pain management strategies with perioperative outcomes and resource utilization: a population-based study. *Anesthesiology*. 2018;128:891–902.
17. Prescott LF. Paracetamol: past, present, and future. *Am J Ther*. 2000;7:143–147.
18. Clarke H, Bonin RP, Orser BA, Englesakis M, Wijeysundera DN, Katz J. The prevention of chronic postsurgical pain using gabapentin and pregabalin: a combined systematic review and meta-analysis. *Anesth Analg*. 2012;115:428–442.
19. Eskandar AM, Ebeid AM. Effect of pregabalin on postoperative pain after shoulder arthroscopy. *Egyptian J Anaesth*. 2013;29:363–367.
20. Bang SR, Yu SK, Kim TH. Can gabapentin help reduce postoperative pain in arthroscopic rotator cuff repair? A prospective, randomized, double-blind study. *Arthroscopy*. 2010;26:S106–S111.
21. Adam F, Ménigaux C, Sessler D, Chauvin M. A single preoperative dose of gabapentin (800 milligrams) does not augment postoperative analgesia in patients given interscalene brachial

plexus blocks for arthroscopic shoulder surgery. *Anesth Analg.* 2006;103:1278–1282.
22. Ong CK, Seymour RA, Lirk P, Merry AF. Combining paracetamol (acetaminophen) with nonsteroidal anti-inflammatory drugs: a qualitative systematic review of analgesic efficacy for acute postoperative pain. *Anesth Analg.* 2010;110:1170–1179.
23. Toivonen J, Pitko VM, Rosenberg PH. Etoricoxib pre-medication combined with intra-operative subacromial block for pain after arthroscopic acromioplasty. *Acta Anaesthesiol Scand.* 2007;51:316–321.
24. Souter AJ, Fredman B, White PF. Controversies in the perioperative use of nonsterodial antiinflammatory drugs. *Anesth Analg.* 1994;79:1178–1190.
25. Virchenko O, Skoglund B, Aspenberg P. Parecoxib impairs early tendon repair but improves later remodeling. *Am J Sports Med.* 2004;32:1743–1747.
26. Dimmen S, Nordsletten L, Madsen JE. Parecoxib and indomethacin delay early fracture healing: a study in rats. *Clin Orthop Relat Res.* 2009;467:1992–1999.
27. Bo J, Sudmann E, Marton PF. Effect of indomethacin on fracture healing in rats. *Acta Orthop Scand.* 1976;47:588–599.
28. Sudmann E, Hagen T. Indomethacin-induced delayed fracture healing. *Arch Orthop Unfallchir.* 1976;85:151–154.
29. Marquez-Lara A, Hutchinson ID, Nuñez F Jr, Smith TL, Miller AN. Nonsteroidal anti-inflammatory drugs and bone-healing: a systematic review of research quality. *JBJS Rev.* 2016;4(3):e4.
30. Romsing J, Møiniche S, Mathiesen O, Dahl JB. Reduction of opioid-related adverse events using opioid-sparing analgesia with COX-2 inhibitors lacks documentation: a systematic review. *Acta Anaesthesiol Scand.* 2005;49:133–142.
31. Nussmeier NA, Whelton AA, Brown MT, et al. Safety and efficacy of the cyclooxygenase-2 inhibitors parecoxib and valdecoxib after non-cardiac surgery. *Anesthesiology.* 2006;104:518–526.
32. Wong I, St John-Green C, Walker SM. Opioid-sparing effects of perioperative paracetamol and nonsteroidal anti-inflammatory drugs (NSAIDs) in children. *Paediatr Anaesth.* 2013;23:475–495.
33. Chou R, Gordon DB, de Leon-Casasola OA, et al. Management of postoperative pain: a clinical practice guideline from the American Pain Society, the American Society of Regional Anesthesia and Pain Medicine, and the American Society of Anesthesiologists' Committee on Regional Anesthesia, Executive Committee, and Administrative Council. *J Pain.* 2016;17:131–157.
34. Schwenk ES, Viscusi ER, Buvanendran A, et al. Consensus guidelines on the use of intravenous ketamine infusions for acute pain management from the American Society of Regional Anesthesia and Pain Medicine, the American Academy of Pain Medicine, and the American Society of Anesthesiologists. *Reg Anesth Pain Med.* 2018;43:456–466.
35. Blaudszun G, Lysakowski C, Elia N, Tramèr MR. Effect of perioperative systemic alpha2 agonists on postoperative morphine consumption and pain intensity: systematic review and meta-analysis of randomized controlled trials. *Anesthesiology.* 2012;116:1312–1322.
36. Ramaswamy S, Wilson J, Colvin L. Non-opioid-based adjuvant analgesia in perioperative care. *Cont Educ Anaesth Crit Care Pain.* 2013;13:152–157.
37. Earls B, Bellil L. Systemic lidocaine: an effective and safe modality for postoperative pain management and early recovery. *APSF Newsletter.* 2018;33:28–30.
38. Thiele RH, Rea KM, Turrentine FE, et al. Standardization of care: impact of an enhanced recovery protocol on length of stay, complications, and direct costs after colorectal surgery. *J Am Coll Surg.* 2015;220:430–443.
39. Nanavati AJ, Prabhakar S. Enhanced recovery after surgery: if you are not implementing it, why not? *Practical Gastroenterol.* 2016;151:46–56.

REVIEW QUESTIONS

(1) A 45-year-old man with a history of diabetes (Hg A1C 5.5) and opioid use disorder undergoes arthroscopic shoulder surgery. He has taken 2 mg/0.5 mg of Suboxone daily over the past year with plans to taper in the coming months. On examination, multiple loose bodies are identified, and the joint is "cleaned up." Concerned with postoperative pain management, the surgeon places a continuous intra-articular catheter infusing 0.2% bupivacaine at 8 mL/hour. The patient has an uneventful immediate postoperative course. Eleven months later, he returns with increasing pain and stiffness in the operative joint. His radiograph demonstrates a reduction in the joint space. He states that he has been compliant with his physical therapy and limits extremes of range of motion as suggested by his therapist. What is the most likely cause of his pathology?

A. Chronic pain and inappropriate postoperative pain management
B. Frozen shoulder related to his diabetes mellitus
C. Re-injury/overuse performing automotive repair
D. Intra-articular chondrolysis

(2) A patient with opioid use disorder and on Suboxone is scheduled for a shoulder arthroscopy. The interview reveals that he has idiopathic vocal cord paralysis on the side of the surgery. What analgesic modality should be used?

A. Multimodal analgesia and continuous interscalene infusion catheter with 0.2% bupivacaine
B. Multimodal analgesia and continuous intra-articular infusion catheter with 0.2% bupivacaine
C. Patient-controlled analgesia
D. Increase the patient's Suboxone dose

3. In the post-anesthesia care unit, a patient who has undergone shoulder arthroplasty with an interscalene block has a dry, droopy, irritated eye, as well as sweating on the opposite side of the face. What is the likely cause and how could this be avoided?

A. Horner's syndrome; placement of the interscalene catheter proximal to the C5 nerve root
B. Improper eye protection; use paper tape and goggles intraoperatively.
C. Horner's syndrome; place an upper trunk catheter with a low-volume continuous infusion of local anesthetic.
D. Corneal abrasion; perform an interscalene block with 0.5% bupivacaine and perform the surgery with the patient awake.

(4) An 82-year-old morbidly obese man has uncontrolled right shoulder pain and decreased mobility. The orthopedic surgeon evaluated him and found that he has significant osteoarthritis of the shoulder and a rotator cuff tear. His medical history includes a body mass index of 60, obstructive sleep apnea on continuous positive airway pressure, poorly controlled chronic obstructive pulmonary disease (COPD) on a 2-L nasal cannula, left hemidiaphragmatic paralysis from a car accident, chronic kidney disease with a creatinine of 2.2, and diabetes mellitus (Hg A1C 6.5). As the orthopedic surgeon, you need to advise the patient on which

surgery he needs. What is your recommendation given his pathology?

A. Hemiarthroplasty
B. Resurfacing hemiarthroplasty
C. Anatomical total shoulder replacement
D. Reverse total shoulder arthroplasty

(5) An 82-year-old morbidly obese male with obstructive sleep apnea, oxygen-dependent COPD, diabetes mellitus, chronic kidney disease, and contralateral hemidiaphragmatic paralysis undergoes a total shoulder arthroplasty. What type of regional pain block would this patient benefit from?

A. Continuous interscalene block
B. Single-shot distal superior trunk block
C. Suprascapular nerve block
D. Local infiltration by the surgeon

(6) An 82-year-old morbidly obese male with obstructive sleep apnea, oxygen-dependent COPD, diabetes mellitus, and chronic kidney disease undergoes a total shoulder arthroplasty. What multimodal pain control medications would this patient benefit from?

A. 1000 mg of acetaminophen every 6 hours, 200 mg of Celebrex every 12 hours, 300 mg of gabapentin three times a day, lidocaine infusion
B. 1000 mg of acetaminophen every 8 hours, 100 mg of Celebrex every 12 hours, 100 mg of gabapentin every night at bedtime, ketamine
C. 1000 mg of acetaminophen every 8 hours, 200 mg of Celebrex every 12 hours, 300 mg of gabapentin three times a day, lidocaine infusion
D. 1000 mg of acetaminophen every 6 hours, 100 mg of Celebrex every 12 hours, 100 mg of gabapentin every night at bedtime, ketamine

ANSWERS

(1) **D.** This condition is likely related to intra-articular chondrolysis given the onset, symptoms, and radiographic findings. Patients may benefit transiently from repeat arthroscopy but if the pathology is advanced, an arthroplasty is the next step. Chronic pain exacerbation is unlikely given the presentation and findings. Frozen shoulder is a possibility, but the patient had an acceptable A1C.

Reference

Anderson SL, Buchko JZ, Taillon MR, Ernst MA. Chondrolysis of the glenohumeral joint after infusion of bupivacaine through an intra-articular pain pump catheter: a report of 18 cases. *Arthroscopy*. 2010;26:451–461.

(2) **A.** A continuous interscalene catheter is the best option for this patient. For shoulder arthroscopy, anesthetizing the nerves supplying the shoulder with a concentrated local anesthetic such as 0.2% bupivacaine will provide analgesia to the shoulder joint. The patient can continue on Suboxone, thereby avoiding the complicated process of tapering. An intra-articular catheter is not recommended due to risks of chondrolysis. Patient-controlled anesthesia alone would likely be insufficient given his opioid use disorder as well as his perioperative continuation of Suboxone.

(3) **C.** A continuous perineural catheter placed near the upper trunk, with a low volume of local anesthetic, would likely avoid a recurrence of Horner's and provide excellent analgesia. Horner's syndrome is related to anesthetizing the ipsilateral sympathetic trunk, resulting in transient ptosis, myosis, and anhydrosis. Horner's typically occurs with higher volumes of local anesthetic which spreads around the anterior scalene muscle behind the carotid artery and internal jugular vein toward the longus colli muscle. This results in blockade of the cervical ganglion (Horner syndrome) and phrenic nerve, which are located in this area. Providers should use caution when blocking at the nerve root level, as subarachnoid injection into the neural foramen is possible.

Reference

Stasiowski M, Zuber M, Marciniak R, et al. Risk factors for the development of Horner's syndrome following interscalene brachial plexus block using ropivacaine for shoulder arthroscopy: a randomised trial. *Anaesthesiol Intensive Ther.* 2018;50(3):215–220.

(4) **D.** The patient would benefit from a reverse total shoulder arthroplasty given his age, significant arthritis, and rotator cuff tear. He is older than 80, meaning that a reverse total shoulder offers a better outcome for shoulder mobility and pain. Hemiarthroplasties and resurfacing hemiarthroplasties are performed most often on young patients. An anatomical total shoulder requires an intact rotator cuff.

Reference

Sanchez-Sotelo J. Total shoulder arthroplasty. *Open Orthop J.* 2011;5:106–114.

(5) **C.** The patient would benefit from a suprascapular nerve block given the high risk of phrenic nerve block. He has contralateral hemidiaphragmatic paralysis, severe COPD, and is morbidly obese, which puts him at high risk of respiratory insufficiency if his phrenic nerve were to be inadvertently anesthetized on the right side. Multimodal analgesia and a nerve block will help decrease opioid consumption.

References

Caleffi-Pereira M, Pletsch-Assunção R, Cardenas LZ, et al. Unilateral diaphragm paralysis: a dysfunction restricted not just to one hemidiaphragm. *BMC Pulm Med.* 2018;18:126.
Burckett-St Laurent D, Chan V, Chin KJ. Refining the ultrasound-guided interscalene brachial plexus block: the superior trunk approach. *Can J Anaesth.* 2014;61:1098–1102.
Cros Campoy J, Domingo Bosch O, Pomés J, Lee J, Fox B, Sala-Blanch X. Upper trunk block for shoulder analgesia with potential phrenic nerve sparing: a preliminary anatomical report. *Reg Anesth Pain Med.* 2019. pii: rapm-2019-100404. doi:10.1136/rapm-2019-100404.
Kang R, Jeong JS, Chin KJ, et al. Superior trunk block provides noninferior analgesia compared with interscalene brachial plexus block in arthroscopic shoulder surgery. *Anesthesiology.* 2019;131:1316–1326.

(6) **B.** Due to patient age and chronic kidney disease, the doses of acetaminophen and NSAID should be adjusted. Gabapentin should be given at night given the risk of drowsiness, and ketamine would be a great adjunct. Given this patient's age, it is

advisable to decrease the acetaminophen dose to 3 g per 24 hours. His NSAID dose should be reduced because of his history of chronic kidney disease with an elevated creatinine value. Because gabapentin can cause drowsiness and dizziness, a low night dose should be the starting dose. Ketamine would be a great adjunct to this patient's multimodal plan given the risk of a continuous interscalene block.

References

American Society of Anesthesiologists Task Force on Acute Pain Management. Practice guidelines for acute pain management in the perioperative setting: an updated report by the American Society of Anesthesiologists Task Force on Acute Pain Management. *Anesthesiology*. 2012;116:248–273.

Bang SR, Yu SK, Kim TH. Can gabapentin help reduce postoperative pain in arthroscopic rotator cuff repair? A prospective, randomized, double-blind study. *Arthroscopy*. 2010;26:S106–S111.

Memtsoudis SG, Poeran J, Zubizarreta N, et al. Association of multimodal pain management strategies with perioperative outcomes and resource utilization: a population-based study. *Anesthesiology*. 2018;128:891–902.

Souter AJ, Fredman B, White PF. Controversies in the perioperative use of nonsterodial antiinflammatory drugs. *Anesth Analg*. 1994;79:1178–1190.

24.

ARTERIOVENOUS FISTULA CREATION

Peter Dienhart and Michael Kushelev

STEM CASE AND KEY QUESTIONS

A 35-year-old woman with a past medical history of long-standing and progressively worsening type 1 diabetes mellitus and hypertension has developed end-stage renal disease (ESRD) that requires hemodialysis to be started. The patient is brought to the preoperative area and is assessed by the anesthesiologist. Consent is obtained and the anesthetic plan comprises a supraclavicular nerve block with 0.5% ropivacaine, followed by intraoperative sedation by the anesthesia team. Thirty minutes after the supraclavicular block is completed, the patient is taken to the operating room, where intraoperative ultrasound demonstrates adequate arterial and venous vessel patency at both the elbow and the wrist. The vascular surgeon, in accordance with the "fistula first" initiative, proceeds with radiocephalic arteriovenous (AV) fistula formation rather than the previously planned AV graft placement for the initiation of hemodialysis.

(1) WHAT ARE THE OPTIONS FOR INITIATING HEMODIALYSIS?

The three mainstays of initiating hemodialysis are AV fistulas (AVF), AV grafts (AVG), and central venous catheters (CVC). The majority of patients begin on dialysis through a CVC that can be easily placed outside of the operating room by a number of medical providers. An AVG, sometimes referred to as a bridge graft, uses a synthetic tube as an indirect connection between artery and vein. An AVF creates a direct connection between the artery and vein.

(2) WHAT IS THE "FISTULA FIRST INITIATIVE"?

The "fistula first" initiative prioritizes the use of AVFs over AVGs and CVCs for the initiation of hemodialysis to decrease infection rates as well as overall morbidity and mortality.

(3) WHAT TYPES OF AVFS ARE COMMONLY USED? IS ONE PREFERRED OVER OTHERS?

Three broad surgical categories of AVF are radiocephalic, brachiocephalic, and brachiobasilic fistulas. According to the National Kidney Foundation, the preferred site for an initial AVF is a distal site on the non-dominant arm. As distal vessels become inaccessible for cannulation, preferred placement moves proximally in the arm. Brachiobasilic fistulas attempt to access the deeper basilic vein, which typically has not been exposed to previous venipuncture. While these proximal fistulas generally remain accessible for an extended period of time, the surgical approach is more complex, and rates of infection and bleeding complications are higher.

(4) WHAT CAUSES AVF FAILURE AND WHAT DEFINES A SUCCESSFUL AVF?

Nearly one-third of AVFs become nonfunctional in the first 4 months following surgical placement. Distal fistula sites such as radiocephalic fistulas, which rely on small caliber vessels, fail at a higher rate. Fistula failure is frequently multifactorial, but often involves inadequate fistula flow and avoiding thrombosis. The scientific literature is inconsistent and at times defines success of an AVF by secondary markers, such as a bruit or thrill, instead of by effective hemodialysis. A standardized definition for a successful fistula is based on fistula flow, vessel caliber, and proximity to the skin for ease of cannulation.

(5) IS REGIONAL ANESTHESIA (RA) SAFER THAN GENERAL ANESTHESIA (GA) FOR ACCESS CASES?

RA and GA offer distinct risks and benefits for AVF creation. In this patient population that frequently suffers from cardiopulmonary disease, GA may be poorly tolerated and has been shown to lead to a higher mortality rate compared to RA during AVF cases. GA may also be associated with a higher rate of bleeding and infectious complications at the fistula site. RA may minimize hemodynamic disturbances during AVF procedures and may considerably improve fistula blood flow. No definitive trial has demonstrated the overall improved safety of RA over GA.

(6) ARE ALL APPROACHES TO BRACHIAL PLEXUS BLOCK (BPB) EQUALLY EFFICACIOUS FOR AVF?

RA via a BPB can be performed in various ways with similar results. When choosing an approach, the main factor to consider is the anatomic positioning of the planned AVF, as well as the possible need to extend the incision intraoperatively based on vessel caliber. Patients on dialysis frequently experience platelet dysfunction and are often taking antiplatelet medications for various cardiovascular conditions. Therefore, performing a thorough ultrasound examination and choosing a compressible site with a clear needle path that minimizes vessel trauma may decrease the potential bleeding risk of the procedure. Frequently used approaches include supraclavicular, infraclavicular, and axillary, while interscalene blockade is somewhat less common because of the higher rate of phrenic nerve palsy and the sparing of the lower segment of the brachial plexus.

(6) WHAT IS THE MOST COMMON PERIPHERAL NERVE BLOCK FOR AVF PLACEMENT?

Supraclavicular and infraclavicular approaches are likely preferable in providing an adequate sympathectomy while limiting the risk of phrenic nerve palsy that may be poorly tolerated with an interscalene block and the highly vascular area with an axillary approach.

(7) HOW DOES A REGIONAL BLOCK IMPROVE AVF SURVIVAL?

RA, either through a BPB or stellate ganglion block, induces a time-dependent sympathectomy that results in decreased arterial resistance and increased venous diameter. This improves primary patency, but has mixed results in improving long-term AVF survival. In addition, the increase in venous diameter may make a previously unavailable small vein easier to identify and access intraoperatively. Blocks of the brachial plexus, by increasing vessel caliber, allow for placement of a fistula more distal than was thought possible during preoperative planning.

(8) IS THE TOXICITY OF LOCAL ANESTHETIC DIFFERENT IN ESRD?

Patients with ESRD have complex physiologic differences that may affect the plasma concentration of commonly used local anesthetics. Metabolic acidosis and hyperdynamic circulation are offset by an increase in α-1-acid glycoprotein production that binds local anesthetics. The systemic toxicity of ropivacaine seen in patients with renal dysfunction appears to be similar to that in patients with normal kidney function, and similar results have been seen with mepivacaine, bupivacaine, and levobupivacaine. Hemodialysis's effect on blood volume, extremes of age, and other comorbidities must be considered when deciding on the dose of local anesthetic for individual patients.

DISCUSSION

The prevalence of ESRD is increasing worldwide, with approximately 10%–14% of the world population affected by kidney disease.[1,2] Of the 600,000 patients with renal failure in the United States, 450,000 are on dialysis, at an estimated cost of approximately $100 billion (USD) per year, paid by Medicaid. This represents a significant direct and indirect economic burden with an approximate annual cost per patient of up to $180,000.[1] Further, the increased prevalence of multiple comorbidities, such as cardiovascular disease, diabetes, stroke, infection, and coagulation disorders, among others, greatly complicates the evaluation of the medical economic impact. This makes estimating the future costs and complexity of medically managing ESRD more difficult.

One of the mainstays for managing end-stage renal failure is dialysis. The vast majority of the approximately 120,000 new patients who begin dialysis yearly in the United States receive hemodialysis, with only about 10% being treated with peritoneal dialysis. Patients and providers must consider several hemodialysis access options, including AVFs versus AVGs versus tunneled CVCs. Large studies have demonstrated that, nationwide, nearly 80% of patients are initiated on hemodialysis through a tunneled CVC, with the majority remaining on catheter dialysis indefinitely.[3,4] The consequence of this practice is a 30% increase in infection rates and a doubling in mortality.[4] When comparing AVF to AVG, there is a 6-fold reduction in the risk of systemic sepsis of AVF over AVG.[5-7] AVF has lower all-cause and cardiovascular mortality compared to other dialysis access options, while sustaining future access sites.[7,8] In 2003 a collaboration between Centers for Medicare & Medicaid Services and the End Stage Renal Disease Networks encouraged AVF as the preferred vascular access site for dialysis patients. This initiative, known as the National Vascular Access Improvement Initiative and subsequently renamed the Fistula First Breakthrough Initiative, was in response to the significantly lower rate of AVF use by the medical community in the United States compared to other developed countries. Its primary goals were (1) to increase the use of AVF for hemodialysis beyond the Kidney Disease Outcomes Quality Initiative (KDOQI) Clinical Practice Guidelines of 50% AVF use for hemodialysis; and (2) to collect and analyze data on AVF use to track and improve outcomes. This program quickly achieved the aforementioned goals and in 2009 increased the goal AVF rate for hemodialysis to nearly 70%.[9–12]

FISTULA FAILURE

One of the most common causes of complications related to hemodialysis access is early fistula failure, which can reach 25%.[13] Early fistula failure is defined as needing a revision of vascular access within the first 120 days through endovascular techniques such as stenting, angioplasty, or thrombectomy versus open surgical repair. Failure rates are particularly high for radiocephalic fistulas, which are formed by using the small distal vessels at the wrist that account for one-third of AVF target sites.[14,15] Not only do these failures result in the need for another invasive medical intervention with its inherent risks, but they are an economic burden. It is estimated that the United States spends up to $1 billion per year on declotting and revision procedures related to fistula failure.[16]

One significant limitation in the literature regarding fistula failure is the variable definitions of AVF success and inconsistent time frames that define "primary failure."[17] Studies have used variables such as the presence of a thrill or bruit in the AVF to denote success without evaluating whether a patient can be effectively dialyzed. Fistula failure has been defined by AVF as thrombosis, hematoma, infection, ischemia, or failure to cannulate. Prior to 2006, there was no single universal definition for successful fistula maturation, which therefore limited examination of long-term outcomes. In 2006, the National Kidney Foundation Kidney Disease Outcomes Quality Initiative (NKF-KDOQI) updated its guidelines and provided a definition of a functional and mature AVF that has since been adopted as the gold standard. KDOQI introduced the "rule of sixes" to define maturation (flow of 600 mL/min, AVF located less than 6 mm from the skin surface to facilitate successful repeated cannulation, and a minimal vein diameter of 6 mm).[18] Blood flow through a mature fistula should be, at a minimum, 300–400 mL/min, with an ideal of 600 mL/min, to meet hemodialysis needs. A clinically efficacious AVF should allow for consistent cannulation, whereas the exact depth and diameter may be variable and may not always meet the ideal as described by the KDOQI rule of sixes. Creating a successful fistula requires adequate preexisting vessel diameter, suitable postoperative blood flow through the newly created shunt, and proper maturation to an appropriate vessel diameter and flow for hemodialysis.

AVF PHYSIOLOGY

Causes of early fistula malfunction can be separated into thrombosis, insufficient vascular flow, and failure of maturation. The exact cause of an AVF failure often cannot be determined and is a consequence of several interrelated factors. One common etiology of early fistula failure is a result of thrombosis with a subsequent failure of adequate vascular flow. However, this oversimplifies the mechanism at play. Thrombosis of a hemodialysis fistula or graft often occurs as a consequence of vascular stenosis, leading to severely compromised blood flow. The most likely determinant of newly created access stenosis and consequent failure of AVF maturation is likely the response of both the feeding artery and the draining vein to the increase in shear stress that occurs after an AV anastomosis is created.[19–22] Shear stress acting on the newly formed access vessel has been defined mathematically by the formula $4\eta Q/\pi r3$, where η is blood viscosity (a constant), Q is blood flow, and r is vessel radius.[21] Conceptually, this stress rate is an indicator of the difference in velocity of the blood flow between the center of the vessel and the boundary layer or the luminal wall, where flow would be close to zero. Therefore, the shear stress will go up proportionally to the laminar flow of the blood and will conversely decrease in areas where there is a low flow velocity or where multidirectional flow with eddies exists. The importance of shear stress is that physiologically the vessel attempts to regain homeostasis by achieving a similar level of shear stress at the luminal interface as was seen pre-anastomosis. Because shear stress is inversely related to the radius of the lumen, the vessels dilate to attempt to regain the desired pre-anastomosis level. Following fistula formation, high shear stress results in endothelial proliferation, alignment of endothelial cells in the direction of flow, and the secretion of substances such as nitric oxide and prostacyclin to promote vasodilation and inhibit thrombosis and platelet aggregation. This mechanism allows for the eventual reduction of shear forces to pre-anastomosis levels by allowing for an increase in luminal diameter, as well as the needed wall hypertrophy to provide a eutrophic wall diameter relative to pre-anastomotic levels.[20,23–25] In contrast, if early fistula flow is reduced for one reason or another, there is a marked reduction in shear stress on the luminal interface, resulting in endothelial activation and proliferation with the secretion of prothrombotic and vasoconstrictive substances such as thromboxane in an attempt to increase blood velocity to regain pre-anastomosis wall sheer forces.[22,26,27] This has the opposite of the desired clinical effect. Although the luminal flow now approximates pre-anastomotic shear stress, it is ineffective for a functioning hemodialysis fistula. Therefore, the pathogenesis of vascular stenosis is driven by the downstream mechanical and biologic impacts wrought by the changes in shear stress as it relates to the AVF anastomotic site.[28] This results in vessel dilation with *appropriate* intimal hyperplasia via smooth muscle proliferation, or *excessive* intimal hyperplasia that achieves the presurgery luminal shear forces.[19–21,29] A review of the literature from the past four decades demonstrates common identifiable risk factors that impact this modulation at the vessel lumen. We will briefly examine the non-anesthetic as well as anesthetic-related variables that can be used to optimize the chances of successful AVF development in the context of "normalizing" luminal sheer forces.

RISK FACTORS FOR FISTULA FAILURE

Factors such as female gender, increasing age, diabetes mellitus, vascular disease, smoking, and previous cannulation may all decrease AVF patency.[30] Each individual patient's vascular anatomy, including preoperative and postoperative arterial and venous diameters, preoperative arterial inflow, and early postoperative blood flow through the newly created fistula, can play a role in fistula maturation. Improving fistula flow and using antiplatelet medications may decrease the risk of fistula thrombosis but do not necessarily connote long-term cannulation success for hemodialysis.[31,32] Surgical skill and experience may also play significant roles.[33,34] Anesthetic technique may influence all of the vascular parameters mentioned above by altering perioperative blood flow and venous and arterial dilatation.

ANESTHESIA FOR AVF

For the anesthesia provider, consideration should be given to the type of anesthetic that is available and whether provider choice in anesthetic may influence fistula survival and medical complications. There are three broad anesthetic categories for successful surgical fistula formation: (1) GA; (2) RA with or without adjunct anesthetic; and (3) local anesthetic (LA), which is frequently combined with monitored anesthetic care (MAC). It is important to understand that patients who undergo vascular surgical procedures are at high risk for perioperative vascular spasm from surgical manipulation. Higher rates of coexisting arterial calcifications place patients with ESRD at higher risk for vascular spasms compared to the general population.[35] Enhanced sympathetic tone as well as the local handling of the vessel by the surgeon results in decreased vessel size and impaired blood flow through the anastomotic site. These factors predispose to conditions that favor more turbulent flow with a concomitant reduction in blood flow velocities and an increased risk of thrombosis and early anastomosis failure.

GENERAL ANESTHESIA (GA)

Historically, GA has been the most common method to facilitate surgical AVF placement, and has been used in up to 85% of all AVF cases.[36,37] Since the placement of the first AV access in the United States by Belding Scribner in 1960 and the subsequent first autologous AVF by Michael Bresicia in 1966, GA has been the predominant method for anesthetizing patients undergoing these procedures.[12] GA eliminates involuntary movement by the patient that can be detrimental to achieving successful vascular surgical results. GA provides some transient increase in fistula blood flow by increasing blood velocity, but not at the level of a BPB, and quickly returns to baseline.[36,38] GA results in a 2- to 5-fold higher risk for postoperative death and cardiovascular events in those with chronic kidney disease than in those without.[37,39–41] In fact, at least one investigation has demonstrated an increase in mortality when AVF was performed under GA compared to RA.[37] In addition, using GA compared RA is not as effective in blocking the adrenergic stress response, with subsequent platelet hyperaggregability ultimately decreasing blood flow and increasing the risk of thrombosis in the newly formed graft.[42,43]

As it is familiar and prevalent in both community and academic practices, GA is an appealing modality in facilitating surgical procedures such as fistula placements. Most anesthesia practitioners are comfortable in providing GA and are familiar with the pathophysiologic changes common in ESRD patients. GA does not require additional expertise or subspecialty skill training. Several studies have shown decreased operative times for GA relative to RA.[3,37] Siracuse et al. found that there appeared to be an approximately 15-minute addition to total procedural/operative time for fistula creation when using RA.[37] The potential increase in procedural time must be weighed against long-term considerations such as fistula survival and patient outcomes. Conversely, findings are also available demonstrating shorter operating room times for AVF performed under RA over GA, as well as decreased perioperative stays.[44–46]

In terms of long-term outcomes, a large study by Beaulieu et al. argued the benefits of GA over LA/RA in decreasing AVG failure. The study was a database retrospective review of 31,028 patients identified by accessing the Vascular Quality Initiative hemodialysis data set between 2011 and 2017 for AVF and AVG creation. Patients were grouped by mode of anesthesia (GA vs. LA/RA) in comparing fistula and graft failure within the first 120 days. Secondary outcomes included procedural complications such as swelling, hemorrhage, steal, and wound infection as well as in-hospital and 30-day postoperative rates. The researchers found that patients undergoing access creation with RA had higher early failure rates for both AVG (26.2% vs. 23%; $P = 0.04$) and AVF (22.3% vs. 20.6%; $P = 0.04$) compared to GA. When controlling for confounding variables, higher failure rates with RA remained for AVG but not for AVF. Despite the possibility of worsening fistula maturation rates with RA, the AVF group that had used GA during access creation had a 26% increase in bleeding complications and a 3.4-fold increase in wound infection rates relative to RA. One potential explanation that the authors provide to explain higher graft failure rates is to speculate that by performing the procedure under RA/LA, surgeons limit themselves in vessel selection by avoiding more proximal vessels for AVF formation, as this may involve territory not traditionally covered by BPB. Of particular interest, the study found that the mode of anesthesia chosen might have been influenced by the type of hemodialysis access planned by the surgeon. Of the 31,028 cases, 77.5% (24,067) received AVF, while only 22.5% (6961) patients were given an AVG for their hemodialysis access.[3] The study population's higher deployment rate of AVF over AVG mirrored the goals defined by the most recent guidelines of "fistula first" for vascular access for patients on dialysis.[10,12] This increased rate of AVF over AVG may be correlated to a higher dependence on RA in the study population compared to the historical rate of 85% of access procedures performed under GA.[36,37] The study by Beaulieu et al. deserves particular attention because of its large patient population and relatively recent data collection. The conclusions leave a mixed picture of some survival benefit of AVG with GA, but a higher medical complication rate with GA over RA. In addition, this is one of the few investigations that have demonstrated the superiority of GA over RA in a subset of patients undergoing dialysis access procedures. Other investigations showed relative equivalence between anesthetic techniques in terms of long-term AVF survival. Solomonson et al. wrote one of the larger, but still underpowered, retrospective reviews of patients from 1986 to 1991 at the Mayo Clinic, assessing 406 patients who underwent fistula creation using GA versus LA versus RA with a BPB and found no difference in maturation rates or outcomes measures.[47]

LOCAL ANESTHESIA (LA)

In the surgical literature, a distinct anesthetic option for AVF is LA. The majority of these procedures, especially in the United States, are not performed solely with LA as injected by the surgeon but are accompanied by MAC. For most patients to achieve acceptable surgical conditions, the surgeon frequently has to inject LA repeatedly while the anesthesia team provides deep sedation. Often, the level of sedation approaches that of GA with resultant need for some level of airway and hemodynamic support. Although using LA/MAC may avoid the need for more invasive airway instrumentation, in many other ways it approaches GA. Specifically comparing GA and LA/MAC for AVF creation, a recent retrospective single-institution study by Son et al. looked at 253 fistula surgeries performed on 224 patients and showed no significant differences in maturation and complication rates when fistula creation was done under GA with general endotracheal anesthesia versus GA with laryngeal mask airway versus LA with MAC.[48] Vascular access cases performed under LA are complicated more frequently by arterial and venous vasospasms compared to GA or RA.[49] LA infiltration by the surgeon at the operative site does not provide the beneficial sympathectomy provided by a BPB.[13,50] One of the larger randomized prospective trials by Aitken et al. compared RA (supraclavicular or axillary block) vs. LA for AVF on medium-term postoperative fistula patency.[15] The authors found that at 3 months, the primary patency rate was higher for BPB compared to LA (84.1% vs. 61.9%, OR 3.3, $P = 0.005$). The beneficial effect was most pronounced for radiocephalic AVF and corresponded to an increase in vascular flow and vasodilation in the perioperative time period. In addition, using a BPB facilitated modification of the operative plan to a more favorable distal AVF.[15] Similar benefits to RA were shown in an Indian patient population in a randomized study comparing supraclavicular BPB with LA infiltration. Patients in the RA group demonstrated enhanced primary patency as well as improved vascular diameter and flow at all time periods studied, extending to 6 weeks postoperatively.[51] Although LA may spare a vulnerable patient population from requiring GA, LA frequently does require additional sedation and does not provide the added benefits of RA.

REGIONAL ANESTHESIA (RA)

Two significant factors for successful AVF maturation are preserving blood flow and maintaining vascular diameter to offset the anticipated intraoperative vascular spasm caused by sympathetic stimulation and manual manipulation by the surgeon. RA using a BPB promotes stable patient hemodynamics with the additional benefit of improved vessel size for anastomosis via a sympathectomy-like effect that leads to enhanced perioperative blood flow and decreased early thrombosis rates, thereby increasing fistula survival rates.[13,50] Numerous investigations have found supportive evidence to prioritize RA as the anesthetic of choice to maximize outcomes for AVF placement.[15,36,50,51] There appears to be a trend in the literature, as well as clinically, toward a growing reliance on RA over GA and LA.[3,36,52,52] In addition, patients undergoing AVF creation using RA may experience improved postoperative pain control and report higher satisfaction, as seen with many other surgical procedures.

REGIONAL TECHNIQUE BASED ON SURGICAL APPROACH

AVF surgeries fall into three main operative sites in order of preference as designated by the National Kidney Foundation.[5] First, a radiocephalic fistula involves a distal incision on the forearm anastomosing the radial artery to the cephalic vein. The anterior forearm is innervated by the lateral cutaneous nerve of the forearm (C5 and C6), a terminal branch of the musculocutaneous nerve, and the medial antebrachial cutaneous nerve (C8 and T1). Second, the brachiocephalic fistula is created at the antecubital fossa and involves linking the brachial artery to the end of the cephalic vein. This is accomplished by one or several incisions on the ventral side of the elbow that is innervated by the same nerves as the radiocephalic fistula, with the addition of the radial nerve (C5 and C6) and potentially the intercostobrachial nerve (T2) if the incision is extended into the medial proximal arm. Third, the brachiobasilic fistula requires connecting the brachial artery to the transposed basilic vein that is elevated from its deeper position. This approach typically involves a longer incision on the ventral aspect of the upper arm that approaches the axilla, more invasive dissection into the arm, and, frequently, longer operation times. The proximal arm is innervated by a combination of radial (C5 and C6), axillary (C5 and C6), medial cutaneous (C8 and T1), and intercostobrachial nerves (T2). Formation of a brachiobasilic fistula, typically used following multiple distal AVF failures as previous venipuncture of the deeper basilic vein is rare, is associated with an increased rate of infection and bleeding complications.[5]

After considering the anticipated surgical plan, an appropriate regional anesthetic approach may be chosen. While an anatomic review of brachial plexus and sympathetic chain anatomy is beyond the scope of this chapter, certain anatomical implications of individual regional techniques for patients undergoing AVF repair should be considered. Interscalene block (ISB) allows for significant deposition of local anesthetic in close proximity to the stellate ganglion and the remainder of the sympathetic chain while achieving a consistent blockade of C5, C6, and C7. ISB may not be as reliable in blocking the lower segments of the brachial plexus (C8 and T1) and thus the medial antebrachial cutaneous nerve. In addition, the nearly 100% incidence of phrenic nerve palsy may be poorly tolerated in a patient with ESRD with concomitant cardiovascular and pulmonary pathophysiology.[54] Supraclavicular block and infraclavicular block are the most common approaches for achieving a regional block in radiocephalic and brachiocephalic AVF repairs. Supraclavicular block may have a greater rate of sparing the lower parts of the brachial plexus (C8 to T1) compared to infraclavicular block, which may contribute to greater block failure.[55] The risk of phrenic nerve palsy from BPB decreases with more distal approaches but still remains a significant consideration with infraclavicular block and can be as high as 25%.[56] Axillary block provides a distal approach to the brachial plexus, minimizing the risk for phrenic nerve palsy and pneumothorax while providing a superficial target even in extremes of body habitus. The musculocutaneous nerve, which is not located perivascularly to the brachial artery, must be blocked separately, especially for radiocephalic and brachiocephalic AVF. Axillary approaches may have a shorter duration of action compared to other BPB blocks, which can be beneficial depending on the anesthetic goals for each individual patient.[57] Individual nerve blocks in the upper arm may allow for a more targeted block (specifically, the musculocutaneous and medial antebrachial cutaneous nerves for radiocephalic AVF), may decrease the total dose of local anesthetic, and may provide an earlier return of motor function, thereby improving patient satisfaction.[58] Sparing the blockade of other nerves of the brachial plexus potentially minimizes nerve injury and allows for near full sensation in the hand, thus letting a responsive patient notify medical providers of steal syndrome, a known risk factor of AVF.[59] Avoiding the brachial plexus completely, Yildirim et al. demonstrated that a selective stellate ganglion block can improve fistula maturation rates.[60] Although the entirety of the sympathetic chain is not consistently blocked by this approach, preemptive blockade of the stellate ganglion has been shown to blunt vascular spasms, arterial dilation, and improve fistula flow.[60] The investigation by Yildirim et al. is particularly notable because the study design selected patients to receive a stellate ganglion block on 7 consecutive days following AVF placement. Considering that the end result of repeated single injections may be more easily accomplished with a continuous catheter technique, the outcomes of this study raise the question of whether continuous nerve blockade potentially creates greater benefits in fistula flow and long-term survival compared to single-shot techniques. Outside of peripheral nerve blocks, intravenous RA (Bier block) has also been reported to provide vascular vasodilation and a bloodless field to facilitate AVF creation.[61] While there has been no conclusive study that has compared different regional techniques in maximizing the duration and magnitude of the sympathectomy, all RA approaches discussed here have reported some level of sympathectomy, with corresponding increases in vascular flow and providing surgical anesthesia, allowing the patient to be minimally sedated during AVF creation.

RA for more proximal fistula sites requires, in addition to BPB, accounting for the intercostobrachial nerve, which provides innervation to the medial proximal arm extending into the axilla.[46] The intercostobrachial nerve, a cutaneous branch of the second intercostal nerve, pierces the serratus anterior muscle and crosses the axilla to the medial side of the arm, and joins with the medial antebrachial cutaneous nerve. It provides sensation to the medial upper extremity from the axilla to the elbow or sometimes even just distal to the elbow, a distribution that often is found in the surgical field with the creation of brachiocephalic and brachiobasilic fistulas.[62] While patients can undergo brachiobasilic fistula creation under RA, a more proximal incision into the axilla and the longer anticipated operative times may require additional anesthetic coverage.[46] A variety of options have been presented to achieve blockade of the intercostobrachial nerve, ranging from direct infiltration, ultrasound-guided intercostal block, pectoralis nerve blocks, serratus plane blocks, and thoracic paravertebral blocks.[63] Specifically for proximal arm AVF procedures, Moustafa et al. demonstrated that an injection of 6 mL of 0.25% bupivacaine between the serratus anterior and pectoralis minor at the third rib had a 100% success rate in avoiding GA and a 91% success rate in blocking the intercostobrachial nerve.[64]

CHOICE OF LOCAL ANESTHETICS

Similar to the lack of consensus on any specific regional approach, there is no definitive literature to guide selection of LAs for BPB during AVF creation. One telling investigation by Ginosar et al. examined the level of sympathectomy created by lumbar epidural administration of various volumes and concentrations of bupivacaine.[65] The authors concluded that the concentration of bupivacaine was more important than total dose in maximizing sympathectomy.[65] Based on investigations of neuraxial blockade, one cannot presume that a similar relationship exists for dose of LA used for BPBs and level of sympathectomy created. Specifically for patients with ESRD, complex physiologic changes may alter LA pharmacodynamics and pharmacokinetics as a result of a number of factors, including hypoalbuminemia, elevated cardiac output, metabolic acidosis, hyperkalemia, and the presence of an underlying neuropathy. Additional factors in ESRD include the liver's increasing production of α-1-acid glycoprotein that binds LAs and thus decreases free plasma concentration[66] and the fact that most clinically used LAs are metabolized by the liver and are therefore minimally altered by changes in renal function. Various investigations have demonstrated similar clinical efficacy and side effect profile for bupivacaine, levobupivacaine, mepivacaine, and ropivacaine when performing BPBs in patients with ESRD compared to those with normal renal physiology.[67–70] Pere et al. examined the pharmacokinetics of ropivacaine in healthy volunteers compared to patients with moderate to severe kidney dysfunction, concluding that although there are ropivacaine metabolites (most significantly, pipecoloxylidide) that may be affected by decreased renal clearance, their systemic toxicity profile is relatively insignificant.[71] Because there are no specific recommendations for the ideal LA type, volume, or concentration, the practitioner must weigh the complex physiology of ESRD, the patient's age and weight, and specific anesthetic goals on a case-by-case basis.

BENEFITS OF REGIONAL ANESTHESIA (RA)

It is believed that a BPB facilitates vasodilation by inducing a sympathectomy-like effect. The sympathetic chain runs ventral to the vertebral transverse processes in close proximity to the longus colli and anterior scalene muscles. Blockade of the sympathetic chain at the stellate ganglion, positioned at the junction of the first rib and thoracic vertebral body, may not provide a consistent sympathectomy due to the presence of other sympathetic fibers traveling along intercostal nerves and directly adjacent to the brachial plexus itself.[72] The presence of a sympathetically mediated blockade can be intimated by the presence of Horner's syndrome and the corresponding temperature change. The sympathectomy that is induced by BPB creates more significant venous dilation compared to the application of a proximal tourniquet.[50] Shemesh et al. showed that performing a supraclavicular block decreased the pulsatility index, a marker of arterial resistance, and increased the basilic vein diameter by 25%, which lasted at least 5 hours.[36] Lo Monte et al. demonstrated a significant decrease in pulsatility index and an increase in venous vessel diameter, leading to improved laminar flow in patients who received axillary nerve blocks compared to patients who received LA.[73] Similar to supraclavicular and axillary blocks, interscalene and infraclavicular BPB approaches allow for a concomitant sympathectomy with corresponding vasodilation.[73–75] While there is no investigation dictating which peripheral nerve block produces the most profound sympathectomy in AVF patients, it is logical that the distance between the site of injection and the stellate ganglion may correspond to the level of sympathectomy achieved.

Achieving a sympathectomy allows for easier intraoperative identification and access of vessels, as well as temporary enhancement of peripheral blood flow with the downstream effect of improving rates of maturation and early patency.[36,38,41] Sympathetically mediated increases in blood flow as a result of spinal anesthesia and epidural anesthesia has also been shown to decrease failure for infrainguinal arterial bypass grafts.[76–78] A recent review and meta-analysis by Cerneviciute et al. confirmed the advantage of RA for AVF.[79] The review examined four randomized control trials with a total of 286 patients undergoing primary radiocephalic AVFs to establish dialysis access. The study showed a lower failure rate with RA (12/143) versus LA (36/143) (OR 0.28, 95% CI 0.14–0.57).[79] The authors note that the studies included did have significant methodological failings, such as low overall AVF failure rates, questionable blinding and randomization, and inadequate follow-up, and were single-center investigations.[79] The findings of this study can be contrasted to a similar-sized meta-analysis by Ismail et al. demonstrating that RA improved blood flow and initial patency but did not show a difference in primary failure rate.[52] Although no well-designed, adequately powered, large randomized controlled trial is available to definitively support the benefit of RA over GA and LA, numerous studies have demonstrated improvements in patient outcomes and improved AVF survival.[13,15,36,38,44,50,79]

In addition to a regional anesthetic's ability to decrease fistula failure, using RA may allow the operative plan to be favorably altered, allowing for access at a more distal AVF site and selection of an AVF over AVG. Prior to undergoing attempts at AVF creation, patients may undergo preoperative vessel mapping using ultrasound, venograms, and contrast-enhanced spiral computed tomography to facilitate the identification of vessel targets for surgery.[80–82] The goal of this preoperative planning is to identify vein diameters greater than 2.5 mm, as smaller vein selection may lead to a greater than 80% failure rate.[4,5] There does not appear to be a consensus on the utility and cost-effectiveness of this preoperative planning on fistula maturation rates.[80] While preoperative vascular mapping has had mixed results, a number of investigations have demonstrated that using a BPB provides for venous dilation past the minimum threshold, thus allowing for a more favorable distal AVF site in up to one-half of cases.[83–86] This is particularly useful for distal radiocephalic fistulas that use small-caliber vessels. One of the most recent examinations studied 65 patients with ESRD undergoing a dialysis access procedure using a BPB (supraclavicular or infraclavicular nerve block at the discretion of the anesthesiologist). Forty-six percent of patients underwent a more favorable distal AVF procedure than planned, with six patients able to undergo AVF rather than the prior anticipated AVG. The primary patency and functional access rates of these unanticipated distal fistula sites was comparable to those previously reported in the literature.[87] While a regional anesthetic's ability to ultimately influence fistula maturity is somewhat mixed, it does appear to provide a benefit to patients with relatively small vessel caliber in allowing for selection of a more distal fistula site.

CONCLUSION

Although the literature fails to categorically define which anesthetic modality provides better overall outcomes when taking into account perioperative complications, fistula maturation rates, and economic costs, RA continues to grow in popularity.[3] The lack of well-designed and powered prospective randomized controlled trials, inconsistent definitions for fistula maturation and success, and the prominence of physiologic variables in the days and weeks following fistula creation on AVF maturation all limit definitive demonstration of the superiority of RA over GA and/or LA. Despite the paucity of clear proof, the past two decades have seen an evolution of anesthetic approaches for AVF surgery. Familiarity and proficiency with regional techniques continue to improve, providing continued growth in the body of evidence suggesting improvements in fistula survival and maturation, as well as a reduction in the potential risks of GA in patients with ESRD. This has resulted in the beginnings of a paradigm shift from the traditional GA-predominant system to more consideration being given to RA via BPB for the creation of dialysis access. Anesthetic options must account for multiple factors, including surgical time, cost, comorbidities, expertise, and surgical preferences. While no one peripheral nerve block technique has been demonstrated as superior for this patient population, decision-making includes weighing the assessment of potential complications such as hematoma formation, pneumothorax, and phrenic nerve palsy with the benefits on vascular flow from the resulting sympathectomy. Ultimately, the goal is to provide patient comfort and safety while optimizing surgical success in long-term AVF creation.

REFERENCES

1. Wang V, Vilme H, Maciejewski ML, Boulware LE. The economic burden of chronic kidney disease and end-stage renal disease. *Semin Nephrol.* 2016;36:319–30.
2. Himmelfarb J, Shankland SJ. Creating research infrastructure and functionality to address chronic kidney disease: the Kidney Research Institute. *Semin Nephrol.* 2009;29:457–466.
3. Beaulieu RJ, Locham S, Nejim B, Dakour-Aridi H, Woo K, Malas MB. General anesthesia is associated with reduced early failure among patients undergoing hemodialysis access. *J Vasc Surg.* 2019;69:890–897 e895.
4. Arhuidese IJ, Orandi BJ, Nejim B, Malas M. Utilization, patency, and complications associated with vascular access for hemodialysis in the United States. *J Vasc Surg.* 2018;68:1166–1174.
5. Vascular Access 2006 Work Group. Clinical practice guidelines for vascular access. *Am J Kidney Dis.* 2006;48(Suppl 1):S248–273.
6. Goh MA, Ali JM, Iype S, Pettigrew GJ. Outcomes of primary arteriovenous fistulas in patients older than 70 years. *J Vasc Surg.* 2016;63:1333–1340.

7. Bray BD, Boyd J, Daly C, et al. Vascular access type and risk of mortality in a national prospective cohort of haemodialysis patients. *QJM.* 2012;105:1097–1103.
8. Thomson PC, Stirling CM, Geddes CC, Morris ST, Mactier RA. Vascular access in haemodialysis patients: a modifiable risk factor for bacteraemia and death. *QJM.* 2007;100:415–422.
9. The University of Texas MD Anderson Cancer Center. *Fistula First Catheter Last.* Available at https://www.kidney.org/patients/pfc/DialysisEducation. Accessed June 30, 2020.
10. Lynch JR, Wasse H, Armistead NC, McClellan WM. Achieving the goal of the Fistula First breakthrough initiative for prevalent maintenance hemodialysis patients. *Am J Kidney Dis.* 2011;57:78–89.
11. Ikizler, T. Alp et al. KDOQI Clinical Practice Guideline for Nutrition in CKD: 2020 Update. *Am J Kidney Dis.* 2020;76(3):S1–S107.
12. Lee T. Fistula first initiative: historical impact on vascular access practice patterns and influence on future vascular access care. *Cardiovasc Eng Technol.* 2017;8:244–254.
13. Malinzak EB, Gan TJ. Regional anesthesia for vascular access surgery. *Anesth Analg.* 2009;109:976–980.
14. Golledge J, Smith CJ, Emery J, Farrington K, Thompson HH. Outcome of primary radiocephalic fistula for haemodialysis. *Br J Surg.* 1999;86:211–216.
15. Aitken E, Jackson A, Kearns R, et al. Effect of regional versus local anaesthesia on outcome after arteriovenous fistula creation: a randomised controlled trial. *Lancet.* 2016;388:1067–1074.
16. Feldman HI, Kobrin S, Wasserstein A. Hemodialysis vascular access morbidity. *J Am Soc Nephrol.* 1996;7:523–535.
17. Lee T, Mokrzycki M, Moist L, et al. Standardized definitions for hemodialysis vascular access. *Semin Dial.* 2011;24:515–524.
18. Gilmore J. KDOQI clinical practice guidelines and clinical practice recommendations: 2006 updates. *Nephrol Nurs J.* 2006;33:487–488.
19. Corpataux JM, Haesler E, Silacci P, Ris HB, Hayoz D. Low-pressure environment and remodelling of the forearm vein in Brescia-Cimino haemodialysis access. *Nephrol Dial Transplant.* 2002;17:1057–1062.
20. Ballermann BJ, Dardik A, Eng E, Liu A. Shear stress and the endothelium. *Kidney Int Suppl.* 1998;67:S100–108.
21. Papaioannou TG, Stefanadis C. Vascular wall shear stress: basic principles and methods. *Hellenic J Cardiol.* 2005;46:9–15.
22. Paszkowiak JJ, Dardik A. Arterial wall shear stress: observations from the bench to the bedside. *Vasc Endovascular Surg.* 2003;37:47–57.
23. Joannides R, Haefeli WE, Linder L, et al. Nitric oxide is responsible for flow-dependent dilatation of human peripheral conduit arteries in vivo. *Circulation.* 1995;91:1314–1319.
24. Tohda K, Masuda H, Kawamura K, Shozawa T. Difference in dilatation between endothelium-preserved and -desquamated segments in the flow-loaded rat common carotid artery. *Arterioscler Thromb.* 1992;12:519–528.
25. Tronc F, Wassef M, Esposito B, et al. Role of NO in flow-induced remodeling of the rabbit common carotid artery. *Arterioscler Thromb Vasc Biol.* 1996;16:1256–1262.
26. Berceli SA, Davies MG, Kenagy RD, Clowes AW. Flow-induced neointimal regression in baboon polytetrafluoroethylene grafts is associated with decreased cell proliferation and increased apoptosis. *J Vasc Surg.* 2002;36:1248–1255.
27. Qin F, Dardik H, Pangilinan A, et al. Remodeling and suppression of intimal hyperplasia of vascular grafts with a distal arteriovenous fistula in a rat model. *J Vasc Surg.* 2001;34:701–706.
28. Kamiya A, Togawa T. Adaptive regulation of wall shear stress to flow change in the canine carotid artery. *Am J Physiol.* 1980;239:H14–H21.
29. Rekhter M, Nicholls S, Ferguson M, Gordon D. Cell proliferation in human arteriovenous fistulas used for hemodialysis. *Arterioscler Thromb.* 1993;13:609–617.
30. Smith GE, Gohil R, Chetter IC. Factors affecting the patency of arteriovenous fistulas for dialysis access. *J Vasc Surg.* 2012;55:849–855.
31. Dember LM, Beck GJ, Allon M, et al. Effect of clopidogrel on early failure of arteriovenous fistulas for hemodialysis: a randomized controlled trial. *JAMA.* 2008;299:2164–2171.
32. Viecelli AK, Polkinghorne KR, Pascoe EM, et al. Fish oil and aspirin effects on arteriovenous fistula function: secondary outcomes of the randomised omega-3 fatty acids (Fish oils) and Aspirin in Vascular access OUtcomes in REnal Disease (FAVOURED) trial. *PLoS One.* 2019;14:e0213274.
33. O'Hare AM, Dudley RA, Hynes DM, et al. Impact of surgeon and surgical center characteristics on choice of permanent vascular access. *Kidney Int.* 2003;64:681–689.
34. Fassiadis N, Morsy M, Siva M, et al. Does the surgeon's experience impact on radiocephalic fistula patency rates? *Semin Dial.* 2007;20:455–457.
35. Nakamura S, Ishibashi-Ueda H, Niizuma S, et al. Coronary calcification in patients with chronic kidney disease and coronary artery disease. *Clin J Am Soc Nephrol.* 2009;4:1892–1900.
36. Shemesh D, Olsha O, Orkin D, et al. Sympathectomy-like effects of brachial plexus block in arteriovenous access surgery. *Ultrasound Med Biol.* 2006;32:817–822.
37. Siracuse JJ, Gill HL, Parrack I, et al. Variability in anesthetic considerations for arteriovenous fistula creation. *J Vasc Access.* 2014;15:364–369.
38. Mouquet C, Bitker MO, Bailliart O, et al. Anesthesia for creation of a forearm fistula in patients with endstage renal failure. *Anesthesiology.* 1989;70:909–914.
39. Mathew A, Devereaux PJ, O'Hare A, et al. Chronic kidney disease and postoperative mortality: a systematic review and meta-analysis. *Kidney Int.* 2008;73:1069–1081.
40. Higgins TL, Estafanous FG, Loop FD, et al. Stratification of morbidity and mortality outcome by preoperative risk factors in coronary artery bypass patients: a clinical severity score. *JAMA.* 1992;267:2344–2348.
41. Howell SJ, Sear YM, Yeates D, et al. Risk factors for cardiovascular death after elective surgery under general anaesthesia. *Br J Anaesth.* 1998;80:14–19.
42. Naesh O, Haljamae H, Hindberg I, et al. Epidural anaesthesia prolonged into the postoperative period prevents stress response and platelet hyperaggregability after peripheral vascular surgery. *Eur J Vasc Surg.* 1994;8:395–400.
43. Liu S, Carpenter RL, Neal JM. Epidural anesthesia and analgesia: their role in postoperative outcome. *Anesthesiology.* 1995;82:1474–1506.
44. Shoshiashvili V, Tataradze A, Beglarishvili L, Managadze L, Chkhotua A. Influence of type of anesthesia on hemodynamic parameters and outcome of dialysis arteriovenous fistula operations. *Georgian Med News.* 2015 Dec;(249):20–27.
45. Mariano ER, Chu LF, Peinado CR, Mazzei WJ. Anesthesia-controlled time and turnover time for ambulatory upper extremity surgery performed with regional versus general anesthesia. *J Clin Anesth.* 2009;21:253–257.
46. Cole NM, Vlassakov K, Brovman EY, Heydarpour M, Urman RD. Regional anesthesia for arteriovenous fistula surgery may reduce hospital length of stay and reoperation rates. *Vasc Endovascular Surg.* 2018;52:418–426.
47. Solomonson MD, Johnson ME, Ilstrup D. Risk factors in patients having surgery to create an arteriovenous fistula. *Anesth Analg.* 1994;79:694–700.
48. Son A, Mannoia K, Herrera A, et al. Dialysis access surgery: does anesthesia type affect maturation and complication rates? *Ann Vasc Surg.* 2016;33:116–119.
49. Konner K, Nonnast-Daniel B, Ritz E. The arteriovenous fistula. *J Am Soc Nephrol.* 2003;14:1669–1680.
50. Hingorani AP, Ascher E, Gupta P, et al. Regional anesthesia: preferred technique for venodilatation in the creation of upper extremity arteriovenous fistulae. *Vascular.* 2006;14:23–26.
51. Meena S, Arya V, Sen I, Minz M, Prakash M. Ultrasound-guided supraclavicular brachial plexus anaesthesia improves arteriovenous fistula flow characteristics in end-stage renal disease patients. *Southern African J Anaesth Analg.* 2015;21:131–134.
52. Ismail A, Abushouk AI, Bekhet AH, et al. Regional versus local anesthesia for arteriovenous fistula creation in end-stage renal disease: a systematic review and meta-analysis. *J Vasc Access.* 2017;18:177–184.

53. Al-Jaishi AA, Oliver MJ, Thomas SM, et al. Patency rates of the arteriovenous fistula for hemodialysis: a systematic review and meta-analysis. *Am J Kidney Dis.* 2014;63:464–478.
54. Bergmann L, Martini S, Kesselmeier M, et al. Phrenic nerve block caused by interscalene brachial plexus block: breathing effects of different sites of injection. *BMC Anesthesiol.* 2016;16:45.
55. Neal JM, Gerancher JC, Hebl JR, et al. Upper extremity regional anesthesia: essentials of our current understanding, 2008. *Reg Anesth Pain Med.* 2009;34:134–170.
56. Macfarlane A, Anderson K. Infraclavicular brachial plexus blocks. *BJA Educ.* 2009;9:139–143.
57. Arnuntasupakul V, Leurcharusmee P, Chora De La Garza D, et al. A randomized trial comparing axillary block versus targeted intracluster injection supraclavicular block for upper limb surgery. *Can J Anaesth.* 2015;62:1287–1294.
58. Zhu W, Zhou R, Chen L, et al. The ultrasound-guided selective nerve block in the upper arm: an approach of retaining the motor function in elbow. *BMC Anesthesiol.* 2018;18:143.
59. Matsuda H, Oka Y, Takatsu S, et al. Ultrasound-guided block of selective branches of the brachial plexus for vascular access surgery in the forearm: a preliminary report. *J Vasc Access.* 2016;17:284–290.
60. Yildirim V, Doganci S, Yanarates O, et al. Does preemptive stellate ganglion blockage increase the patency of radiocephalic arteriovenous fistula? *Scand Cardiovasc J.* 2006;40:380–384.
61. Kazemzadeh G-H, Bameshki A, Fathi M, et al. Intravenous regional anesthesia (Bier bock) method for arteriovenous fistula creation in patients with end stage renal disease. *J Surg Trauma.* 2013;1:11–15.
62. Loukas M, Hullett J, Louis RG, Jr., Holdman S, Holdman D. The gross anatomy of the extrathoracic course of the intercostobrachial nerve. *Clin Anat.* 2006;19:106–111.
63. Seidel R, Gray AT, Wree A, Schulze M. Surgery of the axilla with combined brachial plexus and intercostobrachial nerve block in the subpectoral intercostal plane. *Br J Anaesth.* 2017;118:472–474.
64. Moustafa MA, Kandeel AA. Randomized comparative study between two different techniques of intercostobrachial nerve block together with brachial plexus block during superficialization of arteriovenous fistula. *J Anesth.* 2018;32:725–730.
65. Ginosar Y, Weiniger CF, Kurz V, et al. Sympathectomy-mediated vasodilatation: a randomized concentration ranging study of epidural bupivacaine. *Can J Anaesth.* 2009;56:213–221.
66. Svensson CK, Woodruff MN, Baxter JG, Lalka D. Free drug concentration monitoring in clinical practice. Rationale and current status. *Clin Pharmacokinet.* 1986;11:450–469.
67. Pere P, Salonen M, Jokinen M, et al. Pharmacokinetics of ropivacaine in uremic and nonuremic patients after axillary brachial plexus block. *Anesth Analg.* 2003;96:563–569, table of contents.
68. Rice AS, Pither CE, Tucker GT. Plasma concentrations of bupivacaine after supraclavicular brachial plexus blockade in patients with chronic renal failure. *Anaesthesia.* 1991;46:354–357.
69. Crews JC, Weller RS, Moss J, James RL. Levobupivacaine for axillary brachial plexus block: a pharmacokinetic and clinical comparison in patients with normal renal function or renal disease. *Anesth Analg.* 2002;95:219–223, table of contents.
70. Mojica V, Nieuwveld D, Herrera AE, et al. Axillary brachial plexus block duration with mepivacaine in patients with chronic renal failure: case-control study. *Rev Esp Anestesiol Reanim.* 2017;64:192–197.
71. Pere PJ, Ekstrand A, Salonen M, et al. Pharmacokinetics of ropivacaine in patients with chronic renal failure. *Br J Anaesth.* 2011;106:512–521.
72. Stevens RA, Stotz A, Kao TC, et al. The relative increase in skin temperature after stellate ganglion block is predictive of a complete sympathectomy of the hand. *Reg Anesth Pain Med.* 1998;23:266–270.
73. Lo Monte AI, Damiano G, Mularo A, et al. Comparison between local and regional anesthesia in arteriovenous fistula creation. *J Vasc Access.* 2011;12:331–335.
74. Lehtipalo S, Winso O, Koskinen LO, Johansson G, Biber B. Cutaneous sympathetic vasoconstrictor reflexes for the evaluation of interscalene brachial plexus block. *Acta Anaesthesiol Scand.* 2000;44:946–952.
75. Sahin L, Gul R, Mizrak A, et al. Ultrasound-guided infraclavicular brachial plexus block enhances postoperative blood flow in arteriovenous fistulas. *J Vasc Surg.* 2011;54:749–753.
76. Chamberlain DP, Chamberlain BD. Changes in the skin temperature of the trunk and their relationship to sympathetic blockade during spinal anesthesia. *Anesthesiology.* 1986;65:139–143.
77. Malmqvist LA, Bengtsson M, Bjornsson G, Jorfeldt L, Lofstrom JB. Sympathetic activity and haemodynamic variables during spinal analgesia in man. *Acta Anaesthesiol Scand.* 1987;31:467–473.
78. Singh N, Sidawy AN, Dezee K, et al. The effects of the type of anesthesia on outcomes of lower extremity infrainguinal bypass. *J Vasc Surg.* 2006;44:964–968; discussion 968–970.
79. Cerneviciute R, Sahebally SM, Ahmed K, et al. Regional versus local anaesthesia for haemodialysis arteriovenous fistula formation: a systematic review and meta-analysis. *Eur J Vasc Endovasc Surg.* 2017;53:734–742.
80. Wong CS, McNicholas N, Healy D, et al. A systematic review of preoperative duplex ultrasonography and arteriovenous fistula formation. *J Vasc Surg.* 2013;57:1129–1133.
81. Huber TS, Ozaki CK, Flynn TC, et al. Prospective validation of an algorithm to maximize native arteriovenous fistulae for chronic hemodialysis access. *J Vasc Surg.* 2002;36:452–459.
82. Smits JH, Bos C, Elgersma OE, et al. Hemodialysis access imaging: comparison of flow-interrupted contrast-enhanced MR angiography and digital subtraction angiography. *Radiology.* 2002;225:829–834.
83. Laskowski IA, Muhs B, Rockman CR, et al. Regional nerve block allows for optimization of planning in the creation of arteriovenous access for hemodialysis by improving superficial venous dilatation. *Ann Vasc Surg.* 2007;21:730–733.
84. Reynolds TS, Kim KM, Dukkipati R, et al. Pre-operative regional block anesthesia enhances operative strategy for arteriovenous fistula creation. *J Vasc Access.* 2011;12:336–340.
85. Schenk WG 3rd. Improving dialysis access: regional anesthesia improves arteriovenous fistula prevalence. *Am Surg.* 2010;76:938–942.
86. Renaud CJ, Leong CR, Bin HW, Wong JC. Effect of brachial plexus block-driven vascular access planning on primary distal arteriovenous fistula recruitment and outcomes. *J Vasc Surg.* 2015;62:1266–1272.
87. Hui SH, Folsom R, Killewich LA, et al. A comparison of preoperative and intraoperative vein mapping sizes for arteriovenous fistula creation. *J Vasc Surg.* 2018;67:1813–1820.

REVIEW QUESTIONS

(1) A 67-year-old woman with a past medical history of diabetes mellitus and tobacco use has developed end-stage renal disease that requires hemodialysis. Which of the patient factors below places her at increased risk of AVF failure?

A. Age
B. Diabetes mellitus
C. Smoking
D. Female gender

(2) A 49-year-old man with a past medical history of hypertension and diabetes mellitus requires fistula creation for initiation of dialysis. In his preadmission testing visit with the anesthesiologist, the patient asks about the potential benefits of receiving a brachial plexus block compared to local anesthesia infiltration offered by the surgeon. Which of the following are NOT benefits of brachial plexus block over local anesthesia infiltration?

A. Vascular access under local anesthesia is more frequently complicated by vascular spasm.

B. Brachial plexus block achieves significantly better pain control following the procedure and less frequent conversion to general anesthesia.
C. Brachial plexus block provides a greater level of sympathectomy compared to local anesthesia infiltration.
D. The primary patency at 3 month is higher for patients who have arteriovenous fistula under brachial plexus block compared to local anesthesia.

(3) Which regional anesthesia techniques may be an appropriate choice for creation of a radiocephalic arteriovenous fistula?

A. Interscalene block
B. Supraclavicular block
C. Bier block
D. All of the above

(4) While performing a supraclavicular block for an arteriovenous fistula creation for a patient with end-stage renal disease, what dosage of ropivacaine should be used?

A. Increase volume
B. Decrease concentration
C. Decrease concentration
D. None of the above

ANSWERS

(1) **C.** Although female patients present with smaller caliber vasculature, the 1-year patency rate is similar to male patients. Advanced age (defined as 50–70 years old) is correlated to an increased rate of primary radiocephalic fistula failures. Diabetes may decrease arteriovenous fistula patency, which may be offset by using a more proximal arteriovenous fistula location. Smoking has been consistently shown to increase both early and late fistula failure.

Reference

Smith GE, Gohil R, Chetter IC. Factors affecting the patency of arteriovenous fistulas for dialysis access. *J Vasc Surg.* 2012;55:849–855.

(2) **B.** Local anesthetic (LA) infiltration has been shown to have similar postoperative pain control to BPB for AVF creation. Manipulation of small-caliber vessels by the surgeon under LA causes vascular spasms that can be offset by brachial plexus block (BPB) and, to a smaller degree, by general anesthesia, but not by LA. Radiocephalic fistulas have a greater primary patency rate (at 3 months) when performed using a BPB compared to LA. The benefits appear to be related to improved vascular flow secondary to a sympathectomy for patients receiving a BPB.

References

Aitken E, Jackson A, Kearns R, et al. Effect of regional versus local anaesthesia on outcome after arteriovenous fistula creation: a randomised controlled trial. *Lancet.* 2016;388:1067–1074.
Konner K, Nonnast-Daniel B, Ritz E. The arteriovenous fistula. *J Am Soc Nephrol.* 2003;14:1669–1680.
Hingorani AP, Ascher E, Gupta P, et al. Regional anesthesia: preferred technique for venodilatation in the creation of upper extremity arteriovenous fistulae. *Vascular.* 2006;14:23–26.

(3) **D.** An interscalene block provides a consistent blockade of the C5, C6, and C7 nerve roots, but may not be as effective for proximal arteriovenous fistula creation. Supraclavicular and infraclavicular brachial plexus block are two of the most commonly studied regional techniques for arteriovenous fistula and have been shown to be highly successful in providing optimal intraoperative conditions and potentially improved fistula survival. A Bier block can provide satisfactory anesthesia while achieving vasodilation. No definitive evidence exists that identifies any one optimal regional anesthetic that provides reliable intraoperative anesthesia while allowing for improved intermediate and long-term fistula survival.

Reference

Kazemzadeh G-H, Bameshki A, Fathi M, et al. Intravenous regional anesthesia (Bier bock) method for arteriovenous fistula creation in patients with end stage renal disease. *J Surg Trauma.* 2013;1:11–15.

(4) **D.** Patients with end-stage renal disease experience multiple potentially offsetting physiologic changes that can alter the pharmacokinetics and pharmacodynamics of ropivacaine. These may include hypoalbuminemia, elevated cardiac output, metabolic acidosis, underlying neuropathy, and increased levels of α-1-acid glycoprotein that bind local anesthetics. More generally, most commonly used local anesthetics are metabolized by the liver and are minimally altered by isolated changes in renal function. Similar to other regional anesthetics, the dose chosen is specific to each individual situation and should be limited to the minimal effective volume and concentration.

25.

HAND INJURY AND DIGIT REIMPLANTATION

Jennifer Matos and Sylvia H. Wilson

STEM CASE AND KEY QUESTIONS

A 28-year-old, right-hand-dominant fisherman presents to the trauma bay after suffering a severe injury to his right upper extremity. The patient was working on a shrimp boat when his right hand was trapped by a cable and partially drawn into the winch mechanism. In the accident, his thumb was amputated (Figure 25.1).

He also suffered a crush injury to his mid-forehand and a mid-shaft radius fracture. His amputated digit was recovered and brought in on ice with the patient via emergency medical services. The plan is to bring the patient to the operating room in an expedited fashion. You are the anesthesiologist assigned to the room and are called to manage this patient's reimplantation operation.

The patient is brought to the holding area for preoperative preparation and evaluation. The hand surgeon alerts you that the patient is experiencing severe pain. The surgeon asks if you can perform a regional technique to help with pain control and graft survival. You evaluate the patient for any contraindications to the different approaches to the brachial plexus. The patient shows no signs of respiratory compromise and his history is otherwise unremarkable. You deem him eligible to receive a supraclavicular nerve block for pain control and improved graft viability.

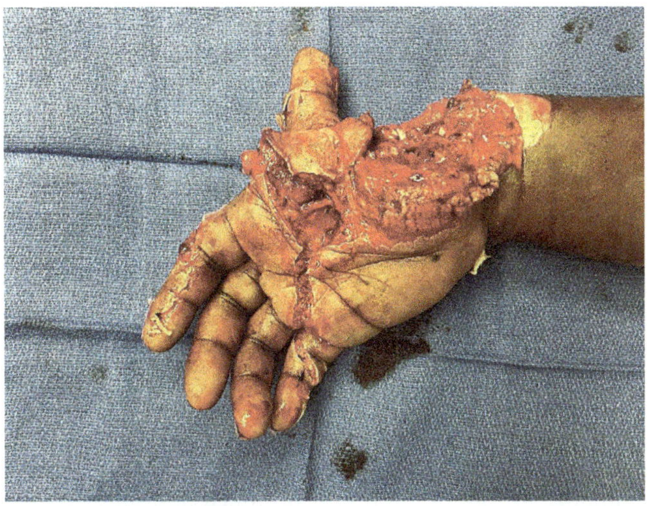

Figure 25.1. Photo of hand injury.

You perform an ultrasound-guided supraclavicular nerve block and leave a catheter for continuous local anesthetic administration. Brachial plexus nerve blocks result in vasodilation of the vasculature supplying the arm and hand and consequently improve blood flow in the vascular anastomoses. Single-injection regional techniques can be performed; however, a perineural catheter provides a continuous infusion of local anesthetic at the target site. Perineural catheters produce a prolonged sympathectomy, resulting in arterial and venous vasodilation and avoidance of vasospasm. Analgesia offered by the perineural catheter also helps with decreasing anxiety and a stress response that can promote vasoconstriction.[1]

In the operating room, standard American Society of Anesthesiologists monitors are placed, and general anesthesia is induced.

Over the next few hours, the patient's blood pressure begins to slowly decline. He has been receiving only maintenance IV fluids. His urine output is marginal, and its appearance is markedly darker. This observation, combined with a high degree of variability on the pulse oximetry waveform, leads you to believe that the patient is intravascularly volume depleted. Thus, you administer an IV 500-mL bolus of an isotonic crystalloid (Plasmalyte) to increase intravascular volume and blood pressure. The patient's blood pressure improves to low-normal levels (90s/60s). You increase his maintenance of IV fluids to improve blood pressure and minimize vasopressor use, which could lead to vasoconstriction and worsening graft perfusion. Your goal is to maintain euvolemia in this patient, as microvascular anastomosis for free flaps have been shown to be subject to interstitial edema in the setting of hypervolemia.

The operating room personnel note that the room is warm and decrease the ambient room temperature from 72°F to 65°F because the patient's core temperature is 36.5°C. However, the patient's temperature lowers to 36.1°C over 20 minutes. You notice this temperature change and find that the forced-air warmer was unplugged for the surgeon's head lamp. You immediately reconnect the forced-air warmer and rewarm the room to optimize vasodilation of the anastomotic site.

At the end of the operation, the surgeon expresses concern about the functional viability of the replantation. She attributes this to the profound extent of the crush injury, which necessitated significant debridement of tissue, extensive microvascular anastomosis and repair, and a prolonged warm ischemic time prior to complete reimplantation. After the patient emerges from general anesthesia, he is moved to his hospital bed with the operative extremity elevated above his heart to aid in venous drainage.

To optimize his postoperative management, the surgical team places detailed orders for his postoperative care. He requires continuous pulse oximetry monitoring measurements on the injured extremity and a warm room. He needs hourly Doppler flowmeter/neurological checks for the first 12 hours and then every 2 hours thereafter. His dressings require regular assessment to ensure that they are not constricting the surgical site and leading to decreased blood flow from compression of the microvasculature. Subcutaneous heparin is initiated for thrombotic prophylaxis.

Given the fractures and extensive crush injury to the operative extremity, the surgical team is concerned that the patient may develop compartment syndrome. The team asks you if the continuous brachial plexus nerve block will mask compartment syndrome should it develop. You concur that compartment syndrome is a very serious potential complication. Increased intracompartmental pressures can lead to diminished blood flow with irreversible damage to muscles and nerves. Treatment requires prompt recognition and emergent surgical decompression and debridement. However, multiple case reports have found that continuous peripheral nerve blocks do not mask an evolving compartment syndrome. These published reports have shown that an increasing severity of pain in the setting of a functioning peripheral nerve block (motor and sensory blockade) is a hallmark of compartment syndrome. You advise the surgeon and the patient's nurse to alert the regional anesthesia pain team for further assessment if the patient has symptoms concerning the development of compartment syndrome. Specifically, they should call if the patient develops increased pain that is not controlled with medications, requires escalated doses of pain medications, or experiences amplified pain with a passive stretch of the extremity.

The acute pain service rounds on the patient daily and manages the supraclavicular catheter. On postoperative day 3, the patient complains of increased pain to his hand. He has motor blockade of the extremity, evidenced by his inability to abduct his arm at the shoulder. He also has an extensive dressing covering his hand, forearm, elbow, and distal humerus. Thus, you are able to assess sensory blockade only at the mid-humerus (proximal to the dressing) and at the distal fifth digit (distal to the dressing). He is unable to distinguish sharp sensations in these areas. However, he does complain of sharp pains and intense pressure in the hand and replanted digit that has worsened significantly over the last several hours. Your resident asks whether the patient may be experiencing tachyphylaxis to the local anesthetic. While that is a possibility, the literature supporting tachyphylaxis to local anesthetics is not as well-defined as it is for other medications. Some earlier investigators found it in a large proportion of their subjects, whereas others have found it in very few or none, making its incidence and mechanism unclear. Newer meta-analyses have confirmed the rarity of tachyphylaxis to local anesthetics, calling into question the clinical significance of the condition.

You are more concerned with graft failure causing tissue ischemia and necrosis, given that analgesic peripheral nerve blocks using low concentrations of local anesthetics do not mask pain from ischemia. However, surgical anesthetic blocks may delay the signs and symptoms of ischemic pain. The precise mechanism of action of ischemic pain is poorly understood, and it has been suggested that it should be classified differently than nociceptive pain to heat/cold or neuropathic pain. Ischemic pain may involve pathways not blocked by perineural blockade. Clinically, patients who undergo a surgical peripheral nerve block show signs of discomfort, including elevated blood pressure and heart rate, 1–1.5 hours after tourniquet inflation (ischemic time). Similarly, one case report described a patient who underwent ankle reconstruction under regional anesthesia and experienced worsened pain 90 minutes after cast placement. The cast caused compression and ischemia of the medial side of his ankle, and immediate pain relief occurred with cast removal.

You immediately page the surgeon and discuss your concerns. She arrives at the bedside quickly, assesses the patient, and agrees with your diagnosis. The operating room is called to have an emergent room set up for revision surgery. Unfortunately, while the patient is being transported to the operating room and moved to the operating room table, the supraclavicular catheter becomes inadvertently dislodged.

The anesthesia and surgical teams discuss possible replacement of the brachial plexus nerve block. Some team members express concern that the brachial plexus block may mask recognition of compartment syndrome and graft failure. You explain that the patient was successfully diagnosed with graft failure secondary to increasing pain despite having the peripheral nerve block in place; therefore, this should not prohibit perineural catheter replacement. Additionally, as brachial plexus nerve blocks promote graft survival by improving blood flow and reducing vasospasm, it is prudent to replace the brachial plexus catheter for this patient. The surgeon agrees and an infraclavicular catheter is placed in the post-anesthesia recovery area.

The patient's pain is well controlled postoperatively. On postoperative day 2 after his reoperation, he asks about the overall plan for pain control for his hand in the hospital and longer term. You discuss the general course of acute pain healing and the potential for chronic pain to develop after trauma. As the fisherman depends on his hands for his livelihood, he is very concerned about the possibility of developing chronic pain and requests more information.

CPSP syndrome, or chronic (persistent) postsurgical pain, is defined as pain lasting over 3–6 months after surgery. The incidence of CPSP varies widely. While some publications report some degree of pain or discomfort in 10%–30% of patients after 1 year, other reports describe CPSP in 5%–85%, depending on the surgery.[2,3] This incidence increases after traumas that involve nerve injury. The patient is noticeably apprehensive about the potential for developing CPSP due to his risk factors. To allay some of his fears, you inform him that the acute pain team and his surgical team have collaborated to minimize his risk of CPSP. Uncontrolled postoperative pain can lead to central sensitization, leading to an amplified pain response and long-term potentiation of the pain response. The plan is for him to use a multimodal analgesic regimen, which includes his peripheral nerve block combined with oral and IV pain medications, to decrease the risk of CPSP. Given that the most consistent risk factor for CPSP is the duration of severe postoperative pain, aggressively managing his pain in the immediate postsurgical period is the best method to minimize his risk of developing CPSP.[4]

(1) WHAT REGIONAL TECHNIQUES HELP WITH PAIN MANAGEMENT IN A PATIENT WITH CRUSH INJURY TO THE HAND AND FOREARM?

Brachial plexus nerve blocks below the level of the interscalene can be used for pain control for injury to the hand and forearm. Supraclavicular, infraclavicular, and axillary approaches have been used in these patients with good effect.

(2) IS THERE A RISK OF TACHYPHYLAXIS IN A PATIENT RECEIVING A CONTINUOUS INFUSION OF LOCAL ANESTHETIC THROUGH A REGIONAL ANESTHETIC CATHETER?

Given that tachyphylaxis is a rare occurrence, there is a low risk of tachyphylaxis with continuous infusions of local anesthetics. It is an unproven phenomenon and may contribute much less to rebound pain than previously described.

(3) WHAT IS THE IMPACT OF BRACHIAL PLEXUS NERVE BLOCK ON VASCULAR TONE?

Brachial plexus nerve blocks result in a sympathectomy to the extremity which leads to decreased vascular tone (reduced vasospasm) and improved blood flow.

(4) WHAT ARE ANESTHETIC CONSIDERATIONS THAT IMPACT GRAFT SURVIVAL?

Anesthetic considerations for graft survival include blood pressure and euvolemic intravascular volume status to maintain appropriate blood flow to the extremity, ambient temperature (as cold leads to vasoconstriction and decreased perfusion), and appropriate pain and anxiety control to decrease the stress response and resulting vasoconstriction.

(5) WHAT ARE THE RISK FACTORS FOR THE DEVELOPMENT OF CHRONIC POSTSURGICAL PAIN (CPSP)?

Risk factors for CPSP are injuries resulting in nerve injury, uncontrolled perioperative pain, anxiety or catastrophizing psychological personality, longer surgical duration, younger patients, female patients, and certain surgical procedures (amputations, thoracotomy, breast surgery, and cardiac surgery).

DISCUSSION

According to the US Centers for Disease Control and Prevention, the most commonly injured body sites are the wrist, hand, and fingers. Over 1 million patients with hand traumas visit the emergency department annually.[5] Amputations, partial amputations, crush injuries, and fractures account for 15% of these injuries.[6] Amputations and partial amputations of digits or hands result in significant functional loss, pain, and psychological trauma. Reimplantation of amputated digits leads to decreased pain, better patient satisfaction and appearance, and improvement in functional outcome, as evidenced by decreased disability scores.[7] Such reimplantations should be performed at institutions that specialize in microvascular surgery and have appropriate surgical and support staff.[8] In many institutions that perform reimplantations, intraoperative anesthesia usually consists of a combination of general anesthesia and regional anesthesia to optimize analgesia, immobilization (minimizes movement that can cause further damage to joints, bones, tissues, and vessels to optimize future function), and vascular tone. In the postoperative period, a surgical block is not required to achieve the desired decreased motor function. For example, low concentrations of local anesthetic can provide motor and sensory blockade of the peroneal nerve.[9] Well-placed perineural catheters should be able to decrease motor function with less-concentrated local anesthetics.

BRACHIAL PLEXUS ANATOMY AND REGIONAL ANESTHESIA TECHNIQUES

The brachial plexus arises from the ventral rami of C5 to T1 and provides innervation to almost all upper extremity dermatomes and all osteotomes. These rami combine to form three trunks (superior, middle, and inferior) that then divide into anterior and posterior divisions. The divisions then unite into three cords (lateral, posterior, and medial) before dividing into terminal branches of individual peripheral nerves. The main peripheral nerves stemming from the brachial plexus include the axillary, median, musculocutaneous, radial, and ulnar nerves; however, numerous other terminal nerves also arise, including the medial brachial and antebrachial cutaneous, the medial and lateral pectoral, and the suprascapular nerve. Notably, the intercostal brachial nerve supplies innervation to the medial upper arm but arises from the T2 intercostal nerve and is not part of the brachial plexus.

Regional anesthesia of the brachial plexus is commonly achieved with four approaches: interscalene, supraclavicular, infraclavicular, and/or axillary (Table 25.1). The interscalene approach targets the roots/trunks as they pass between the anterior and middle scalene muscles. It is used to anesthetize the shoulder and proximal third of the humerus and is associated with sparing the ulnar nerve. Because the phrenic nerve passes in proximity, ipsilateral phrenic nerve blockade and consequent ipsilateral diaphragmatic paralysis should be anticipated with all interscalene nerve blocks. Recurrent laryngeal nerve blockade, although less common, may also occur. The supraclavicular approach blocks the plexus trunks/

Table 25.1 SUMMARY OF BRACHIAL PLEXUS BLOCKS

APPROACH	LEVEL	COVERAGE	BENEFITS	CONSIDERATIONS
Interscalene	Roots/trunks	Shoulder and proximal humerus	Superficial location	Phrenic nerve blockade; possible SLN blockade; ulnar sparing
Supraclavicular	Trunks/divisions	Mid-humerus and distal	Superficial location; compact nerve arrangement	Concern for pneumothorax; possible phrenic nerve blockade; possible SLN blockade
Infraclavicular	Cords	Mid-humerus and distal	Low risk for phrenic or superior laryngeal nerve blockade	Deep location
Axillary	Terminal branches	Distal humerus and beyond	Superficial location	Does not block axillary nerve

SLN = Superior laryngeal nerve.

divisions and is an appropriate choice for surgeries or injuries distal to the mid-humerus. In this approach, the brachial plexus is compact, superficial, and easily located by ultrasonography posterolateral to the subclavian artery in the midclavicular line as the subclavian artery passes over the first rib. These features allow for a quick and well-tolerated approach to anesthetize the brachial plexus. Potential complications to the supraclavicular approach include the pneumothorax and phrenic nerve blockades. Although historically the rate of pneumothorax with the supraclavicular approach is quoted to be 0.5%–6% with nerve stimulation, a 0% pneumothorax rate was more recently reported in a review of ultrasound-guided blocks at a training institution.[10,11] Compared to the interscalene approach, phrenic nerve block is less common (36%–67%) but must still be considered in patients with preexisting pulmonary disease.[12] The infraclavicular block is placed below the clavicle at the level of the brachial plexus cords and is appropriate for surgeries distal to the mid-humerus. In terms of block success and density, the infraclavicular block is equivalent to the supraclavicular approach and is associated with reduced tourniquet pain compared to the axillary approach. However, the deeper location and nearby coracoid and clavicle necessitate an acute angle of needle insertion. Consequently, infraclavicular block placement is often more challenging compared to other approaches.

The axillary approach to the brachial plexus targets four terminal nerves: musculocutaneous, median, radial, and ulnar. It does not anesthetize the axillary nerve, which has already branched off the posterior cord. Ultrasonography is frequently used to visualize the nerves because they surround the axillary artery in the axilla or deltopectoral groove. The musculocutaneous nerve is often located further from the artery and is easily found between the biceps and coracobracialis muscles or within the coracobracialis muscle. Although this approach is appropriate for surgeries beyond the distal humerus, some minor nerve branches (e.g., the medial brachial cutaneous) are not blocked at this location. These nerves supply sensory innervation only and may be blocked individually; however, they may be difficult to identify. In addition, because the nerves are more spread out compared with supra- or infraclavicular approaches, the axillary approach may be less effective for continuous perineural techniques. However, the superficial location and lack of impact on the phrenic and recurrent laryngeal nerves make the axillary approach extremely useful in medically complicated and/or morbidly obese patients.

The brachial plexus is commonly targeted distal to the roots for trauma injuries to the elbow, forearm, and/or hand. Supraclavicular brachial plexus blocks have been effective for hand trauma and reimplantation of digits. The compact nerve arrangement and superficial location of the supraclavicular approach allow for straightforward ultrasound visualization to aid in block placement; however, its superficial location may increase the risk of catheter dislodgement. Conversely, the infraclavicular block may be especially useful in trauma patients when a supraclavicular approach is impeded by a cervical collar or contraindicated by potential hemidiaphragmatic paresis. As the needle traverses the pectoralis major and minor muscle, perineural catheters are also well anchored, decreasing the risk of inadvertent displacement. Case series have also reported success with axillary brachial plexus blocks. In a case series of 18 patients, Su et al. examined the survival of crushed digits after reimplantation and skin temperature (as an index of tissue perfusion).[13] They found a trend toward increased skin temperature in the group with the continuous axillary brachial plexus block and attributed their findings to improved tissue perfusion. Similarly, in a series of 5 patients, Berger et al. found that continuous axillary brachial plexus blocks help with healing and graft survival in patients undergoing reimplantation of digits and toe–finger transfers.[14]

BRACHIAL PLEXUS NERVE BLOCKS AND VASCULAR TONE

Nerve blocks targeting the brachial plexus cause sympathetic blockade of the vasculature in the upper extremity. This sympathetic inhibition results in arterial and venous vasodilation, improved blood flow, and reduced vasospasm.[15,16] Following arteriovenous fistula creation, sympathectomy and vessel dilation have been found immediately after brachial plexus block placement.[14] Consequently, regional blockade of the brachial plexus has led to better patency rates of the vessels in arteriovenous fistula creation.[16]

It is also notable that sympathectomy occurs regardless of the approach to the brachial plexus. Several reports have described these results with supraclavicular nerve blocks, and Breschan et al. described similar results with an axillary brachial plexus block.[15–17] In this case report, a single-injection technique was used in a neonate with severe forearm and hand ischemia after radial and ulnar arterial catheterization. Successful regional blockade produced regression of the blanching and discoloration of the forearm and forehand, which was attributed to improved vasodilation and decreased vasospasm.

REGIONAL ANESTHESIA AND GRAFT SURVIVAL

Brachial plexus nerve blocks have been used to improve analgesia and tissue perfusion for decades. The digits of the hand are more vulnerable to ischemia during microvascular anastomosis as the digital vessels are susceptible to vasospasm. Consequently, continuous perineural blockade has been used for its sympatholytic property to avoid vasospasm and has been shown to aid in the survival of replanted and revascularized digits.[1,18] In the 1980s, Berger et al. published a series of 5 patients who underwent finger replantation, toe–finger transfers, or finger–finger transfers with the aid of axillary plexus catheters.[14] The patients showed improved pain control, improved vascular flow, and decreased muscle activity, helping the digits to heal. In a larger study by Su et al., patients underwent general anesthesia for the replantation of crushed digits and received ultrasound-guided axillary brachial plexus blocks with ropivacaine infusions.[13] Temperature measurement was used as a marker of graft perfusion, and the authors found a trend toward increased skin temperature in patients with continuous nerve blocks. They concluded that increased tissue perfusion leads to improved graft survival of transplanted fingers. Vascular Doppler is also commonly used to assess the presence of blood flow following hand trauma.

OTHER CONSIDERATIONS IMPACTING GRAFT SURVIVAL

Successful graft survival is influenced by anesthetic considerations and surgical/non-anesthetic conditions.

NON-ANESTHETIC CONSIDERATIONS

An important factor influencing graft survival is the ischemic time of the transplanted digit. The time between amputation and reimplantation should be minimized as much as possible. For the reimplantation of digits, the warm ischemia time should be kept to 12 hours or less, whereas cold ischemia time can be up to 24 hours.[7] In addition to the ischemic time, the functional recovery of the replantation depends on successful microvascular anastomosis, coupled with the appropriate debridement of tissues and adequate repair of bone, tendon, skin, and nervous tissue.[7]

ANESTHETIC CONSIDERATIONS

The anesthetic goals for these patients are to provide optimum anesthesia and analgesia while avoiding circumstances that can lead to anastomotic impairment and vasoconstriction. Notably, pain and anxiety can cause a stress response and trigger vasoconstriction, which further emphasizes the importance of aggressive analgesic management.[1]

Hemodynamic Management

The use of vasoconstrictors for microvascular hand surgery is debated. Vasoconstrictors, specifically alpha-adrenergic receptor agonists (phenylephrine), can theoretically lead to decreased blood flow to the graft tissue, causing poor perfusion and graft failure. However, this theoretical concern has been questioned in the literature. For example, intraoperative vasopressor use was not associated with complications or the failure rate of free tissue transfers in head and neck surgery.[19] Nonetheless, many institutions and surgeons performing microvascular surgical techniques of this type try to avoid phenylephrine administration.[20] Dopamine is administered as an alternative for these patients because its inotropic and chronotropic effects can increase cardiac output and blood pressure. Regardless of the methods used, it is imperative that patients remain euvolemic. Because hypervolemia has been linked to extravasation and increased interstitial fluid, a blood pressure management plan cannot simply involve fluid administration. In this regard, prior studies have suggested algorithms for fluid and vasopressor administration involving minimally invasive cardiac output monitoring devices.

Intraoperative Access and Monitoring

In addition to standard American Society of Anesthesiologists monitors, adequate IV access must be obtained in patients undergoing microvascular surgery. For hand surgery, this access is obtained on the contralateral upper extremity and, less desirably, in the lower extremities if needed. If patients have extensive trauma to both upper extremities or have numerous traumatic injuries, further access may be obtained centrally.

POSTOPERATIVE CONCERNS FOLLOWING HAND TRAUMA

COMPARTMENT SYNDROME

Compartment syndrome is a serious complication of trauma to an extremity that can have devastating consequences. While normal compartment pressures vary between 0 and 25 mmHg, osseo-fascial swelling from trauma can lead to increased pressures within a confined myofascial compartment.[21] Without decompression, elevated pressures cause capillary bed collapse. This leads to decreased tissue perfusion and results in ischemia, necrosis, and nerve damage. These complications are compounded by increased capillary permeability and interstitial leakage into the compartment, which further raises compartment pressures.[21] If it is not promptly recognized, compartment syndrome can lead to the loss of the affected limb or even death. Amputation rates from compartment syndrome range from 11% to 21%, with mortality rates of 11%–15%.

Risk factors for compartment syndrome include male gender, age younger than 35 years old, and fracture of the tibia or forearm. Compartment syndrome is most likely to occur in the forearm and lower leg, with compartment syndrome of the hand being relatively uncommon.[22,23] Compartment syndrome is most common in lower extremity trauma, with an incidence of 1.5%–29% in closed tibial fractures and 1.2%–10.2% in open tibial fractures.[24]

Diagnosis is often based on clinical suspicion. Patients often report pain out of proportion to what is expected with the injury, which is exacerbated with passive stretching.[25] Frequent patient evaluation and an elevated index of suspicion are essential to recognize compartment syndrome early and to minimize sequelae. Measurement of compartment pressures may also be used in certain patients for early detection. These measurements may be obtained using a hand-held manometer, a simple needle manometer system, or a slit catheter technique. Regardless of which method is used, accuracy depends on properly calibrating the measuring device, along with proper placement of the needle and transducer. The needle should be placed within 5 cm of the fracture or reimplanted site; accuracy decreases the further away the measurement is taken. Conversely, measurements may be inaccurately elevated if they are immediately adjacent to the site. Absolute pressures or a Δ pressure (diastolic blood pressure–compartment pressure) may be used. An absolute pressure greater than 25–30 mmHg or a Δ pressure of less than 35 mmHg is suggestive of compartment syndrome and has been used as a cutoff for fasciotomy. However, a single normal reading does not rule out acute compartment syndrome. These measurements may need to be taken serially and correlated with the patient's clinical picture. Because few studies have examined compartment measurements, the specificity and sensitivity of these measurements are not truly known. In addition, most of the published data are on lower extremity trauma, specifically tibial fractures, and may not be applicable to other muscle compartments.

Specific to upper extremity trauma, the most common sign of compartment syndrome is hand swelling. Patients report tightness, weakness or paralysis, and paresthesias in the affected limb, and pain is often out of proportion to the injury.[25] Once diagnosed, immediate fasciotomy is indicated to prevent worsening muscle and nerve damage. This is a time-sensitive process. While muscle and nerve damage occurs in all patients with compartment syndrome, this injury is often reversible, even after 4 hours of elevated compartment pressures. However, irreversible damage may occur within 8 hours of elevated compartment pressures, necessitating prompt operative intervention for the release of high compartment pressures and debridement of necrotic tissue.

Regional analgesic techniques for trauma patients at risk for compartment syndrome remain controversial. Although published case reports have highlighted that peripheral nerve blocks will not mask compartment syndrome, vigilance is paramount.[26,27] Patients should be assessed frequently. Because awareness is needed from all healthcare team members, nurses caring for trauma patients should also receive education regarding compartment syndrome and be encouraged to expeditiously notify anesthesia and surgical teams in the event of a dramatic increase in pain.

POSTOPERATIVE GRAFT FAILURE AND REOPERATION

The goal of reimplantation surgery is to perform optimal tissue debridement and effective microvascular anastomosis so that reoperation is not necessary. However, graft failure can occur because of arterial or venous insufficiency, clot formation, or external constriction of the appendage. To avoid thrombosis of the digital arteries, some institutions have introduced an anticoagulation protocol such as an IV infusion of heparin, subcutaneous low-molecular-weight heparin, or oral aspirin therapy. Because there have been no randomized studies on the use of anticoagulation, or specific anticoagulation therapies, this is not a standard regimen at centers performing microvascular anastomosis for hand reimplantation, and protocols may vary.

Digital vessels are highly susceptible to vasospasm, resulting in decreased blood flow and ischemia. These injured and amputated digits have poorer graft survival rates and worse functional outcomes. In a recent paper by Chinta et al., the authors found an overall reoperative rate of 25% for patients undergoing initial replantation or amputation surgery.[28] The success rate for patients requiring reoperation is 9%–89%.[29] Given the significant decline in functional success of these reoperative cases, steps should be taken to maximize graft survival potential for the initial surgery.

Multiple studies have shown improvement in blood flow and prevention of neurally mediated vasospasm with brachial plexus blocks.[1,13,15,18] Therefore, it is prudent to maintain these blocks in the perioperative period for these patients. Brachial plexus blockade provides analgesia and promotes vasodilation. With such benefits, it is imperative that their replacement be considered if perineural catheters are dislodged early in the perioperative period.

TACHYPHYLAXIS

Tachyphylaxis is the rapid appearance of a progressive decrease in the response to a pharmacologically or physiologically active substance after repetitive administration. Whether these changes are caused by alterations in pharmacodynamics or pharmacokinetics is unclear. Depletion of neurotransmitters has been implicated in certain medications such as amphetamines, antidepressants, and ephedrine.

The question of tachyphylaxis to local anesthetics has been debated for decades. Some authors have reported that it did occur in their study populations, whereas other authors have noted the condition in a few to the majority of their examined subjects. Given the wide variation in findings, there is disagreement on the mechanisms for tachyphylaxis and its true prevalence. Scott et al. questioned whether local anesthetics lead to tachyphylaxis. The study postulated that an observed decrease in local anesthetic effectiveness may occur with an increase in the anatomic distribution of the local anesthetic or an escalation of the underlying pain severity, such as breakthrough pain from worsening ischemia not blocked by a peripheral nerve block.[30]

CHRONIC POSTSURGICAL PAIN (CPSP)

CPSP is defined as pain that persists over 3–6 months postoperatively or after normal healing of tissues has occurred (Table 25.2). This chronic pain may be severe 2%–10% of the time for patients.[31] Although the incidence of CPSP varies after several common surgical procedures, surgeries with the highest incidence of CPSP are amputations, thoracotomies, breast surgery, and cardiac surgery.[31] Furthermore, over 20% of patients in pain clinics reported surgery as the precipitating event for their chronic pain.[32] Over 20% of all surgical patients develop chronic pain, but 22%–96% of trauma patients experience chronic pain.[33,34] In one study, 69% of patients who experience major trauma reported pain 6 years after the trauma, and 24% of these patients said they had severe pain.[33] The severity of the trauma was correlated with the frequency of developing chronic pain. In addition to surgical type, other risk factors for developing CPSP include the presence of inadequately treated preoperative pain, psychological characteristics of anxiety or catastrophizing, female gender, younger patients, surgical approach with increased risk of nerve damage (e.g., stretching, transection), increased surgical duration, and the intensity of pain in the immediate postoperative period.[4] Specifically, patients who experience uncontrolled pain in the first few days after surgery have an increased risk of developing CPSP. The prevention of CPSP relies on a multimodal approach to pain management.

Table 25.2 CHARACTERISTICS OF CHRONIC POSTSURGICAL PAIN

Description	Pain lasting over 3–6 months after surgery Also called persistent postsurgical pain
Incidence	Highly variable: All surgical patients: 10%–30%[2] to 5%–85%[3] Trauma patients: 22%–96%[33,34] (incidence increased with increased severity of trauma)
Risk factors[4]	Inadequately treated preoperative pain Psychological characteristics of anxiety or catastrophizing Female gender Younger patient age Surgical approach with increased risk of nerve damage (e.g., stretching, transection) Surgical type: amputations, thoracotomies, breast surgery, and cardiac surgery[30] Increased surgical duration Intense pain in the immediate postoperative period

COMPLEX REGIONAL PAIN SYNDROME (CRPS)

CRPS is a chronic neurologic disorder that usually occurs after minor trauma or nerve injury. The hallmarks of CRPS are pain, vasomotor changes, swelling, sudomotor changes, and changes in motor function of the affected limb. The pain is debilitating and out of proportion to the severity of the inciting injury.[35]

CRPS is separated into two types: CRPS1 and CRPS2. CRPS1 is the result of trauma but without a confirmed nerve injury. CRPS2 occurs in patients who have a defined nerve injury. The reasons that certain patients develop CRPS while others do not are poorly understood. Regardless of the type of CRPS, treatment modalities are similar and include rehabilitation with physical therapy, psychotherapy, and medications (nonsteroidal anti-inflammatory medications, steroids, gabapentinoids, NMDA receptor antagonists, and topical creams). Sympathectomy by brachial plexus nerve blockade can provide short-term relief, while more invasive procedures (e.g., neural stimulation or intrathecal drugs devices) are reserved for unrelieved pain.

CONCLUSIONS

- In patients with hand trauma, brachial plexus blocks offer the benefits of analgesia, coupled with sympathetic inhibition and improved vascular blood flow.
- The brachial plexus may be blocked by supraclavicular, infraclavicular, or axillary approaches when injuries are distal to the mid-humerus.
- Aggressive postoperative pain management that includes a multimodal approach with a brachial plexus perineural catheter may reduce rates of patients developing chronic pain.
- As compartment syndrome is associated with significant morbidity and mortality, patients with forearm injuries receiving brachial plexus blocks require a care team with close and clear communication and collaboration with nursing staff to minimize patient risk and allow early detection of possible compartment syndrome.

REFERENCES

1. Kurt E, Ozturk S, Isik S, Zor F. Continuous brachial plexus blockade for digital replantations and toe-to-hand transfers. *Ann Plast Surg*. 2005;54:24–27.
2. Bruce J, Quinlan J. Chronic post surgical pain. *Rev Pain*. 2011;5:23–29.
3. Macrae WA. Chronic post-surgical pain: 10 years on. *Br J Anaesth*. 2008;101:77–86.
4. Thapa P, Euasobhon P. Chronic postsurgical pain: current evidence for prevention and management. *Korean J Pain*. 2018;31:155–173.

5. Pitts SR, Niska RW, Xu J, Burt CW. National hospital ambulatory medical care survey: 2006 emergency department summary. *Natl Health Stat Report*. 2008;(7):1–38.
6. Welch LS, Hunting KL, Murawski JA. Occupational injuries among construction workers treated in a major metropolitan emergency department in the United States. *Sand J Work Environ Health*. 2005;31 Suppl 2:11–21.
7. Maricevich M, Carlsen B, Mardini SM. Upper extremity and digital replantation. *Hand (NY)*. 2011;6:356–363.
8. Jazayeri L, Klausner JQ, Chang J. Distal digital replantation. *Plast Reconstr Surg*. 2013;132:1207–1217.
9. Christiansen CB, Hadsen MH, Rothe C, Andreasen AM, Lundstrøm LH, Lange KHW. Volume of ropivacaine 0.2% and common peroneal nerve block duration: a randomized, double-blind cohort trial in healthy volunteers. *Anaestheasia*. 2018;73:1361–1367.
10. Kumari A, Gupta R, Bhardwaj A, Madan D. Delayed pneumothorax after supraclavicular block. *J Anaesthesiol Clin Pharmacol*. 2011;27:121–122.
11. Kakazu C, Tokhner V, Li J, Ou R, Simmons E. In the new era of ultrasound guidance: is pneumothorax from supraclavicular block a rare complication of the past? *Br J Anaesth*. 2014;113:190–191.
12. Bigeleisen PE. Anatomical variations of the phrenic nerve and its clinical implication for supraclavicular block. *Br J Anaesth*. 2003;91:916–917.
13. Su HH, Lui PW, Yu CL, et al. The effects of continuous axillary brachial plexus block with ropivacaine infusion on skin temperature and survival of crushed fingers after microsurgical replantation. *Chang Gung Med J*. 2005:28:567–574.
14. Berger A, Tizian C, Zenz M. Continuous plexus blockade for improved circulation in microvascular surgery. *Ann Plast Surg*. 1985;14:16–19.
15. Shemesh D, Raikhinstein Y, Goldin I, Olsha O. General, regional or local anesthesia for successful radial cephalic arteriovenous fistula. *J Vas Access*. 2017;18(Suppl 1):24–28.
16. Aitken E, Jackson A, Kearns R, et al. Effect of regional versus local anaesthesia on outcome after arteriovenous fistula creation: a randomised controlled trial. *Lancet*. 2016;388:1067–1074.
17. Breschan C, Kraschl R, Jost R, Marhofer P, Likar R. Axillary brachial plexus block for the treatment of severe forearm ischemia after arterial cannulation in an extremely low birth-weight infant. *Paediatr Anaesth*. 2004;14:681–684.
18. Taras JS, Behrman MJ. Continuous peripheral nerve block in replantation and revascularization. *J Reconstr Microsurg*. 1998;14:17–21.
19. Hand WR, McSwain JR, McEvoy MD, et al. Characteristics and intraoperative treatments associated with head and neck free tissue transfer complications and failures. *Otolaryngol Head Neck Surg*. 2015;152:480–487.
20. Lang RS, Gorantla VS, Esper S, et al. Anesthetic management in upper extremity transplantation: the Pittsburgh experience. *Anesth Analg*. 2012;115:678–688.
21. Oak NR, Abrams RA. Compartment syndrome of the hand. *Orthop Clin North Am*. 2016;47:609–616.
22. McQueen MM, Gaston P, Court-Brown CM. Acute compartment syndrome: who is at risk? *J Bone Joint Surg Br*. 2000;82: 200–203.
23. Choi JJ, Lin E, Gasden J. Regional anesthesia for trauma outside the operating theatre. *Curr Opin Anaesthesiol*. 2013;26:495–500.
24. Heemskerk J, Kitslaar P. Acute compartment syndrome of the lower leg: retrospective study on prevalence, technique, and outcome of fasciotomies. *World J Surg*. 2003;27:744–747.
25. Mehta V, Chowdhary V, Lin C, Jbara M, Hanna S. Compartment syndrome of the hand: a case report and review of the literature. *Radiol Case Rep*. 2018;13:212–215.
26. Walker BJ, Noonan KJ, Bosenberg AT. Evolving compartment syndrome not masked by continuous peripheral nerve block: evidence-based case management. *Reg Anesth Pain Med*. 2012;37:393–397.
27. Rauf J, Iohom G, O'Donnell B. Acute compartment syndrome and regional anesthesia: a case report. *Rom J Anaesth Intensive Care*. 2015;22:51–54.
28. Chinta M, Wilkens SC, Vlot MA, Chen NC, Eberlin KR. Secondary surgery following initial replantation/revascularization or completion amputation in the hand or digits. *Plast Reconstr Surg*. 2018;142:709–716.
29. Pederson WC. Replantation. *Plast Reconstr Surg*. 2001;107:823–841.
30. Kucera TJ, Boezaart AP. Regional anesthesia does not consistently block ischemic pain: two further cases and a review of the literature. *Pain Med*. 2014;15:316–319.
31. Correll D. Chronic postoperative pain: recent findings in understanding and management. *F1000Res*. 2017;6:1054.
32. Reddi D, Curran N. Chronic pain after surgery: pathophysiology, risk factors and prevention. *Postgrad Med J*. 2014;90:222–227.
33. Kolstadbraaten KM, Spreng UJ, Wisloeff-Aase K, Gaarder C, Naess PA, Raeder J. Incidence of chronic pain 6 y after major trauma. *Acta Anaesthesiol Scand*. 2019;63:1074–1078.
34. Daoust R, Paquet J, Moore L, et al. Early factors associated with the development of chronic pain in trauma patients. *Pain Res Manag*. 2018;2018:7203218.
35. Albazaz R, Wong YT, Homer-Vanniasinkam S. Complex regional pain syndrome: a review. *Ann Vasc Surg*. 2008;22:297–306.

REVIEW QUESTIONS

(1) Regional anesthesia is planned for a patient undergoing operative fixation of a distal radius fracture. Which of the following approaches to the brachial plexus is most likely to provide adequate surgical coverage?

A. Axillary
B. Infraclavicular
C. Supraclavicular
D. All the above

(2) A 20-year-old woman presents following a motor vehicle collision in which she suffered crush injuries to her left hand and wrist. She also has a left radial artery transection. Her family requests a perineural brachial plexus catheter to minimize postoperative opiates. Which of the following variables is the strongest indication for brachial plexus blockade in the acute, perioperative period?

A. History of anxiety
B. History of smoking
C. Radial artery transection
D. Radius fracture

(3) A brachial plexus perineural catheter is requested for a morbidly obese patient undergoing digit reimplantation. Which of the following best describes a benefit of the supraclavicular approach to brachial plexus blockade over the infraclavicular approach?

A. Muscles anchor the perineural catheter
B. Proximity to lungs
C. Superficial block location
D. Widespread nerve arrangement

(4) Which of the following is a benefit of brachial plexus blockade after hand trauma?

A. Arterial vasodilation
B. Improved analgesia
C. Reduced vasospasm
D. All the above

(5) The surgery team is concerned that an 83-year-old man with a distal radius fracture and an indwelling infraclavicular catheter (0.2% ropivacaine at 7 mL/h) may be developing compartment syndrome. Which of the following is most likely to be present on examination of the patient's hand if he is developing compartment syndrome?

A. Erythema
B. Paresthesias
C. Swelling
D. Weakness

(6) Compartment syndrome is diagnosed in a patient with a tibial fracture. How long after compartment pressures are elevated may irreversible tissue damage occur?

A. 1 hour
B. 3 hours
C. 6 hours
D. 10 hours

(7) An infraclavicular perineural catheter is placed for a patient in the intensive care unit with severe forearm and hand ischemia after radial and ulnar arterial catheterization. The patient is currently intubated and sedated. Which is the best way to assess successful brachial plexus blockade?

A. Electromyography evaluation
B. Frequent neurological examinations
C. Hand color changes
D. Vascular Doppler assessment

(8) A 70-year-old man undergoes fifth finger amputation caused by necrosis from peripheral vascular disease. Surgery lasts 30 minutes. Which of the following increases this patient's risk for chronic postsurgical pain (CPSP) syndrome?

A. Patient age
B. Patient gender
C. Surgical duration
D. Surgical procedure

(9) Which of the following patients, based on their risk factors, is most likely to experience CPSP?

A. A 40-year-old woman who underwent lumpectomy for early-stage breast cancer who received paravertebral blocks for postoperative pain control.
B. A 57-year-old woman who underwent pulmonary resection via thoracotomy who had refused a thoracic epidural and failed intercostal nerve blocks, resulting in elevated pain scores on postoperative days 0 to 4.
C. A 72-year-old man who underwent total knee arthroplasty with postoperative adductor canal block but no posterior knee analgesia.
D. A 29-year-old male smoker who underwent exploratory laparotomy with epidural analgesia for postoperative pain control.

(10) A 27-year-old day laborer presents to the trauma bay after having both hands caught in a hay bailer. He has suffered significant crush injury and digital amputations of both hands along with radius fractures bilaterally. The surgical team is concerned with pain control and adequate perfusion in the postoperative period for this patient. You are consulted for a regional technique to assist with bilateral upper extremities. What perineural catheter(s) would be appropriate to perform?

A. Interscalene
B. Supraclavicular
C. Infraclavicular
D. All of the above

ANSWERS

(1) **D.** Supraclavicular, infraclavicular, and axillary approaches to brachial plexus blockade are all appropriate regional anesthesia choices for trauma to the hand, wrist, or forearm. An interscalene approach should be selected for traumas or surgeries involving the shoulder or proximal one-third of the humerus.

Reference

Taras JS, Behrman MJ. Continuous peripheral nerve block in replantation and revascularization. *J Reconstr Microsurg*. 1998;14:17–21.

(2) **C.** Brachial plexus nerve blocks result in vasodilation of the vasculature supplying the arm and hand. As this patient has a radial artery transection, vasodilation helps with the vascular anastomosis. Single-injection regional techniques can be performed and are a valid option; however, a perineural catheter provides a continuous infusion of local anesthetics at the target site. This produces a prolonged sympathectomy, resulting in arterial and venous vasodilation and avoidance of vasospasm. Analgesia offered by the perineural catheter also helps with decreasing anxiety and the stress response that can promote vasoconstriction. Nicotine also causes vasoconstriction and should be avoided.

Because this patient's young age, female gender, and preoperative anxiety increase her risk of CPSP syndrome, a perineural brachial plexus catheter is an ideal component of her perioperative analgesic management. However, the most immediate advantage is vasodilation.

References

Berger A, Tizian C, Zenz M. Continuous plexus blockade for improved circulation in microvascular surgery. *Ann Plast Surg*. 1985;14:16–19.

Aitken E, Jackson A, Kearns R, et al. Effect of regional versus local anaesthesia on outcome after arteriovenous fistula creation: a randomised controlled trial. *Lancet*. 2016;388:1067–1074.

Breschan C, Kraschl R, Jost R, Marhofer P, Likar R. Axillary brachial plexus block for the treatment of severe forearm ischemia after arterial cannulation in an extremely low birth-weight infant. *Paediatr Anaesth*. 2004;14:681–684.

Taras JS, Behrman MJ. Continuous peripheral nerve block in replantation and revascularization. *J Reconstr Microsurg*. 1998;14:17–21.

(3) **C.** Supraclavicular, infraclavicular, and axillary approaches to brachial plexus blockade are all appropriate following hand trauma. The compact nerve arrangement and superficial location of the supraclavicular approach allow for straightforward ultrasound visualization to aid in block placement. This can be a great benefit in obese and morbidly obese patients.

However, the proximity of the supraclavicular approach to the lung makes pneumothorax a potential complication. Although the infraclavicular approach to the brachial plexus has a deeper location, the perineural catheter transverses the pectoral muscles, which may assist in anchoring the catheter and preventing dislodgement.

Reference

Kakazu C, Tokhner V, Li J, Ou R, Simmons E. In the new era of ultrasound guidance: is pneumothorax from supraclavicular block a rare complication of the past? *Br J Anaesth.* 2014;113:190–191.

(4) **D.** Brachial plexus nerve blocks improve analgesia and cause sympathetic blockade of the vasculature in the territory supplied by the brachial plexus. Sympathectomy results in both arterial and venous vasodilation, creating improved blood flow and reduced vasospasm.

References

Su HH, Lui PW, Yu CL, et al. The effects of continuous axillary brachial plexus block with ropivacaine infusion on skin temperature and survival of crushed fingers after microsurgical replantation. *Chang Gung Med J.* 2005:28:567–574.

Berger A, Tizian C, Zenz M. Continuous plexus blockade for improved circulation in microvascular surgery. *Ann Plast Surg.* 1985;14:16–19

(5) **C.** The most common sign of compartment syndrome of the upper extremity is hand swelling. Patients may also report tightness, weakness or paralysis, and paresthesias in the affected limb. Notably, pain is often out of proportion to the injury and exacerbated with passive stretching. Diagnosis is often based on clinical suspicion; however, the measuring of compartment pressures can help in diagnosis. Weakness and paresthesias may be expected with a brachial plexus nerve block. Erythema would be concerning for infection.

References

Oak NR, Abrams RA. Compartment syndrome of the hand. *Orthop Clin North Am.* 2016;47:609–616.

McQueen MM, Gaston P, Court-Brown CM. Acute compartment syndrome: who is at risk? *J Bone Joint Surg Br.* 2000;82:200–203.

Heemskerk J, Kitslaar P. Acute compartment syndrome of the lower leg: retrospective study on prevalence, technique, and outcome of fasciotomies. *World J Surg.* 2003;27:744–747.

Mehta V, Chowdhary V, Lin C, Jbara M, Hanna S. Compartment syndrome of the hand: a case report and review of the literature. *Radiol Case Rep.* 2018;13:212–215.

(6) **C.** Diagnosis of compartment syndrome is often based on clinical suspicion. Once compartment syndrome is diagnosed, immediate fasciotomy is indicated to prevent further muscle and nerve damage. This is a time-sensitive process. Muscle and nerve damage is often reversible within 4 hours of elevated compartment pressures. However, irreversible damage may occur in 8 hours or less.

Reference

Mehta V, Chowdhary V, Lin C, Jbara M, Hanna S. Compartment syndrome of the hand: a case report and review of the literature. *Radiol Case Rep.* 2018;13:212–215.

(7) **D.** Vascular Doppler is also commonly used to assess the presence of blood flow following hand trauma and extremity ischemia. A successful brachial plexus block will result in vasodilation and improved vascular blood flow. Temperature measurements are also used to assess block success. However, the rise in temperature is caused by the increased blood flow. As infection could also cause increased temperature, monitoring of vascular blood flow is a more reliable monitor. Last, erythema can also result from increased perfusion. However, this can also be associated with infection.

Reference

Kurt E, Ozturk S, Isik S, Zor F. Continuous brachial plexus blockade for digital replantations and toe-to-hand transfers. *Ann Plast Surg.* 2005;54:24–27.

(8) **D.** Chronic postsurgical pain (CPSP) syndrome is defined as pain that persists over 3–6 months postoperatively or after the normal healing of tissues should have occurred. Surgeries with the highest incidence of CPSP are amputations, thoracotomies, breast surgery, and cardiac surgery. Other factors that increase the risk of CPSP include the presence of inadequately treated preoperative pain, psychological characteristics of anxiety or catastrophizing, female gender, younger patients, surgical approach with increased risk of nerve damage (e.g., stretching, transection), increased surgical duration, and the intensity of pain in the immediate postoperative period. This patient is older, male, and had a brief operative procedure duration. Therefore, only the surgical procedure (amputation) increases his risk for CPSP.

References

Thapa P, Euasobhon P. Chronic postsurgical pain: current evidence for prevention and management. *Korean J Pain.* 2018;31:155–173.

Correll D. Chronic postoperative pain: recent findings in understanding and management. *F1000Res.* 2017;6:1054.

(9) **B.** The feature most associated with the development of CPSP is duration of severe postoperative pain. Given that this patient was unable to receive an epidural and had inadequate pain control from the intercostal nerve blocks, coupled with known nerve transection and stretching resulting from thoracotomy, she is most at risk for developing CPSP. Another significant risk factor for CPSP is inadequately controlled pain preoperatively. Other risk factors for CPSP include young age, female gender, and preoperative anxiety.

Reference

Thapa P, Euasobhon P. Chronic postsurgical pain: current evidence for prevention and management. *Korean J Pain.* 2018;31:155–173.

(10) **C.** Bilateral infraclavicular perineural catheters would be most appropriate for this patient. Continuous perineural catheters will result in both analgesia and sympathectomy. Bilateral interscalene catheters are not reliable in providing analgesia to his hands or to the radial fractures given the distal nature of the injuries. Also, it is highly likely that bilateral interscalene catheters would result in bilateral phrenic nerve palsy and respiratory failure. The distribution of analgesia

from supraclavicular brachial plexus nerve blocks is adequate for this patient; however, supraclavicular brachial plexus nerve blocks also confer upward of a 50% risk of phrenic nerve palsy and can lead to respiratory failure. These risks make the supraclavicular approach an inappropriate choice if bilateral blocks are required. The infraclavicular approach to brachial plexus blockade provides analgesia and sympathectomy to the distal arm and entire forearm with the least risk of phrenic nerve palsy. Therefore, the infraclavicular approach is the most appropriate choice for the patient. Axillary catheters are less optimal because the terminal branches of the nerves are not tightly packed in a single location, resulting in many missed nerve distributions.

References

Kakazu C, Tokhner V, Li J, Ou R, Simmons E. In the new era of ultrasound guidance: is pneumothorax from supraclavicular block a rare complication of the past? *Br J Anaesth.* 2014;113:190–191.

Bigeleisen PE. Anatomical variations of the phrenic nerve and its clinical implication for supraclavicular block. *Br J Anaesth.* 2003;91: 916–917.

SECTION 7

LOWER EXTREMITY

Nabil Elkassabany

26.

HIP FRACTURE AND REGIONAL ANESTHESIA

Jason B. Ochroch and Mark D. Neuman

STEM CASE AND KEY QUESTIONS

You are covering the acute pain service and are called to the emergency department to evaluate an 83-year-old woman for right lower leg pain. She has a history significant for hypertension and a 50 pack-year smoking history. The patient describes having had a witnessed mechanical fall and noticed immediate pain around her right hip and inability to walk. Vital signs are notable for a heart rate of 104, a blood pressure of 157/89 mmHg, and an oxygen saturation of 93% on room air. On exam the right hip is painful to palpation, the right leg appears shorter than the left and externally rotated, and there is no bruising or swelling present. Plain radiographs of the hip reveal a mildly displaced femoral neck fracture. The patient's children are at the bedside and visibly worried. How would you address them?

(1) WHAT IS A HIP FRACTURE?

Hip fracture is an umbrella term that applies to a fracture of the femur in the area of the bone immediately distal to the articular cartilage of the hip to an area about 5 cm below the lower border of the lesser trochanter.

(2) HOW IS THE HIP INNERVATED?

Hip innervation includes the femoral nerve, obturator nerve, and sciatic nerve. The lateral femoral cutaneous nerve innervates the skin in the lateral part of the thigh, often the site of the surgical incision.

(3) WHAT LEVEL OF SPINAL ANESTHESIA IS REQUIRED FOR HIP SURGERY?

Spinal anesthesia needs to cover up to T10 for hip surgery.

(4) WHICH ANESTHETIC TECHNIQUE IS PREFERRED IN HIP FRACTURE SURGERIES?

There is currently no consensus on general versus neuraxial anesthesia as the optimal anesthetic technique, but several large multicenter pragmatic-design prospective randomized controlled trials are currently underway.

(5) WHAT ARE THE REGIONAL ANESTHESIA OPTIONS FOR HIP SURGERY?

Epidural analgesia, femoral nerve block, fascia iliaca compartment block, lumbar plexus block, pericapsular nerve group (PENG) block, obturator nerve block, quadratus lumborum block, and local infiltration.

(6) WHAT IS FASCIA ILIACA COMPARTMENT BLOCK?

The fascia iliaca compartment block (FICB) is a plane block that targets the femoral, obturator nerves. There are two approaches to fascia iliaca block: the infrainguinal and the suprainguinal approach.

In hip fracture patients, FICBs have been shown to be effective in reducing pain scores, opioid consumption, opioid related side effects, the development of delirium and other adverse events, and overall improvements in patient satisfaction. They have also been shown to facilitate positioning for neuraxial anesthesia prior to surgery.

(7) IS THE LATERAL FEMORAL CUTANEOUS NERVE BLOCK IMPORTANT IN HIP FRACTURE SURGERY?

Blockade of the lateral femoral cutaneous nerve (LFCNB) is intended to cover the surgical incision on the lateral thigh. The sole blockade of LFCNB for hip fractures is not useful as it does not supply the joint. Its value is only to supplement other blocks.

(8) WHAT IS PERICAPSULAR NERVE GROUP (PENG) BLOCK?

The pericapsular nerve group (PENG) block is intended to block the articular branches of both the femoral and obturator nerves, theoretically sparing motor weakness.

DISCUSSION

TYPES OF HIP FRACTURES

Hip fracture is an umbrella term that applies to a fracture of the femur in the area of the bone immediately distal to the articular cartilage of the hip to an area about 5 cm below the lower border of the lesser trochanter.[1]

Hip fractures are further classified anatomically in relation to the hip capsule.[2] Intracapsular fractures occur at the femoral head and neck; extracapsular fractures are classified as either intertrochanteric or subtrochanteric fractures. Intertrochanteric fractures occur at or between the greater and lesser trochanter, whereas subtrochanteric fractures occur in the region up to 5 cm distal to the lesser trochanter.[2] The fracture itself can also be classified as nondisplaced or displaced, depending on the separation of the bone at the fracture site.

THE SCOPE OF THE PROBLEM

Hip fractures occur in up to 300,000 people each year in the United States alone, and the annual incidence is expected to surpass 6 million people worldwide by the year 2050.[3] Hip fractures primarily affect older adults and may have long-lasting effects on health and functional independence.[4] Mortality rates at 1 month approach 10% and at 1 year range from 12% to 37%, with approximately one-half of previously independent individuals being unable to regain their ability to live independently.[4–6] Pooled data have shown that the relative hazard for all-cause mortality at 3 months after hip fracture is 5.75 and 7.95 for women and men, respectively.[7]

Hip fractures also account for an annual estimated cost in the United States between $10–15 billion due to costs of hospitalization, post-acute care, and supportive services for individuals who develop new functional limitations.[8]

RISK FACTORS FOR HIP FRACTURES

There are a variety of factors that increase someone's risk of sustaining a hip fracture. The most commonly cited contributors are age, fall risk, and osteoporosis.[9] Hip fractures are often considered a disease of older adults, with the rate of occurrence increasing greatly with age.[9] Additionally, falls account for over 90% of hip fractures in older adults.[10] Osteoporosis, which weakens bone strength, has also been shown to be a leading risk factor for bone fractures, particularly of the hip.[9] Another commonly cited risk factor is female sex. Women, likely due to their higher rates of osteoporosis, have a 2.3-fold increase in having a hip fracture in their lifetime, with an incidence of 957.3 per 100,000 vs. 414.4 per 100,000 in men.[3]

Frailty, a syndrome of aging that involves progressive decline across multiple organ systems, has also been identified as a risk factor for sustaining a hip fracture.[11] While frailty is beyond the scope of this chapter, it is important to recognize that many of its accompanying symptoms, such as inactivity, decreased strength, and weight loss, may be associated with an increased likelihood of falls and fractures.[12]

Additional risks also involve a variety of physiologic, social, and environmental factors. These risk factors include the presence of preexisting cardiovascular or neurocognitive disease, polypharmacy, having a history of a prior hip fracture, smoking status, poor nutrition, low body mass index, low socioeconomic status, and decreased mobility.[9]

TREATMENT OF HIP FRACTURES

For most patients, the standard of care for hip fracture is surgical treatment to treat pain, allow mobilization, and maximize the chances of functional recovery. Non-surgical management of hip fracture may be associated with an increased risk of cardiovascular, pulmonary, thrombotic, infectious, and bleeding complications that can result in death.[2] One recent study found that mortality for patients with hip fractures who chose non-operative treatment was 4-fold at 1 year compared to those who had surgical repair.[13]

Despite this, non-surgical management of hip fracture may be appropriate in limited contexts, such as when patients or their family members refuse surgical treatment, in moribund patients, in patients with long-standing fractures that have already begun to heal, and in patients who lack prospects for meaningful functional recovery and whose pain can be controlled adequately via non-surgical approaches.[14] The decision to operate therefore needs to be carefully discussed with the patient and their family regarding the risks and benefits of the surgery and overall goals of care.

Surgical options vary depending on the nature of the fracture, and may include internal fixation by reducing the fracture with bone screws and/or side plates, hemiarthroplasty, or total arthroplasty.[2,15]

HIP JOINT INNERVATION

Hip innervation is complex and involves several nerves. The femoral nerve, obturator nerve, and sciatic nerve innervate the superior and anterolateral, anteromedial, and posterior and inferior portions of the joint capsule, respectively.[16] However, of all these nerves, nociceptive fibers are predominantly present on the anterolateral and superior aspects of the capsule.[17] Of note, the lateral femoral cutaneous nerve innervates the skin in the lateral part of the thigh, often the site of the surgical incision.[16]

HOW DO THESE PATIENTS TYPICALLY PRESENT?

Hip fractures predominantly affect older adults, with a median age of 83 years.[5] Patients will often present with a history of a fall and the sudden onset of hip pain and the inability to walk. The injured leg may appear shortened and externally rotated.

Intracapsular fractures at the femoral head or neck are relatively avascular and will present with little bruising, whereas extracapsular fractures at the intertrochanteric and subtrochanteric regions will often have swelling and significant ecchymosis. A large volume of blood can be lost into the thigh for extracapsular fractures. While plain radiographs of the hip will typically provide the diagnosis, MRIs can be also be used.

TIMING OF SURGERY

Once the decision is made to operate, surgery should be performed as soon as possible. Studies have shown that earlier evaluations and surgeries confer improved outcomes. Several studies have found that surgery within 72 hours has not only shown a 19% reduction in mortality, but also decreased postoperative pain and overall length of stay.[18,19] Additionally, a separate meta-analysis found that surgery within 48 hours reduces 30-day and 1-year all-cause mortality by as much as 41% and 32%, respectively.[20] Another recent pilot study of 60 patients found that surgery within 6 hours is not only feasible, but resulted in improved perioperative 30-day complications.[21] However, these findings were not found when expanded to a large international trial of 2970 patients, which found that those randomized into an accelerated pathway (6 hours) did not have any significantly lower risk of mortality or major complications compared to standard care (24 hours).[22]

As a final point, while earlier surgery has been shown to improve outcomes in hip fracture patients, it is important to recognize a potential bias in preoperative comorbidities. Sicker patients who may have worse outcomes will need additional workups and optimization that exclude them from surgery within these time frames.[2]

PREOPERATIVE PREPARATION

The anesthesiologist can have a major role in caring for these patients outside of the operating room. Preoperative evaluations and medical optimization are essential components in helping to minimize complications and improve long-term outcomes and focuses on three specific goals (Box 26.1).[23]

This can be a particularly challenging process, especially given the heterogeneity of the geriatric population, prevalence of polypharmacy, and overall higher incidence of comorbidities.[23]

Initial steps will include stabilizing the patient, assessing for additional injuries, and determining the underlying cause of the hip fracture.[24] As these patients await surgery, prolonged immobilization can predispose them to several complications, including pressure ulcers, pneumonias, urinary tract infections, or venous thromboembolisms, that will all need to be addressed.[25] Medical optimization can also include beginning the treatment for any contributory risk factors, including managing osteoporosis, malnutrition, or smoking cessation education.[26] Some centers have also successfully employed routine preoperative echocardiography in patients with undiagnosed heart murmurs.[27]

Box 26.1 **GOALS FOR PREOPERATIVE EVALUATION IN HIP FRACTURE PATIENTS**

- Define patient comorbidities and physiological changes that may affect or alter perioperative management.
- Determine if medical optimization or further preoperative testing for preexisting conditions is necessary prior to surgery.
- Stratify patient risk and determine an appropriate and safe anesthetic plan.

WHAT ABOUT PREOPERATIVE PAIN CONTROL?

Pain is a universal complication of hip fractures. Unfortunately, pain is often undertreated in older patients, which is not only inhumane but also increases the risk of delirium.[28] Delirium has been shown to occur in 13%–55% of patients with hip fracture.[29] Undertreated perioperative pain has also been shown to result in longer hospital stays, persistent pain, and disability in locomotion at 6 months after surgery.[30,31]

Current guidelines by the American Academy of Orthopedic Surgeons endorse "strong" recommendations to employ a multimodal analgesic regimen, including the use of a preoperative peripheral nerve block.[32] These regimens should be tailored to each individual's unique medical conditions.[23]

INTRAOPERATIVE ANESTHETIC OPTIONS

Broadly speaking, the anesthetic options for surgery include general anesthesia or neuraxial anesthesia. For adequate coverage for hip surgery, neuraxial blockade can occur at either the epidural or intrathecal space and requires a T10 level.[5] While peripheral nerve blockade alone will not provide reliable surgical anesthesia, it can be placed preoperatively as a perioperative analgesic.

Single-shot intrathecal injections are the most commonly used technique, although epidural catheter, combined spinal-epidural, or continuous spinal techniques have also been described for high-risk patients who cannot tolerate the accompanying sympathectomy with spinal anesthesia and need a slower titration of effect. Hypotension, however, can occur with all modalities, including general anesthesia, and has been associated with increased mortality.[33]

During the preoperative evaluation, certain factors may exclude neuraxial anesthesia as an option. For example, absolute contraindications for spinal anesthesia include patient refusal, allergy to the local anesthetic, infection at the site of injection, and increased intracranial pressure. Relative contraindications include coagulopathy, sepsis, fixed cardiac output states, and indeterminate neurological disease.

WHICH INTRAOPERATIVE TECHNIQUE IS BEST (GA VS. NEURAXIAL)?

The optimal approach to intraoperative anesthesia management for hip fracture surgery is a complex topic and is reviewed only briefly here. Many studies have looked at various outcomes comparing general versus neuraxial anesthesia for hip fracture surgery with varying results. While several large nonrandomized studies have found reductions in mortality in those receiving neuraxial anesthesia,[34–37] others have not.[1,33,38–41] Unfortunately, few large-scale randomized controlled trials exist that fully address the current issues that employ clinically relevant protocols or outcomes.[42]

Available studies suggest an association between neuraxial anesthesia and postoperative thromboembolic events,[1,36,37,43,44] pulmonary complications,[34–36] and postoperative delirium[37] after hip fracture, but these findings have been variable across studies.[1,45–47] Additional hypothesized benefits of neuraxial anesthesia include reduced transfusion requirements,[36,43,44] reduced urinary tract infections,[44] shorter operating room times,[43] reduced rates of ICU admissions,[35,48] shorter hospital length of stays,[35,38,39] and lower overall costs of hospitalization,[35] although the presence and magnitude of observed associations between anesthesia type and these outcomes have also varied across studies.[1,39,49]

It should be noted that most recent studies of anesthesia type for hip fracture care have been observational and thus are limited in their ability to control for confounding due to baseline differences in health between patients who receive neuraxial versus general anesthesia for hip fracture.[1,5] To this end, multiple large multicenter pragmatic-design prospective randomized controlled trials are underway to compare differences in outcomes with spinal versus general anesthesia for hip fracture surgery.[42,50,51]

DO PERIPHERAL NERVE BLOCKS IMPROVE OUTCOMES IN HIP FRACTURE PATIENTS?

Peripheral nerve blocks can be administered as either a single-shot or by continuous infusion through a catheter. Several systematic reviews have found that pain treatment strategies incorporating peripheral nerve blockade result in better outcomes, including decrease in pain scores, opioid consumption, postoperative delirium, and time to first mobilization, as well as improved patient satisfaction.[52,53]

One recent Cochrane review found that peripheral nerve blockade reduced pain by as much as 3.4 points on a 0–10 scale within 30 minutes of block performance.[52] Interestingly, this study did not find consistent differences in pain scores deeper into the postoperative period, perhaps due to the heterogeneity in both surgical and block techniques.

Peripheral nerve blocks for hip fractures resulted in better pain control in the emergency department and allowed for positioning for neuraxial anesthesia.[54] It also resulted in lower opioid consumption and less incidence of opioid-related side effects, such as nausea, pruritis, and constipation.[55]

Also, these blocks may have benefits well beyond the duration of the local anesthetic. One study by Morrison and colleagues found that patients who received a single-shot femoral block and fascia iliaca catheter upon admission had not only improved perioperative pain scores and ambulatory status, but also had significantly greater independence in walking at 6 weeks postoperatively than those treated with opioids alone.[56] Whether these benefits can also confer improved long-term cardiopulmonary or mortality outcomes remains to be seen.[52]

These blocks are also relatively easy to teach and are low-cost interventions, particularly when a single-shot block is administered.[52,57]

Performing these blocks is not without risk, however. Complications can still occur, such as causing or worsening preexisting nerve injury, hematoma, local anesthetic systemic toxicity, or block failure.[23] Additionally, unintended motor blockade of the lower extremities may lead to increased weakness and a theoretical increased risk of falls, although this can be minimized with proper safety precautions and has not been shown to be the case.[52]

Recent guidelines from the American Academy of Orthopedic Surgeons have made a "strong" recommendation that all hip fracture patients receive a preoperative nerve block as a component of their pain treatment.[32] Not only has this been endorsed by the American Geriatrics Society and the American Society of Anesthesiologists, but these recommendations have also been in alignment with major organizations in other countries as well.[58–60] Despite these guideline recommendations, there is significant underutilization. A recent retrospective cohort study by our group found that only 3.0% of hip fracture patients between 2004 and 2016 received a nerve block for pain control.[61]

REGIONAL ANESTHESIA OPTIONS FOR HIP SURGERY

The hip is primarily innervated from the femoral, obturator, and sciatic nerves, with additional cutaneous coverage laterally by the lateral femoral cutaneous nerve, all of which arise from the lumbosacral plexus. As such, a variety of blocks have been developed to target some or all of these nerves or their spinal origins at a variety of locations.

These blocks can be placed during any phase of perioperative care and should be considered regardless of the type of intraoperative anesthetic administered. Unfortunately, many of these blocks are technically harder in hip fracture patients than in non-trauma settings. Proper positioning may be difficult due to the hip fracture or arthritis, and older adults generally have poorer tissue echogenicity on ultrasound. Furthermore, injection volumes should also be carefully considered as serum protein levels can be lower in frailer patients, predisposing this patient population to local anesthetic systemic toxicity.[23]

Absolute contraindications to peripheral nerve blocks include patient refusal, allergy to the local anesthetic, or infection at the site of injection, and relative contraindications include anticoagulation (depending on the superficial or deep nature of the block) or any pertinent medical history such as preexisting nerve disease.[5]

Block choice for hip fracture is also driven by user experience, patient cooperativity, block site compressibility, and the pharmacologic anticoagulation needs of the patient.[16] Additionally, based on timing and expected postoperative needs, these blocks can be done as a single shot or with the placement of a catheter to prolong its effect. While single-shot blocks are limited in duration, it should be noted that indwelling catheters may pose an increased infection risk or become inadvertently removed.[62]

While there are numerous nerve blocks available to cover hip innervation, we here focus on those blocks most commonly used for hip fracture patients while also providing an overview of the less common blocks and an introduction to newer blocks.

EPIDURAL ANALGESIA

Epidurals have been shown to not only decrease pain scores and opioid consumption in the hip fracture population, but also reduce the number of perioperative cardiac events without significantly impairing motor function for rehabilitation when titrated appropriately.[63] However, these neuraxial blocks are non-selective for unilateral surgery, have stricter anticoagulation guidelines, and altogether have a more complex side effects and complication profile than peripheral blockade.[64] For these reasons, the use of epidurals for the sole purpose of analgesia is rare.

FASCIA ILIACA COMPARTMENT BLOCK

The fascia iliaca compartment block (FICB) is a plane block that targets the femoral, obturator, and lateral femoral cutaneous nerves by depositing large volumes of dilute local anesthetic underneath the fascia iliaca, with the goal that the injectate diffuses proximally to these nerves.[16]

A common ultrasound-guided technique utilizes a lateral-to-medial approach at the infrainguinal region (Figure 26.1), whereas a newer suprainguinal caudal-to-cranial approach has also been described to inject the same plane and enhance proximal spread (Figure 26.2).[65] These ultrasound-guided approaches can be used as an alternative to the original loss-of-resistance "double-pop" technique as the needle penetrates through the fascia lata and fascia iliaca.

The FICB is considered a relatively safe and easy block to perform.[16] It is our opinion that the infrainguinal approach is considered safer than the suprainguinal approach as it is more compressible and the injection site is lateral from the femoral vessels. Studies have shown that an ultrasound-guided FICB will achieve complete sensory blockade of all three nerves at a proximal level at least 82% of the time.[66]

In hip fracture patients, FICBs have been shown to be effective in reducing pain scores, opioid consumption, opioid-related side effects, the development of delirium and other adverse events, and in overall improvements in patient satisfaction.[53,67–71] They have also been shown to facilitate positioning for neuraxial anesthesia prior to surgery.[72] And while single-shot techniques are the most common, placing a continuous catheter has also been associated with improved postoperative cognitive outcomes, side effect profiles, and ambulation.[56,73]

FEMORAL NERVE BLOCK

A femoral nerve block (FNB) is very common for hip fractures, because, like the FICB, it is relatively safe, easy to perform, and effective, particularly with ultrasound-guidance.[16,74] An ultrasound probe is placed transverse in the femoral crease distal to the inguinal ligament, identifying the nerve lateral to the femoral artery (Figure 26.3).

Multiple studies and reviews have found that the use of FNB has resulted in improved outcomes such as decreased pain scores and opioid consumption.[54,75] These favorable outcomes have also been found in continuous catheters; however, some studies have found conflicting results.[76–79]

At present, there is no clear consensus in the literature whether FICBs are more effective than FNBs. When the two blocks are compared directly, there are often mixed results.[80,81]

LUMBAR PLEXUS BLOCK

Lumbar plexus blocks (LPBs) target the femoral, obturator, and lateral femoral cutaneous nerves as they run within the psoas major muscle. It can be performed in the posterior approach using both nerve stimulation and ultrasound-guided techniques.[82]

LPBs have been shown to reduce pain scores and opioid consumption and to improve patient satisfaction, and have even been shown to be effective alternatives to neuraxial anesthesia as an intraoperative anesthetic.[83,84] However, this is

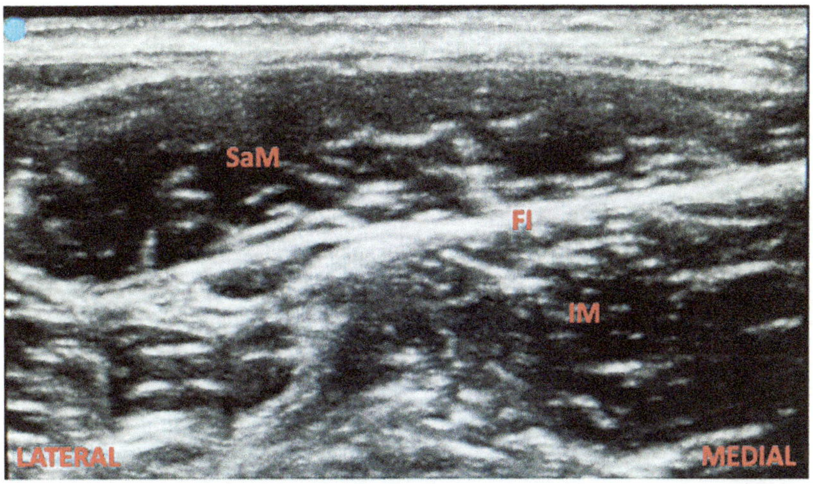

Figure 26.1. Infrainguinal fascia iliaca compartment block. Ultrasound anatomy of the infrainguinal approach to the fascia iliaca compartment block. Local anesthetic is deposited deep to the fascia iliaca (FI) between the sartorius muscle (SaM) and iliopsoas muscle (IM).

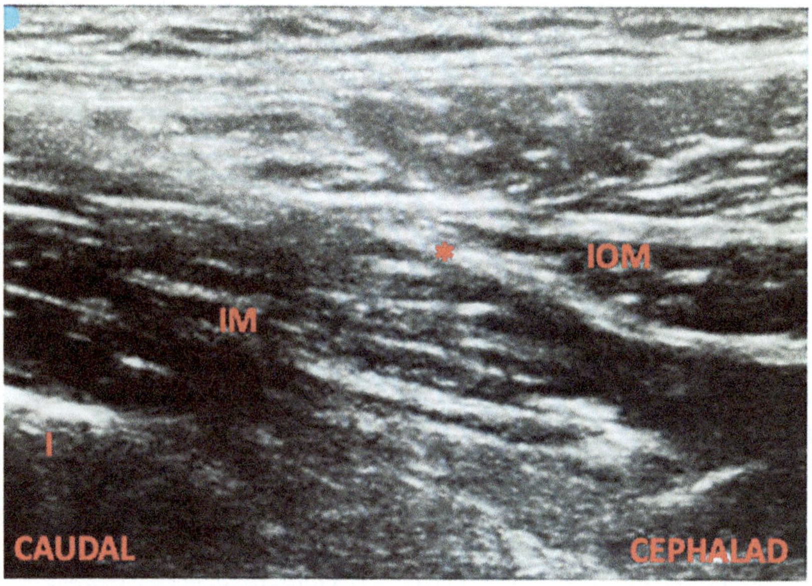

Figure 26.2. Suprainguinal fascia iliaca compartment block. Ultrasound anatomy of the suprainguinal approach to the fascia iliaca compartment block. Local anesthetic is deposited in the plane (*) between the iliacus (IM) and internal oblique muscles (IOM). Ileum (I).

considered an advanced block due to its relative depth, stricter anticoagulation considerations, and risk of local anesthetic spread to the epidural space.[16] Because of these issues, other blocks such as FNBs and FICBs which have been shown to have comparable analgesic outcomes and relatively safer profiles, have become more popular.[85,86]

LATERAL FEMORAL CUTANEOUS NERVE BLOCK

Blockade of the lateral femoral cutaneous nerve (LFCNB) is intended to cover the surgical incision on the lateral thigh, since it does not innervate the hip joint. However, this nerve has a highly variable distribution and may not always reliably block the area of interest. Because of this variability, the use of an ultrasound-guided technique is preferred.[16] There is limited utility of LFCNB as a sole nerve block for hip fractures, but some studies have found improved outcomes when used as to supplement other blocks.[87,88]

OBTURATOR NERVE BLOCK

The obturator nerve descends through the obturator canal to innervate the hip joint and thigh, and can be selectively targeted by ultrasound medial to the femoral vessels.[16] Similar to the LFCNB, it is still unclear if the obturator nerve block (ONB) alone can significantly improve pain for hip surgeries.[89] As such, it is more common to block this nerve more proximal and in conjunction with other nerve blocks (i.e., FICB).

QUADRATUS LUMBORUM BLOCK

The quadratus lumborum block (QLB) refers to blockade of the low thoracic and high lumbar spinal nerves (typically T6–L2)

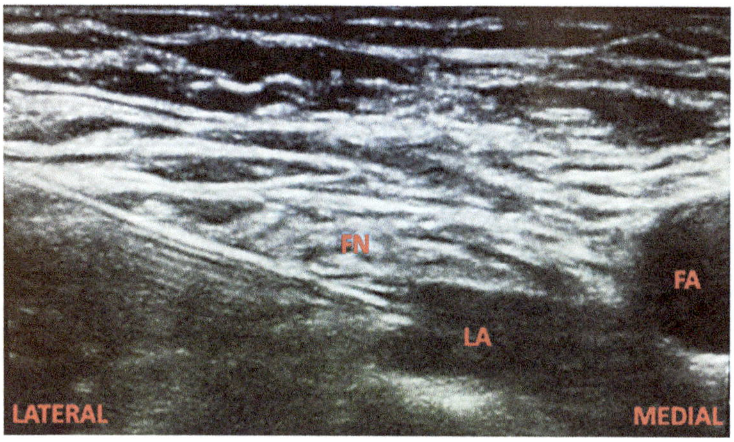

Figure 26.3. Femoral nerve block. Ultrasound anatomy of the femoral nerve block. Local anesthetic (LA) is deposited adjacent to the femoral nerve (FN). Femoral artery (FA).

at or around the quadratus lumborum muscle, with possible spread to the paravertebral space.[16,90] Because of this coverage, QLBs have mostly been described for abdominal surgery, but recently studies have looked at hip surgery. To our knowledge, only one randomized control trial has evaluated the efficacy of QLB in the hip fracture population, which resulted in greater reductions in pain scores and opioid consumption while still providing similar motor function and patient satisfaction compared to FNBs.[91] The QLB also has been tentatively shown to improve outcomes in the hip arthroplasty population, although more studies are needed.[92–94] The QLB is considered a deep block, and appropriate safety measures must be taken.

PERICAPSULAR NERVE GROUP (PENG) BLOCK

The pericapsular nerve group (PENG) block was first described in 2018 to block the articular branches of both the femoral and obturator nerves, theoretically sparing motor weakness.[95] A curvilinear low-frequency ultrasound probe can be placed obliquely over the anterior inferior iliac spine and iliopubic eminence. The PENG block bears some similarity to a separate novel block, the iliopsoas plane block, described elsewhere.[96] Despite being a relatively new block with only a few case series published thus far, outcomes are promising.[97,98]

LOCAL INFILTRATION ANALGESIA

Local infiltration analgesia (LIA) is a technique performed by surgeons that involves directly infiltrating the wound during surgery with a large volume of a dilute local anesthetic and typically with the addition of adjuvants such as opioids and possibly with the placement of an indwelling catheter.[16] LIA has been shown to improve pain scores and opioid consumption, mobilization, and hospital length of stay in the hip fracture populations, although there have been mixed results.[99–101] Recently, there has been renewed interest in this technique using liposomal bupivacaine (Exparel, Pacira Inc., Parsippany, NJ) to augment multimodal therapy in the hip fracture population, but more studies are still needed.[102]

CONCLUSIONS

- Hip fractures carry significant risk of premature mortality and comorbidities, including pain, delirium, increased hospital length of stay, decreased ambulatory status, and loss of independent living.
- There is currently no consensus on general vs. neuraxial anesthesia as the optimal anesthetic technique, but several large multicenter pragmatic-design prospective randomized controlled trials are currently underway.
- Current specialty and national guidelines recommend using peripheral nerve blockade in conjunction with multimodal analgesic regimens, which has been shown to improve multiple outcomes in the hip fracture population.
- The hip is primarily innervated from the femoral, obturator, and sciatic nerves. A variety of blocks have been developed to target these nerves, with the most common procedures including ultrasound-guided femoral nerve and fascia iliaca compartment blocks.

REFERENCES

1. Guay J, Parker MJ, Gajendragadkar PR, Kopp S. Anaesthesia for hip fracture surgery in adults. *Cochrane Database Syst Rev.* 2016;2:CD000521.
2. Bhandari M, Swiontkowski M. Management of acute hip fracture. *N Engl J Med.* 2017;377(21):2053–2062.
3. Brauer CA, Coca-Perraillon M, Cutler DM, Rosen AB. Incidence and mortality of hip fractures in the United States. *JAMA.* 2009;302(14):1573–1579.
4. Bentler SE, Liu L, Obrizan M, et al. The aftermath of hip fracture: discharge placement, functional status change, and mortality. *Am J Epidemiol.* 2009;170(10):1290–1299.
5. Dawe H. Modernising hip fracture anaesthesia. *Open Orthop J.* 2017;11:1190–1199.
6. Panula J, Pihlajamäki H, Mattila VM, et al. Mortality and cause of death in hip fracture patients aged 65 or older: a population-based study. *BMC Musculoskelet Disord.* 2011;12:105.
7. Haentjens P, Magaziner J, Colón-Emeric CS, et al. Meta-analysis: excess mortality after hip fracture among older women and men. *Ann Intern Med.* 2010;152(6):380–390.
8. Dy CJ, McCollister KE, Lubarsky DA, Lane JM. An economic evaluation of a systems-based strategy to expedite surgical treatment of hip fractures. *J Bone Joint Surg Am.* 2011;93(14):1326–1334.
9. Marks R. Hip fracture epidemiological trends, outcomes, and risk factors, 1970–2009. *Int J Gen Med.* 2010;3:1–17.
10. Hayes WC, Myers ER, Robinovitch SN, Van Den Kroonenberg A, Courtney AC, McMahon TA. Etiology and prevention of age-related hip fractures. *Bone.* 1996;18(1 Suppl):77S–86S.
11. Ensrud KE, Ewing SK, Taylor BC, et al. Frailty and risk of falls, fracture, and mortality in older women: the study of osteoporotic fractures. *J Gerontol A Biol Sci Med Sci.* 2007;62(7):744–751.
12. Rolland Y, Abellan van Kan G, Bénétos A, et al. Frailty, osteoporosis and hip fracture: causes, consequences and therapeutic perspectives. *J Nutr Health Aging.* 2008;12(5):335–346.
13. Tay E. Hip fractures in the elderly: operative versus nonoperative management. *Singapore Med J.* 2016;57(4):178–181.
14. Parker M, Johansen A. Hip fracture. *BMJ.* 2006;333(7557):27–30.
15. Mears SC. Classification and surgical approaches to hip fractures for nonsurgeons. *Clin Geriatr Med.* 2014;30(2):229–241.
16. Bugada D, Bellini V, Lorini LF, Mariano ER. Update on selective regional analgesia for hip surgery patients. *Anesthesiol Clin.* 2018;36(3):403–415.
17. Gerhardt M, Johnson K, Atkinson R, et al. Characterisation and classification of the neural anatomy in the human hip joint. *Hip Int.* 2012;22(1):75–81.
18. Simunovic N, Devereaux PJ, Sprague S, et al. Effect of early surgery after hip fracture on mortality and complications: systematic review and meta-analysis. *CMAJ.* 2010;182(15):1609–1616.
19. Orosz GM, Magaziner J, Hannan EL, et al. Association of timing of surgery for hip fracture and patient outcomes. *JAMA.* 2004;291(14):1738–1743.
20. Shiga T, Wajima Z, Ohe Y. Is operative delay associated with increased mortality of hip fracture patients? Systematic review, meta-analysis, and meta-regression. *Can J Anaesth.* 2008;55(3):146–154.
21. Hip Fracture Accelerated Surgical Treatment and Care Track (HIP ATTACK) Investigators. Accelerated care versus standard care among patients with hip fracture: the HIP ATTACK pilot trial. *CMAJ.* 2014;186(1):E52–60.

22. Investigators HA. Accelerated surgery versus standard care in hip fracture (HIP ATTACK): an international, randomised, controlled trial. *Lancet.* 2020;395(10225):698–708.
23. Cai L, Liu J, Elkassabany N. Anesthesia and pain management in geriatric fractures. In: Pignolo R, Ahn J, eds. *Fractures in the Elderly: Aging Medicine.* Cham: Humana Press; 2018.
24. Agarwal S, Azocar R. Trauma and the geriatric patient. In: Barnett S, ed. *Manual of Geriatric Anesthesia.* New York: Springer; 2013:193–202.
25. Beaupre LA, Jones CA, Saunders LD, Johnston DW, Buckingham J, Majumdar SR. Best practices for elderly hip fracture patients: a systematic overview of the evidence. *J Gen Intern Med.* 2005;20(11):1019–1025.
26. American Academy of Orthopaedic Surgeons Management of Hip Fractures in Older Adults EvidenceBased Clinical Practice Guideline. https://www.aaos.org/hipfxcpg. Published 12/03/2021.
27. Heyburn G, McBrien ME. Pre-operative echocardiography for hip fractures: time to make it a standard of care. *Anaesthesia.* 2012;67(11):1189–1193.
28. Morrison RS, Magaziner J, Gilbert M, et al. Relationship between pain and opioid analgesics on the development of delirium following hip fracture. *J Gerontol A Biol Sci Med Sci.* 2003;58(1):76–81.
29. Yang Y, Zhao X, Dong T, Yang Z, Zhang Q, Zhang Y. Risk factors for postoperative delirium following hip fracture repair in elderly patients: a systematic review and meta-analysis. *Aging Clin Exp Res.* 2017;29(2):115–126.
30. Morrison RS, Magaziner J, McLaughlin MA, et al. The impact of post-operative pain on outcomes following hip fracture. *Pain.* 2003;103(3):303–311.
31. Morrison RS, Flanagan S, Fischberg D, Cintron A, Siu AL. A novel interdisciplinary analgesic program reduces pain and improves function in older adults after orthopedic surgery. *J Am Geriatr Soc.* 2009;57(1):1–10.
32. Brox WT, Roberts KC, Taksali S, Wright DG, Wixted JJ, et al. The American Academy of Orthopaedic Surgeons Evidence-Based Guideline on Management of Hip Fractures in the Elderly. *J Bone Joint Surg Am.* 2015 Jul 15;97(14):1196–1199. doi:10.2106/JBJS.O.00229. PMID: 26178894; PMCID: PMC6948785.
33. White SM, Moppett IK, Griffiths R, et al. Secondary analysis of outcomes after 11,085 hip fracture operations from the prospective UK Anaesthesia Sprint Audit of Practice (ASAP-2). *Anaesthesia.* 2016;71(5):506–514.
34. Neuman MD, Silber JH, Elkassabany NM, Ludwig JM, Fleisher LA. Comparative effectiveness of regional versus general anesthesia for hip fracture surgery in adults. *Anesthesiology.* 2012;117(1):72–92.
35. Chu CC, Weng SF, Chen KT, et al. Propensity score-matched comparison of postoperative adverse outcomes between geriatric patients given a general or a neuraxial anesthetic for hip surgery: a population-based study. *Anesthesiology.* 2015;123(1):136–147.
36. Rodgers A, Walker N, Schug S, et al. Reduction of postoperative mortality and morbidity with epidural or spinal anaesthesia: results from overview of randomised trials. *BMJ.* 2000;321(7275):1493.
37. Luger TJ, Kammerlander C, Gosch M, et al. Neuroaxial versus general anaesthesia in geriatric patients for hip fracture surgery: does it matter? *Osteoporos Int.* 2010;21(Suppl 4):S555–572.
38. Neuman MD, Rosenbaum PR, Ludwig JM, Zubizarreta JR, Silber JH. Anesthesia technique, mortality, and length of stay after hip fracture surgery. *JAMA.* 2014;311(24):2508–2517.
39. O'Donnell CM, McLoughlin L, Patterson CC, et al. Perioperative outcomes in the context of mode of anaesthesia for patients undergoing hip fracture surgery: systematic review and meta-analysis. *Br J Anaesth.* 2018;120(1):37–50.
40. White SM, Moppett IK, Griffiths R. Outcome by mode of anaesthesia for hip fracture surgery: an observational audit of 65 535 patients in a national dataset. *Anaesthesia.* 2014;69(3):224–230.
41. Patorno E, Neuman MD, Schneeweiss S, Mogun H, Bateman BT. Comparative safety of anesthetic type for hip fracture surgery in adults: retrospective cohort study. *BMJ.* 2014;348:g4022.
42. Neuman MD, Ellenberg SS, Sieber FE, et al. Regional versus General Anesthesia for Promoting Independence after Hip Fracture (REGAIN): protocol for a pragmatic, international multicentre trial. *BMJ Open.* 2016;6(11):e013473.
43. Basques BA, Bohl DD, Golinvaux NS, Samuel AM, Grauer JG. General versus spinal anaesthesia for patients aged 70 years and older with a fracture of the hip. *Bone Joint J.* 2015;97-B(5):689–695.
44. Fields AC, Dieterich JD, Buterbaugh K, Moucha CS. Short-term complications in hip fracture surgery using spinal versus general anaesthesia. *Injury.* 2015;46(4):719–723.
45. Wright SP, Hall Brown TS, Collier SR, Sandberg K. How consumer physical activity monitors could transform human physiology research. *Am J Physiol Regul Integr Comp Physiol.* 2017;312(3):R358–R367.
46. Patel V, Champaneria R, Dretzke J, Yeung J. Effect of regional versus general anaesthesia on postoperative delirium in elderly patients undergoing surgery for hip fracture: a systematic review. *BMJ Open.* 2018;8(12):e020757.
47. Sieber FE, Neufeld KJ, Gottschalk A, et al. Effect of depth of sedation in older patients undergoing hip fracture repair on postoperative delirium: the STRIDE randomized clinical trial. *JAMA Surg.* 2018;153(11):987–995.
48. Seitz DP, Gill SS, Bell CM, et al. Postoperative medical complications associated with anesthesia in older adults with dementia. *J Am Geriatr Soc.* 2014;62(11):2102–2109.
49. Whiting PS, Molina CS, Greenberg SE, Thakore RV, Obremskey WT, Sethi MK. Regional anaesthesia for hip fracture surgery is associated with significantly more peri-operative complications compared with general anaesthesia. *Int Orthop.* 2015;39(7):1321–1327.
50. Li T, Yeung J, Li J, et al. Comparison of regional with general anaesthesia on postoperative delirium (RAGA-delirium) in the older patients undergoing hip fracture surgery: study protocol for a multicentre randomised controlled trial. *BMJ Open.* 2017;7(10):e016937.
51. Kowark A, Adam C, Ahrens J, et al. Improve hip fracture outcome in the elderly patient (iHOPE): a study protocol for a pragmatic, multicentre randomised controlled trial to test the efficacy of spinal versus general anaesthesia. *BMJ Open.* 2018;8(10):e023609.
52. Guay J, Parker MJ, Griffiths R, Kopp S. Peripheral nerve blocks for hip fractures. *Cochrane Database Syst Rev.* 2017;5:CD001159.
53. Steenberg J, Møller AM. Systematic review of the effects of fascia iliaca compartment block on hip fracture patients before operation. *Br J Anaesth.* 2018;120(6):1368–1380.
54. Ritcey B, Pageau P, Woo MY, Perry JJ. Regional nerve blocks for hip and femoral neck fractures in the emergency department: a systematic review. *CJEM.* 2016;18(1):37–47.
55. Ilfeld BM, Enneking FK. Continuous peripheral nerve blocks at home: a review. *Anesth Analg.* 2005;100(6):1822–1833.
56. Morrison RS, Dickman E, Hwang U, et al. Regional nerve blocks improve pain and functional outcomes in hip fracture: a randomized controlled trial. *J Am Geriatr Soc.* 2016;64(12):2433–2439.
57. Carvalho B, Yun R, Mariano E. Continuous versus single-injection peripheral nerve blocks: a prospective cohort study comparing procedural time and estimated personnel cost. *Open Anesth J.* 2015;9:1–5.
58. Australian and New Zealand Hip Fracture Registry. Annual report of hip fracture care 2022. September 2022. https://anzhfr.org/wp-content/uploads/sites/1164/2022/08/ANZHFR-2022-Annual-Report-Print-version-v2.pdf
59. *Scottish Intercollegiate Guidelines Network: Management of Hip Fracture in Older People.* 2009. https://www.sign.ac.uk/our-guidelines/management-of-hip-fracture-in-older-people/
60. National Clinical Guideline Centre (UK). The Management of Hip Fracture in Adults [Internet]. London: Royal College of Physicians (UK); 2011. PMID: 22420011.
61. Neuman MD, Elkassabany NM, Ochroch J, et al. Nerve block use after hip fracture versus elective hip or knee arthroplasty: retrospective analysis. *J Am Geriatr Soc.* 2020;68(4):835–840.
62. Jeng CL, Torrillo TM, Rosenblatt MA. Complications of peripheral nerve blocks. *Br J Anaesth.* 2010;105 Suppl 1:i97–107.
63. Foss NB, Kristensen MT, Kristensen BB, Jensen PS, Kehlet H. Effect of postoperative epidural analgesia on rehabilitation and pain after hip fracture surgery: a randomized, double-blind, placebo-controlled trial. *Anesthesiology.* 2005;102(6):1197–1204.

64. Rawal N. Current issues in postoperative pain management. *Eur J Anaesthesiol.* 2016;33(3):160–171.
65. Hebbard P, Ivanusic J, Sha S. Ultrasound-guided supra-inguinal fascia iliaca block: a cadaveric evaluation of a novel approach. *Anaesthesia.* 2011;66(4):300–305.
66. Dolan J, Williams A, Murney E, Smith M, Kenny GN. Ultrasound guided fascia iliaca block: a comparison with the loss of resistance technique. *Reg Anesth Pain Med.* 2008;33(6):526–531.
67. Amin NH, West JA, Farmer T, Basmajian HG. Nerve blocks in the geriatric patient with hip fracture: a review of the current literature and relevant neuroanatomy. *Geriatr Orthop Surg Rehabil.* 2017;8(4):268–275.
68. Groot L, Dijksman LM, Simons MP, Zwartsenburg MM, Rebel JR. Single fascia iliaca compartment block is safe and effective for emergency pain relief in hip-fracture patients. *West J Emerg Med.* 2015;16(7):1188–1193.
69. Callear J, Shah K. Analgesia in hip fractures: do fascia-iliac blocks make any difference? *BMJ Qual Improv Rep.* 2016;5(1):u210130.w4147.
70. Rashiq S, Vandermeer B, Abou-Setta AM, Beaupre LA, Jones CA, Dryden DM. Efficacy of supplemental peripheral nerve blockade for hip fracture surgery: multiple treatment comparison. *Can J Anaesth.* 2013;60(3):230–243.
71. Ridderikhof ML, De Kruif E, Stevens MF, et al. Ultrasound guided supra-inguinal fascia iliaca compartment blocks in hip fracture patients: an alternative technique. *Am J Emerg Med.* 2020;38(2):231–236.
72. Diakomi M, Papaioannou M, Mela A, Kouskouni E, Makris A. Preoperative fascia iliaca compartment block for positioning patients with hip fractures for central nervous blockade: a randomized trial. *Reg Anesth Pain Med.* 2014;39(5):394–398.
73. Odor PM, Chis Ster I, Wilkinson I, Sage F. Effect of admission fascia iliaca compartment blocks on post-operative abbreviated mental test scores in elderly fractured neck of femur patients: a retrospective cohort study. *BMC Anesthesiol.* 2017;17(1):2.
74. Tran Q, Salinas FV, Benzon HT, Neal JM. Lower extremity regional anesthesia: essentials of our current understanding. *Reg Anesth Pain Med.* 2019:rapm-2018-000019.
75. Hartmann FV, Novaes MR, de Carvalho MR. Femoral nerve block versus intravenous fentanyl in adult patients with hip fractures: a systematic review. *Braz J Anesthesiol.* 2017;67(1):67–71.
76. Chaudet A, Bouhours G, Rineau E, et al. Impact of preoperative continuous femoral blockades on morphine consumption and morphine side effects in hip-fracture patients: a randomized, placebo-controlled study. *Anaesth Crit Care Pain Med.* 2016;35(1):37–43.
77. Rowlands M, Walt GV, Bradley J, et al. Femoral Nerve Block Intervention in Neck of Femur Fracture (FINOF): a randomised controlled trial. *BMJ Open.* 2018;8(4):e019650.
78. Riddell M, Ospina M, Holroyd-Leduc JM. Use of femoral nerve blocks to manage hip fracture pain among older adults in the emergency department: a systematic review. *CJEM.* 2016;18(4):245–252.
79. Arsoy D, Huddleston JI, Amanatullah DF, Giori NJ, Maloney WJ, Goodman SB. Femoral nerve catheters improve home disposition and pain in hip fracture patients treated with total hip arthroplasty. *J Arthroplasty.* 2017;32(11):3434–3437.
80. Newman B, McCarthy L, Thomas PW, May P, Layzell M, Horn K. A comparison of pre-operative nerve stimulator-guided femoral nerve block and fascia iliaca compartment block in patients with a femoral neck fracture. *Anaesthesia.* 2013;68(9):899–903.
81. Yu B, He M, Cai GY, Zou TX, Zhang N. Ultrasound-guided continuous femoral nerve block vs continuous fascia iliaca compartment block for hip replacement in the elderly: a randomized controlled clinical trial (CONSORT). *Medicine (Baltimore).* 2016;95(42):e5056.
82. Nielsen MV, Bendtsen TF, Børglum J. Superiority of ultrasound-guided Shamrock lumbar plexus block. *Minerva Anestesiol.* 2018;84(1):115–121.
83. Ahamed ZA, Sreejit MS. Lumbar plexus block as an effective alternative to subarachnoid block for intertrochanteric hip fracture surgeries in the elderly. *Anesth Essays Res.* 2019;13(2):264–268.
84. Amiri HR, Zamani MM, Safari S. Lumbar plexus block for management of hip surgeries. *Anesth Pain Med.* 2014;4(3):e19407.
85. Amiri HR, Safari S, Makarem J, Rahimi M, Jahanshahi B. Comparison of combined femoral nerve block and spinal anesthesia with lumbar plexus block for postoperative analgesia in intertrochanteric fracture surgery. *Anesth Pain Med.* 2012;2(1):32–35.
86. Antonopoulou E, Papaioannou K, Stertsou E, Karamoulas B, Itsiopoulos I. Continuous psoas compartment block versus continuous femoral block in elderly patients with hip fractures. *Eur J Anaesthesiol.* 2010;27(47):141.
87. Segado Jiménez MI, Bayón Gago M, Arias Delgado J, et al. [Efficacy of obturator and femoral cutaneous nerve blocks for postoperative analgesia in hip surgery]. *Rev Esp Anestesiol Reanim.* 2009;56(10):590–597.
88. Vandebroek A, Vertommen M, Huyghe M, Van Houwe P. Ultrasound guided femoral nerve block and lateral femoral cutaneous nerve block for postoperative pain control after primary hip arthroplasty: a retrospective study. *Acta Anaesthesiol Belg.* 2014;65(1):39–44.
89. Nielsen ND, Runge C, Clemmesen L, et al. An obturator nerve block does not alleviate postoperative pain after total hip arthroplasty: a randomized clinical trial. *Reg Anesth Pain Med.* 2019:rapm-2018-100104.
90. Elsharkawy H, El-Boghdadly K, Barrington M. Quadratus lumborum block: anatomical concepts, mechanisms, and techniques. *Anesthesiology.* 2019;130(2):322–335.
91. Parras T, Blanco R. Randomised trial comparing the transversus abdominis plane block posterior approach or quadratus lumborum block type I with femoral block for postoperative analgesia in femoral neck fracture, both ultrasound-guided. *Rev Esp Anestesiol Reanim.* 2016;63(3):141–148.
92. Stuart Green M, Ryan Hoffman C, Iqbal U, Olabisi Ives O, Hurd B. Transmuscular quadratus lumborum block reduces length of stay in patients receiving total hip arthroplasty. *Anesth Pain Med.* 2018;8(6):e80233.
93. Ueshima H, Yoshiyama S, Otake H. The ultrasound-guided continuous transmuscular quadratus lumborum block is an effective analgesia for total hip arthroplasty. *J Clin Anesth.* 2016;31:35.
94. Adhikary SD, Short AJ, El-Boghdadly K, Abdelmalak MJ, Chin KJ. Transmuscular quadratus lumborum versus lumbar plexus block for total hip arthroplasty: a retrospective propensity score matched cohort study. *J Anaesthesiol Clin Pharmacol.* 2018;34(3):372–378.
95. Girón-Arango L, Peng PWH, Chin KJ, Brull R, Perlas A. Pericapsular nerve group (PENG) block for hip fracture. *Reg Anesth Pain Med.* 2018;43(8):859–863.
96. Nielsen ND, Greher M, Moriggl B, et al. Spread of injectate around hip articular sensory branches of the femoral nerve in cadavers. *Acta Anaesthesiol Scand.* 2018;62(7):1001–1006.
97. Tran J, Agur A, Peng P. Is pericapsular nerve group (PENG) block a true pericapsular block? *Reg Anesth Pain Med.* 2019:rapm-2018-100278. doi:10.1136/rapm-2018-100278.
98. Fusco P, Di Carlo S, Paladini G, et al. Could the combination of PENG block and LIA be a useful analgesic strategy in the treatment of postoperative pain for hip replacement surgery? *Reg Anesth Pain Med.* 2019:rapm-2018-100277. doi:10.1136/rapm-2018-100277.
99. Harrison WD, Lees D, A'Court J, Ankers T, Harper I, Inman D, Reed MR. Local anaesthetic infiltration and indwelling postoperative wound catheters for patients with hip fracture reduce death rates and length of stay. *Surg Res Pract.* 2015;2015:316817.
100. Bech RD, Lauritsen J, Ovesen O, Emmeluth C, Lindholm P, Overgaard S. Local anaesthetic wound infiltration after internal fixation of femoral neck fractures: a randomized, double-blind clinical trial in 33 patients. *Hip Int.* 2011;21(2):251–259.
101. Aprato A, Audisio A, Santoro A, et al. Fascia-iliaca compartment block vs intra-articular hip injection for preoperative pain management in intracapsular hip fractures: a blind, randomized, controlled trial. *Injury.* 2018;49(12):2203–2208.

102. Amin NH, Hutchinson HL, Sanzone AG. Infiltration techniques for local infiltration analgesia with liposomal bupivacaine in extracapsular and intracapsular hip fracture surgery: expert panel opinion. *J Orthop Trauma.* 2018;32(Suppl 2):S5–S10.

REVIEW QUESTIONS

(1) The suprainguinal approach to the fascia iliaca compartment block has become increasingly popular compared to the infrainguinal approach because:

A. It is more compressible in the event of vascular injury.
B. The approach is purported to enhance proximal spread.
C. It can be done with loss-of-resistance technique and does not require ultrasound.
D. Local anesthetic will spread to the sacral plexus and cause a "4-in-1" block.

(2) The American Academy of Orthopedic Surgeons supports the placement of a peripheral nerve block during which part of perioperative care of someone with hip fracture?

A. Preoperative
B. Intraoperative
C. Postoperative
D. This is not a recommendation.

(3) In the recovery room after a hemiarthroplasty for hip fracture under general anesthesia, your patient complains of medial pain in the upper thigh. The patient weighs 43 kg and you want to limit her exposure to local anesthetic and deliver as targeted block as possible. Which procedure will you perform?

A. Epidural catheter
B. Fascia iliaca compartment block
C. Femoral nerve block
D. Obturator nerve block

(4) A 97-year-old man with a hip fracture presents for preoperative evaluation in the ED. He is bedbound, has a history of Alzheimer's dementia, and prostate cancer metastatic to the lumbar spine. His chart is listed as DNR/DNI. The exam is notable for hip pain and a newfound systolic heart murmur. What is your next step?

A. Obtain consent from the patient and proceed immediately to the operating room.
B. Obtain an echocardiogram to evaluate the systolic heart murmur, but plan to proceed with neuraxial anesthesia to avoid intubation.
C. Discuss the risks and benefits of surgery with the family and surgeon and decide if surgical intervention is appropriate for this patient's goals of care.
D. Do not give analgesics as this may worsen his cognitive dysfunction.

(5) When performing an anterior quadratus lumborum block (QLB 3), local anesthetic is deposited between the quadratus lumborum muscle and what structure?

A. Erector spinae muscles
B. Transverse process
C. Psoas major muscle
D. Perinephric fat

(6) You are called to evaluate an otherwise healthy 76-year-old female who will be undergoing open reduction and internal fixation of an intertrochanteric fracture. You explain the various anesthetic options and she asks you which option carries the least perioperative mortality, to which you reply:

A. General anesthesia with an endotracheal tube
B. Neuraxial anesthesia with a single-shot intrathecal injection
C. Monitored anesthesia care with peripheral nerve blockade providing analgesic coverage
D. This is a complex question with no "textbook" answer, and the anesthetic plan will therefore be tailored to the needs of the patient and anesthesiologist and hospital practice.

(7) Femoral neck fractures are not typically associated with ecchymosis because:

A. This is an intracapsular fracture with relatively little blood supply that will not reach the skin.
B. Internal bleeding occurs that tracks up into the pelvis.
C. The stress response of hip fracture causes peripheral vasoconstriction preventing ecchymosis.
D. Ecchymosis is a pathognomonic finding for femoral neck fractures.

(8) Which of the following is an absolute contraindication to spinal anesthesia?

A. Moderate aortic stenosis
B. Patient refusal
C. History of L3–L5 laminectomy and fusion
D. Allergy to procaine

ANSWERS

(1) **B.** The suprainguinal approach to the fascia iliaca compartment block is via a caudal-to-cranial injection that is thought to aid in the proximal spread of the local anesthetic to the lumbar plexus. It will still block the same femoral, obturator, and lateral femoral cutaneous nerve distributions and does not spread to the sacral plexus. This approach is considered a deeper block since it is posterior to the inguinal ligament and requires ultrasound assistance.

Reference

Hebbard P, Ivanusic J, Sha S. Ultrasound-guided supra-inguinal fascia iliaca block: a cadaveric evaluation of a novel approach. *Anaesthesia.* 2011;66(4):300–305.

(2) **A.** The American Academy of Orthopedic Surgeons (AOS) guidelines on the management of hip fractures in the elderly make a "strong" recommendation supporting peripheral nerve blockades to improve preoperative pain control.

Of note, the majority of studies cited for this recommendation included either femoral nerve or fascia iliaca compartment blocks.

Reference

American Academy of Orthopaedic Surgeons Management of Hip Fractures in Older Adults Evidence Based Clinical Practice Guideline. https://www.aaos.org/hipfxcpg. Published 12/03/2021.

(3) **D.** The hip joint is innervated from the lumbosacral plexus, with the femoral, obturator, and sciatic nerves innervating the superior and anterolateral, anteromedial, and posterior and inferior portions of the joint capsule, respectively. Medial pain will be selectively covered with an obturator nerve block. While an epidural or fascia iliaca compartment block will also cover this nerve, they will do so nonselectively and with greater local anesthetic volumes necessary.

Reference

Yoshida T, Nakamoto T, Kamibayashi T. Ultrasound-guided obturator nerve block: a focused review on anatomy and updated techniques. *Biomed Res Int.* 2017;2017:7023750.

(4) **C.** For most patients, the standard of care for hip fracture is surgical treatment. However, non-surgical treatment may be appropriate in limited contexts such as patient refusal and unlikelihood of a meaningful recovery. Given the patient's history, it would be reasonable to discuss goals of care with all parties before proceeding directly to the OR. Echocardiography may be indicated for a newfound unexplained systolic heart murmur, particularly before surgery.

References

Tay E. Hip fractures in the elderly: operative versus nonoperative management. *Singapore Med J.* 2016;57(4):178–181.

Parker M, Johansen A. Hip fracture. *BMJ.* 2006;333(7557):27–30.

5 C The quadratus lumborum block can be performed at various points relative to the muscle due to the continuity of the enveloping thoracolumbar fascia. For the anterior approach, local anesthetic is deposited between the quadratus lumborum and the psoas major muscle, whereas the posterior approach involves the erector spinae muscles.

Reference

Elsharkawy H, El-Boghdadly K, Barrington M. Quadratus lumborum block: anatomical concepts, mechanisms, and techniques. *Anesthesiology.* 2019;130(2):322–335.

(6) **D.** Hip fracture surgery is invasive and will not be adequately covered with peripheral nerve blockade and sedation alone; it will require a general or neuraxial anesthetic. However, the optimal plan is a complex topic, with multiple studies yielding conflicting results. Unfortunately, few of these studies are large-scale randomized controlled trials that employ clinically relevant protocols or outcomes. However, many such trials are currently underway, including the REGAIN, iHOPE, and RAGA-Delirium studies.

References

Neuman MD, Ellenberg SS, Sieber FE, et al. Regional versus General Anesthesia for Promoting Independence after Hip Fracture (REGAIN): protocol for a pragmatic, international multicentre trial. *BMJ Open.* 2016;6(11):e013473.

Li T, Yeung J, Li J, et al. Comparison of regional with general anaesthesia on postoperative delirium (RAGA-delirium) in the older patients undergoing hip fracture surgery: study protocol for a multicentre randomised controlled trial. *BMJ Open.* 2017;7(10):e016937.

Kowark A, Adam C, Ahrens J, et al. Improve hip fracture outcome in the elderly patient (iHOPE): a study protocol for a pragmatic, multicentre randomised controlled trial to test the efficacy of spinal versus general anaesthesia. *BMJ Open.* 2018;8(10):e023609.

(7) **A.** The hip joint is primarily supplied by medial and lateral circumflex arteries, which arise from the deep femoral artery. However, the intracapsular femoral neck area has relatively little cancellous bone and a poor blood supply, especially compared to the intertrochanteric region. As such, fractures in this area do not tend to be associated with a lot of bleeding but do have higher rates of nonunion or malunion and are more likely to lead to avascular necrosis.

Reference

LaValle DG. Fractures and dislocations of the hip. In: Campbell WC, Canale ST, Beaty JH, eds. *Campbell's Operative Orthopaedics.* 11th ed. Phildelphia: Mosby/Elsevier; 2008:3237–3283.

(8) **B.** There are relatively few absolute contraindications to spinal anesthesia, and they include patient refusal, allergy, and infection at the site of injection. Allergies to aminoester local anesthetics does not preclude the use of aminoamides as there is little cross reactivity. Further, remote surgery at the site of injection may make the procedure more challenging but is not a contraindication. Relative contraindications include coagulopathies, sepsis, neurological disease, and fixed cardiac output states. Moderate aortic stenosis is a fixed cardiac output state and is relatively contraindicated; this can still be a viable option if neuraxial blockade is titrated slowly via a catheter, for example.

Reference

Brull R, Macfarlane A, Chan V. Spinal, epidural, and caudal anesthesia. In Gropper MA, Miller RD, eds. *Miller's Anesthesia.* Ninth ed. Philadelphia PA: Elsevier; 2020:1413–1449.e9

27.

REGIONAL ANESTHESIA AND PAIN MANAGEMENT FOR TOTAL HIP ARTHROPLASTY

Bradley H. Lee, Marko Mamic, and Jiabin Liu

STEM CASE AND KEY QUESTIONS

A 72-year-old female is scheduled for primary total hip replacement. Past medical history is significant for hypertension, coronary artery disease, asthma, and gastroesophageal reflux. Surgical history includes lumbar laminectomy. Her functional capacity is excellent (>4 METS). She has no known drug allergies and her BMI is 32 kg/m^2. She has taken oxycodone 5 mg twice daily for the past 2 years for chronic hip and back pain.

Patient states that she had a hard time coming out of anesthesia after her lumbar laminectomy and is inquiring whether there are other options for anesthesia you can offer. She also mentions that she felt terrible when she received morphine after her back surgery. She felt very nauseous and recalls that one night she saw elephants moving on the wall.

(1) WHAT ARE INDICATIONS FOR TOTAL HIP REPLACEMENT (THR)?

The most common indication for total hip replacement is osteoarthritis (approximately 90%).[1] Other indications are femoral neck fracture (5%), avascular necrosis (2%), dysplasia (2%), and inflammatory arthritis (1%)[1]. The etiology of hip osteoarthritis is typically multifactorial, involving factors such as genetics, age, sex, trauma, and joint morphology.[1]

(2) WHAT ARE THE DIFFERENT APPROACHES FOR HIP REPLACEMENT?

There are multiple surgical approaches for THR: anterior, lateral, and posterior. Surgical approach and patient positioning should be considered as we design the plan for anesthesia and postoperative analgesia for each patient.

(3) WHAT ARE THE DIFFERENT OPTIONS FOR ANESTHESIA FOR THR? WHAT ARE THE ADVANTAGES OF EACH OPTION?

Options for anesthesia for THR include general anesthesia and neuraxial anesthesia. The latter can be spinal, epidural, or combined spinal and epidural anesthesia. Compared with general anesthesia, neuraxial anesthesia may be associated with lower risk of perioperative complications, including decreased incidence of pneumonia, acute renal failure, blood loss, thromboembolic events, infection, and mortality.[2] Combining general with neuraxial anesthesia may also confer benefits with regard to the previously mentioned outcomes, though likely to a lesser degree than with the use of neuraxial anesthesia alone.[2] Risk of urinary retention with neuraxial anesthesia is not reduced versus general anesthesia.[2]

(4) WHAT ARE THE DIFFERENT OPTIONS FOR ANALGESIA AFTER THR?

Multimodal analgesia for THR is defined as the use of two or more analgesics of different classes of medication.[3] These medications act synergistically to improve analgesia while minimizing side effects.[3] Multimodal analgesia protocols often include the use of epidural analgesia, peripheral nerve blocks, or periarticular local anesthetic infiltration.

(5) WHAT ARE THE DIFFERENT TYPES OF NERVE BLOCKS THAT CAN BE USED FOR ANALGESIA AFTER THR?

Nerve blocks used for analgesia after THR include: lumbar plexus block, fascia iliaca compartment block (FICB), and femoral nerve block (FNB). More recently, quadratus lumborum block (QLB) and pericapsular nerve group (PENG) block have been used with varying degrees of success.[4–9]

DISCUSSION

THR is one of the most commonly performed procedures, with a projection of at least 2 million performed per year.[10] It is indicated when conservative treatment for degenerative arthritis fails. Different surgical approaches for THR include anterior, lateral, and posterior approaches, with each approach differing in terms of patient positioning, surgical exposure, dislocation rates, and muscle-sparing.

In the *anterior approach*, the patient is positioned supine, and surgical incision is typically made lateral to anterior superior iliac spine and extended distally.[11] Potential advantages of this approach include sparing of muscle and low dislocation rates.[11] With a *lateral approach*, surgery takes place in the lateral decubitus position, and femoral neck osteotomy is performed to access acetabulum and proximal femur.[11] The advantages of the direct lateral approach are good surgical exposure and low dislocation rates.[11] The *posterior approach* is the most common surgical approach.[12] The patient is positioned in lateral decubitus position, and skin incision is made distal to the greater trochanter and extended toward posterior superior iliac spine.[11] The posterior approach provides adequate visualization of both the acetabulum and femur for hip replacement surgery, and it also spares the abductor muscles during surgical exposure.[13]

The hip joint is innervated by nerves arising from the lumbar and sacral plexuses. The anterior capsule of the hip is innervated by the femoral nerve (anterolaterally), obturator nerve (anteromedially), and accessory obturator nerve.[14–16] The posterior and inferior hip joint capsule is supplied by the sacral plexus, including branches from the sciatic and superior gluteal nerves.[15,16] The nerve supply to the inferior and posterior parts of the hip capsule, however, are primarily mechanoreceptors;[17] therefore, the main mediators of nociceptive pain from the hip joint are the femoral, obturator, and accessory obturator nerves.[15,18] The incision for the various surgical approaches typically lies in the distribution of the lateral femoral cutaneous nerve.[11,15] With an anterior approach, the incision may extend into the cutaneous distributions of the femoral or genitofemoral nerves.[11,15]

Options for anesthesia for THR include general anesthesia and neuraxial anesthesia (spinal, epidural, or combined spinal and epidural anesthesia). The advantage of epidural and combined spinal/epidural anesthesia is the use of the epidural catheter for postoperative pain management. Risk of post-dural puncture headache after spinal versus epidural for THR is unclear. Spinal and epidural anesthesia are associated with lower risk of perioperative complications of pneumonia, acute renal failure, blood loss, thromboembolic events, infection, and mortality relative to general anesthesia.[2] The risk of urinary retention with spinal and epidural anesthesia is not reduced compared with general anesthesia.[2]

A number of regional anesthesia techniques have been described for addressing postoperative pain in THR patients. Epidural analgesia improves pain at rest and with movement compared with systemic analgesia, while causing less sedation.[19] However, epidural analgesia is more likely to result in urinary retention, pruritis, and hypotension.[19] Another limitation is the motor weakness caused by epidural analgesia that impairs ambulation.[20] Lumbar plexus block provides effective analgesia comparable to epidural analgesia, while allowing earlier ambulation,[21,22] However, it also can also cause motor weakness.[22]

Femoral nerve blocks (FNBs) have shown analgesic efficacy in patients undergoing THR.[23,24] FNB and epidural analgesia provide similar pain control, while FNB is less likely to cause hypotension.[25] FNB does, however, cause significant quadriceps weakness, which limits ambulation to a greater degree than LPB.[24] Fascia iliaca compartment block (FICB) is a similar technique that also causes quadriceps weakness,[26] and appears to provide similar pain control as FNB.[27]

Quadratus lumborum block (QLB) and pericapsular nerve group (PENG) blocks are newer techniques that are being investigated for hip surgery. QLB is potentially motor-sparing, though evidence for QLB is limited and exists mostly in the form of case reports showing analgesia and minimal opioid use.[4,5,28] At this time, there are no randomized controlled trials comparing QLB to other techniques. PENG block is also motor-sparing, and case reports demonstrate analgesia for hip dislocations, arthroscopy, and arthroplasty, though randomized controlled trials are lacking.[7,8,29]

EPIDURAL ANALGESIA

WHAT ARE THE OPTIONS FOR EPIDURAL ANALGESIA?

Analgesia after hip replacement can be achieved with lumbar epidural catheter placement.[19,20,30] Local anesthetics and opioids are used most commonly and can be administered through continuous infusion or patient-controlled analgesia.[20,30,31] When used in combination, local anesthetics and opioids act synergistically and provide improved analgesia.[31]

HOW DOES EPIDURAL ANALGESIA COMPARE WITH SYSTEMIC ANALGESIA?

Epidural analgesia may improve pain at rest in the first 4–6 hours after surgery compared with systemic analgesia.[19] Patients receiving epidural analgesia also have less pain with movement after surgery.[19] Sedation occurs less frequently with epidural analgesia.[19] There does not appear to be a difference in the incidence of nausea, vomiting, or respiratory depression.[19]

HOW DOES EPIDURAL ANALGESIA COMPARE WITH OTHER REGIONAL TECHNIQUES?

Studies have shown that intra-articular injection may provide similar pain relief to epidural analgesia, while reducing side effects such as vomiting and urinary retention.[20,32] Intra-articular injection is also less likely to cause motor weakness and therefore facilitates postoperative ambulation compared with epidural analgesia.[20] Lumbar plexus blocks seem to provide improved analgesia, while also allowing earlier postoperative ambulation.[21,22] In a study by Singelyn et al., continuous FNB and epidural analgesia provided similar pain control with no difference in hip flexion or time to ambulation, though the epidural group experienced more frequent hypotension and catheter-related problems.[25]

WHAT ARE THE LIMITATIONS OF EPIDURAL ANALGESIA?

Compared with systemic analgesia, epidural analgesia is more likely to result in urinary retention, itching, and hypotension.[19] Epidural analgesia may also result in motor weakness, which hinders postoperative ambulation.[20] Use of thromboprophylaxis and epidural catheter removal must be coordinated in order to minimize risk of bleeding-related complications.[19,31]

LUMBAR PLEXUS BLOCK (LPB)

The lumbar plexus is formed by ventral rami of nerve roots L1–L4, also with contributions from T12 and L5, and descends along the psoas muscle.[33] Lumbar plexus block (LPB) is also commonly referred to as "psoas compartment block" and targets femoral, obturator, lateral femoral cutaneous, iliohypogastric, ilioinguinal, and genitofemoral nerves.[33]

HOW IS THE LUMBAR PLEXUS BLOCK PERFORMED?

Patients can be placed in either seated or lateral decubitus position to perform the block. Both nerve stimulation and ultrasound-guided techniques have been described.[33–35] LPB is typically performed by approaching the plexus posteriorly between L3 and L5 with the block needle inserted a few cm lateral to the spinous process.[33,36,37] After contacting the transverse process, the needle is directed either cephalad or caudad and advanced no more than 2 cm beyond the transverse process. With nerve stimulation, motor response of the quadriceps muscle is used as an endpoint for block placement. Ultrasound can be used to identify structures, including transverse process, psoas muscle, and quadratus lumborum muscle (Figure 27.1), though its use has not necessarily improved block success, likely due to depth of the plexus and varying image quality.[34,35]

WHAT IS THE EVIDENCE FOR POSTOPERATIVE ANALGESIA WITH LUMBAR PLEXUS BLOCK?

Lumbar plexus block has demonstrated efficacy for postoperative analgesia as a single injection.[38] Continuous infusions through catheters are also effective and extend the duration of analgesia beyond 24 hours.[36] Compared with epidural analgesia, lumbar plexus catheters may lead to similar analgesia while allowing earlier ambulation.[21,22]

Because LPB is a deep block, concerns related to anticoagulant use and bleeding complications for neuraxial anesthesia also apply to LPB.[39–41] During block placement, it is possible to have contralateral spread with injection, as well as epidural spread.[42,43] There are also reports of injection or catheter placement in subarachnoid, epidural, and subdural spaces given proximity to these areas.[43–45] It may therefore be prudent to consider use of a test dose when performing LPB.[45] Finally, LPB can cause motor weakness likely related to femoral nerve blockade, which may impair ambulation and potentially increase risk of falls postoperatively.[43]

FEMORAL NERVE BLOCK (FNB)

HOW IS THE FEMORAL NERVE BLOCKADE PERFORMED?

Femoral nerve block (FNB; see also Chapter 26) is a relatively safe and reliable block technique that has demonstrated analgesic efficacy for total hip replacement.[25,46] The femoral artery can be located either with palpation or ultrasound in the inguinal region, and the femoral nerve lies lateral to the artery between the iliacus muscle and fascia iliaca[15] (Figure 27.2).

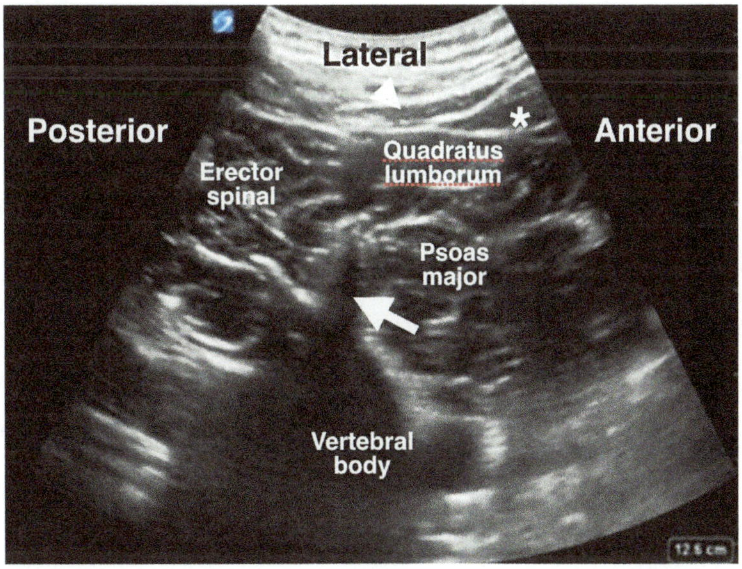

Figure 27.1. Anatomy of lumbar plexus and quadratus lumborum block. Ultrasound image with curvilinear probe placed in transverse position just above iliac crest. Structures are labeled.
Arrowhead = latissimus dorsi; * = abdominal muscles; arrow = transverse process.

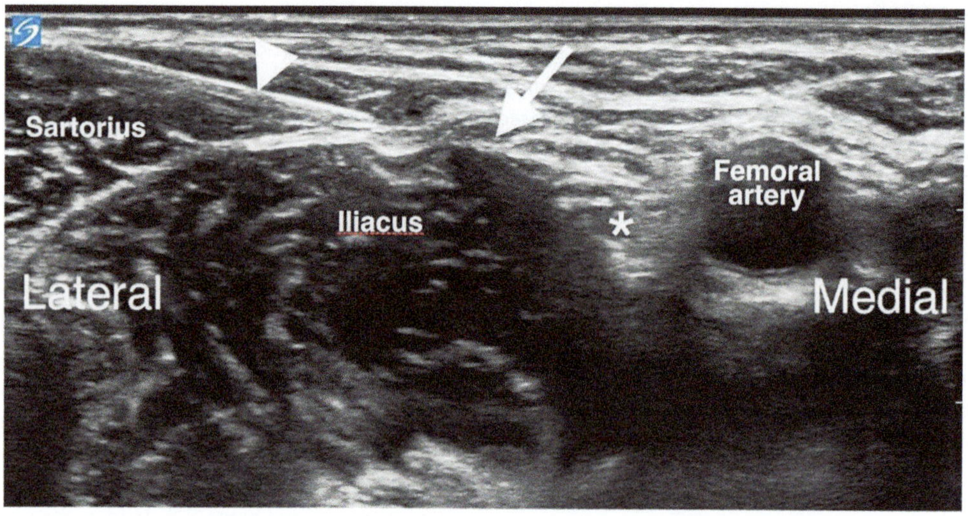

Figure 27.2. Fascia iliaca block. Ultrasound image with linear probe placed in transverse position near level of inguinal crease. Structures are labeled. Arrowhead = needle; arrow = fascia iliaca; * = femoral nerve.

WHAT IS THE EVIDENCE FOR ANALGESIA FOR HIP FRACTURE?

Compared to opioids, FN Block provides improved analgesia while minimizing systemic complications.[47–49] Additionally, the pain relief can help facilitate radiologic examinations and traction placement when necessary[50] (see Chapter 26 for further details).

THE ROLE OF FEMORAL NERVE BLOCK FOR HIP REPLACEMENT SURGERY

Femoral nerve block as a single injection may provide short-term analgesia after hip replacement.[51,52] Patients with FN Block experience lower pain scores and reduced opioid consumption in the initial 24 hours after surgery.[52] Femoral nerve block is also amenable to catheter placement that provides continuous infusions and longer duration of analgesia.[23] Compared to epidural analgesia, continuous FN Block provides similar pain control with fewer complications of hypotension and catheter-related problems.[25] Continuous fascia iliaca and continuous FNBs appear to have similar analgesic efficacy.[27]

An effective FNB results in quadriceps weakness which has implications for postoperative ambulation[53]. Continuous femoral nerve and psoas compartment blocks demonstrated similar analgesic efficacy; however, patients receiving psoas compartment blocks were more likely to ambulate greater distances compared to those receiving FNB[24].

FASCIA ILIACA COMPARTMENT BLOCK (FIC) BLOCK)

WHAT IS THE FASCIA ILIACA COMPARTMENT?

The fascia iliaca compartment describes the space formed by the iliac fascia and the psoas and iliacus muscles that it covers.[54] Nerves that originate from the lumbar plexus, including the femoral, lateral femoral cutaneous, and obturator nerves, lie posterior to the iliac fascia, and injection beneath this fascia is postulated to block these nerves.[54,55]

DESCRIBE THE ULTRASOUND-GUIDED APPROACH TO FIC BLOCK

FICB is commonly performed using ultrasound guidance with probe placement either transverse or longitudinal relative to the inguinal ligament.[54,56] In the transverse image, the femoral artery, femoral nerve, and iliac and sartorius muscles can be visualized, and the needle is advanced until it penetrates the fascia iliaca near the junction of the iliac and sartorius muscles[54] (Figure 27.2). Ultrasound-guided block can also be performed by placing the probe in longitudinal position at the lateral third of inguinal ligament with internal oblique muscle seen superiorly and sartorius muscle inferiorly with iliacus muscle deep to it.[57,58] Although the classic FICB is usually performed below the inguinal ligament, others have described supra-inguinal approaches with various probe orientation.[58,59] The supra-inguinal approaches may result in more proximal spread to cover more lumbar plexus, and therefore result in better anesthesia and analgesia.[54,60]

HOW EFFECTIVE IS FIC BLOCK FOR PROVIDING ANALGESIA FOR HIP REPLACEMENT?

Case series, meta-analyses, and randomized controlled trials have demonstrated effective analgesia from FICB for total hip arthroplasty,[27,59,61–63] though there are also conflicting studies that do not show such an effect.[64] The difference in results may possibly be attributed to variations in block technique.[54] In a recent meta-analysis, preoperative FICB was found to lower pain scores with movement compared to opioids and to reduce overall opioid consumption. FICB did not, however, demonstrate a postoperative advantage in analgesic consumption compared with other peripheral nerve blocks.[65] Also, in patients with intracapsular hip fracture, it appears that intra-articular hip injection may provide better analgesia than FICB.[66]

WHAT ARE THE ADVANTAGES OF FICB AS A REGIONAL TECHNIQUE?

FICB theoretically has less concern for direct nerve trauma or nerve injury because injection occurs in a fascial plane rather than in close proximity to nerves.[56] Continuous FICB can also be performed by using catheters in the fascia iliaca compartment.[27] Preoperative FICB may improve analgesia for positioning patients with hip fracture for spinal anesthesia.[65,67]

WHAT ARE THE LIMITATIONS TO FICB?

The primary disadvantage of the FICB is the associated motor weakness of the quadriceps muscle that occurs due to blockade of the femoral nerve, which may affect postoperative ambulation after hip replacement.[26]

QUADRATUS LUMBORUM BLOCK (QL BLOCK)

HOW DOES QL BLOCK PROVIDE POSTOPERATIVE ANALGESIA FOR HIP REPLACEMENT?

The quadratus lumborum block (QLB) is an interfascial plane block most effectively performed under ultrasound guidance[28,68] (Figure 27.1). The proposed mechanism is spread of local anesthetic along the thoracolumbar fascia, possibly into the paravertebral space.[28,68] Spread of local anesthetic is believed to block various nerves, including subcostal, iliohypogastric, and ilioinguinal nerves and possibly genitofemoral and lateral femoral cutaneous nerves, as well.[28,69]

APPROACHES TO QUADRATUS LUMBORUM BLOCK

Lateral QLB involves injection of local anesthetic on the lateral border of the quadratus lumborum muscle near its junction with the transversalis fascia where the transversus abdominis muscle tapers into its aponeurosis.[28,68,70] Posterior QLB involves injection posterior to the quadratus lumborum muscle in the plane between the muscle and middle thoracolumbar fascia just anterior to the latissimus dorsi.[28,68,70] Transmuscular or anterior QLB is performed by advancing the needle through the quadratus lumborum muscle to inject local anesthetic between the quadratus lumborum and psoas major muscles.[28,68,70]

WHAT IS THE EVIDENCE FOR POSTOPERATIVE ANALGESIA WITH QLB?

There is limited evidence demonstrating analgesia with QLB for hip surgery. Most of the evidence is in the form of case reports or case series.[4–6,71,72] These case reports demonstrate that patients who underwent hip arthroplasty with QLB experienced effective analgesia while minimizing opioid use.[5,6,71] To date, however, there are no randomized controlled trials demonstrating improved analgesia with QLB compared with other techniques.

WHAT IS THE ADVANTAGE OF UTILIZING QLB FOR ANALGESIA?

Because QLB is an interfascial plane block, there is minimal concern for risk of direct nerve injury or trauma.[28] Also, QLB may be a motor-sparing block and therefore should not inhibit ambulation and rehabilitation after surgery.[28]

WHAT ARE THE POTENTIAL DOWNSIDES OF USING QLB FOR ANALGESIA?

Although in most cases the QLB should be motor-sparing, there is the rare possibility of quadriceps weakness, and this risk may be increased with injection into the psoas major muscle.[28,73] Another concern is that the block is relatively deep in a non-compressible area; therefore, the presence of any coagulopathy and associated risk of hematoma should be carefully considered. Lastly, hypotension has been previously noted with QLB, potentially related to paravertebral spread of local anesthetic.[68,74]

PERICAPSULAR NERVE GROUP (PENG) BLOCK

WHAT IS THE AREA OF LOCAL ANESTHETIC INJECTION WHEN PERFORMING PENG BLOCK?

Pericapsular nerve group (PENG) block describes a novel regional technique that has demonstrated analgesic efficacy for hip fracture and hip surgery.[7–9] It is typically performed with ultrasound guidance, and local anesthetic is injected in the plane between the psoas tendon (anteriorly) and pubic ramus (posteriorly) near the level of the anterior inferior iliac spine (Figure 27.3).[9]

HOW DOES PENG BLOCK PROVIDE ANALGESIA?

Local anesthetic in this plane should block the articular branches of the femoral and accessory obturator nerves which innervate the anterior hip capsule, which is the more highly innervated part of the hip joint.[9] The posterior capsule of the hip is primarily innervated by the sciatic nerve, which is not affected by the PENG block.[9,15,16,75]

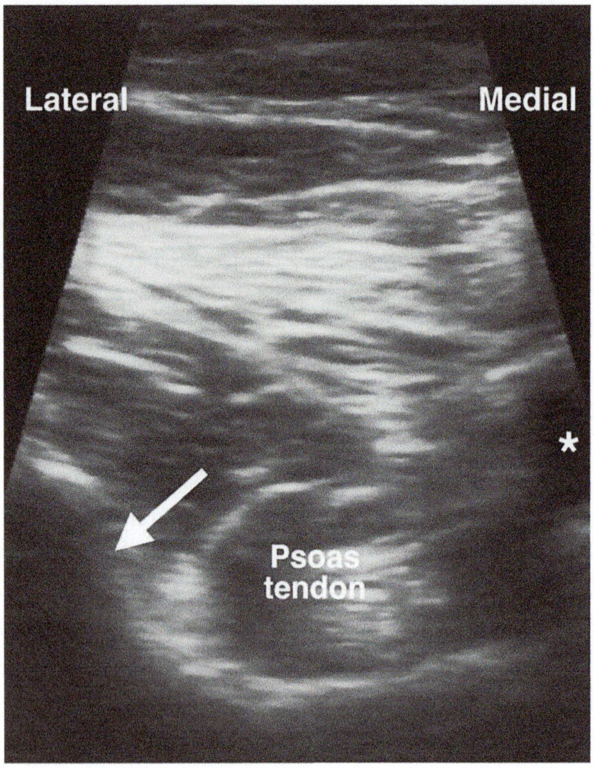

Figure 27.3. Ultrasound image with probe placed in transverse position below level of inguinal crease. Structures are labeled. Arrow = anterior inferior iliac spine, * = femoral artery

WHAT EVIDENCE EXISTS FOR ANALGESIA USING PENG BLOCK FOR HIP SURGERY?

PENG block was shown to reduce pain at rest and with movement in a case series of 5 patients who suffered various hip fractures.[9] There are other case reports and case series that demonstrate analgesic effects of PENG block for hip dislocations, hip arthroscopy, and hip arthroplasty.[7,8,29] There are no randomized controlled trials that have investigated the effects of PENG block for hip surgery, however.

WHAT ARE THE ADVANTAGES OF PENG BLOCK?

Because injection occurs in a plane, there is theoretically less risk for direct nerve injury or nerve trauma compared with block techniques that target specific nerves. Also, the PENG block occurs near the joint capsule and therefore is motor-sparing, which may provide analgesia while allowing for early ambulation.[9]

WHAT ARE THE POTENTIAL RISKS WITH PENG BLOCK?

In spite of the proposed motor-sparing effects of the block, depending on the needle placement and volume of local anesthetic, it is possible for local anesthetic to affect the femoral nerve and its motor branches, which may result in quadriceps weakness.[76]

MULTIMODAL ANALGESIA

WHAT ARE THE OPTIONS FOR MULTIMODAL ANALGESIA FOR HIP REPLACEMENT?

There is an extensive list of analgesic agents that are available for use in hip replacement surgery. The most commonly used modes of analgesic medications are presented here. Regional techniques are often regarded as part of multimodal analgesia, but will not be included because they are discussed elsewhere in the chapter.

ACETAMINOPHEN

What Is the Mechanism of Action for Acetaminophen?

Acetaminophen is a well-known analgesic with minimal side effects. Its mechanism of action is not entirely understood, though it is believed to act in a similar manner to nonsteroidal anti-inflammatory drugs (NSAIDs) by inhibiting cyclooxygenase enzymes.[3,77,78] It is available in both parenteral and oral formulations, and oral administration has reliable onset within 30–45 minutes with up to 79%–87% bioavailability.[3]

What Is the Evidence for Postoperative Analgesia Using Acetaminophen?

Recent meta-analyses have found that acetaminophen improved analgesia and reduced opioid consumption after hip arthroplasty compared with placebo.[79,80] A randomized controlled trial also demonstrated that acetaminophen has improved efficacy versus placebo in reducing pain and opioid consumption.[81] There does not appear to be a difference in efficacy between oral and parenteral forms, though the parenteral formulation is significantly more expensive.[82–85]

NSAIDS

What Is the Mechanism of Action for NSAIDs?

Nonsteroidal anti-inflammatory drugs act by inhibiting cyclooxygenase 1 and cyclooxygenase 2, which reduces prostaglandins that mediate pain and inflammation.[3,78] There are numerous NSAIDs that vary in onset, duration, route of administration, efficacy, and side effects. NSAIDs can be administered via oral, intravenous (IV), topical, and rectal routes.

What Are Potential Side Effects or Risks Associated with NSAID Use?

These medications can cause some degree of platelet dysfunction, gastrointestinal mucosal injury, and renal dysfunction, and should be used cautiously in patients with underlying impairment to these systems. There are also agents that selectively inhibit cyclooxygenase-2, such as parecoxib and celecoxib.[78] COX-2 inhibitors maintain gastric mucosal integrity, though there may be cardiovascular risks with long-term use.[86]

What Evidence Exists for Using NSAIDs for Postoperative Analgesia in Hip Replacement Surgery?

There is evidence that NSAIDs are effective as part of multimodal analgesia after hip replacement.[87] Compared with placebo, patients who received celecoxib perioperatively had improved pain, less opioid use, and earlier ambulation after hip replacement.[87] Elderly patients who received parecoxib after hip surgery experienced less pain, morphine use, and incidence of delirium relative to the control placebo group.[88] There is some evidence that NSAIDs may have improved efficacy over acetaminophen for analgesia as part of multimodal regimen.[89,90]

GABAPENTINOIDS

What Are Gabapentinoids?

This class includes gabapentin and pregabalin, which are structural analogs of gamma-aminobutyric acid, though they do not exert any activity on gamma-aminobutyric acid receptors.[91] Gabapentinoids actually bind to the alpha-2 delta subunit of presynaptic voltage-gated calcium channels and thereby modulate the release of excitatory neurotransmitters from activated nociceptors.[91]

What Are the Side Effects of Gabapentinoids?

Gabapetinoids are generally safe and well tolerated, with the most common reported side effects of sedation, dizziness, headache, and visual disturbances.[91,92] Patients taking gabapentin may experience peripheral edema, as well.[91,93]

How Effective Are Gabapentinoids in Providing Analgesia After Hip Replacement?

There is limited evidence that gabapentinoids compared with placebo reduce opioid consumption after hip replacement, though it also results in increased sedation.[94–96] It is unclear whether the addition of gabapentinoids to a postoperative multimodal regimen that includes acetaminophen and NSAID will necessarily result in improved analgesia.[97]

STEROIDS

How Do Steroids Provide Analgesia?

By binding intracellular glucocorticoid receptors, steroids affect the expression of various genes, including pro-inflammatory cytokines that mediate pain.[98] Potential concerns related to steroid use include hyperglycemia, effects on wound healing, infection, and suppression of the hypothalamic-pituitary axis, though most of these concerns are due to long-term use.[98,99]

What Evidence Exists for Steroid Use and Postoperative Analgesia?

Dexamethasone is a commonly used corticosteroid and has demonstrated analgesic efficacy.[100,101] A single dose of dexamethasone given preoperatively resulted in reduced dynamic pain after hip replacement, and repeated dosing of dexamethasone starting preoperatively and continued after surgery led to improved pain and less opioid consumption.[100,101]

OTHER AGENTS

Ketamine and magnesium sulfate function as antagonists of the N-methyl D-aspartate (NMDA) receptor and therefore inhibit nociception.[3,78,84] Clonidine and dexmedetomidine are alpha-2 agonists that can also reduce pain transmission.[3,102] Although these agents have analgesic effects, studies investigating efficacy in patients undergoing hip replacement are limited.

WHAT ARE THE ADVANTAGES OF MULTIMODAL ANALGESIA?

Overall, there is growing evidence for the advantages of multimodal analgesia including both improved analgesia, reduced opioid consumption, and possibly even shorter hospital stays and lower direct medical costs.[87,89,103–106] It is recommended that multimodal analgesia be utilized when possible for hip replacement surgery.[89,103,104]

WHAT ARE POTENTIAL NERVE-RELATED COMPLICATIONS ASSOCIATED WITH HIP REPLACEMENT?

The overall prevalence of nerve injury is estimated to be around 1%.[107] With lateral approach, there is 2.2%–42.5% incidence of superior gluteal nerve injury which can result in abductor insufficiency.[108,109] The lateral femoral cutaneous nerve can be injured in up to 15%–80% of surgeries through the anterior approach.[110] Sciatic nerve injury is highest with the posterior approach, with estimated incidence of 1.3%.[111] With all three approaches, there is risk for femoral nerve palsy ranging from 0.1% to 2.4%.[107,112]

WHAT IS THE RISK OF NERVE INJURY WITH REGIONAL ANESTHESIA?

In many cases, fortunately, neurapraxias are transient and improve over time. Regarding regional anesthesia, an evaluation of patients over a 20-year period undergoing hip replacement did not identify an increase in risk of perioperative nerve injury with use of neuraxial anesthesia or peripheral nerve blockade.[113]

REFERENCES

1. Ferguson RJ, Palmer AJ, Taylor A, Porter ML, Malchau H, Glyn-Jones S. Hip replacement. *Lancet*. 2018;392(10158):1662–1671. doi: 10.1016/S0140-6736(18)31777-X.
2. Memtsoudis SG, Cozowicz C, Bekeris J, et al. Anaesthetic care of patients undergoing primary hip and knee arthroplasty: consensus recommendations from the International Consensus on Anaesthesia-Related Outcomes after Surgery group (ICAROS) based on a systematic review and meta-analysis. *Br J Anaesth*. 2019;123(3):269–287. doi: 10.1016/j.bja.2019.05.042.

3. Tang R, Evans H, Chaput A, Kim C. Multimodal analgesia for hip arthroplasty. *Orthop Clin North Am*. 2009;40(3):377–387. doi: 10.1016/j.ocl.2009.04.001.
4. Ueshima H, Yoshiyama S, Otake H. The ultrasound-guided continuous transmuscular quadratus lumborum block is an effective analgesia for total hip arthroplasty. *J Clin Anesth*. 2019;31(2016):35. doi: 10.1016/j.jclinane.2015.12.033.
5. La Colla L, Uskova A, Ben David B. Single-shot quadratus lumborum block for postoperative analgesia after minimally invasive hip arthroplasty: a new alternative to continuous lumbar plexus block? *Reg Anesth Pain Med*. 2017;42(1):125–126.
6. Hocket MM, Hembrador S, Lee A. Continuous quadratus lumborum block for postoperative pain in total hip arthroplasty: a case report. *A A Case Rep*. 2016;7(6):129–131.
7. Pascarella G, Costa F, Del Buono R, et al.; collaborators. Impact of the pericapsular nerve group (PENG) block on postoperative analgesia and functional recovery following total hip arthroplasty: a randomised, observer-masked, controlled trial. *Anaesthesia*. 2021 Nov;76(11):1492–1498. doi: 10.1111/anae.15536. Epub 2021 Jul 1. PMID: 34196965; PMCID: PMC8519088.
8. Morrison C, Brown B, Lin DY, Jaarsma R, Kroon H. Analgesia and anesthesia using the pericapsular nerve group block in hip surgery and hip fracture: a scoping review. *Reg Anesth Pain Med*. 2021 Feb;46(2):169–175. doi: 10.1136/rapm-2020-101826. Epub 2020 Oct 27. Erratum in: Reg Anesth Pain Med. 2022 May;47(5):e1. PMID: 33109730.
9. Girón-Arango L, Peng PWH, Chin KJ, et al. Pericapsular nerve group (PENG) block for hip fracture. *Reg Anesth Pain Med*. 2018;43(8):859–863.
10. Kremers HM, Larson DR, Crowson CS, et al. Prevalence of total hip and knee replacement in the United States. *J Bone Jt Surg Am Vol*. 2014;97(17):1386–1397. doi: 10.2106/JBJS.N.01141.
11. Petis S, Howard JL, Lanting BL, Vasarhelyi EM. Surgical approach in primary total hip arthroplasty: anatomy, technique and clinical outcomes. *Can J Surg*. 2015;58(2):128–139. doi: 10.1503/cjs.007214.
12. Chechik O, Khashan M, Lador R et al. Surgical approach and prosthesis fixation in hip arthroplasty worldwide. *Arch Orthop Trauma Surg*. 2013;133:1595–1600.
13. Hoppenfeld S, DeBoer P, Buckley R. *Surgical Exposures in Orthopaedics: The Anatomic Approach*. Philadelphia: Lippincott Williams and Wilkins; 2009.
14. Short AJ, Barnett JJG, Gofeld M, et al. Anatomic study of innervation of the anterior hip capsule. *Reg Anesth Pain Med*. 2017;43(2):1. doi: 10.1097/aap.0000000000000701.
15. Bugada D, Bellini V, Lorini LF, Mariano ER. Update on selective regional analgesia for hip surgery patients. *Anesthesiol Clin*. 2018;36(3):403–415. doi: 10.1016/j.anclin.2018.04.001.
16. Birnbaum K, Prescher A, Hessler S, et al. The sensory innervation of the hip joint: an anatomical study. *Surg Radiol Anat*. 1997;19(6):371–375.
17. Gerhardt M, Johnson K, Atkinson R, et al. Characterisation and classification of the neural anatomy in the human hip joint. *Hip Int*. 2012;22(1):75–81.
18. Nielsen TD, Moriggl B, Soballe K, et al. A cadaveric study of ultrasound-guided subpectineal injectate spread around the obturator nerve and its hip articular branches. *Reg Anesth Pain Med*. 2017;42(3):357–361.
19. Choi PT, Bhandari M, Scott J, Douketis J. Epidural analgesia for pain relief following hip or knee replacement. *Cochrane Database Syst Rev*. 2003;(3):CD003071. doi: 10.1002/14651858.CD003071. PMID: 12917945.
20. Andersen KV, Pfeiffer-Jensen M, Haraldsted V, Søballe K. Reduced hospital stay and narcotic consumption, and improved mobilization with local and intraarticular infiltration after hip arthroplasty: a randomized clinical trial of an intraarticular technique versus epidural infusion in 80 patients. *Acta Orthop*. 2007;78(2):180–186. doi: 10.1080/17453670710013654.
21. Harvey NR, Wolf BJ, Bolin ED, Wilson SH. Comparison of analgaesia with lumbar epidurals and lumbar plexus nerve blocks in patients receiving multimodal analgaesics following primary total hip arthroplasty: a retrospective analysis. *Int Orthop*. 2017;41(11):2229–2235. doi: 10.1007/s00264-017-3465-7.
22. Wilson SH, Wolf BJ, Algendy AA, Sealy C, Demos HA, McSwain JR. Comparison of lumbar epidurals and lumbar plexus nerve blocks for analgesia following primary total hip arthroplasty: a retrospective analysis. *J Arthroplasty*. 2017;32(2):635–640. doi: 10.1016/j.arth.2016.07.042.
23. Arsoy D, Huddleston JI, Amanatullah DF, Giori NJ, Maloney WJ, Goodman SB. Femoral nerve catheters improve home disposition and pain in hip fracture patients treated with total hip arthroplasty. *J Arthroplasty*. 2017;32(11):3434–3437. doi: 10.1016/j.arth.2017.05.047.
24. Ilfeld BM, Mariano ER, Madison SJ, et al. Continuous femoral versus posterior lumbar plexus nerve blocks for analgesia after hip arthroplasty: a randomized, controlled study. *Anesth Analg*. 2011;113(4):897–903.
25. Singelyn FJ, Ferrant T, Malisse MF, Joris D. Effects of intravenous patient-controlled analgesia with morphine, continuous epidural analgesia, and continuous femoral nerve sheath block on rehabilitation after unilateral total-hip arthroplasty. *Reg Anesth Pain Med*. 2005;30(5):452–457. doi: 10.1016/j.rapm.2005.05.008.
26. Gasanova I, Alexander JC, Estrera K, Wells J, Sunna M, Minhajuddin A JG. Ultrasound-guided suprainguinal fascia iliaca compartment block versus periarticular infiltration for pain management after total hip arthroplasty: a randomized controlled trial. *Reg Anesth Pain Med*. 2019;44(2):206–211.
27. Yu B, He M, Cai GY, Zou TX, Zhang N. Ultrasound-guided continuous femoral nerve block vs continuous fascia iliaca compartment block for hip replacement in the elderly: A randomized controlled clinical trial (CONSORT). *Med (United States)*. 2016;95(42):1–5. doi: 10.1097/MD.0000000000005056.
28. Akerman M, Pejčić N, Veličković I. A Review of the Quadratus Lumborum Block and ERAS. *Front Med (Lausanne)*. 2018;5:44. doi: 10.3389/fmed.2018.00044. PMID: 29536008; PMCID: PMC5834926.
29. Orozco S, Muñoz D, Jaramillo S, Herrera AM. Pericapsular nerve group (PENG) block for perioperative pain control in hip arthroscopy. *J Clin Anesth*. 2019;4(59):3–4.
30. Jules-Elysee KM, Goon AK, Westrich GH, et al. Patient-controlled epidural analgesia or multimodal pain regimen with periarticular injection after total hip arthroplasty: a randomized, double-blind, placebo-controlled study. *J Bone Jt Surg Am 2*. 2015;97(10):789–798.
31. Horlocker TT, Kopp SL, Pagnano MW, Hebl J. Analgesia for total hip and knee arthroplasty: a multimodal pathway featuring peripheral nerve block. *J Am Acad Orthop Surg*. 2006;14(3):126–135.
32. Pandazi A, Kanellopoulos I, Kalimeris K, et al. Periarticular infiltration for pain relief after total hip arthroplasty: a comparison with epidural and PCA analgesia. *Arch Orthop Trauma Surg 2*. 2013;133(11):1607–1612.
33. Awad IT, Duggan EM. Posterior lumbar plexus block: anatomy, approaches, and techniques. *Reg Anesth Pain Med*. 2005;30(2):143–149. doi: 10.1016/j.rapm.2004.11.006.
34. Kirchmair L, Entner T, Kapral S, et al. Ultrasound guidance for the psoas compartment block: an imaging study. *Anesth Analg*. 2002;94(3):706–710.
35. Karmakar MK, Li JW, Kwok WH, et al. Ultrasound-guided lumbar plexus block using a transverse scan through the lumbar intertransverse space: a prospective case series. *Reg Anesth Pain Med2*. 2015;40(1):75–81.
36. Capdevila X, Macair P, Dadure C, et al. Continuous psoas compartment block for postoperative analgesia after total hiph arthroplasty: new landmarks, technical guidelines, and clinical evaluation. *Anesth Analg*. 2002;94:1606–1613.
37. Chayen D, Nathan H, Chayen M. The psoas compartment block. *Anesthesiology*. 1976;45:95–99.
38. Stevens RD, Van Gessel E, Flory N, et al. Lumbar plexus block reduces pain and blood loss associated with total hip arthroplasty. *Anesthesiology*. 2000;93(1):115–121.

39. Aida S, Takahashi H, Shimoji K. Renal subcapsular hematoma after lumbar plexus block. *Anesthesiology*. 1996;84:452–455.
40. Klein SM, D'Ercole F, Greengrass RA, et al. Enoxaparin associated with psoas hematoma and lumbar plexopathy after lumbar plexus block. *Anesthesiology*. 1997;87(1576–1579).
41. Horlocker TT, Vandermeuelen E, Kopp SL, et al. Regional anesthesia in the patient receiving antithrombotic or thrombolytic therapy: American Society of Regional Anesthesia and Pain Medicine evidence-based guidelines (fourth edition). *Reg Anesth Pain Med*. 2018;43(3):263–309.
42. Gadsden JC, Lindenmuth DM, Hadzic A, et al. Lumbar plexus block using high-pressure injection leads to contralateral and epidural spread. *Anesthesiology*. 2008;109(4):683–688. doi: 10.1097/ALN.0b013e31818631a7
43. YaDeau JT, Tedore T, Goytizolo EA, et al. Lumbar plexus blockade reduces pain after hip arthroscopy. *Anesth Analg*. 2012;115(4):968–972. doi: 10.1213/ane.0b013e318265bacd.
44. Litz RJ, Vicent O, Wiessner D, et al. Misplacement of a psoas compartment catheter in the subarachnoid space. *Reg Anesth Pain Med*. 2004;29(1):60–64.
45. Bradley H. Lee, Matthias Braehler. Use of test dose allows early detection of subdural local anesthetic injection with lumbar plexus block. *J Clin Anesth*. 2017;37:111–113.
46. Nishio S, Fukunishi S, Juichi M, et al. Comparison of continuous femoral nerve block, caudal epidural block, and intravenous patient-controlled analgesia in pain control after total hip arthroplasty: a prospective randomized study. *Orthop Rev (Pavia)*. 2014;6(1):15–19. doi: 10.4081/or.2014.5138.
47. Singh AP, Kohli V, Bajwa S. Intravenous analgesia with opioids versus femoral nerve block with 0.2% ropivacaine as preemptive analgesic for fracture femur: a randomized comparative study. *Anesth Essays Res*. 2016;10(2):338–342.
48. Hartmann FV, Novaes MR, de Carvalho MR. Femoral nerve block versus intravenous fentanyl in adult patients with hip fractures: a systematic review. *Brazilian J Anesthesiol*. 2017;67(1):67–71. doi: 10.1016/j.bjan.2016.10.008.
49. Hsu YP, Hsu CW, Chu KCW, et al. Efficacy and safety of femoral nerve block for the positioning of femur fracture patients before a spinal block: a systematic review and meta-analysis. *PLoS One*. 2019;14(5):e0216337.
50. Somvanshi M, Tripathi A, Meena N. Femoral nerve block for acute pain relief in fracture shaft femur in an emergency ward. *Saudi J Anaesth*. 2015;9(4):439–441.
51. Fournier R, Van Gessel E, Gaggero G, Boccovi S, Forster A, Gamulin Z. Postoperative analgesia with "3-in-1" femoral nerve block after prosthetic hip surgery. *Can J Anaesth*. 1998;45(1):34–38. doi: 10.1007/BF03011989.
52. Wiesmann T, Steinfeldt T, Wagner G, Wulf H, Schmitt J, Zoremba M. Supplemental single shot femoral nerve block for total hip arthroplasty: impact on early postoperative care, pain management and lung function. *Minerva Anestesiol*. 2014;80(1):48–57.
53. Charous MT, Madison SJ, Suresh PJ, et al. Continuous femoral nerve blocks: varying local anesthetic delivery method (bolus versus basal) to minimize quadriceps motor block while maintaining sensory block. *Anesthesiology*. 2011;115(4):774–781.
54. Desmet M, Balocco AL, Van Belleghem V. Fascia iliaca compartment blocks: different techniques and review of the literature. *Best Pr Res Clin Anaesthesiol*. 2019;33(1):57–66.
55. Dalens B, Vanneuville G, Tanguy A. Comparison of the fascia iliaca compartment block with the 3-in-1 block in children. *Anesth Analg*. 1989;69(6):705–713.
56. Dolan J, Williams A, Murney E, et al. Ultrasound guided fascia iliaca block: a comparison with the loss of resistance technique. *Reg Anesth Pain Med*. 2008;33(6):526–531.
57. Hebbard P, Ivanusic J SS. Ultrasound-guided supra-inguinal fascia iliaca block: a cadaveric evaluation of a novel approach. *Anaesthesia*. 2011;66(4):300–305.
58. Singh H, Jones D. Hour-glass pattern recognition simplifies fascia iliaca compartment block. *Reg Anesth Pain Med*. 2013;38(5):467–468.
59. Bullock WM, Yalamuri SM, Gregory SH, et al. Ultrasound-guided suprainguinal fascia iliaca technique provides benefit as an analgesic adjunct for patients undergoing total hip arthroplasty. *J Ultrasound Med*. 2017;36(2):433–438.
60. Vermeylen K, Desmet M, Leunen I, et al. Supra-inguinal injection for fascia iliaca compartment block results in more consistent spread towards the lumbar plexus than an infra-inguinal injection: a volunteer study. *Reg Anesth Pain Med*. 2019;44:483–491.
61. Cai L, Song Y, Wang Z, et al. The efficacy of fascia iliaca compartment block for pain control after hip arthroplasty: a meta-analysis. *Int J Surg*. 2019;66:89–98.
62. Desmet M, Vermeylen K, Van Herreweghe I, et al. A longitudinal supra-inguinal fascia iliaca compartment block reduces morphine consumption after total hip arthroplasty. *Reg Anesth Pain Med*. 2017;42(3):327–333.
63. Gao Y, Tan J, Sun R, et al. Fascia iliaca compartment block reduces pain and opioid consumption after total hip arthroplasty: a systematic review and meta-analysis. *Int J Surg*. 2019;65:70–79.
64. Shariat AN, Hadzic A, Xu D, et al. Fascia iliaca block for analgesia after hip arthroplasty: a randomized double-blind, placebo-controlled trial. *Reg Anesth Pain Med*. 2013;38(3):201–205.
65. Steenberg J, Møller AM. Systematic review of the effects of fascia iliaca compartment block on hip fracture patients before operation. *Br J Anaesth*. 2018;120(6):1368–1380.
66. Aprato A, Audisio A, Santoro A, et al. Fascia-iliaca compartment block vs intra-articular hip injection for preoperative pain managemenet in intracapsular hip fractures: a blind, randomized, controlled trial. *Injury*. 2018;49(12):2203–2208.
67. Kacha NJ, Jadeja CA, Patel PJ, et al. Comparative study for evaluating efficacy of fascia iliaca compartment block for alleviating pain of positioning for spinal anesthesia in patients with hip and proximal femur fractures. *Indian J Orthop*. 2018;52(2):147–153.
68. Elsharkawy H. Quadratus lumborum blocks. *Adv Anesth*. 2017;35(1):145–157. doi: 10.1016/j.aan.2017.07.007.
69. Carline L, Mcleod GA, Lamb C. A cadaver study comparing spread of dye and nerve involvement after three different quadratus lumborum blocks. *Br J Anaesth*. 2016;117(3):387–394. doi: 10.1093/bja/aew224.
70. Ueshima H, Otake H, Lin JA. Ultrasound-guided quadratus lumborum block: an updated review of anatomy and techniques. *Biomed Res Int*. 2017;2017(2752876).
71. Bak H, Bang S, Yoo S, et al. The continuous quadratus lumborum block for multimodal analgesia after total hip arthroplasty. *Korean J Anesth*. 2019;doi: 10.40. 28154824; PMCID: PMC5244003.
72. Sato M, Hara M, Uchida O. An antero-lateral approach to ultrasound-guided lumbar plexus block in supine position combined with quadratus lumborum block using single-needle insertion for pediatric hip surgery. *Paediatr Anaesth*. 2017;27(10):1064–1065.
73. Wikner M. Unexpected motor weakness following quadratus lumborum block for gynaecological laparoscopy. *Anaesthesia*. 2017;72(2):230–232
74. Sa M, Cardoso JM, Reis H, et al. Quadratus lumborum block: are we aware of its side effects? A report of 2 cases. *Rev Bras Anaestesiol*. 2018;68(4):396–399.
75. Short AJ, Barnett JJG, Gofeld M, et al. Anatomic study of innervation of the anterior hip capsule: implication for image-guided intervention. *Reg Anesth Pain Med*. 2018;43(2):186–192.
76. Yu HC, Moser JJ, Chu AY, et al. Inadvertent quadriceps weakness following the pericapsular nerve group (PENG) block. *Reg Anesth Pain Med*. 2019;44(5):611–613.
77. Graham GG, Davies MJ, Day RO, et al. The modern pharmacology of paracetamol: therapeutic actions, mechanism of action, metabolism, toxicity and recent pharmacological findings. *Inflammaopharmacology*. 2013;21(3):201–232.
78. Beverly A, Kaye AD, Ljungqvist O, Urman RD. Essential elements of multimodal analgesia in enhanced recovery after surgery (ERAS) guidelines. *Anesthesiol Clin*. 2017;35(2):e115–e143. doi: 10.1016/j.anclin.2017.01.018.

79. Liang L, Cai Y, Li A, Ma C. The efficiency of intravenous acetaminophen for pain control following total knee and hip arthroplasty: A systematic review and meta-analysis. *Med (United States)*. 2017;96(46):e8586.
80. Yang L, Du S, Sun Y. Intravenous acetaminophen as an adjunct to multimodal analgesia after total knee and hip arthroplasty: a systematic review and meta-analysis. *Int J Surg*. 2017;47:135–146.
81. Takeda Y, Fukunishi S, Nishio S, Yoshiya S, Hashimoto K, Simura Y. Evaluating the effect of intravenous acetaminophen in multimodal analgesia after total hip arthroplasty: a randomized controlled trial. *J Arthroplasty*. 2019;34(6):1155–1161. doi: 10.1016/j.arth.2019.02.033.
82. Westrich GH, Birch GA, Muskat AR, et al. Intravenous vs oral acetaminophen as a component of multimodal analgesia after total hip arthroplasty: a randomized, blinded trial. *J Arthroplasty*. 2019 Jul;34(7S):S215–S220.
83. Sun L, Zhu X, Zou J, et al. Comparison of intravenous and oral acetaminophen for pain control after total knee and hip arthroplasty: a systematic review and meta-anlysis. *Med*. 2018;97(6):e9751.
84. Pitchon DN, Dayan AC, Schwenk ES, Baratta JL, Viscusi ER. Updates on multimodal analgesia for orthopedic surgery. *Anesthesiol Clin*. 2018;36(3):361–373. doi: 10.1016/j.anclin.2018.05.001.
85. Gallipani A, Mathis AS, Lee Ghin, et al. Adverse effect profile comparison of pain regimens with and without intravenous acetaminophen in total hip and knee arthroplasty patients. *SAGE Open Med*. 2017;5:2050312117699146.
86. Martin Arias LH, Martin Gonzalez A, Sanz Fadrique R, et al. Cardiovascular risk of nonsteroidal anti-inflammatory drugs and classical and selective cyclooxygenase-2 inhibitors: a meta-analysis of observational studies. *J Clin Pharmacol*. 2019;59(1):55–73.
87. Chen J, Zhu W, Zhang Z, et al. Efficacy of celecoxib for acute pain management following total hip arthroplasty in elderly patients: a prospective, randomized, placebo-control trial. *Exp Ther Med*. 2015;10(2):737–742. doi: 10.3892/etm.2015.2512.
88. Mu DL, Zhang DZ, Wang DX, et al. Parecoxib supplementation to morphine analgesia decreases incidence of delirium in elderly patients after hip or knee replacement surgery: a randomized controlled trial. *Anesth Analg*. 2017;124(6):1992–2000. doi: 10.1213/ANE.0000000000002095.
89. Cozowicz C, Poeran J, Zubizarreta N, et al. Non-opioid analgesic modes of pain management are associated with reduced postoperative complications and resource utilisation: a retrospective study of obstructive sleep apnoea patients undergoing elective joint arthroplasty. *Br J Anaesth*. 2019;122(1):131–140.
90. Thybo KH, Hägi-Pedersen D, Dahl JB, et al. Effect of combination of paracetamol (acetaminophen) and ibuprofen vs either alone on patient-controlled morphine consumption in the first 24 hours after total hip arthroplasty: the PANSAID Randomized clinical trial. *JAMA*. 2019;321(6):562–571. doi: 10.1001/jama.2018.22039.
91. Schmidt PC, Ruchelli G, Mackey SC, Carroll IR. Perioperative gabapentinoids. *Anesthesiology*. 2013;119(5):1215–1221. doi: 10.1097/aln.0b013e3182a9a896.
92. Zhang J, Ho KY, Wang Y. Efficacy of pregabalin in acute postoperative pain: a meta-analysis. *Br J Anaesth*. 2011;106(4):454–462.
93. Parsons B, Tive L, Huang S. Gabapentin: a pooled analysis of adverse events from three clinical trials in patients with postherpetic neuralgia. *Am J Geriatr Pharmacother*. 2004;2(3):157–162.
94. Mao Y, Wu L, Ding W. The efficacy of preoperative administration of gabapentin/pregabalin in improving pain after total hip arthroplasty: a meta-analysis. *BMC Musculoskelet Disord*. 2016;17(1):373.
95. Mathiesen O, Jacobsen LS, Holm HE, et al. Pregabalin and dexamethasone for postoperative pain control: a randomized controlled study in hip arthroplasty. *Br J Anaesth*. 2008;101(4):535–541.
96. Clarke H, Page GM, McCartney CJ, et al. Pregabalin reduces postoperative opioid consumption and pain for 1 week after hospital discharge, but does not affect function at 6 weeks or 3 months after total hip arthroplasty. *Br J Anaesth*. 2015;115(6):903–911.
97. Clarke H, Pereira S, Kennedy D, et al. Adding gabapentin to a multimodal regimen does not reduce acute pain, opioid consumption or chronic pain after total hip arthroplasty. *Acta Anaesthesiol Scand*. 2009;53(8):1073–1083.
98. Czock D, Keller F, Rasche FM, Häussler U. Pharmacokinetics and pharmacodynamics of systemically administered glucocorticoids. *Clin Pharmacokinet*. 2005;44(1):61–98. doi: 10.2165/00003088-200544010-00003.
99. Bartlett R, Hartle AJ. Routine use of dexamethasone for postoperative nausea and vomiting: the case against. *Anaesthesia*. 2013;68(9):892–896. doi: 10.1111/anae.12309.
100. Kardash KJ, Sarrazin F, Tessler MJ, Velly AM. Single-dose dexamethasone reduces dynamic pain after total hip arthroplasty. *Anesth Analg*. 2008;106(4):1253–1257. doi: 10.1213/ANE.0b013e318164f319.
101. Backes JR, Bentley JC, Politi JR, Chambers BT. Dexamethasone reduces length of hospitalization and improves postoperative pain and nausea after total joint arthroplasty: a prospective, randomized controlled trial. *J Arthroplasty*. 2013;28(8 Suppl):11–17. doi: 10.1016/j.arth.2013.05.041.
102. Grape S, Kirkham KR, Fraunknecht J, et al. Intra-operative analgesia with remifentanil vs. dexmedetomidine: a systematic review and meta-analysis with trial sequential analysis. *Anaesthesia*. 2019;74(6):793–800.
103. Golladay GJ, Balch KR, Dalury DF, Satpathy J, Jiranek WA. Oral multimodal analgesia for total joint arthroplasty. *J Arthroplasty*. 2017;32(9):S69–S73. doi: 10.1016/j.arth.2017.05.002.
104. Soffin EM, Wu CL. Regional and multimodal analgesia to reduce opioid use after total joint arthroplasty: a narrative review. *HSS J*. 2019;15(1):57–65. doi: 10.1007/s11420-018-9652-2.
105. Duncan CM, Long KH, Warner DO, Hebl JR. The economic implications of a multimodal analgesic regimen for patients undergoing major orthopedic surgery: a comparative study of direct costs. *Reg Anesth Pain Med*. 2009;34(4):301–307. doi: 10.1097/AAP.0b013e3181ac7f86.
106. Maheshwari AV, Blum YC, Shekhar L, Ranawat AS, Ranawat CS. Multimodal pain management after total hip and knee arthroplasty at the ranawat orthopaedic center. *Clin Orthop Relat Res*. 2009;467(6):1418–1423. doi: 10.1007/s11999-009-0728-7.
107. Schmalzried TP, Noordin S, Amstutz HC. Update on nerve palsy associated with total hip replacement. *Clin Orthop Relat Res*. 1997;344(344):188–206.
108. Oldenburg M, Müller RT. The frequency, prognosis and significance of nerve injuries in total hip arthroplasty. *Int Orthop*. 1997;21:1–3.
109. Ramesh M, O'Byrne J, McCarthy N, et al. Damage to the superior gluteal nerve after the Hardinge approach to the hip. *J Bone Jt Surg Br*. 1996;78:903–906.
110. Bhargava T, Goytia R, Jones L, et al. Lateral femoral cutaneous nerve impairment after direct anterior approach for total hip arthroplasty. *Orthopedics*. 2010;33:472.
111. Farrell CM, Springer B, Haidukewych G, et al. Motor nerve palsy following primary total hip arthroplasty. *J Bone Jt Surg Am*. 2005;87:2619–2625.
112. Fox AJ, Bedi A, Wanivenhaus F, et al. Femoral neuropathy following total hip arthroplasty: review and management guidelines. *Acta Orthop Belg*. 2012;78:145–151.
113. Jacob AK, Mantilla CB, Sviggum HP, Schroeder DR, Pagnono MW, Hebl JR. Perioperative nerve injury after total hip arthroplasty. *Surv Anesthesiol*. 2013;57(2):94. doi: 10.1097/sa.0b013e318287da38.

REVIEW QUESTIONS

(1) Which nerve does not supply the anterior capsule of the hip?

A. Femoral nerve
B. Genitofemoral nerve
C. Obturator nerve
D. Accessory obturator nerve

(2) The lumbar plexus forms from ventral rami of nerve roots L1–L4 and descends along which muscle?

A. Psoas
B. Quadratus lumborum
C. Internal oblique
D. Paraspinal

(3) What is the expected motor response when performing lumbar plexus block with nerve stimulation?

A. Foot dorsiflexion
B. Foot eversion
C. Quadriceps twitch
D. Gluteus maximus twitch

(4) Which is true regarding epidural analgesia for hip replacement?

A. Epidural analgesia provides improved analgesia compared with intra-articular injection while reducing side effects such as nausea and urinary retention.
B. Epidural analgesia is less likely to result in motor weakness compared with intra-articular injection.
C. Systemic analgesia is more likely to result in urinary retention and itching than epidural analgesia.
D. Lumbar plexus block provides improved analgesia and earlier ambulation compared with epidural analgesia.

(5) Which is true regarding femoral nerve block for hip replacement?

A. Femoral nerve block provides similar pain control as epidural analgesia with fewer complications including hypotension.
B. Femoral nerve blockade results in weakness of the adductor muscles.
C. Femoral nerve block generally results in earlier ambulation than lumbar plexus block.
D. Femoral nerve block does not significantly reduce opioid consumption in the first 24 hours.

(6) In the ultrasound-guided longitudinal approach to fascia iliaca compartment block (FICB), which muscles are visualized?

A. Vastus medialis inferiorly, transversus abdominis superiorly
B. Sartorius muscle inferiorly, internal oblique superiorly
C. Rectus femoris inferiorly, internal oblique superiorly
D. Adductor magnus inferiorly, external oblique superiorly

(7) In the anterior or transmuscular approach to quadratus lumborum block (QLB), local anesthetic is injected between which layers?

A. Quadratus lumborum and psoas major muscles
B. Quadratus lumborum and transversus abdominis muscles
C. Quadratus lumborum and latissimus dorsi muscles
D. Quadratus lumborum and erector spinae muscles

(8) Pericapsular nerve group (PENG) block targets the articular branches of which nerves?

A. Femoral
B. Obturator
C. Accessory obturator
D. All of the above

(9) Which of the following is true regarding NSAID use after hip replacement?

A. Acetaminophen provides improved analgesia compared with NSAIDs.
B. NSAIDs are contraindicated after hip replacement due to platelet dysfunction.n
C. NSAIDs result in less pain and lower incidence of delirium compared with placebo.
D. NSAIDs do not significantly reduce opioid consumption compared with placebo.

(10) What is the approximate risk of femoral nerve palsy after hip replacement in the absence of nerve blockade?

A. 0.1% to 2.4%
B. 3.5% to 5%
C. 6.3% to 7.8%
D. 8.7% to 9.9%

ANSWERS

(1) **A.** The anterior capsule of the hip is supplied by the following nerves: femoral, obturator, accessory obturator.

Reference

Short AJ, Barnett JJG, Gofeld M, et al. Anatomic study of innervation of the anterior hip capsule. *Reg Anesth Pain Med*. 2017;43(2):1. doi: 10.1097/aap.0000000000000701.

(2) **A.** The nerves from the lumbar plexus descend along the psoas muscle. Lumbar plexus block is also commonly referred to as "psoas compartment block."

Reference

Awad IT, Duggan EM. Posterior lumbar plexus block: anatomy, approaches, and techniques. *Reg Anesth Pain Med*. 2005;30(2):143–149. doi: 10.1016/j.rapm.2004.11.006.

(3) **C.** Lumbar plexus block performed with nerve stimulation should result in quadriceps twitch.

Reference

Awad IT, Duggan EM. Posterior lumbar plexus block: anatomy, approaches, and techniques. *Reg Anesth Pain Med*. 2005;30(2):143–149. doi: 10.1016/j.rapm.2004.11.006.

(4) **D.** Lumbar plexus block provides better analgesia and earlier ambulation than epidural analgesia.

References

Harvey NR, Wolf BJ, Bolin ED, Wilson SH. Comparison of analgaesia with lumbar epidurals and lumbar plexus nerve blocks in patients receiving multimodal analgaesics following primary total hip arthroplasty: a retrospective analysis. *Int Orthop*. 2017;41(11):2229–2235. doi: 10.1007/s00264-017-3465-7.

Wilson SH, Wolf BJ, Algendy AA, Sealy C, Demos HA, McSwain JR. Comparison of lumbar epidurals and lumbar plexus nerve blocks for analgesia following primary total hip arthroplasty: a retrospective analysis. *J Arthroplasty*. 2017;32(2):635–640. doi: 10.1016/j.arth.2016.07.042.

(5) **A.** Femoral nerve block provides similar analgesia as epidural catheter with fewer complications. Femoral nerve blockade results in quadriceps weakness.

Reference

Singelyn FJ, Ferrant T, Malisse MF, Joris D. Effects of intravenous patient-controlled analgesia with morphine, continuous epidural analgesia, and continuous femoral nerve sheath block on rehabilitation after unilateral total-hip arthroplasty. *Reg Anesth Pain Med*. 2005;30(5):452–457. doi: 10.1016/j.rapm.2005.05.008.

(6) **B.** In the ultrasound-guided longitudinal approach to fascia iliaca compartment block (FICB), the sartorius muscle is visualized inferiorly and the internal oblique muscle superiorly.

References

Hebbard P, Ivanusic J SS. Ultrasound-guided supra-inguinal fascia iliaca block: a cadaveric evaluation of a novel approach. *Anaesthesia*. 2011;66(4):300–305.

Singh H, Jones D. Hour-glass pattern recognition simplifies fascia iliaca compartment block. *Reg Anesth Pain Med*. 2013;38(5):467–468.

(7) **A.** Anterior or transmuscular quadratus lumborum block (QLB) involves injection of local anesthetic between the quadratus lumborum and psoas major muscles.

References

Akerman M, Pejčić N, Veličković I. A Review of the Quadratus Lumborum Block and ERAS. *Front Med (Lausanne)*. 2018 Feb 26;5:44. doi: 10.3389/fmed.2018.00044.

Elsharkawy H. Quadratus lumborum blocks. *Adv Anesth*. 2017;35(1):145–157. doi: 10.1016/j.aan.2017.07.007.

(8) **D.** PENG block targets articular branches of the femoral, obturator, and accessory obturator nerves.

Reference

Girón-Arango L, Peng PWH, Chin KJ, et al. Pericapsular nerve group (PENG) block for hip fracture. *Reg Anesth Pain Med*. 2018;43(8):859–863.

(9) **C.** Nonsteroidal anti-inflammatory drugs (NSAID) use results in less pain and lower risk of delirium after hip replacement compared with placebo.

Reference

Mu DL, Zhang DZ, Wang DX, et al. Parecoxib supplementation to morphine analgesia decreases incidence of delirium in elderly patients after hip or knee replacement surgery: a randomized controlled trial. *Anesth Analg*. 2017;124(6):1992–2000. doi: 10.1213/ANE.0000000000002095.

(10) **A.** Approximate risk of femoral nerve palsy after hip replacement without nerve blockade is 0.1% to 2.4%.

References

Schmalzried TP, Noordin S, Amstutz HC. Update on nerve palsy associated with total hip replacement. *Clin Orthop Relat Res*. 1997;344(344):188–206.

Fox AJ, Bedi A, Wanivenhaus F, et al. Femoral neuropathy following total hip arthroplasty: review and management guidelines. *Acta Orthop Belg*. 2012;78:145–151.

28.

ANALGESIA FOR KNEE ARTHROSCOPY AND ANTERIOR CRUCIATE LIGAMENT RECONSTRUCTION

Michael Feduska and Colin Feduska

STEM CASE AND QUESTIONS

A 28-year-old male professional basketball player presents for anterior cruciate ligament (ACL) reconstruction at an outpatient surgery center. The patient has a past medical history significant for spontaneous deep vein thrombosis (DVT), and a family history of substance abuse. His current home medications include Eliquis (apixaban) 5 mg BID and ibuprofen 800 mg TID. The patient is visibly anxious in the preoperative holding area, and the nurse reports he experienced a vasovagal episode with placement of the peripheral intravenous (IV) line. The patient states that he has had difficulty with postoperative pain control and required postoperative admission following prior shoulder arthroscopy under general anesthesia. He states that he is very concerned about the anesthetic plan for today's surgery. Additionally, he comments that his team was eliminated from the playoffs due to his injury and absence, and he wishes to return to competitive play as soon as possible. He is concerned about the success of the operation and any long-term effects that may affect his ability to play at a high level.

The patient is eager to begin rehabilitation as quickly as possible after the procedure. He is concerned about the use of opioids postoperatively, and would like to avoid them entirely, if possible, as he has seen the issues they have caused in his family members. The surgeon is also concerned that postoperative pain may prevent him from early rehabilitation exercises and enhanced recovery. The patient and surgeon would like to discuss what options are available for both intraoperative and postoperative analgesia. After discussing with the patient and surgeon, the decision is made to perform an adductor canal nerve block under ultrasound guidance for postoperative pain management. Fifteen milliliters of 0.5% ropivacaine is given as a bolus. The patient is brought to the operating room, induced with general anesthesia, and a laryngeal mask airway (LMA) is placed. The surgeon mentioned that he will do local infiltration for the graft harvest site.

The operation is uneventful, and the patient is brought to the recovery area. He appears mildly uncomfortable and is complaining of pain on the medial aspect of his knee and distal thigh. The physical therapists arrive to help begin recovery exercises, but when the patient stands he reports weakness in his operative knee, and has difficulty maintaining his balance. The patient refuses to continue therapy until his pain has improved. An obturator nerve block is performed to assist with medial knee pain.

The patient reports his pain is significantly better controlled after the block, but he continues to report weakness in his operative leg, preventing him from participating in therapy. He is discharged from the surgery center. The following day the patient is contacted and he states that his pain has increased significantly, and he is currently unable to move his leg due to extreme discomfort. The patient states that he anticipated longer pain relief and is disappointed with his current pain level. He discusses treatment options with the current prescription and agrees to contact the orthopedic team to adjust his pain management protocol or report to the emergency room if he feels that his pain is too severe.

Three weeks later, the patient complains of decreased sensation in the anterior aspect of his knee and medial aspect of his calf. The orthopedic surgeon states that the surgery was uncomplicated and has told the patient that the "anesthesia" is likely responsible for the sensory deficit. The patient plays professional basketball and is concerned about nerve damage and his ability to perform at his previous elite level.

Thankfully, the patient's deficit spontaneously resolves a few weeks later, and he eventually returns to practice with his team. Ten months later the patient is celebrating a historically successful season, capped off by a league championship. As he raises the championship trophy, he gives a special thank you to the anesthesia team who cared for him during his surgery and rehabilitation.

(1) THE PATIENT AND SURGEON ARE CONCERNED ABOUT POSTOPERATIVE PAIN CONTROL. WHAT ARE YOUR OPTIONS?

The anterior cruciate ligament (ACL) is the most injured knee ligament, with most injuries occurring in young athletes participating in non-contact sports.[1] Options for postoperative analgesia include multimodal analgesia, which may feature the use of lower extremity nerve blocks and/or local infiltration in addition to analgesic medications from different classes.

(2) THE SURGEON HAS CHOSEN TO USE A GRACILIS TENDON AUTOLOGOUS GRAFT FOR THIS PROCEDURE. HOW DOES THIS AFFECT THE ANESTHETIC PLAN?

The anesthesiologist will have to consider the nociceptive stimuli generated at the harvest site if autograft is chosen. Local anesthetic infiltration or targeted nerve blocks can be used if the pain at the harvest site is severe enough to warrant an additional intervention.

(3) IS REGIONAL ANESTHESIA CONTRAINDICATED IN THIS PATIENT? IS PRIMARY REGIONAL ANESTHESIA AN OPTION FOR THIS CASE?

Primary neuraxial anesthetic is not an option for the patient as he is on Eliquis 5 mg twice daily for prophylaxis against DVT and he did not stop it within 72 hours before placement of neuraxial anesthesia, as listed in the American Society of Regional Anesthesia and Pain Medicine (ASRA) guidelines on neuraxial anesthesia in patients receiving anticoagulant medications.[2] However, if the plan is to do the case with peripheral nerve blocks as a primary anesthetic, consideration would include whether the planned blocks are superficial or deep and whether the target nerves are located in a compressible area.[3] Other contraindications for regional anesthesia (infection, preexisting nerve damage, allergies) should be also considered. Primary regional anesthesia for knee surgery can be accomplished with blockade of the sciatic, femoral, obturator, and lateral femoral cutaneous nerve of the thigh ("quadruple nerve block").[4]

(4) WHAT CLINICAL ADVANTAGE DOES AN ADDUCTOR CANAL BLOCK (ACB) PROVIDE? IS FEMORAL OR ADDUCTOR CANAL APPROACH AT HIGHER RISK FOR NERVE DAMAGE?

An ACB is preferred for ACL reconstruction, due to its tendency to cause less quadriceps muscle weakness compared to femoral nerve blocks (FNBs).[5] Early recovery of quadriceps function may facilitate early ambulation and enhanced recovery. Multiple factors can contribute to nerve injury in the context of surgery and regional anesthesia. These factors include direct mechanical injury from needle trauma, surgery-related factors, and neurotoxicity of local anesthetics. The rate of nerve injury seems to be stable regardless of the type of block performed, ACB or FNB. There are data that suggest the possibility of quadriceps muscle weakness 3–6 months post-procedure.[6]

(5) WHAT ARE SOME COMMONLY USED LOCAL ANESTHETICS IN LOWER EXTREMITY NERVE BLOCKS? ARE THERE OPTIONS TO INCREASE THE EFFECTIVE LENGTH OF ANALGESIA? WHAT IS LIPOSOMAL BUPIVACAINE? CAN LIPOSOMAL BUPIVACAINE BE USED WITH OTHER LOCAL ANESTHETICS?

Bupivacaine and ropivacaine are probably the most commonly used local anesthetics for lower extremity nerve blocks. Volume and concentration will vary according to the nerve to be blocked, whether the block is needed for primary surgical anesthesia or for postoperative analgesia, and the practice norms of the institution. If prolonged analgesia is needed beyond the duration of action of local anesthetic, the anesthesiologist may consider perineural continuous catheter or additive to local anesthetics that will prolong the duration of sensory analgesia and/or motor nerve blocks. These additives include dexamethasone, buprenorphine, clonidine, and dexmedetomidine. Liposomal bupivacaine has a DepoFoam multivesicular liposome technology that will allow slow release of bupivacaine from its stores over a longer period. Currently, it is only approved for local infiltration and interscalene block.[7]

(6) HOW WOULD YOU DIFFERENTIATE BETWEEN THE MECHANISMS OF INJURY? WHAT DIAGNOSTIC TEST(S) SHOULD BE DONE, AND WHEN SHOULD IT OCCUR?

The patient calls the surgery center to discuss his symptoms with his anesthesiologist. The anesthesiologist explains to him again that nerve injury is an inherent risk for peripheral nerve blocks (PNBs), but the risk of nerve block–related nerve injury is very low. Patient- and surgery-related risk factors can contribute to nerve injury. Adequate history and physical examination and documentation of the extent of the sensory and motor deficits are key components. The patient did not have any preexisting nerve deficits or symptoms on examination the day of surgery and was an ideal candidate for regional anesthesia. The anesthesiologist explains that nerve injury can resolve spontaneously, and the best option is to monitor the current deficit. Nerve conduction studies 4–6 weeks after the initial insult are diagnostic for nerve damage. At this time the patient is complaining of a purely sensory deficit consistent with a saphenous nerve injury. Nerve injury in this distribution could be related to the PNB or surgical trauma. The patient is instructed to continue rehabilitation and to return for nerve conduction studies in a few weeks if symptoms persist. The patient appears satisfied with the explanation and plan.

DISCUSSION

Surgical repair of the ACL can be accomplished via knee arthroscopy using donor allografts or patient autografts. The most used sites for autografts are the mid-third of the patellar tendon, the medial hamstrings, or the quadriceps tendon.

Other graft materials available include cadaver allografts and synthetic grafts. ACL repair using an autograft is typically reserved for young patients and athletes due to a possible risk of re-rupture associated with allografts in this patient population. The procedure involves the insertion of an arthroscopic camera through small incisions in the knee and injection of a sterile solution to assist with visualization of the joint structures. The torn ligament is then removed, and small holes are created through the femur and the tibia into the joint space. The graft material is threaded through these holes and anchored on the exterior surfaces of the femur and tibia, with enough tension to mimic the original ligament. The incisions are closed with sutures and dressed sterilely. Rehabilitation of the knee begins as soon as possible, often in the recovery area with simple exercises, and continues for approximately 6 months after the surgery (Figures 28.1 and 28.2).

A multimodal analgesia approach is commonly employed for patients undergoing ACL reconstruction, with the primary analgesic being a lower extremity nerve block, when clinically appropriate. Options for PNBs include femoral nerve block (FNB) and adductor canal block (ACB).[8] The choice of the nerve block is mainly based on the institutional culture and practice norms. An ACB is preferred for ACL reconstruction, due to its tendency to cause less muscle weakness compared to FNBs (.[9,10] Early recovery of quadriceps function may facilitate early ambulation and enhanced recovery. FNB had previously been the gold standard for ambulatory knee surgery and may theoretically provide better overall pain control, as it might

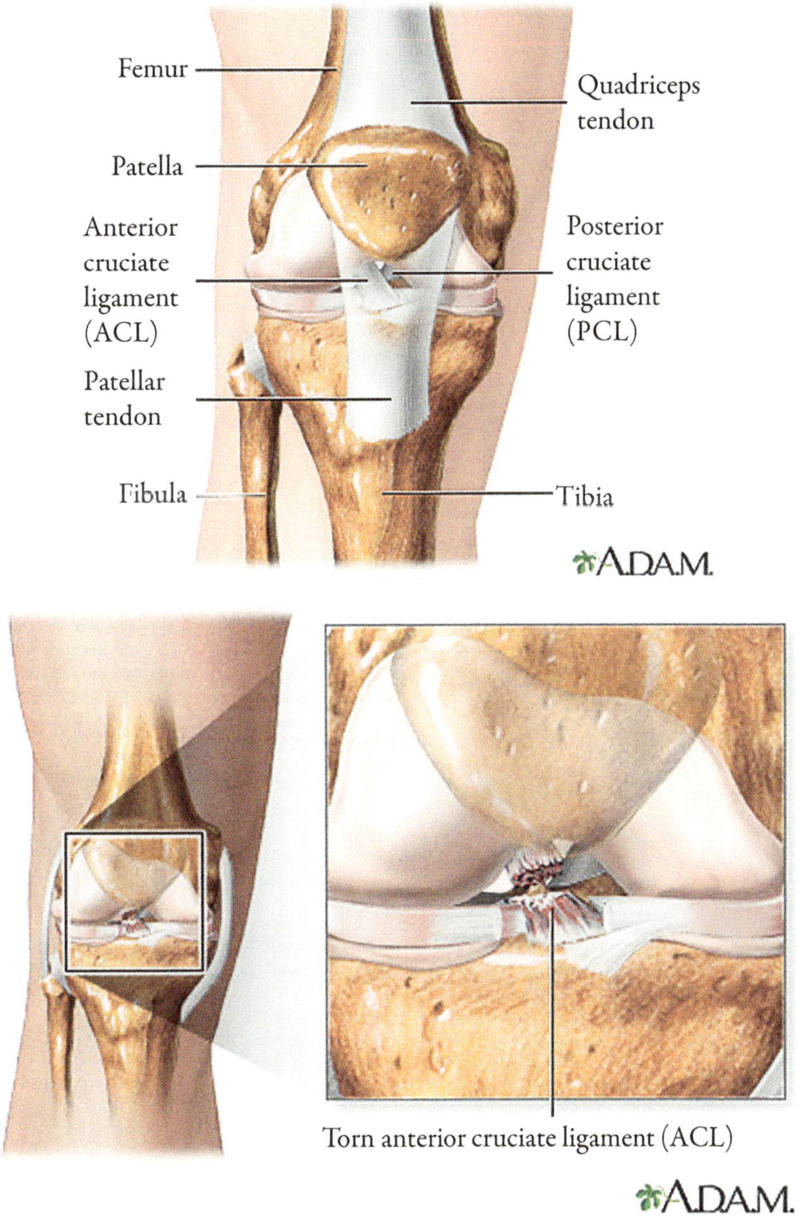

Figure 28.1. Anatomy of the cruciate ligaments.
Courtesy of MedlinePlus from the National Library of Medicine.

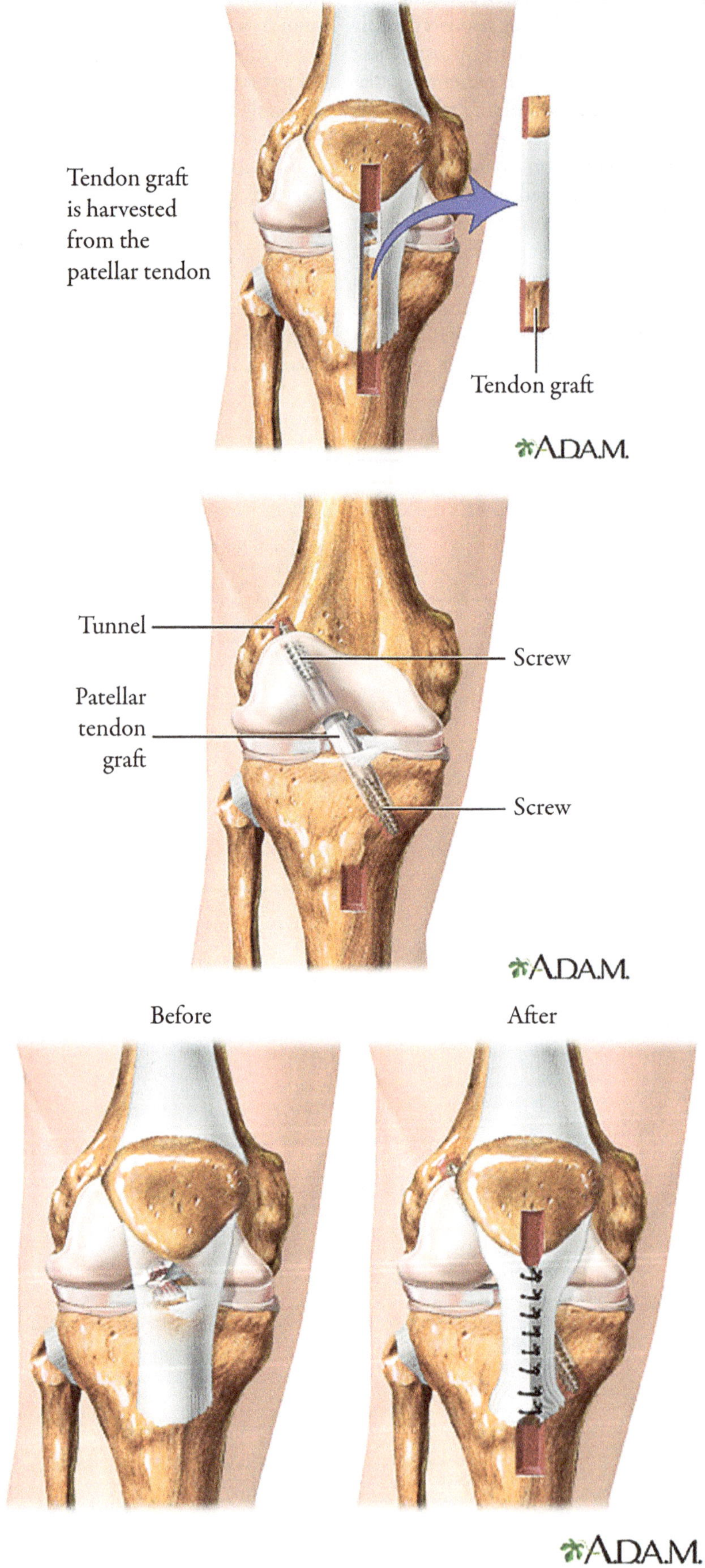

Figure 28.1. Continued

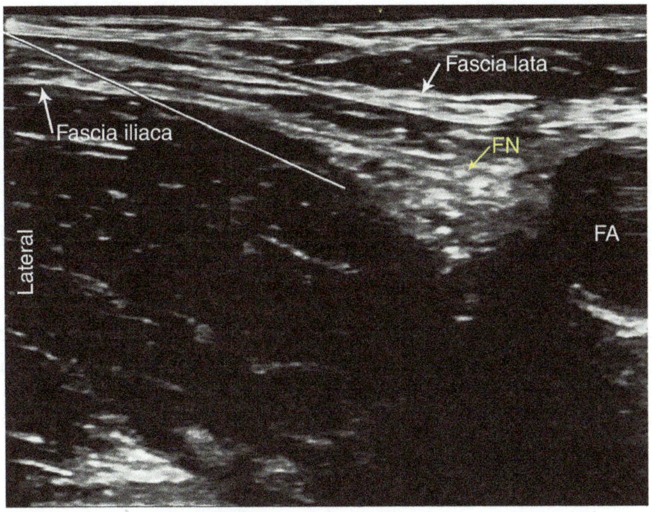

Figure 28.2. Torn anterior cruciate ligament.
From https://medlineplus.gov/ency/article/001074.htm

encompass some additional coverage for nerve branches before they branch more distally. However, if the patient uses a knee immobilizer, and is instructed to be non-weight bearing, then either femoral or adductor canal nerve blocks may be utilized. The ACB has been shown to be non-inferior in postoperative pain management compared to FNB.[10] If a lower extremity block is not an option or is contraindicated (patient refusal, or local anesthetic allergy, etc.) other, more traditional, analgesic regimens can be utilized. These include a multimodal approach using medications such as systemic (parenteral or oral) opioids, acetaminophen, or nonsteroidal anti-inflammatory drugs (NSAIDs). In fact, recent data even suggest that FNB does not provide superior analgesia to multimodal analgesic protocols.[10] Additionally, the surgeon can inject local anesthetic and opioid directly into the joint space to provide analgesia. Local infiltration has shown to have a significant effect on the reduction of opioid use postoperatively.[11] Intra-articular injection, coupled with local infiltration at the arthroscopic port sites, can be used as the primary analgesic modality for knee arthroscopy. A mixture of 20–30 mL of long-acting local anesthetic, sometimes mixed with 10 mg of morphine, is administered at our institution for both standard knee arthroscopy and ACL repair.

The use of cadaveric (allograft) or autograft carries with it not only differences in surgical technique and length of recovery, but may have anesthetic and analgesic implications as well. Use of an autograft is typically reserved for younger patient populations and athletes. The use of an autograft harvested from the gracilis tendon requires an additional incision site on the medial aspect of the knee. The skin over that site is innervated by the obturator nerve, a branch of the lumbar plexus. Therefore, if an FNB is utilized, it is possible that this additional site may be a source of postoperative pain, as the femoral nerve typically covers the anterior aspect of the knee. An autograft from the semitendinosus tendon requires a lateral or posterior lateral incision involving the sensory input from branches of the sciatic nerve. Sciatic nerve blockade would be required to achieve a primary regional anesthetic and may be used to improve postoperative analgesia for this surgical approach. Utilizing general anesthesia with a FN Block or AC Block for ACL repair with an autograft provides adequate operating conditions for the case, but may require additional analgesic options for the harvest site incisions. Harvesting of the hamstring (semitendinosus tendon or gracilis tendon) for tissue grafting has a strong association with postoperative saphenous nerve injury and should be considered when diagnosing a postoperative sensory deficit.[12]

The primary contraindication for using neuraxial anesthesia for this patient is his use of the anticoagulant Eliquis (apixaban). This medication should be stopped for at least 72 hours before attempting any neuraxial procedure.[2,3] Both femoral and adductor canal nerve blocks are considered superficial blocks, and as such carry a lower risk of neurovascular compromise should bleeding be encountered. Therefore, either block can be utilized in patients on anticoagulation. Absolute contraindications to femoral or adductor canal blocks include allergy to local anesthetics, inability to cooperate, or patient refusal. Other relative contraindications include large inguinal lymph nodes or tumor, local infection, peritoneal infection, and preexisting neuropathy. Clinical judgment and patient education should be exercised to avoid patient harm.

Recovery time from a neuraxial anesthetic can limit its effectiveness in the setting of ambulatory surgery, but it can be used as a primary anesthetic in an appropriate setting for certain knee procedures.[13,14] If spinal anesthesia is chosen, using a short-acting local anesthetic such as mepivacaine should be considered to decrease post-anesthesia recovery time.[13] While FNB is useful for postoperative analgesia, its use as a primary anesthetic for ACL reconstruction is suboptimal.[15] Port incisions at the knee joint, an anchor incision at the tibia, and potential autograph incisions along the medial (gracilis tendon) or lateral (semitendinosus tendon) require anesthesia of multiple nerves. The innervation of the knee is primarily supplied by the femoral nerve. The skin overlying the tibia and the posterior aspect of the knee is supplied by terminal branches from the sciatic nerve. Cutaneous innervation of the medial aspect of the knee varies according to different investigators but is commonly innervated by the obturator nerve.[8] Therefore, a femoral or adductor canal nerve block would likely be insufficient as a primary anesthetic. Sciatic nerve block can be used to supplement a lumbar plexus or an FNB to achieve a regional primary anesthetic.[4] Normal anatomic variation may lead to analgesic sparing and require additional local infiltration. In addition, given this patient's baseline anxiety about the anesthesia and pain control, it is unlikely that he would be able to tolerate the manipulation of the knee during the procedure. Any movement could compromise the surgery and put the patient at increased risk for surgical failure or collateral damage.

The femoral nerve is the largest branch of the lumbar plexus, and is made up by the dorsal divisions of the anterior rami of the L2, L3, and L4 spinal nerves. The femoral nerve enters the thigh under the inguinal ligament, at which point it divides into multiple terminal branches. During its course down the thigh, the nerve remains deep to the fascia lata and fascia iliaca and can be found immediately lateral and slightly posterior to the femoral artery. Utilizing a nerve stimulator with an output current set between 0.3 and 0.5 mA to elicit the quadriceps muscle contraction, causing a patellar snap, indicates proper positioning of the needle tip next to the femoral nerve. Ultrasound guided identification of the femoral artery, femoral vein, fascia lata, and fascia iliaca should help with proper block placement. The femoral nerve courses lateral to the vascular structures and beneath the fascia layers. Perineural injection around the large hyperechoic nerve bundle will achieve a successful block.

When performing an ACB, the landmarks that should be identified on ultrasound are the sartorius muscle, the trapezoid shaped muscle that forms the "roof" over the adductor canal, the vastus medialis laterally and the adductor longus (proximal) or magnus (distal) medially. On ultrasound, the saphenous nerve is typically seen as a hyperechoic structure anterolateral to the artery. Peri-arterial injection of local anesthetic under the sartorius muscle plane should achieve an adequate block if the saphenous nerve is not clearly visible. The saphenous nerve is a terminal sensory branch of the femoral nerve, and stimulation with low amperage will not elicit a motor response. Paresthesia in the distribution of the saphenous can be seen when applying current to the nerve. Optimal needle placement occurs at the mid-thigh level, proximal thigh injection may lead to blockade of branches of the femoral nerve to the vastus lateralis and can potentially lead to postoperative motor weakness.

Nerve injury is an inherent risk when performing PNBs; however, the incidence is relatively low. Preexisting nerve damage may increase the risk of further complications and a risk/benefit analysis should be discussed with the patient. The reported incidence of femoral nerve palsy following FNB has been reported to be as low as 0.1%–1%, while other complications, such as chronic pain syndromes, carry an even lower risk.[16,17] Nerve injury typically occurs because of intraneural injection or direct needle trauma, while direct needle trauma without injection results in a lesser degree of injury.[18] High injection pressures (25–45 psi) into the intra-fascicular space can cause endoneurial ischemia.[19,20] Concentration of the local anesthetic appears to be directly related to neural toxicity, with higher concentrations being more neurotoxic.[21,22] While nerve injury may spontaneously resolve, the healing process may take several months due to the slow regeneration of peripheral nerves. There appears to be no difference in the risk of developing neuropathy between the two blocks, FNB and ACB.[23] Nerve injury may occur following an uneventful regional anesthetic. Ultrasound guidance and patient participation during the procedure may give the provider the sense of risk mitigation; however, nerve injury may occur despite our best efforts. Diagnosis of nerve injury should start with identification of the motor or sensory deficit and corresponding anatomic structure. Perioperative events unrelated to regional anesthesia often contribute to postoperative nerve palsy. Patient positioning, tourniquet placement, intraoperative limb manipulation, and direct surgical injury to neurovascular structures are some of the causes that may contribute to nerve injury. Careful postoperative examination is key to identifying if the regional anesthetic could be responsible for the injury. Briefly, there are three major considerations when determining peripheral nerve injury: (1) Is there an active process, such as compressive neuropathy secondary to hematoma or compartment syndrome, causing the injury that can be treated? (2) Is the injury related to intraoperative surgical manipulation? (3) Can the nerve deficit be localized?[8] Further diagnostic testing or consultation may be warranted; evaluation of nerve injury will be covered in more detail in Chapter 50. As mentioned above, the risk for saphenous nerve injury in ACL repair with autograft from the hamstring is a well-described complication. Semitendinosis or gracilis harvesting for autograft repair can cause direct injury to the infrapatellar branch of the saphenous nerve and has been a documented complication in as high as 88% of surgeries.[12] Injury to the infrapatellar branch is thought to be caused by perpendicular transection of the nerve by use of a vertical incision.[12] The sartorial branch of the saphenous nerve is also at risk and is thought to be injured by the tendon stripper used to harvest the graft. Use of both the semitendinosus and gracilis tendon may increase the risk for nerve alteration to one or both branches of the saphenous nerve.[24]

Local anesthetics commonly used include 0.125%–0.5% bupivacaine, or 0.2%–0.5% ropivacaine. Dosing for the various local anesthetics is based on the patient's total body weight (Table 28.1). Total volume of injection will depend on the local anesthetic used, its concentration, and the patient's total body weight, but typically averages 10–20 mL for femoral or adductor canal nerve blocks. Adjunct medications such as buprenorphine, clonidine, dexamethasone, dexmedetomidine, and tramadol have been suggested as additives to prolong the duration of action of local anesthetic or increase its analgesic potency, as they are used for PNBs by acting on different nociceptive pathways.[25,26]

Liposomal bupivacaine is a multivesicular formulation of bupivacaine. It is currently approved only for administration

Table 28.1 THE MAXIMUM ALLOWED DOSE OF LOCAL ANESTHETIC IN MG/KG AND THE EXPECTED DURATION OF ACTION

LOCAL ANESTHETIC	MAXIMUM SINGLE DOSE WITHOUT VASOCONSTRICTOR (MG/KG)	ANTICIPATED LENGTH OF ANALGESIA
Lidocaine	3–4.5	2–4 hrs
Mepivacaine	4.5–5 Not to exceed 400 mg per dose Maximum 1000 mg/24h	2–3 hrs
Bupivacaine	2–2.5 Not to exceed 175 mg per dose Maximum 400 mg/24h	8–16 hrs
Ropivacaine	2–3 Not to exceed 225 mg per dose	8–16 hrs
Liposomal bupivacaine	133 mg (10 mL)	72 hours

into the surgical site via local infiltration, but has been used off label for peripheral nerve injections as well. Liposomal bupivacaine (266 mg) has been shown to result in modestly lower pain scores when used in FNBs for other knee procedures (such as total knee arthroplasty).[27] It is recommended that additional use of local anesthetics should be avoided within 96 hours following administration of liposomal bupivacaine. It is also recommended to wait at least 20 minutes to inject liposomal bupivacaine after local infiltration with lidocaine, as this may cause an increased release of bupivacaine due to lysis of the multivesicular liposome. Dosing for local anesthetics is weight based and typically expressed in milligrams per kilogram (see Table 28.1). The commonly used local anesthetics (e.g., lidocaine, ropivacaine, bupivacaine, mepivacaine) have varying degrees of toxicity, and their maximum doses can be changed with the use of vasoconstrictors (e.g., epinephrine).

In pediatric and adolescent populations (patients 18 years and younger), there is evidence that FNB for postoperative analgesia after ACL reconstruction can impact lower extremity strength months after the procedure. Furthermore, those patients who receive an FNB may be less likely to meet criteria for clearance to return to sports 6 months after the procedure.[6] Similar evidence regarding weakness 6 months after the block was performed was found in a retrospective study of an older population (average age 21), but did not show a significant delay in return to sports.[28] This is in contrast to a study that showed no statistically or clinically significant difference in quadriceps strength at 3 and 6 months postoperatively in patients who received ACBs or FNBs for ACL reconstruction.[29] While these findings may not be critical to the general population, they may have significant impact on younger athletes performing at high levels of competition. The decision for which block to perform should be multifactorial in this population and take into consideration elements such as patient satisfaction, cost-effectiveness analysis, or patient/surgeon preference.

CONCLUSION

- The femoral nerve is the largest branch of the lumbar plexus, and is made up by the dorsal divisions of the anterior rami of the L2, L3, and L4 spinal nerves.
- Femoral nerve and adductor canal blocks provide similar analgesia with no difference in complication rate.
- Femoral nerve blocks (FNBs) are associated with quadriceps weakness and have a higher risk of falls postoperatively.
- Intra-articular joint injection is an alternative analgesic method that has been shown to decrease postoperative opioid use.
- The femoral nerve provides sensory innervation to the anterior knee, but does not cover the medial or lateral aspects.
- The obturator nerve is a branch of the lumbar plexus that innervates the medial aspect of the thigh and the medial cutaneous surface of the knee.
- Absolute contraindications to femoral or adductor canal blocks include allergy to local anesthetics, inability to cooperate, and patient refusal.
- Relative contraindications to femoral or adductor canal include large inguinal lymph nodes or tumor, local infection, peritoneal infection, and preexisting neuropathy.
- The borders of the adductor canal are made up of the sartorius muscle, the vastus medialis, and the adductor longus (proximal) or magnus (distal) medially.
- Adductor canal and femoral nerve blocks have a very high safety profile. Nerve injury typically occurs as a result of intraneural injection rather than direct needle trauma.
- Total volume of local anesthetics used for peripheral nerve blocks (PNBs) is based on anesthetic concentration and patient total body weight.
- Use of local anesthetics should be avoided within 96 hours following administration of liposomal bupivacaine.
- Postoperative weakness at 6 months following regional anesthesia has been noted in some studies, though data are conflicting.

REFERENCES

1. Dordevic M, Hirschmann MT Injury Mechanisms of ACL Tear. In: R Siebold, D Dejour, S Zaffagnini, eds., *Anterior Cruciate Ligament Reconstruction*. Springer, Berlin, Heidelberg. https://doi.org/10.1007/978-3-642-45349-6
2. Horlocker TT, Vandermeulen E, Kopp SL, Gogarten W, Leffert LR, Benzon HT. Regional anesthesia in the patient receiving antithrombotic or thrombolytic therapy. *Reg Anesth Pain Med.* 2018;43(3):263–309.
3. Tsui BCH, Kirkham K, Kwofie MK, et al. Practice advisory on the bleeding risks for peripheral nerve and interfascial plane blockade: evidence review and expert consensus. *Can J Anaesth.* (2019) Nov; 66(11). 1356–1384
4. Baverel L, Cucurulo T, Lutz C, et al.; French Arthroscopic Society. Anesthesia and analgesia methods for outpatient anterior cruciate ligament reconstruction. *Orthop Traumatol Surg Res.* 2016 Dec;102(8S):S251–S255.
5. Muraskin SI, Conrad B, Zheng N, Morey TE, Enneking FK. Falls associated with lower-extremity-nerve blocks: A pilot investigation of mechanisms. *Reg Anesth Pain Med.* 2007;32:67–72.
6. Luo TD, Ashraf A, Dahm DL, Stuart MJ, McIntosh AL. Femoral nerve block is associated with persistent strength deficits at 6 months after anterior cruciate ligament reconstruction in pediatric and adolescent patients. *Am J Sports Med.* 2015;43(2):331–336.
7. Vandepitte C, Kuroda M, Witvrouw R, et al. Addition of liposome bupivacaine to bupivacaine HCl versus bupivacaine HCl alone for interscalene brachial plexus block in patients having major shoulder surgery. *Reg Anesth Pain Med.* 2017 May/Jun;42(3):334–341.
8. Hadzic A, Balocco AL. *Hadzic's Textbook of Regional Anesthesia and Acute Pain Management: Self-Assessment and Review.* New York: McGraw-Hill Education; 2019.
9. Grevstad U, Mathiesen O, Valentiner LS, Jaeger P, Hilsted KL, Dahl JB. Effect of adductor canal block *versus* femoral nerve block on quadriceps strength, mobilization, and pain after total knee arthroplasty: a randomized, blinded study. *Reg Anesth Pain Med.* 2015;40:3–10.

10. Faraj WA, Whelan DB, Chan VW, et al. Adductor canal block provides noninferior analgesia and superior quadriceps strength compared with femoral nerve block in anterior cruciate ligament reconstruction. *Anesthesiology*. 2016;124(5):1053–1064.
11. Abdallah FW, Brull R, Joshi GP; Society for Ambulatory Anesthesia (SAMBA). Pain Management for Ambulatory Arthroscopic Anterior Cruciate Ligament Reconstruction: Evidence-Based Recommendations From the Society for Ambulatory Anesthesia. *Anesth Analg*. 2019;128(4):631–640.
12. Papastergiou SG, Voulgaropoulos H, Mikalef P, Ziogas E, Pappis G, Giannakopoulos I. Injuries to the infrapatellar branch(es) of the saphenous nerve in anterior cruciate ligament reconstruction with four-strand hamstring tendon autograft: vertical versus horizontal incision for harvest. *Knee Surg Sports Traumatol Arthrosc*. 2005;14(8):789–793.
13. Mulroy MF, Larkin KL, Hodgson PS, Helman JD, Pollock JE, Liu SS. A comparison of spinal, epidural, and general anesthesia for outpatient knee arthroscopy, *Anesth Analg*. 2000 Oct;91(4):860–864.
14. Black AS, Newcombe GN, Plummer JL, McLeod DH, Martin DK. Spinal anaesthesia for ambulatory arthroscopic surgery of the knee: a comparison of low-dose prilocaine and fentanyl with bupivacaine and fentanyl. *Br J Anaesth*. 2011 Feb;106(2):183–188.
15. Mall NA, Wright RW. Femoral nerve block use in anterior cruciate ligament reconstruction surgery. *Arthroscopy*. 2010;26:404–416.
16. Auroy Y, Benhamou D, Bargues L, et al. Major complications of regional anesthesia in France: the SOS Regional Anesthesia Hotline Service. *Anesthesiology*. 2002;97:1274–1280.
17. Kaufman BR, Nystrom E, Nath S, et al. Debilitating chronic pain syndromes after presumed intraneural injections. *Pain*. 2000;85:283–286.
18. Enneking FK, Chan V, Greger J, et al. Lower-extremity peripheral nerve blockade: essentials of our current understanding. *Reg Anesth Pain Med*. 2005;30:4–35.
19. Borgeat A. Regional anesthesia, intraneural injection, and nerve injury: beyond the Epineurium. Anesthesiology. 2006;105:647–648.
20. Hadzic A, Dilberovic F, Shah S, et al. Combination of intraneural injection and high injection pressure leads to fascicular injury and neurologic deficits in dogs. *Reg Anesth Pain Med*. 2004;29:417–423.
21. Fremling MA, Mackinnon SE. Injection injury to the median nerve. *Ann Plast Surg*. 1996;37:561–567.
22. Selander D. Neurotoxicity of local anesthetics: animal data. *Reg Anesth*. 1993;18:461–468.
23. Seo SS, et al. Comparison of the effect of continuous femoral nerve block and adductor canal block after primary total knee arthroplasty. *Clin Orthop Surg*. 2017;9(3):303–309. doi: 10.4055/cios.2017.9.3.303.
24. Ochiai S, Hagino T, Senga S, et al. Injury to infrapatellar branch of saphenous nerve in anterior cruciate ligament reconstruction using vertical skin incision for hamstring harvesting: risk factors and the influence of treatment outcome. *J Orthop Surg Res*. 2017;12(1):101.
25. Knight JB, Schott NJ, Kentor ML, Williams BA. Neurotoxicity of common peripheral nerve block adjuvants. *Curr Opin Anaesthesiol*. 2015;28(5):598–604. doi: 10.1097/ACO.0000000000000222\.
26. Sousa AM, Ashmawi HA, Costa LS, Posso IP, Slullitel A. Percutaneous sciatic nerve block with tramadol induces analgesia and motor blockade in two animal pain models. *Braz J Med Biol Res*. 2012;45(2):147–152. doi: 10.1590/s0100-879x2011007500164.
27. Hadzic A, Minkowitz HS, Melson TI, et al. Liposome bupivacaine femoral nerve block for postsurgical analgesia after total knee arthroplasty. *Anesthesiology*. 2016;124(6):1372–1383.
28. Krych A, Arutyunyan G, Kuzma S, et al. Adverse effect of femoral nerve blockade on quadriceps strength and function after ACL reconstruction. *J Knee Surg*. 2015;28(1):83–88.
29. Runner RP, Boden SA, Godfrey WS, et al. Quadriceps strength deficits after a femoral nerve block versus adductor canal block for anterior cruciate ligament reconstruction: a prospective, single-blinded, randomized trial. *Orthop J Sports Med*. 2018;6(9):2325967118797990.

REVIEW QUESTIONS

(1) Which of the following nerves provide innervation to the anterior aspect of the knee?

A. Femoral nerve
B. Sciatic nerve
C. Obturator nerve
D. Tibial nerve

(2) Which of the following anatomic structures does NOT constitute a border of the adductor canal?

A, Vastus medialis
B. Adductor longus
C. Vastus lateralis
D. The sartorius

(3) Which of the following is an absolute contraindication for femoral nerve block (FNB)?

A. Infection at the surgical site
B. Use of Eliquis (apixaban) within 24 hours
C. Patient refusal
D. Bilateral lower extremity neuropathy

(4) Which of the following injection pressures indicates intraneural needle placement may lead to severe fascicular injury?

A. <4 psi
B. 4–10 psi
C. 10–20 psi
D. 25–45 psi

(5) Surgical injury to which of the following nerves is associated with ACL repair with an autologous graft?

A. Saphenous nerve
B. Peroneal nerve
C. Lateral femoral cutaneous nerve
D. Tibial nerve

(6) Which of the following local anesthetics provides the longest duration of analgesia?

A. Chloroprocaine
B. Lidocaine
C. Mepivacaine
D. Bupivacaine

(7) ACL repair using autograft of the gracilis tendon may require additional analgesia in which nerve distribution?

A. Popliteal nerve
B. Superficial femoral artery
C. Lateral femoral cutaneous nerve
D. Obturator nerve

(8) Which of the following procedures is contraindicated in a patient currently taking a factor Xa inhibitor?

A. Adductor canal block
B. Fascia iliaca block
C. Popliteal nerve block
D. Lumbar plexus block

ANSWERS

(1) **A.** Femoral nerve provides innervation to the anterior aspect of the knee.

Reference

Hadzic A. *Hadzic's Textbook of Regional Anesthesia and Acute Pain Management.* New York: McGraw-Hill Education; 2017.

(2) **C.** The anatomical structure of the adductor canal includes the vastus medialis laterally, the adductor longus medially, and the sartorius forms the roof of the adductor canal.

Reference

Hadzic, A. *Hadzic's Textbook of Regional Anesthesia and Acute Pain Management.* New York: McGraw-Hill Education; 2017.

(3) **C.** Patient refusal is an absolute contraindication to any procedure.

Reference

Butterworth JF, Mackey DC, Wasnick JD, Morgan GE, Mikhail MS. *Morgan & Mikhail's Clinical Anesthesiology.* Sixth ed. New York: McGraw-Hill Education; 2018.

(4) **D.** An intraneural injection pressure of 25–45 psi indicates intraneural needle placement and may lead to severe intrafascular injury.

Reference

Hadzic A, Dilberovic F, Shah S, et al. Combination of intraneural injection and high injection pressure leads to fascicular injury and neurologic deficits in dogs. *Reg Anesth Pain Med.* 2004;29:417–423.

(5) **A.** Harvesting of the hamstring (semitendinosus tendon or gracilis tendon) for tissue grafting has a strong association with postoperative saphenous nerve injury and should be considered when diagnosing a postoperative sensory deficit.

Reference

Papastergiou SG, Voulgaropoulos H, Mikalef P, Ziogas E, Pappis G, Giannakopoulos I. Injuries to the infrapatellar branch(es) of the saphenous nerve in anterior cruciate ligament reconstruction with four-strand hamstring tendon autograft: vertical versus horizontal incision for harvest. *Knee Surg Sports Traumatol Arthrosc.* 2005;14(8):789–793.

(6) **D.** Bupivacaine is longer acting local anesthetic than lidocaine, mepivacaine, and chloroprocaine. Chloroprocaine lasts from 40–90 minutes, lidocaine analgesic effect lasts from 2–4 hs, while mepivacaine is 2–3 hs and bupivacaine is 8–16 hs. https://www.medicine.com/drug/chloroprocaine/hcp. Accessed October 21, 2021.

Reference

Butterworth JF, Mackey DC, Wasnick JD, Morgan G,E Mikhail MS. *Morgan & Mikhail's Clinical Anesthesiology.* Sixth ed. New York: McGraw-Hill Education; 2018.

(7) **D.** The use of an autograft harvested from the gracilis tendon requires an additional incision site on the medial aspect of the knee. The skin over that site is innervated by the obturator nerve, a branch of the lumbar plexus.

Reference

Sakura S, Hara K, Ota J, Tadenuma S. Ultrasound-guided peripheral nerve blocks for anterior cruciate ligament reconstruction: effect of obturator nerve block during and after surgery. *J Anesth.* 2010;24(3):411–417.

29.

ENHANCED RECOVERY AFTER TOTAL KNEE REPLACEMENT

Jamie-Lee Metesky and Meg A. Rosenblatt

STEM CASE AND KEY QUESTIONS

A 76-year-old man presents for a right total knee replacement (TKR). He is 3 years s/p percutaneous coronary intervention (PCI), during which time he received a stent in his left anterior descending coronary. He currently denies chest pain, but physical activity is limited by his knee pain. His medications include clopidogrel, baby aspirin, metoprolol, and atorvastatin. He lives with his wife in an apartment with no stairs and desires to be discharged to home as early as possible postoperatively. You speak with the surgeon about an enhanced recovery after surgery (ERAS) pathway for this patient, but the surgeon insists that injecting liposomal bupivacaine into the joint space at the conclusion of the procedure will be adequate. The patient explains that his wife had a unicondylar (partial) knee replacement and wonders if that is an option for him. The surgeon explains that all the details will be worked out during his preoperative joint education class and testing that he must attend prior to surgery.

During the pre-admission testing, the patient meets with an anesthesiologist to be evaluated for the upcoming surgery. The patient asks what type of anesthesia will be used and is adamant that "he wants to be completely asleep" during the entirety of the surgery. The options of neuraxial anesthesia (NA) and general anesthesia (GA) are explained and the patient is amenable to NA with deep sedation for the maintenance of the case. The patient also asks if there is anything that can be done to decrease his risk for a need for blood transfusion. The anesthesiologist inquires as to why the patient is still taking clopidogrel, given it has been 3 years since his cardiac stent placement, but the patient is unsure and says, "I take what the doctor tells me to." The patient is then instructed to stop taking clopidogrel 5 days prior to his surgery. The surgeon is adamant about the patient receiving 2 doses of tranexamic acid (TXA) during the case. You feel that, given his history of cardiac stent, the risk of in-stent thrombosis is greater than the benefit of decreased blood loss. You and the surgeon finally agree that TXA will be administered topically, rather than intravenously. The patient is also instructed to drink a bottle of sports drink before leaving for the hospital and to be prepared to receive several oral medications to take with a sip of water on the morning of surgery.

The patient remembers from the joint class that he heard about the options for peripheral nerve blocks and started asking the anesthesiologist whether he will be getting a nerve block to help him with his pain after surgery. The anesthesiologist explained to the patient that these nerve blocks will only cover pain in the front and the inside of the knee, but will not cover the back of the knee. The anesthesiologist went on to explain that an additional IPACK (infiltration between popliteal artery and capsule of the knee) block can be performed with the either the femoral or adductor canal block to allow total knee pain coverage. In addition, the surgeon can inject local anesthetic around the knee joint during surgery, and oral pain medications can be given postoperatively for any breakthrough pain.

Prior to the scheduled surgery, the anesthesiologist meets with the surgeon to discuss intraoperative and postoperative care plan. The surgeon insists on administering liposomal bupivacaine for periarticular infiltration during the case, but after discussing the recent literature he is amenable to using an alternative "cocktail" for periarticular infiltration. The surgeon asks what else can be offered to this patient to provide analgesia and facilitate early discharge from the hospital.

(1) WHAT IS THE DIFFERENCE BETWEEN A PARTIAL AND TOTAL KNEE REPLACEMENT (TKR)?

Partial arthroplasty is used for disease processes that are too severe for arthroscopic management, but not severe enough for TKR, as degeneration is limited to one condyle. Unicondylar arthroplasty is done through a smaller incision and is associated with less pain, blood loss, and recovery time. However, a TKR may be necessary in the future, if the healthy condyle degenerates.

(2) ARE THERE SPECIFIC PROTOCOLS THAT ALLOW PATIENTS TO UNDERGO TKR AND BE DISCHARGED TO HOME THE SAME DAY?

Enhanced recovery after surgery (ERAS) protocol is used. It is a multimodal, multidisciplinary approach to optimizing perioperative care and recovery following surgery. It includes preoperative, intraoperative and postoperative components.

Preoperative:

- Preoperative assessment, optimization, and education
- Preoperative fasting: a carbohydrate load via a clear carbohydrate drink 2–3 hours before surgery is recommended.
- Multimodal analgesia that includes: acetaminophen, nonsteroidal anti-inflammatory drugs (NSAID), and gabapentinoids.

Intraoperative:

- Anesthesia technique is tailored to each patient; NA is usually used.
- The surgeon uses periarticular local anesthetic infiltration.
- Normothermia and optimal fluid balance are maintained.
- The use of tranexamic acid has been shown to reduce intraoperative blood loss and rate of blood transfusion.

Postoperative:

- Multimodal opioid-sparing analgesic techniques that include a nerve block that is placed pre- or postoperatively
- Early immobilization and rehabilitation.

(3) WHAT IS A "PREOPERATIVE JOINT EDUCATION CLASS"?

The joint class is a preoperative education. This may occur online or in person, where the patient may meet members of the surgical, anesthesia, medical, nutrition, social work, physical therapy, discharge planning, and floor nurse teams.

(4) WHAT ARE THE ADVANTAGES/ DISADVANTAGES OF GENERAL ANESTHESIA (GA)?

GA may be a better option in patients with severe coagulopathies, history of extensive spine surgery, an inability to lie still due to neurologic disease, and failed NA. The disadvantages are postoperative nausea, vomiting, and delirium.

(5) WHAT ARE THE ADVANTAGES/ DISADVANTAGES OF NEURAXIAL ANESTHESIA (NA)?

NA anesthesia uses less medications, avoids intubation, and results in less postoperative nausea and vomiting (PONV). Drawbacks are intraoperative hypotension and postoperative urinary retention.

(6) IS TRANEXAMIC ACID (TXA) CONTRAINDICATED IN THIS PATIENT, GIVEN HIS CARDIAC HISTORY?

The current literature does not suggest increased risk. However, larger studies in sicker patients with a history of thrombotic disease are needed.

(7) WHAT IS THE EVIDENCE FOR ANALGESIC EFFECTIVENESS OF LIPOSOMAL BUPIVACAINE AFTER TKR?

When compared to periarticular injection, it showed either no difference or some benefit. However, the cost is prohibitive.

(9) WHAT AGENTS PROVIDE ANALGESIA WHEN ADMINISTERED INTRA-ARTICULARLY? WHAT IS THE UTILITY OF INTRA-ARTICULAR INJECTIONS?

The most commonly used drugs for periarticular injections include local anesthetics (ropivacaine or bupivacaine), morphine, ketorolac, epinephrine, and steroids. Intra-articular injections have been shown to decrease postoperative need for narcotics following TKA.

(10) WHAT PERIPHERAL NERVE BLOCK TECHNIQUES (PNB) WILL PROVIDE ANALGESIA POST-TKR?

Femoral nerve block provides good analgesia but with quadriceps weakness; adductor canal block is more motor sparing, and infiltration between popliteal artery and capsule of the knee (IPACK) helps to cover the posterior part.

(11) WHAT IS THE ROLE FOR A CONTINUOUS ANESTHETIC TECHNIQUE AFTER TKR?

Continuous peripheral nerve blocks can provide prolonged analgesia. They may allow procedures to be performed on an ambulatory basis, and the local anesthetics injected can be more dilute than agents used in single-shot injections.

DISCUSSION

Currently there are more than 700,000 TKRs performed annually in the United States, and this number is increasing with an aging population.[1] Total knee replacement is one of the most commonly performed procedures worldwide. The volume of TKR is projected to be 1.28 million by the year 2030.[2] Knee replacement is usually the last resort for degenerative arthritis of the knee, and can be either a partial or TKR.

Unicondylar arthroplasty is used for disease process that is too severe for arthroscopic management, but not severe enough for TKR, as degeneration is limited to one condyle. Unicondylar arthroplasty is done through a smaller incision and is associated with less pain, blood loss, and recovery time. However, a TKR may be necessary in the future, if the healthy condyle degenerates.[3]

For a TKR, a vertical skin incision is made over the knee and the patella is rotated away to allow access to the knee joint. No muscles are cut through in order to enter the joint capsule, although in order for the femur and tibia to be resurfaced, the anterior cruciate ligament (ACL) and posterior cruciate ligament (PCL) must be cut. Once the femur and tibia are resurfaced, prostheses are implanted with cement. The ACL

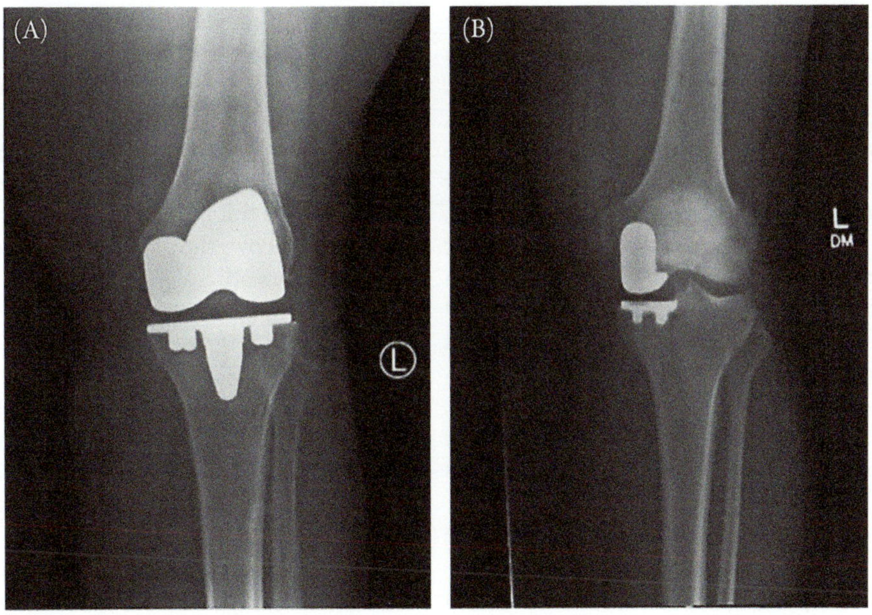

Figure 29.1. (A) X-ray of total knee arthroplasty; (B) X-ray of partial (unicondylar) arthroplasty.

and PCL are not usually reattached, but some specific hardware allows for their reattachment. For a unicondylar arthroplasty, neither muscles nor cruciate ligaments are cut, and only one femoral condyle and half of the tibia are resurfaced and implanted (Figure 29.1).

ERAS PROTOCOLS AFTER TKR

ERAS is a multimodal, multidisciplinary approach to optimizing perioperative care and recovery following surgery. ERAS consists of a protocol developed from evidence-based techniques which aim to expedite the recovery process through reducing surgical and postoperative stress, having adequate pain control, reducing complications, improving outcomes, and decreasing length of stay. The ERAS pathway was originally developed for colorectal surgery, but has since been expanded to incorporate many different procedures, including total joint replacement. Each institution can alter the generic ERAS protocol to align with their specific patient population needs; however, the overall goals remain the same.

PRE-ADMISSION TESTING AND PREOPERATIVE PATIENT EDUCATION CLASS

Before total joint surgery, every patient should have some type of perioperative education. This may occur online or in person as the patient attends a pre-admission testing clinic or specific class, where they may meet members of the surgical, anesthesia, medical, nutrition, social work, physical therapy, discharge planning, and floor nurse teams. The overall goals of this education are to set expectations, answer questions, and minimize any confusion that may arise during the perioperative process. After completing a medical history, physical, and lab work, the patient may meet with the anesthesiologist to go over the anesthetic plan. Each plan is tailored to account for any comorbid conditions a patient may have. This time allows the anesthesiologist to stratify whether patients would benefit from NA vs. GA, what pre-medications should be administered, to introduce the PNBs that might be appropriate, and to identify any chronic pain patients who may pose challenges with their postoperative pain management.

During this session, patients are able to complete necessary paperwork, receive instructions regarding NPO status and medication guidelines, receive instructions about the use of antimicrobial scrub, and begin to develop a plan for discharge following surgery. At the conclusion of any type of educational session, all questions should be answered and patients should feel comfortable and prepared for the upcoming surgery.

ANESTHETIC OPTIONS FOR TKR

GENERAL ANESTHESIA

General anesthesia (GA) has been used as the primary anesthetic technique for TKR for years. However, overwhelming literature has more recently favored the transition to NA and PNB techniques, either in place of GA or in addition to it.[4] The lower extremity location for TKR allows for more flexibility in the type of anesthesia that can be used. While beneficial to have multiple options, a disparity in research outcomes and methods has led to equivocal information in regard to which type of anesthesia is considered safest to use for TKR. In addition, with the moving trend toward ambulatory total joint replacement and the push toward quick ambulation after surgery, there are even more variables to consider when choosing the anesthetic type.

GA may still be a better option in certain patients. Severe coagulopathies, history of extensive spine surgery, an inability to lie still due to neurologic disease, and failed NA attempts are instances where GA may be a more reasonable choice over NA. Memtsoudis and colleagues showed that compared with GA, NA was associated with overall fewer complications, including fewer thromboembolic events, blood transfusions, infections, acute renal failure, respiratory complications, critical care admissions, and hospital readmissions, and shorter length of hospital stay. However, the association was weak, and they also showed that in regard to stroke, cardiovascular complications, and mortality there was no difference between the groups.[5] In addition, Johnson and colleagues reviewed 29 studies, including 10,500 patients undergoing TKR or total hip replacement, and found no statistically significant differences between NA and GA for mortality, surgical duration, surgical site or chest infections, nerve palsies, PONV, or thromboembolic disease when antithrombotic prophylaxis was used.[6]

While more research studies continue to evaluate the effectiveness of GA vs. NA, it is best to evaluate and formulate a plan specific to each patient. If GA is used, attentiveness to heart rate, hematocrit, and avoidance of potential sympathetic stress response will help prevent an increased oxygen demand.[7] GA may result in postoperative nausea, vomiting, and delirium.[8] In addition, the use of systemic opioids as part of a balanced anesthetic may result in increased atelectasis with hypoventilation post-surgery.

NEURAXIAL ANESTHESIA (NA)

Major surgery increases the risk of both minor complications and serious life-threatening events. However, the debate is ongoing on whether GA or NA can better mitigate some of the complications. NA has been steadily gaining popularity for anesthetic choice during lower extremity total joint replacement surgery. In patients with multiple comorbid conditions, NA may cause less disruptions in certain, potentially limited or failing organ systems. NA causes a sympathectomy resulting in a decreased stress response with resultant vasodilation allowing more perfusion to and from tissues, increased oxygenation, and decreased venous stasis.[9] However, with the sympathectomy comes hypotension which, if not treated accordingly, can result in decreased coronary perfusion pressure with resultant myocardial ischemia.[10] In addition, there may be a global lower pressure of oxygen in all tissues. Factors contributing to lower subcutaneous oxygen tension include obesity, hypothermia, and smoking.[11,12] Literature has shown an inverse relationship between surgical infections and partial pressure of oxygen in tissue.[13,14]

The stress of surgery causes a hypercoagulable state, with the complication of venous thromboembolism (VTE), which includes deep venous thrombosis (DVT) and pulmonary embolism (PE). VTE complications are associated with high morbidity and increased hospital costs.[15] Multiple studies suggest that NA lowers the incidence of VTE. A systemic review by Rodgers and colleagues found an association between NA and a decrease in DVT, PE, transfusion requirement, pneumonia, and respiratory depression. Overall mortality of patients with NA was also reduced by approximately one-third compared to those who received GA.[16] However, more recent studies suggest that this relationship exists, but is not as strong as previously thought.[17]

With the advent of ERAS, specifically early ambulation with PT, one must consider what type and dose of LA to use for NA that corresponds with the type of surgery (total vs. partial knee replacement) and the speed of the surgeon. The goal is to have full motor recovery in the post-anesthesia care unit, which allows the patient to ambulate once the anesthetic sedation wears off.

USE OF ANTI-FIBRINOLYTICS IN TKR

Tranexamic acid (TXA) is a synthetic lysine analogue which reversibly binds to plasminogen, causing a reduction in the conversion of plasminogen to plasmin and ultimately impairing fibrin degradation.[18] Through a decrease in fibrin degradation, there is a stronger fibrin clot and bleeding is decreased. The side-effect profile includes thromboembolic risk, seizures, hypersensitivity reactions, visual disturbances, and dizziness.

TXA can be administered via intravenous, oral, or topical routes. Zhang and colleagues examined oral TXA vs. no TXA and found that TXA prevented hemoglobin drop, decreased 24-hour blood loss, and decreased need for blood transfusion.[19] The optimal oral dosing regimen is still being investigated, but Wang and colleagues showed that multiple postoperative doses of oral TXA reduced blood loss to a greater extent, when compared to a single oral dose.[20] A randomized clinical trial comparing IV to topical TXA (1 gram of IV TXA given prior to tourniquet inflation and 1 gram at closure vs. 3 grams diluted in normal saline and applied topically after cementation), showed that IV TXA was associated with less overall blood loss and drain output, but that transfusion rates and VTE complications did not differ.[21] While recent literature has shown that intravenous TXA is effective at reducing blood loss and need for transfusion when compared to placebo,[22] a lack of evidence has been presented regarding TXA use in patients with a higher risk of thromboembolic events. Most studies exclude ASA physical status 3 and 4 patients, making it difficult to assess the safety of TXA in the sicker patient population. Whiting and colleagues were able to show that IV TXA reduced the need for transfusion and did not increase thromboembolic events in high-risk patients (prior DVT, PE, MI, CVA, CABG, coronary stent, or prothrombotic conditions).[23–25] Until stronger studies are performed, one should still use caution when administering IV TXA to high-risk patients. The oral and topical forms of TXA may be beneficial in this patient population.

MULTIMODAL ANALGESIA

Multimodal analgesia is used as part of ERAS protocols to minimize postoperative pain that promotes ambulation and early discharge. The overall objective is to combine analgesics with different mechanisms of action as a means to synergistically maximize pain control while minimizing the use of opioids. Postoperative pain, including chronic neuropathic pain, can be lessened through preemptive analgesia.[26]

Given the national opioid epidemic, this multimodal approach to pain control is quickly gaining popularity. Since 2000, the rate of deaths from opioids has seen a 200% increase and is predicted to continue climbing.[27] Opioid-related adverse effects include respiratory depression, delirium, ileus, paradoxical worsening of pain with higher opioid doses, and opioid-induced respiratory depression with subsequent hypoxia, hypercapnia, and cardiorespiratory arrest. Further complicating the issue is that many patients presenting for TKR are already on some type of pain medication. Kim and colleagues showed that preoperative chronic opioid users were at an increased risk of needing opioids, even 6 months following surgery. Characteristics that were predictive of persistent opioid use included male gender, prior injury or surgery to the ipsilateral knee, current tobacco smoking status, and a history of psychiatric disorder.[28] It is therefore even more important in this patient population to use multimodal analgesia in hopes of decreasing the need for chronic opioid therapy.

Premedication can include oral administration of opioids and non-opioid analgesics, including selective and nonselective anti-inflammatory drugs (NSAIDs), acetaminophen, and gabapentinoids.

Nonsteroidal Anti-inflammatory Drugs (NSAIDs)

NSAIDs are used extensively as the mainstay treatment for pain caused by inflammation. They exert their anti-inflammatory effect through inhibition of cyclooxygenase enzymes (COX-1 and/or COX-2). Through inhibition of COX-1 and COX-2 there is decreased conversion of arachidonic acid to prostaglandins, which play a key role in the generation of the inflammatory response, and their biosynthesis is significantly increased in inflamed tissue.[29] Most NSAIDs, such as aspirin, ibuprofen, and naproxen, are nonselective, which means both COX-1 and COX-2 enzymes are inhibited. Prostaglandins are essential in maintaining homeostasis in many organ systems.

Gastrointestinal

At the level of the stomach, COX-1 enzyme controls the production of prostaglandins PGE_2 and PGI_2, which regulate the production of bicarbonate, mucus, and blood flow in the stomach, ultimately protecting the stomach lining from acid production. With the use of nonselective NSAIDs, the inhibition of COX-1 can result in dyspepsia, gastroduodenal ulcers, GI bleeding, and perforation.

Renal

At the level of the kidney, COX-1 and COX-2 enzyme production of prostaglandin PGE_2 selectively vasodilates the afferent arterioles in the glomerulus, which results in increased glomerular filtration rate (GFR). When prostaglandin synthesis is decreased or inhibited, it can lead to acute kidney injury through a reduction in GFR and overall decreased renal perfusion. NSAID-induced nephrotoxicity includes acute kidney injury (AKI), electrolyte imbalances, decreased GFR, acute interstitial nephritis, edema, renal papillary necrosis, and possible chronic kidney disease if left untreated.[30]

Cardiovascular

At the level of the heart, COX-1 and COX-2 enzymes control the production of prostacyclin (PGI_2) and thromboxane A_2 (TXA_2), which regulate vasodilation and platelet aggregation. TXA_2 production is mainly controlled by COX-1, while PGI_2 production is mediated by COX-2. TXA_2 acts as a vasoconstrictor and platelet aggregator, while PGI_2 has opposite effects, acting as a vasodilator and inhibitor of platelet aggregation, together maintaining vascular homeostasis. When COX-2 is selectively inhibited, the pro-thrombotic activity of TXA_2 can result in myocardial infarction, stroke, and DVT.[31]

Selective COX-2 Inhibitors

Selective COX-2 inhibitor (celecoxib) was designed with the intent of minimizing the GI side-effect profile of the nonselective NSAIDs, while still achieving the anti-inflammatory and pain control effect. Other selective coxibs have been withdrawn from the market due to concerns for cardiovascular complications, mainly myocardial infarction and stroke.[32] When used chronically, one must weigh the GI risk factors versus the cardiovascular risk factors to determine which NSAID is most appropriate.

Acetaminophen

Acetaminophen has been widely used for its analgesic and antipyretic activity and is administered via IV, PO, and PR routes. The exact mechanism of action is unclear, but research suggests that acetaminophen effects are primarily mediated through a combination of eicosanoid and serotonin pathways.[33] Similar to NSAIDs, inhibition of COX-1 and COX-2 enzymes results in decreased prostaglandin synthesis and inflammatory response.

Acetaminophen primarily acts within the CNS and thus it will not provide the peripheral decrease in inflammation that one would expect from NSAIDs, but it does result in a decrease in central mediated prostaglandin effects. Although generally considered safe, hepatotoxicity can occur with doses exceeding 4 grams daily.[34]

Acetaminophen can be administered via multiple routes and current research is ongoing to find the most effective and cost-efficient dosing regimen. A small clinical trial compared the use of IV vs. oral formulations and found no analgesic difference between the two groups, but stronger studies need to be done.[35]

Pregabalin and Gabapentin

Pregabalin and gabapentin bind the $\alpha 2\delta$ subunit of voltage-gated calcium channels in the spinal cord and brain. Both drugs are used for treatment of neuropathic pain and seizures. It is thought that the $\alpha 2\delta$ calcium channel subunit binding results in a reduction in the release of neurotransmitters such as glutamate and substance P, which allows suppression of neuronal excitability, ultimately decreasing pain transmission.[36]

While some studies show decreased pain and morphine consumption with use of pregabalin for TKA;[37] other studies suggest the side-effect profile, including sedation, dizziness, and ataxia, may limit the future use of these drugs. Yadeau and colleagues showed that pregabalin did not reduce pain at rest or with ambulation in TKA and that pregabalin actually increased sedation and drowsiness while decreasing patient satisfaction. Although the side effect profile may not adversely affect younger patients, caution should be used in the older population already prone to postoperative delirium.[38]

N-methyl-D-aspartate (NMDA) Receptor Antagonist

Ketamine primarily functions as an NMDA antagonist and is used for analgesia, amnesia, and psychomimetic effects. It also acts to modulate opioid, monoaminergic, cholinergic, and nicotinic receptors. Ketamine can be administered via intravenous, intramuscular, oral, nasal, transdermal, subcutaneous, and rectal routes, making it a versatile drug.

Ketamine is a sympathomimetic drug that stimulates the cardiovascular system, resulting in an increase in heart rate, blood pressure, and cardiac output. In healthy patients, the sympathetic effects are beneficial to counteract the hemodynamics changes from the induction of both GA and NA. However, in critically ill patients, endogenous catecholamines are depleted and may result in unexpected negative inotropic effects and can result in cardiovascular compromise. Another useful application of ketamine is its ability to preserve airway reflexes and produce bronchial smooth muscle relaxation.[39]

The NMDA receptor is an excitatory glutamatergic receptor present in spinal and supraspinal sites and is involved in afferent transmission of nociceptive signals. In chronic pain states, prolonged nociceptive signal transmission causes upregulation and activation of the NMDA receptor at dorsal horn synapses, resulting in central sensitization and hyperexcitability.[40]

In patients undergoing knee arthroplasty, a low-dose infusion of ketamine reduced morphine requirements and decreased the time to achieve 90 degrees of active flexion.[41] Other studies further showing ketamine administered in subanesthetic doses is effective in reducing morphine requirements in the first 24 hours after surgery.[42]

While useful in pain control, the side-effect profile, including psychotomimetic effects (hallucinations, nightmares, vivid dreams) and increased salivation, may limit its use.

Local Anesthetic Infiltration Analgesia (LIA)

Liposomal Bupivacaine

Using multivesicular liposomal delivery technology, bupivacaine is placed in numerous aqueous chambers surrounded by naturally occurring lipids. As the lipids on the surface reorganize in the patient's body and break down, the bupivacaine is released. This sustained release of local anesthetic is supposed to provide continuous and prolonged pain relief. Orthopedic surgeons have been using liposomal bupivacaine infiltration, in an off-label use of the product, after total joint replacements, but to date there is no convincing evidence of its superiority to standard local anesthetic formulations. Currently liposomal bupivacaine is only FDA approved for infiltrative analgesia and interscalene plexus blocks.

Hyland et al., in a prospective, randomized, single-blinded, controlled trial, compared liposomal bupivacaine to periarticular injection with 0.2% ropivacaine, 10 mg morphine, 30 mg ketorolac, and 40 mg methylprednisolone in patients enrolled in an ERAS protocol which included an adductor canal block (ACB). There was no significant difference in the number of physical therapy sessions to achieve discharge readiness, nor were there differences in total opioid consumption, average VAS pain scores, or unplanned readmissions between the 2 groups.[43] Three recent meta-analyses of random controlled trials showed similar findings. Zhao et al. looked at 12 studies that compared liposomal bupivacaine with standard periarticular injections in patients undergoing total joint arthroplasties. They found that although the liposomal bupivacaine group had significantly decreased opioid consumption, both groups had similar pain control, functional recovery, length of stay, and VAS scores at 24 and 48 hours.[44] Looking at data from 88,830 TKAs, of which liposomal bupivacaine was used in 18,717 (21.2%), the liposomal bupivacaine was not associated with significant reductions in opioid use, length of stay, or decreased odds for opioid-related complications.[45] Finally, in an analysis of 11 studies comparing liposomal bupivacaine to periarticular injection of at least 2 agents, liposomal bupivacaine was as effective as injection with respect to VAS at 24, 48, and 72 hours, total opioid consumption, range of motion, length of stay, PONV, and ambulation distance. Those authors concluded that considering the cost of liposomal bupivacaine and the outcomes achieved, they could not recommend its use.[46]

Other Medications Used for Periarticular Infiltration

Intra-articular multimodal drug injections have been steadily gaining popularity for TKA. It is hypothesized that there are abundant concentrations of nociceptors present in the knee joint (infrapatellar fat pad, fibrous capsule, ligament insertion sites, periosteum, and bone).[47]

Intra-articular injections have been shown to decrease postoperative need for narcotics following TKA.[48–50] However, neither the optimal composition of (agents and dosages) nor techniques of injection have been established, and there is still disagreement over its influence on reduced opioid consumption. A small retrospective analysis revealed that intra-articular injection of high-dose local anesthetics provided similar analgesic efficacy as FNB and was associated with early ambulation.[51]

The most commonly used drugs for periarticular injections include local anesthetics (ropivacaine or bupivacaine), morphine, ketorolac, epinephrine, and steroids. While steroids lengthen the duration of the periarticular injection, caution should be used in patients with high infection risks, such as diabetes or advanced age.[52]

PERIPHERAL NERVE BLOCK TECHNIQUES (PNB)

Femoral Nerve Block (FNB)

The femoral nerve is the major nerve supplying the anterior compartment of the thigh and arises from the lumbar plexus dorsal divisions of L2, L3, L4. The femoral nerve travels posterior to the inguinal ligament and then traverses to enter the femoral triangle (Scarpa's triangle).

Borders of the femoral triangle:

- Superiorly = inguinal ligament
- Medial wall = adductor longus muscle
- Lateral wall = sartorius muscle.

Within this anatomic location, the femoral nerve will lie lateral to the femoral artery. The orientation moving lateral to medial is "NAVEL" (femoral **N**erve, **A**rtery, **V**ein, **E**mpty space, **L**ymphatics).

Motor innervation is to the anterior thigh muscles that flex the hip joint (pectineus, iliacus, sartorius) and extend the knee quadriceps femoris (rectus femoris, vastus lateralis, vastus medialis, and vastus intermedius).

Sensory innervation is to the anterior cutaneous branches of the femoral and saphenous nerves. The saphenous nerve is a terminal sensory branch that travels within the adductor canal and gives sensory innervation to the medial thigh down to the medial malleolus.

An FNB can be performed as a single-shot block or a continuous catheter. While providing excellent pain coverage for the TKR, the use of an FNB has fallen out of favor due to its association with quadriceps weakness, which makes early ambulation difficult and puts the patients at risk of falling. However, other research has shown that the use of a continuous FNB with dilute bupivacaine (0.125%) and knee immobilizer does not prevent early ambulation.[53,54]

Technique

The patient is placed in a supine position with hip slightly abducted and leg externally rotated. A linear ultrasound probe (6–13 MHz) is placed at or slightly below the inguinal ligament. The femoral artery is identified, usually lateral to the femoral vein. Occasionally, the deep artery of the thigh (a branch of the femoral artery) is also seen, giving the appearance of two arteries. The probe should be moved proximal until only the femoral artery is seen. The femoral nerve will be lateral to the femoral artery and appears as a hyperechoic bundle. Using an in-plane technique, a 22-gauge echogenic needle is inserted and directed in a lateral to medial direction. The needle is advanced until the fascia iliaca covering the femoral nerve is reached. The location of injection should ideally occur between the fascia iliaca and the femoral nerve. If a nerve stimulator is used, one should see quadriceps twitch and a patellar snap with the correct location. After aspirating to rule out intravascular needle placement, 20 mL of local anesthetic is injected.

Adductor Canal Block (ACB)

Adductor canal block (ACB) aims to anesthetize the saphenous nerve distal to its innervation of the quadriceps muscles, although occasionally it blocks the nerve to vastus medialis, which can result in quadriceps weakness. Sensory distribution includes medial and anteromedial aspects of the lower extremity from the mid/distal thigh to the medial malleolus. Both single-shot and continuous techniques have been used for analgesia after TKR.

The adductor canal is an aponeurotic tunnel extending from the apex of the femoral triangle to the adductor hiatus or opening of the adductor magnus. The contents include: superficial femoral artery, femoral vein, saphenous nerve, and nerve to vastus medialis.

Borders of the adductor canal:

- Anterior wall = sartorius muscle
- Posterior wall = adductor longus and Magnus muscles
- Medial wall = vastus medialis muscle.

Technique

The block is performed usually at the mid-thigh level, but can be done anywhere along the adductor canal tract. Using a linear ultrasound probe (6–13 MHz), the femur is identified first; the probe is then moved medially until the femoral artery is identified. The femoral artery usually lies underneath the sartorius muscle, with the femoral vein beneath the artery. The saphenous nerve lies lateral to the artery and is identified as a hyperechoic structure. Using an in-plane technique, a 22-gauge echogenic needle is inserted and directed toward the lateral border of the femoral artery at the 5 o'clock position. Once in the correct location, 10–20 mL of local anesthetic is injected (Figure 29.2).

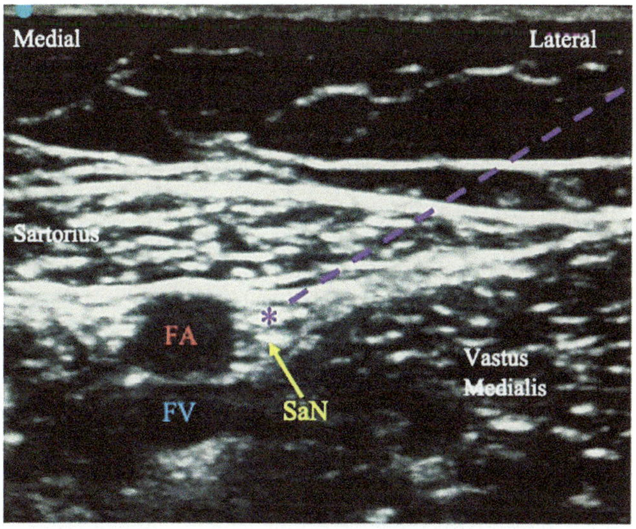

Figure 29.2. Adductor canal block.

INJECTION BETWEEN THE POPLITEAL ARTERY AND POSTERIOR COMPARTMENT OF THE KNEE (IPACK) BLOCK

Analgesia to the posterior aspect of the knee has been achieved using the IPACK block. This block targets the deep genicular nerves of the posterior knee, providing selective sensory blockade without involvement of tibial and common peroneal motor branches.

IPACK block allows for early ambulation in accordance with ERAS protocols. When performed in conjunction with an ACB, it has been shown that pain control is superior and patients have better knee range of motion and ambulatory ability as compared to the use of an ACB alone.[55]

Posterior knee pain is a common complaint postoperatively, and due to location it is not adequately controlled with use of an ACB.

The posterior knee joint capsule is innervated by articular branches from the posterior division of the tibial and obturator nerves. Due to anatomic variations, some also have articular branch contributions from the common peroneal and sciatic nerves, though less commonly seen. The tibial nerve component supplies the entire posterior capsule, with overlapping coverage from the obturator nerve (superomedial portion), and common peroneal (superolateral portion) when present.[56]

If the main trunks of the tibial and common peroneal nerves are anesthetized, one can expect to see weakness in foot plantar flexion, dorsiflexion, eversion, and inversion. This weakness will likely prevent the patient from participating in physical therapy and may delay discharge.

Supine (Proximal) Technique

Patient is placed in a supine position with the knee flexed and hip slightly abducted. A low frequency curvilinear probe (2–5MHz) is placed transversely over the anteromedial thigh about 1–2 fingerbreadth superior to the patella. The probe is then moved cephalad until the shaft of the femur is seen, with the popliteal artery located posterior/deeper in relation to the femoral shaft.

Using an in-plane technique, a 22-gauge echogenic needle is advanced in an anterior to posterior direction until the tip of the needle lies in the interspace between the popliteal artery and distal femoral shaft. After aspiration, 20 mL of local anesthetic is injected as the needle is withdrawn.

This technique offers the advantage that the ACB can also be performed with this approach, minimizing the need to reposition the patient (Figure 29.3A).

Prone (Distal) Technique

The patient is placed in a prone position and a low frequency curvilinear probe (2–5 MHz) is placed transversely at the popliteal crease. The popliteal artery is placed in the center of the screen with the hyperechoic femoral condyles on each side. The popliteal vein may or may not be seen, depending on pressure applied. The tibial and common peroneal nerves can be seen by adjusting the tilt of the probe and are usually located superior and lateral to the popliteal artery. The articular branches supplying the posterior capsule are found deeper in the space between the popliteal artery and femur, which is where the injection will occur.[57]

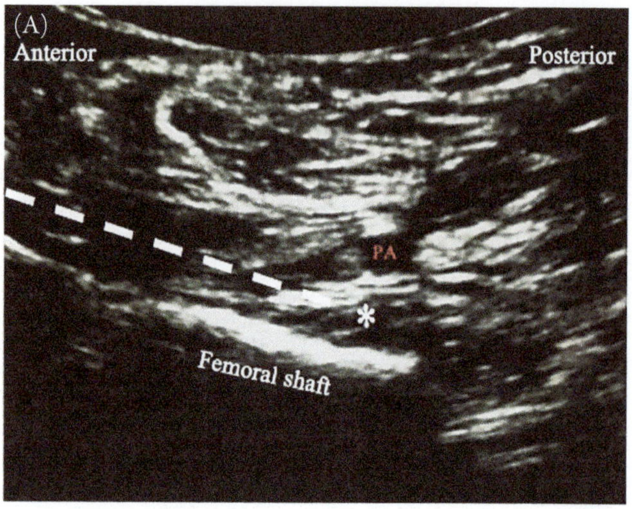

Figure 29.3A. Proximal IPACK.

Using an in-plane technique, a 22-gauge echogenic needle is advanced from medial to lateral into the space between the popliteal artery and femur. The needle is advanced until it reaches past the lateral border of the popliteal artery. After aspiration, 20 mL is injected as the needle is withdrawn (Figure 29.3B).

THE ROLE FOR CONTINUOUS NERVE BLOCKS AFTER TKR

The advantages of using single-shot peripheral nerve blocks are numerous, including prolonged analgesia, avoidance of GA, low cost, and ease of performance. Prolonged dense sensory

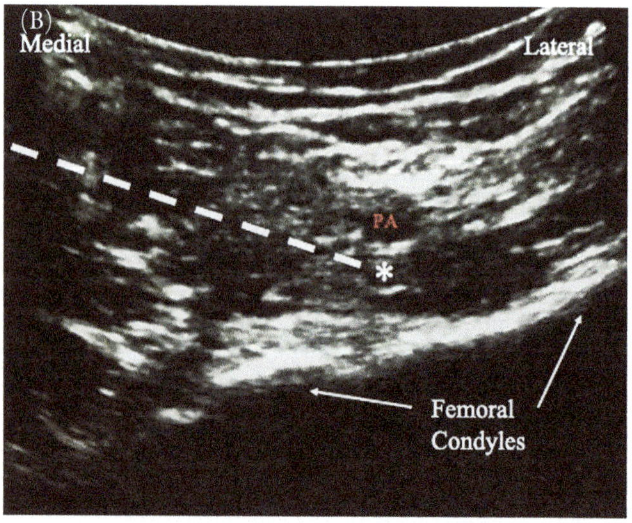

Figure 29.3B. Distal IPACK.

analgesia may not be desirable postoperatively, and may interfere in ambulation. Adjuvants, like dexamethasone and dexmedetomidine, can prolong block duration, but they are not FDA approved and their effects are finite. Furthermore, there is evidence that rebound pain can be significant when a block resolves. Continuous peripheral nerve blocks can provide effective analgesia for several days. They may allow procedures to be performed on an ambulatory basis, and the local anesthetics injected can be more dilute than agents used intraoperatively.

Salinas looked at the effect of single-injection FNB vs. continuous FNB after TKR, in patients whose primary anesthetic was a ropivacaine spinal. Patients who received the continuous block had less morphine use, lower VAS scores, both resting and with physical activity, and identical milestones of flection and independent function at 12 weeks.[58] More recently, Turner et al. compared single-injection adductor canal block (SACB) with adjuvants (20 mL of 0.25% bupivacaine, 1.67 mcg/mL of clonidine, 2 mg of dexamethasone, 150 mcg of buprenorphine, and 2.5 mcg/mL of epinephrine) to continuous adductor canal block (CACB) (20 mL 0.25% of bupivacaine injection with 2.5 mcg/mL of epinephrine, followed by an 8 mL/h infusion of 0.125% bupivacaine continued through postoperative day 2). All numeric rating scale of pain (NRS) scores were equivalent until 36 hours after block placement, but the CACB provided superior analgesia after 42 hours.[59] A meta-analysis of 4 randomized controlled trials comparing SACB with CACB concluded similarly. It showed that the SACB and CACB provided similar analgesia for the first 24 hours postoperatively, but the analgesia provided by the CACB was better over 48 hours.[60]

Continuous nerve blocks have their own issues. They may be more challenging to place than single-shot blocks. They also require 24/7 coverage to respond to calls about, and not limited to, analgesia, leakage, dislocation, and local anesthetic systemic toxicity. For organizations with the ability to insert, maintain, and follow up, the continuous anesthetic techniques have advantages extending past the second postoperative day, but for those unable to provide service or coverage, single-shot blocks with adjuvants can provide excellent analgesia through the first postoperative day.

CONCLUSION

Total knee replacement surgery continues to be one of the most common procedures performed in the United States, and numbers are only expected to rise. While we have various options for anesthesia, not all plans and medications are fit for every patient. The advent of ERAS protocols has led us to examine what anesthetic interventions will allow for an efficient, yet cost-effective, perioperative course. In addition, with an overall sicker and aging population, we must find the safest way to control pain. Through using a multimodal analgesic approach in combination with peripheral nerve blocks, we may be able to achieve adequate pain control without unwanted complications.

REFERENCES

1. Kurtz S, Ong K, Lau E, Mowat F, Halpern M. Projections of primary and revision hip and knee arthroplasty in the United States from 2005 to 2030. *J Bone Joint Surg (American)*. 2007;89(4):780–785. doi: 10.2106/jbjs.f.00222.
2. *AAOS*: *Volume of Primary and Revision Total Joint Replacement in U.S. Projected to Grow by Triple Digits*. PPM. http://www.phillipsmedicraft.com/2018/03/14/aaos-volume-of-primary-and-revision-total-joint-replacement-in-u-s-projected-to-grow-by-triple-digits/. Published January 1, 1970. Accessed April 21, 2020.
3. Orthoinfo.org. *Total Joint Replacement—OrthoInfo—AAOS*. 2019. Available at: https://www.orthoinfo.org/en/treatment/total-joint-replacement. Accessed September 24, 2019.
4. Turnbull ZA, Sastow D, Giambrone GP, Tedore T. Anesthesia for the patient undergoing total knee replacement: current status and future prospects. *Local Reg Anesth*. 2017 Mar 8;10:1–7. doi: 10.2147/LRA.S101373.
5. Memtsoudis SG, Cozowicz C, Bekeris J, et al. Anaesthetic care of patients undergoing primary hip and knee arthroplasty: consensus recommendations from the International Consensus on Anaesthesia-Related Outcomes after Surgery group (ICAROS) based on a systematic review and meta-analysis. *Br J Anaesth*. 2019;123(3):269–287. doi: 10.1016/j.bja.2019.05.042.
6. Johnson R, Kopp S, Burkle C, et al. Neuraxial vs general anaesthesia for total hip and total knee arthroplasty: a systematic review of comparative-effectiveness research. *Br J Anaesth*. 2016;116(2): 163–176. doi: 10.1093/bja/aev455.
7. Warltier DC, Pagel PS, Kersten JR. Approaches to the prevention of perioperative myocardial ischemia. *Anesthesiology*. 2000;92(1):253. doi: 10.1097/00000542-200001000-00038.
8. Pugely AJ, Martin CT, Gao Y, Mendoza-lattes S, Callaghan JJ. Differences in short-term complications between spinal and general anesthesia for primary total knee arthroplasty. *J Bone Joint Surg AM*. 2013;95(3):193–199.
9. Butterworth JF IV, Mackey DC, Wasnick JD, eds. *Morgan & Mikhail's Clinical Anesthesiology*. 6th ed. New York: McGraw-Hill. http://accessmedicine.mhmedical.com/content.aspx? Bookid=2444&sectioned=189634642. Accessed September 24, 2019.
10. Warltier DC, Pagel PS, Kersten JR. Approaches to the prevention of perioperative myocardial ischemia. *Anesthesiology*. 2000;92(1):253. doi: 10.1097/00000542-200001000-00038.
11. Kabon B, Nagele A, Reddy D, et al. Obesity decreases perioperative tissue oxygenation. *Anesthesiology*. 2004;100(2):274–280.
12. Jonsson K, Jensen JA, Goodson WH 3rd, et al. Tissue oxygenation, anemia, and perfusion in relation to wound healing in surgical patients. *Ann Surg*. 1991;214(5):605–613. doi: 10.1097/00000658-199111000-00011
13. Hopf HW, Hunt TK, West JM, et al. Wound tissue oxygen tension predicts the risk of wound infection in surgical patients. *Arch Surg*. 1997; 132: 997–1004; discussion 1005.
14. Treschan TA, Taguchi A, Ali SZ, et al. The effects of epidural and general anesthesia on tissue oxygenation. *Anesth Analg*. 2003;96(6):1553–1557.
15. Moheimani F, Jackson DE. Venous thromboembolism: classification, risk factors, diagnosis, and management. *ISRN Hematol*. 2011;2011:124610. doi: 10.5402/2011/124610.
16. Rodgers A, Walker N, Schug S, et al. Reduction of postoperative mortality and morbidity with epidural or spinal anaesthesia: results from overview of randomised. *BMJ*. 2000;321(7275):1493–1493. doi: 10.1136/bmj.321.7275.1493.
17. Turan A, Bajracharya GR, Leung S, et al. Association of neuraxial anesthesia with postoperative venous thromboembolism after noncardiac surgery: a propensity-matched analysis of ACS-NSQIP database. *Anesth Analg*. *2019*;128(3):494–501. doi: 10.1213/ANE.0000000000003394
18. McCormack PL. Tranexamic acid. *Drugs*. 2012;72(5):585–617. doi: 10.2165/11209070-000000000-00000.

19. Zhang LK, Ma JX, Kuang MJ, et al. The efficacy of tranexamic acid using oral administration in total knee arthroplasty: a systematic review and meta-analysis. *J Orthop Surg Res*. 2017 Oct 27;12(1):159. doi:10.1186/s13018-017-0660-6
20. Wang D, Wang H-Y, Luo Z-Y, et al. Finding the optimal regimen for oral tranexamic acid administration in primary total hip arthroplasty. *J Bone Joint Surg*. 2019;101(5):438–445. doi: 10.2106/jbjs.18.00128.
21. Abdel MP, Chalmers BP, Taunton MJ, et al. Intravenous versus topical tranexamic acid in total knee arthroplasty. *J Bone Joint Surg. 2018*;100(12):1023–1029. doi: 10.2106/jbjs.17.00908.
22. Fillingham YA, Ramkumar DB, Jevsevar DS, et al. Tranexamic acid use in total joint arthroplasty: the clinical practice guidelines endorsed by the American Association of Hip and Knee Surgeons, American Society of Regional Anesthesia and Pain Medicine, American Academy of Orthopaedic Surgeons, Hip Society, and Knee Society. *J Arthroplasty*. 2018;33(10):3065–3069. doi: 10.1016/j.arth.2018.08.002.
23. Whiting DR, Gillette BP, Duncan C, et al. Preliminary results suggest tranexamic acid is safe and effective in arthroplasty patients with severe comorbidities. *Clin Orthop Relat Res*. 2014;472(1):66–72. doi: 10.1007/s11999-013-3134-0.
24. Porter SB, White LJ, Osagiede O, Robards CB, Spaulding AC. Tranexamic acid administration is not associated with an increase in complications in high-risk patients undergoing primary total knee or total hip arthroplasty: a retrospective case-control study of 38,220 patients. *J Arthroplasty*. 2020 Jan;35(1):45–51.e3. doi: 10.1016/j.arth.2019.08.015.
25. Poeran J, Chan JJ, Zubizarreta N, Mazumdar M, Galatz LM, Moucha CS. Safety of Tranexamic Acid in Hip and Knee Arthroplasty in High-risk Patients. *Anesthesiology*. 2021 Jul 1;135(1):57–68.
26. Woolf CJ, Chong M-S. Preemptive analgesia: treating postoperative pain by preventing the establishment of central sensitization. *Anesth Analg*. 1993;77(2):362–379. doi: 10.1213/00000539-199308000-00026.
27. Rudd RA, Aleshire N, Zibbell JE, Gladden RM. Increases in drug and opioid overdose deaths: United States, 2000–2014. *Am J Transplant*. 2016;16(4):1323–1327. doi: 10.1111/ajt.13776.
28. Kim KY, Anoushiravani AA, Chen KK, Roof M, Long WJ, Schwarzkopf R. Preoperative chronic opioid users in total knee arthroplasty: which patients persistently abuse opiates following surgery? *J Arthroplasty*. 2018;33(1):107–112. doi: 10.1016/j.arth.2017.07.041.
29. Ricciotti E, Fitzgerald GA. Prostaglandins and inflammation. *Arterioscler Thromb Vasc Biol*. 2011;31(5):986–1000. doi: 10.1161/atvbaha.110.207449.
30. Wongrakpanich S, Wongrakpanich A, Melhado K, Rangaswami J. A comprehensive review of non-steroidal anti-inflammatory drug use in the elderly. *Aging Dis*. 2018;9(1):143. doi: 10.14336/ad.2017.0306.
31. Smyth EM, Grosser T, Wang M, Yu Y, Fitzgerald GA. Prostanoids in health and disease. *J Lipid Res*. 2008;50(Suppl). doi: 10.1194/jlr.r800094-jlr200.
32. Cairns JA. The coxibs and traditional nonsteroidal anti-inflammatory drugs: a current perspective on cardiovascular risks. *Can J Cardiol*. 2007;23(2):125–131. doi: 10.1016/s0828-282x(07)70732-8.
33. Graham GG, Davies MJ, Day RO, Mohamudally A, Scott KF. The modern pharmacology of paracetamol: therapeutic actions, mechanism of action, metabolism, toxicity and recent pharmacological findings. *Inflammopharmacology*. 2013;21(3):201–232. doi: 10.1007/s10787-013-0172-x.
34. Candiotti KA, Bergese SD, Viscusi ER, Singla SK, Royal MA, Singla NK. Safety of multiple-dose intravenous acetaminophen in adult inpatients. *Pain Med*. 2010 Dec;11(12):1841–1848. https://doi.org/10.1111/j.1526-4637.2010.00991.x
35. Politi JR, Davis RL, Matrka AK. Randomized prospective trial comparing the use of intravenous versus oral acetaminophen in total joint arthroplasty. *J Arthroplasty*. 2017;32(4):1125–1127. doi: 10.1016/j.arth.2016.10.018.
36. Coderre TJ, Kumar N, Lefebvre CD, Yu JSC. Evidence that gabapentin reduces neuropathic pain by inhibiting the spinal release of glutamate. *J Neurochemistry*. 2005;94(4):1131–1139. doi: 10.1111/j.1471-4159.2005.03263.x.
37. Lubis AMT, Rawung RBV, Tantri AR. Preemptive analgesia in total knee arthroplasty: comparing the effects of single dose combining celecoxib with pregabalin and repetition dose combining celecoxib with pregabalin: double-blind controlled clinical Trial. *Pain Res Treat*. 2018;2018:3807217. doi:10.1155/2018/3807217.
38. Yadeau J, Lin Y, Mayman D, et al. Pregabalin and pain after total knee arthroplasty: a double-blind, randomized, placebo-controlled, multidose trial. *Br J Anaesth*. 2015;115(2):285–293. doi: 10.1093/bja/aev217.
39. Kurdi MS, Theerth KA, Deva RS. Ketamine: current applications in anesthesia, pain, and critical care. *Anesth Essays Res*. 2014;8(3):283–290. doi: 10.4103/0259-1162.143110.
40. Yam MF, Loh YC, Tan CS, Khadijah Adam S, Abdul Manan N, Basir R. General pathways of pain sensation and the major neurotransmitters involved in pain regulation. *Int J Mol Sci*. 2018 Jul 24;19(8):2164. doi: 10.3390/ijms19082164.
41. Adam F, Chauvin M, Du Manoir B, Langlois M, Sessler DI, Fletcher D. Small-dose ketamine infusion improves postoperative analgesia and rehabilitation after total knee arthroplasty. *Anesth Analg*. 2005;100(2):475–480. doi: 10.1213/01.ANE.0000142117.82241.DC.
42. Bell RF, Dahl JB, Moore RA, Kalso E. Perioperative ketamine for acute postoperative pain. *Cochrane Database System Rev*. 2006;(1):CD004603. doi: 10.1002/14651858.CD004603.pub2. Update in: Cochrane Database Syst Rev. 2015;7:CD004603. PMID: 16437490.
43. Hyland SJ, Deliberato DG, Fada RA, et al. Liposomal bupivacaine versus standard periarticular injection in total knee arthroplasty with regional anesthesia: a prospective, randomized controlled trial. *J Arthroplasty*. 2019;34: 488–494.
44. Zhao B, Ma X, Zhang J, Ma J, Cao Q. The efficacy of local liposomal bupivacaine infiltration on pain and recovery after total joint arthroplasty: a systematic review and meta-analysis of randomized controlled trials. *Medicine (Baltimore)*. 2019 Jan;98(3):e14092. doi: 10.1097/MD.0000000000014092.
45. Pichler L, Poeran, J, Zubizarreta N, et al. Liposomal bupivacaine does not reduce inpatient opioid prescription or related complications after knee arthroplasty. *Anesthesiology*. 2018;129:689–689.
46. Kuang MJ, Du Y, Ma JX, et al. The efficacy of liposomal bupivacaine using periarticular injection in total knee arthroplasty: a systematic review and meta-analysis. *J Arthroplasty*. 2017;32:1395–1402.
47. Ross JA, Greenwood AC, Sasser P, Jiranek WA. Periarticular injections in knee and hip arthroplasty: where and what to inject. *J Arthroplasty*. 2017;32(9S):S77–S80. doi: 10.1016/j.arth.2017.05.003.
48. Badner NH, Bourne RB, Rorabeck CH, Macdonald SJ, Doyle JA. Intra-articular injection of bupivacaine in knee-replacement operations. results of use for analgesia and for preemptive blockade. *J Bone Joint Surg*. 1996;78(5):734–738. doi: 10.2106/00004623-199605000-00013.
49. Lombardi AV, Berend KR, Mallory TH, Dodds KL, Adams JB. Soft tissue and intra-articular injection of bupivacaine, epinephrine, and morphine has a beneficial effect after total knee arthroplasty. *Clin Orth Rel Res*. 2004;428:125–130. doi: 10.1097/01.blo.0000147701.24029.cc.
50. Sadigursky D, Simões DP, de Albuquerque RA, Silva MZ, Fernandes RJC, Colavolpe PO. Local periarticular analgesia in total knee arthroplasty. *Acta Ortop Bras*. 2017;25(2):81–84. doi: 10.1590/1413-785220172502151116.
51. Kao S, Lee H, Cheng C, Lin C, Tsai H. Pain control after total knee arthroplasty: comparing intra-articular local anesthetic injection with femoral nerve block. *BioMed Res Int*. 2015;2015:649140. doi: 10.1155/2015/649140.
52. Korean Knee Society. Guidelines for the management of postoperative pain after total knee arthroplasty. *Knee Surg Relat Res*. 2012;24(4):201–207. doi: 10.5792/ksrr.2012.24.4.201.
53. Elkassabany NM, Antosh S, Ahmed M, et al. The risk of falls after total knee arthroplasty with the use of a femoral nerve block versus an adductor canal block. *Anesth Analg*. 2016;122(5):1696–1703. doi: 10.1213/ane.0000000000001237.

54. Beebe MJ, Allen R, Anderson MB, Swenson JD, Peters CL. Continuous femoral nerve block using 0.125% bupivacaine does not prevent early ambulation after total knee arthroplasty. *Clin Orth Rel Res*. 2013;472(5):1394–1399. doi: 10.1007/s11999-013-3164-7.
55. Sankineani SR, Reddy ARC, Eachempati KK, Jangale A, Gurava Reddy AV. Comparison of adductor canal block and IPACK block (interspace between the popliteal artery and the capsule of the posterior knee) with adductor canal block alone after total knee arthroplasty: a prospective control trial on pain and knee function in immediate postoperative period. *Eur J Orthop Surg Traumatol*. 2018 Oct;28(7):1391–1395.
56. Tran J, Peng PWH, Gofeld M, Chan V, Agur AMR. Anatomical study of the innervation of posterior knee joint capsule: implication for image-guided intervention. *Reg Anesth Pain Med*. 2019;44:234–238.
57. American Society of Regional Anesthesia and Pain Medicine. *ASRA News—How I Do It: Infiltration Between Popliteal Artery and Capsule of Knee (iPACK)*. 2019. [online] *Asra.com*. https://www.asra.com/asra-news/article/158/how-i-do-it-infiltration-between-poplite. Accessed September 25, 2019.
58. Salinas FV, Liu SS, Mulroy MF. The effect of single-injection femoral nerve block versus continuous femoral nerve block after total knee arthroplasty on hospital length of stay and long-term functional recovery within an established clinical pathway. *A&A* 2006; 102:1234–1239.
59. Turner J, Dobson S, Henshaw D, et al. Single-injection adductor canal block with multiple adjuvants provides equivalent analgesia when compared with continuous adductor canal blockade for primary total knee arthroplasty: a double-blinded, randomized, controlled, equivalency trial. *J Arthroplasty*. 2018;33(10):3160–3166.e1.
60. Zhang L, Zhang B, Quan R, Xu H, Sun Y, Zhou J. Single shot versus continuous technique adductor canal block for analgesia following total knee arthroplasty: a PRISMA-compliant meta-analysis. *Medicine (Baltimore)*. 2019 May;98(20):e15539. doi: 10.1097/MD.0000000000015539.

REVIEW QUESTIONS

(1) Which of the following criteria is associated with increased success of same-day discharge following TKR?

A. Preoperatively use of an aid to walk
B. Residing with a spouse
C. Living in an apartment with stairs
D. Daily opioid use

(2) Liposomal bupivacaine has FDA approval for use in which of the following procedures?

A. TKR
B. Interscalene block
C. IPACK block
D. ACB

(3) Which of the following medications may be associated with somnolence in an elderly patient?

A. Ketamine
B. Gabapentin
C. Acetaminophen
D. Ketorolac

(4) Which of the following quadriceps muscles may be blocked during the performance of an ACB?

A. Rectus femoris
B. Vastus medialis
C. Vastus intermedius
D. Vastus lateralis

(5) What is the medial border of the femoral triangle?

A. Inguinal ligament
B. Adductor longus muscle
C. Sartorius muscle
D. Fascia iliaca

(6) Inhibition of COX-2 was associated with which of the following conditions?

A. Stroke
B. GI bleed
C. Dyspepsia
D. Increased GFR

(7) Which of the following nerves does not supply any sensory innervation to the posterior capsule of the knee?

A. Tibial
B. Femoral
C. Obturator
D. Common peroneal

(8) Common complications of continuous catheters include all of the following EXCEPT:

A. Rebound pain
B. Leakage
C. Dislocation
D. Dense block

(9) TXA reduces intraoperative bleeding by what activity?

A. Strengthening of fibrin clot
B. Activation of platelets
C. Stimulation of prothrombin production
D. Formation of tissue factor-activated factor VIIa complex

ANSWERS

(1) **B.** Patients who have a support system at home and good functional status prior to surgery tend to be better candidates for same-day discharge.

Reference

Scully RD, Kappa JE, Melvin JS. Outpatient: same-calendar-day discharge hip and knee arthroplasty. *J Am Acad Orthopaed Surg*. October 15, 2020 Oct 15; 28(20):e900–e909.

(2) **B.** Currently, liposomal bupivacaine is only FDA approved for infiltrative analgesia and interscalene blocks.

Reference

Food and Drug Administration Web site. https://www.accessdata.fda.gov/drugsatfda_docs/label/2018/022496s9lbl.pdf Accessed January,11, 2023 .

(3) **B.** While multimodal analgesia is important, gabapentin and pregabalin tend to have an undesirable side-effect profile consisting of sedation and drowsiness, which is seen mainly in

the elderly population. The benefit/risk profile of each drug should be considered and tailored to each specific patient.

Reference

Yadeau J, Lin Y, Mayman D, et al. Pregabalin and pain after total knee arthroplasty: a double-blind, randomized, placebo-controlled, multidose trial. *Br J Anaesth*. 2015;115(2):285–293. doi: 10.1093/bja/aev217.

(4) **B.** ACB aims to anesthetize the saphenous nerve distal to its innervation of the quadriceps muscles, although occasionally it blocks the nerve to vastus medialis, which can result in quadriceps weakness.

Reference

Nada E, Elmansoury A, Elkassabany N, Whitney ER. Location of the entry point of the muscular branch of the nerve to vastus medialis. *Br J Anaesth*. 2021 Aug;127(2):e58–e60.

(5) **B.** Borders of the femoral triangle:

- Superiorly = inguinal ligament
- Medial wall = adductor longus muscle
- Lateral wall = sartorius muscle.

Reference

Bendtsen TF, Moriggl B, Chan V, Borglum J. The optimal analgesic block for total knee arthroplasty. *Reg Anesth Pain Med*. 2016;41(6):711–719.

(6) **A.** Thromboxane A2 (TXA_2) acts a vasoconstrictor and platelet aggregator and is blocked by cyclo-oxygenase-1 (COX-1). Prostaglandin I_2 (PGI_2) acts as a vasodilator and inhibitor of platelet aggregation and is blocked by COX-2. When COX-2 is selectively inhibited, the pro-thrombotic activity of TXA_2 can result in myocardial infarction, stroke, and deep-vein thrombosis (DVT).

Reference

Smyth EM, Grosser T, Wang M, Yu Y, FitzGerald GA. Prostanoids in health and disease. *J Lipid Res*. 2009 Apr;50 Suppl(Suppl):S423–S428.

(7) **B.** The posterior knee is innervated by articular branches from the posterior division of the tibial, obturator, and common peroneal nerves—the deep genicular nerves. The femoral nerve gives sensory innervation to the medial thigh down to the medial malleolus via its terminal sensory branch, the saphenous nerve.

Reference

Tran J, Peng PWH, Gofeld M, Chan V, Agur AMR. Anatomical study of the innervation of posterior knee joint capsule: implication for image-guided intervention. *Reg Anesth Pain Med*. 2019;44:234–238.

(8) **A.** Rebound pain occurs after a nerve block wears off. Catheters mitigate the rebound pain, but are prone to leakage, dislocation, and causing a block that is too dense.

Reference

Muñoz-Leyva F, Cubillos J, Chin KJ. Managing rebound pain after regional anesthesia. *Korean J Anesthesiol*. 2020;73(5):372–383. doi: 10.4097/kja.20436.

(9) **A.** TXA is an anti-fibrinolytic that reduces the conversion of plasminogen to plasmin, which in turn decreases fibrin degradation to fibrinogen and ultimately stabilizes the clot.

Reference

McCormack PL. Tranexamic acid. *Drugs*. 2012;72(5):585–617.

30.

REGIONAL ANESTHESIA FOR ISCHEMIC PAIN

BELOW KNEE AMPUTATION AND ABOVE KNEE AMPUTATION

Shanthi Reddy, Cameron Sumner, and James Kim

STEM CASE AND KEY QUESTIONS

A 67-year-old female with peripheral vascular disease presents to the emergency department with severe right foot pain. On exam, the fourth and fifth toes of her right foot are deeply erythematous and exquisitely tender to palpation. She has undergone multiple prior interventions including lower extremity angiograms, femoral stents, and most recently, a femoral-popliteal bypass. Doppler exam reveals profoundly diminished dorsalis pedis and posterior tibial pulses, suggesting graft failure. She is admitted to the hospital for pain control and vascular surgery evaluation. The vascular surgery team explains that despite their best efforts to salvage her forefoot, all options for revascularization have been exhausted. The vascular surgeon strongly recommends surgery, but the patient continues to vehemently refuse an amputation at this time. The team now shifts their focus to management of her ischemic pain. Over the hospital course, the patient's toes become black and the erythema now extends just proximal to her ankle. Despite increasing the dose and frequency of opioids and the trial of multiple pharmacologic adjuvants, her pain has only marginally improved. The vascular surgery team has decided it is time to revisit the discussion of amputation. The patient now decides to proceed with a below the knee amputation (BKA).

After undergoing BKA a few weeks ago, the patient presents to the vascular surgery clinic for a postoperative follow-up appointment. On exam, the patient appears unwell and is found to be febrile with purulent secretions draining from her surgical site. The vascular surgeon admits the patient to the hospital for further evaluation. The ischemia has continued to worsen and this patient now requires an above the knee amputation (AKA).

(1) WHAT IS CRITICAL LIMB ISCHEMIA (CLI)?

Critical limb ischemia (CLI) is a severe manifestation of peripheral artery disease that results from poor perfusion of a limb.[1] CLI is characterized by chronic (≥2 weeks) ischemic pain at rest, non-healing wounds, ulcers, or gangrene attributable to objectively proven arterial occlusive disease.[2] One year after diagnosis, there is a 25% mortality in CLI patients, while 30% live with amputations, 20% have ongoing symptoms, and 25% experience symptom resolution.[3]

(2) WHAT PHARMACOLOGIC OPTIONS ARE AVAILABLE FOR PALLIATIVE MANAGEMENT OF ISCHEMIC PAIN?

Opioids remain the cornerstone for the management of severe pain. Despite the lack of definitive recommendations, small studies looked at the use of adjuvants like gabapentin, ketamine, and lidocaine.

(3) WHICH PERIPHERAL NERVE BLOCKS ARE MOST APPROPRIATE FOR LEG AMPUTATION?

In order to provide surgical anesthesia below the knee, a distal sciatic nerve block in the popliteal fossa and a femoral/saphenous nerve block are required for above knee amputation; a proximal sciatic in addition to femoral nerve block is needed; a lateral femoral cutaneous and an obturator nerve block results in complete block.

(4) WHAT IS THE RELEVANT ANATOMY AND TECHNIQUE FOR SCIATIC NERVE BLOCKADE AT THE LEVEL OF THE POPLITEAL FOSSA?

The sciatic nerve divides into two branches: the tibial (TN) and the common peroneal nerve (CPN). The TN, which is usually the largest branch, lies more medially, closely related to the vessels, while the CPN lies laterally and more superficially. Using a needle from the lateral side of the thigh, directed medially under ultrasound guidance, the nerve is recognized and local anesthetics are injected and seen to spread circumferentially around the nerve. A subparaneural technique targets the nerve at its bifurcation between the paraneural sheath and epineurium. This technique is associated with a faster onset and longer duration than when each branch is blocked separately and does not require multiple readjustments.

(5) WHAT IS THE RELEVANT ANATOMY FOR LUMBAR PLEXUS?

The lumbar plexus is formed from the ventral rami of L1–L4 with variable contributions from T12 and L5. The lumbar plexus gives off 6 nerves that supply the lower abdomen and upper leg. These nerves are the femoral, obturator, lateral femoral cutaneous, ilioinguinal, iliohypogastric, and genitofemoral nerves.

(6) WHAT ARE THE COMPLICATIONS OF THE LUMBAR PLEXUS BLOCK?

The lumbar plexus block (LPB) is an advanced, deep block with the potential for serious complications. The most common complications are epidural spread resulting in a high neuraxial anesthesia, hypotension, and local anesthetic toxicity. A retroperitoneal hematoma can result from this block due to the deep incompressible location.

(7) DESCRIBE THE LABAT APPROACH TO SCIATIC NERVE BLOCKADE.

A line is drawn from the greater trochanter to the posterior superior iliac spine; another line is drawn from the greater trochanter to the sacral hiatus. A third line is drawn perpendicular to the midpoint of the first line to its intersection with the second line; the needle is inserted at the latter point.

(8) WHAT ARE THE ANATOMIC LANDMARKS OF THE SUBGLUTEAL APPROACH TO THE SCIATIC NERVE?

It is the middle of a line drawn from the ischial tuberosity to the greater trochanter of the femur.

(9) WHAT IS PHANTOM LIMB PAIN?

Phantom limb pain is the most widely known post-amputation syndrome and is typically felt in the distal extremity of the absent limb. Phantom limb pain occurs in up to 80% of amputees. At least 75% of patients who develop phantom limb pain do so within the first week after amputation.

(10) WHAT ARE RISK FACTORS FOR DEVELOPMENT OF PHANTOM PAIN?

While there are no definitive predisposing factors, the presence of certain circumstances increases the likelihood of developing phantom pain, such as severe preoperative pain, bilateral amputation, stump pain, repeated limb surgeries, and increasing age.

DISCUSSION

PATHOPHYSIOLOGY OF ISCHEMIC LIMB PAIN

While there is a nociceptive element, it is the substantial neuropathic component of ischemic limb pain that is difficult to treat. Neuropathic mechanisms play a major role in this type of pain due to ischemia or direct damage to the nerve (via a distal axonopathy that affects nerve fibers of all sizes). It is well accepted that inflammation leads to neuropathic pain.[2] It may result from the N-methyl-D-aspartate (NMDA) receptor-mediated increase in synaptic excitability of the spinal cord, clinically manifested as hyperalgesia and allodynia.

PHARMACOLOGIC OPTIONS FOR MANAGEMENT OF ISCHEMIC PAIN

The data are limited regarding the most effective therapies available to treat ischemic pain in patients with CLI without options for limb salvage. Opioids remain the cornerstone for the management of severe pain. The use of adjuvants in addition to opioids to relieve this pain has been studied. These adjuvants include gabapentin, ketamine, and lidocaine.[2]

Gabapentin has anti-nociceptive and anti-neuropathic effects. It is thought to act by binding to calcium channels and modulating calcium influx, which results in analgesic, anti-epileptic, and sedative effects.[2] In a prospective observational study of patients with non-reconstructible CLI, gabapentin significantly reduced pain scores, improved sleep, and in some, reduced opioid requirements with no documented side effects.[3] Many pain specialists extrapolate positive studies in other surgical cohorts and utilize gabapentin in the peri-amputation period. Gabapentin has become an integral element of enhanced recovery pathways due to its opioid-sparing effects. It is practical to include gabapentin to the analgesic plan early because it requires a period of titration. Sedation, dizziness, respiratory depression, and visual changes have been reported with gabapentin use.[4]

Ketamine has antagonist effects at the NMDA receptor, which plays a major role in neuroplasticity and excitotoxicity.[5] It is not known if ketamine can prevent the transition from acute to chronic pain by virtue of its NMDA antagonist and opioid-sparing properties.[6]

Intravenous lidocaine generates most of its analgesic action by blocking high-voltage sodium channels through nerve cell membranes. Frohlich et al. studied the effect of intravenous lidocaine in a group of 14 healthy volunteers and found that lidocaine had an inhibitory effect on ischemic pain, producing a sustained analgesic state in ischemic pain induced by the tourniquet technique.[7] These results suggest that lidocaine may be beneficial in treating acute pain. The more recent study by Vahidi et al. was the first trial conducted in patients with CLI and showed that intravenous lidocaine provides a considerable analgesia in this patient population.[8] Compared with morphine, intravenous lidocaine significantly decreased pain scores 30 minutes after administration, and the lidocaine group became pain-free earlier than those in the morphine group.[8] Compared to opioids, lidocaine has limited side effects and can generate a faster and more efficient analgesic state without the need to repeat opioid doses. Lidocaine may be beneficial for the short-term relief of ischemic pain in non-reconstructible CLI, particularly in emergency conditions.

Patients with CLI have an increased incidence of coronary artery disease, renal insufficiency, and advanced age. As such, dosing adjustments should be made based on the burden of comorbidities, with extra caution exercised in renal disease given drug excretion.[9] Opioids are often not well tolerated in this population due to increased sensitivity to their side effects related to end-stage renal disease. Gabapentin and systemic lidocaine also require dose adjustments in renal failure while ketamine does not.

An antidepressant (i.e., serotonin and norepinephrine reuptake inhibitor or low-dose tricyclic antidepressants) may be added, especially if depression is present or suspected. Due to its opioid and anti-neuropathic effects, methadone may also be beneficial.

REGIONAL ANESTHESIA FOR LOWER EXTREMITY AMPUTATION

Peripheral nerve blocks provide surgical anesthesia with better cardiorespiratory stability when compared to central neuraxial blockade, which often causes hypotension and bradycardia.[10] For isolated limb surgery, the introduction of ultrasound guidance has shifted the practice of anesthesia away from general anesthesia and neuraxial techniques to peripheral nerve blocks.[11,12]

In order to provide surgical anesthesia below the knee, a distal sciatic nerve block in the popliteal fossa and a femoral nerve block are required.[13] The majority of the sensory and motor innervation of the lower limb below the knee, except the medial leg and foot, is provided by the sciatic nerve.[14] The popliteal block is a more distal approach to blockade of the sciatic nerve. As such, it has the advantage of preserving hamstring motor function (as compared to more proximal approaches). The saphenous nerve (a branch of the femoral nerve) provides only sensory innervation to the medial leg and foot. The use of ultrasound allows real-time visualization of the nerves and deposition of local anesthetic, which increases the likelihood of successful nerve blockade.

SCIATIC NERVE BLOCKADE AT THE LEVEL OF THE POPLITEAL FOSSA

The sciatic nerve in the popliteal fossa is bordered superolaterally by the long head of the biceps femoris muscle, superomedially by the semimembranosus (SMM) and semitendinosus (STM) muscles, and inferiorly by the lateral and medial heads of the gastrocneumius.[15] The tibial nerve (TN) and common peroneal nerve (CPN) components of the sciatic nerve are two distinct functional entities, surrounded by a single epineurial sheath (within the sciatic nerve).[16] Further discussion of the sciatic nerve in the popliteal fossa can be found in Chapter 31 on regional anesthesia for ankle fractures.

Technique

Place the patient in the supine position with the knee in 45° flexion. Place the ultrasound probe transversely and parallel to the popliteal crease.[16] At about 6–8 cm from the popliteal crease, the sciatic nerve is seen as a round hyperechoic shadow that will appear superficial and lateral to the artery. Move the transducer proximally while keeping the popliteal artery in view at all times. If two hyperechoic structures are viewed, the probe needs to be moved to a more proximal location on the leg.[16] The larger and medial branch is the tibial nerve, while the CPN lies laterally and more superficially.[17] Both nerves are highly anisotropic (they appear bright when the probe is perpendicular to them, but become indistinct with a change in the angle of the probe). Aligning the transducer beam caudally toward the foot brings the angle of incidence of the beam with the nerve at 90° (Figure 30.1A, B).

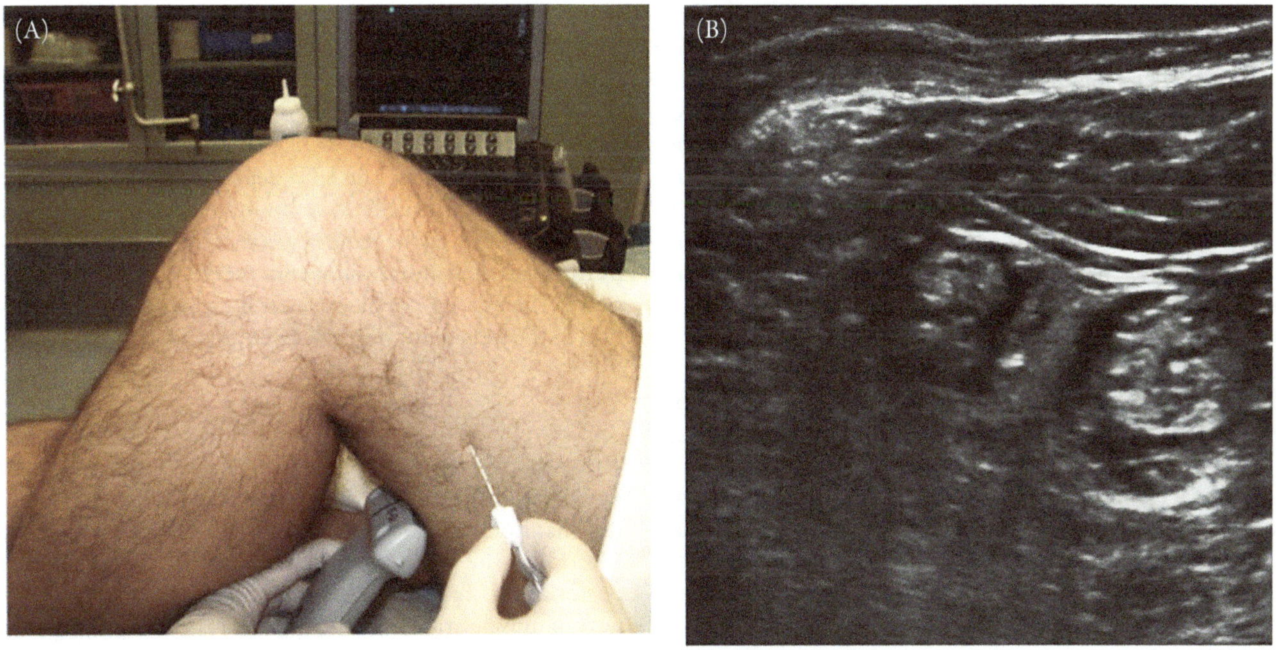

Figure 30.1. (A) Ultrasound guided popliteal nerve block in the supine position. (B) Ultrasonic image of the tibial (larger nerve) and common peroneal (smaller nerve) after local anesthetics are injected.
CPN = Common Peroneal Nerve; TN = Tibial Nerve; PA = Popliteal Artery.
From: Canales M, Huntley H, Reiner M, Ehredt DJ, Razzante M. The popliteal nerve block in foot and ankle surgery: an efficient and anatomical technique. *J Anesth Clin Res*. 2015;6:8. License CC BY.

Using an in-plane approach, the needle is inserted from a lateral to medial direction to avoid the popliteal artery. The local anesthetic is seen to spread circumferentially as a hypoechoic solution around the nerve ("donut sign").

Paraneural Approach

Using ultrasound, the hyperechoic paraneural sheath is identified.[17] it is usually recognizable at the point at the bifurcation of the sciatic nerve, so the needle tip is inserted at this point (space between the paraneural sheath and epineurium).[17] Then the local anesthetic will be seen spreading around the two nerves. Importantly, this technique results in faster onset and longer duration than when the CPN and TN are blocked separately and has the advantage of avoiding multiple readjustments of the needle.[17]

ADDUCTOR CANAL NERVE BLOCK

The adductor canal is bordered by the sartorius muscle, adductor longus, and vastus medialis. The sartorius muscle forms a "roof" over the adductor canal in the lower half of the thigh.[18] The sides of the triangular canal are formed by the vastus medialis laterally and the adductor longus or magnus medially.[18] Within the adductor canal lies the saphenous nerve and nerve to vastus medialis. The saphenous nerve block (SNB) should be performed at the most distal level where the artery still lies immediately deep to the sartorius muscle, thus minimizing the amount of motor block of the vastus medialis.[19] The adductor canal block (ACB) is performed with the patient in the supine position with the thigh abducted and externally rotated to allow access to the medial thigh.[18] The transducer is placed transverse and oriented anteromedially at the junction between the middle and distal third of the thigh.[18] The needle is inserted in-plane and directed anterior to the superficial femoral artery, deep to the sartorius muscle, and to deposit up to 20 mL of local anesthetic.[19] It is not necessary to visualize the nerve for this block because the saphenous nerve is not always well imaged. During needle advancement, it is important to penetrate two layers of fascia/membrane to enter the adductor canal. The first layer is the fascia surrounding the sartorius muscle and the deeper layer is the vastoadductor membrane.

REGIONAL ANESTHETIC TECHNIQUES FOR AMPUTATIONS

A neuraxial technique can be used to achieve surgical anesthesia, and a lumbar epidural can be used for postoperative analgesia. Pisansky et al. compared perioperative outcomes after neuraxial/regional vs. general anesthesia for above the knee amputations. The results showed no difference in 30-day mortality or other secondary outcomes, including length of stay, cardiac, pulmonary, infectious, and bleeding complications.[20] If there are contraindications to neuraxial anesthesia, peripheral techniques are available. The lumbar plexus block (LPB) combined with the posterior approach to the sciatic nerve (L4–S3) provides complete anesthesia of the lower extremity. The entire lumbar plexus can be blocked via a posterior approach (also known as the psoas compartment block).[21] Alternatively, the individual nerves of the lumbar plexus—the femoral nerve (L2–L4), obturator nerve (L2–L4), and lateral femoral cutaneous nerve (L2–L3)—can be accessed and blocked via an anterior approach.[21]

LUMBAR PLEXUS BLOCK (LPB)

The patient is placed in the lateral decubitus position. A line is drawn at the level of the iliac crest starting at the midline and extending to the posterior superior iliac spine (PSIS). The line is then divided into thirds. The junction of the lateral and middle thirds is the point of needle insertion and is typically 5 cm lateral from the midline in most patients.[21]

Nerve Stimulator Technique

With a nerve stimulator set to deliver a current intensity of 1.2–1.5 mA, a needle is advanced; once bone is contacted (usually the transverse process of L4), withdraw the needle and redirect it caudally to "walk off" the process. The plexus should be stimulated at a depth of no more than 2 cm beyond the transverse process. Beyond 2 cm, the risk of injury to retroperitoneal structures is increased. Once quadriceps twitches are obtained, the current should be decreased to obtain stimulation between 0.5 and 1.0 mA. If the twitch remains evident with the decreased current, proceed with injection of local anesthetic. Obtaining twitches with currents less than 0.5 mA may indicate the placement of the needle inside the dural sleeve. An injection inside this sheath can result in the spread of local anesthetic toward the epidural or subarachnoid space. In most adults, 30–40 mL of local anesthetic with frequent aspiration is sufficient to block the lumbar plexus.[21] Successful lumbar plexus blockade depends on the deposition of the local anesthetic in the fascial plane (psoas muscle) where the roots of the plexus are situated.

The onset time for the LPB depends on the type of local anesthetic, but is usually 15–25 minutes. Following an injection at the L4 level, the femoral nerve is blocked first, followed by the lateral femoral cutaneous nerve and the obturator nerve. The first sign of block onset is usually the loss of sensation in the saphenous nerve distribution.[21]

Ultrasound Guided Block

The patient's flank is scanned to identify the anatomical structures surrounding the lumbar plexus. A helpful sign is the shamrock sign, which is made up of the psoas muscle anterior to the transverse process, the erector spinae muscle posterior to the transverse process, and the quadratus lumborum muscle attached to the apex of the transverse process of L4. The lumbar plexus can be visualized within the psoas muscle, roughly 2 cm anterior to the transverse process. By advancing the needle in-plane and perpendicular to the ultrasound beam, the needle tip can be guided beside the plexus.[22]

Complications

The most common complication is the epidural spread with a risk of high neuraxial anesthesia, spinal anesthesia, local anesthetic toxicity, or iliopsoas or retroperitoneal hematoma. Epidural spread results in a unilateral sympathectomy and may result in significant hypotension and occurs in up to 15% of patients. The plasma concentrations of local anesthetics are not significantly higher after LPB relative to other peripheral nerve blocks, but toxicity can happen due to the large local anesthetic volumes and intramuscular injection. Because this is a deep block in a non-compressible area, it should be avoided in anticoagulated patients.

SCIATIC NERVE BLOCK

CLASSIC (LABAT) APPROACH

Labat's posterior technique (first described in 1924) has the advantage of also blocking the posterior femoral cutaneous nerve, which provides sensory innervation to the gluteus and uppermost medial and posterior thigh. Blockade of the posterior femoral cutaneous nerve is important when thigh tourniquets are used for lower extremity procedures of long duration.[23]

Technique

The patient is positioned in the lateral decubitus position with the operative side up while the leg is flexed at the knee.[23] A line is drawn from the greater trochanter (GT) to the posterior superior iliac spine (PSIS). A second line is drawn from the greater trochanter to the sacral hiatus. Then another line is drawn perpendicular to the midpoint to the first one to intersect the lower line; the point of intersection with the lower line is the point of needle introduction.[24] With the nerve stimulator set to 1.0–1.5 mA, insert the needle perpendicular to all planes. Stimulation of the gluteus maximus muscle can happen along the way to the sciatic nerve. The appearance of plantar flexion and/or inversion (tibial nerve) or dorsiflexion and/or eversion (common peroneal nerve) with 0.5 mA or less of current denotes proximity to the nerve. Plantar flexion of the foot (tibial nerve stimulation) was found to result in shorter onset time and more frequent success of the block as compared to dorsiflexion (common peroneal nerve stimulation). In most adults, 20–30 mL of local anesthetic is sufficient to block the sciatic nerve.

PARASACRAL APPROACH

Parasacral sciatic nerve blocks sensations from the posterior thigh, hamstrings, and biceps femoris muscles; part of the hip and knee joint; and the entire leg below the knee except the medial cutaneous skin of the lower leg.

Landmarks: a line is drawn between the posterior superior iliac spine (PSIS) and the ischial tuberosity (IT). The needle insertion point lies 6 cm caudal to the PSIS on this line.

SUBGLUTEAL APPROACH

The patient is in the lateral decubitus position with the operative side up. The sciatic nerve bisects the midpoint of a line from the greater trochanter and the ischial tuberosity. An ultrasound probe is placed transversely along this line between the ischial tuberosity medically and the greater trochanter laterally. The sciatic nerve appears as a hyperechoic elliptical structure between these two landmarks. The sciatic nerve lies in between the gluteus maximus muscle and the quadratus femoris muscle (Figure 30.2).

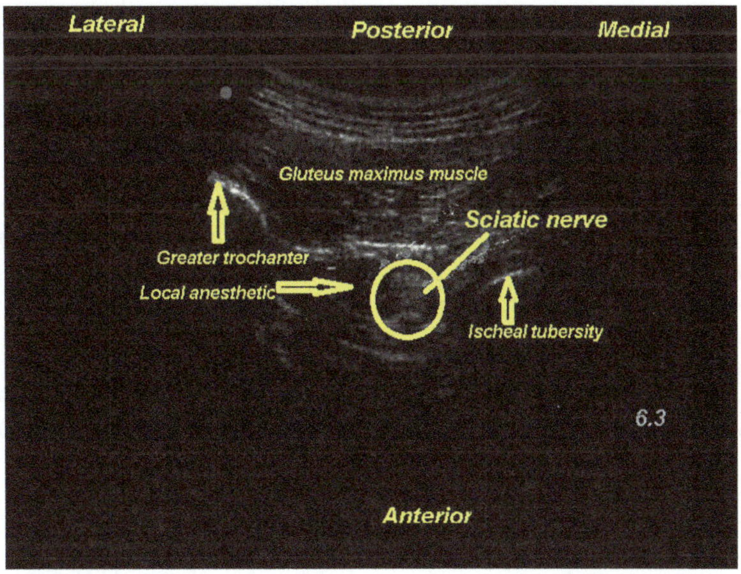

Figure 30.2. Subgluteal sciatic nerve block.
From: Eldegwy, Negm. Adductor canal block combined with sciatic nerve block vs. local analgesic infiltration for pain control after total knee arthroplasty. *J Anesth Clin Res*. 2018;9:1. License Creative Common Attribution License CC BY.

Because it is a deeper block, a low-frequency (2–5 MHz) curvilinear is used. Lateral needle insertion is preferred to medial insertion because the inferior gluteal artery is located medial to the nerve and may be in the needle path with needle advancement. At this level, the sciatic nerve is located between the gluteus maximus muscle and the quadratus femoris muscle. Injection and spread of 20–30 mL of local anesthetic is usually required.

PHANTOM LIMB PAIN

Phantom limb pain is the most widely known post-amputation syndrome and is typically felt in the distal extremity of the absent limb.[25] Pain characteristics vary, but are often described as being crampy, burning, or shooting in nature. If severe limb pain exists prior to surgery, the same pain will frequently be experienced after removal of the limb. Phantom limb pain tends to be episodic in nature, occurring in short bursts ranging from a few seconds to many hours.

Phantom limb pain occurs in up to 80% of amputees.[25] At least 75% of patients who develop phantom limb pain do so within the first week after amputation. Some cases are resolved completely, while many patients suffer phantom pain for life.

The presence of certain circumstances increases the likelihood of developing phantom pain, such as severe preoperative pain, bilateral amputation, stump pain, repeated limb surgeries, and increasing age.

TREATMENT OF PHANTOM LIMB PAIN

Opioids, particularly intravenous or oral morphine, have been shown to reduce phantom limb pain. A cross sectional study found that acetaminophen and NSAIDs were the most common medications used in the treatment of phantom limb pain.[26] NSAIDs are cyclooxygenase inhibitors that block the synthesis of prostaglandin and decrease both peripheral and central nociception.[27]

Some studies have shown that 6 weeks of gabapentinoids after amputation are better than placebo in relieving postamputation phantom limb pain. There were no significant differences in mood, sleep interference, or activities of daily living, but VAS pain scores were better in patients who received gabapentin.[28] Due to its side effect profile, which includes drowsiness, dizziness, ataxia, blurred vision, respiratory depression when combined with other medications, as well as its pharmacokinetic properties involving renal excretion, starting with low doses and slow titration is advised.

A limited number of studies on ketamine in the setting of phantom limb pain have shown that it does not decrease opioid consumption or acute pain as compared to other systemic analgesics.

Current evidence suggests that a severed nerve after an amputation triggers a complex interaction between the dynamic peripheral and central nervous systems. Injury to peripheral nerves provokes changes in the spinal cord, dorsal root ganglia, thalamus, and cerebral cortex, also known as neuronal plasticity.[29] At the level of the spinal cord, reorganization of neuronal activity may result in sensitization, leading to responses to peripheral stimulation that may cause exaggerated responses to both painful (hyperalgesia) and non-painful (allodynia) stimuli.[30] Studies using functional magnetic resonance imaging (fMRI) have demonstrated a correlation between phantom limb pain and cortical reorganization, with the most intense phantom pain provoking the greatest cortical changes.[31] Interestingly, when peripheral nerve blocks were administered and afferent input to the central nervous system was blocked, a few of the patients had complete resolution of their pain, and the previous cortical changes reverted back to normal.[32] This demonstrates that phantom limb pain and the cortical changes may be reversible and may depend largely on signaling from the peripheral nervous system. These results suggest that patients undergoing lower limb amputations may benefit from continuous peripheral nerve blocks, which may be beneficial for both acute pain and decreasing the incidence of developing chronic pain.[33,34]

Overall, implementing regional anesthetic techniques along with multimodal pharmacologic agents is an elegant and effective approach to managing postoperative amputation pain and phantom limb pain. Aside from providing superior postoperative analgesia, peripheral nerve blocks are very useful for providing surgical anesthetics, especially for patients with severe comorbidities that make them poor candidates for general anesthesia. Aside from the lumbar plexus block, the peripheral nerve blocks mentioned in this chapter are also great options when neuraxial anesthesia is contraindicated due to anticoagulation. Peripheral nerve stimulation is a newer modality that holds promise in reduction of the incidence of phantom limb pain and may improve disability in patients with chronic neuropathic post-amputation pain.[35]

CONCLUSION

The perioperative management of critical limb ischemia, lower limb amputation, and phantom limb pain may be challenging, but with current multimodal pharmacologic agents and regional anesthetic techniques, patients experience improved pain relief both in the acute and chronic setting. Providing adequate analgesia by applying a multimodal approach in the perioperative setting is extremely important and beneficial for patients' short- and long-term pain outcomes. Multimodal analgesia, which combines analgesic drugs from different classes and employs analgesic techniques that target different mechanisms of pain, is recommended in the perioperative setting of critical limb ischemia and postoperative phantom limb pain. Regional anesthesia, along with multimodal pharmacologic agents, is an effective approach to managing postoperative amputation pain and phantom limb pain.

REFERENCES

1. Laoire ÁN, Murtagh FEM. Systematic review of pharmacological therapies for the management of ischaemic pain in patients with non-reconstructable critical limb ischaemia. *BMJ Support Palliat Care.* 2018;8:400–410.

2. Norgren L, Hiatt WR, Dormandy JA, et al. Inter-Society Consensus for the management of peripheral arterial disease (TASC II). *J Vasc Surg*. 2007;45 Suppl S:S5–S67.
3. Morris-Stiff G, Lewis MH. Gabapentin (Neurontin®) improves pain scores of patients with critical limb ischaemia: an observational study. *Int J Surg*. 2010;8(3):212–215.
4. Woelk CJ. Management of critical limb ischemia. *Can Fam Physician*. 2012;58(9):960–963.
5. Kent ML, Hsia H-LJ, Van de Ven TJ, Buchheit TE. Perioperative pain management strategies for amputation: a topical review. *Pain Med*. 2017 Mar;18(3):504–519.
6. Schwenk ES, Viscusi ER, et al. Consensus guidelines on the use of intravenous ketamine infusions for acute pain management from the American Society of Regional Anesthesia and Pain Medicine, the American Academy of Pain Medicine, and the American Society of Anesthesiologists. *Reg Anesth Pain Med*. 2018 Jul;43(5):456–466.
7. Froelich MA, McKeown JL, Worrell MJ, et al. Intravenous lidocaine reduces ischemic pain in healthy volunteers. *Reg Anesth Pain Med*. 2010;35:249–254.
8. Vahidi E, Shakoor D, Aghaie Meybodi M, Saeedi M. Comparison of intravenous lidocaine versus morphine in alleviating pain in patients with critical limb ischaemia. *Emerg Med J*. 2015 Jul;32(7):516–519. doi: 10.1136/emermed-2014-203944. Epub 2014 Aug 21. PMID: 25147364.
9. De Jong R, Shysh AJ. Development of a multimodal analgesia protocol for perioperative acute pain management for lower limb amputation. *Pain Res Manag*. 2018 Jun 3;2018:5237040.
10. Tantry TP, Kadam D, Shetty P, Bhandary S. Combined femoral and sciatic nerve blocks for lower limb anaesthesia in anticoagulated patients with severe cardiac valvular lesions. *Indian J Anaesth*. 2010;54:235–238.
11. Mansour A. Femoral nerve block versus spinal anesthesia for lower limb peripheral vascular surgery. *AJAIC*. 2006;9:1.
12. Malik S, Krishna D, Malik S. Combined psoas compartment and sciatic nerve block for lower limb surgery: an alternative anesthetic option in high-risk geriatric patients. *Karnataka Anaesth J*. 2015;1:85–88.
13. Tomaszewski KA, Graves MJ, Henry BM, et al. Surgical anatomy of the sciatic nerve: a meta-analysis. *J Orthop Res*. 2016;34:1820–1827.
14. Sala-Blanch X, Reina MA, Ribalta T, Prats-Galino A. Sciatic nerve structure and nomenclature: epineurium to paraneurium: is this a new paradigm? *Reg Anesth Pain Med*. 2013;38:463–465.
15. Karmakar MK, Shariat AN, Pangthipampai P, et al. High-definition ultrasound imaging defines the paraneural sheath and the fascial compartments surrounding the sciatic nerve at the popliteal fossa. *Reg Anesth Pain Med*. 2013;38:447–451.
16. Perlas A, Wong P, Abdallah F, et al. Ultrasound-guided popliteal block through a common paraneural sheath versus conventional injection: a prospective, randomized, double-blind study. *Reg Anesth Pain Med*. 2013;38:218–225.
17. Choquet O, Brault Noble G, Abbal B, et al. Subparaneural versus circumferential extraneural injection at the bifurcation level in ultrasound-guided popliteal sciatic nerve blocks: a prospective, randomized, double-blind study. *Reg Anesth Pain Med*. 2014;39:306–311.
18. Sahin L, Sahin M, Isikay N. A different approach to an ultrasound-guided saphenous nerve block. *Acta Anaesthesiol Scand*. 2011;55:1030–1031.
19. Bendtsen TF, Moriggl B, Chan V, Børglum J. Basic topography of the saphenous nerve in the femoral triangle and the adductor canal. *Reg Anesth Pain Med*. 2015;40(4):391–392.
20. Pisansky AJB, Brovman EY, Kuo C, Kaye AD, Urman RD. Perioperative outcomes after regional versus general anesthesia for above the knee amputations. *Ann Vasc Surg*. 2018;48:53–66.
21. Mannion S, O'Callaghan S, Walsh M, et al. In with the new, out with the old? Comparison of two approaches for psoas compartment block. *Anesth Analg*. 2005;101:259–264.
22. Sauter AR, Ullensvang K, Niemi G, et al. The Shamrock lumbar plexus block: a dose-finding study. *Eur J Anaesthesiol*. 2015;31:764–770.
23. Franco CD, Choksi N, Rahm an A, Voronov G, Almachnouk M. A subgluteal approach to the sciatic nerve in adults at 10 cm from the midline. *Reg Anesth Pain Med*. 2006; 31:215–220.
24. Di Benedetto P, Bertini L, Casati A, et al. A new approach to the sciatic nerve block: a prospective, randomized comparison with the classic posterior approach. *Anesth Analg*. 2001;93:1040–1044.
25. Hanley MA, Ehde DM, Campbell KM, Osborn B, Smith DG. Self-reported treatments used for lower-limb phantom pain: descriptive findings. *Arch Phys Med Rehab*. 2006;87(2):270–277.
26. Smith HS. Potential analgesic mechanisms of acetaminophen. *Pain Physician*. 2009;12(1):269–280.
27. Hallivis R, Derksen TA, Meyr AJ. Peri-operative pain management. *Clin Podiatr Med Surg*. 2008;25(3):443–463.
28. Bone M, Critchley P, Buggy DJ. Gabapentin in postamputation phantom limb pain: a randomized, double-blind, placebo-controlled, cross-over study. *Reg Anesth Pain Med*. 2002;27(5):481–486.
29. Von Plato H, Kontinen V, Hamunen K. Efficacy and safety of epidural, continuous perineural infusion and adjuvant analgesics for acute postoperative pain after major limb amputation: a systematic review. *Scand J Pain*. 2018;18(1):3–17.
30. Woolf CJ, Mannion RJ. Neuropathic pain: aetiology, symptoms, mechanisms, and management. *Lancet*. 1999;353:1959–1964.
31. Flor H. Phantom-limb pain: characteristics, causes, and treatment. *Lancet Neurol*. 2002;1:182–189.
32. Nikolajsen L, Ilkjaer S, Jensen TS. Relationship between mechanical sensitivity and postamputation pain: a prospective study. *Eur J Pain*. 2000;4:327–334.
33. Flor H, Elbert T, Knecht S, et al. Phantom-limb pain as a perceptual correlate of cortical reorganization following arm amputation. *Nature*. 1995;375:482–484.
34. Birbaumer N, Lutzenberger W, Montoya P, et al. Effects of regional anesthesia on phantom limb pain are mirrored in changes in cortical reorganization. *J Neurosci*. 1997;17:5503–5508.
35. Gilmore C, Ilfeld B, Rosenow J, et al. Percutaneous peripheral nerve stimulation for the treatment of chronic neuropathic postamputation pain: a multicenter, randomized, placebo-controlled trial. *Reg Anesth Pain Med*. 2019 Jun;44(6):637–645.

REVIEW QUESTIONS

(1) Which of the pharmacologic adjuncts can be used for managing ischemic pain?

A. Gabapentinoids
B. NMDA antagonists
C. Intravenous Local anesthetics
D. All of the above

(2) Which of the following is true regarding the anatomic location of the sciatic nerve at the level of the popliteal fossa?

A. The sciatic nerve is bordered superomedially to the biceps femoris muscle.
B. The sciatic nerve is bordered inferomedially by both the semimembranosus and semitendinosus muscles.
C. The sciatic nerve is bordered inferiorly by the lateral and medial heads of the gastrocnemius.
D. The tibial nerve and common peroneal nerve components of the sciatic nerve are encased in separate epineurial sheaths.

(3) A sciatic nerve block utilizing the sub-paraneural technique is associated with a more predictable block, faster onset, and longer duration than when the tibial nerve and the

common peroneal nerve are blocked with conventional separate circumferential spread.

A. True
B. False

(4) Which of the following is NOT true regarding the anatomic location of the adductor canal when performing an ultrasound-guided saphenous block?

A. The adductor canals is bordered laterally by the vastus lateralis.
B. The adductor canals is bordered laterally by the vastus medialis.
C. The adductor canals is bordered superiorly by the sartorius muscle.
D. The adductor canals is bordered medially by the adductor longus or magnus.

(5) Which is true regarding the saphenous nerve?

A. It provides both sensory and motor innervation to the medial aspect of the lower leg.
B. It is a purely sensory nerve.
C. It is a purely motor nerve.
D. High concentrations of local anesthetic are required for an adequate surgical block.

(6) Which of the following is NOT true regarding lumbar plexus blockade?

A. The entire lumbar plexus can be blocked via a posterior approach (also known as the psoas compartment block).
B. It is important to contact the L4 transverse process before entering into the lumbar plexus.
C. There are minimal complications associated with lumbar plexus blocks.
D. The obturator, femoral, and lateral femoral cutaneous nerves make up the lumbar plexus.

(7) You are attempting to perform a lumbar plexus block using nerve stimulation when you begin to get stimulation of the hamstring muscles. What needle adjustment is needed for adequate blockade?

A. Adjust needle more caudal and medial.
B. Adjust needle more cephalad and medial.
C. Adjust needle more caudal and lateral.
D. Adjust needle more cephalad and lateral.

(8) Which of the following nerves are blocked in addition to the sciatic nerve during the Labat's posterior approach to sciatic nerve blockade?

A. Posterior femoral cutaneous nerve
B. Pudendal nerve
C. Cuneal nerve
D. Lateral femoral cutaneous nerve

(9) Which of the following is not used as a landmark for performing Labat's posterior approach to sciatic nerve blockade?

A. Greater trochanter
B. Sacral hiatus
C. Posterior superior iliac spine (PSIS)
D. Anterior superior iliac spine (ASIS)

(10) Which of the following are risk factors for development of severe acute and/or persistent pain?

A. History of anxiety and/or depression
B. Preoperative opioid use and/or opioid tolerance
C. Significant preoperative pain
D. Complicated surgical intervention (infection, prolonged closure)
E. All of the above

(11) Which of the following is NOT true regarding phantom limb pain?

A. Phantom limb pain tends to be episodic in nature.
B. Occurs in <25% of amputees
C. Bilateral amputation is a risk factor for development of phantom limb pain.
D. Most patients who develop phantom limb pain do so within the first week after amputation.

ANSWERS

(1) **D.** Gabapentin has been shown to reduce pain scores, improve sleep, and in some, reduced opioid requirements. NMDA antagonists may help reduce transition from acute to chronic pain. Intravenous lidocaine can produce a sustained analgesic state for ischemic pain.

References

Morris-Stiff G, Lewis MH. Gabapentin (Neurontin®) improves pain scores of patients with critical limb ischaemia: an observational study. *Int J Surg*. 2010;8(3):212–215.
De Jong R, Shysh AJ. Development of a multimodal analgesia protocol for perioperative acute pain management for lower limb amputation. *Pain Res Manag*. 2018 Jun 3;2018:5237040.

(2) **C.** The biceps femoris muscle is superolateral, while the semimembranosus and semitendinosus muscles are superomedial, and the lateral and medial heads of the gastrocnemius are inferior to the sciatic nerve the popliteal fossa. The two branches of the sciatic nerve at the popliteal fossa are encased in one paraneural sheath that allows the spread of injectate to the two nerves.

References

Karmakar MK, Shariat AN, Pangthipampai P, et al. High-definition ultrasound imaging defines the paraneural sheath and the fascial compartments surrounding the sciatic nerve at the popliteal fossa. *Reg Anesth Pain Med*. 2013;38:447–451.
Perlas A, Wong P, Abdallah F, et al. Ultrasound-guided popliteal block through a common paraneural sheath versus conventional injection: a prospective, randomized, double-blind study. *Reg Anesth Pain Med*. 2013;38:218–225.

(3) **A.** The sub-paraneural technique is associated with a more predictable, faster onset, and longer duration block than when the tibial nerve and the common peroneal nerve are blocked separately.

Reference

Perlas A, Wong P, Abdallah F, et al. Ultrasound-guided popliteal block through a common paraneural sheath versus conventional injection: a prospective, randomized, double-blind study. *Reg Anesth Pain Med.* 2013;38:218–225.

(4) **A.** The adductor canal is bordered superiorly by the sartorius muscle, laterally by the vastus medialis, and medially by the adductor longus or magnus depending on the ultrasound probe location.

Reference

Sahin L, Sahin M, Isikay N. A different approach to an ultrasound-guided saphenous nerve block. *Acta Anaesthesiol Scand.* 2011;55:1030–1031.

(5) **B.** The saphenous nerve is a purely sensory nerve, and high concentrations of local anesthetic are not required for an adequate nerve block.

Reference

Sahin L, Sahin M, Isikay N. A different approach to an ultrasound-guided saphenous nerve block. *Acta Anaesthesiol Scand.* 2011;55:1030–1031.

(6) **C.** The lumbar plexus block has the potential for serious complications, including retroperitoneal bleeding, high neuraxial anesthesia, hypotension, local anesthetic toxicity, and spinal anesthesia.

Reference

Mannion S, O'Callaghan S, Walsh M, et al. In with the new, out with the old? Comparison of two approaches for psoas compartment block. *Anesth Analg.* 2005;101:259–264.

(7) **D.** Hamstring stimulation suggests sacral plexus stimulation (sciatic nerve) and indicates that the needle tip is too caudal and medial.

Reference

loka J, Tsai T, Hadzic A. Lumbar plexus block. In: AHadzic, ed. *New York School of Regional Anesthesia. Hadzic's Textbook of Regional Anesthesia and Acute Pain Management.* Second ed. New York: McGraw-Hill Education; 2017:1380–1387.

(8) **A.** The Labat's posterior approach to the sciatic nerve also blocks the posterior femoral cutaneous nerve which provides sensory innervation to the gluteus and uppermost medial and posterior thigh, which can be advantageous when thigh tourniquets are used for lower extremity procedures.

Reference

Madison SJ, Ilfeld BM. Peripheral nerve blocks. In: JF Butterworth, DC Mackey, JD Wasnick JD. *Morgan & Mikhail's Clinical Anesthesiology 6e.* 6th ed. New York, NY: McGraw-Hill Education LLC; 2018.

(9) **D.** When using landmarks to perform Labat's posterior approach to sciatic nerve blockade, a line is drawn from the greater trochanter to the PSIS, a second line is drawn from the greater trochanter to the sacral hiatus, and a third line is drawn perpendicular to the midpoint of the first line to its intersection with the second line. The ASIS is not a relevant landmark.

Reference

Madison SJ, Ilfeld BM. Peripheral nerve blocks. In: JF Butterworth, DC Mackey, JD Wasnick, eds. *Morgan & Mikhail's Clinical Anesthesiology 6e.* 6th ed. New York, NY: McGraw-Hill Education LLC; 2018.

(10) **E.** The risk factors for development of post-amputation pain are significant preoperative pain, preoperative opioid use and/or opioid tolerance, anxiety and/or depression, catastrophizing, and complicated surgeries (infection, prolonged closure).

Reference

Dijkstra PU, Geertzen JH, Stewart R, van der Schans CP. Phantom pain and risk factors: a multivariate analysis. *J Pain Symptom Manage.* 2002 Dec;24(6):578–585.

(11) **B.** Phantom limb pain occurs in up to 80% of amputees, and 75% of patients who develop phantom limb pain will do so within the first week after amputation.

Reference

Hanley MA, Ehde DM, Campbell KM, Osborn B, Smith DG. Self-reported treatments used for lower-limb phantom pain: descriptive findings. *Arch Phys Med Rehab.* 2006;87(2):270–277.

31.

REGIONAL ANESTHESIA FOR OPEN REDUCTION AND INTERNAL FIXATION OF AN ANKLE FRACTURE

Maryam Nilforoshan, Stephanie Huang, and Nabil Elkassabany

STEM CASE AND KEY QUESTIONS

A 24-year-old presents to the emergency room immediately after a fall while playing soccer. He complains of severe pain and inability to bear weight on his left ankle. Examinations reveals significant swelling, deformity of his ankle, and tenderness to palpation along the lateral and medial malleoli. Orthopedic surgery is consulted for further evaluation.

What other information should be obtained in the history and physical examination?

Gathering history on the mechanism and timing of injury will provide information on the nature of the injury (e.g., soft tissue or ligament damage, complex fracture, preexisting neuropathy). During the examination, identify evidence of open injury, dislocation, or neurovascular compromise. Palpation along the malleoli and bones of the foot for tenderness will help identify bony injuries. Examination of this patient by the orthopedic surgeon suggests a closed dislocated bimalleolar fracture. Posterior tibial and dorsalis pedis pulses are strong and palpable; swelling is evident, but capillary refill is normal. There are no gross sensorimotor deficits. The patient's pain is controlled with oral analgesics.

(1) WHAT ARE THE NEXT STEPS IN DIAGNOSIS?

The patient undergoes an ankle x-ray series to further evaluate his injury, which confirms a dislocated bimalleolar fracture. X-ray imaging is the primary mode of radiographic evaluation in patients with traumatic ankle injuries. If the patient had tenderness along the proximal leg, full length tibia/fibula films should be obtained. Computed tomography (CT) and magnetic resonance imaging (MRI) are not routinely indicated for acute assessment of ankle fractures, but they can be used in more complex cases to better assess the various bones of the ankle joint, the soft tissue structures, and the cartilaginous and ligamentous structures.

(2) WHAT ARE THE INITIAL STEPS FOR TREATMENT? IS SURGERY INDICATED?

Due to the dislocation, the patient undergoes manual axial traction and splinting in the emergency room. Decision is made to undergo open reduction and internal fixation (ORIF) surgery when the swelling has reduced. Indications for surgery include open fractures, unstable (bimalleolar, bimalleolar-equivalent, or trimalleolar) fractures, significantly displaced fractures, and patients with neurovascular compromise.

(3) WHAT ARE THE ANESTHETIC OPTIONS FOR SURGERY?

Patient undergoes surgery a week after the initial injury. He is offered sciatic and saphenous peripheral nerve blocks as either a primary anesthetic or for postoperative analgesia to supplement spinal or general anesthesia.

As previously discussed, popliteal sciatic block must sometimes be supplemented with a saphenous nerve block, depending on the surgical site. Questions have been raised regarding the necessity of saphenous nerve block supplementation for ankle surgery, particularly ankle surgery without a medial incision. Anatomical studies examining the role of the saphenous nerve have demonstrated that the saphenous nerve innervates the periosteum of the distal tibia and the talocrural joint capsule. These results suggest that saphenous nerve blocks are necessary for effective analgesia following ankle surgery—even surgery without a medial skin incision.[10]

(4) WHAT NERVE BLOCK IS DONE FOR ANKLE SURGERY?

Sciatic block must sometimes be supplemented with a saphenous nerve block.

(5) WHAT IS THE SAPHENOUS NERVE SUPPLY OF THE ANKLE AREA?

The saphenous nerve innervates the periosteum of the distal tibia and the talocrural joint capsule.

(6) WHERE DOES THE SCIATIC NERVE BIFURCATE?

Although the nerve divides at a mean distance of 60 mm above the popliteal crease, studies have demonstrated that this division can occur at a wide range of 0–115 mm above the popliteal crease.

(7) WHAT IS THE LANDMARK OF THE SCIATICA POPLITEAL NERVE?

The tibial nerve should be visualized as a hyperechoic structure superficial and lateral to artery, with the common peroneal nerve superficial and lateral to the tibial nerve. The artery and nerves are framed laterally by the biceps femoris muscle and medially by the semimembranosus and semitendinosus muscles.

(8) HOW EFFECTIVE IS EPIDURAL ANESTHESIA/ANALGESIA IN ANKLE SURGERY?

Beyond these side effects and complications, epidural anesthesia is also an unreliable technique for foot and ankle surgery, as the L5–S1 segments have demonstrated resistance to epidural blockade and frequently remain unblocked.

(9) WHAT IS THE INNERVATION OF ILIAC CREST?

The periosteum of the iliac crest is innervated by the subcostal, ilioinguinal, and iliohypogastric, and lateral femoral cutaneous nerves.

(10) WHAT IS THE MOST COMMON SITE FOR COMPARTMENT SYNDROME?

The tibial shaft is the most common site for compartment syndrome in orthopedic procedures.

DISCUSSION

Ankle injuries commonly occur, leading to greater than 5 million emergency department (ED) visits per year;[1] 15% of these ankle injuries are ankle fractures, with ankle sprains contributing to the remaining 85% of ankle injuries.[1] Ankle fractures account for 9% of all fractures, with the ankle fracture being the most common intra-articular fracture of a weight-bearing joint.[1] Overall, ankle fractures have an incidence of up to 187 cases per 100,000 person-years.[2] Regression models have indicated that, if current trends continue, there will be a rapid rise in the incidence of ankle fractures, particularly low-trauma ankle fractures in the elderly population.[3]

EPIDEMIOLOGY

The incidence of ankle fractures is slightly higher in men (210 per 100,000 person-years) as compared to women (172 per 100,000 person-years).[2] The average age of patients in the adult ankle fracture population is 45 years old, but there is a bimodal distribution; the highest age-specific incidence in men is seen between the ages of 15 and 24, while the highest age-specific incidence in women occurs between 75 and 84 years of age.[4]

Fractures due to severe trauma and sports-related injuries are seen more frequently in men than women. Meanwhile, fractures due to moderate trauma are seen more frequently in older women.[2] Overall, falls are the most common cause of ankle fracture, accounting for 37.5% of ankle fractures. This is followed by inversion injuries (31.5%) and sports-related injuries (10.2%).[5] Of the sports-related ankle fractures, soccer injuries are the leading cause (75%), followed by rugby injuries (11%).[4]

ANKLE JOINT ANATOMY

The ankle, or talocrural joint, is a hinge joint that plays a crucial role in facilitating upright posture and ambulation. Its bony components include the junction of the distal portions of the tibia and fibula and the trochlea of the talus. The posterior aspect of the distal tibial articular surface, the tibial plafond, is referred to as the posterior malleolus; the medial distal tibia and the distal fibula are referred to as the medial malleolus and lateral malleolus, respectively.[6] Associated ligaments contribute to the maintenance of ankle joint stability against stress. These ligaments include the lateral ligament complex and the deltoid ligament.[6]

Ankle joint anatomy has important biomechanical implications. Among the body's weight-bearing joints, the ankle joint has the smallest surface area.[6] At the same time, ambulation exposes the ankle to forces ranging from 1.25 to 5.5 times normal body weight.[7] This small surface area, combined with large stresses, leads to the talar dome supporting more weight per unit area than any other surface and leaves the ankle particularly vulnerable to injury and degenerative changes.[6,7]

ANKLE AND FOOT INNERVATION

There are a number of nerves that cross the ankle, providing innervation of the ankle and foot (Figure 31.1). The medial aspect of the ankle and foot is innervated by the saphenous nerve, a terminal branch of the femoral nerve. The remainder of the ankle and foot is innervated by branches of the sciatic nerve. The sural nerve supplies the lateral lower ankle, lateral heel, and lateral border of the foot. The medial heel is supplied by the medial calcaneal nerve. The medial and lateral plantar nerves innervate the sole of the foot. The superficial peroneal nerve provides sensation for the majority of the dorsum of the ankle and foot. The deep peroneal nerve innervates the dorsal web space between the great and second toes.[7] A thorough understanding of the ankle joint's sensory innervation is important for identifying the neuronal components that must be anesthetized to achieve surgical anesthesia and postoperative analgesia.

CLINICAL PRESENTATION AND PHYSICAL EVALUATION

Patients with ankle fracture will classically present with a history of trauma to the ankle, followed by painful swelling, possible gross deformity in the ankle region, as well as inability to bear weight on the affected ankle. In evaluating the patient, it is vital to obtain a complete history. Gathering history regarding the mechanism of injury provides important information

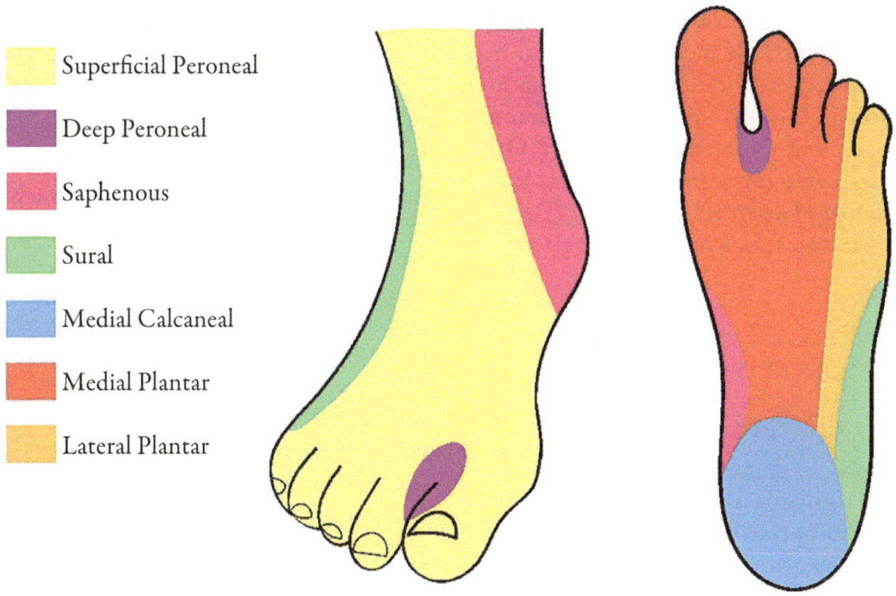

Figure 31.1. Ankle and foot innervation.

regarding the anticipated nature of the injury; for example, fractures produced by large forces such as falling from a height are likely to be associated with soft tissue damage and complex fracture patterns.[7] Additional elements of the history, such as a patient who is unsure as to how they were injured or a patient who walked on the injured limb for several days before presenting, are suggestive of underlying pathology such as diabetic neuropathy.[7]

During the initial examination, it is crucial to identify any evidence of open injury, dislocation, or neurovascular compromise, as each of these would be an indication for immediate orthopedic consultation and treatment. Inspection that reveals grossly visible deformity or malposition of the joint is suggestive of a dislocated fracture; ankle fractures associated with dislocation must be emergently reduced with manual axial traction.[8] Prompt anatomic alignment is crucial for minimizing the risk of future arthritic sequelae.[7] A vascular examination may consist of palpation of posterior tibial and dorsalis pedis pulses, inspection for pallor suggestive of ischemia, and measurement of capillary refill in order to ensure sufficient perfusion.[7] Neurologic exam can be performed by gross sensorimotor examination of the foot.[7,8]

Although certain findings such as swelling, hematoma formation, and tenderness to palpation over the medial and lateral malleolus are indicators of possible ankle fractures, some nondisplaced fractures may have only minimal swelling and no obvious deformity. In addition to palpation along the medial malleolus and lateral malleolus, one should palpate the talus, calcaneus, navicular bone, mid-tarsal joint, and base of the fifth metatarsal bone for tenderness suggestive of further associated bony injuries.

RADIOGRAPHIC EVALUATION

Radiographic evaluation in patients with traumatic ankle pain often necessitates an x-ray series. The Ottawa ankle rules should be applied in order to provide guidance regarding which patients require an ankle imaging series. Per these guidelines, an ankle x-ray series is only required if pain in the malleolar zone is accompanied by one of the following: bone tenderness at the posterior edge or tip of the lateral malleolus, bone tenderness at the posterior edge or tip of the medial malleolus, or inability to bear weight both immediately and in the ED. Studies have shown that this rule is 100% sensitive and 40.1% specific for detecting malleolar fractures; application of this rule demonstrated a reduction of 36% of ankle x-ray series ordered.[9]

Computer tomography (CT) can provide further information, as it depicts a cross-section of the ankle joint that clearly demonstrates the relationship between the tibia and fibula, and the state of soft tissue structures of the ankle. Magnetic resonance imaging (MRI) can be a useful tool for the assessment of cartilaginous or ligamentous injuries.[7]

ANKLE FRACTURE CLASSIFICATION

There are several classification systems used to describe ankle fractures. While some of these are purely descriptive, others correlate pathophysiologic findings with particular injury patterns and patient positioning. These classification systems are useful for a better understanding of fracture anatomy and possibly deciding on the most appropriate course of treatment.

Percival Pott's Classification System

The first classification system was developed by Percival Pott. He described the injury by the number of malleoli involved, terming ankle injuries either *unimalleolar*, *bimalleolar*, or *trimalleolar* ankle fractures.[6] Unimalleolar fractures are the most common (approximately 70%) and entail either an isolated medial malleolar or isolated lateral malleolar fracture. Bimalleolar fractures, also called

Pott's fractures, are the second most common (11%–19%) and involve a fracture of both the medial and lateral malleoli. Trimalleolar fractures, also called Cotton fractures, are the least common (7%–12%) and involve a fracture of the medial, lateral, and posterior malleoli.[2,4] Other classifications for ankle fractures include: Danis-Weber Classification and Lauge-Hansen Classification. Detailed description of these classifications is beyond the scope of this chapter.

TREATMENT

The primary goals of ankle fracture management are to establish anatomical alignment and ankle stability.[6] Whenever a fracture is suspected, the ankle joint must be stabilized with a splint until fracture is ruled out.[8] Once an ankle fracture is confirmed, the clinician must pursue either conservative treatment or surgical management, depending on ankle joint stability and the congruency of the tibiotalar joint. This is assessed by evaluation of joint tenderness and the displacement of the tibiotalar joint visualized on x-ray.[6] Stress view x-rays to evaluate joint stability may be necessary if the evidence of displacement is equivocal or difficult to assess.

CONSERVATIVE (NON-OPERATIVE) TREATMENT

Stable fractures with non-displaced or minimally displaced fragments can be managed conservatively, by being splinted in a leg splint or boot with the ankle positioned at 90 degrees for at least 6 weeks, with weight bearing as tolerated.[7,8]

OPERATIVE TREATMENT

Unstable fractures should be managed surgically. Indications for surgery include open fractures, unstable (bimalleolar or bimalleolar-equivalent and trimalleolar) fractures, fractures with significant displacement, and fractures in patients with neurovascular compromise.[6] Surgery is also indicated for posterior malleolus fractures involving greater than 25% of the articular surface.[6]

Surgical intervention timing is also of importance. If surgery is performed in the setting of soft tissues swelling, excessive tension may be required to close the wound, leading to an increased risk of wound infection and wound-edge necrosis. As a result, surgery is typically delayed until soft tissue swelling has resolved.[8] Surgical management usually entails open reduction and internal fixation (ORIF) using plates and screws. Complex fractures, certain open fractures, and high-energy fractures (e.g., pilon fractures) sometimes require alternative techniques, such as the use of external fixators.[6,9] Surgery is usually performed with the patient supine under either general or regional anesthesia. Postoperatively, the patients remain non-weight-bearing for at least s6 weeks.

REGIONAL ANESTHESIA FOR ANKLE SURGERY

Ankle surgery typically results in severe, prolonged postoperative pain.[10] Patients after ankle surgery tend to require large doses of systemic opioids[11] which may result in development of opioid-related side effects such as nausea and vomiting.[12] Uncontrolled pain in the postoperative period impairs mobilization, has an adverse impact on patient satisfaction, and has been shown to be a strong risk factor in developing chronic pain after surgery.[10,12,13] Furthermore, pain management impacts postoperative stay and hospital readmission and is associated with significant increase in healthcare costs.[13] Regional anesthesia techniques have demonstrated significant value in improving pain control in the postoperative period following ankle surgery. There is ample evidence that popliteal sciatic block combined with a saphenous nerve block provides both excellent anesthesia and postoperative analgesia for patients undergoing foot and ankles surgeries.[13,14]

REGIONAL ANESTHESIA FOR POSTOPERATIVE ANALGESIA

Placement of a single-injection popliteal sciatic block and saphenous nerve block prior to foot and ankle surgery has been shown to minimize postoperative pain for up to 24 hours.[15] Studies have shown that patients receiving a popliteal sciatic block following major foot and ankle operations reported 95% satisfaction; 96% of patients who had had prior foot or ankle surgery reported that the popliteal block provided superior pain control compared to their prior analgesic regimen.[13] Peripheral nerve catheters can further extend the analgesic benefit of these nerve blocks. Continuous nerve blocks have been shown to result in decreased pain and opioid use postoperatively, improved patient satisfaction scores, earlier patient discharge, and decreased hospitalization costs.[15]

REGIONAL ANESTHESIA AS A PRIMARY ANESTHETIC TECHNIQUE

Regional techniques can also be successfully used as a primary anesthetic technique. Hansen et al. used a popliteal fossa sciatic nerve block combined with a saphenous nerve block as the sole anesthetic for 48 patients undergoing foot and ankle surgeries including ORIF, ankle ligament repair, ankle arthroscopy, hardware removal, and Achilles tendon repair. This block method was successful in 95% of patients, with 5% requiring a supplemental saphenous nerve block at the ankle, and no patients requiring conversion to general anesthesia.[14] Regional anesthesia as a sole anesthetic for ankle surgery allows one to avoid the risks and systemic complications associated with general anesthesia, making regional anesthesia an appealing alternative for patients with multiple comorbidities.

POPLITEAL SCIATIC BLOCK

The sciatic nerve is responsible for much of the motor and sensory innervation of the lower extremity. Regional anesthetic blockade of the sciatic nerve can be performed at numerous locations, including the sacral plexus, transgluteal approach, subgluteal approach, and popliteal approach. Compared to more proximal sciatic nerve block approaches, the popliteal sciatic block offers the advantage of sparing hamstring motor function.[16] Popliteal sciatic block anesthetizes the lower extremity distal to the knee with the exception of the medial leg, which derives its cutaneous innervation from the saphenous nerve.[16,17] Therefore, a popliteal block sometimes requires supplementation with a saphenous nerve block depending on the surgical site.

Indications

The popliteal sciatic nerve block can be utilized to provide analgesia and/or anesthesia of the lower extremities, particularly in patients presenting with foot and ankle pathology. More specifically, it can be used in the setting of foot and ankle fractures, corrective foot surgery, Achilles tendon repair, dislocation reduction, exploration for foreign bodies, bedside incision and drainage procedures, and wound debridements.[18] Depending on the volume and concentration of the local anesthetic used to perform the blockade, the block can provide postoperative analgesia or it can be used as a primary regional anesthetic for surgical procedures, which may be beneficial in patients with significant comorbidities.

Sciatic Nerve Anatomy

The lower extremities are innervated by nerves that originate from the lumbosacral plexus which is formed by the ventral rami of L1 to S5; it gives rise to many branches, including the sciatic and femoral nerves.[19] The sciatic nerve leaves the pelvis through the greater sciatic foramen and travels down the gluteal region and posterior compartment of the thigh until it reaches the posterior compartment of the knee. It gives away muscular branches to innervate the hamstring muscles.[19]

In the popliteal fossa, the sciatic nerve runs lateral and superficial to the popliteal artery and vein. Near the apex of the popliteal fossa, the sciatic nerve separates into its tibial and common peroneal nerve trunks, which are encapsulated by a common paraneural sheath. This division of the sciatic nerve occurs at a variable distance from the popliteal crease. Although the nerve divides at a mean distance of 60 mm above the popliteal crease, studies have demonstrated that this division occurred at a wide range of 0–115 mm above the popliteal crease. This has important implications for the popliteal block, suggesting that needle placement 100 mm above the popliteal crease (rather than 50–70 mm above the popliteal crease as classically taught) will increase the likelihood of needle placement proximal to the division of the sciatic nerve.[20]

The tibial nerve descends into the posterior compartment of the leg. It travels posterior to the medial malleolus and divides into its terminal cutaneous branches—medial and lateral plantar nerves that supply sensation to the sole of the foot. Collateral branches of the tibial nerve give rise to the cutaneous sural nerve (which provides sensation to the lateral aspect of the calf and foot) and the cutaneous calcaneal nerves (which provide sensation to the heel). The tibial nerve's muscular branches innervate the calf muscles responsible for plantar flexion of the ankle, as well as the muscles responsible for adduction, abduction, and flexion of the toes.[19]

The common peroneal nerve descends laterally along the fibula. It divides into its terminal branches, the superficial and deep peroneal nerves. The superficial peroneal nerve has muscular branches that are responsible for eversion of the ankle, while its cutaneous branches supply sensation along the dorsal aspect of the ankle and foot. The deep peroneal nerve has muscular branches that are responsible for dorsiflexion of the ankle, inversion of the ankle, and extension of the toes. Its cutaneous branches supply sensation to the dorsum of the foot between the first and second toes.[19]

Ultrasound Anatomy and Technique

The popliteal sciatic block is performed by depositing local anesthetic within the sciatic nerve sheath (Vloka's sheath), which contains both the tibial and common peroneal nerves. Ultrasound allows for visualization of sufficient local anesthetic spread within Vloka's sheath; as a result, ultrasound techniques can usually achieve successful blocks with smaller volumes of local anesthetic than nerve stimulator techniques. The particular type and concentration of local anesthetic should be selected based on whether the block is intended for primary regional anesthesia or postoperative analgesia.[16]

First, the ultrasound transducer is placed along the popliteal crease, and the popliteal artery is found. The tibial nerve should be visualized as a hyperechoic structure superficial and lateral to artery, with the common peroneal nerve superficial and lateral to the tibial nerve (Figure 31.2). The artery and nerves should be framed laterally by the biceps femoris muscle and medially by the semimembranosus and semitendinosus muscles. Next, one should scan proximally to identify the point where the tibial and common peroneal nerves converge to form the sciatic nerve. The needle tip should be localized within Vloka's sheath, between the tibial and common peroneal nerves. If local anesthetic injection results in the separation of the two nerves and results in proximal spread of local anesthetic within the sheath, this confirms successful block performance.[16]

There are several approaches to the popliteal sciatic block, including the posterior approach and the lateral approach. Catheter placement is feasible in both approaches. For the posterior (intertendinous) approach, described by Duane Keith Rorie, the patient is positioned prone. For an ultrasound-guided block, the needle can be inserted in-plane (from lateral to medial) or out of plane.[16] For the lateral (popliteal) approach, described by Jerry Vloka, the patient is positioned supine.[17] Supine positioning is an advantage of the lateral approach, particularly in the case of obese, pregnant, and trauma patients who cannot conveniently be positioned prone. However, although the lateral approach is equally

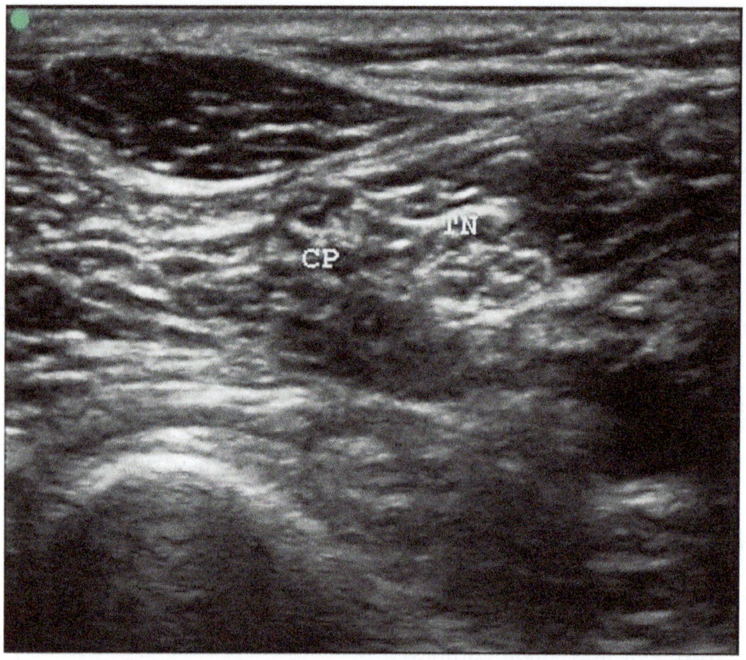

Figure 31.2. Ultrasound image of the tibial nerve (TN) and common peroneal nerve (CP) encapsulated in Vloka's sheath within the popliteal fossa.

effective, its primary disadvantage is the fact that it often takes longer to perform and necessitates more attempts as compared to the posterior approach.[12] For an ultrasound-guided block, the needle is inserted in plane on the lateral aspect of the thigh, 2–3 cm above the lateral edge of the transducer.[16]

CONTINUOUS POPLITEAL BLOCK

Single-injection nerve blocks are limited in their ability to offer sufficient analgesia beyond 24 hours. Continuous popliteal sciatic nerve blocks offer better postoperative analgesia compared to intramuscular (IM) opioids and intravenous patient-controlled analgesia (IV PCA).[11] More specifically, in patients undergoing ORIF of the ankle, continuous popliteal sciatic nerve block with an infusion of ropivacaine 0.2% at 10 mL/hr for 48 hours showed an impressive 29% and 62% decrease in morphine use during postoperative days 1 and 2, respectively.[21]

The continuous popliteal sciatic block requires that a peripheral nerve catheter be positioned in Vloka's sheath. First, correct needle placement is verified by injection of a small amount of local anesthetic. Then, the peripheral nerve catheter is inserted 2–4 cm beyond the needle tip.[16] It has been demonstrated that directing the needle slightly cephalad aids in catheter insertion.[17] When placing a catheter, the lateral approach offers an advantage over the prone approach as the catheter is anchored through the biceps femoris muscle, reducing the risk of catheter dislodgement.[16]

Side Effects and Complications

Potential complications of popliteal nerve blocks, whether single-injection or continuous nerve blocks, include incomplete anesthesia, paresthesia or pain during nerve localization, difficult catheter insertion, allergic reaction, systemic local anesthetic toxicity, hematoma or bleeding, infection at the site of injection, and peripheral nerve deficit. These complications are relatively uncommon, with an overall incidence of 0%–10%.[22] The most common complications include incomplete anesthesia, infection, and neuropraxia.[18] A retrospective study of 157 popliteal nerve blocks performed for foot surgery demonstrated partial block failure in 10%, complete block failure in 4%, and persistent postoperative peripheral neuropathy in 1.26%.[22] A study of 400 continuous popliteal nerve catheters for postoperative analgesia showed an incidence of severe neuropathy in 0.5% and infection in 0.25%.[23]

SAPHENOUS BLOCK

The saphenous nerve is a sensory branch of the femoral nerve. It supplies sensation to the medial aspect of the lower extremity from the knee down to the medial malleolus and as far distal as the first metatarsophalangeal joint.[12,24] Its articular branches innervate the knee joint.[24] Thus, the combination of a sciatic nerve block and saphenous nerve block will provide total anesthesia of the lower extremity distal to the knee. Due to the fact that the saphenous nerve is a purely sensory nerve, the saphenous nerve block offers the advantage of no loss of muscle strength, as compared to the femoral nerve block.

Regional anesthetic blockade of the saphenous nerve can be performed at several anatomic locations. Approaches to saphenous nerve block (from proximal to distal along the course of the saphenous nerve) include perifemoral, subsartorial at the femoral triangle, subsartorial at the adductor canal (adductor canal block), block at the medial femoral condyle, below the knee field block, the paravenous approach, and block at the medial malleolus.[24] The transsartorial saphenous nerve block is highly successful (80% success rate), as compared to the below the knee field block and femoral paracondylar field block approaches (success rates of 65% and 40%, respectively). Additionally, the transsartorial approach provided complete anesthesia of the medial malleolus in 94% of subjects, while the other methods provided complete medial malleolus coverage in less than 40% of successful blocks.[25] In discussing saphenous nerve block technique, we will focus primarily on the proximal transsartorial approach.

Indications

The saphenous nerve block can be utilized in conjunction with the popliteal nerve block to provide complete surgical anesthesia for the lower extremity, thus allowing for vascular, orthopedic, and podiatric procedures involving the medial aspect of the lower leg to be performed under primary regional anesthetic. Such procedures may include saphenous vein harvesting, ORIF of the ankle, and medial foot surgery.[24]

The saphenous nerve block can also be used for postoperative analgesia in patients undergoing knee surgery, such as total knee arthroplasty (TKA). Studies have demonstrated that in the setting of TKA, adductor canal blocks provide comparable pain relief to femoral nerve blocks while simultaneously minimizing motor blockade of the quadriceps muscle.[26] Such studies highlight the important role that saphenous nerve blocks can play in decreasing the risk of falls and facilitating early mobilization after knee surgery.

Saphenous Nerve Anatomy

In the femoral triangle, the femoral nerve gives off two main cutaneous branches: the anterior division of the femoral nerve branches off into the anterior femoral cutaneous nerve that provides sensation to the anterior thigh, while the posterior division of the femoral nerve branches off into the saphenous nerve that supplies sensation to the medial aspect of the calf and foot.[19]

The saphenous nerve, accompanied by the femoral artery and vein, travels down the triangular adductor canal. The adductor canal is formed by the vastus medialis laterally and the adductor longus/magnus medially, with the sartorius muscle functioning as the "roof" of the canal.[24] The saphenous nerve then descends down the medial aspect of the knee and tibia.[24] In approximately 10% of individuals, the saphenous nerve extends beyond the medial malleolus to the first metatarso-phalangeal joint.[12]

Ultrasound Anatomy and Technique

The proximal transsartorial approach to saphenous nerve block is typically performed with the patient supine, with the lower extremity abducted and externally rotated. The ultrasound transducer should be placed transverse on the anteromedial thigh, at mid-thigh level. The femoral artery should be identified and followed distally until it passes through the adductor hiatus. The saphenous nerve may be visualized as a hyperechoic structure just lateral and superficial to the artery, which lies superficial to the femoral vein.[24]

The needle should be inserted in-plane in the lateral to medial direction until the needle tip is anterolateral to the femoral artery. Successful saphenous nerve block is confirmed when local anesthetic injection results in local anesthetic spread lateral to the femoral artery and deep to the sartorius muscle.[24] Continuous saphenous nerve blocks add significant value when used for postoperative analgesia following foot and ankle surgery. When used in conjunction with continuous popliteal block, patients reported less pain, more satisfaction with pain control, and required significantly less opioid medication postoperatively compared to patients with popliteal catheters and single-injection saphenous nerve blocks.[15]

Side Effects and Complications

Saphenous nerve blocks, just as with popliteal and other lower extremity nerve blocks, have the potential for various complications. While uncommon, these possible complications include incomplete anesthesia, allergic reaction to the local anesthetic, vascular damage at the injection site, hematoma, risk of intravascular injection, infection, and mechanical damage to the nerve at the injection site.[15]

One important potential side effect of proximal saphenous nerve blocks is the potential for partial quadriceps weakness. The mechanism for this weakness can be explained by spread of the local anesthetic proximally to involve the muscular branches of the femoral nerve. The likelihood of this side effect can be minimized by performing the saphenous block using a more distal approach.[24]

Necessity of Saphenous Block for Ankle Surgery

As previously discussed, popliteal sciatic block must sometimes be supplemented with a saphenous nerve block, depending on the surgical site. Questions have been raised regarding the necessity of saphenous nerve block supplementation for ankle surgery, particularly ankle surgery without a medial incision. Anatomical studies examining the role of the saphenous nerve have demonstrated that the saphenous nerve innervates the periosteum of the distal tibia and the talocrural joint capsule. These results suggest that saphenous nerve blocks are necessary for effective analgesia following ankle surgery—even surgery without a medial skin incision.[10]

EPIDURAL ANESTHESIA FOR FOOT AND ANKLE SURGERY

Neuraxial regional anesthesia, such as spinal or epidural anesthesia, has been used for ankle and foot surgery.[14] However, while these methods achieve superior analgesia compared to parenteral opioids, they have numerous undesirable side effects and potential complications. Neuraxial anesthesia can be complicated by sympathetic blockade with hypotension, urinary retention, and prolonged sensory blockade.[12,14] Neuraxial anesthesia is also associated with bilateral lower extremity weakness, resulting in motor impairment and immobilization, which is important for all patients requiring postoperative rehabilitation.[12]

Beyond these side effects and complications, epidural anesthesia is also an unreliable technique for foot and ankle surgery, as the L5–S1 segments have demonstrated resistance to epidural blockade and frequently remain unblocked.[11] Ponhold et al. demonstrated the high failure rate and lack of reliability of epidural anesthesia for foot surgery. Among patients in the horizontal supine position, injection of 20 mL 2% lidocaine into a lumbar epidural catheter at the L2/3 or L3/4 levels resulted in adequate anesthesia for foot surgery in only 13% of subjects.[27]

ILIAC CREST BONE GRAFT

Occasionally, challenging fractures and bone defects necessitate autologous bone grafting. The most common donor site for autologous bone grafts is the iliac crest, as it is both easy to access and a plentiful source of both cancellous and cortical bone.[28] However, the major disadvantage to use of autologous iliac crest bone graft is graft-site morbidity. Iliac crest bone grafting is associated with major complications, such as chronic pain, nerve injury, arterial injury, infection, pelvic instability, and abdominal organ herniation. Minor complications of the procedure include temporary pain, scar dysesthesia, local numbness and tenderness, hypertrophic scars, superficial seromas/hematomas, temporary ambulation difficulty, stitch abscesses, and prolonged drainage.[28] Acute postoperative pain is of significant concern, potentially leading to delays in ambulation and developing into chronic pain.[29] One study showed that 48 months after iliac crest bone graft, 26.1% of patients reported persistent pain at the donor site and 11.2% chronically used pain medication.[30] It is vital to optimize perioperative analgesia for iliac crest bone grafts in order to minimize the likelihood of these chronic pain sequelae.

Iliac Crest Innervation

The periosteum of the iliac crest is mainly innervated by the subcostal, ilioinguinal, and iliohypogastric, and lateral femoral cutaneous nerves.[29] Regional anesthesia techniques providing coverage to these nerves can aid in postoperative analgesia following iliac crest bone graft.

FASCIA TRANSVERSALIS BLOCK (TYPE 1 QUADRATUS LUMBORUM BLOCK)

The fascia transversalis block is a truncal fascial plane block indicated for analgesia following iliac crest bone graft. It aims to block the ilioinguinal, iliohypogastric, and subcostal (T12–L1) nerves at the point when they are between the transversalis fascia and fascia of the transversus abdominis muscle, thus blocking them proximal to where they innervate the anterior iliac crest.

COMPARTMENT SYNDROME

Acute compartment syndrome (ACS) is a concern with many acute orthopedic trauma injuries. The syndrome is defined as an increase in pressures within a closed myofascial compartment that results in compromised tissue perfusion and subsequent ischemic and necrotic injury to the muscles, nerves, and other organs of that compartment. When treatment is delayed or not administered, ACS can lead to catastrophic permanent injury including loss of a limb or death. The most common cause of ACS is trauma, and the most common compartment of the body for ACS to occur is the lower leg, with tibial shaft fractures making up 40% of all trauma-related ACS.[31] Diagnosis relies heavily on clinical suspicion and repeated exams. "Pain out of proportion to the injury," specifically pain on passive stretching of the involved compartment, has a specificity of 97% and negative predictive value of 98%, albeit a low sensitivity and positive predictive value.[31]

Discussion with the surgical team is necessary to determine if ACS is a concern perioperatively. Fortunately, ACS is extremely rare in isolated ankle fractures with the available documented cases limited to case reports.[32–41] Joseph et al.'s review found no common ankle fracture pattern that was more likely to lead to compartment syndrome.[36]

CONCLUSIONS AND KEY POINTS

- Ankle fractures are commonly occurring orthopedic injuries impacting both men and women across a broad age range, from adolescents to the elderly. The incidence of ankle fractures is anticipated to increase.
- The ankle, a weight-bearing hinge joint, refers to the junction of the tibia, fibula, and talus. The ankle's small surface area, juxtaposed with its exposure to large forces, results in vulnerability to ankle injuries.
- The majority of the ankle, with the exception of the medial aspect, is innervated by various branches of the sciatic nerve: the medial and lateral plantar nerves, sural nerve, calcaneal nerves, and superficial and deep peroneal nerves. The medial aspect of the ankle is innervated by the saphenous nerve.
- Proper ankle injury evaluation involves obtaining a history, performing a physical examination, and in some cases, radiographic evaluation.
    - o History should include details such as mechanism and time frame of ankle injury.
    - o Physical exam findings such as swelling, hematoma formation, and tenderness to palpation are suggestive of possible fracture.
    - o The Ottawa ankle rules provide highly sensitive guidelines as to the subset of patients who should undergo an ankle x-ray series.
- Ankle fractures can be classified as unimalleolar, bimalleolar, or trimalleolar. Some stable ankle fractures can be managed conservatively with a boot. However, unstable

(bimalleolar and trimalleolar) fractures, open fractures, and fractures with significant displacement require surgical treatment, usually an ORIF.

- Ankle surgery is associated with significant postoperative pain. Regional anesthesia in the form of a popliteal sciatic block combined with a saphenous nerve block has been shown to significantly improve pain control and patient satisfaction following ankle surgery.
- Ankle surgery can be performed under general anesthesia, neuraxial anesthesia, or regional anesthesia in the form of a popliteal sciatic nerve block and saphenous nerve block as a primary anesthetic technique. Regional anesthesia offers the advantage of avoiding the systemic complications and risks associated with general and neuraxial anesthesia, making it an appealing alternative for patients with comorbidities.
- The popliteal sciatic block anesthetizes the lower extremity distal to the knee with the exception of the medial leg. It is used for foot and ankle surgeries such as fracture repair and Achilles tendon repair. It involves the deposition of local anesthetic within Vloka's sheath, resulting in local anesthetic spread around the tibial and common peroneal nerves.
- The saphenous nerve block anesthetizes portions of the knee joint as well as the medial aspect of the lower extremity from the knee down to the medial malleolus. The saphenous nerve block can be used for analgesia in knee surgery, as well as surgeries involving the medial aspect of the lower leg. The transsartorial approach to saphenous nerve block is particularly effective and involves deposition of local anesthetic deep to the sartorius muscle and lateral to the femoral artery, where the saphenous nerve lies.
- Popliteal sciatic blocks and saphenous blocks are accompanied by a risk of complications including incomplete anesthesia, local anesthetic allergic reactions, hematoma, and infection. These complications are relatively uncommon.
- Acute compartment syndrome (ACS), defined as increases in pressure within a closed myofascial compartment resulting in tissue ischemia and necrosis, most commonly occurs in the lower leg in the setting of trauma and tibial shaft fractures. However, ACS is extremely rare in isolated ankle fractures.
- The fascia transversalis block (Type 1 quadratus lumborum block) is a truncal fascial plane block that aids in postoperative analgesia following iliac crest bone graft.

REFERENCES

1. Mandi DM. Ankle fractures. *Clin Podiatr Med Surg.* 2012; 29(2):155–186.
2. Daly PJ, Fitzgerald RH Jr, Melton LJ, Ilstrup DM. Epidemiology of ankle fractures in Rochester, Minnesota. *Acta Orthopaed Scand.* 1987;58(5):539–544.
3. Kannus P, Palvanen M, Niemi S, Parkkari J, Jrvinen M. Increasing number and incidence of low-trauma ankle fractures in elderly people: Finnish statistics during 1970–2000 and projections for the future. *Bone.* 2002;31(3):430–433.
4. Court-Brown CM, McBirnie J, Wilson G. Adult ankle fractures—an increasing problem? *Acta Orthopaed Scand.* 1998;69(1):43–47.
5. Court-Brown CM, Caesar B. Epidemiology of adult fractures: a review. *Injury.* 2006;37(8):691–697.
6. Seewoonarain S, Prempeh M, Shakokani M, Magan A. Ankle fractures: review article. *J Arthritis.* 2016;5:188. doi: 10.4172/2167-7921.1000188.
7. Carr JB, Gebhard F. Malleolar fractures and soft tissue injuries of the ankle. In: BD Browner BD, Jupiter JB, Krettek C, Anderson P, eds. *Skeletal Trauma: Basic Science, Management, and Reconstruction.* 5th ed. Philadelphia: Saunders; 2014:2189–2249.
8. Goost H, Wimmer MD, Barg A, Kabir K, Valderrabano V, Burger C. Fractures of the ankle joint: investigation and treatment options. *Deutsch Ärztebl Int.* 2014;111(21):377–388.
9. Stiell IG, Greenberg GH, McKnight RD, Nair RC, McDowell I, Worthington JR. A study to develop clinical decision rules for the use of radiography in acute ankle injuries. *Ann Emerg Med.* 1992;21(4):384–390.
10. Bjørn S, Wong WY, Baas J, et al. The importance of the saphenous nerve block for analgesia following major ankle surgery: a randomized, controlled, double-blind study. *Reg Anesth Pain Med.* 2018;43(5):474–479.
11. Singelyn FJ, Aye F, Gouverneur JM. Continuous popliteal sciatic nerve block: an original technique to provide postoperative analgesia after foot surgery. *Anesth Analg.* 1997;84:383–386.
12. Kopka A, Serpell MG. Distal nerve blocks of the lower limb. *Cont Educ Anesth Crit Care Pain.* 2005;5(5):166–170.
13. Rongstad K, Mann RA, Prieskorn D, Nichelson S, Horton G. Popliteal sciatic nerve block for postoperative analgesia. *Foot Ankle Int.* 1996;17(7):378–382.
14. Hansen E, Eshelman MR, Cracchiolo A III. Popliteal fossa neural blockade as the sole anesthetic technique for outpatient foot and ankle surgery. *Foot Ankle Int.* 2000;21(1):38–44.
15. Jarrell K, McDonald E, Shakked R, Nicholson K, Kasper V, Raikin SM. Combined popliteal catheter with single-injection vs continuous-infusion saphenous nerve block for foot and ankle surgery. *Foot Ankle Int.* 2018;39(3):332–337.
16. Hadzic A, Lopez AM, Vandepitte C, Sala-Blanch X. Ultrasound-guided popliteal sciatic block. In: Hadzic A, ed. *Hadzic's Textbook of Regional Anesthesia and Acute Pain Management.* 2nd ed. New York: McGraw-Hill; 2017:628–635.
17. Vloka JD, Hadzic A. Block of the sciatic nerve in the popliteal fossa. In: Hadzic A, ed. *Hadzic's Textbook of Regional Anesthesia and Acute Pain Management.* 2nd ed. New York: McGraw-Hill; 2017:1418–1426.
18. Canales MB, Huntley H, Reiner M, Ehredt DJ, Razzante M. The popliteal nerve block in foot and ankle surgery: an efficient and anatomical technique. *J Anesth Clin Res.* 2015;6(8). doi: 10.4172/2155-6148.1000553.
19. Carrera A, Lopez AM, Sala-Blanch X, Kapur E, Hasanbegovic I, Hadzic A. Functional regional anesthesia anatomy. In: Hadzic A, ed. *Hadzic's Textbook of Regional Anesthesia and Acute Pain Management.* 2nd ed. New York: McGraw-Hill; 2017:39–70.
20. Vloka J, Hadžić A, April E, Thys D. The division of the sciatic nerve in the popliteal fossa: anatomical implications for popliteal nerve blockade. *Anesth Analg.* 2001;92(1):215–217.
21. Chelly JE, Greger J, Casati A, Al-Samsam T, McGarvey W, Clanton T. Continuous lateral sciatic blocks for acute postoperative pain management after major ankle and foot surgery. *Foot Ankle Int.* 2002;23(8):749–752.
22. Hajek V, Dussart C, Klack F, et al. Neuropathic complications after 157 procedures of continuous popliteal nerve block for hallux valgus surgery: a retrospective study. *Orthopaed Traumatol Surg Res.* 2012;98(3):327–333.

23. Compère V, Rey N, Baert O, et al. Major complications after 400 continuous popliteal sciatic nerve blocks for post-operative analgesia. *Acta Anaesthesiol Scand*. 2009;53:339345.
24. Bendtsen TF, Lopez AM, Clark TB. Ultrasound-guided saphenous (subsartorius/adductor canal) nerve block. In: Hadzic A, ed. *Hadzic's Textbook of Regional Anesthesia and Acute Pain Management*. 2nd ed. New York: McGraw-Hill; 2017:615–619.
25. van der Wal M, Lang SA, Yip RW. Transsartorial approach for saphenous nerve block. *Can J Anesth*. 1993;40(6):542–546.
26. Kim DH, Lin Y, Goytizolo EA, et al. Adductor canal block versus femoral nerve block for total knee arthroplasty: a prospective, randomized, controlled trial. *Anesthesiology*. 2014;120(3):540–550.
27. Ponhold H, Kulier AH, Rehak PH. 30 degree trunk elevation of the patient and quality of lumbar epidural anesthesia: effects of elevation in operations on the lower extremities. *Anaesthesist*. 1993;42(11):788–792.
28. Lementowski PW, Lucas P, Taddonio RF. Acute and chronic complications of intracortical iliac crest bone grafting versus the traditional corticocancellous technique for spinal fusion surgery. *Orthopedics*. 2010;33(4). doi: 10.3928/01477447-20100225-08.
29. Sondekoppam RV, Ip V, Johnston DF. Ultrasound-guided lateral-medial transducer quadratus lumborum block for analgesia following anterior iliac crest bone graft harvesting: a clinical and anatomical study. *Can J Anesth*. 2018;65:178–187.
30. Silber J, Anderson D, Daffner S, et al. Donor site morbidity after anterior iliac crest bone harvest for single-level anterior cervical discectomy and fusion. *Spine*. 2003;28(2):134–139.
31. McMillan TE, Gardner WT, Schmidt AH, Johnstone AJ. Diagnosing acute compartment syndrome-where have we got to? *Int Orthop*. 2019 Nov;43(11):2429–2435. doi: 10.1007/s00264-019-04386-y.
32. Horne G. Pes cavovarus following ankle fracture: a case report. *Clin Orthop Relat Res*. 1984;184:249–250.
33. Luk K, Pun W. Unrecognised compartment syndrome in a patient with tourniquet palsy. *J Bone Joint Surg Br*. 1987;69:97–99.
34. Hawkins B, Bays P. Catastrophic complication of simple cast treatment: case report. *J Trauma*. 1993;34:760–762.
35. Ashworth M, Patel N. Compartment syndrome following ankle fracture-dislocation: a case report. *J Orthop Trauma*. 1998;12:67–68.
36. Joseph J, Giannoudis P, Hinshce A, et al. Compartment syndrome following isolated ankle fracture. *Int Orthop*. 2000;24:173–175.
37. Young Szalay M, Roberts J. Compartment syndrome after Bosworth fracture-dislocation of the ankle: a case report. *J Orthop Trauma*. 2001;15:301–303.
38. Beekman R, Watson J. Bosworth fracture-dislocation and resultant compartment syndrome: a case report. *J Bone Joint Surg Am*. 2003;85:2211–2214.
39. Zachariah S, Taylor L, Kealey D. Isolated lateral compartment syndrome after Weber C fracture dislocation of the ankle: a case report and literature review. Injury. 2005;36:345–346.
40. Seyahi A, Uludag S, Akman S, et al. Unrecognized anterior compartment syndrome following ankle fracture surgery. *J Amer Pod Med Assoc*. 2009;99:438–442.
41. Starr AM, Swan KG Jr, Swan KG. Isolated anterior compartment syndrome after a bimalleolar ankle fracture in a collegiate football player. *Sports Health*. 2011 Nov;3(6):560–563.

REVIEW QUESTIONS

(1) An 18-year-old otherwise healthy male presents to the emergency department complaining of a painful, swollen right ankle following injury sustained during a soccer game. He endorses difficulty bearing weight on his right leg. Which of the following physical examination findings would NOT be an indication for IMMEDIATE orthopedic consultation and surgical treatment?

A. Grossly visible malposition of the joint
B. Laceration and visible bony structures on the medial aspect of the ankle
C. X-ray imaging revealing trimalleolar fracture
D. Decreased sensitivity to touch on the plantar aspect of the foot

(2) A 56-year-old female presents to the emergency department after slipping on ice, twisting her left ankle, and falling on the ice. On physical exam, her left ankle and foot are significantly swollen. An x-ray series of her left ankle reveals a medial malleolar fracture with 2 mm talar shift. What is the appropriate course of treatment?

A. Splint the left ankle with the ankle positioned at 90 degrees for at least 6 weeks with weight bearing as tolerated
B. Schedule the patient for an ORIF today
C. Split the left ankle and schedule an ORIF once the left ankle swelling has subsided
D. Perform a reduction of the ankle in the emergency department

(3) A 32-year-old male was diagnosed with a right ankle bimalleolar-equivalent fracture 1 week ago, having fractured his lateral malleolus and having injured his deltoid ligament. His right ankle was splinted and today he presents for ORIF of his right ankle. He is interested in regional anesthesia and is looking forward to decreased pain allowing him to engage in physical therapy. Which peripheral block(s) would be the most appropriate choice for this patient?

A. Transgluteal sciatic + saphenous nerve
B. Popliteal sciatic + saphenous nerve
C. Popliteal sciatic + femoral nerve
D. Popliteal sciatic

(4) From which levels of the lumbosacral plexus does the sciatic nerve originate?

A. L2–L4
B. L2–S3
C. L4–S2
D. L4–S3

(5) Which of the following is an accurate description of the structures forming the borders of the adductor canal?

A. Vastus medialis laterally, adductor magnus medially, sartorius as the "roof"
B. Adductor magnus laterally, vastus medialis medially, sartorius as the "roof"
C. Gracilis laterally, adductor magnus medially, sartorius as the "roof"
D. Adductor magnus laterally, gracilis medially, sartorius as the "roof"

(6) Which of the following patients would be an inappropriate candidate for a saphenous nerve block?

A. 75-year-old ASA 3 male undergoing total knee arthroplasty

B. 59-year-old ASA 4 female undergoing saphenous vein harvesting
C. 62-year-old ASA 3 undergoing amputation of the second digit of his right lower extremity
D. 18-year-old ASA 1 undergoing ORIF for left ankle trimalleolar fracture

(7) A 44-year-old female presents to the hospital for right ankle ORIF. She prefers that the procedure be done under epidural anesthesia. The anesthesiologist places an L3–L4 epidural and boluses 20 mL of 2% lidocaine. After 10 minutes, the patient continues to report full sensation in her feet. The anesthesiologist boluses another 10 mL of 2% lidocaine. After 20 minutes, the surgeons make incision. A few minutes into the surgical procedure, the patient is unable to tolerate the procedure and the case is converted to general anesthesia. What is the most likely reason for failure of epidural anesthesia in this case?

A. The surgical team did not give enough time for the local anesthetic to take effect.
B. The patient required greater volume of local anesthetic.
C. Resistance of the L5–S1 segments to epidural blockade.
D. The patient required a higher concentration of local anesthetic.

ANSWERS

(1) **C.** Grossly visible malposition of the joint is suggestive of dislocated fracture, which must be emergently reduced. Decreased sensitivity to touch in the plantar aspect of the foot indicates possible neural compromise. Along with dislocation, neurovascular compromise and open injury are indications for immediate orthopedic consultation.

Reference

Seewoonarain S, Prempeh M, Shakokani M, Magan A. Ankle fractures: review article. *J Arthritis.* 2016;5:188. doi: 10.4172/2167-7921.1000188.

(2) **A.** The patient presents with a stable fracture, a unimalleolar fracture without significant talar shift (less than 4 mm). Treatment for stable fractures is conservative (non-operative). The ankle should be splinted for 6 weeks with weight bearing as tolerated.

Reference

Seewoonarain S, Prempeh M, Shakokani M, Magan A. Ankle fractures: review article. *J Arthritis.* 2016;5:188. doi: 10.4172/2167-7921.1000188.

(3) **B.** The popliteal sciatic will anesthetize the entire calf, tibia, fibula, ankle, and foot with the exception of the medial leg, which derives its cutaneous innervation from the saphenous nerve. Thus the saphenous nerve must be blocked in order to provide complementary coverage of the medial aspect of the leg. Femoral nerve block would result in significant quadriceps muscle weakness, and transgluteal sciatic nerve block would result in hamstring weakness, making those blocks less than ideal.

Reference

Hansen E, Eshelman MR, Cracchiolo A III. Popliteal fossa neural blockade as the sole anesthetic technique for outpatient foot and ankle surgery. *Foot Ankle Int.* 2000;21(1):38–44.

(4) **D.** The sciatic nerve at the popliteal fossa consists of the junction of the tibial nerve and the common peroneal nerve. The common peroneal nerve originates from the anterior division of the ventral rami of L4 to S2, while the tibial nerve originates from the anterior division of the ventral rami of L4 to S3. The femoral nerve, on the other hand, originates from L2–L4.

Reference

Carrera A, Lopez AM, Sala-Blanch X, Kapur E, Hasanbegovic I, Hadzic A. Functional regional anesthesia anatomy. In: Hadzic A, ed. *Hadzic's Textbook of Regional Anesthesia and Acute Pain Management.* 2nd ed. New York: McGraw-Hill; 2017:39–70. http://accessanesthesiology.mhmedical.com/content.aspx?

(5) **A.** The adductor canal, which houses the saphenous nerve, is formed by the vastus medialis laterally and the adductor longus/magnus medially, with the sartorius muscle functioning as the "roof" of the canal.

Reference

Bendtsen TF, Lopez AM, Clark TB. Ultrasound-guided saphenous (subsartorius/adductor canal) nerve block. In: Hadzic A, ed. *Hadzic's Textbook of Regional Anesthesia and Acute Pain Management.* 2nd ed. New York: McGraw-Hill; 2017:615–619.

(6) **C.** A saphenous nerve block would not provide coverage for the amputation of a second toe; rather than the saphenous nerve, the second toe derives its cutaneous innervation from branches of the sciatic nerve. However, the saphenous nerve is indicated for knee surgery, saphenous vein harvesting, and ankle surgery (although for ankle surgery the saphenous block would need to be used in conjunction with a sciatic block).

Reference

Kopka A, Serpell MG. Distal nerve blocks of the lower limb. *Cont Educ Anesth Crit Care Pain.* 2005;5(5):166–170.

(7) **C.** L5–S1 segments demonstrate resistance to epidural blockade and frequently remain unblocked, making epidural anesthesia unreliable for foot and ankle surgery.

Reference

Ponhold H, Kulier AH, Rehak PH. 30 degree trunk elevation of the patient and quality of lumbar epidural anesthesia: effects of elevation in operations on the lower extremities. *Anaesthesist.* 1993;42(11):788–792.

32.

REGIONAL ANESTHESIA FOR BUNIONECTOMY

Daniel Abraham

STEM CASE AND KEY QUESTIONS

A 75-year-old female with a history of rheumatoid arthritis has had progressive foot pain with ambulation and difficulty finding appropriate shoes to fit. She suffers from joint pain in her ankle and in all her toes and has noted that her big toe is off-centered. She has poorly controlled diabetes, and complains of bilateral burning foot pain. After consultation with a podiatrist, she was diagnosed with a hallux valgus deformity, commonly known as a bunion of the great toe.

In conjunction with her primary physician, she is treated and managed for her diabetes and starts taking gabapentin for her neuropathy. She gets sent for foot and ankle radiographic studies and returns a few months later with continued pain on the medial aspect of her foot and occasional difficulty with ambulation.

Due to her continued pain, the podiatrist suggests operative management. The patient is scheduled for a bunionectomy and Chevron osteotomy at an ambulatory surgical center.

In preparation for her surgery, she presents to a preoperative clinic with her daughter. She is on a single antihypertensive medication and under good control. Her diabetes is now under better control but she still complains of burning pain in both feet. She has chronic stage 3 kidney disease. Her electrocardiogram (EKG) demonstrates left ventricular hypertrophy. She has radiographic evidence of hallux valgus deformity. She states that she tolerates anesthesia well, but her daughter interjects that she is often very slow to wake up after anesthesia.

The patient and her daughter have a discussion about the risks and benefits of the different anesthetic options, as well as her history of delayed emergence from anesthesia. A plan is formulated to avoid general anesthesia that focuses on a peripheral nerve block and mild sedation titrated to the patient's comfort level in the operating room (OR).

The patient presents a few days later for her bunionectomy and would still like to avoid a general anesthetic, wishing to proceed with a block and sedation. You explain to the patient that you will be performing an ankle block, which involves multiple injections into the ankle. You also explained to her the additional risk of nerve injury associated with nerve blocks and added that numbness from the nerve block will be transient and will resolve; however, you cannot guarantee that the nerve block will not make the burning pain in her feet any worse. She agreed and stated that while she would like to feel relaxed during block placement, she is willing to remain responsive to voice during the surgery as long as she feels no discomfort.

The patient is taken back to the OR without any need for pre-procedure sedation.

After American Society of Anesthesiologists (ASA) monitors are placed on the patient, she receives some fentanyl and you start an ankle block. The patient cries out in pain and is unable to keep the leg steady. Given the subcutaneous infiltration of the block and the need for multiple injections, you decide to start a propofol infusion that will continue after the block as a sedative.

The patient is resting comfortably on a low-level propofol infusion and goes to sleep when left alone, but arouses upon hearing her name called. Before starting to operate, the surgeon tests out the block, stimulating the patient in the operative field. During the test, she reports some retained sensation in her first metatarsal. The surgeon states that they will supplement with a Mayo block. Postoperatively, she is placed in a hard cast and then into a surgical boot. She has an uneventful stay in the recovery room, with no need for postoperative opioids.

(1) WHAT IS A BUNION AND HOW IS IT DIAGNOSED?

A hallux valgus deformity, or a bunion, is a complex anatomical deformity of the big toe, often presenting with pain and disfigurement. It is most commonly diagnosed with a physical exam and a corroborating medical history. Initial management after a diagnosis is conservative therapy, including being fitted for cushioned insoles and easily fitted shoes.[1]

(2) WHAT ARE THE INDICATIONS AND OPTIONS FOR OPERATIVE MANAGEMENT?

- Limitations of activity due to foot pain
- Chronic inflammation and swelling
- Toe deformity[1]

(3) WHAT ARE THE ANESTHETIC OPTIONS AND CONSIDERATIONS FOR A BUNIONECTOMY?

Regional anesthesia options include a peripheral nerve block, or a neuraxial block. Options for a block at the level of foot and ankle include the Mayo block and the ankle block. More proximal blocks include a sciatic nerve block at the level of the popliteal fossa or above, plus or minus a saphenous nerve or femoral nerve block.[2,3]

(4) WHAT IS THE RISK OF PERFORMING A REGIONAL ANESTHETIC IN A PATIENT WITH DIABETIC NEUROPATHY? PERIPHERAL VASCULAR DISEASE? INFECTION?

The nerves in a patient with diabetic neuropathy are at risk of neural ischemia due to vascular changes in the nerve, and therefore epinephrine should be avoided as an additive in these patients, as well as patients with peripheral vascular disease.

Diabetic neuropathy can cause microvascular changes in the nerve bundle, leaving those nerves at risk for ischemia. In patients with peripheral vascular disease, ischemia to the nerve is also a concern.[4]

The risk of infection is always present due to the immunocompromised situation or a nearby infection.

(5) WHAT IS THE RELEVANT ANATOMY AND NERVES THAT ARE INVOLVED TO PROVIDE A REGIONAL ANESTHETIC FOR A BUNIONECTOMY?

Five peripheral nerves innervate the foot: the superficial and deep peroneal nerves, posterior tibial nerve, sural nerve, and the saphenous nerve. The saphenous nerve innervates the medial aspect of the ankle and the upper half of the medial aspect of the foot. All other nerves are distal branches of the sciatic nerve. The lateral aspect of the foot is innervated by the sural nerve. The deep ventral structures, muscles, and sole of the foot are innervated by the posterior tibial nerve. The dorsal side of the foot is innervated by the superficial peroneal nerve. The deep dorsal structures and the 1st web space (between 1st and 2nd toe) are innervated by the deep peroneal nerve.

(6) HOW CAN AN ULTRASOUND BE USED IN PERFORMING AN ANKLE BLOCK?

An ultrasound can be helpful in visualizing the deep peroneal nerve and the posterior tibial nerve, especially due to their proximity to arteries. The posterior tibial nerve can be visualized at the level of the medial malleolus. The posterior tibial nerve can be seen posterior to the artery. The deep peroneal nerve can be seen alongside the anterior tibial artery. The nerve can be lateral, medial, or even divided on both sides of the artery. The saphenous and superficial peroneal are subcutaneous nerves.

(7) HOW CAN AN ANKLE NERVE BLOCK BE PROLONGED?

The use of perineural additives like dexamethasone and dexmedetomidine, buprenorphine, epinephrine, and clonidine, in addition to local anesthetics, help prolong the duration of the block.[5]

DISCUSSION

ANATOMICAL CONSIDERATIONS OF A BUNION

Normal anatomy of the first toe consists of two phalanges connected to the metatarsal bone at the first metatarsophalangeal (MTP) joint. The stability of the first MTP joint is provided by collateral ligaments and the joint capsule, with added stability by the abductor hallucis and adductor hallucis muscles as they insert along the medial and lateral side of the first metatarsal head. It is important to note that no muscles originate from the first metatarsal bone and insert into the phalanx to stabilize the MTP joint, and therefore, the metatarsal is basically suspended in a sling of muscles and tendons. Consequently, any asymmetrical force pushing the proximal phalanx laterally, or the metatarsal head medially, can cause a deformity.

A bunion, or hallux valgus deformity, is a distortion of the great toe. Hallux is another name for the great toe. Valgus denotes the oblique displacement away from midline. The deformity is characterized by the progressive lateral deviation of the proximal phalanx and medial deviation of the metatarsal bone (see Figure 32.1) As the proximal phalanx drifts laterally, it pulls the distal metatarsal toward the lateral direction, making the metatarsal head prominent on the medial side of the foot. These deviations typically take place in the transverse plane. As the phalanx moves further laterally, the capsule and its associated ligaments become further strained and the joint capsule may burst. In these situations, the lateral forces (adductor hallucis muscle) can act unopposed, further worsening the deformity. Additionally, rotation of the toe in the frontal plane can cause the nail to face medially.[1]

DIAGNOSIS AND ETIOLOGY OF A BUNION

The development of a bunion is likely multifactorial, and involves a progression of forces on the MTP joint.[6] Any derangement in the mechanics of the MTP joint can be compounded over time and made worse with gait as the foot attempts to compensate. The hallux valgus deformity is more likely to occur in women than men, and it is more common in people wearing shoes. The current belief is that inappropriate shoes can exacerbate underlying bony or mechanical issues, leading to a higher incidence. Additional factors that are associated with bunions include: familial history of bunions, bilateral involvement, female gender, a longer first ray, an oval or curved MTP joint, abnormal foot mechanics affecting the MTP joint, spasticity, and rheumatoid arthritis.[7]

The most common complaint is pain over the medial prominence of the foot, created by the lateralized metatarsal head in the transverse plane. Occasionally, patients also complain of pain in the first MTP joint, as well as pain in the second MTP joint (due to the new pressure exerted from the hallux valgus). Initial evaluation involves physical examination of the joints and gait, including special attention to the skin over the medial prominence, as well as pulses. Although

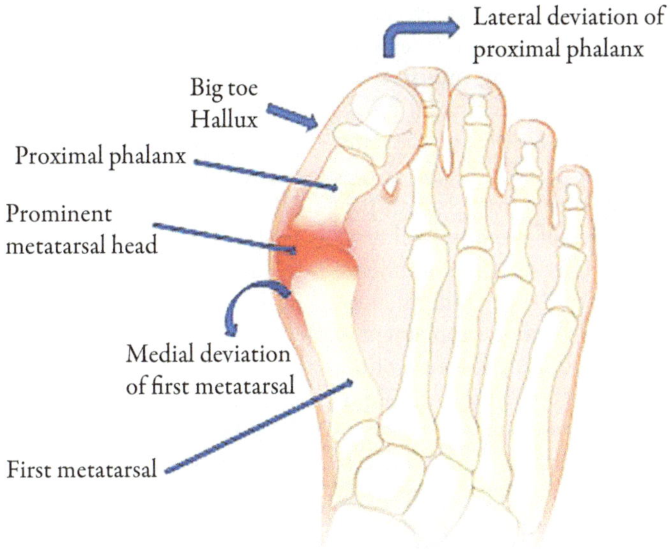

Figure 32.1. Hallux valgus deformity. The deformity, which involves the big toe, is characterized by lateral deviation of the proximal phalanx and medial deviation of the first metatarsal.

the deformity may be recognized by clinical exam and history, x-ray of the joint can also be very helpful in determining the type and severity of the deformity. The hallux valgus angle, or the angle created by the proximal phalanx and first metatarsal, can help gauge severity if the angle is greater than 15 degrees. The first MTP joint is assessed for congruency, which is the lateral subluxation of the proximal phalanx on the metatarsal head. The joint can also be assessed for arthrosis, sclerosis, and osteophyte formation.

MANAGEMENT OF A BUNION: CONSERVATIVE AND OPERATIVE

Conservative management starts with appropriate shoes and/or infills within a shoe. Shoes should fit well and comfortably, and patients can consider wider, low-heeled shoes. In some cases, specific orthotic shoes may provide the best results; studies have shown that when orthotic shoes were compared to no treatment, patients wearing orthotics demonstrated improved pain scores.[8] Additional padding over the medial prominence of the bunion or under the MTP joint can help with the pain at these sites. Padding can also be placed in the first web space between the first and second toe to gently splint the first toe back into its anatomical position. This splinting can also be performed overnight. Lastly, using ice locally can help reduce swelling, and nonsteroidal anti-inflammatory drugs (NSAIDs) can help with pain and inflammation if there is no contraindication.

The most common reason for operative management is continued pain or dysfunction after the failure of conservative management. There are many different surgical approaches to the correction of the hallux valgus deformity, and the patient's symptoms, physical signs, and radiographic findings should be taken into account for a surgical plan. Surgical correction typically involves one or more of the following: soft tissue reconstruction, bunionectomy (removing the medial prominence of the metatarsal head), osteotomy (cutting the first metatarsal), or arthrodesis (fusing the MTP joint). Most surgical approaches are open and involve a medial incision of 3–5 cm.

If a soft tissue procedure is the plan, then an incision in the first interspace allows for releasing the soft tissue contracture (lateral joint capsule, adductor hallucis tendon, ligaments) on the lateral side of the joint. A second incision on the medial side of the foot exposes the joint so that proper alignment can be done and affixed. Postoperatively, the patient is maintained in a firm compression dressing and allowed to ambulate with a postoperative shoe. The Chevron osteotomy procedure is the most common surgical solution to bunion correction. It involves removal of the medial eminence of the bunion through a medial incision by cutting the prominent portion of the metatarsal. The metatarsal head is translated laterally and the medial joint capsule is plicated. The osteotomy site is then fixed with a pin or screw. Postoperatively, the patient is maintained in a firm compression dressing for 6–8 weeks and allowed to ambulate with a postoperative shoe. In severe cases of deformity, or with a failed surgical attempt at correction, arthrodesis of the first MTP joint becomes indicated. A dorsal longitudinal incision is made to expose and remove the joint. A dorsal plate and screws then stabilize the MTP joint. Postoperatively, the patient is sometimes maintained in a short leg walking cast, with gradual progression toward weight bearing.

ANESTHETIC CONSIDERATIONS FOR BUNIONECTOMY

There are a number of anesthetic options for a patient undergoing a bunionectomy. Given the unilateral and distal location of the surgery, strong consideration should be given to using a local anesthetic to complement any anesthetic plan.

Peripheral nerve blocks or subcutaneous infiltration can be performed by the surgeon or the anesthesiologist. If regional anesthesia is delivered by the anesthesiologist, multiple targets for a peripheral nerve block, or even neuraxial block, are available. Options for a block at the level of foot and ankle include the Mayo block and the ankle block. If it is necessary to block proximally, the anesthesiologist can perform a sciatic nerve block at the level of the popliteal fossa or above, plus or minus a saphenous nerve or femoral nerve block. If a higher level is needed, a spinal or epidural anesthetic is an option. These blocks can then be supplemented by a monitored sedation. When determining location of the block, consideration should be given to the patient's physical exam of the foot, with attention to any areas of neuropathy, swelling, infection, and altered anatomy. Additionally, surgical details should be considered, such as location of incision, use of tourniquet, presumed pain level postoperatively, ambulation plan postoperatively, and postoperative destination. Alternatively, general anesthesia is an option if a secured airway is desired, with or without the use of local anesthetics for postoperative pain control. Barring any serious cardiopulmonary considerations or comorbidities of the patient precluding them from being performed in an outpatient setting, bunionectomies are safe to be performed as a same-day surgery.[9]

Bunionectomies are typically done using a tourniquet to minimize bleeding and to maximize operating conditions for the surgeon. Ankle tourniquets are typically tolerated better than mid-calf or thigh, and with appropriate sedation only about 3% of patients complain of tourniquet pain.[10–12] A propofol infusion titrated to maintain spontaneous respiration should offer appropriate sedation for these cases with a block, though each monitored sedation should be tailored to each patient's comorbidities and situation.

PERFORMING A NERVE BLOCK IN A PATIENT WITH DIABETIC NEUROPATHY/PERIPHERAL VASCULAR DISEASE/INFECTION

The concern for a patient with preexisting neuropathy is that the local anesthetic in or near a nerve can result in a new or worsening neurologic deficit. It is possible that these patients may be at a higher risk of further neurological injury simply because they already have some damage to their nerves, a notion known as the double crush phenomenon.[13–15] Although animal studies have demonstrated that nerves may be more susceptible to injury in diabetic models, it is not clear if this extends to diabetic patients after nerve block.[16,17] While it is likely that the nerves of a diabetic are more susceptible to the effects of local anesthetic, the severity and toxicity are not fully understood. The decision, therefore, to use local anesthetics in the diabetic patient population should be made on an individual basis and after discussion with the patient about the risks and benefits of this technique.

Diabetic neuropathy can cause microvascular changes in the nerve bundle, leaving those nerves at risk for ischemia. In patients with peripheral vascular disease, ischemia to the nerve is also a concern. While diabetic neuropathy also affects the nerves themselves, the concerns for a patient with peripheral vascular disease are still similar, due to possible preexisting nerve ischemia and its effect on the susceptibility of the nerve to local anesthetics. The same individualized approach to a plan in conjunction with the patient should be employed here, as well as an avoidance of any vasoconstrictor to the injectate to further worsen ischemia and blood flow to the compromised area.

Since bunionectomies are routinely done with a tourniquet, it can be challenging to discern whether a neurological complication is a result of the tourniquet, the block, or even the combination. That being said, the risk of neurological complications is typically very low.[12]

If a patient has a local infection in the area of the desired injection, a block is not recommended. Placing a needle through any infected tissue could further spread any subcutaneous infection deeper. Additionally, the acidic environment of an infection will render a local anesthetic ineffective. Options include placement of a block more proximal in the leg or performing a general anesthetic.

ANKLE BLOCK ANATOMY AND CONSIDERATIONS

An ankle block provides anesthesia to the foot distal to the level of the ankle by anesthetizing five distinct peripheral nerves at the level of the malleoli: superficial and deep peroneal nerves, posterior tibial nerve, sural nerve, and the saphenous nerve. The saphenous nerve is a sensory nerve that is the continuation of the femoral nerve and innervates the medial aspect of the ankle and the upper half of the medial aspect of the foot. All other nerves are distal branches of the sciatic nerve. The lateral aspect of the foot is innervated by the sural nerve. The deep ventral structures, muscles, and sole of the foot are innervated by the posterior tibial nerve. The dorsal side of the foot is innervated by the superficial peroneal nerve. The deep dorsal structures and the 1st web space (between 1st and 2nd toe) are innervated by the deep peroneal nerve. The saphenous nerve, the superficial peroneal nerve, and the sural nerve are all relatively superficial and course through subcutaneous tissue at the level of the malleoli. The posterior tibial nerve passes alongside the posterior tibial artery, posterior to the medial malleolus and deep to the flexor retinaculum. The deep peroneal nerve travels alongside but lateral to the anterior tibial artery on the anterior surface of the ankle into the foot, also deep to the flexor retinaculum. All of these nerves can be approached and blocked at the level of the malleoli in the ankle, and this can be performed as a landmark-based approach, with ultrasound guidance, or a combination of both. It is also worth noting that ankle and forefoot blocks all require more than one injection and subcutaneous infiltration, which can cause discomfort and are not always well tolerated by an awake patient. A plan for sedation should include increasing levels of medications titrated to comfort for blocks in the ankle or foot.

IS A SAPHENOUS NERVE BLOCK NEEDED FOR A BUNIONECTOMY?

The saphenous nerve provides sensation to the medial ankle and has variable innervation to the medial foot. While one study found that the saphenous nerve innervation does not extend beyond the midfoot in 97% of patients, an anatomical study has demonstrated that branches of the saphenous nerve reach the first metatarsal in 28% of specimens.[18,19] Given the variation in the innervation of the saphenous nerve, and its relative ease of blocking with subcutaneous infiltration, it is beneficial to make sure this nerve is blocked for a bunionectomy, especially if the block is used as the primary anesthetic.

PERFORMING A LANDMARK-BASED ANKLE BLOCK

With the patient in the supine position, place a bump or pillow under the calf to elevate the foot slightly. There are five distal nerves to block for a complete ankle block. The major landmarks to identify are the lateral and medial malleoli. Starting just proximal to the posterior side to the medial malleoli and anterior to the Achilles tendon, inject subcutaneously and circumferentially from medial malleoli around to the lateral malleoli, using a total of 10–20 cc of local anesthetic and a small needle. By circumferentially injecting, every subsequent insertion of the needle can be done in an area that already has local anesthetic and can therefore decrease discomfort. This subcutaneous ring running from the medial to the lateral malleolus will block the saphenous, superficial peroneal, and sural nerves. The best landmark for the deep peroneal nerve can be seen if the great toe is extended, revealing the extensor hallucis tendon. Insert needle immediately lateral to the tendon until bone is hit and then inject 5 cc of local anesthetic after negative aspiration. The best landmark for the posterior tibial nerve is the palpated pulse of the posterior tibial artery. Insert needle just posterior to the pulse until it contacts bone, then slightly withdraw and inject 5 cc of local anesthetic after negative aspiration. If the artery is not palpable, then a point midway between the medial malleolus and the anterior edge of the Achilles tendon can be the insertion point. Again, advance until bone is hit and inject local anesthetic after negative aspiration.

ULTRASOUND-ASSISTED ANKLE BLOCK

An ultrasound can be helpful in visualizing the deep peroneal nerve and the posterior tibial nerve, especially due to their proximity to arteries. While the saphenous, the superficial peroneal, and the sural nerves can be visualized under ultrasound as well, they are all subcutaneous and not as easily found and identified. Given the ease with which they can be anesthetized with a subcutaneous ring injection, it might be easier to use a combination of ultrasound guidance and subcutaneous injection when considering the ankle block. The posterior tibial nerve can be visualized at the level of the medial malleolus, with the linear transducer placed in the transverse plane just posterior to the medial malleolus. The posterior tibial artery is the best landmark to use as it can be identified easily and with the help of color Doppler flow. The posterior tibial nerve can be seen posterior to the artery and typically appears hyperechoic and with honeycomb pattern (see Figure 32.2A and B). The deep peroneal nerve can be seen alongside the anterior tibial artery when the linear probe is placed in the transverse plane on the anterior surface of the ankle in between the medial and lateral malleolus. It is easiest to first identify the anterior tibial artery by looking for pulsatile flow with help of the color Doppler. The nerve can be lateral, medial, or even divided on both sides of the artery. It is hyperechoic and has a honeycomb appearance (see Figure 32.3A and B).

CONSIDERATIONS IN CHOOSING A LOCAL ANESTHETIC AND ADDITIVES FOR A BUNIONECTOMY

Considerations involve the duration of the surgery and the degree of postoperative pain. In the case of a bunionectomy, longer pain relief postoperatively is a desired outcome. Using

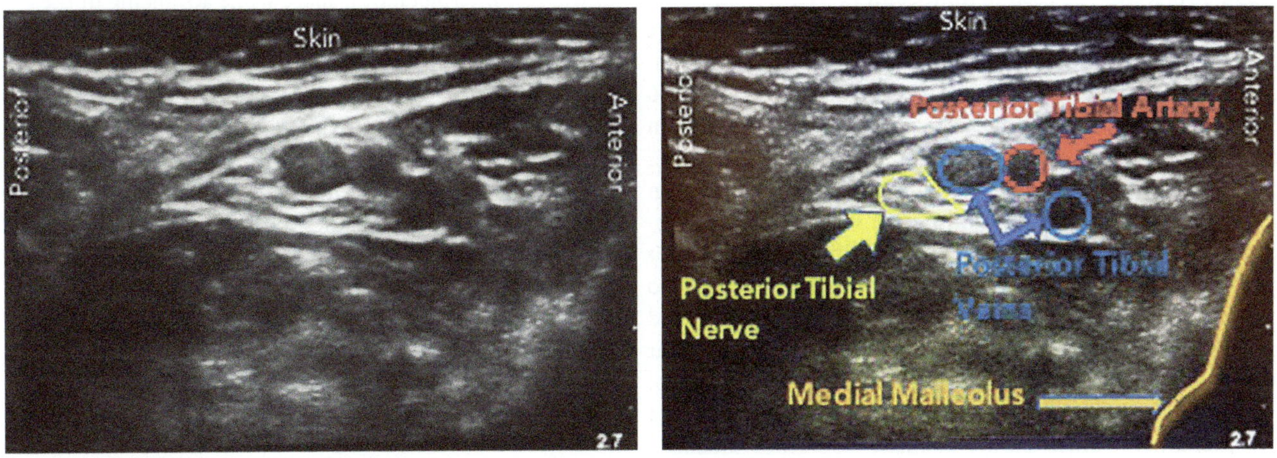

Figure 32.2 (A) Ultrasound image of the tibial nerve and surrounding anatomical structures; (B) annotated ultrasound image of anatomy of the tibial nerve.

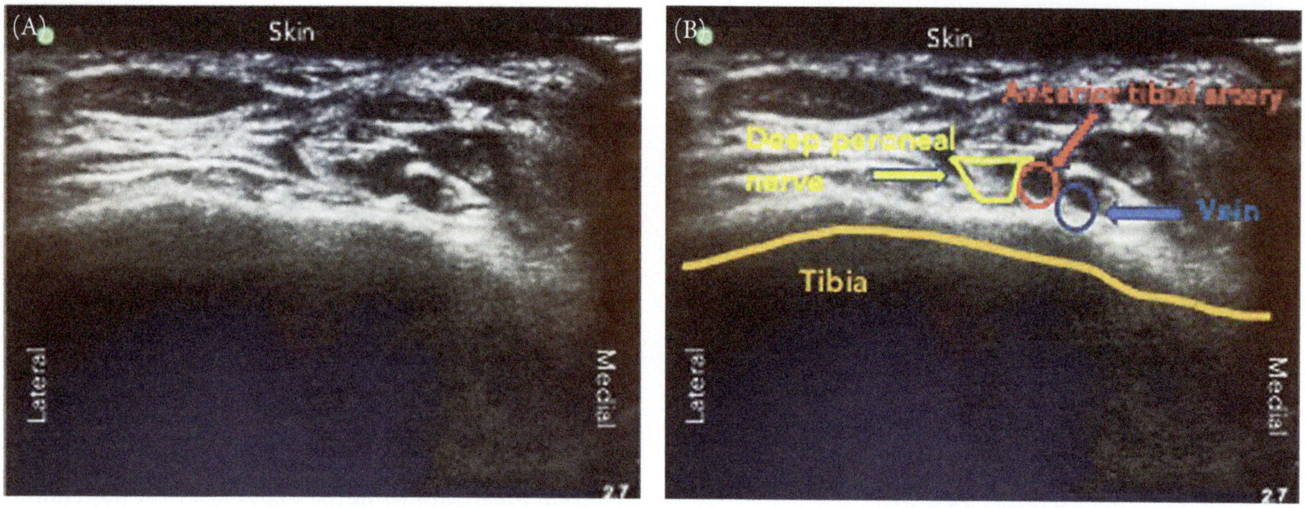

Figure 32.3 (A) Ultrasound image of the deep peroneal nerve and related anatomical structures; (B) annotated ultrasound image of anatomy of the deep peroneal nerve.

an intermediate-length local anesthetic like bupivacaine or ropivacaine can provide longer pain relief than using lidocaine. At least 0.5% bupivacaine or ropivacaine is needed if this block is to be the primary anesthetic. Using these intermediate duration of action local anesthetics necessitates some time for the block to effectively take place, and they should be performed at least 20 minutes prior to incision for best success.[20]

The use of epinephrine as an additive for ankle blocks is controversial due to concerns for distal vessel constriction and cutting off end vascular supply in the foot. While epinephrine should be avoided in patients with peripheral vascular disease and compromised circulation to the foot, it can be safely used in an ankle block in most patients.[21,22] That being said, it should be avoided in any patient where there are concerns that systemic uptake can result in hypertension and tachycardia. The nerves in a patient with diabetic neuropathy are at risk of neural ischemia due to vascular changes in the nerve, and therefore epinephrine should be avoided as an additive in these patients, as well as patients with peripheral vascular disease.[23] If epinephrine is used, a dilute concentration, at least 1:200,000, should be used to limit complications.

A number of other additives have been studied with nerve blocks, but the data for additives to local anesthetics specifically for ankle blocks are limited. A study published in 1996 demonstrated that clonidine added to local anesthetic for an ankle block can prolong the duration of the block.[24] There is conflicting information about the use of dexamethasone as an additive for ankle blocks. While some studies have demonstrated a benefit,[25,26] others have seen no difference.[27] A recent study comparing the use of a single injection of bupivacaine to bupivacaine with 3 additives (buprenorphine, clonidine, and dexamethasone) in foot and ankle surgery demonstrated that additives can prolong the block but carry higher incidence of neuropathy post-block.[28] The decision to use additives in a peripheral nerve block should be made on an individualized basis, with careful consideration being given to the patient's comorbid conditions and the desired length of the block.

Liposomal bupivacaine is a special formulation of bupivacaine encapsulated by liposomes that provides a slow and controlled release of bupivacaine from its location of injection. A clinical trial performed in 2012 involved the use of liposomal bupivacaine for bunionectomy, but the study was used to determine the safety and efficacy of the drug. A limited number of studies involve using liposomal bupivacaine for ankle surgery, but speak mostly to its safety profile.[29,30] While these studies demonstrate that it is safe to use, they do not speak to the length or success of its use in an ankle block. Given that liposomal bupivacaine is not currently approved for use in ankle blocks, more studies need to be performed before recommending its use.

FOREFOOT BLOCKS FOR A BUNIONECTOMY

A Mayo block is a block of the forefoot done at the level of the MTP joint. It involves up to 4 injections of infiltration of local anesthetic in a ring shape around the first metatarsal. The first step is to inject 5 cc of local anesthetic on the dorsal aspect of the first intermetatarsal space while advancing in the plantar direction. The needle is then withdrawn and advanced in the medial direction, injecting subcutaneously. The needle is withdrawn to the skin, and then advanced in the lateral direction, continuing to inject subcutaneously. Lastly, the needle is withdrawn and reinserted on the medial side of the foot, directed plantarly under the first metatarsal bone. Injecting medial to lateral in this plane, another 5 cc of local anesthetic is injected. The four injections of the block are meant to encircle the entire first metatarsal bone. This block should anesthetize all surgical sites of the bunionectomy.

CONCLUSION

- A hallux valgus deformity, or a bunion, is a relatively common and painful condition that involves the big toe.

- Bunions are easily diagnosed and initially treated with conservative measures. Subsequent steps involve surgical correction.
- Appropriate preoperative assessment and risk stratification are critical as these patients typically present with multiple comorbidities.
- A number of anesthetic options exist for this surgery; this author recommends the use of regional anesthesia for a bunionectomy.
- Ankle blocks can be performed using a landmark approach and/or with ultrasound guidance. Further, a Mayo block can be performed distally, at the level of the first MTP joint to add further anesthesia to the first metatarsal.
- Benefits of peripheral nerve blockade for bunionectomy include the avoidance of general anesthesia, adequate analgesia in the postoperative period, and decreased use of opioids.

REFERENCES

1. Mann JA, Chou LB, Ross SDK. Foot and ankle surgery. In: Skinner HB, McMahon PJ, eds. *Current Diagnosis & Treatment in Orthopedics*, 5th ed. New York: McGraw-Hill Education; 2014.
2. Vandepitte C, Lopez AM, Boxstael SV, Jalil H. Ultrasound-guided ankle block. In: Hadzic A, ed. *Hadzic's Textbook of Regional Anesthesia and Acute Pain Management.* 2nd ed. New York: McGraw-Hill Education; 2017:636–641.
3. Kay J, Delmonte R, Greenberg PM. Ankle block. In: Hadzic A, ed. *Hadzic's Textbook of Regional Anesthesia and Acute Pain Management.* 2nd ed. New York: McGraw-Hill Education; 2017:1427–1434.
4. Jacob AK, Kopp SL, Hebl JR. Regional anesthesia in the patient with preexisting neurological disease. In: Hadzic A, ed. *Hadzic's Textbook of Regional Anesthesia and Acute Pain Management.* 2nd ed. New York: McGraw-Hill Education; 2017:910–920.
5. McCartney CJL, Choi S. Analgesic adjuvants in the peripheral nervous system. In: Hadzic A, ed. *Hadzic's Textbook of Regional Anesthesia and Acute Pain Management.* 2nd ed. New York: McGraw-Hill Education; 2017:147–156.
6. Nix SE, Vicenzino BT, Collins NJ, Smith MD. Characteristics of foot structure and footwear associated with hallux valgus: a systematic review. *Osteoarthritis Cartilage.* 2012;20:1059.
7. Coughlin MJ, Jones CP. Hallux valgus: demographics, etiology, and radiographic assessment. *Foot Ankle Int.* 2007;28:759.
8. Torkki M, Malmivaara A, Seitsalo S, Hoikka V, Laippala P, Paavolainen P. Surgery vs orthosis vs watchful waiting for hallux valgus: a randomized controlled trial. *JAMA.* 2001;285:2474.
9. Galois L, Serwier JM, Arashvand AD. Surgery of the hallux valgus in an ambulatory setting: a liability risk? *Eur J Orthop Surg Traumatol.* 2017;27(4):545–548.
10. McGlamry DE, Banks AS, Downey M. Ankle block. In McGlamry DE, Banks AS, Downey M, eds. *Comprehensive Textbook of Foot Surgery.* 2nd ed. Philadelphia: Williams & Wilkins; 1992:243–244.
11. Lichtenfeld NS. The pneumatic ankle tourniquet with ankle block anesthesia for foot surgery. *Foot Ankle.* 1992;13:344–349.
12. Derner R, Buckholz J. Surgical hemostasis by pneumatic ankle tourniquet during 3027 podiatric operations. *J Foot Ankle Surg.* 1995;34:236–246.
13. Upton AR, McComas AJ. The double crush in nerve entrapment syndromes. *Lancet.* 1973;2:359–362.
14. Osterman AL. The double crush syndrome. *Orthop Clin North Am.* 1988;19:147–155.
15. Neal JM, Barrington MJ, Brull R, et al. The second ASRA practice advisory on neurologic complications associated with regional anesthesia and pain medicine: executive summary 2015. *Reg Anesth Pain Med.* 2015;40(5):401–430.
16. Blumenthal S, Borgeat A, Maurer K, et al. Preexisting subclinical neuropathy as a risk factor for nerve injury after continuous ropivicaine administration through a femoral nerve catheter. *Anesthesiology.* 2006;105:1053–1056.
17. Kroin JS, Buvanendran A, Williams DK, et al. Local anesthetic sciatic nerve block and nerve fiber damage in diabetic rats. *Reg Anesth Pain Med.* 2010;35:343–350.
18. Marsland D, Dray A, Little NJ, Solan MC. The saphenous nerve in foot and ankle surgery: its variable anatomy and relevance. *Foot Ankle Surg.* 2013;19(2):76–79.
19. Lopez AM, Sala-Blanch X, Magaldi M, Poggio D, Asuncion J, Franco CD. Ultrasound-guided ankle block for forefoot surgery: the contribution of the saphenous nerve. *Reg Anesth Pain Med.* 2012;37(5):554–557.
20. Rudkin GE, Rudkin AK, Dracopoulos GC. Ankle block success rate: a prospective analysis of 1,000 patients. *Can J Anesth.* 2005;52:209–210.
21. Roth RD. Utilization of epinephrine-containing anesthetic solutions in the toes. *J Am Podiatr Med Assoc.* 1981;71:189–199.
22. Nielsen LJ, Lumholt P, Hölmich LR. Local anaesthesia with vasoconstrictor is safe to use in areas with end-arteries in fingers, toes, noses and ears. *Ugeskr Laeger.* 2014 Oct 27;176(44):V04140238. Danish. PMID: 25354008.
23. Williams BA, Murinson BB, Grable BR, Orebaugh SL. Future considerations for pharmacologic adjuvants in single-injection peripheral nerve blocks for patients with diabetes mellitus. *Reg Anesth Pain Med.* 2009;34:445–457.
24. Reinhart DJ, Wang W, Stagg KS, et al. Postoperative analgesia after peripheral nerve block for podiatric surgery: clinical efficacy and chemical stability of lidocaine alone versus lidocaine plus clonidine. *Anesth Analg.* 1996;83(4):760–765.
25. Marty P, Rontes O, Chassery C, et al. Perineural versus systemic dexamethasone in front-foot surgery under ankle block: a randomized double-blind study. *Reg Anesth Pain Med.* 2018;43(7):732–737.
26. Alzeftawy AE, Elsheikh NA. The effect of preemptive ankle block using ropivicaine and dexathemasone on postoperative analgesia in foot surgery. *Anesth Essays Res.* 2017;11(2):372–375.
27. Dawson RL, McLeod DH, Koerber JP, Plummer JL, Dracopoulos GC. A randomized controlled trial of perineural vs intravenous dexamethasone for foot surgery. *Anaesthesia.* 2016;71(3):285–290.
28. Dang DY, McGarry SM, Melbihess EJ. Comparison of single-agent versus 3-additive regional anesthesia for foot and ankle surgery. *Foot Ankle Int.* 2019 Oct;40(10):1195–1202.
29. Ilfeld BM, Viscusi ER, Hadzic A, et al. Safety and side effect profile of liposomal bupivicaine (exparel) in peripheral nerve blocks. *Reg Anesth Pain Med.* 2015;40(5):572–582.
30. Hamilton TW, Athanassoglou V, Trivella M, et al. Liposomal bupivacaine peripheral nerve block for the management of postoperative pain. *Cochrane Database Syst Rev.* 2016;8.

REVIEW QUESTIONS

(1) A 56-year-old male presenting for a bunionectomy requests regional anesthesia for his procedure, stating that he would like to avoid general anesthesia. Upon exam, you notice that the patient has a rash over the skin at the level of the ankle that the patient believes is from a new detergent. The surgeon would like to proceed with the case and is not concerned with the infectious nature of the redness. Which of the following is your best course of action?

A. Perform general anesthesia for the case as the best option for the patient.
B. Perform an ankle block as the surgeon does not think it is infectious.
C. Perform nerve blocks more proximal in the leg.
D. Cancel the case due to concern for infection.

(2) A patient presents for an ankle surgery, and regional anesthesia is your primary plan. Roughly 30 minutes after you have performed a popliteal sciatic nerve block using 20 mL of 0.5% ropivicaine, an incision is made on the medial aspect of the ankle, and the patient cries out in pain. Which of the following is the most likely reason?

A. The block has not had enough time to set up.
B. Not enough local anesthetic was used for the block.
C. The concentration of local anesthetic was not high enough.
D. The saphenous nerve was not blocked.

(3) Which of the following nerves that innervate the ankle can be found as a result of its proximity to an artery?

A. Posterior tibial nerve
B. Sural nerve
C. Saphenous nerve
D. Superficial peroneal nerve

(4) With which of the following populations are bunions associated?

A. The male sex
B. People who wear shoes
C. Sedentary people
D. Athletes

(5) What is needed to diagnose a bunionectomy?

A. Blood test markers
B. Radiographic evidence
C. Physical exam and clinical story
D. It is a diagnosis of exclusion.

(6) Which of the following areas are innervated by the posterior tibial nerve?

A. Dorsum of the foot
B. Heel and sole of the foot
C. Lateral aspect of the foot
D. Web space between the first and second toe

(7) Which of the following is an appropriate injectate for a patient with poorly controlled diabetes who is getting an ankle block as the primary anesthetic?

A. 0.25% bupivacaine, plain
B. 0.5% bupivacaine, with epinephrine 1:100,000
C. 0.5% ropivacaine, with dexamethasone
D. 0.5% ropivacaine, plain

(8) What is the anatomical reason that a bunion is a deformity seen only in the 1st toe?

A. The first metatarsal is kept aligned by a series of muscles and tendons.
B. The first metatarsal has the weakest bone structure of the toes.
C. The first toe is made up of only two phalanges.
D. This deformity can exist in any of the toes.

ANSWERS

(1) **C.** This patient has already stated that he would like to avoid general anesthesia if possible, so strong consideration should be made for a regional anesthetic technique. A new rash at the site of needle insertion should be avoided due to the possibility that it might be infectious in nature. Despite the surgeon's lack of concern of the rash, a lack of a proper diagnosis should sway the anesthesiologist away from using a needle at that site. Given that the most distal site of nerve blockade, the ankle block, is contraindicated due to possible infection at the skin, the next thing that can be offered to the patient is a more proximal block. The patient is not presenting with signs of a new systemic infection (fevers, chills) and the surgeon is not concerned with the local rash, therefore canceling the case is not the appropriate action here.

Reference

Capdevila X, Bringuier S, Borgeat A. Bruno riou; infectious risk of continuous peripheral nerve blocks. *Anesthesiology,* 2009;110:182–188.

(2) **D.** The saphenous nerve is the distal continuation of the femoral nerve, and is the only nerve innervating the ankle that comes from the lumbar plexus. All other peripheral nerves innervating the ankle come from the sciatic nerve, which stems from the sacral plexus. In this situation, given the medial location of incision and the patient response, it is likely that this patient has saphenous innervation at the level of surgery. The block had been performed with an appropriate amount of time for it to have taken effect, as well as an appropriate concentration and volume. Therefore, in this clinical situation, it is likely that the saphenous nerve should have also been blocked.

Reference

Marsland D, Dray A, Little NJ, Solan MC. The saphenous nerve in foot and ankle surgery: its variable anatomy and relevance. *Foot Ankle Surg.* 2013;19(2):76–79.

(3) **A.** The posterior tibial nerve is the only option here that can be found next to an artery. The sural, saphenous, and superficial peroneal are all superficial nerves found in the subcutaneous layer and not seen traveling alongside an artery.

Reference

Vandepitte C, Lopez AM, Boxstael SV, Jalil H. Ultrasound-guided ankle block. In Hadzic A, ed. *Hadzic's Textbook of Regional Anesthesia and Acute Pain Management.* 2nd ed. New York: McGraw-Hill Education; 2017:636–641.

(4) **B.** There is a strong association between the development of a bunion and someone who wears shoes. This relationship has led to the suggestion that shoes should fit well and be

cushioned as a conservative treatment. Women are much more likely than men to develop a bunion. Bunions are not associated with sedentary or active lifestyles as a sole contributor.

Reference

Coughlin MJ, Jones CP. Hallux valgus: demographics, etiology, and radiographic assessment. *Foot Ankle Int.* 2007;28:759.

(5) **C.** While radiographic evidence of a bunion can be very helpful in understanding the severity of the deformity and helpful in guiding operative management, it is not necessary for a diagnosis. An appropriate clinical history and physical exam are typically all that is necessary. There are no blood test markers for a bunionectomy, and it is not a diagnosis of exclusion.

Reference

Coughlin MJ, Jones CP. Hallux valgus: demographics, etiology, and radiographic assessment. *Foot Ankle Int.* 2007;28:759.

(6) **B.** The posterior tibial nerve innervates the deep structures of the foot and the sole. The dorsum of the foot is innervated by the superficial peroneal nerve. The lateral aspect of the foot is innervated by the sural nerve. The first web space is innervated by the deep peroneal nerve.

Reference

Vandepitte C, Lopez AM, Boxstael SV, Jalil H. Ultrasound-guided ankle block. In: Hadzic A, ed. *Hadzic's Textbook of Regional Anesthesia and Acute Pain Management.* 2nd ed. New York: McGraw-Hill Education; 2017:636–641.

(7) **D.** In a patient with poorly controlled diabetes, preexisting peripheral neuropathy must always be a concern. Diabetic patients may be more susceptible to further nerve injury, and therefore a primary regional anesthetic must always be preceded by a discussion with the patient about the risks and benefits of this approach. The vasculature within the nerve bundle may be compromised secondary to diabetic changes, and therefore epinephrine should be avoided in this population due to concerns of ischemia to the nerve. Dexamethasone, as an additive, is also not appropriate in a diabetic as it causes hyperglycemia. Lastly, if the ankle block will serve as the primary anesthetic, the local anesthetic must be at a high enough concentration for full anesthesia. 0.25% bupivacaine is a great option if analgesia alone is the intention, but not strong enough as a primary regional anesthetic.

Reference

Jacob AK, Kopp SL, Hebl JR. Regional anesthesia in the patient with preexisting neurological disease. In: Hadzic A, ed. *Hadzic's Textbook of Regional Anesthesia and Acute Pain Management.* 2nd ed. New York: McGraw-Hill Education; 2017:910–920.

(8) **A.** The hallux valgus deformity, commonly known as the bunion, is literally translated as "an oblique great toe." This deformity is not seen in any of the other toes and is unique to the first metatarsal. The first metatarsal is attached to the distal phalange at the MTP joint, and no muscle originates on the metatarsal to the phalange to stabilize this connection. The first metatarsal is suspended and splint into its location by the reversing forces of muscles and tendons. Consequently, any asymmetrical force pushing the proximal phalanx laterally, or the metatarsal head medially, can cause a deformity. While the first toe does indeed have two phalanges, this is not the reason for the deformity. There is nothing different in the bone structure of the first metatarsal as compared to the others.

Reference

Coughlin MJ, Jones CP. Hallux valgus: demographics, etiology, and radiographic assessment. *Foot Ankle Int.* 2007;28:759.

SECTION 8

OBSTETRIC ANESTHESIA

Eman Nada

33.

EPIDURAL FOR LABOR IN A MORBIDLY OBESE PATIENT AND NEURAXIAL ULTRASOUND

Manuel C. Vallejo

STEM CASE AND KEY QUESTIONS

A 35-year-old, 5′5″ (162 cm), 350 lb. (159 kg), G-3, P-2 parturient at 38 weeks gestation and 5 cm cervical dilatation is requesting analgesia for labor pain. She is presently receiving pitocin for labor augmentation.

The patient is extremely anxious and nervous. Upon further questioning of her past medical history, she tells you that for her first child, the epidural catheter never worked, and she had to deliver with medications that were given intravenously for pain. She also tells you that her most recent delivery ended up as a stat cesarean under general anesthesia because the epidural once again failed to work, and she developed a severe post-dural puncture headache (PDPH) afterward.

In exploring the etiology of her PDPH, she says she was "poked" multiple times in her back and had a severe headache after delivery, lasting for over 2 weeks. She remains very anxious and nervous because she wants pain relief but doesn't want another devastating headache.

At a recent conference, you heard about the successful placement of labor epidural catheters using ultrasound. The obstetric anesthesiologist assigned to labor and delivery is an ultrasound expert and the resident is very interested in learning the technique and asks many questions. The resident would like to perform the next labor epidural catheter insertion with the use of ultrasound and wants the attending to teach him the process.

The resident, under the guidance of the obstetric anesthesiologist, successfully places the epidural under ultrasound, providing satisfactory labor analgesia after dosing the catheter with local anesthesia. The patient reports adequate pain relief with a T-10 bilateral dermatome block level to pin prick.

Her labor progresses and the fetus is noted to have severe variable decelerations lasting over several minutes. The obstetrician decides to proceed with a cesarean section. The patient tells you she would like to be awake for the delivery and doesn't want general anesthesia if possible, because of the traumatic experience of her last delivery. The fetal decelerations improve, and you decide to use her existing epidural and dose the epidural catheter with 2% lidocaine with 1:200,000 epinephrine in 5 ml increments. Upon transporting the patient from the gurney to the operating room table, the epidural catheter gets caught on the side of the bed and is pulled out. You decide to perform a spinal anesthetic as the obstetrician is in agreement.

You successfully place the spinal anesthetic using 10.5 mg (1.4 mL) of 0.75% bupivacaine with 0.2 mg of preservative-free morphine, you place the patient on a continuous infusion of intravenous phenylephrine to prevent hypotension. Cesarean delivery proceeds uneventfully and a baby is delivered with Apgar scores of 7 and 9 at 1 and 5 minutes. On postoperative rounds, the patient is extremely satisfied and thanks you for the excellent care you provided for her delivery.

(1) WHAT ADDITIONAL INFORMATION (IF ANY) WOULD YOU REQUIRE AT THIS TIME?

It is important to conduct a focused history and physical examination before providing anesthesia. This consists of asking about pertinent allergies, medications, past medical history, past surgical history, obstetrical history, conducting a focused physical examination, and obtaining significant laboratory results.

(2) WHAT LABORATORY EXAMINATION(S) WOULD YOU REQUIRE (IF ANY) AT THIS TIME?

In an otherwise healthy parturient, a laboratory examination is not needed. A platelet count would be useful in the diagnosis of hypertensive disorders of pregnancy, such as preeclampsia; hemolysis, elevated liver enzymes, and low platelet count syndrome; and other conditions associated with coagulopathy.

(3) WHAT TYPES OF REGIONAL ANALGESIA CAN BE OFFERED FOR RELIEF OF HER LABOR PAIN?

Regional blocks for labor analgesia include epidural (continuous, patient controlled epidural analgesia [PCEA], programmed intermittent epidural boluses [PIEB]), spinal, continuous spinal epidural (CSE), caudal, lumbar sympathetic block, paracervical, pudendal, caudal, and local anesthesia infiltration.

(4) WOULD YOU OFFER LABOR EPIDURAL ANALGESIA AT THIS TIME?

Yes, after providing informed verbal and written consent with discussion of the potential complications.

(5) WHAT QUESTIONS WOULD YOU ASK HER IN ORDER TO EXPLORE THE REASON BEHIND THE EPIDURAL NOT WORKING A SECOND TIME?

Questions include finding out about the clinical experience of the previous provider (trainee, faculty) who placed her epidural catheters previously, any possible patient anatomic variations (back surgery), medical conditions (spina bifida occulta, Marfan syndrome), time-period surrounding delivery events (quick delivery without appropriate block time), or any other events that could explain her dysfunctional epidurals.

(6) WHAT ADDITIONAL INFORMATION WOULD YOU NEED TO EXPLORE THE EXTENT AND SEVERITY OF HER PREVIOUS POST-DURAL PUNCTURE HEADACHE (PDPH)?

Explore the signs and symptoms associated with a PDPH. For example, did she experience a postural component (worse sitting up), photophobia, diplopia, nausea, dizziness, tinnitus, emesis, neck stiffness, and/or cephalgia?

(7) WHAT MAY BE THE REASON(S) FOR HER FAILED LABOR EPIDURAL ANALGESIA?

Reasons include the catheter not being in the epidural space resulting in a failed block, unilateral one-sided block, incomplete patchy analgesia, bilateral sensory level below T-10 providing inadequate analgesia, inadequate second-stage labor analgesia, and catheter displacement.

(8) WHAT SPECIFIC TECHNIQUE(S) IF ANY COULD YOU EMPLOY TO PREVENT A PDPH THIS TIME AROUND?

Have the epidural catheter placed by the most experienced anesthesiologist and consider the use of point of care preprocedure neuraxial ultrasound imaging.

(9) WHAT ARE THE AMERICAN SOCIETY OF ANESTHESIOLOGISTS (ASA) TASK FORCE ON OBSTETRIC ANESTHESIA RECOMMENDATIONS FOR FETAL HEART RATE (FHR) MONITORING FOR NEURAXIAL ANESTHESIA?

The Task Force recommends that fetal heart rate patterns should be monitored by a qualified individual before and after administration of neuraxial analgesia for labor.

(10) WHAT ARE THE ASA TASK FORCE ON OBSTETRIC ANESTHESIA RECOMMENDATIONS FOR INTRAVENOUS ACCESS AND MATERNAL MONITORING FOR NEURAXIAL ANESTHESIA?

Before neuraxial anesthesia is provided, the patient should have intravenous access with external blood pressure measurement every 2 to 3 minutes with continuous pulse oximetry.

(11) WHAT SPECIFIC EQUIPMENT IS REQUIRED FOR PLACEMENT OF THE EPIDURAL CATHETER UNDER ULTRASOUND?

Point of care ultrasound machine, ultrasound gel, curved array transducer probe, in addition to the epidural kit.

(12) DESCRIBE THE TECHNIQUE FOR PLACING AN EPIDURAL CATHETER USING ULTRASOUND ASSISTANCE.

Three views (longitudinal paramedian oblique, longitudinal median, and transverse median) are used to visualize and determine the best lumbar intervertebral interspace, the distance from the skin to the epidural space, midline, and optimal epidural needle angle for insertion.

(13) THE PATIENT IS PLACED ON A PATIENT CONTROLLED EPIDURAL ANALGESIA (PCEA) INFUSION. WHAT MEDICATION, DOSE, RATE, AND LOCKOUT INTERVAL DO YOU CHOOSE FOR THE PCEA?

At our institution we use 0.125% bupivacaine with fentanyl 2 mcg/ml at a rate of 10 mL/hr.; 4 mL bolus every 15 minutes; 26 mL maximum dose over 1 hour.

(14) WOULD YOU USE HER EXISTING LABOR EPIDURAL FOR CESAREAN DELIVERY?

Yes, provided the epidural was functioning appropriately during labor and there was enough time (15–20 minutes) to dose the epidural catheter to ensure adequate surgical anesthesia.

(15) IF NOT, WHAT TYPE OF ANESTHETIC WOULD YOU CONSIDER?

If the patient had to have a stat or emergent cesarean, I would consider alternative techniques to provide surgical anesthesia, such as spinal in an experienced provider's hands or general anesthesia in some circumstances (e.g., profound fetal bradycardia, ruptured uterus, severe hemorrhage, and severe placental abruption).

(16) WHAT COMPLICATIONS CAN OCCUR FROM PLACING A SPINAL ANESTHETIC AFTER DOSING AN EPIDURAL CATHETER?

The most serious complication that can occur is a high spinal (total spinal), especially if given after dosing an epidural catheter within 30 minutes of the spinal anesthetic. A high spinal can result in apnea, severe hypotension, cardiovascular collapse, and loss of consciousness.

(17) WHAT DOSE OF SPINAL ANESTHETIC WOULD YOU GIVE?

A typical spinal dose is 12–15 mg of 0.75% bupivacaine. To avoid a high spinal (total spinal) after epidural analgesia, it is recommended to decrease the dose 20%–30%, which is enough to provide surgical anesthesia.

(18) HOW WOULD YOU PREVENT HYPOTENSION AS A RESULT OF YOUR NEURAXIAL ANESTHETIC?

Techniques used to prevent hypotension include intravenous pre/co-loading, intravenous vasopressor (ephedrine, phenylephrine, norepinephrine) use, and/or prophylactic background vasopressor infusion.

(19) WHAT ARE SOME ADVANTAGES OF POINT OF CARE PRE-PROCEDURE NEURAXIAL ULTRASOUND IMAGING COMPARED TO THE STANDARD EPIDURAL TECHNIQUE?

Advantages include determination of midline, deciding the optimal vertebral interspace level in those with normal and difficult anatomy, finding the optimal insertion point, locating the best angle for needle insertion, and determination of epidural needle depth for catheter placement.

(20) YOU PLAN TO PLACE THE EPIDURAL CATHETER USING ULTRASOUND GUIDANCE. WHAT PROBE IS INDICATED FOR NEURAXIAL ULTRASOUND? WHAT DEPTH ON THE ULTRASOUND MACHINE IS INDICATED FOR DEPTH VISUALIZATION?

The curved array probe is best used for ultrasound visualization set initially to a depth of 7–8 cm. During scanning, the depth, focus, and gain settings of the ultrasound machine can be adjusted as needed during the scanning process to produce an optimal image.

(21) WHAT ARE THE LUMBAR NEURAXIAL ULTRASOUND VIEWS THAT ARE HELPFUL TO DETERMINE THE EPIDURAL DEPTH?

Three views (longitudinal paramedian oblique, longitudinal median, and transverse median) are used for visualization.

(22) HOW DO YOU PERFORM THE TRANSVERSE MEDIAN VIEW? AND HOW CAN YOU OPTIMIZE THE IMAGE?

The probe is placed on the lumbar spine horizontally, perpendicular to the long axis of the spine in the intervertebral space. The probe can then be angled up or down to provide the best visual image of the epidural space.

(23) WHAT ARE THE STRUCTURES YOU SEE IN THE TRANSVERSE MEDIAN VIEW?

In this view, the spinous process, laminae, articular process, transverse process, ligamentum flavum, posterior dura mater, intrathecal space, anterior dura mater, posterior longitudinal ligament, and vertebral body can be identified.

(24) WHAT ARE THE STRUCTURES YOU SEE IN THE LONGITUDINAL MEDIAN VIEW?

The structures that can be identified include the articular process, ligamentum flavum and posterior dura mater, intrathecal space anterior dura mater, posterior longitudinal ligament, the sacrum and vertebral bodies.

(25) WHAT IS THE ANTERIOR AND THE POSTERIOR COMPLEX?

Both can be seen on neuraxial ultrasound. The anterior complex includes the anterior dura, posterior longitudinal ligament, and posterior aspect of the vertebral body or the intervertebral disc. The posterior complex includes the ligamentum flavum, epidural space, and posterior dura.

(26) WHAT IS THE SAW SIGN?

In the longitudinal paramedian oblique, the spinous processes can be seen as a series of hyperechoic lines with upward convexity and posterior acoustic shadowing. These spinous processes (saw teeth) represent the "saw sign."

(27) WHAT IS THE EQUAL SIGN?

In the transverse median, the longitudinal paramedian oblique, and the longitudinal median ultrasound views, an "equal sign" (=) can be seen where the upper and lower parallel lines represent the ligamentum flavum/posterior dura and vertebral body/posterior longitudinal ligament/anterior dura, respectively.

DISCUSSION

PHYSIOLOGICAL CHANGES OF PREGNANCY RELATED TO NEURAXIAL ANATOMY

The physiological and anatomical changes associated with pregnancy present several unique considerations for anesthesia management. Pregnancy is associated with generalized tissue edema, weight gain, and an exaggerated lordosis that can alter the pharmacokinetic and pharmacodynamic properties of medications. In addition, most medications can cross from the placenta into the fetus, necessitating fetal concerns as well.

Regarding neuraxial placement, the hormonal changes of pregnancy can make palpation and identification of anatomic landmarks challenging. The ligaments generally soften and the interspinal ligaments develop laxity, which can alter the tactile sensation of the dural ligament. Because of this, the epidural space can be harder to identify and cause a false loss of resistance.[1,2,3,4] Furthermore, the physiological changes of pregnancy narrow the epidural space, causing the intrathecal space to become smaller, increasing the risk for inadvertent dural puncture.[5,6] Parturients may have difficulty achieving and maintaining adequate flexion of the lumbar spine for neuraxial insertion due to the gravid uterus and/or severe pain from contractions, which is often worsened from repeated needle insertions and redirections due to the inability to locate the neuraxial space.[5,6,7]

LABOR ANALGESIA OPTIONS

Labor analgesia options include non-pharmacologic methods, systemic analgesia, and neuraxial analgesia.

Non-Pharmacologic

Antenatal childbirth education, emotional support (provided by family or doula), massage therapy, audio-therapy, and acupuncture have been used to alleviate pain and anxiety during childbirth. Transcutaneous electrical nerve stimulation (TENS) is the application of low-intensity, high-frequency electrical impulses to the lower back and is widely used in Europe for labor analgesia. Hydrotherapy is the immersion of the parturient in warm water to cover the abdomen only during labor. Intradermal water injection consists of the injection of sterile water in the lower back/sacral area and is supposed to relieve the back pain during labor. Hypnosis during childbirth is a labor-intensive technique and requires prenatal training of the mother and her partner.[8]

Systemic Labor Analgesia

This can be provided using inhalational agents or systemic opioid administration. Systemic analgesia is used widely in institutions around the world that lack facilities for the provision of safe neuraxial analgesia. It is useful in women who refuse regional anesthesia or have contraindications (e.g., coagulopathy) for provision of neuraxial blocks.

Inhalational Agents

Nitrous oxide provides both anxiolysis and mild analgesia when provided by the currently commercially available 50% nitrous/50% oxygen intermittent delivery system. The pain relief of nitrous oxide is inferior to labor epidural analgesia.[9] However, maternal satisfaction scores for labor analgesia are not different among women who receive nitrous oxide analgesia, neuraxial analgesia, or those who transition from nitrous to neuraxial analgesia.[9] Special scavenging equipment is necessary to prevent contamination of the environment and when properly operated, reduces levels well below the NIOSH standard of 25 ppm. Nitrous oxide adverse effects are mild in nature, with a reported nausea incidence of 13%, dizziness (3%–5%) and drowsiness (4%).[9] Nitrous oxide is reported to show no adverse effects on uterine activity, the first and second stages of labor, operative (cesarean) delivery rates, and neonatal Apgar scores.[9,10] Instruction must be given to inspire at the beginning of a contraction so that peak brain concentrations of nitrous oxide coincide with the peak of contraction pain. The risk of hypoxemia exists with concomitant use of parenteral opioids and faulty equipment. There has been an interest in use of volatile anesthetic agents for labor analgesia due to availability of agents with low blood-gas solubility (e.g., sevoflurane).[11] However, these agents can cause maternal sedation and adversely affect uterine tone and their use is currently not accepted as standard of clinical care.

Systemic Opioids

Parenteral opioids (Table 33.1) can be used for providing analgesia during childbirth as intermittent bolus doses or as patient controlled analgesia (PCA). Side effects are nausea, vomiting, delayed gastric emptying, dysphoria, drowsiness, and respiratory depression. These medications blunt the pain but do not provide complete analgesia. All opioids easily cross the placenta and can cause neonatal respiratory depression as well as neurobehavioral changes, depending on the dose and timing of drug administration. Trained personnel to care for the newborn in the immediate postpartum period should be available and made aware about the risk of neonatal respiratory depression due to maternally administered opioids. Commonly used parenteral opioids are meperidine, fentanyl, butorphanol, nalbuphine, remifentanil (Table 33.1).[12]

The advantages of PCA are better pain relief with lower drug doses, lesser side effects, and higher patient satisfaction, as the mother can adjust the administration of opioid as per her individual needs (Table 33.2).

Remifentanil is an ultra-short-acting synthetic opioid with rapid onset (blood-brain equilibration time 1.2–1.4

Table 33.1 PARENTERAL OPIOIDS FOR INTERMITTENT BOLUS USE DURING LABOR

OPIOID	IV DOSE	IM DOSE	ONSET OF ACTION (MIN)	DURATION
Meperidine	25–50 mg	50–100 mg	5–10 IV; 40–45 IM	2–3 hrs.
Fentanyl	25–50 mcg	100 mcg	2–3 IV; 10 IM	30–60 min
Butorphanol	1–2 mg	1–2 mg	5–10 IV; 10–30 IM	3–4 hrs.
Nalbuphine	10–20 mg	10–20 mg	2–3 IV; 15 IM	3–6 hrs.
Morphine	2–5 mg	5–10 mg	3–5 IV; 20–40 IM	3–4 hrs.

IV = intravenous; IM= intramuscular; mcg = microgram.

Table 33.2 **PARENTERAL OPIOIDS FOR PATIENT CONTROLLED LABOR ANALGESIA**

OPIOID	PATIENT CONTROLLED DOSE (IV)	LOCKOUT INTERVAL
Meperidine	10–15 mg	8–20 min
Nalbuphine	1–3 mg	6–10 min
Fentanyl	10–25 mcg	5–12 min
Remifentanil (bolus only)*	0.4–0.5 mcg/kg	2–3 min

*Remifentanil (background infusion + bolus): Infusion rate 0.05 mcg/kg/min with lockout interval 2–3 min and bolus dose of 0.25 mcg/kg.

min) and short duration of action (metabolized by plasma and tissue esterases).[13] The effective analgesic half-time is 6 minutes. It is a popular agent for use in labor PCA. As with all other opioids, careful patient monitoring is required to avoid excessive sedation and respiratory depression. Ketamine and benzodiazepines can be used as adjuncts to systemic opioids for labor analgesia, but because of adverse side effects, these medications are avoided in favor of neuraxial blocks and PCA techniques.

Neuraxial Analgesia/Anesthesia

Neuraxial anesthesia offers analgesia and anesthesia for labor, vaginal delivery, cesarean section, and is considered the gold standard because of its limited effects on both the mother and fetus.[5] Neuraxial anesthesia for labor and delivery includes continuous epidural, combined spinal epidural (CSE), continuous spinal and caudal blocks. Caudal blocks are infrequently used in present-day obstetric anesthesia. Continuous spinal analgesia may be used in cases of unintentional dural puncture but is not practical in most parturients. Single-shot spinal techniques are typically not very useful due to the long and unpredictable nature of labor. Neuraxial analgesia/anesthesia relies primarily on the palpation of anatomical landmarks, which can be obscured in the setting of obesity, edema, and anatomical variation.[5,7]

Advantages of neuraxial labor analgesia include: (1) complete analgesia that prevents pain and stress-induced maternal catecholamine surge and hyperventilation; (2) maternal participation in the process of childbirth due to lack of sedation; (3) no neonatal sedation or respiratory depression; (4) continuous analgesia with catheter techniques can be used to provide surgical anesthesia in eventuality of an emergency cesarean section, avoiding the need for general anesthesia.

Disadvantages of neuraxial labor analgesia include: (1) it requires a skilled anesthesia provider; (2) it may prolong the second stage of labor, increasing the chances of an instrumental vaginal delivery; (3) an associated sympathectomy that typically causes maternal hypotension; (4) it may reduce utero-placental circulation with associated FHR changes; and (5) the possibility of a patchy or failed block.

Absolute contraindications to neuraxial analgesia include patient refusal, maternal coagulopathy, infection at puncture site, and allergy to local anesthetic agents. Relative contraindications include maternal hypovolemia, lumbar spine pathology, and untreated systemic infection.

Initiation of neuraxial labor anesthesia should begin with a pre-anesthesia evaluation, along with informed consent about the benefits and complications of the procedure. The caregiver must confirm availability of the resuscitation equipment and medications. Basic monitoring should include noninvasive blood pressure measurement (NIBP), pulse oximetry, and continuous FHR record. Non-reassuring FHR patterns are associated with neuraxial blocks due to the hypotension following sympathectomy and intrathecal opioid administration. The American Society of Anesthesiologists (ASA) Task Force on Obstetric Anesthesia recommends monitoring of the FHR before and after initiation of regional analgesia for labor pain management.[14] Intravenous access should be established, and maternal hydration started with a non-dextrose-containing balanced salt solution (lactated ringer's) before block initiation. Aseptic precautions must be maintained during block placement.

LUMBAR EPIDURAL BLOCK

TECHNIQUE

The lumbar epidural space (usually L2–L3/ L3–L4) is identified using a 17- or 18-gauge Tuohy/Husted needle, with the mother in sitting or lateral position. A 19- or 20-gauge flexible catheter is passed into the epidural space to provide continuous labor analgesia. An epidural test dose consisting of lidocaine 1.5% with epinephrine 5 mcg/mL (1:200,000) to a total volume of 3 mL is given to recognize an unintentional intravascular or subarachnoid placement. An increase in the maternal heart rate by 20 bpm within one minute and motor blockade in 3–5 minutes indicates intravascular and intrathecal placement, respectively. After ruling out a malpositioned catheter, epidural analgesia is initiated using a bolus injection of the anesthetic agents and maintained with intermittent boluses or a continuous infusion. The epidural catheter is removed after delivery when the parturient is stable enough to be sent to the postpartum unit.

COMBINED SPINAL EPIDURAL BLOCK (CSE)

TECHNIQUE

This is usually performed as a needle-through-needle technique. After the lumbar epidural space is identified as described above, a long 25- or 27-gauge spinal needle is introduced through the Tuohy/Husted needle. Intrathecal agent is injected after the dura is punctured and the spinal needle is withdrawn. A catheter is then threaded into the epidural space, fixed to skin, and used for continuous analgesia

Advantages of the CSE technique include: (1) a faster onset of analgesia as compared to the epidural block alone; (2) an intrathecal injection of an opioid alone, without a local anesthetic agent, in early labor allows for good pain relief without motor blockade; (3) a combination of an opioid with local anesthesia in an advanced rapidly progressing labor provides good sacral analgesia within minutes; and (4) a lower dose of an opioid is required as compared to a systemic or epidural dose.

Disadvantages of this technique include: (1) a higher incidence of maternal pruritus and fetal heart rate (FHR) changes noted after intrathecal administration of opioids; (2) dural puncture is required, although the incidence of post-dural puncture headache (PDPH) is not any higher as compared to epidural analgesia; (3) after initiation of CSE, it is difficult to evaluate functioning of the epidural catheter for 1–2 hours until the effect of intrathecally administered medications wears off; and (4) it may not be a practical option when an adequately functioning epidural catheter has to be ensured (e.g., difficult airway, FHR changes with high possibility of urgent cesarean section).

PRE-PROCEDURE ULTRASOUND IMAGING FOR LABOR ANALGESIA

The failure rate for labor epidural analgesia is reported to range from 1.5% to 20%.[3,15,16] Morbidly obese parturients have an even higher incidence of initial failure rate, with reports as high as 42%.[17] Ultrasound imaging is relatively cheap, compact, readily available for point of care testing, involves no radiation, and supplements the relevant anatomical information already obtained using standard palpation techniques.[5,7] As a result, ultrasound imaging is becoming increasingly popular and is now recognized as the clinical gold standard to facilitate nerve block placement because it improves success rates and increases efficiency.[3,5,18]

Advantages of the use of ultrasonography are included in Boxes 33.1 and 33.2.[3,4,5,15,17,19]

In the experienced clinician, point-of-care ultrasound imaging can be of particular benefit in parturients with difficult anatomy and/or landmarks.

In a systemic review and meta-analysis, Perlas et al.[20] determined that ultrasound-assisted lumbar neuraxial ultrasound for spinal and epidural anesthesia provides accurate measurement of the depth of the epidural and intrathecal space and improves efficacy of neuraxial anesthesia, increases accuracy of identification of lumbar interspaces, and can improve neuraxial anesthesia safety. The technique has also proven useful with the combined spinal epidural (CSE) technique.[5,21]

Disadvantages of point-of-care ultrasound imaging include that slight differences (± 0.1 cm) in depth measurement are to be expected. These differences can be attributed to: (1) the ultrasound probe and epidural needle placed at different angles to the skin (optimal correlation occurs when both the probe and epidural needle are placed perpendicular to the skin); (2) the epidural needle being off midline in trajectory; and (3) the blunt epidural needle causing tissue deformation.[3,15,22]

Box 33.1 AVAILABLE DATA OBTAINED FROM NEURAXIAL ULTRASOUND

- Interspace identification
- Establishment of midline
- Estimate depth to the epidural space
- Determine optimal interspace and best insertion space
- Angulation of the Tuohy/Husted needle insertion

TECHNIQUE

Understanding vertebral anatomy is helpful in understanding spinal sonanatomy. Figure 33.1A, 33.1B. Ultrasound guidance for neuraxial placement is most commonly performed before the procedure to establish landmarks and orientation (Figure 33.2). Scanning of the lower back is usually performed in the longitudinal paramedian, longitudinal median, and transverse median planes (Figures 33.2, 33.3, 33.4). Since ultrasound measurements in these planes have high clinical Pearson's correlation coefficients (longitudinal median plane = 0.914, transverse plane = 0.909), the averaging of multiple measurements in each plane is not necessary.[3]

A low-frequency (2–5 MHz) curved array transducer probe (the same transducer used by obstetricians for fetal scanning of the uterus) with a depth of 15 cm is used for scanning.[3,5,23,24] The low-frequency probe allows for deeper penetration of tissues but sacrifices resolution and precision of the image. An initial depth setting of 7–8 cm is appropriate for most patients, but the depth, focus, and gain settings of the ultrasound machine should be adjusted as needed during the scanning process to produce an optimal image.[5,24]

LONGITUDINAL PARAMEDIAN OBLIQUE VIEW

The structures identified in this view include the sacrum, articular process, ligamentum flavum and posterior dura mater, intrathecal space, anterior dura, posterior longitudinal ligament, vertebral bodies.

Box 33.2 IMPROVED EFFICACY OF NEURAXIAL ULTRASOUND

- Reduces the number of epidural attempts, redirects, and levels attempted
- Decreases epidural catheter replacements
- Improved analgesia
- Higher maternal satisfaction
- Improved learning curve in resident trainees

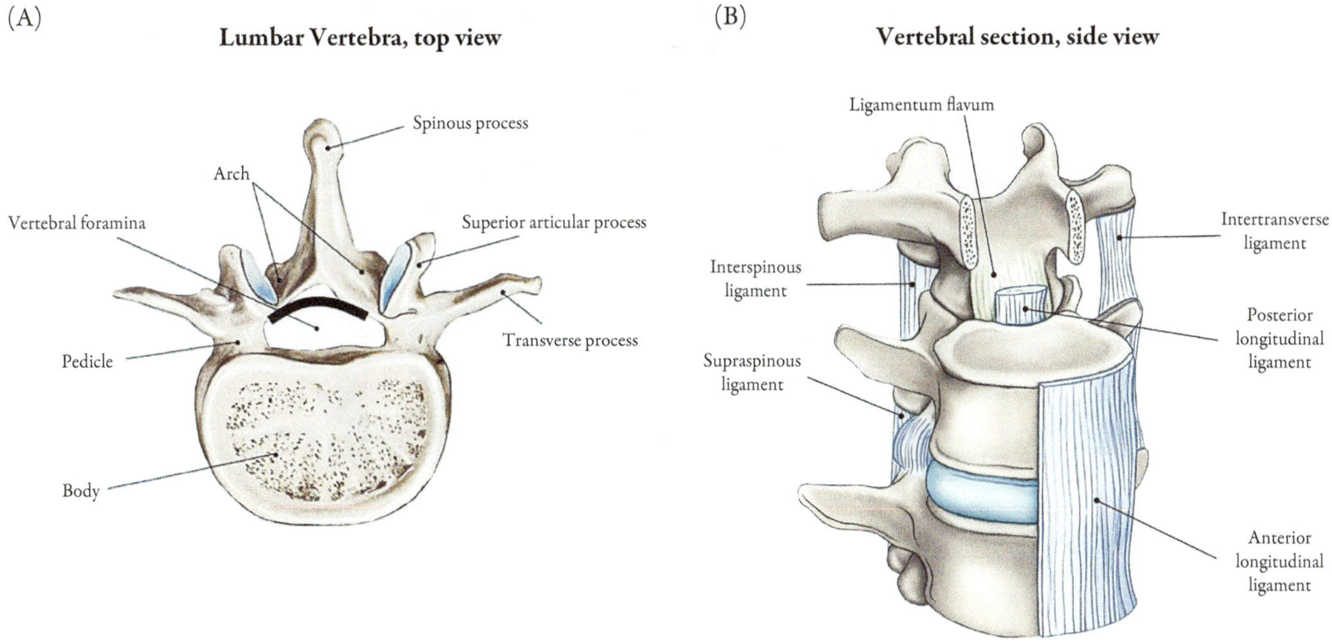

Figure 33.1 (A) Top view of the lumbar vertebra showing anatomical structures identified with ultrasound including the spinous process and transverse processes. * Concave shape ⌒ in lumbar vertebral foramen denotes the posterior dura/ligamentum flavum/epidural space.

(B) Vertebral section side view. Ligaments of the lumbar vertebrae. Ligaments the epidural needle traverse using the midline technique include the supraspinatus, the interspinatus, and the ligamentum flavum. In the paramedian technique, only the ligamentum flavum is traversed.

The ligamentum flavum, epidural space, and posterior dura appear as a single linear hyperechoic structure, which is termed the posterior complex.[5,24] Similarly, the anterior dura, posterior longitudinal ligament, and posterior aspect of the vertebral body or the intervertebral disc also appear as a single linear hyperechoic structure and are collectively referred to as the anterior complex.[5,24] The transducer is positioned vertically 1–2 cm lateral to the spinous process and the ultrasound beam is directed obliquely toward the midline. The spinal canal is visible between the interlaminar spaces. The delineating structures are the ligamentum flavum and dura mater posteriorly and the posterior vertebral body cortex and posterior longitudinal ligament anteriorly. The epidural space appears as a thin hypoechoic line between two hyperechoic lines produced by the ligamentum flavum extending between the laminae and the posterior dura mater, located at a deeper level (Figure 33.2).

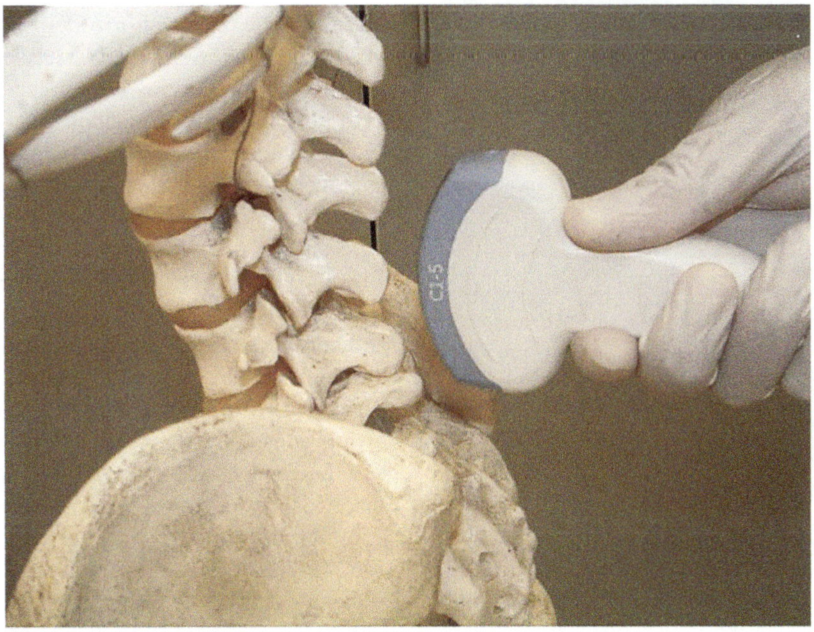

Figure 33.2 Position of the ultrasound probe in the skeletal longitudinal (para-median position).

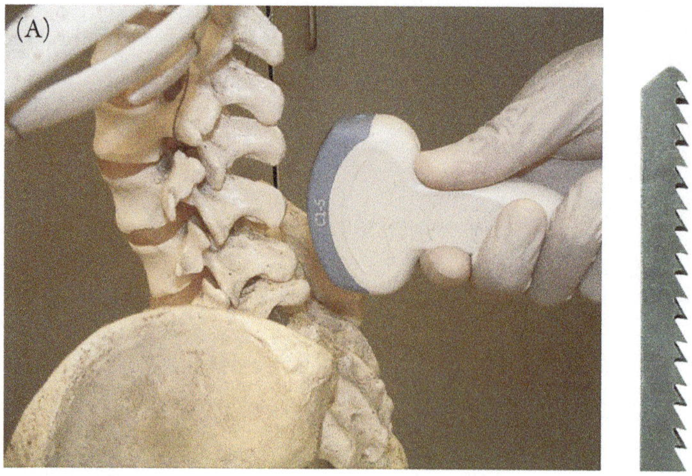

Figure 33.3A. Position of the ultrasound probe in the skeletal longitudinal median plane (midline position). Saw-teeth appearance showed on the right side of the image.

LONGITUDINAL MEDIAN VIEW

This view visualizes the spinous processes and identifies the vertebral levels (Figures 33.3 A, B, C. The structures identified include the sacrum, articular process, ligamentum flavum and posterior dura mater, anterior dura mater, posterior longitudinal ligament, and vertebral bodies. The transducer is placed on the midline, along the spinous processes, in the longitudinal direction. The spinous processes are seen as a series of hyperechoic lines with upward convexity and posterior acoustic shadowing. A "saw" sign, which represents the spinous processes (saw teeth), and the hyperechoic band at the base of the saw waere confirmed (Figure 33.3A, B, C).[3] The sacrum is seen as a flat continuous hyperechoic line compared to the more convex spinous processes.

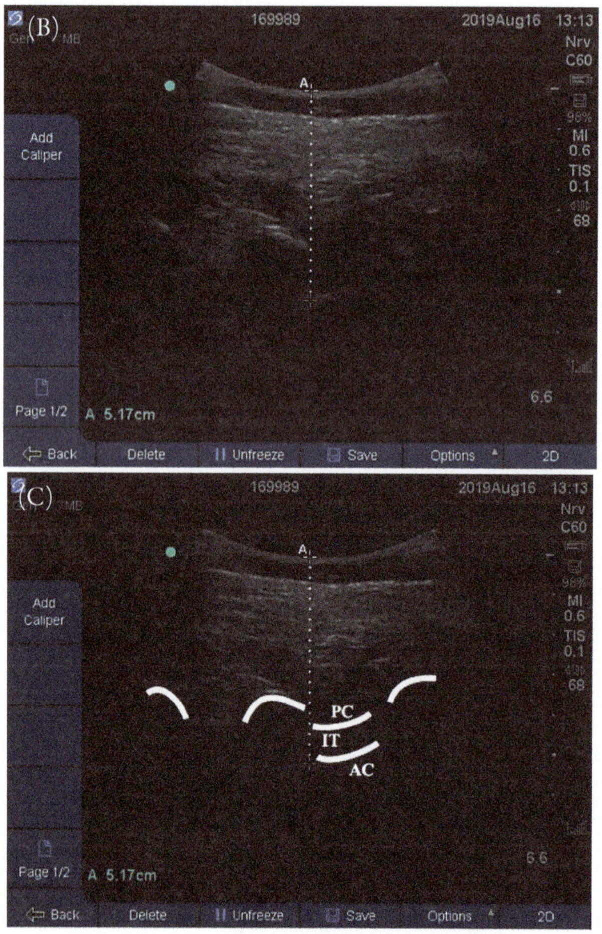

Figure 33.3B and C. Ultrasound image in the longitudinal median plane. "A" represents the distance from the skin to the AC = anterior complex (anterior dura, posterior longitudinal ligament, and posterior aspect of the vertebral body or intervertebral disc), seen in left lower corner as 5.17 cm. PC = posterior complex (ligamentum flavum, epidural space, and posterior dura. IT = intrathecal space.

TRANSVERSE MEDIAN VIEW

In this view, the spinous process, laminae, articular process, transverse process, ligamentum flavum, posterior dura mater, anterior dura mater, posterior longitudinal ligament, and vertebral body can be identified (Figure 33.4A, B).[5,6] The probe is placed on the midline horizontally, perpendicular to the long axis of the spine in the intervertebral space (Figure 33.4A).

The spinous process is seen as a convex hyperechoic line with posterior acoustic shadowing. On either side of, or deep to the spinous process, the laminae produce two horizontal hyperechoic lines with posterior acoustic shadowing. These two oblique hyperechoic lines correspond to the transverse processes. In the midline and within the vertebral interspace, an equal sign (=) can be seen where the upper and lower parallel lines represent the ligamentum flavum/posterior dura and vertebral body/posterior longitudinal ligament/anterior dura, respectively (Figure 33.4C). Positioning the transducer between two spinous processes eliminates the acoustic shadowing, thus allowing visualization of the spinal canal, which is bounded by two hyperechoic parallel lines. The epidural space is above the dura mater, which is seen as a hyperechoic line. The deepest line is the posterior longitudinal ligament and posterior cortex of the vertebral body. The direction and angle of the probe used for transverse plane visualization that provides the best image is the same angle and direction that should be used for epidural and spinal needle placement.[3,5]

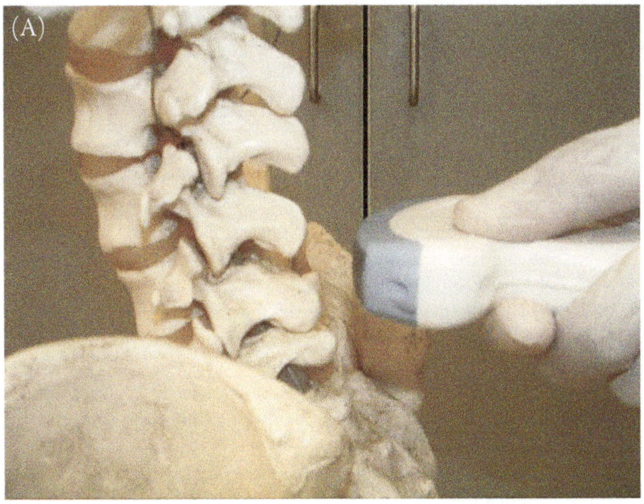

Figure 33.4A. Position of the ultrasound probe in the skeletal median transverse plane.

Once an optimal view has been obtained, the depth from skin surface to the posterior complex may be measured using the electronic caliper built into the ultrasound machine (Figure 33.4B, C).[3,5,24]

REAL-TIME ULTRASOUND VISUALIZATION

Real-time ultrasound guidance for neuraxial procedures is not commonly utilized by practitioners but is becoming more popular as technology and needle-guide devices are being developed.[5,6] Currently, ultrasound probe dimensions, as well as the need to use two hands in securing and placing the needle, makes real-time ultrasound needle placement technically challenging for the single user.[5,23] However, automated loss-of-resistance syringes and needle-guide systems have facilitated performance by the single operator.[5,6]

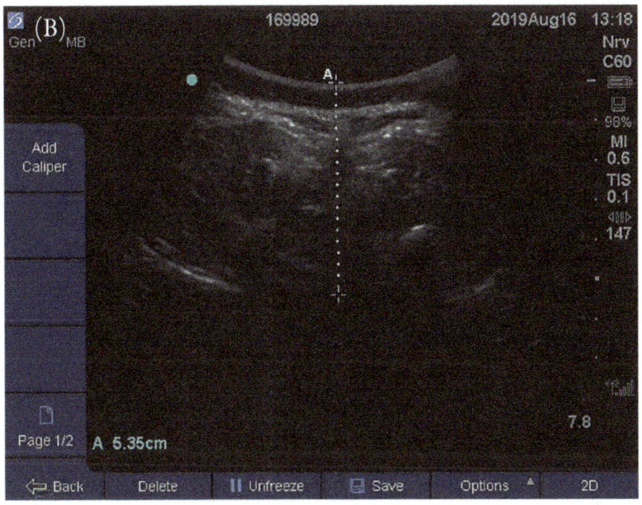

Figure 33.4B. Ultrasound image in the median transverse plane.

"A" represents the distance from the skin to the epidural space (seen in left lower corner as 5.35 cm).

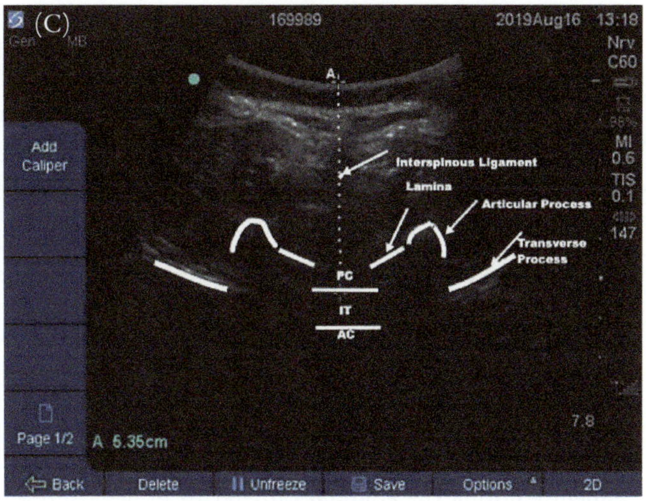

Figure 33.4C. Ultrasound image in the median transverse plane with labels.

Skeletal anatomy superimposed. Note the equal sign (=) where the upper and lower parallel lines represent the ligamentum flavum/posterior dura and vertebral body/posterior longitudinal ligament/anterior dura. PC = posterior complex (ligamentum flavum, epidural space, and posterior dura), AC = anterior complex (anterior dura, posterior longitudinal ligament, and posterior aspect of the vertebral body or intervertebral disc). IT = intrathecal space.

SPINAL AFTER EPIDURAL ANALGESIA

Single-shot spinal anesthesia after a failed epidural can provide fast onset and reliable surgical anesthesia. However, the possibility of an unpredictably high or total spinal anesthesia can occur, especially if the epidural catheter is dosed within 30 minutes of the spinal anesthetic.[25,26] Einhorn et al.[26] retrospectively searched their perioperative database for women with a labor epidural who received spinal or combined spinal-epidural anesthesia for cesarean delivery due to the inadequacy of the existing epidural. They had 263 patients in their analysis; 29 (11%) had failed spinals and 9 (3%) had high spinals. Of the 9 patients with a high spinal, 56% (n = 5) had to be converted to general anesthesia due to weakness, altered mentation, or respiratory distress, and 44% (n = 4) had recorded block levels ≥T1 without conversion to general anesthesia.[26] The mechanism of a high spinal after epidural analgesia is thought to be compression of the dural sac by residual anesthetic in the epidural space, resulting in cephalad displacement of the intrathecal dose within the cerebrospinal fluid (CSF).[26] Similarly, the Society for Obstetric Anesthesia and Perinatology developed a Serious Complication Repository (SCORE) project to establish the incidence of serious complications related to obstetric anesthesia and to identify risk factors associated with each of these complications.[27] Most patients in the SCORE project who developed a high neuraxial block from spinal and epidural anesthesia had known risk factors, the most frequent of which were obesity and the administration of spinal anesthetic after a failed epidural anesthetic.[27]

Measures to prevent a high spinal (total spinal) after single-shot spinal anesthesia after failed epidural include using a lower intrathecal dose (20%–30%), limiting top-up doses to greater than 30 minutes prior to spinal administration, delaying supine positioning for at least 1 minute following spinal placement, and having a low threshold to supplement the patient with an intravenous vasopressor (ephedrine, phenylephrine, norepinephrine) and/or start a background prophylactic vasopressor infusion.[25,26]

Another technique that can be utilized to prevent a high spinal is a combined spinal epidural (CSE) using a decreased spinal dose (1 mL = 7.5 mg of 0.75% bupivacaine) and subsequently dosing the epidural catheter to provide surgical anesthesia. Administration of a lower spinal dose would reduce the risk of a high spinal, and the epidural catheter would provide the ability to extend the block. However, a CSE can be more time-consuming compared with a single-shot spinal, especially if there is urgency to the cesarean delivery.

CONCLUSIONS

Pre-procedure ultrasound imaging allows for greater accuracy and fewer needle passes by providing reliable and accurate information for successful neuraxial placement, such as determination of the midline, deciding the optimal vertebral interspace level in those with normal and difficult anatomy, finding the optimal insertion point, locating the best angle for needle insertion, and accurately determining the proper depth for needle advancement. These advantages can enhance the parturient's overall comfort, experience, and satisfaction, by reducing the risk of failed or traumatic lumbar punctures and epidural catheterizations, the number of insertion attempts, and needle redirections.

REFERENCES

1. Balki M. Locating the epidural space in obstetric patients-ultrasound a useful tool: continuing professional development. *Can J Anaesth*. 2010;57(12):1111–1126.
2. Ellison M, Ranganathan P, Wang H, Vallejo MC. Ultrasound and the pregnant patient. *Curr Anesthesiol Rep*. 2017;7(1):76–83.
3. Vallejo MC, Phelps AL, Singh S, Orebaugh SL, Sah N. Ultrasound decreases the failed labor epidural rate in resident trainees. *Int J Obstet Anesth*. 2010;19(4):373–378.
4. Blair JM, Hill DA, Fee JPH. Patient-controlled analgesia for labour using remifentanil: a feasibility study. *Br J Anaesth*. 2001;87(3):415–420.
5. Vallejo MC. Pre-procedure neuraxial ultrasound in obstetric anesthesia. *J Anesth Perioper Med*. 2018;5(2):85–91.
6. Lee A. Ultrasound in obstetric anesthesia. *Semin Perinatol*. 2014;38(6):349–358.
7. Shaikh F, Brzezinski J, Alexander S, Arzola C, Carvalho JCA, Beyene J. Ultrasound imaging for lumbar punctures and epidural catheterisations: systematic review and meta-analysis. *BMJ*. 2013;346:f1720.
8. Wong CA. Advances in labor analgesia. *Int J Womens Health*. 2009;1:139–154.
9. Likis FE, Andrews JC, Collins MR, et al. Nitrous oxide for the management of labor pain: a systematic review. *Anesth Analg*. 2014;118(1);153–167.
10. Vallejo MC, Phelps AL, Shepherd CJ, Kaul B, Mandell GL, Ramanathan S. Nitrous oxide anxiolysis for elective cesarean section. *J Clin Anesth*. 2005:17(7):543–548.
11. Yeo ST, Holdcroft A, Yentis SM, Stewart A. Analgesia with sevoflurane during labour: i. determination of the optimum concentration. *Br J Anaesth*. 2007;98(1):105–109.
12. Vallejo MC. Principles of obstetric anesthesia. Retrieved from Dr. Vallejo's academic website: http://www.drvallejo.net/documents. Accessed March 27, 2020.
13. Grau T, Leipold RW, Horter J, Conradi R, Martin E, Motsch J. The lumbar epidural space in pregnancy: visualization by ultrasonography. *Br J Anaesth*. 2001;86(6):798–804.
14. Practice guidelines for obstetric anesthesia: an updated report by the American Society of Anesthesiologists Task Force on Obstetric Anesthesia and the Society for Obstetric Anesthesia and Perinatology. *Anesthesiology*. 2016;124(2):270–300.
15. Grau T, Leipold RW, Conradi R, Martin E, Motsch J. Efficacy of ultrasound imaging in obstetric epidural anesthesia. *J Clin Anest*. 2002;14(3):169–175.
16. Pan PH, Bogard TD, Owen MD. Incidence and characteristics of failures in obstetric neuraxial analgesia and anesthesia: a retrospective analysis of 19,259 deliveries. *Int J Obstet Anesth*. 2004;13(4):227–233.
17. Singh S, Wirth KM, Phelps AL, et al. Epidural catheter placement in morbidly obese parturients with the use of an epidural depth equation prior to ultrasound visualization. *Scientific World Journal*. 2013 Jul 25;2013:695209.
18. Hopkins PM. Ultrasound guidance as a gold standard in regional anaesthesia. *Br J Anaesth*. 2007;98(3);299–301.
19. Grau T, Bartusseck E, Conradi R, Martin E, Motsch J. Ultrasound imaging improves learning curves in obstetric epidural anesthesia: a preliminary study. *Can J Anaesth*. 2003;50(10):1047–1050.
20. Perlas A, Chaparro LE, Chin KJ. Lumbar neuraxial ultrasound for spinal and epidural anesthesia: a systematic review and meta-analysis. *Reg Anesth Pain Med*. 2016;41(2):251–260.
21. Nassar M, Abdelazim IA. Pre-puncture ultrasound guided epidural insertion before vaginal delivery. *J Clin Monit Comput*. 2015;29(5):573–577.
22. Currie JM. Measurement of the depth to the extradural space using ultrasound. *Br J Anaesth*. 1984;56(4):345–347.
23. Darrieutort-Laffite C, Hamel O, Glémarec J, Maugars Y, Le Goff B. Ultrasonography of the lumbar spine: sonoanatomy and practical applications. *Joint Bone Spine*. 2014;81(2):130–136.
24. Chin KJ, Karmakar MK, Peng P. Ultrasonography of the adult thoracic and lumbar spine for central neuraxial blockade. *Anesthesiology*. 2011;114(6):1459–1485.
25. Portnoy D, Vadhera RB. Mechanisms and management of an incomplete epidural block for cesarean section. *Anesthesiol Clin North Am*. 2003;21(1):39–57.
26. Einhorn LM, Habib AS. Evaluation of failed and high blocks associated with spinal anesthesia for cesarean delivery following inadequate labour epidural: a retrospective cohort study. *Can J Anaesth*. 2016;63(10):1170–1178.
27. D'Angelo R, Smiley RM, Riley ET, Segal S. Serious complications related to obstetric anesthesia: the serious complication repository project of the society for obstetric anesthesia and perinatology. *Anesthesiology*. 2014;120(6):1505–1512.

REVIEW QUESTIONS

(1) Which of the following parenteral opioids is ultra-short-acting with a rapid onset and short duration?

A. Fentanyl
B. Butorphanol
C. Remifentanil
D. Nalbuphine

(2) A disadvantage of conventional labor epidural analgesia without the use of ultrasound is

A. Complete analgesia that prevents pain and stress induced maternal catecholamine surge and hyperventilation
B. Labor epidural analgesia failure rates from 1.5%–20%
C. Minimal to no neonatal sedation or respiratory depression
D. Continuous analgesia with the ability to provide surgical anesthesia in eventuality of an emergency cesarean section, avoiding the need for general anesthesia

(3) Which of the following anatomic structures is not part of the "anterior complex"?

A. Ligamentum flavum
B. Anterior dura
C. Vertebral body
D. Posterior longitudinal ligament

(4) Which of the following anatomic structures is not part of the "posterior complex"?

A. Ligamentum flavum
B. Epidural space
C. Posterior dura
D. Vertebral body

(5) Which transducer probe is best used for neuraxial ultrasound visualization?

A. Curved array
B. Linear array
C. Phased array
D. All are equally useful for neuraxial ultrasound visualization.

(6) How much should the intrathecal dose be reduced in a patient undergoing a single-shot spinal anesthetic for cesarean delivery after a failed epidural bolus catheter dose within 30 minutes of the surgical procedure?

A. 10% to 20%
B. 20% to 30%
C. 30% to 40%
D. 40% to 50%

(7) Data not obtained from the use of neuraxial ultrasound is:

A. Exact/accurate depth to the epidural space
B. Interspace identification
C. Establishment of midline
D. Determination of the best needle-insertion space

(8) Which of the following is not a benefit of neuraxial ultrasound?

A. Reduces the number of epidural needle attempts, needle redirections, and levels attempted
B. Decreases the number of epidural catheter replacements
C. Better maternal analgesia
D. Improved Apgar scores

(9) The "equal sign" can be seen in which of the following neuraxial ultrasound views?

A. Longitudinal paramedian oblique view
B. Longitudinal median view
C. Transverse median view
D. All the above

(10) The "saw sign" cannot be seen in which neuraxial ultrasound view?

A. Longitudinal paramedian oblique view
B. Longitudinal median view
C. Transverse median view
D. All the above

ANSWERS

(1) **C.** Remifentanil is an ultra-short acting synthetic opioid with rapid onset (blood-brain equilibration time 1.2–1.4 min) and short duration of action (metabolized by plasma and tissue esterases).

Reference

Grau T, Leipold RW, Horter J, Conradi R, Martin E, Motsch J. The lumbar epidural space in pregnancy: visualization by ultrasonography. *Br J Anaesth*. 2001;86(6):798–804.

(2) **B.** The failure rate for labor epidural analgesia is reported to range from 1.5% to 20%.

References

Vallejo MC, Phelps AL, Singh S, Orebaugh SL, Sah N. Ultrasound decreases the failed labor epidural rate in resident trainees. *Int J Obstet Anesth*. 2010;19(4):373–378.

Grau T, Leipold RW, Conradi R, Martin E, Motsch J. Efficacy of ultrasound imaging in obstetric epidural anesthesia. *J Clin Anest*. 2002;14(3):169–175.

Pan PH, Bogard TD, Owen MD. Incidence and characteristics of failures in obstetric neuraxial analgesia and anesthesia: a retrospective analysis of 19,259 deliveries. *Int J Obstet Anesth*. 2004;13(4):227–233.

Vallejo MC, Phelps AL, Singh S, Orebaugh SL, Sah N. Ultrasound decreases the failed labor epidural rate in resident trainees. *Int J Obstet Anesth*. 2010;19(4):373–378.

(3) **A.** The anatomic structures seen with the use of neuraxial ultrasound in the "anterior complex" include the anterior dura, posterior longitudinal ligament, and posterior aspect of the vertebral body or the intervertebral disc.

References

Vallejo MC. Pre-procedure neuraxial ultrasound in obstetric anesthesia. *J Anesth Perioper Med*. 2018;5(2):85–91.

Chin KJ, Karmakar MK, Peng P. Ultrasonography of the adult thoracic and lumbar spine for central neuraxial blockade. *Anesthesiology*. 2011;114(6):1459–1485.

(4) **D.** The anatomic structures seen with the use of neuraxial ultrasound in the "posterior complex" include the ligamentum flavum, epidural space, and posterior dura.

References

Vallejo MC. Pre-procedure neuraxial ultrasound in obstetric anesthesia. *J Anesth Perioper Med.* 2018;5(2):85–91.

Chin KJ, Karmakar MK, Peng P. Ultrasonography of the adult thoracic and lumbar spine for central neuraxial blockade. *Anesthesiology.* 2011;114(6):1459–1485.

(5) **A.** A low-frequency (2–5 MHz) curved array transducer probe (the same transducer used by obstetricians for fetal scanning of the uterus) with a depth of 15 cm is used for scanning. The low-frequency probe allows for deeper penetration of tissues but sacrifices resolution and precision of the image. An initial depth setting of 7–8 cm is appropriate for most patients, but the depth, focus, and gain settings of the ultrasound machine should be adjusted as needed during the scanning process to produce an optimal image.

References

Vallejo MC, Phelps AL, Singh S, Orebaugh SL, Sah N. Ultrasound decreases the failed labor epidural rate in resident trainees. *Int J Obstet Anesth.* 2010;19(4):373–378.

Vallejo MC. Pre-procedure neuraxial ultrasound in obstetric anesthesia. *J Anesth Perioper Med.* 2018;5(2):85–91.

Chin KJ, Karmakar MK, Peng P. Ultrasonography of the adult thoracic and lumbar spine for central neuraxial blockade. *Anesthesiology.* 2011;114(6):1459–1485.

Darrieutort-Laffite C, Hamel O, Glémarec J, Maugars Y, Le Goff B. Ultrasonography of the lumbar spine: sonoanatomy and practical applications. *Joint Bone Spine.* 2014;81(2):130–136.

(6) **B.** The technique of providing a single-shot spinal anesthetic after epidural analgesia can be a safe alternative provided appropriate precautions and modifications are taken. These modifications include limiting the amount of epidural local anesthetic administered when diagnosing a nonfunctioning epidural and decreasing the dose of intrathecal local anesthetic by 20% to 30%. Other measures to prevent a high spinal (total spinal) include having the patient remain in the sitting position for up to 1 minute after the spinal anesthetic to allow the block to set, having a low threshold to supplement the patient with an intravenous vasopressor (ephedrine, phenylephrine, norepinephrine) and/or start a background prophylactic vasopressor infusion. Another technique that can be utilized to prevent a high spinal after epidural analgesia includes providing a combined spinal epidural (CSE) technique using a decreased spinal dose (1 mL = 7.5 mg of 0.75% bupivacaine) and subsequently dosing the epidural catheter to provide surgical anesthesia.

Reference

Portnoy D, Vadhera RB. Mechanisms and management of an incomplete epidural block for cesarean section. *Anesthesiol Clin North Am.* 2003;21(1):39–57.

(7) **A.** Slight differences (± 0.1 cm) are expected to occur in ultrasound depth measurement. These differences can be attributed to: (1) the ultrasound probe and epidural needle placed at different angles to the skin (optimal correlation occurs when both the probe and epidural needle are placed perpendicular to the skin), (2) the epidural needle being off midline in trajectory, and (3) the blunt epidural needle causing tissue deformation.

References

Vallejo MC, Phelps AL, Singh S, Orebaugh SL, Sah N. Ultrasound decreases the failed labor epidural rate in resident trainees. *Int J Obstet Anesth.* 2010;19(4):373–378.

Grau T, Leipold RW, Conradi R, Martin E, Motsch J. Efficacy of ultrasound imaging in obstetric epidural anesthesia. *J Clin Anest.* 2002;14(3):169–175.

Currie JM. Measurement of the depth to the extradural space using ultrasound. *Br J Anaesth.* 1984;56(4):345–347.

(8) **D.** Benefits of neuraxial ultrasound include reduced needle attempts, reduced number of needle redirects and levels attempted, decreased epidural catheter replacements, improved analgesia, higher maternal satisfaction, and improved ultrasound technique learning curve in resident trainees. Improved Apgar scores are not a benefit.

References

Ellison M, Ranganathan P, Wang H, Vallejo MC. Ultrasound and the pregnant patient. *Curr Anesthesiol Rep.* 2017;7(1):76–83.

Vallejo MC, Phelps AL, Singh S, Orebaugh SL, Sah N. Ultrasound decreases the failed labor epidural rate in resident trainees. *Int J Obstet Anesth.* 2010;19(4):373–378.

Chin KJ, Karmakar MK, Peng P. Ultrasonography of the adult thoracic and lumbar spine for central neuraxial blockade. *Anesthesiology.* 2011;114(6):1459–1485.

Grau T, Leipold RW, Conradi R, Martin E, Motsch J. Efficacy of ultrasound imaging in obstetric epidural anesthesia. *J Clin Anest.* 2002;14(3):169–175.

Grau T, Bartusseck E, Conradi R, Martin E, Motsch J. Ultrasound imaging improves learning curves in obstetric epidural anesthesia: a preliminary study. *Can J Anaesth.* 2003;50(10):1047–1050.

Singh S, Wirth KM, Phelps AL, et al. Epidural catheter placement in morbidly obese parturients with the use of an epidural depth equation prior to ultrasound visualization. *Scientific World Journal.* 2013 Jul 25;2013:695209.

(9) **D.** In the transverse median, the longitudinal paramedian oblique, and the longitudinal median ultrasound views, an "equal sign" (=) can be seen where the upper and lower parallel lines represent the posterior complex (PC = ligamentum flavum, epidural space, posterior dura) and anterior complex (AC = anterior dura, posterior longitudinal ligament, and posterior aspect of the vertebral body/intervertebral disc), respectively.

Reference

Vallejo MC. Pre-procedure neuraxial ultrasound in obstetric anesthesia. *J Anesth Perioper Med.* 2018;5(2):85–91.

(10) **C.** In the transverse median view, the "saw sign" cannot be seen. However, the "saw sign" can be seen in both the longitudinal paramedian oblique view and the longitudinal median ultrasound views.

Reference

Vallejo MC. Pre-procedure neuraxial ultrasound in obstetric anesthesia. *J Anesth Perioper* Med. *2018;*5(2):85–91.

34.

INADEQUATE LABOR EPIDURAL ANALGESIA

Mohamed Ibrahim and Rakesh Vadhera

STEM CASE AND KEY QUESTIONS

A 27-year-old gravida 2 para 1 parturient in active labor is admitted to labor and delivery suite. The pre-anesthesia evaluation shows no significant past medical or surgical history. On physical exam, she had a Mallampati 3 airway classification and within normal range vital signs. The patient reports that she was not happy about her previous labor epidural analgesia. Despite multiple attempts to bolus the catheter with local anesthetics, she felt significant pain on left side of her abdomen. Eventually, it was replaced, but unfortunately a wet tap happened during replacement, and she had severe headache after delivery that necessitated a blood patch. On this admission, her cervical examination showed 6 cm dilation, 100% effacement, −1 station, and her membranes ruptured before arrival to the hospital. Shortly after, her nurse reports that the patient is starting to complain of severe pelvic pain and is requesting an epidural placement.

(1) WHY DID SHE GET A UNILATERAL EPIDURAL COVERAGE PREVIOUSLY?

Unilateral epidural coverage can happen due to several reasons, such as excessive length of the catheter in epidural space. It may lead to transforaminal migration of catheter tip into the paravertebral space or its extension into anterior epidural space. Other anatomical factors, such as the presence of anatomical barriers within epidural space, e.g., dorsal median connective tissue band and scoliosis, may limit the flow of local anesthetic to one side of epidural space.

(2) THE PATIENT IS BECOMING RESTLESS, AND IN SEVERE PAIN; YOU DECIDE THAT YOU ARE GOING TO PROCEED WITH THE COMBINED SPINAL EPIDURAL (CSE) TECHNIQUE. WHAT BENEFITS DOES THE CSE TECHNIQUE CARRY OVER LABOR EPIDURAL ANALGESIA?

Both labor epidural analgesia and CSE have been shown to manage labor pain effectively. Studies have shown that the CSE technique has a quicker onset of analgesia, and increased incidence of maternal satisfaction, but showed no difference regarding labor outcome, incidence of post-dural puncture headache (PDPH), or rescue analgesia requirement.

(3) WOULD YOU HAVE PREFERRED A DURAL PUNCTURE EPIDURAL (DPE) OVER CSE OR LABOR EPIDURAL?

In comparison to traditional epidural technique, DPE carries the benefits of early onset and better sacral coverage; it decreases the incidence of a unilateral block and requires fewer physician interventions. Though CSE provides quicker analgesia compared to epidural or DPE, DPE has shown to decrease the incidence of hypotension, pruritis, and uterine hypertonus, thus decreasing the risk of fetal bradycardia that has been attributed to CSE technique.

(4) YOU PLAN TO PLACE A CSE. HOWEVER, YOU FIND THAT YOU RAN OUT OF THE CSE KITS. WHAT WILL YOU DO?

In case of absence of the preassembled kits, a 25–27 g of 12.7 cm (5 inch) long can be passed through an epidural needle of 9 cm (3.5 in.) long. Attempting to pass the desired spinal needle through the epidural needle is recommended before the start of the procedure, as it has been noted that different spinal and epidural needle hubs may not fit properly into each other, thus decreasing the spinal needle length that extends beyond the epidural needle tip (Figure 34.1).

(5) AFTER SUCCESSFULLY PLACING THE SPINAL MEDICATIONS AND TRYING TO THREAD THE EPIDURAL CATHETER, BLOOD IS OBSERVED FLOWING BACK IN THE CATHETER. HOW WILL YOU PROCEED?

The epidural catheter can be carefully withdrawn 1 cm back and flushed with saline prior to aspiration again. If blood aspiration persists, replacement of epidural catheter at a different level is warranted.

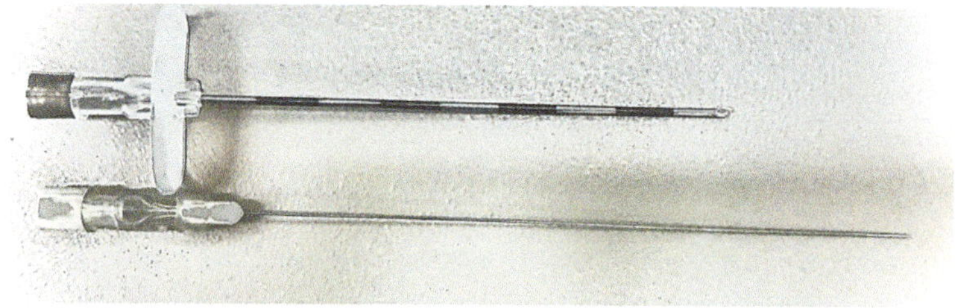

Figure 34.1. An assembled CSE kit: a 17G × 3 1/2″ epidural needle and a 27G × 4 11/16″ pencil point spinal needle.

(6) YOU MANIPULATED THE CATHETER AS BEFORE, AND NO MORE BLOOD WAS COMING. THEN YOU TEST THE CATHETER BY INJECTING LIDOCAINE WITH EPINEPHRINE. HOW ACCURATE ARE THE NEGATIVE ASPIRATION AND TEST DOSE IN CONFIRMING A LACK OF INTRAVASCULAR CANNULATION IN PREGNANT PATIENTS?

Aspiration through the epidural catheter cannot be the only test to exclude intravascular catheter placement. The development of soft-tip and multi-orifice catheters has improved the sensitivity of aspiration test compared to the stiff and single lumen catheters. Still, false-negative testing has been reported even with soft-tip and multi-orifice catheters, mostly when catheters are withdrawn back from the initial placement site.[1] While the epinephrine in test dose has been shown to have very high sensitivity (some studies report 100% sensitivity), it lacks specificity, as it is difficult to distinguish between the maternal tachycardia secondary to positive test dose and that secondary to pain during uterine contraction, causing false-positive test results.

(7) ASSUMING THERE WAS NO INTRAVASCULAR CANNULATION, AND THREADING THE CATHETER WAS UNEVENTFUL, AND THE SPINAL BLOCK IS WORKING WELL, WILL YOU TEST THE EPIDURAL? WHY?

Yes, I will test the catheter after the spinal component has worn off to rule out intravascular or intrathecal placement. If the patient is comfortable after the intrathecal injection of 2.5 mg bupivacaine and 15 mcg of fentanyl, I would still do the test dose after 45–60 minutes to avoid motor weakness that might take place secondary to the cumulative effect of epidural and intrathecal local anesthetics. The epinephrine component of the epidural test dose would exclude the possibility of intravascular catheter placement.

(8) SHORTLY AFTER CSE PLACEMENT, THE PATIENT BECOMES VERY COMFORTABLE. HOWEVER, SHE BECOMES MILDLY HYPOTENSIVE, AND THE FETUS BECOMES BRADYCARDIC. HOW WOULD YOU EVALUATE AND MANAGE THE PATIENT?

The subarachnoid opioid injection may cause fetal bradycardia that usually resolves within a few minutes with or without obstetric interventions. Management of maternal hypotension or fetal bradycardia will include left uterine displacement, 100% oxygen by facemask, and intravenous fluid boluses. Blood pressure support with phenylephrine or ephedrine might be warranted. Meanwhile, the anesthesia provider should be assessing the level of sensory block.

(9) AFTER A NEGATIVE EPIDURAL TEST DOSE, HOW WILL YOU RUN YOUR EPIDURAL?

Continuous epidural infusion (CEI) with patient-controlled epidural analgesia (PCEA) is the most common maintenance regimen. CEI of diluted bupivacaine concentration (0.0625%–0.125%) and fentanyl (2–3 mcg/ml) at 8–12 mL/hour would maintain continuous analgesia, thus maintaining hemodynamic stability. PCEA of 4–8 mL with 10–20 minutes lockout interval would better control breakthrough pain with less physician intervention.

(10) THE LABOR PROGRESSES WELL; HOWEVER, 3 HOURS LATER THE NURSE INFORMS YOU THAT THE PATIENT IS INCREASINGLY COMPLAINING OF LOWER BACK PAIN DESPITE THE PCEA USE. HOW CAN YOU MANAGE?

Part of the management is setting the patient's pain expectations right from the start. This is done by explaining that there might be some periods when the pain becomes uncontrolled. In this case, the epidural catheter can be bloused using a higher concentration of local anesthetic, e.g. 5 mL of 0.25% bupivacaine or 1% lidocaine in a semi-sitting position. Also, a 50–100 mcg fentanyl bolus can be given if the local anesthetic bolus did not provide relief. In general, combined spinal-epidural and dural puncture epidural techniques decrease the incidence of sacral sparing by providing quicker sacral coverage.

(10) AFTER SUCCESSFULLY CONTROLLING THE PELVIC PAIN, WOULD YOU HAVE CONSIDERED THE PROGRAMMED INTERMITTENT EPIDURAL INFUSION (PIEB) FROM THE START?

PIEB ensures using smaller volumes of local anesthetics and opioids, less incidence of breakthrough pain, decreases the incidence of motor block, and results in a better spread of local anesthetic in the epidural space. However, its use is still controversial compared to continuous epidural analgesia regimen.

Table 34.1 EPIDURAL FAILURE REASONS

• Subcutaneous • Intrathecal • Intravascular • Subdural • Transforaminal/Paravertebral space • Anterior epidural space	• Neuraxial anatomy distortion (e.g., epidural space scarring after spine surgery) • Neuraxial anatomy abnormality (e.g., scoliosis) • Dorsal median connective tissue band • Midline fat patches	• Single orifice end catheter (higher risk of a unilateral block) • Catheter obstruction (e.g., knot, clot, debris) • Improper connection with the injection port • Inadequate infusion rate, PCA dose or concentration • Precipitous labor • Low pain threshold or high patient expectation

(11) YOU CHECK ON THE PATIENT SEVERAL TIMES, AND SHE IS COMFORTABLE AND HAPPY. SHE DELIVERS A HEALTHY BABY AND IS VERY SATISFIED. WHAT ARE THE FACTORS THAT MAKE LABORING WOMEN LESS SATISFIED WITH EPIDURAL ANALGESIA?

Multiple factors may lead to patient dissatisfaction with epidural analgesia, low analgesic effectiveness, and post-epidural pain that will cause patient dissatisfaction. Instrument-assisted vaginal delivery, epidural catheter replacement, late epidural placement compared to its placement in early labor are important causes of disatisfaction.[2] Complications secondary to neuraxial anesthesia would increase the risk of dissatisfaction, e.g., post-dural puncture headache, back pain, and nerve injuries.

DISCUSSION

INTRODUCTION

In 2018, a retrospective study that included more than 2.6 million deliveries has shown that neuraxial analgesia was used in 73.1% of those deliveries.[3] Similarly, the U.S. national vital statistics report on the epidural and spinal use during labor in 2009 has shown that there were 2.7 million vaginal deliveries in the United States; neuraxial anesthesia was used in 61% of those deliveries.[4]

A large retrospective study that included 19,259 deliveries has shown that labor epidural failure rate is about 12%. Of those, 46% were fixed by simple manipulations, while 7.1% required epidural catheter replacement, and 1.9% required more than one replacement.[5] Different reasons have been attributed to epidural failure to provide adequate analgesia (Table 34.1). However, even with successful epidural catheter placement in the epidural space, the patient can present with a unilateral block or present with perineal pain/pressure during the second stage of labor secondary to sacral sparing. The anesthesia provider needs to find the cause of the failed epidural analgesia in order to be able to troubleshoot it correctly.

BREAKTHROUGH PAIN IN PROPERLY SITED EPIDURAL ANALGESIA

Some parturients with a good working labor epidural may experience breakthrough pain that requires supplemental medications or even additional interventions. The incidence of such breakthrough pain has been reported to be as high as 25%.[6] Breakthrough pain may result from obstetric or anesthetic issues or a combination of the two. A unilateral pain may suggest a problem with the epidural catheter or its location within the epidural space; abdominal pain with a good block in a patient undergoing a trial of labor may suggest uterine rupture, while increasing perineal pain may indicate the onset of the second stage of labor with inadequate sacral block. More common predictors of breakthrough pain are nulliparity, heavier fetal weight, and epidural catheter placement at an early cervical dilation.[7] All these predictors usually increase the length of labor. Other possible factors for breakthrough pain are augmentation of labor with oxytocin leading to stronger contractions, large body mass index (BMI), catheter migration, unfavorable epidural catheter tip position in epidural space, known scoliosis or spinal surgery, or patient lying on one side. Sacral sparing is a more common phenomenon with the epidural than a combined spinal epidural (CSE).[8]

CAUSES OF BREAKTHROUGH PAIN IN A CORRECTLY SITED EPIDURAL

Epidural Catheter Migration

It has been shown that tips of epidural catheters are not always in the midline in the epidural space in normally working epidural catheters.[9] However, the catheter tip may migrate through the intervertebral foramina into the paravertebral space and result in unilateral epidural analgesia. This problem can be reduced by limiting threading the catheter into epidural space to 4–5 cm. Threading it to less that 3 cm in the epidural space may risk subcutaneous migration. This is especially noted in higher BMI patients, where patient movement can cause outward migration of the catheter outside the epidural space. Inward migration of the epidural catheter can happen with the change of position from the flexed spine to the upright position during insertion. The provider is advised to allow the patient to sit upright before fixing the epidural.

Another reason for unilateral epidural coverage can be due to anterior epidural space catheter location. These cases will require a bigger volume of a local anesthetic to spread along the longitudinal axis (cephalocaudal), laterally then circumferentially to posterior epidural space, to be able to provide proper coverage and adequate analgesia.[10]

Epidural Anatomical Barriers

Other reasons for unilateral block have been described, including the presence of a dorsal median connective tissue band that limits the local anesthetic to one side of epidural space. However, it has been described to be usually incomplete membrane that usually does not prevent uniform spread of local anesthetic in the epidural space.[11] Hogan failed to detect a complete septum in his cadaver studies by microtome; however, the ligamenta flava were fused in the midline to a variable degree. He also suggested that the midline structure is a vascular structure attached to the epidural fat in posterior epidural space [12] Some other studies and case reports has seen a midline structure that prevented uniform bilateral contrast spread[11,13] (Figure 34.2). Another study has suggested that the midline membrane can be disrupted by the epidural needle or injecting saline with high pressure through the needle or catheter tip.[14]

Spinal Epidural Lipomatosis

Spinal epidural lipomatosis (SEL) is the abnormal accumulation of adipose tissue in epidural space. Most patients with SEL are asymptomatic and diagnosed as an incidental finding on magnetic resonance imaging (MRI).[15] Symptomatic patients may present with sensory or motor deficits secondary to the adipose tissue compression effect on the dural sac. SEL can be idiopathic or secondary to Cushing disease, chronic steroid use, obesity, or the use of retroviral protease inhibitors in HIV patients. SEL is characterized by the unpredictability of the distribution of medication in the intrathecal/epidural space. Multiple patterns of distribution have been described; it has been associated with failure of numerous epidural attempts,[16] while other reports have shown normal function of epidural;[17] a study described high sensory level up to C3–C4 level with sacral sparing despite multiple boluses given.[18] The presence of adipose tissue in epidural space may create difficulty for the provider locating the epidural space, increasing the risk of nerve damage.

Though SEL is a relative contraindication to neuraxial anesthesia, multiple case reports have reported successful epidural placement in SEL patients.[15,16] Caution is advised during placement to avoid nerve injury, accidental dural puncture, or during bolusing the epidural to avoid a high level of sympathetic, sensory, or motor block.

Intravascular Placement

Another possible aberrant site for the epidural catheter is intravascular placement. The incidence of intravascular catheter placement is 3%–7%; it is usually identified by observation of blood in the catheter or during aspiration before the injection of the test dose, but still, this simple step has a high false-negative rate.[19,20] During pregnancy, the gravid uterus compresses the inferior vena cava and leads to engorgement of epidural venous plexus, increasing the risk of intravenous injection of local anesthetic compared to the non-pregnant patient, especially if the rigid nylon catheter is used. Intravenous injection of local anesthetic will provide no analgesia and will present as local anesthetic systemic toxicity manifestations. [21] Incidence of intravascular catheter placement can be decreased by placing the epidural in a lateral position, using a soft-tipped catheter, and limiting the length of the epidural catheter to 4–5 cm.[22,23]

Sacral Sparing

The first stage of labor is characterized by visceral pain, transmitted via T10–L1 nerve roots innervating the uterus

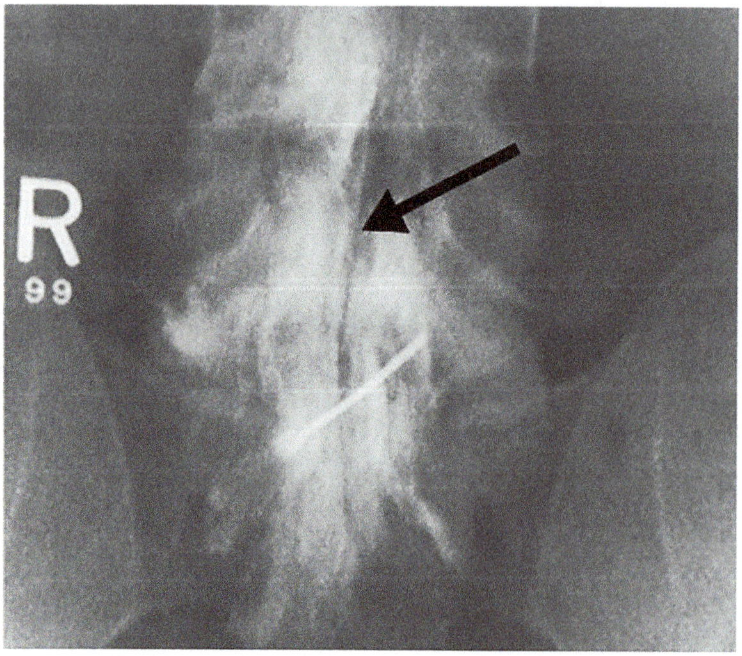

Figure 34.2. An AP view of a lumbosacral epidurogram. The arrow is pointing to the plica mediana dorsalis. Notice also the uneven distribution of the contrast dye.

and cervix. In contrast, in the second stage of labor, the pain is primarily somatic, transmitted via S2–S4 nerve roots that innervate the perineum. Arendt and Segal[8] explained that the reason of sacral sparing is due to the sacral nerve roots being larger in diameter, covered with thicker dura and relatively further from the tip of the epidural catheter at the lumbar region. Moreover, the tendency of the lumbar epidural infusion is to spread more cephalad, which may result in less coverage of sacral nerves. The incidence is reduced when the CSE technique is used. When it happens with epidural-only techniques, the epidural catheter can be bolused in the semi-sitting position.

MANAGEMENT OF BREAKTHROUGH PAIN DURING LABOR

Common strategies for troubleshooting breakthrough pain are as follows: additional bolus of dilute local anesthetics is indicated when the sensory level is below T10 level with mild pain; additional bolus with a higher concentration of a local anesthetic solution is indicated for pain despite an adequate sensory level at T10; and top-up in lateral position with the painful side down with or without withdrawal of epidural catheter by 1–2 cm if feasible[24] (Table 34.2A and B).

The following techniques and modalities have been suggested to either reduce the incidence or treat the breakthrough pain, as well as improve the efficacy and reliability of epidurals. These include CSE, DPE, and automated mandatory bolus (AMB) or program intermittent epidural bolus (PIEB), and computer-integrated patient-controlled epidural analgesia (CIPCEA).

For persistent pain, after 2 clinician boluses, it is a good strategy to replace the epidural and consider other techniques, such as CSE or DPE with or without PIB or CIPCEA.[25]

COMBINED SPINAL EPIDURAL TECHNIQUE

Techniques

1. The needle-through-needle–single-interspace technique:

Table 34.2A **INITIATION OF EPIDURAL CHECK LIST**

Test dose after negative aspiration: • Give 1.5% lidocaine with 1:200.000 epinephrine × 3mL • Do not give the test dose during contraction	
• HR increase >10 beats/minute • Ringing in ears • Numbness around the mouth • Palpitations	May indicate intravascular injection
• Pain relief in less than 2 minutes • Acute leg numbness or heaviness	Possible intrathecal injection
Loading: Begin by giving 3–5mL of bupivacaine and fentanyl solution incrementally, to a total of 10–12 mL Start continuous epidural pump infusion for maintenance	

Table 34.2B **TROUBLESHOOTING INADEQUATE LABOR EPIDURAL ANALGESIA**

Check:	• The insertion site and the depth of catheter at the skin • The epidural catheter and tubing connections • The pump for malfunction • If the patient has been using the bolus button
Test the block level bilaterally:	• Motor on Bromage Scale • Sensory by using ice
• Bilateral sensory level below T10 during the first stage	Use 5–10 mL bolus from the epidural bag, assess in 20 min for level If level rising but still below T10, consider giving second 5 mL bolus Consider increasing baseline epidural infusion 1–2mL/hour
• Unilateral block	1. Check the depth of the catheter at the skin and compare it to the initial placement depth. If catheter >5 cm in epidural space, under sterile conditions, consider withdrawing catheter 1 cm or until depth in space = 4–5 cm 2. Place the patient with the failed block side down and bolus 5–10 mL from the epidural bag and reassess sensory level in 20 min.
• Patchy block/ Window of inadequate analgesia	1. Bolus 5–10 mL of 0.125%–0.25% bupivacaine; while the patient is lying on the side of the patchy block, recheck level in 20 min. 2. Consider using 50–100 mcg fentanyl. Do not use in case of fetal distress. 3. If the above steps yield equivocal or negative results, consider testing the epidural with a definitive dose of LA 5 mL of 1% lidocaine with or without epinephrine.
When bolusing, evaluate the patient for at least 30 minutes to ensure adequate analgesia and monitor the vital signs In general, consider early replacement of epidural catheter, if 2 interventions fail to control pain.	

This is the most popular technique of placing CSE, using either a preassembled kit, or an epidural needle and spinal needle in the absence of a preassembled kit. In an average-sized patient, an epidural needle (9 cm or 3.5 in.) and a longer (12.7 cm or 5 in.) 25- or 27-gauge spinal needle are used (Figure 34.3).

2. The double-needle–double interspace technique:

The epidural needle and catheter are inserted at one space, and spinal injection is done at another space. However, the double technique can be side by side on the same interspace.

Combined Spinal Epidural Analgesia versus Epidural Analgesia

Both the CSE and traditional epidural techniques have been used as effective measures to provide adequate labor analgesia. Simmons et al.[26] reviewed clinical trials involving 3274 laboring patients, comparing CSE techniques to the traditional epidural technique. They found that the CSE technique has

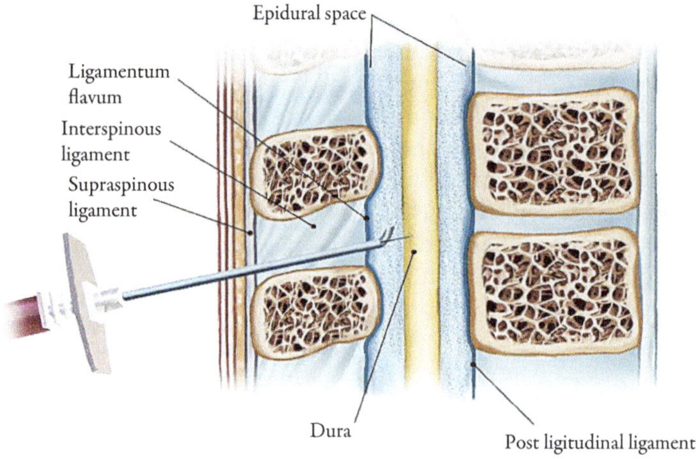

Figure 34.3. Combined spinal-epidural technique.

decreased the time to reaching maternal analgesia, needed less top-up doses, resulted in lower incidence of urinary retention, and less instrumental delivery. However, no difference was shown between both techniques regarding the need for labor augmentation, cesarean section rate, post-dural puncture headache (PDPH) incidence, maternal hypotension, umbilical arterial pH, or neonatal Apgar scores.[26]

A drawbacks of CSE analgesia compared to epidural is that it has shown to increase the incidence of pruritis secondary to intrathecal opioid injection. A study reported an incidence of 41% for CSE compared to 1.3% in epidural.[27] It also increased the incidence of high spinal/epidural, which may lead to maternal hypotension and neonatal bradycardia. Additionally, it needs a relatively longer time to set up the equipment and the additional medications.[28] While both CSE and epidural provide adequate maternal analgesia, the outcomes are greatly affected by the concentration and total dosage of different medications used.

Intrathecal Medications

Intrathecal Opioids

Intrathecal opioid injection can be sufficient for first-stage labor pain but cannot cover the entire process of labor. For second-stage analgesia, using a combination of local anesthetic and opioid is recommended. The intrathecal injection reduces the dose of local anesthetic and opioids needed and will provide better analgesia as both components interact synergistically together.[29] Fentanyl 15–25 μg and sufentanil of 5–10 μg can provide adequate analgesia, but pruritis and respiratory depression can be seen if higher doses are used. However, if added to a local anesthetic, the opioid dosage can be reduced to 1.5–2.5 μg for sufentanil and 10–15 μg for fentanyl. Morphine 150–250 μg has also been described with and without the combination of local anesthetics and short-acting opioids. It has the advantages of less breakthrough pain and longer duration of action, thus decreasing the postpartum analgesic requirement but with increased risk of postpartum nausea.[30]

Intrathecal Local Anesthetics

Bupivacaine is the most common local anesthetic used; a dose of 1.25–2.5 mg would achieve adequate analgesia if used with opioids. Similarly, intrathecal ropivacaine can be used as it causes less motor blockade than bupivacaine (3.6 mg of ropivacaine is equipotent to 2.4 mg of bupivacaine).[31]

Intrathecal Additives

Several additives have been described aiming to provide better and prolonged analgesic effects. Epinephrine addition to the bupivacaine-opioid combination is known to prolong the duration of the mixture by 15–40 minutes. Different doses have been described as small as 2.5 μg and up to 200 μg. However, Gurbet et al.[32] did not show a difference in the quality of analgesia when 12.5 μg vs. 100 μg of epinephrine was used as an additive. Clonidine and neostigmine have been shown to prolong the duration of analgesia· Clonidine has been shown to cause maternal sedation and hypotension, fetal heart rate, rhythm abnormalities, while neostigmine has been shown to cause severe nausea.[33]

Effect of CSE on Labor

Tsen et al.[34] have reported that the first stage of labor was shorter in patients with CSE in a study done on 50 laboring patients; a possible explanation is that the rapid decrease of epinephrine level after injection of intrathecal fentanyl provides quicker maternal analgesia, allowing an improvement of uterine contraction pattern and cervical dilation.[35] A randomized clinical trial conducted by Norris et al.[36] that included 2183 laboring patients, comparing CSE to epidural techniques, showed no difference in the mode of delivery or duration of labor. However, they were directly correlated with the patient's parity and late induction of labor analgesia (>5 cm cervical dilation).

Fetal heart rate changes may happen after induction of analgesia via epidural catheter or subarachnoid opioid injection; it usually resolves within 5–8 minutes with or without obstetric interventions.[37] Fetal bradycardia following CSE and intrathecal opioid injection might be secondary to the sudden decrease in circulating epinephrine levels. This imbalance of plasma epinephrine concentration is thought to cause uterine hypertonus, impairing uteroplacental circulation, and fetal bradycardia.[38] Multiple studies failed to show a higher incidence of cesarean delivery with CSE technique.[36,39,40] Norris et al.[36] looked at neonatal outcomes and found that umbilical arterial blood pH values were slightly more acidic in the CSE group compared to the epidural group, but the results were clinically insignificant.

As regards the PDPH, a large study of 2183 patients by Norris et al.[36] did not support that the CSE has a higher incidence of PDPH; in addition, the needle-through-needle technique was associated with lower probability of failed epidural catheter placement and is one of best practices to check correct epidural positioning.

Maternal end-tidal carbon dioxide ($ETCO_2$) was shown to rise after intrathecal opioid injection and it might be attributed to the rostral spread within CSF, risking respiratory depression, or respiratory arrest. The increase $ETCO_2$ can happen with doses as low as 5 ug of sufentanil and with any dose of fentanyl that can provide labor analgesia.[41,42] It is recommended to monitor the patient for 20–30 minutes after intrathecal opioid injection.

Epidural Test Dose in a CSE Procedure

Using of the epidural test dose in CSE following intrathecal injection has been controversial. The opinion opposing using it believes that the addition of the epidural test dose following the intrathecal injection of bupivacaine and fentanyl would cause motor weakness for 30–60 minutes, and with possible weakening of the pelvic muscles, making spontaneous vaginal delivery challenging.[43] On the other hand, epidural test dose advocates believe that the negative blood aspiration through the catheter is not sensitive enough to identify an intravascular catheter. However, the epinephrine in the test dose is sensitive enough to identify intravascular placement. While the low concentrations of local anesthetic and opioid in epidural analgesia might be safe if no test dose is used, if an emergency cesarean section is warranted, a large bolus of local anesthetic will be needed, thus carrying the risk of local anesthetic systemic toxicity if intravascular placement was not ruled out previously.

DURAL PUNCTURE EPIDURAL TECHNIQUE

DPE is a technique that depends on creating a hole in the dura matter, thus creating a conduit through which the diffusion of the drug from epidural space to subarachnoid space can take place. In 1988, Leach et al.[44] injected contrast in an epidural catheter that was replaced at a higher level after an inadvertent dural puncture and noted the spread of contrast dye to the subarachnoid space. Comparing DPE with CSE in labor, Chau and Tsen[45] found that DPE had a more rapid onset and higher incidence of sacral coverage, with a lower incidence of unilateral or motor block and fewer physician interventions in comparison to labor epidural. In contrast to CSE, DPE showed less incidence of maternal hypotension, pruritus, uterine hypertonus, and subsequent conversion of fetal heart rate category I to category II. In contrast, CSE had more rapid onset of analgesia, and labor epidural had the highest incidence of motor blockade. In both DPE and CSE, the CSF flow through the spinal needle can be a confirmatory test for proper positioning of the Tuohy needle in epidural space.

Factors Affecting the Success of DPE Technique

A 2019 systematic review of labor DPE by Layera et al.[46] showed that the onset of analgesia and spread in patients receiving DPE depends on multiple factors, including size of the hole, transmeningeal drug diffusion, and total drug mass injected into epidural space. Cappiello et al.[47] showed improved sacral spread using a 25-gauge Whitacre needle, while Thomas et al.[48] were not able to show that DPE using 27-gauge Whitacre needle improved labor analgesia. As different drugs will have different transmeningeal diffusion rates, the drugs with low diffusion rates will benefit from the physical hole.[49]

Layera's systematic review[46] found inconclusive results of the benefits of the DPE. They thought that small (i.e., 26- or 27-gauge) spinal needles seem to confer minimal benefits in the first 10 minutes, while using 25 G needle was better in improving sacral root blockade and resulted in a lower incidence of unilateral/asymmetric block compared to LEA.

Another controversial result shown by Chau et al.[45] is that fewer physician interventions were needed in DPE technique (25-gauge Whitacre needle) compared to CSE or labor epidural. Goodman et al.[50] did not show any difference in physician intervention (using 27-gauge Whitacre needle) in DPE compared to CSE, which might be related to the smaller size needle used. Chau et al.[45] explained that using the CSE technique might require more physician interventions secondary to the transition from the initial superior relief following spinal analgesia to maintenance epidural analgesia, which is not as potent as the initial spinal analgesia, or it might be secondary to starting CSE early in labor leading to stronger uterine contractions as labor progresses, thus increasing analgesic requirements.[34,51]

PROGRAMMED INTERMITTENT EPIDURAL BOLUS ANALGESIA MODE (PIEB)

PIEB with patient-controlled epidural analgesia (PCEA) for maintenance of labor analgesia has been shown to result in less use of local anesthetic and opioid, less breakthrough pain, less incidence of motor block, and less instrumental vaginal delivery, and increased maternal satisfaction without increasing risks of nausea, vomiting, hypotension, or pruritis in comparison to CEI + PCEA[52,53] (Table 34.3). The reason PIEB provides better analgesia and less local anesthetics is because of the sensory regression due to tachyphylaxis that necessitates the need for rescue medications

Table 34.3 **COMMON SETTINGS OF PIEB**

PIEB bolus interval: 15 min–60 min	**PCEA lockout interval: 10–15 min**
PIEB volume: 2.5–10 mL	**PCEA volume 5–15 mL**

in CEI.[54,55] However, other experts may disagree with the advantages of PIEB. Ojo et al.'s[56] randomized clinical trial failed to show any benefits with PIEB regimen when compared to CEI, except for less motor block. Similarly, Tien et al.'s[57] retrospective study that included 528 patients failed to show a difference in the amount of local anesthetic consumption, mode of delivery, and degree of motor block. Moreover, Riley et al.[58] acknowledge the benefits of PIEB mode over CEI but suggest that differences between modes are very modest and with limited clinical benefits, especially when recognizing that the adoption of new PIEB mode will include more costs and will require logistical changes. The optimum PIEB settings are still debatable; PIEB requires new pump programs and the education of the anesthesia and nursing team.

Onuoha[59] noted that most of the PIEB versus PCEA studies were conducted on nulliparous women, suggesting that women with expected longer duration of labor would benefit more from the PIEB technique. More studies are needed to evaluate further differences between PIEB and CEI, e.g., in multiparous women, in the second stage of labor, or to measure the failure rate in operative delivery situations.

Why Would PIEB Provide Better Analgesia?

In 2002, Hogan et al.[60] studied the distribution of solutions in epidural space in cadavers using the cryomicrotome section; they showed that an uneven distribution of solution is affected by the pressures applied and suggested that better spread in epidural space happens with large volumes at high pressure. Wong et al.[61] described the contributing factors to optimize the time interval and bolus regimen, e.g., the concentration of local anesthetic, components of the epidural solution, duration of labor, and rate of administration of the programmed bolus dose. Fegley et al.'s[62] study has shown that a bolus through a multi-orifice catheter will provide better spread in comparison to continuous infusion that may exit through the proximal orifice. An interesting study by Capogna et al.[63] identified the status of equilibrium between intraneural and extraneural local anesthetic concentration as the key difference between CEI and PIEB effectiveness. In CEI mode, the extraneural concentration continues to be higher than intraneural, and thus continues to diffuse intraneuronal along the diffusion gradient until motor fibers get blocked. However, in PIEB mode, the local anesthetic concentration fluctuates up and down, depending on the programmed dosage and lockout interval, and the diffusion gradient shifts into and out of the nerve fibers, thus decreasing the risk of motor fibers being blocked (Figure 34.4A, B).

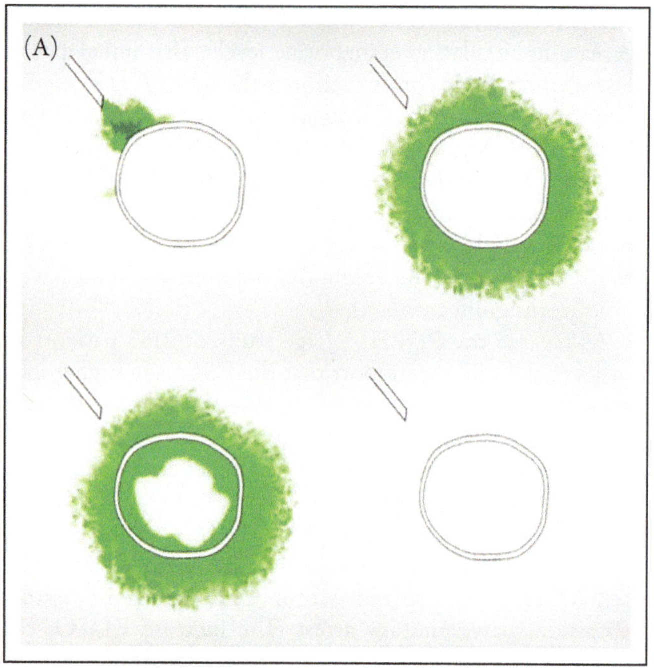

Figure 34.4A. Analgesia and motor block are produced by the movement of local anesthetic from the extraneural space into the nerve along a diffusion gradient. Over time, the extraneural concentration equals the intraneural concentration of local anesthetic, establishing a steady state. Nerve blockade is eventually overcome when the intraneural concentration exceeds the extraneural concentration, and the diffusion gradient is reversed. If low concentrations of local anesthetic are given in intermittent boluses, blockade of motor fibers is unlikely, as the total amount of local anesthetic inside the nerve is insufficient.

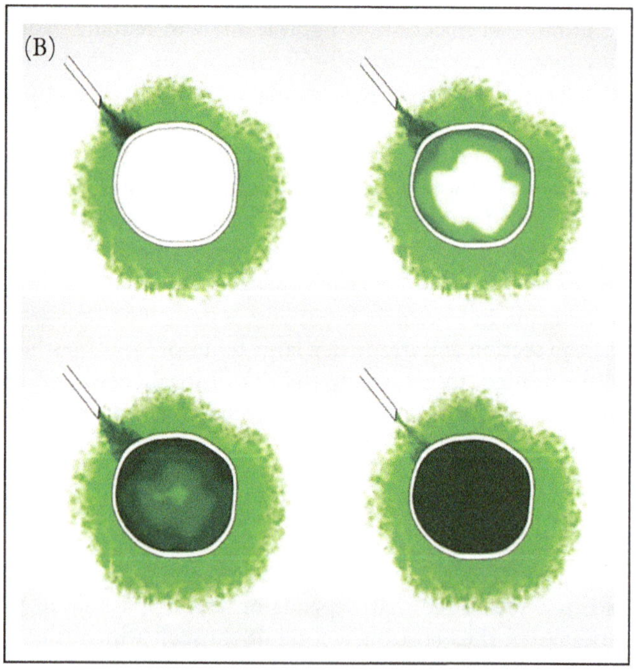

Figure 34.4B. In the case of continuous infusion, the extraneural concentration of local anesthetic is generally persistently higher than in the intraneural space, and the total concentration inside the nerve is increased and may reach the threshold for motor fiber block. This may explain the frequent occurrence and intensification of the motor block during continuous infusion. Figures 34.4A and B: Reprinted from: Capogna G, Stirparo S. Techniques for the maintenance of epidural labor analgesia. *Curr Opin Anesthesiol.* 2019;26(14), copyright 2019, with permission from Elsevier.

REFERENCES

1. Norris MC, Fogel ST, Dalman H, Borrenpohl S, Hoppe W, Riley A. Labor epidural analgesia without an intravascular "test dose." *Anesthesiology.* 1998;88(6):1495–1501.
2. Tan DJA, Sultana R, Han NLR, Sia ATH, Sng BL. Investigating determinants for patient satisfaction in women receiving epidural analgesia for labour pain: a retrospective cohort study. *BMC Anesthesiol.* 2018;18(1):50.
3. Butwick AJ, Bentley J, Wong CA, Snowden JM, Sun E, Guo N. United States state-level variation in the use of neuraxial analgesia during labor for pregnant women. *JAMA Netw Open.* 2018;1(8):e186567.
4. Osterman MJ, Martin JA. Epidural and spinal anesthesia use during labor: 27-state reporting area, 2008. *Natl Vital Stat Rep.* 2011;59(5):1–13, 16.
5. Pan PH, Bogard TD, Owen MD. Incidence and characteristics of failures in obstetric neuraxial analgesia and anesthesia: a retrospective analysis of 19,259 deliveries. *Int J Obstet Anesth.* 2004;13(4): 227–233.
6. Tan HS, Sng BL, Sia ATH. Reducing breakthrough pain during labour epidural analgesia: an update. *Curr Opin Anaesthesiol.* 2019;32(3):307–314.
7. Hess PE, Pratt SD, Lucas TP, et al. Predictors of breakthrough pain during labor epidural analgesia. *Anesth Analg.* 2001;93(2):414–418.
8. Arendt K, Segal S. Why epidurals do not always work. *Rev Obstet Gynecol.* 2008;1(2):49–55.
9. Hogan Q. Epidural catheter tip position and distribution of injectate evaluated by computed tomography. *Anesthesiology.* 1999;90(4):964–970.
10. Usubiaga JE, dos Reis A Jr, Usubiaga LE. Epidural misplacement of catheters and mechanisms of unilateral blockade. *Anesthesiology.* 1970;32(2):158–161.
11. Savolaine ER, Pandya JB, Greenblatt SH, Conover SR. Anatomy of the human lumbar epidural space: new insights using CT-epidurography. *Anesthesiology.* 1988;68(2):217–220.
12. Hogan QH. Lumbar epidural anatomy: a new look by cryomicrotome section. *Anesthesiology.* 1991;75(5):767–775.
13. Nada EM, Turan MA, Mohamed MN. Some epidurographic explanations for incomplete epidural analgesia coverage in the absence of a catheter. *J Clin Anesth.* 2013;25(7):565–571.
14. Blomberg R. A method for epiduroscopy and spinaloscopy: presentation of preliminary results. *Acta Anaesthesiol Scand.* 1985;29(1):113–116.
15. Theyskens NC, Paulino Pereira NR, Janssen SJ, Bono CM, Schwab JH, Cha TD. The prevalence of spinal epidural lipomatosis on magnetic resonance imaging. *Spine J.* 2017;17(7):969–976.
16. Lang SA, Korzeniewski P, Buie D, Du Plessis S, Paterson K, Morris G. Repeated failure of epidural analgesia: an association with epidural fat? *Reg Anesth Pain Med.* 2002;27(5):494–500.
17. Ali H, Huang J. A case of epidural management in a pregnant patient with spinal epidural lipomatosis. *Cureus.* 2019;11(9):e5553.
18. Smith MK, Martin R, Robblee J, Shore EM. A case of epidural lipomatosis in pregnancy: management during labour and caesarean section. *J Obstet Gynaecol Can.* 2018;40(9):1182–1185.
19. Paech MJ, Godkin R, Webster S. Complications of obstetric epidural analgesia and anaesthesia: a prospective analysis of 10,995 cases. *Int J Obstet Anesth.* 1998;7(1):5–11.
20. Collier CB. Accidental subdural injection during attempted lumbar epidural block may present as a failed or inadequate block: radiographic evidence. *Reg Anesth Pain Med.* 2004;29(1):45–51.
21. Corman SL, Skledar SJ. Use of lipid emulsion to reverse local anesthetic-induced toxicity. *Ann Pharmacother.* 2007;41(11):1873–1877.
22. Mhyre JM, Greenfield ML, Tsen LC, Polley LS. A systematic review of randomized controlled trials that evaluate strategies to avoid epidural vein cannulation during obstetric epidural catheter placement. *Anesth Analg.* 2009;108(4):1232–1242.
23. Lubenow T, Keh-Wong E, Kristof K, Ivankovich O, Ivankovich AD. Inadvertent subdural injection: a complication of an epidural block. *Anesth Analg.* 1988;67(2):175–179.
24. Beilin Y, Zahn J, Bernstein HH, Zucker-Pinchoff B, Zenzen WJ, Andres LA. Treatment of incomplete analgesia after placement of an epidural catheter and administration of local anesthetic for women in labor. *Anesthesiology.* 1998;88(6):1502–1506.
25. Sng BL, Sia ATH. Maintenance of epidural labour analgesia: the old, the new and the future. *Best Pract Res Clin Anaesthesiol.* 2017;31(1):15–22.
26. Simmons SW, Taghizadeh N, Dennis AT, Hughes D, Cyna AM. Combined spinal-epidural versus epidural analgesia in labour. *Cochrane Database Syst Rev.* 2012;10:CD003401.
27. Arkoosh VA, Cooper M, Norris MC, et al. Intrathecal sufentanil dose response in nulliparous patients. *Anesthesiology.* 1998;89(2):364–370.
28. Hepner DL, Gaiser RR, Cheek TG, Gutsche BB. Comparison of combined spinal-epidural and low dose epidural for labour analgesia. *Can J Anaesth.* 2000;47(3):232–236.
29. Ngan Kee WD, Khaw KS, Ng FF, Ng KK, So R, Lee A. Synergistic interaction between fentanyl and bupivacaine given intrathecally for labor analgesia. *Anesthesiology.* 2014;120(5):1126–1136.
30. Vasudevan A, Snowman CE, Sundar S, Sarge TW, Hess PE. Intrathecal morphine reduces breakthrough pain during labour epidural analgesia. *Br J Anaesth.* 2007;98(2):241–245.
31. Camorcia M, Capogna G, Columb MO. Minimum local analgesic doses of ropivacaine, levobupivacaine, and bupivacaine for intrathecal labor analgesia. *Anesthesiology.* 2005;102(3):646–650.
32. Gurbet A, Turker G, Kose DO, Uckunkaya N. Intrathecal epinephrine in combined spinal-epidural analgesia for labor: dose-response relationship for epinephrine added to a local anesthetic-opioid combination. *Int J Obstet Anesth.* 2005;14(2):121–125.
33. D'Angelo R, Dean LS, Meister GC, Nelson KE. Neostigmine combined with bupivacaine, clonidine, and sufentanil for spinal labor analgesia. *Anesth Analg.* 2001;93(6):1560–1564.
34. Tsen LC, Thue B, Datta S, Segal S. Is combined spinal-epidural analgesia associated with more rapid cervical dilation in nulliparous patients when compared with conventional epidural analgesia? *Anesthesiology.* 1999;91(4):920–925.
35. Cascio M, Pygon B, Bernett C, Ramanathan S. Labour analgesia with intrathecal fentanyl decreases maternal stress. *Can J Anaesth.* 1997;44(6):605–609.
36. Norris MC, Fogel ST, Conway-Long C. Combined spinal-epidural versus epidural labor analgesia. *Anesthesiology.* 2001;95(4):913–920.
37. Clarke VT, Smiley RM, Finster M. Uterine hyperactivity after intrathecal injection of fentanyl for analgesia during labor: a cause of fetal bradycardia? *Anesthesiology.* 1994;81(4):1083.
38. Albright GA, Forster RM. Does combined spinal-epidural analgesia with subarachnoid sufentanil increase the incidence of emergency cesarean delivery? *Reg Anesth.* 1997;22(5):400–405.
39. Mardirosoff C, Dumont L, Boulvain M, Tramèr MR. Fetal bradycardia due to intrathecal opioids for labour analgesia: a systematic review. *BJOG.* 2002;109(3):274–281.
40. Sharma SK, Alexander JM, Messick G, et al. Cesarean delivery: a randomized trial of epidural analgesia versus intravenous meperidine analgesia during labor in nulliparous women. *Anesthesiology.* 2002;96(3):546–551.
41. Hays RL, Palmer CM. Respiratory depression after intrathecal sufentanil during labor. *Anesthesiology.* 1994;81(2):511–512.
42. Mackey DC, Carpenter RL, Thompson GE, Brown DL, Bodily MN. Bradycardia and asystole during spinal anesthesia: a report of three cases without morbidity. *Anesthesiology.* 1989;70(5):866–868.
43. Calimaran AL, Strauss-Hoder TP, Wang WY, McCarthy RJ, Wong CA. The effect of epidural test dose on motor function after a combined spinal-epidural technique for labor analgesia. *Anesth Analg.* 2003;96(4):1167–1172.
44. Leach A, Smith GB. Subarachnoid spread of epidural local anaesthetic following dural puncture. *Anaesthesia.* 1988;43(8):671–674.
45. Chau A, Bibbo C, Huang CC, et al. Dural puncture epidural technique improves labor analgesia quality with fewer side effects compared with epidural and combined spinal epidural techniques: a randomized clinical trial. *Anesth Analg.* 2017;124(2):560–569.

46. Layera S, Bravo D, Aliste J, Tran Q. A systematic review of DURAL puncture epidural analgesia for labor. *J Clin Anesth.* 2019;53:5–10.
47. Cappiello E, O'Rourke N, Segal S, Tsen LC. A randomized trial of dural puncture epidural technique compared with the standard epidural technique for labor analgesia. *Anesth Analg.* 2008;107(5):1646–1651.
48. Thomas JA, Pan PH, Harris LC, Owen MD, D'Angelo R. Dural puncture with a 27-gauge Whitacre needle as part of a combined spinal-epidural technique does not improve labor epidural catheter function. *Anesthesiology.* 2005;103(5):1046–1051.
49. Bernards CM, Kopacz DJ, Michel MZ. Effect of needle puncture on morphine and lidocaine flux through the spinal meninges of the monkey in vitro. Implications for combined spinal-epidural anesthesia. *Anesthesiology.* 1994;80(4):853–858.
50. Goodman SR, Smiley RM, Negron MA, Freedman PA, Landau R. A randomized trial of breakthrough pain during combined spinal-epidural versus epidural labor analgesia in parous women. *Anesth Analg.* 2009;108(1):246–251.
51. Wong CA, Scavone BM, Peaceman AM, et al. The risk of cesarean delivery with neuraxial analgesia given early versus late in labor. *N Engl J Med.* 2005;352(7):655–665.
52. George RB, Allen TK, Habib AS. Intermittent epidural bolus compared with continuous epidural infusions for labor analgesia: a systematic review and meta-analysis. *Anesth Analg.* 2013;116(1):133–144.
53. Xu J, Zhou J, Xiao H, et al. A systematic review and meta-analysis comparing programmed intermittent bolus and continuous infusion as the background infusion for parturient-controlled epidural analgesia. *Sci Rep.* 2019;9(1):2583.
54. Fettes PD, Moore CS, Whiteside JB, McLeod GA, Wildsmith JA. Intermittent vs continuous administration of epidural ropivacaine with fentanyl for analgesia during labour. *Br J Anaesth.* 2006;97(3):359–364.
55. Mogensen T, Hjortso NC, Bigler D, Lund C, Kehlet H. Unpredictability of regression of analgesia during the continuous postoperative extradural infusion of bupivacaine. *Br J Anaesth.* 1988;60(5):515–519.
56. Ojo OA, Mehdiratta JE, Gamez BH, Hunting J, Habib AS. Comparison of programmed intermittent epidural boluses with continuous epidural infusion for the maintenance of labor analgesia: a randomized, controlled, double-blind study. *Anesth Analg.* 2020;130(2):426–435.
57. Tien M, Allen TK, Mauritz A, Habib AS. A retrospective comparison of programmed intermittent epidural bolus with continuous epidural infusion for maintenance of labor analgesia. *Curr Med Res Opin.* 2016;32(8):1435–1440.
58. Riley ET, Carvalho B. Programmed intermittent epidural boluses (pieb) for maintenance of labor analgesia: a superior technique to continuous epidural infusion? *Turk J Anaesthesiol Reanim.* 2017;45(2):65–66.
59. Onuoha OC. Epidural analgesia for labor: continuous infusion versus programmed intermittent bolus. *Anesthesiol Clin.* 2017;35(1):1–14.
60. Hogan Q. Distribution of solution in the epidural space: examination by cryomicrotome section. *Reg Anesth Pain Med.* 2002;27(2):150–156.
61. Wong CA, McCarthy RJ, Hewlett B. The effect of manipulation of the programmed intermittent bolus time interval and injection volume on total drug use for labor epidural analgesia: a randomized controlled trial. *Anesth Analg.* 2011;112(4):904–911.
62. Fegley AJ, Lerman J, Wissler R. Epidural multiorifice catheters function as single-orifice catheters: an in vitro study. *Anesth Analg.* 2008;107(3):1079–1081.
63. Capogna G, Stirparo S. Techniques for the maintenance of epidural labor analgesia. *Curr Opin Anaesthesiol.* 2013;26(3):261–267.

REVIEW QUESTIONS

(1) The incidence of epidural failure rate in parturient during labor is:

A. 5%–6%
B. 8%–12%
C. 15%–20%
D. 1%–2%

(2) Which dermatomes mediate the second stage of labor pain?

A. T10–L1
B. T10–S2
C. L1–S4
D. S2–S4

(3) All of the following are known causes for asymmetric or failure of epidural analgesia EXCEPT:

A. Catheter tip in anterior epidural space
B. Change of patient position after catheter placement
C. Prolonged labor
D. Precipitous labor

(4) All the following statements regarding the risk of intravascular catheter placement are true EXCEPT:

A. Placement in sitting position decreases the incidence of intravenous catheter placement.
B. Risk increases in the pregnant patient.
C. Rigid nylon catheter increases the risk of intravascular placement.
D. Limiting catheter to 4–5 cm of depth beyond the loss of the resistance decreases the incidence of intravascular placement.

(5) All of the following methods are recommended to lessen the incidence of sacral sparing, EXCEPT:

A. Combined spinal epidural (CSE)
B. Dural puncture epidural (DPE)
C. A bolus of 0.5% bupivacaine while patient is in semi-sitting position
D. 50 mcg fentanyl bolus

(6) When comparing CSE technique to epidural technique for labor analgesia, all of the following are correct EXCEPT:

A. CSE has shown to increase maternal analgesia and maternal satisfaction.
B. Most studies agree that CSE does not affect the mode of delivery.
C. CSE may cause an imbalance of epinephrine level, causing uterine hypertonus and fetal bradycardia.
D. Increase the incidence of cesarean delivery secondary to fetal bradycardia.

(7) When CSE is compared to continuous epidural analgesia (CEA), it increases the followings EXCEPT:

A. The risk of pruritis
B. The incidence of post-dural puncture headache
C. Maternal end-tidal carbon dioxide level with intrathecal fentanyl doses as low as 15 mcg
D. Maternal hypotension and fetal bradycardia

(8) When comparing the programmed intermittent epidural (PIEB) infusion to continuous epidural technique (CEI) infusion, all the following statements are true except

A. Higher maternal satisfaction
B. Sensory block regression due to bupivacaine level fluctuation.
C. Decreased incidence of motor block and instrumental delivery
D. Decreased incidence of fetal respiratory depression

(9) All of the following have been shown to affect the optimum PIEB regimen EXCEPT:

A. The concentration of local anesthetics
B. The mixture of opioid and local anesthetics
C. Duration of labor
D. More effectiveness is observed in multiparous women.

(10) Compared to CEI, the PIEB results in less motor weakness because of:

A. Higher concentration of local anesthetics in the extraneural tissues
B. Less total amount of local anesthetics given
C. Injection under pressure will ensure uniform spread of local anesthetics in the epidural space.
D. Regardless of the concentration, PIEB does not result in motor blockade.

(11) All the following statements about dural puncture epidurals (DPE) are accurate EXCEPT:

A. Slower onset of analgesia compared to CSE
B. Quicker onset of analgesia compared to epidural
C. Less incidence of maternal hypotension and fetal bradycardia
D. DPE needs more physician interventions for breakthrough pain compared to CSE.

ANSWERS

(1) **B.** Different reasons for epidural failure include misplacement of epidural catheters (e.g., intrathecal, intravascular, subcutaneous), or abnormal anatomy (e.g., lumbar scoliosis, scarring epidural space, etc.). On average, the epidural failure rate had been reported to be between 8% and 12%.

Reference

Arendt K, Segal S. Why epidurals do not always work. *Rev Obstet Gynecol.* 2008;1(2):49–55.

(2) **D.** It is essential to understand the labor pain pathways to provide adequate analgesia. The pain of first stage of labor is mainly of visceral origin. It is transmitted via T10–L1 nerve roots innervating the uterus and cervix. During the second stage of labor, the pain is primarily somatic and is transmitted via S2–S4 pudendal nerve roots that innervate the perineum.

Reference

Brownridge P. The nature and consequences of childbirth pain. *Eur J Obstet Gynecol Reprod Biol.* 1995;59:S9–S15.

(3) **C.** The presence of the catheter outside of the posterior epidural space will lead to the failure of epidural analgesia. During placement of the catheter, the change of flexed spine position to supine may cause the catheter to migrate deeper than intended and the presence of anatomical barriers. At the same time, patients with precipitous labor will not have enough time for epidural analgesia to build up, leading to failure of establishing adequate analgesia.

References

Savolaine ER, Pandya JB, Greenblatt SH, Conover SR. Anatomy of the human lumbar epidural space: new insights using CT-epidurography. *Anesthesiology.* 1988;68(2):217–220

Usubiaga JE, dos Reis A Jr, Usubiaga LE. Epidural misplacement of catheters and mechanisms of unilateral blockade. *Anesthesiology.* 1970;32(2):158–161.

(4) **A.** Incidence of intravascular catheter placement can be decreased by placing in lateral position (to alleviate compression on inferior vena cava and epidural veins during sitting position), using a soft-tipped catheter, and limiting the depth of epidural catheter to 4–5 cm.

Reference

Mhyre JM, Greenfield ML, Tsen LC, Polley LS. A systematic review of randomized controlled trials that evaluate strategies to avoid epidural vein cannulation during obstetric epidural catheter placement. *Anesth Analg.* 2009;108(4):1232–1242.

(5) **C.** CSE and DPE are both techniques that provide better sacral analgesia. Medications like fentanyl 0.125% and 0.25% bupivacaine in a semi-sitting position can treat sacral sparing; while bupivacaine 0.5% might treat sacral sparing, it is not used as it will cause surgical anesthesia rather than epidural analgesia only.

Reference

Arendt K, Segal S. Why epidurals do not always work. *Rev Obstet Gynecol.* 2008;1(2):49–55.

(6) **D.** CSE has been shown to provide adequate maternal analgesia and maternal satisfaction. But it was hypothesized that following intrathecal injection and providing adequate pain relief, the imbalance of epinephrine level may cause uterine hypertonus and fetal bradycardia lasting a few minutes. But none of the studies has shown increased cesarean delivery following CSE techniques.

Reference

Hughes D, Simmons SW, Brown J, Cyna AM. Combined spinal-epidural versus epidural analgesia labor. *Cochrane Database Syst Rev.* 2003;4:CD003401.

(7) **B.** CSE may cause pruritis, and most studies using different opioid doses have shown to increase the end-tidal carbon dioxide even with the smallest amount of opioids, but failed to prove correlation with post-dural puncture headache.

References

Norris MC, Grieco WM, Borkowski M, et al. Complications of labor analgesia: epidural versus combined spinal epidural techniques. *Anesth Analg*. 1994;79:529–537.

Hays RL, Palmer CM. Respiratory depression after intrathecal sufentanil during labor. *Anesthesiology*. 1994;81(2):511–512.

(8) **B.** When compared to CEI, PIEB has shown to provide higher maternal satisfaction, and less total amount of local anesthetic was needed. This caused a decrease in the incidence of motor block and instrumental delivery, while some studies have shown the regression of sensory block with CEI technique, not with PIEB.

References

Capogna G, Stirparo S. Techniques for the maintenance of epidural labor analgesia. *Curr Opin Anaesthesiol*. 2013;26(3):261–267.

George RB, Allen TK, Habib AS. Intermittent epidural bolus compared with continuous epidural infusions for labor analgesia: a systematic review and meta-analysis. *Anesth Analg*. 2013;116(1):133–144.

(9) **D.** Epidural local anesthetics mixtures and concentrations affect the efficiency of PIEB mode. However, most studies have been done on nulliparous women, suggesting a longer duration is needed for laboring women to get pain relief.

References

Wong CA, McCarthy RJ, Hewlett B. The effect of manipulation of the programmed intermittent bolus time interval and injection volume on total drug use for labor epidural analgesia: a randomized controlled trial. *Anesth Analg*. 2011;112(4):904–911.

Onuoha OC. Epidural analgesia for labor: continuous infusion versus programmed intermittent bolus. *Anesthesiol Clin*. 2017;35(1):1–14.

(10) **B.** PIEB mode will provide a less total amount of local anesthetic compared to CEI mode so that motor fibers will not get blocked, while in CEI mode there is a high extraneural local anesthetic level that diffuses intraneural and causes the motor fibers blockade. In PIEB mode, the set volume under high injectate pressure will ensure uniform spread but does not explain why less motor blockade is affected.

Reference

Capogna G, Stirparo S. Techniques for the maintenance of epidural labor analgesia. *Curr Opin Anaesthesiol*. 2013;26(3):261–267.

(11) **D.** Dural puncture epidurals (DPE) will provide a quicker onset of analgesia compared to epidural. When compared to CSE, it provides a slower onset due to lack intrathecal injection of opioids or local anesthetics. However, this results in less incidence of maternal hypotension and fetal bradycardia. DPE also needs less physician interventions for treating breakthrough pain contrary of CSE after fading of the spinal component and transition to the epidural maintenance.

References

Chau A, Bibbo C, Huang CC, et al. Dural puncture epidural technique improves labor analgesia quality with fewer side effects compared with epidural and combined spinal epidural techniques: a randomized clinical trial. *Anesth Analg*. 2017;124(2):560–569.

Layera S, Bravo D, Aliste J, Tran Q. A systematic review of DURAL puncture epidural analgesia for labor. *J Clin Anesth*. 2019;53:5–10.

35.

REGIONAL ANESTHESIA AND ANALGESIA FOR CESAREAN DELIVERY

Caroline Martinello, Matthew Williams, and Jill M. Mhyre

STEM CASE AND KEY QUESTIONS

A 29-year-old female with a history of 2 prior cesarean deliveries presents for repeat cesarean delivery (CD) with bilateral tubal ligation. The patient has a history of heroin abuse and is currently on suboxone therapy. You decide to place a combined spinal epidural for the procedure in case the spinal block wears off before the surgery is finished and for help with postoperative pain management. The patient reports she had severe nausea during her last CD and spent 3 hours in the post-anesthesia care unit (PACU) before she could move her legs again.

(1) WHAT SPINAL DOSE DO YOU CHOOSE, AND HOW LONG DO YOU EXPECT THE SPINAL BLOCK TO LAST? WHY IS THE DOSE REQUIRED FOR SURGICAL BLOCKADE SMALLER IN PREGNANT PATIENTS?

Bupivacaine is the most commonly used local anesthetic. The dose for CD ranges from 7.5 mg to 15 mg, with the specific dose depending on: (1) the anesthetic technique used (combined spinal epidural vs. single shot spinal); (2) the addition of adjuvants to spinal solution; (3) the expected duration of surgery (higher doses are associated with prolonged block); (4) the surgical technique (uterine exteriorization requires higher doses); (5) and the patient's demographic factors such as gestational age, extremes of height (<5 ft or >6 ft) and high BMI (>50 kg/m^2).[1,2]

(2) ANTICIPATING A PROLONGED SURGERY TIME FROM ADHESIONS DUE TO PRIOR CD, ALONG WITH THE ADDITION OF A BILATERAL TUBAL LIGATION, YOU DECIDE ON A COMBINED SPINAL EPIDURAL (CSE) ANESTHETIC. ATTEMPTING TO MINIMIZE POTENTIAL SIDE EFFECTS, YOU SELECT A LOWER DOSE INTRATHECAL BUPIVACAINE (9 MG HYPERBARIC BUPIVACAINE) WITH 15 MCG OF FENTANYL, AND PLAN TO BOLUS EPIDURAL IF NEEDED. THE CSE BLOCKADE IS PLACED SUCCESSFULLY, AND 10 MINUTES AFTER PLACEMENT THE PATIENT EXPERIENCES NAUSEA AND VOMITING AND PROCEEDS TO REPORT FEELING NUMBNESS IN HER THUMBS BILATERALLY. WHAT IS THE SIGNIFICANCE OF THESE SYMPTOMS, AND WHAT IS THE APPROPRIATE TREATMENT?

Nausea and vomiting during CD has multifactorial cause. In this scenario, immediately following spinal anesthesia administration, it is most likely related to sympathectomy with resultant hypotension.

The sensation of numbness in the thumbs after a spinal anesthetic indicates high spinal block, or more specifically, anesthetic sensory block extension to the C6 dermatome. Treatment consists of hemodynamic support, limiting further cephalad spread of local anesthetic by raising the patient's back or reverse Trendelenburg position. Respiratory support is indicated if the block extends to C3–C5, blocking diaphragmatic function.

(3) THE PATIENT'S SYSTOLIC BLOOD PRESSURE IS NOTED TO BE 20% LOWER THAN BASELINE. SHE HAS PRESERVED STRENGTH IN UPPER EXTREMITIES BILATERALLY BUT REPORTS DIFFICULTY BREATHING. YOU ELEVATE THE BACK OF THE BED 20 DEGREES AND ADMINISTER VASOPRESSORS WHILE ENSURING LEFT UTERINE DISPLACEMENT. AFTER NECESSARY TREATMENT IS PROVIDED, THE PATIENT'S NAUSEA IMPROVES QUICKLY, AND PATIENT REPORTS THAT HER BREATHING IS IMPROVED. THE PROCEDURE TAKES LONGER THAN ANTICIPATED AND THE PATIENT STARTS COMPLAINING OF PAIN AS THE SPINAL IS WEARING OFF. HOW WOULD YOU BOLUS THE EPIDURAL?

You administer 2% lidocaine with epinephrine 1:200,000 epidurally, and after a few minutes the patient reports that her pain has improved.

(4) THE SURGEONS REPORT UTERINE ATONY AND PERFORM VIGOROUS UTERINE MASSAGE. YOU ADMINISTER INTRAVENOUS OXYTOCIN, INFUSED AT 0.5 IU/MIN. AFTER 8 MINUTES, THE UTERUS IS STILL ATONIC, SO THE OBSTETRICIAN ASKS YOU TO GIVE ANOTHER AGENT. WHAT AGENT WILL YOU GIVE?

Considering the patient has received a total of 4 IU of oxytocin through the infusion with no response, you agree with administering a second uterotonic agent. In deciding which second uterotonic would be preferable, you take into consideration the side-effect profile of each medication. Contraindications to methyergonovine include hypertension, preeclampsia, and cardiovascular disease, while contraindications to carboprost include reactive airway disease and pulmonary hypertension. This patient does not have contraindications to either agent, so you decide to administer methylergonovine 200 mcg intramuscularly. Uterine tone is still not adequate, but because methylergonovine should not be repeated before 2–4 hours, a third agent is requested. You administer carboprost 250 mcg intramuscularly. After 15 minutes, uterine tone is still inadequate, so you repeat carboprost administration (can be repeated Q 15 min up to 2 mg total dose) and uterine tone finally improves.

(5) THE NURSE CALLS YOU TO THE PACU AS THE PATIENT HAS QUESTIONS ABOUT POSTOPERATIVE PAIN CONTROL. THE PATIENT REQUESTS TO KEEP HER EPIDURAL FOR PAIN MANAGEMENT. WHAT ARE SOME OF THE REASONS THAT A LUMBAR EPIDURAL IS GOOD FOR POST-CESAREAN PAIN CONTROL, AND WHAT ARE SOME REASONS WHY IT IS NOT?

During discussion with the patient, she reveals that she is worried about postoperative pain due to her history of opioid use disorder and Suboxone treatment. However, she also reveals a history of deep vein thrombosis and pulmonary embolism postoperatively following her last CD. Due to concern about leg weakness from a lumbar epidural, immobility, and need for thromboprophylaxis with the epidural in place, you decide to remove the catheter.

(6) YOU ADMINISTER EPIDURAL MORPHINE AND THEN REMOVE THE EPIDURAL CATHETER. WHAT DOSE DO YOU CHOOSE, AND HOW LONG DO YOU EXPECT THE EFFECTS TO LAST? WHAT ARE SOME OF THE SIDE EFFECTS OF EPIDURAL MORPHINE?

A bolus of 3.0 mg of morphine is administered through epidural catheter prior to removal. One hour later, patient reports itching. You treat it with 5 mg of intravenous nalbuphine with complete resolution of symptoms. You instruct the nurses on the postpartum unit to periodically monitor the patient for any evidence of respiratory depression given that she received neuraxial morphine.

(7) THE PATIENT CONTINUES TO COMPLAIN OF PAIN. YOU ASK YOUR REGIONAL ANESTHESIA COLLEAGUE ABOUT WHAT NERVE BLOCK WOULD HELP HER PAIN, AND THEY SUGGEST A TRANSVERSE ABDOMINUS PLANE (TAP) BLOCK OR A QUADRATUS LUMBORUM BLOCK (QLB). WHAT IS A QLB, AND HOW DOES IT COMPARE TO TAP BLOCKS IN RELATION TO POSTOPERATIVE PAIN FROM CD?

After discussing with you colleague, you learn that both TAP block and QLB are most beneficial in improving postoperative pain control in the absence of intrathecal morphine administration. You decide to perform a posterior QLB, as it may result in wider and longer sensory blockade when compared to TAP block. With the patient in supine position, the transducer is placed in transverse orientation at the midaxillary line at the L2–L4 level. The posterior aspect of the quadratus lumborum muscle is identified. The needle is inserted in-plane with ultrasound in an anterolateral to posteromedial direction until reaching the posterior border of the quadratus lumborum muscle, where 15 mL of 0.125% bupivacaine is injected. The procedure is then repeated on the opposite side. Thirty minutes later, the patient reports her pain is improving.

(8) YOU ROUND ON THE PATIENT THE NEXT DAY AND SHE REPORTS THAT SHE IS GENERALLY COMFORTABLE, WITH OCCASIONAL PAIN WHEN SHE TRIES TO GET OUT OF BED. SHE ADDS THAT THE NURSE HAS BEEN OFFERING HER AS NEEDED INTRAVENOUS HYDROMORPHONE, BUT SHE DECLINES IT DUE TO CONCERN OF PASSING IT TO THE BABY IN THE BREAST MILK. WHAT CAN YOU TELL HER?

You explain to the patient that hydromorphone is transferred to breast milk, where it does have a prolonged half-life and therefore should be used with caution. However, the use of small spaced-out doses is likely safe for her and her baby. It would be preferable to use other adjuvant pain medications with more favorable breastfeeding profile, such as scheduled acetaminophen and ibuprofen so as to minimize her need for hydromorphone as much as possible.[3–5]

DISCUSSION

Cesarean delivery (CD) is one of the most common surgical procedures performed in the United States. In 2018, over 1.2 million CDs were performed in the U.S., accounting for 31.9% of the total deliveries. Of these, almost 700,000 represent primary CD.[6] In patients with a history of prior CD, elective repeat CD is frequently selected, given the risk of uterine rupture with trial of labor after cesarean (TOLAC), and the ability to perform tubal ligation at the time of the cesarean. The indications for CD are multiple and are usually divided in (1) maternal indications: such as antepartum and intrapartum hemorrhage, arrest of labor, chorioamnionitis, deteriorating maternal condition, genital herpes with active lesions, multiples gestation, placenta previa, prior classic uterine incision, uterine rupture; and (2) fetal: such as malpresentation, fetal intolerance to labor, fetal macrosomia, and prolapsed umbilical cord. Depending on the indication, the CD will be performed on emergent, urgent, or elective setting.[1]

NEURAXIAL TECHNIQUES FOR CESAREAN DELIVERY

Neuraxial anesthesia for CD is usually preferred over general anesthesia, given less neonatal exposure to anesthetic, better postoperative pain control with use of neuraxial opioids, and avoidance of the maternal complications of general anesthesia such as failed intubation, aspiration, and intraoperative awareness.[7,8] The optimal neuraxial technique depends on the presence of maternal comorbidities and anticipated surgical needs, each of which could affect goals for the onset, spread, and duration of analgesia, as well as the importance of hemodynamic stability:[8] Spinal anesthesia, combined spinal epidural anesthesia, and rarely continuous spinal anesthesia.

Epidural Anesthesia/Analgesia

Advantages of epidural anesthesia include decreased incidence of maternal hypotension, less vasopressor requirements, ability to extend the duration of neuraxial block, and avoidance of deliberate dural puncture. Disadvantages include increased induction to incision time, increased risk of inadequate sacral nerve coverage, increased risk of incomplete block requiring either supplemental analgesia or conversion to general anesthesia, and requirement for larger doses of local anesthetic compared to single-shot spinal anesthesia.[9] Epidural anesthesia is usually appropriate for women with preexisting labor epidural analgesia, for whom extension of epidural analgesia to cesarean anesthesia is frequently faster than establishing a *de novo* neuraxial anesthetic.

Epidural anesthesia for CD is typically performed between the lumbar spaces of L2–L5 The epidural space falls between 3–8 cm in 90% of the patients, with average depth of 5 cm from skin. The block from an epidural is most heavily influenced by the total mass and volume of local anesthetic used.[1,7]

Spinal Anesthesia

Single-shot spinal (SSS) anesthesia is faster to perform than *de novo* epidural anesthesia, decreases operating room time compared to epidural anesthesia, and provides quick, effective and reliable surgical anesthesia with failure rate of <1%.[7] These advantages of spinal anesthesia must be weighed against the risks of more rapid and profound hypotension compared to epidural anesthesia.[8]

The duration of an SSS is variable and is dependent on type and concentration of local anesthetic, as well as the addition of adjuvants to spinal solution (Table 35.1). Commonly used for CD, bupivacaine doses in the range of 10–15 mg result in surgical anesthesia for >90 minutes.[7] Hyperbaric local anesthetic is frequently used to enable modification of block level by changing patient's positioning to either increase or decrease block distribution as needed. Factors most affecting spread of a spinal include the mass of local anesthetic, its baricity, and patient positioning. In general, pregnant patients require smaller doses of spinal local anesthetic than nonpregnant patients due to physiologic changes of pregnancy. Those include smaller cerebrospinal fluid (CSF) volume, a more cephalad movement of hyperbaric local anesthetic in supine position, and a greater sensitivity of nerve fibers to the local anesthetics.[1]

Combined Spinal Epidural (CSE)

The main advantage of CSE placement is that it allows rapid and dense surgical anesthesia with spinal component while retaining the ability to titrate additional local anesthetic via the epidural if operative times are expected to be prolonged.[7] For women with anticipated difficult airway management, a CSE anesthetic may be selected to minimize the risk of needing to convert to general anesthesia. CSE anesthesia can also be considered when labor epidural analgesia is incomplete, and the patient needs cesarean anesthesia; the spinal dose may be deliberately reduced for safety, and the epidural catheter is then used to titrate the anesthetic to the desired height and density.

While a CSE gives the advantage of administering further local anesthetic, it negates some of the technical advantages of performing a spinal anesthetic by increasing the complexity and time to perform the procedure and increasing risk of postdural puncture headache (PDPH).[8] There is some evidence to suggest that using the same dose of intrathecal local anesthetic and performing a CSE results in higher cephalad sensory blockade compared to SSS. Further research is needed, as some literature found no difference in sensory spread comparing CSE and SSS.[10,11] Epidural volume extension is a technique involving administering normal saline in the epidural space after performing a CSE to increase effect of intrathecal block and can provide adequate anesthesia while decreasing intrathecal local anesthetic dose and resulting in faster motor recovery.[12]

CSE using a low-dose spinal component along with epidural lidocaine compared to SSS has been shown to result in decreased incidence of hypotension, nausea, and vomiting. CSE also resulted in less dense motor block and quicker recovery of motor function postoperatively.[13] When maintenance of hemodynamics is essential, a low-dose CSE may provide the best middle ground in obtaining a dense surgical block compared to an epidural and less hypotension compared to SSS.[14,15]

Table 35.1 ADJUVANT AGENTS FOR NEURAXIAL ANESTHESIA

DRUG	SPINAL DOSE	EPIDURAL DOSE	ADVANTAGES	DISADVANTAGES
Opioids[65–68] Fentanyl Sufentanil	10–25 mcg 2.5–5 mcg	50–100 mcg 10–25 mcg	Improve quality of block Reduce incidence of intraoperative nausea and vomiting[a]	Increase incidence of pruritus
Morphine Hydromorphone	50–200 mcg 60–75 mcg	2–4 mg 0.4–1 mg	Improve postoperative pain control	Increase incidence of pruritus and postoperative nausea and vomiting Increase risk for delayed respiratory depression
Epinephrine[67,69,70]	100–200 mcg	5–10 mcg/mL	Improves quality and prolongs duration of block	May increase incidence of nausea Prolongs motor block[b]
Clonidine[68,71–73]	15–150 mcg	400–800 mcg[c]	Improves quality and prolongs duration of block Decreases shivering May decrease peri-incisional hyperalgesia	Increases incidence of hypotension and sedation
Neostigmine[74–77]	12.5–50 mcg	75–300 mcg[c]	Improves postoperative analgesia Decreases incidence of pruritus	Associated with high incidence of postoperative nausea and vomiting[d]

[a] Related to visceral stimulation—such as exteriorization of the uterus or peritoneal closure

[b] Intrathecal administration

[c] Single dose

[d] Markedly associated with spinal administration.

Source: Landau R. Post-cesarean delivery pain: management of the opioid-dependent patient before, during and after cesarean delivery. *Int J Obstetr Anesthes.* 2019 Aug;39:105–116.

Continuous Intrathecal

Deliberate placement of a spinal catheter should be avoided when possible, but in certain situations the benefits of an intrathecal catheter may outweigh the risks of not being able to obtain neuraxial anesthesia, such as an urgent CD in a patient with morbid obesity. Intrathecal catheters allow for a dense and reliable anesthetic that can be titrated as needed but has higher risk for total spinal due to dosing error if unrecognized as well as increased risk of PDPH.[7]

SIDE EFFECTS OF NEURAXIAL TECHNIQUES AND APPROPRIATE MANAGEMENT

Side effects of neuraxial techniques can range from common side effects, such as pruritus, nausea, and hypotension, to rare but potentially life-threatening complications, such as local anesthetic systemic toxicity (LAST) or total spinal anesthetic. Prompt recognition and treatment are important not only for maternal comfort and satisfaction, but also because delays in treatment can potentially increase maternal and fetal morbidity and mortality.[7]

PRURITUS

Pruritus is a common side effect of neuraxial opioid administration, and its etiology is unclear. Postulated mechanisms include the presence of an "itch center" in the central nervous system, medullary dorsal horn activation, and antagonism of inhibitory transmitters, as well as modulation of serotonergic pathways and involvement of prostaglandins. Therefore, a number of drugs have been investigated for prophylaxis and treatment of pruritus, including serotonin receptor antagonists, antihistamines, and propofol. The most effective treatment seems to be central acting mu-receptor antagonists such as naloxone or partial agonist-antagonist such as nalbuphine.[16,17]

NAUSEA AND VOMITING

The etiology of nausea and vomiting during and after CD is multifactorial and includes sympathectomy with resultant hypotension and vagal hyperreactivity, visceral pain, neuraxial opioid administration, and use of uterotonics. Strategies to prevent nausea and vomiting should be aimed at addressing these causes by promptly managing hypotension, improving quality of block, and judicious use of opioids and uterotonics. Prophylaxis with a combination of antiemetics should also be considered.[17,18]

HYPOTENSION

Hypotension is one of most common side effects of spinal anesthesia and can result in maternal discomfort and uteroplacental insufficiency if not treated promptly. The neuraxial-induced sympathectomy causes arterial and venous dilation, resulting in decreased peripheral vascular resistance and decreased venous return. Although the uterus compresses the inferior vena cava in the supine position at term (even in the absence of sympathectomy), aortic compression becomes significant only when systolic blood pressure decreases below 85 mmHg.[19] Potent vasopressor infusion (with phenylephrine or dilute norepinephrine) is the most important strategy to minimize this important and common side effect. Left uterine displacement, fluid loading, and wrapping the lower extremities decrease the amount of vasopressor required to maintain hemodynamic stability. Decreasing the intrathecal local anesthetic dose (<8 mg of bupivacaine) can also modulate spinal hypotension; administration as part of a CSE technique ensures that epidural local anesthetic may be used to rescue spinal anesthesia of insufficient density or duration.[20–23]

HIGH SPINAL/TOTAL SPINAL ANESTHESIA

A high spinal progressing above the level of T4 can cause severe bradycardia, hypotension, mental status changes, and motor block to respiratory muscles. A total spinal resulting in loss of airway reflexes should be treated with supportive measures to restore maternal and fetal oxygenation, ventilation, and circulation, and includes use of vasopressors, endotracheal intubation, respiratory support, and administration of fluids.[7] Risk factors for high spinal include performing spinal following a labor epidural, morbid obesity, and short stature (<60 in).[2,14,24]

INADEQUATE SURGICAL BLOCK

Inadequate surgical block is a complication that can result in increased discomfort to the mother and often necessitates systemic analgesic adjuncts, repeat neuraxial procedures, or conversion to general anesthesia, all of which increase risk for the mother and infant. Leo et al.[25] found the incidence of failed spinal anesthesia requiring conversion to general anesthesia to be 0.5% and inadequate analgesia requiring intravenous or inhalational analgesic supplementation to be 4.1%. The management of inadequate analgesia from neuraxial anesthesia depends on block height and density, and the stage of the operation. Options prior to start of surgery include repeating neuraxial procedure with lower intrathecal dose (potentially as part of a CSE technique), replacement of an epidural catheter, and knee-to-chest or lateral position to facilitate the spread of local anesthetic. Once surgery has started, the options include dosing epidural catheter if present, systemic analgesia, local infiltration by surgeon or conversion to general anesthesia.[14]

OTHER COMPLICATIONS

Other frequently seen complications from neuraxial anesthesia include PDPH, elevated temperature, urinary retention, motor weakness, and prolonged motor block.[7] Found mostly in case reports, rare complications of neuraxial anesthesia include meningitis, spinal nerve or cord injury, neuraxial abscess, and central nervous system hematoma.[7]

POSTOPERATIVE PAIN MANAGEMENT OF CESAREAN DELIVERY

Adequate pain relief is associated with better maternal-infant bonding and early ambulation, which decreases risk of thromboembolism. Inadequate pain coverage both intraoperatively and postoperatively in women undergoing CD has many adverse effects, including delayed functional recovery, disruption to maternal-fetal bonding, increased opioid use, development of chronic pain, and even increased incidence of postpartum depression.[26] Drug transfer into breast milk must also be considered, particularly for systemic medications.

Comprehensive analgesia for cesarean surgery should include neuraxial morphine unless contraindicated, non-opioid adjuncts, regional analgesia, and oral (PO) or intravenous (IV) opioids if there is severe breakthrough pain.[26]

A personalized anesthetic plan for each patient can be enhanced by identifying patients who are at increased risk of experiencing severe pain and having increased analgesic requirements after CD. Simple tools that show potential for clinical use to identify patients who may be at increased risk of severe postoperative pain include assessing the patient's response to local anesthetic infiltration[27] and asking the patient simple questions about anticipated pain and analgesic needs postoperatively.[28] Compared to standard protocols regarding prescribing opioids at discharge, individualized prescribing practices have shown to reduce postoperative opioid consumption and number of prescriptions.[28] These individualized pain treatment protocols should be tailored based on opioid requirement while inpatient and should focus more on maternal satisfaction and scores of physical comfort and independence versus only relying on pain-rating scores.[28,29]

EPIDURAL ANALGESIA

While there are many regional anesthetic techniques available for postoperative CD analgesia, neuraxial anesthesia with addition of opioids has long been the gold standard treatment. A systematic review comparing parenteral opioids to single-dose epidural morphine found that epidural morphine provides better analgesia during the first 24 hours postoperatively. While epidural morphine results in less morphine use and better pain scores postoperatively, there is an increased incidence of opioid-related side effects such as pruritus and nausea compared to parenteral opioids.[30]

Postoperative patient-controlled lumbar epidural analgesia, although highly efficacious, is associated with limited mobility, need to adjust timing of thromboprophylaxis, increased nursing workload, and increased patient and hospital costs. This modality of analgesia should, however, be considered in special circumstances, such as in patients with a history of chronic pain.[26] Since epidural catheters may dislodge, it can be a good strategy to administer neuraxial morphine, and then infuse a local anesthetic-only solution through the epidural catheter. Another option to be considered is the placement of a thoracic epidural for postoperative analgesia. As thoracic epidural will result in less motor block, it is a good option when early ambulation is desired. However, it does share the same other disadvantages of lumbar epidural.[31]

REGIONAL NERVE BLOCKS

The most widely studied and used in clinical practice are the transversus abdominus plane (TAP) block and quadratus lumborum block (QLB). Other options have limited literature currently available and include intraperitoneal instillation and continuous wound infiltration, ilioinguinal-iliohypogastric block, and paravertebral and erector spinae blocks.

Tranversus Abdominis Plane (TAP) Block

TAP block is beneficial for treating incisional pain, in particular if intrathecal opioids were unable to be administered.

In a meta-analysis including 9 studies, Mishriky et al.[32] found lower opioid consumption at 6 hours (h) (reduction by 10.18 mg morphine equivalent dose [MED]), 12 h (−13.83 mg MED) and 24 h (−20.23 mg MED) in the TAP block group when compared to placebo. When TAP block was compared to intrathecal morphine (ITM), they found significantly lower opioid consumption at 24 h in the ITM group (−8.42 mg MED). In women who received ITM, TAP block had a modest effect, which was limited to reducing pain scores on movement in the early postoperative period. Another meta-analysis from Champaneria et al.[33] of TAP blocks in CD similarly showed that while ITM is more effective than TAP block in regard to pain scores and opioid consumption (2.7 mg vs. 7.5 mg of MED between 10–24 h post-delivery[34]), performing a TAP block in addition to ITM has no further opioid-sparing benefit.[33,35] In the absence of ITM, TAP block showed reduction in opioid use at different time points (2h, 6h, 12h, 24h), with pooled results across all time points showing a mean difference of 15.88 mg of MED use.[33] Interestingly, Staker et al.[36] performed ilioinguinal-transversus abdominus plane (I-TAP) block in patients who received ITM as part of multimodal analgesia regimen, and contrary to the prior studies, the patients showed better pain scores and reduced cumulative mean fentanyl use at 24 h from 179.1 mcg to 71.9 mcg when compared to placebo.

The limited benefit of TAP blocks in patients who received ITM could be related to the short duration of analgesia provided by commonly used local anesthetics. Nedeljkovic et al.[37] compared opioid consumption after TAP block with liposomal bupivacaine (LB) plus plain bupivacaine hydrochloride versus TAP block with plain bupivacaine alone in patients receiving ITM for elective CD. The total opioid consumption in MED through 72 hours was reduced by 51.6% in the LB plus bupivacaine group versus that in the bupivacaine alone group.

In summary, available evidence suggests that TAP block is effective when the use of ITM is not possible or desired, but does not offer much improvement of analgesia when combined with ITM and should not replace the use of ITM.[32–35,38]

Quadratus Lumborum Block (QLB)

The QLB is another regional anesthetic technique that gathered attention in recent years. Three variants of ultrasound-guided QLB approach are commonly described, with no consensus on nomenclature. Based on location of needle tip in relation to quadratus lumborum muscle, they can be described as lateral, posterior, and anterior QLB.[39,40] Both posterior and lateral approaches have been studied in obstetrics,[41–44] but there is not enough evidence to recommend one approach over others.

While the posterior TAP blocks somatic pain from neural afferents of the abdominal anterior wall from dermatomes at T10–L1 level,[45,46] the QLB may result in spread of local anesthetic under the thoracolumbar fascia into the paravertebral space, theoretically prolonging the block and achieving visceral pain relief.[41,47] A meta-analysis from Xu et al.[48] confirmed the results of other studies[41,43] and concluded that QLB significantly improved postoperative analgesia with reduction in 12 h pain score both at rest and movement. Additionally, it reduced opioid consumption in women undergoing CD when ITM was not administered (reduced use of MED by 14.1 mg in 24 h and by 20.8 mg in 48 h). Recent meta-analysis from Hussain et al.[49] found no benefit of QLB when compared with or in addition to ITM; however, it did offer analgesic and opioid consumption benefit in absence of ITM (−18 mg MED in 24 h).

Blanco et al.[42] compared posterior QLB with TAP block in a randomized controlled study. Patients who did not receive ITM and received QL Block showed no opioid-sparing benefit on initial 6 hours but had significant benefit at 12, 24, and 48 h postoperatively (the differences were 37.5%, 55%, and 48%, respectively). There were no significant differences in visual analog scale (VAS) pain scores between TAP and QLB groups.[42] However, a systematic review by El-Boghdadly[50] showed no difference in opioid consumption in the first 24 h when comparing QLB and TAP block. In the absence of ITM administration, QLB and TAP block were equivalent and superior in their analgesic efficacy relative to inactive control for up to 48 h, reducing 24 h intravenous morphine consumption by approximately 20 mg. They concluded that the presence of ITM, QLB, and TAP blocks did not provide any additional analgesic benefit.

SYSTEMIC PHARMACOLOGICAL MANAGEMENT

While a multimodal approach for post-cesarean analgesia should include intrathecal morphine and opioids for severe breakthrough pain, conservative non-opioid adjuncts should also be included.

Acetaminophen and Non-Steroidal Anti-Inflammatory Drugs (NSAIDs)

Acetaminophen decreases postoperative opioid use, has a good safety profile at regular doses, and minimal breast milk transfer. Although there is potential benefit of a single preoperative dose of acetaminophen, the most benefit is seen when regular interval dosing is used.[51,52] Meta-analysis of NSAID use versus control showed better pain scores on initial 24 hours, also less opioid use (mean difference of −12.03 mg MED) and less drowsiness/sedation.[53] Given the strong evidence for and the favorable safety profile of these medications, post-CD analgesic protocols should include use of routine scheduled acetaminophen along with NSAIDs.[26,51]

Intravenous Ketamine

The perioperative use of ketamine as adjunct for postoperative analgesia has been extensively studied. For non-obstetric surgery it seems clear the use of ketamine decreases VAS pain score as well as postoperative use of morphine equivalents.[54] Although there are multiple studies on use of sub-anesthetic doses of ketamine as adjunct for post-cesarean pain control after both neuraxial and general anesthesia, the results are not uniform. In a meta-analysis by Heesen et al.[55] 12 studies were included, comprising 953 patients. For the spinal anesthesia subgroup, administration of intravenous ketamine prolonged time for first analgesic request (weighted mean difference of 49.36 min) and decreased VAS pain scores 2 h after surgery. No differences on incidence of significant side effects, including psychomimetic effects, were noted. Those benefits were not confirmed for the general anesthesia subgroup.

Steroids

There is weak evidence that steroids provide an opioid-sparing effect, but given they are effective and routinely used to prevent postoperative nausea and vomiting,[56] it is reasonable to include them in post-cesarean analgesia regimen.

Gabapentin

The literature on gabapentinoids has shown some benefit but at the expense of increased side effects such as sedation, dizziness, and abnormal vision. In addition, breast milk transfer may be of concern.[26,57,58]

Conservative postoperative pain management should focus on opioid-sparing medications, with acetaminophen and nonsteroidal anti-inflammatory medications being prescribed for all women unless contraindicated. In patients at increased risk of severe postoperative pain or women with inadequate pain control, other adjuncts such as gabapentinoids, ketamine, and dexamethasone can be considered.[26,51]

MANAGEMENT OF MEDICATION ASSISTED TREATMENT (MAT) FOR OPIOID USE DISORDER (OUD)

Management of the Parturient on Methadone or Buprenorphine

With a 4-fold increase in pregnant patients with OUD over the last decade and a half,[59] the peripartum management of the opioid-tolerant patient requires consideration, as this patient population often requires higher average doses of opioid medications postoperatively.[60]

Treatment during pregnancy includes administration of either a full opioid agonist such as methadone, or a partial agonist such as buprenorphine, along with behavioral counseling.[61] It is also important to avoid acute maternal withdrawal, as it can result in increased maternal catecholamine release, uterine contractions, and decreased placental blood flow and oxygen supply, along with precipitating fetal withdrawal symptoms. All these events may lead to preterm labor, fetal hypoxia, and even fetal demise. The goal of MAT is to decrease symptoms from cravings and withdrawal as well as to decrease incidence of relapse into illicit opioid use.[59]

While women maintained on morphine and buprenorphine tend to experience similar pain levels intrapartum compared to women not on MAT, they have increased pain postpartum and require more morphine-equivalent doses if undergoing CD.[59,62] Hoflish et al.[60] examined the postoperative pain management of women dependent on opioids and found that patients maintained on methadone or buprenorphine were less likely to receive opioids and were more likely to receive NSAIDs postoperatively. One possibility proposed by the authors of this study was that clinicians for various reasons were hesitant to prescribe opioids to patients with a history of opioid abuse and instead increased NSAID use to attempt to treat pain.[60]

Both buprenorphine and methadone can be safely continued throughout peripartum and postpartum period, and these patients benefit from multimodal analgesia with acetaminophen, NSAIDs, and systemic opioids.[59,63] The addition of epidural clonidine has been shown to be beneficial for this patient population potentially by providing further analgesia by alpha-2 receptor activation as well as providing a local anesthetic-sparing effect. Possible side effects of epidural clonidine include hypotension, maternal sedation, and both fetal and maternal bradycardia.[64] Regional blocks such as TAP or QLB may be helpful if neuraxial anesthesia is unable to be performed or if breakthrough pain is experienced, but no studies have been done to evaluate the benefit of blocks in this patient population. The goal is to manage postoperative pain with neuraxial analgesia, multimodal pain regimen, and judicious opioid administration in a safe manner that provides pain relief and prevents withdrawal.[59]

POSTOPERATIVE PAIN MANAGEMENT AND LACTATION

For mothers looking to breastfeed, effective postoperative analgesia facilitates a better chance of successful breastfeeding, leading to better maternal-neonatal bonding. Many treatment options have the potential to transfer to the breastfeeding infant, and human data regarding the transfer to breast milk remains lacking, likely from the difficulty of conducting randomized control trials in this patient population.[5,26]

The majority of medications transfer to breast milk by passive diffusion at a rate that is proportionate to the maternal plasma concentration of the drug. Pharmacological properties associated with greater transfer of medications into breast milk include low molecular weight, higher pKa, decreased protein binding, and high lipid solubility.[5] To minimize infant analgesic exposure through breast milk, several general principles should be applied, including: use of opioid-sparing multimodal analgesia, utilization of neuraxial opioids when feasible, opting for medications that are highly protein bound, have low oral bioavailability, a short half-life, and inactive metabolites.[4,26]

Acetaminophen, ibuprofen, and ketorolac are commonly used for treatment of post-CD pain. Ibuprofen has some benefits, such as half-life of only 1.8 hours and opioid-sparing effect. Meperidine and codeine should be avoided due to higher risk of neonatal respiratory sedation secondary to variability in half-life and active metabolites, respectively. The half-life of hydromorphone in breast milk is 10.5 hours and therefore should be used cautiously given its potency. Single-dose epidural or intravenous morphine is proven to be safe, as it has low bioavailability and a short half-life in breast milk (3 h); however, repeat dosing should be avoided as it may lead to increased levels of both morphine and its metabolite morphine-6-glucoronide in breast milk, potentially leading to neonatal side effects.

Generally, a woman can resume breastfeeding after general anesthesia once she is awake and alert, as this indicates sedation medications have redistributed from the plasma to the adipose and muscle tissue, and therefore only minimal medication is available in the plasma to transfer to the neonate.[5]

In conclusion, the goal for postoperative management of women wanting to breastfeed should be aimed at adequate analgesia while minimizing neonatal and maternal systemic opioid exposure.[52]

CONCLUSIONS

Benefits of neuraxial anesthesia for CD are multiple, including: (1) less neonatal exposure to anesthetics; (2) better postoperative pain control with use of neuraxial opioids; and (3) avoidance of general anesthesia that poses increased risk for failed intubation, aspiration, and intraoperative awareness. Different neuraxial techniques may be used. Compared to epidural or CSE, spinal anesthesia is faster to perform, results in quicker and denser block, and decreases operating room time; but it results in more profound hypotension and does not allow for repeat neuraxial dosing.

Suboptimal perioperative pain control for CD is associated with increased opioid use and the development of chronic pain, worse maternal-fetal bonding, and increased incidence of postpartum depression. Comprehensive analgesia for cesarean surgery should include neuraxial morphine unless contraindicated, non-opioid adjuncts, regional analgesia, and PO or IV opioids if there is severe breakthrough pain.

Abdominal wall blocks should be considered when neuraxial morphine is not administered. Quadratus lumborum and transverse abdominus blocks have minimal improvement in pain control if neuraxial morphine was administered, but show significant improvement if no neuraxial morphine was given.

Both buprenorphine and methadone can be safely continued throughout peripartum and postpartum period, and patients on MAT benefit from multimodal analgesia with acetaminophen, NSAIDs, and systemic opioids, as well as addition of clonidine to epidural solution.

REFERENCES

1. Tsen L, Bateman B. Anesthesia for cesarean delivery. In: DH Wong, CA Tsen LC, et al. *Chestnut's Obstetric Anesthesia: Principles and Practice*. Sixth ed. Philadelphia, PA: Elsevier; 2020:568–626.
2. Lamon AM, Einhorn LM, Cooter M, Habib AS. The impact of body mass index on the risk of high spinal block in parturients undergoing cesarean delivery: a retrospective cohort study. *J Anesthes.* 2017;31(4):552–558.
3. ACOG. Committee opinion no. 742: postpartum pain management. *Obstet Gynecol.* 2018;132(1):e35–e43.
4. Dalal PG, Bosak J, Berlin C. Safety of the breast-feeding infant after maternal anesthesia. *Paediatr Anaesth.* 2014;24(4):359–371.
5. Cobb B, Liu R, Valentine E, O'nuoha O. Breastfeeding after anesthesia: a review for anesthesia providers regarding the transfer of medications into breast milk: a manuscript. 2015:1–7. Located at: Transl Perioper Pain Med.
6. Martin JA, Hamilton BE, Osterman MJK, Driscoll AK. Births: final data for 2018. *Natl Vital Stat Rep.* 2019;68(13):1–47.
7. Rollins M, Lucero J. Overview of anesthetic considerations for Cesarean delivery. *Br Med Bull.* 2012;101:101–125.
8. Benhamou D, Wong C. Neuraxial anesthesia for cesarean delivery: what criteria define the "optimal" technique? *Anesth Analg.* 2009;109(5):1370–1373.
9. Huang C, Hsieh Y, Wei K, Sun W, Tsao S. A comparison of spinal and epidural anesthesia for cesarean section following epidural labor analgesia: a retrospective cohort study. *Acta Anaesthesiol Taiwanica.* 2015;53(1):7–11.
10. Horstman DJ, Riley ET, Carvalho B. A randomized trial of maximum cephalad sensory blockade with single-shot spinal compared with combined spinal-epidural techniques for cesarean delivery. *Anesth Analg.* 2009;108(1):240–245.
11. Ithnin F, Lim Y, Sia AT, Ocampo CE. Combined spinal epidural causes higher level of block than equivalent single-shot spinal anesthesia in elective cesarean patients. *Anesth Analg.* 2006;102(2):577–580.
12. Lew E, Yeo SW, Thomas E. Combined spinal-epidural anesthesia using epidural volume extension leads to faster motor recovery after elective cesarean delivery: a prospective, randomized, double-blind study. *Anesth Analg.* 2004;98(3):810–814.
13. Choi DH, Ahn HJ, Kim JA. Combined low-dose spinal-epidural anesthesia versus single-shot spinal anesthesia for elective cesarean delivery. *Int J Obstet Anesth.* 2006;15(1):13–17.
14. Javed S, Hamid S, Amin F, Mahmood K. Spinal anesthesia induced complications in caesarean section: a review. *J Pharm Sci and Res.* 2011;3(10):1530–1538.
15. Teoh WH, Thomas E, Tan HM. Ultra-low dose combined spinal-epidural anesthesia with intrathecal bupivacaine 3.75 mg for

cesarean delivery: a randomized controlled trial. *Int J Obstet Anesth.* 2006;15(4):273–278.
16. Alhashemi J, Crosby E, Grodecki W, Duffy P, Hull K, Gallant C. Treatment of intrathecal morphine-induced pruritus following caesarean section. *Can J Anaesth.* 1997;44(10):1060–1065.
17. Szarvas S, Harmon D, Murphy D. Neuraxial opioid-induced pruritus: a review. *J Clin Anesth.* 2003;15(3):234–239.
18. Balki M, Carvalho JC. Intraoperative nausea and vomiting during cesarean section under regional anesthesia. *Int J Obstet Anesth.* 2005;14(3):230–241.
19. Lee AJ, Landau R. Aortocaval compression syndrome: time to revisit certain dogmas. *Anesth Analg.* 2017;125(6):1975–1985.
20. Turhanoglu S, Kaya S, Erdogan H. Is there an advantage in using low-dose intrathecal bupivacaine for cesarean section? *J Anesth.* 2009;23(3):353–357.
21. Lee JE, George RB, Habib AS. Spinal-induced hypotension: Incidence, mechanisms, prophylaxis, and management: Summarizing 20 years of research. *Best Pract Res Clin Anaesthesiol.* 2017;31(1):57–68.
22. Arzola C, Wieczorek PM. Efficacy of low-dose bupivacaine in spinal anaesthesia for caesarean delivery: systematic review and meta-analysis. *Br J Anaesth.* 2011;107(3):308–318.
23. Fitzgerald JP, Fedoruk KA, Jadin SM, Carvalho B, Halpern SH. Prevention of hypotension after spinal anaesthesia for caesarean section: a systematic review and network meta-analysis of randomised controlled trials. *Anaesthesia.* 2020;75(1):109–121.
24. D'Angelo R, Smiley RM, Riley ET, Segal S. Serious complications related to obstetric anesthesia: the serious complication repository project of the Society for Obstetric Anesthesia and Perinatology. *Anesthesiology.* 2014;120(6):1505–1512.
25. Leo S, Sng BL, Lim Y, Sia AT. A randomized comparison of low doses of hyperbaric bupivacaine in combined spinal-epidural anesthesia for cesarean delivery. *Anesth Analg.* 2009;109(5):1600–1605.
26. Sutton CD, Carvalho B. Optimal pain management after cesarean delivery. *Anesthesiology clinics.* 2017;35(1):107–124.
27. Gamez BH, Habib AS. Predicting severity of acute pain after cesarean delivery: a narrative review. *Anesth Analg.* 2018;126(5):1606–1614.
28. Bauchat JR, Weiniger CF, Sultan P, et al. Society for Obstetric Anesthesia and Perinatology consensus statement: monitoring recommendations for prevention and detection of respiratory depression associated with administration of neuraxial morphine for cesarean delivery analgesia. *Anesth Analg.* 2019;129(2):458–474.
29. Lavand'homme P. Postoperative cesarean pain: real but is it preventable? *Curr Opin Anaesthesiol.* 2018;31(3):262–267.
30. Bonnet MP, Mignon A, Mazoit J, Ozier Y, Marret E. Analgesic efficacy and adverse effects of epidural morphine compared to parenteral opioids after elective caesarean section: A systematic review. *Eur J Pain.* 2010;14:e891–894;e899.
31. Leighton BL, Crock LW. Case series of successful postoperative pain management in buprenorphine maintenance therapy patients. *Anesth Analg.* 2017;125(5):1779–1783.
32. Mishriky BM, George RB, Habib AS. Transversus abdominis plane block for analgesia after cesarean delivery: a systematic review and meta-analysis. *Can J Anaesth.* 2012;59(8):766–778.
33. Champaneria R, Shah L, Wilson MJ, Daniels JP. Clinical effectiveness of transversus abdominis plane (TAP) blocks for pain relief after caesarean section: a meta-analysis. *Int J Obstet Anesth.* 2016;28:45–60.
34. Loane H, Preston R, Douglas MJ, Massey S, Papsdorf M, Tyler J. A randomized controlled trial comparing intrathecal morphine with transversus abdominis plane block for post-cesarean delivery analgesia. *Int J Obstet Anesth.* 2012;21(2):112–118.
35. Singh S, Dhir S, Marmai K, Rehou S, Silva M, Bradbury C. Efficacy of ultrasound-guided transversus abdominis plane blocks for post-cesarean delivery analgesia: a double-blind, dose-comparison, placebo-controlled randomized trial. *Int J Obstet Anesth.* 2013;22(3):188–193.
36. Staker JJ, Liu D, Church R, et al. A triple-blind, placebo-controlled randomised trial of the ilioinguinal-transversus abdominis plane (I-TAP) nerve block for elective caesarean section. *Anaesthesia.* 2018;73(5):594–602.
37. Nedeljkovic SS, Kett A, Vallejo MC, et al. Transversus abdominis plane block with liposomal bupivacaine for pain after cesarean delivery in a multicenter, randomized, double-blind, controlled trial. *Anesth Analg.* 2020;131(6):1830–1839.
38. Mitchell KD, Smith CT, Mechling C, Wessel CB, Orebaugh S, Lim G. A review of peripheral nerve blocks for cesarean delivery analgesia. *Reg Anesth Pain Med.* 2019 Oct 25:rapm-2019-100752.
39. Patel SD, Sharawi N, Sultan P. Local anaesthetic techniques for post-caesarean delivery analgesia. *Int J Obstet Anesth.* 2019;40:62–77.
40. Elsharkawy H, El-Boghdadly K, Barrington M. Quadratus lumborum block: anatomical concepts, mechanisms, and techniques. *Anesthesiology.* 2019;130(2):322–335.
41. Krohg A, Ullensvang K, Rosseland LA, Langesaeter E, Sauter AR. The analgesic effect of ultrasound-guided quadratus lumborum block after cesarean delivery: a randomized clinical trial. *Anesth Analg.* 2018;126(2):559–565.
42. Blanco R, Ansari T, Riad W, Shetty N. Quadratus lumborum block versus transversus abdominis plane block for postoperative pain after cesarean delivery: a randomized controlled trial. *Reg Anesth Pain Med.* 2016;41(6):757–762.
43. Mieszkowski MM, Mayzner-Zawadzka E, Tuyakov B, et al. Evaluation of the effectiveness of the quadratus lumborum block type I using ropivacaine in postoperative analgesia after a cesarean section: a controlled clinical study. *Ginekologia polska.* 2018;89(2):89–96.
44. Blanco R, Ansari T, Girgis E. Quadratus lumborum block for postoperative pain after caesarean section: a randomised controlled trial. *Eur J Anaesthesiol.* 2015;32(11):812–818.
45. Canakci E, Gultekin A, Cebeci Z, Hanedan B, Kilinc A. The analgesic efficacy of transverse abdominis plane block versus epidural block after caesarean delivery: which one is effective? TAP block? Epidural block? *Pain Res Manage.* 2018;2018:3562701.
46. Hayaran N, Malhotra R, Tyagi S, Jain A. Transversus abdominis plane block with ilioinguinal-iliohypogastric nerve a viable alternative to provide surgical anesthesia for cesarean delivery: a case report. *A&A Pract.* 2019;12(6):185–186.
47. Ueshima H, Otake H, Lin JA. Ultrasound-guided quadratus lumborum block: an updated review of anatomy and techniques. *Biomed Res Int.* 2017;2017:2752876.
48. Xu M, Tang Y, Wang J, Yang J. Quadratus lumborum block for postoperative analgesia after cesarean delivery: a systematic review and meta-analysis. *Int J Obstet Anesth.* 2020;42:87–98.
49. Hussain N, Brull R, Weaver T, Zhou M, Essandoh M, Abdallah FW. Postoperative analgesic effectiveness of quadratus lumborum block for cesarean delivery under spinal anesthesia. *Anesthesiology.* 2021;134(1):72–87.
50. El-Boghdadly K, Desai N, Halpern S, et al. Quadratus lumborum block vs. transversus abdominis plane block for caesarean delivery: a systematic review and network meta-analysis. *Anaesthesia.* 2021 Mar;76(3):393–403.
51. Hamburger J, Beilin Y. Systemic adjunct analgesics for cesarean delivery: a narrative review. *Int J Obstet Anesth.* 2019 Nov;40:101–118.
52. Carvalho B, Butwick AJ. Postcesarean delivery analgesia. *Best Pract Res Clin Anaesthesiol.* 2017;31(1):69–79.
53. Zeng AM, Nami NF, Wu CL, Murphy JD. The analgesic efficacy of nonsteroidal anti-inflammatory agents (NSAIDs) in patients undergoing cesarean deliveries: a meta-analysis. *Reg Anesth Pain Med.* 2016;41(6):763–772.
54. Brinck EC, Tiippana E, Heesen M, et al. Perioperative intravenous ketamine for acute postoperative pain in adults. *Cochrane Database Syst Rev.* 2018;12(12):CD012033.
55. Heesen M, Böhmer J, Brinck EC, et al. Intravenous ketamine during spinal and general anaesthesia for caesarean section: systematic review and meta-analysis. *Acta Anaesthesiol Scand.* 2015;59(4):414–426.
56. Allen TK, Jones CA, Habib AS. Dexamethasone for the prophylaxis of postoperative nausea and vomiting associated with neuraxial morphine administration: a systematic review and meta-analysis. *Anesth Analg.* 2012;114(4):813–822.
57. El Kenany S, El Tahan MR. Effect of preoperative pregabalin on post-caesarean delivery analgesia: a dose-response study. *Int J Obstet Anesth.* 2016;26:24–31.

58. Monks DT, Hoppe DW, Downey K, Shah V, Bernstein P, Carvalho JC. A perioperative course of gabapentin does not produce a clinically meaningful improvement in analgesia after cesarean delivery: a randomized controlled trial. *Anesthesiology.* 2015;123(2):320–326.
59. Landau R. Post-cesarean delivery pain: management of the opioid-dependent patient before, during and after cesarean delivery. *Int J Obstet Anesth.* 2019 Aug;39:105–116.
60. Hoflich AS, Langer M, Jagsch R, et al. Peripartum pain management in opioid dependent women. *Eur J Pain (London, England).* 2012;16(4):574–584.
61. Jones CW, Terplan M. Pregnancy and naltrexone pharmacotherapy. *Obstetr Gynecol.* 2018;132(4):923–925.
62. Meyer M, Paranya G, Keefer Norris A, Howard D. Intrapartum and postpartum analgesia for women maintained on buprenorphine during pregnancy. *Eur J Pain (London, England).* 2010;14(9):939–943.
63. Vilkins AL, Bagley SM, Hahn KA, et al. Comparison of post-cesarean section opioid analgesic requirements in women with opioid use disorder treated with methadone or buprenorphine. *J Addict Med.* 2017;11(5):397–401.
64. Hoyt MR, Shah U, Cooley J, Temple M. Use of epidural clonidine for the management of analgesia in the opioid addicted parturient on buprenorphine maintenance therapy: an observational study. *Int J Obstet Anesth.* 2018;34:67–72.
65. Dahl JB, Jeppesen IS, Jorgensen H, Wetterslev J, Moiniche S. Intraoperative and postoperative analgesic efficacy and adverse effects of intrathecal opioids in patients undergoing cesarean section with spinal anesthesia: a qualitative and quantitative systematic review of randomized controlled trials. *Anesthesiology.* 1999;91(6):1919–1927.
66. Dahlgren G, Hultstrand C, Jakobsson J, Norman M, Eriksson EW, Martin H. Intrathecal sufentanil, fentanyl, or placebo added to bupivacaine for cesarean section. *Anesth Analg.* 1997;85(6):1288–1293.
67. Tsen L, Bateman B. Anesthesia for cesarean delivery. In: DH Wong CA Tsen LC, et al. *Chestnut's Obstetric Anesthesia: Principles and Practice.* Sixth ed. Philadelphia, PA: Elsevier; 2020:568–626.
68. George R, Carvalho B, Butwick A, Flood P. In: DH Wong CA Tsen LC, et al. *Chestnut's Obstetric Anesthesia: Principles and Practice.* Sixth ed. Philadelphia, PA: Elsevier; 2020:627–669.
69. Tschopp C, Tramèr MR, Schneider A, Zaarour M, Elia N. Benefit and harm of adding epinephrine to a local anesthetic for neuraxial and locoregional anesthesia: a meta-analysis of randomized controlled trials with trial sequential analyses. *Anesth Analg.* 2018;127(1):228–239.
70. Katz D, Hamburger J, Gutman D, et al. The effect of adding subarachnoid epinephrine to hyperbaric bupivacaine and morphine for repeat cesarean delivery: a double-blind prospective randomized control trial. *Anesth Analg.* 2018;127(1):171–178.
71. Crespo S, Dangelser G, Haller G. Intrathecal clonidine as an adjuvant for neuraxial anaesthesia during caesarean delivery: a systematic review and meta-analysis of randomised trials. *Int J Obstet Anesth.* 2017;32:64–76.
72. Lavand'homme PM, Roelants F, Waterloos H, Collet V, De Kock MF. An evaluation of the postoperative antihyperalgesic and analgesic effects of intrathecal clonidine administered during elective cesarean delivery. *Anesth Analg.* 2008;107(3):948–955.
73. Fernandes HS, Bliacheriene F, Vago TM, et al. Clonidine effect on pain after cesarean delivery: a randomized controlled trial of different routes of administration. *Anesth Analg.* 2018;127(1):165–170.
74. Cossu AP, De Giudici LM, Piras D, et al. A systematic review of the effects of adding neostigmine to local anesthetics for neuraxial administration in obstetric anesthesia and analgesia. *Int J Obstet Anesth.* 2015;24(3):237–246.
75. Kaya FN, Sahin S, Owen MD, Eisenach JC. Epidural neostigmine produces analgesia but also sedation in women after cesarean delivery. *Anesthesiology.* 2004;100(2):381–385.
76. Pan PM, Huang CT, Wei TT, Mok MS. Enhancement of analgesic effect of intrathecal neostigmine and clonidine on bupivacaine spinal anesthesia. *Reg Anesth Pain Med.* 1998;23(1):49–56.
77. Chung CJ, Kim JS, Park HS, Chin YJ. The efficacy of intrathecal neostigmine, intrathecal morphine, and their combination for post-cesarean section analgesia. *Anesth Analg.* 1998;87(2):341–346.

REVIEW QUESTIONS

(1) What best describes the mechanism of action of buprenorphine?

A. Full mu receptor agonist
B. Partial mu receptor antagonist
C. Partial mu receptor agonist and kappa receptor antagonist
D. Mu receptor agonist and kappa receptor agonist

(2) Which of the following has not been shown to decrease incidence of postoperative nausea and vomiting (PONV) in cesarean delivery (CD)?

A. Judicious use of opioids
B. Supplemental oxygen
C. Low-dose intrathecal bupivacaine
D. Limiting uterotonic administration

(3) In regard to postoperative pain management for CD, which patient would benefit most from transversus abdominis plane (TAP) block?

A. Patient had single-shot spinal with intrathecal bupivacaine, fentanyl, and morphine.
B. Patient with epidural who underwent emergent CD under general anesthesia and morphine was administered through epidural prior to emergence.
C. Patient had single-shot spinal with intrathecal bupivacaine and fentanyl.
D. Patient underwent emergent CD under general anesthesia, but morphine was administered postoperatively through epidural before catheter was removed.

(4) Which of the following has the least effect on spread of block after spinal anesthetic?

A. Cerebrospinal fluid (CSF) volume
B. Patient positioning
C. Dose of local anesthetic
D. Baricity of local anesthetic

(5) What is the recommended first-line agent in treatment of hypotension during cesarean delivery (CD) after administration of intrathecal local anesthetic?

A. Glycopyrrolate
B. Ephedrine
C. Norepinephrine
D. Phenylephrine

(6) Compared to TAP block, when would you see the most significant opioid-sparing benefit from performing QLB in patients who did not receive intrathecal morphine (ITM)?

A. Immediately postoperatively
B. At the time of PACU discharge
C. At 6 hours postoperative
D. >12 hours postoperative

(7) Which pharmacological property is associated with a greater transfer of medications from maternal circulation to breast milk?

A. High protein binding
B. Low lipid solubility
C. High pKa
D. Increased molecular weight

(8) Which treatment approach would decrease post-CD opioid consumption the most?

A. Single preoperative dose of a gabapentinoid
B. Scheduled acetaminophen along with NSAIDs
C. Intravenous dexamethasone
D. Acetaminophen as needed

(9) Which of the following is not a benefit from medication assisted treatment (MAT) for patients with opioid use disorder (OUD) during pregnancy?

A. Decreased post-CD pain compared to women not on MAT
B. Decreased symptoms from cravings and withdrawal
C. Improved adherence to prenatal care
D. Decreased incidence of relapse into illicit opioid use

ANSWERS

(1) **A.** Buprenorphine is a partial mu opioid receptor agonist and a weak kappa receptor antagonist. Buprenorphine has a high affinity for mu opioid receptors and dissociates slowly from mu receptor, which decreases chance of withdrawal with cessation of medication. Large doses of full mu receptor agonists are required to replace buprenorphine from mu receptors.

Reference

Jones CW, Terplan M. Pregnancy and naltrexone pharmacotherapy. *Obstetr Gynecol.* 2018;132(4):923–925.

(2) **B.** Supplemental oxygen has not been shown to decrease incidence of PONV. Strategies to prevent PONV include avoiding hypotension and treating with vasopressors if needed, judicious use of uterotonics and opioids, low-dose intrathecal anesthetic, and adequate surgical block to decrease surgical stimuli.

Reference

Balki M, Carvalho JC. Intraoperative nausea and vomiting during cesarean section under regional anesthesia. *Int J Obstetr Anesth.* 2005;14(3):230–241.

(3) **C.** While transversus abdominis plane (TAP) block has shown some benefit if neuraxial morphine is administered, the most benefit from TAP block is seen if neuraxial morphine is unable to be administered. Both quadratus lumborum block (QLB) and single-shot epidural anesthesia have shown to be better than postoperative TAP block. Situations in which TAP block is beneficial for postoperative pain is if the provider is unfamiliar with the technique of QLB, neuraxial morphine was not administered, or as rescue adjunct if breakthrough pain is experienced, especially in patient population on opioid-dependence therapy.

References

Mishriky BM, George RB, Habib AS. Transversus abdominis plane block for analgesia after Cesarean delivery: a systematic review and meta-analysis. *Can J Anaesth.* 2012;59(8):766–778.
Champaneria R, Shah L, Wilson MJ, Daniels JP. Clinical effectiveness of transversus abdominis plane (TAP) blocks for pain relief after caesarean section: a meta-analysis. *Int J Obstetr Anesth.* 2016;28:45–60.

(4) **A.** CSF volume has the least effect on the spread of the spinal block. The most important determinants of anesthetic spread after spinal include dose of local anesthetic, baricity of local anesthetic, and initial patient positioning. Other factors that have a minor effect on spread of block include CSF volume, with an increased volume resulting in decreased spread, and abdominal pressure, with increase in pressure causing an increase in spread.

References

Lamon AM, Einhorn LM, Cooter M, Habib AS. The impact of body mass index on the risk of high spinal block in parturients undergoing cesarean delivery: a retrospective cohort study. *J Anesth.* 2017;31(4):552–558.
Javed S, Hamid S, Amin F, Mahmood K. Spinal anesthesia induced complications in caesarean section: a review. *J Pharm Sci and Res.* 2011;3(10):1530–1538.

(5) **D.** Phenylephrine is the first line treatment of hypotension after spinal anesthesia. Glycopyrrolate has not shown to decrease the incidence of hypotension following spinal anesthesia in cesarean section. Norepinephrine has not been shown to be superior to phenylephrine. While ephedrine is effective in treating hypotension, it has shown to cause fetal acidosis compared to phenylephrine.

References

Lee JE, George RB, Habib AS. Spinal-induced hypotension: incidence, mechanisms, prophylaxis, and management: summarizing 20 years of research. *Best Pract Res Clin Anaesthesiol.* 2017;31(1):57–68.
Fitzgerald JP, Fedoruk KA, Jadin SM, Carvalho B, Halpern SH. Prevention of hypotension after spinal anaesthesia for caesarean section: a systematic review and network meta-analysis of randomised controlled trials. *Anaesthesia.* 2020;75(1):109–121.

(6) **D.** When compared to TAP in patients who did not receive ITM, QLB showed no opioid-sparing benefit on initial 6 hours after cesarean delivery, but had significant benefit at 12, 24, and 48 hours postoperatively (the differences were 37.5%, 55%, and 48%, respectively). There were no significant differences in visual analog scale (VAS) pain scores between TAP and QLB groups.

Reference

Blanco R, Ansari T, Riad W, Shetty N. Quadratus lumborum block versus transversus abdominis plane block for postoperative pain after cesarean delivery: a randomized controlled trial. *Reg Anesth Pain Med.* 2016;41(6):757–762.

(7) **C.** Pharmacological properties associated with greater transfer of medications into breast milk include low molecular weight, higher pKa, decreased protein binding, and high lipid solubility.

Reference

Cobb B, Liu R, Valentine E, O'nuoha O. Breastfeeding after anesthesia: a review for anesthesia providers regarding the transfer of medications into breast milk: a manuscript. 2015:1–7. Located at: Transl Perioper Pain Med.

(8) **B.** Acetaminophen decreases postoperative opioid use, has a good safety profile at regular doses, and minimal breast-milk transfer. Although there is potential benefit of a single preoperative dose of acetaminophen, the most benefit is seen when regular interval dosing is used. Meta-analysis of NSAID use versus control showed better pain scores on initial 24 hours, also less opioid use and less drowsiness/sedation. There is only weak evidence that steroids provide an opioid-sparing effect, but given that they are effective and routinely used to prevent PONV, it is reasonable to consider their use. The literature on gabapentinoids has shown some benefit but at the expense of increased side effects such as sedation, dizziness, and abnormal vision.

References

Hamburger J, Beilin Y. Systemic adjunct analgesics for cesarean delivery: a narrative review. *Int J Obstet Anesth*. 2019 Nov;40:101–118.

Monks DT, Hoppe DW, Downey K, Shah V, Bernstein P, Carvalho JC. A perioperative course of gabapentin does not produce a clinically meaningful improvement in analgesia after cesarean delivery: a randomized controlled trial. *Anesthesiology*. 2015;123(2):320–326.

(9) **A.** The goal of medication assisted treatment is to decrease symptoms from cravings and withdrawal, as well as to decrease incidence of relapse into illicit opioid use. Women maintained on morphine and buprenorphine tend to experience similar pain levels intrapartum compared to women not on medication-assisted therapy, but they have increased postpartum pain and require more morphine-equivalent doses if undergoing cesarean delivery.

Reference

Landau R. Post-cesarean delivery pain: management of the opioid-dependent patient before, during and after cesarean delivery. *Int J Obstet Anesth*. 2019 Aug;39:105–116.

36.

POST-DURAL PUNCTURE HEADACHE

Lauren Sayre and Robert Gaiser

CASE

Ms. RH is a 23-year-old G2P1001 at 39 weeks gestation. Her past medical history is notable for migraine headaches. She has not experienced a headache during her pregnancy. Her previous pregnancy resulted in an uncomplicated spontaneous vaginal delivery of a live male infant. The obstetrician is performing an induction of labor because of the ARRIVE Trial (a randomized trial of induction of labor versus expectant management).[1] Twenty-six hours after beginning the induction, her cervical dilation is 5 cm and the pain is 10/10, and she requests epidural analgesia. During epidural placement, she experiences a contraction and moves. The anesthesiologist seemed annoyed by her movement and made a comment about fluid from the epidural needle. She feels a stick at another location and shortly thereafter, she achieves fairly quick relief from the pain and delivers a healthy live female neonate 7 hours later. The following day, she notes a bilateral frontal headache that is positional. She attributes the headache to her migraines and requests Fioricet. She is discharged and is noting difficulty feeding the baby due to a headache with no relief from medications. She calls her obstetrician who refers her to the Department of Anesthesiology. She is diagnosed with a post-dural puncture headache (PDPH) and receives a sphenopalatine ganglion block. There is relief of the headache, with the symptoms returning the following day. After discussion with the anesthesiologist, she agrees to an epidural blood patch. Following the blood patch, she noted immediate relief of the headache; she returned home and was able to care for the baby. She did note some minor back pain, which lasted for approximately 1 month.

(1) WHAT ARE THE CAUSES OF HEADACHE IN THE POSTPARTUM PATIENT IN GENERAL?

The most common cause of a headache after delivery is a tension headache, most likely due to the stress and fatigue accompanying delivery. After tension headache, the second most common reason for a postpartum headache is pre-eclampsia, requiring management of blood pressure to prevent further complications. The third most common cause of headache is post-dural puncture headache (PDPH), following spinal anesthesia with a Quincke needle or accidental dural puncture (ADP) during epidural catheter placement.[2] Not all dural punctures are witnessed; headache may follow epidural catheter placement without seeing cerebrospinal fluid due to nicking of the dura.[3]

(2) WHY DID THIS PATIENT DEVELOP A POST-DURAL PUNCTURE HEADACHE (PDPH)? DOES EVERY PATIENT WHO HAS AN ADP DEVELOP A HEADACHE?

Not all parturients who experience ADP develop a headache. The incidence of PDPH in the parturient after ADP with an epidural needle is 52.1%.[4] This differs from the general surgical population, where the incidence of headache following ADP ranges from 0.5% to 50%.[5] The variability in incidence is related to the age of the patient and the management of the patient postoperatively. In regard to obstetric patients, not all parturients who have an ADP will develop a PDPH. Patient factors influence the risk. These factors include age (older patients less likely) and cesarean delivery (bearing down during the second stage of labor increases the risk). Studies regarding body mass index (BMI) decreasing the risk of PDPH are conflicting. High BMI definitely does not increase the risk.

(3) WHAT IS THE CLINICAL PRESENTATION OF THE PDPH?

A PDPH is a positional headache that worsens with the upright position and improves with the supine position. The headache is generally bilateral and located in the frontal-occipital area. Occasionally, patients present with a non-positional headache or a headache that improves with the upright position (these findings are the exception).[6] Other findings with the traditional positional headache include nausea, neck pain, shoulder pain, diplopia, hypoacusis, and back pain (Box 36.1).

(4) WHAT FACTORS INCREASE OR DECREASE THE INCIDENCE OF DEVELOPING PDPH AFTER DURAL TAP?

Age had a significant inverse relationship with the development of PDPH for spinal anesthesia and for ADP during epidural catheter placement. The type of needle is important, as cutting-edge needles have higher incidences compared to pencil-point needles. Men have approximately half the risk of developing a PDPH compared to non-pregnant women. A higher BMI does not increase the risk of the development of

Box 36.1 CHARACTERISTICS OF POST-DURAL PUNCTURE HEADACHE

Positional
Frontal-occipital
Bilateral
Nausea
Afebrile
Hearing alteration
Diplopia

PDPH and may be protective. The possible protective effect in individuals with greater BMI is controversial. Cesarean delivery in itself may be protective as it avoids the bearing down during the second stage of labor, which has been proposed to increase the size of the rent in the dura. This point is confirmed when considering women who require cesarean delivery after a failed attempt at labor. Women who deliver prior to pushing have a lesser risk of developing a headache as compared to those who push.[7,8]

(5) IS THERE ANYTHING THAT THE ANESTHESIA PROVIDER MAY HAVE DONE TO PREVENT THE PATIENT FROM DEVELOPING A HEADACHE?

At the time of ADP during epidural anesthesia, the provider is confronted with the decision of whether to thread the catheter into the intrathecal space or to reattempt epidural catheter placement at another location. Initially, there was some thought that an intrathecal catheter placed at the time of ADP would prevent or decrease the incidence of PDPH; a well-conducted randomized trial failed to prove a benefit to an intrathecal catheter in regard to PDPH. An intrathecal catheter does spare the patient from a second needle stick and a possible second ADP. The decision of whether or not to place an intrathecal catheter should be based upon the initial difficulty of the attempt as well as the stage in labor for the patient; the decision should not be based upon the risk of developing a PDPH.[9]

(6) WHAT OTHER PROPHYLACTIC OPTIONS THAT CAN PREVENT THE DEVELOPMENT OF PDPH?

The other options that have been proposed for the prevention of a headache following ADP is placement of a prophylactic epidural blood patch or the use of intravenous cosyntropin. Both therapies do have literature to support a possible benefit and are not considered standard treatment for the prevention of PDPH.

(7) WHAT IS THE MECHANISM OF A PDPH?

This loss of cerebrospinal fluid creates intracranial hypotension, which causes a downward descent of the brain, with traction on the meninges in the frontal and occipital areas. This postulated mechanism is the most favored explanation as it easily accounts for the typical symptoms of a PDPH. Another postulated mechanism is the increase in the cerebral blood flow as a contributing factor. An instantaneous headache may occur when ADP occurs during epidural catheter placement when using loss-of-resistance to air. In this situation, air is introduced intrathecally, resulting in a headache that resolves in 24 hours, generally the time frame when PDPH begins.[10]

(8) HOW IS A PDPH DIAGNOSED?

A PDPH should be considered in any patient who complains of a headache after neuraxial anesthesia or lumbar puncture. Many ADPs are not obvious, and no CSF is seen. The diagnosis is based upon symptoms; the headache is positional and located in frontal-occipital area.

When diagnosing PDPH, life-threatening diagnoses should be considered in patients who have a constant, nonpositional headache. If the patient is febrile, a workup for meningitis is warranted. If the headache is consistent with a subdural hematoma or a cerebral venous thrombosis, computed tomography (CT) or magnetic resonance imaging (MRI) is indicated. If the symptoms are consistent with a PDPH, treatment may be initiated. If the patient does not respond to treatment or if there are neurologic abnormalities, imaging of the head with a CT scan or MRI should be considered.

(9) WHAT ARE THE AVAILABLE MEASURES FOR THE MANAGEMENT OF THE PATIENT?

Noninvasive means of treating a PDPH have limited success. Studies found no benefit to bed rest and increased fluid intake. Also, there is no scientific basis to recommend the use of caffeine or theophylline. While both agents are cerebral vasoconstrictors, the headache is more from cerebrospinal fluid loss as compared to cerebral vasodilation. Intravenous neostigmine and atropine have been investigated and may be beneficial for a PDPH accompanying spinal anesthesia; they are not effective for PDPH from epidural catheter placement.

Invasive means for treating PDPH include the sphenopalatine ganglion block and the epidural blood patch.[11]

(10) WHAT IS THE NATURAL HISTORY OF PDPH IF NOT TREATED?

Although the International Headache Society states that a PDPH resolves within 1 week, this occurrence is based upon the assumption that the headache is the result of a dural puncture from a spinal needle. Epidural needles are much larger, and unintentional dural puncture may result in a headache of longer duration. Accidental dural puncture with an epidural needle places the patient at risk of developing a chronic headache which may persist for several months. The actual percentage of those who develop chronic headache is low and it is unclear which factors place the patient at risk for this complication.[12]

(11) WHAT IS SPHENOPALATINE GANGLION BLOCK?

The sphenopalatine ganglion block (SPGB) is a minimally invasive procedure that targets parasympathetic and sympathetic ganglia, as well as sensory innervation of the maxillary distribution of the trigeminal nerve. The block is simple to perform involving a cotton swab soaked with 2%–4% viscous lidocaine, inserted into the nasal cavity until it meets the posterior pharyngeal wall superior to the middle turbinate. After the application has been held in place for 5–10 minutes, it is then removed and repeated in the other nostril. The block is relatively safe with minimal associated side effects, which include bleeding and discomfort during application of the swab. There are not enough prospective randomized studies to prove its beneficial effect as a first-line treatment for PDPH.

(12) WHAT IS AN EPIDURAL BLOOD PATCH? HOW IT IS PERFORMED?

An epidural blood patch (EBP) is a procedure in which autologous blood is injected into the epidural space to "patch" the hole where the dura was punctured. The optimal amount of blood to use for an epidural blood patch is 20 mL. The long-term benefit to an epidural blood patch is the "sealing" of the dural puncture; the immediate relief occurs from compression of the intrathecal space in the lumbar area, forcing cerebrospinal fluid cephalad. To perform an epidural blood patch, the patient is positioned either sitting or lateral. Once the epidural space is accessed, 10 to 20 mL of autologous blood is drawn in an aseptic fashion, and then slowly injected into the epidural space. While it is possible to perform this procedure with one person, a team of two or three individuals is helpful in order to aid in placing the intravenous catheter to retrieve the blood and to position the patient. While there are some studies to suggest a benefit to delaying an epidural blood patch for 24 hours after the development of a headache, these studies are retrospective. An epidural blood patch should be performed once the patient develops a headache and consents for the procedure.[13] An epidural blood patch is partially or completely effective in 90% of the cases. Approximately 10% of individuals receiving an EBP will require a second one (similar volume), which may be repeated within 24 hours. Failure to provide relief requires evaluation by neurology to confirm diagnosis and to prevent patient harm.

DISCUSSION

POST-DURAL PUNCTURE HEADACHE (PDPH)

A PDPH is a positional headache that is worse with the upright position and is improved with the supine position. The headache is generally bilateral and located in the frontal-occipital area and may be accompanied by nausea, neck pain, shoulder pain, and back pain. Cranial nerves are frequently affected; the cranial nerves are III, IV, VI, and VIII. Cranial nerve VI is the most commonly affected due to its long intracranial course; the resulting nerve palsy results in difficulty with eye movement.[14] Cranial nerve VIII is also affected following accidental dural puncture (ADP) with a Quincke needle. When there is cerebrospinal fluid loss from a dural puncture, there is essentially an endolymphatic hydrops through a patent cochlear aqueduct in the inner ear, resulting in hearing loss in the low frequency range.[15]

A meta-analysis was conducted to evaluate the risk of developing PDPH. This analysis included randomized controlled trials, cohort studies, and case series. The most important finding from the study was that the incidence of PDPH in the parturient after ADP with an epidural needle is 52.1%.[4] As such, not all parturients who have an ADP will develop a PDPH. The incidence of headache with lumbar puncture using a Quincke needle, 25-gauge, is 6.2%; it is 2% when using a pencil-point needle regardless of gauge (if headache occurs, it is generally less severe and does not require treatment).[5] In regard to the Quincke needle, the position of the bevel as relative to the spine has an influence on the risk of headache. If the bevel is parallel to the longitudinal axis of the spine, the incidence of headache is 10.9%; turning the needle 90 degrees so that the bevel is perpendicular to the longitudinal axis of the spine results in an incidence of 25.8%.[16] The incidence of PDPH following ADP in the non-obstetric population is influenced by the age of the patient and is reported in the range of 2%–50%, while the incidence of headache from a Quincke needle when used for spinal anesthesia in the non-obstetric population is 2%–25%.[17]

Even if the provider did not see cerebrospinal fluid during epidural catheter placement, it is possible for the patient to develop a headache afterward due to nicking of the dura by the local anesthetic infiltration needle, the epidural needle, or the catheter. When the dura is nicked, there will not be cerebrospinal fluid present in the needle or catheter. The incidence of unrecognized dural puncture is rare. In a series of 18,337 parturients who received epidural catheters, 61 of them developed a PDPH (0.33%).[3] The ability to place an epidural catheter in the parturient is a skill that must be maintained. When the labor floor is covered by those who do not typically do obstetric anesthesia, the risk of accidental dural puncture is increased.

DIFFERENTIAL DIAGNOSIS OF A HEADACHE IN THE POSTPARTUM PERIOD

While it is automatically assumed that a patient who presents with a headache after neuraxial anesthesia that the etiology is the anesthesia, there are other causes of headache in the postpartum patient (Box 36.2). A retrospective review of 95 parturients with a headache after delivery was conducted.[6] The most common cause of a headache after delivery was tension or migraine. This result is not surprising given the stress of childbirth, as well as the lack of sleep and concern for the newborn.

Box 36.2 **DIFFERENTIAL DIAGNOSIS OF HEADACHE IN THE POST-PARTUM PERIOD**

Post-dural puncture headache

Stress

Pre-eclampsia

Migraine

Meningitis

Cortical vein thrombosis

Subdural hematoma

The second leading cause of headache was preeclampsia. Headache is one of the criteria for the diagnosis of preeclampsia. This review highlights that postpartum preeclampsia is a reality and must be considered by all providers. The third leading cause of headache was PDPH. A tension headache is the most common cause of headache after delivery, not post-dural puncture.

Other causes of headache include medications. A woman experienced nausea following her delivery. She was treated with ondansetron 6 mg every 12 hours.[18] After initiating the ondansetron, she developed a headache, consistent with a PDPH. She did not have an accidental dural puncture and did have a normal CT scan. The headache resolved when the ondansetron was discontinued. Other causes of headache include caffeine withdrawal and lack of sleep.

Two important considerations when evaluating a headache in a patient who experienced an ADP is cerebral venous thrombosis and subdural hematoma. Both will present with headaches. Unlike a PDPH, headaches from cerebral venous thrombosis and subdural hematoma tend to be constant and not altered by position. Furthermore, these headaches do not respond to epidural blood patching. The incidence of cerebral venous thrombosis is between 1 in 3,000 to 1 in 10,000 pregnancies.[19] The hypercoagulable state of pregnancy increases the risk. Unlike a PDPH, the headache of a cerebral venous thrombosis is non-positional and has accompanying neurologic signs. It frequently progresses to seizures. PDPH may be a risk factor for its development.[20] A subdural hematoma may occur from the traction on the bridging veins from the intracranial hypotension accompanying the loss of cerebrospinal fluid.[21] It too has been associated with post-dural puncture and is different from PDPH in its constant nature. Finally, anytime there is a puncture of the dura, the patient is at risk for the development of meningitis. It too presents with a constant headache, with the patient being usually febrile and having photophobia. The most common organism in meningitis following accidental dural puncture is *Streptococcus salivarius*.[22]

A headache following an accidental dural puncture with a Tuohy needle or a deliberate dural puncture with a Quincke spinal needle during spinal anesthesia is a result of a loss of cerebrospinal fluid into the epidural space. Magnetic resonance imaging of patients with headache confirms this point.[23,24] This mechanism explains the location of the headache as well as the positional aspects to the headache. Another aspect to the headache is the increase in cerebral blood flow.[25] Transcranial Doppler in patients with a PDPH confirms this increase. This contribution to the headache is less than the downward descent of the brain from intracranial hypotension. Finally, while the use of loss-of-resistance to air for identifying the epidural space may increase the chance of the patient developing a headache if there is an ADP, this headache is different from a traditional PDPH. The headache that occurs when the provider has an ADP when using loss-of-resistance to air is a result of intrathecal air and is rapid in onset and self-limited.[10]

RISK FACTORS FOR THE DEVELOPMENT OF PDPH

Age is one characteristic that has been consistently shown to affect the risk of developing a PDPH. The study which established age as a risk factor was for spinal anesthesia with a Quincke needle and did not examine ADP. In this study of 873 consecutive patients, age had a significant inverse relationship with the development of PDPH.[26] It is fair to conclude that using a Quincke needle increases the risk of PDPH in a young patient. Since its publication, pencil-point needles are relatively uniformly used for spinal anesthesia in obstetric patients and have a lower chance of headache regardless of age.[27] There is a lower incidence of headache following ADP with an epidural needle in the older population, with the effect being not as great as seen for spinal anesthesia.

Gender was suggested as a risk factor for the development of a PDPH and was first postulated by Vandam and Dripps in 1954 when they published their study examining the use of spinal anesthesia.[28] This conclusion suffered from confounding as the authors included parturients who were young; it was unclear whether it was gender versus age. In a meta-analysis of 18 studies, men had a lower odds ratio of developing a PDPH (OR 0.55, CI 0.44–0.67), which means that men have approximately half the risk of developing a PDPH compared to non-pregnant women.[29] Importantly, this analysis excluded studies of parturients to remove the concern of age as a confounding variable. It is unclear why women have the higher risk. Furthermore, this analysis only applied to spinal anesthesia using a Quincke needle. There is no difference in the difference of headache following ADP using a Tuohy needle.

Body mass index (BMI) does not influence the risk of the development of headache following ADP in the obstetric population. Two studies have examined the issue, arriving at different conclusions. The first conducted a retrospective analysis of 18,315 neuraxial procedures (epidural or combined spinal-epidural), identifying 125 ADP.[30] Obesity was defined as a BMI greater than 30 kg/m^2. In this analysis, there was no difference in the incidence of headache, 80%. Another group conducted a retrospective analysis of 97,736 neuraxial procedures and identified 518 ADP. The incidence of headache was approximately 50% but was lower in those parturients with a BMI >31.5 kg/m^2.[31] Considering both studies, one may conclude that a higher BMI does not increase the risk of the development of PDPH and may be protective. These studies are confounded by the fact that obesity increases the risk of cesarean delivery.[32] Cesarean delivery in itself may be protective.

Box 36.3 **PATIENT CHARACTERISTICS INFLUENCING RISK OF DEVELOPING POST-DURAL PUNCTURE HEADACHE**

Age (older age being protective): primarily for spinal, not epidural

Gender (male gender being protective): primarily for spinal, not epidural

Body mass index (does not increase risk)

Cesarean delivery: lower risk for both spinal and epidural

Needle bevel 90° to the longitudinal axis of the spine (applies only to Quincke needle)

Women who deliver prior to pushing have a lesser risk of developing a headache as compared to those who push. In a retrospective analysis of 33 parturients who had an ADP with an 18-gauge Tuohy needle, 23 patients pushed, with 17 of them developing a PDPH. Of the 10 patients who did not push because of cesarean delivery prior to the second stage, only 1 patient developed a headache.[7] Bearing down during the second stage increases the risk of developing a headache following ADP. This point was confirmed in a study examining prophylactic epidural blood patches.[8] While the study demonstrated the lack of benefit to a prophylactic epidural blood patch, it also demonstrated a markedly lower incidence of headache in those parturients who delivered by cesarean section as compared to those delivered vaginally. An explanation for this increase in risk is within the anatomy of the dura mater and the arachnoid mater.[33] The thickness of the dura and arachnoid maters varies; in areas where the dura is particularly thin, bearing down may increase the size of the puncture hole (Box 36.3).

AFTER ACCIDENTAL DURAL PUNCTURE (ADP), WHAT OPTIONS ARE AVAILABLE TO THE PROVIDER?

Initially, it was thought that placement of a catheter into the subarachnoid space at the time of ADP would prevent the patient from developing a PDPH. This supposition was based upon a study in which 3 groups of patients were included: those who had the epidural catheter re-sited at another location; those who had an intrathecal catheter placed with removal immediately after delivery; and those who had an intrathecal catheter placed with removal 24 hours later.[34] In this case series (patients were not randomized to the groups), the placement of an intrathecal catheter reduced the risk of headache to half that of the group who did not receive an intrathecal catheter, while leaving the catheter in place for 24 hours resulted in a 10-fold decrease. The problem with this case series was that no one was able to repeat these impressive results. Patients who had an ADP and received an intrathecal catheter seemed to have a similar risk of developing a headache as those patients who did not. This issue was addressed by a study in which 34 institutions randomized parturients with ADP to 1 of 2 management strategies: place an intrathecal catheter with removal after delivery, or re-site the epidural catheter at another location.[9] Of the final 97 parturients included in the analysis, placing an intrathecal catheter did not prevent a headache or the need for an epidural blood patch. Placing an intrathecal catheter did prevent the patient from experiencing a second ADP and also did prevent delay in analgesia. The major learning point from these results is that an intrathecal catheter may not prevent the patient from developing a headache; it will prevent a second ADP. A recent case series suggests that an intrathecal catheter may have some benefit in preventing PDPH after ADP as compared to re-siting the epidural catheter. While the incidence of PDPH was different, there was no difference in the need for epidural blood patch, suggesting that the difference was not impressive. In this series of 128 patients with ADP, 89 patients received an intrathecal catheter. There was a lower incidence of headache in the intrathecal group (42% compared to 62%).[35] There is the confounding variable of not reporting the mode of delivery in this series, as cesarean delivery has a lower risk of developing headache. An update of a meta-analysis and a trial-sequential analysis examined the role of intrathecal catheters.[36] The conclusion summarized the current thought on intrathecal catheters for the prevention of PDPH: there is no firm evidence that an intrathecal catheter decreases the risk of development of PDPH or of the need for an epidural blood patch. The advantage to an intrathecal catheter is the ability to provide analgesia or anesthesia in a rapid fashion. Also, an intrathecal catheter prevents a possible second ADP. In a small series of 109 patients who had a re-sited epidural catheter or an intrathecal catheter, there was no difference in the incidence of catheter failure.[37] These results are surprising, as the presence of cerebrospinal fluid suggests that the catheter would be functional. Dosing an intrathecal catheter is approximately 10% of the dose one would administer epidurally. If an intrathecal catheter is placed, it must be properly labeled, and all individuals must know that the catheter is located within the intrathecal space.

OTHER OPTIONS FOR PREVENTION OF POST-DURAL PUNCTURE HEADACHE

The other aspect that has been proposed for the prevention of a headache following ADP is placement of a prophylactic epidural blood patch. The concept for a prophylactic epidural blood patch is the performance of a blood patch prior to the patient developing a headache by injecting blood through the catheter before pulling it. In one study, 64 parturients who had an ADP were randomized to receive a prophylactic epidural blood patch or a sham one.[8] A prophylactic epidural blood patch involves injecting blood through a re-sited epidural catheter prior to removal of the catheter. In this study, all patients had an accidental dural puncture. Also, all patients had blood taken from the arm and were placed in the sitting position. Only those patients who were randomized to a prophylactic epidural blood patch received the blood through the epidural catheter. There was no difference in the incidence of headache or in the need for subsequent epidural blood patch between the two groups. While this study suggests no benefit to a prophylactic epidural blood patch, another study demonstrated its benefit in preventing headache.[38] In this study of 109 patients with ADP, 60 of the patients received a prophylactic epidural blood patch (blood injected through the catheter), while 49 received traditional expectant management. The incidence of headache was 18.3% in the prophylactic group and 79.6% in the expectant management group. According to these results, there is a benefit to a prophylactic epidural blood patch. As such, there are two well-conducted studies with conflicting results. The best way to put these studies into clinical context is to consider the risks of prophylactic epidural blood patch, which is primarily infectious (injecting blood through an epidural catheter prior to its removal). If every patient received a prophylactic epidural blood patch, all would be exposed to the risk, even those who would not have developed a headache. A prophylactic epidural blood patch is best for patients with high risk of developing a headache and in whom epidural catheter placement was very difficult.

One other means that may prevent a PDPH after ADP is cosyntropin. Cosyntropin is a synthetic adrenocorticotropic hormone (ACTH) that is used as part of the adrenal stimulation test. ACTH is made in the pituitary and causes the adrenal to release cortisol and epinephrine. Patients who experienced an ADP during epidural catheter placement were randomized to receive either 1 mg cosyntropin or placebo.[39] The incidence of headache in the cosyntropin group was lower (33.3%) than in the placebo group (68.9%). Despite the impressive results, this mode of prevention has not been adopted, and no other investigator has been able to repeat these results. Another study examined the use of cosyntropin for the treatment of a PDPH with some benefit; epidural blood patch still being superior to cosyntropin.[40]

TREATMENT OF POST-DURAL PUNCTURE HEADACHE

Once the headache is determined to be a PDPH, treatment should be initiated. These headaches are usually self-limited; in some individuals, it may develop into a chronic headache. In a case series of 40 patients who had an ADP with a 17-gauge Tuohy needle, 28% of the patients developed a chronic headache.[12] Also, those parturients who develop a PDPH have an increased risk of developing postpartum depression.[20] Given these risks, the treatment of a PDPH is important.

Noninvasive means of treating a PDPH have limited success. There is no benefit to bed rest and increased fluid intake.[41] Studies consistently demonstrate the lack of benefit. In regard to medications, two different medications have been reported: caffeine and neostigmine/atropine. Caffeine has been proposed as a management of PDPH. Caffeine is a cerebral vasoconstrictor. It is hoped that the administration of caffeine would decrease the increase in cerebral blood flow that has been demonstrated following ADP. The problem with this supposition is that the increase in cerebral blood flow is a small component of a PDPH. In a review of the literature examining the use of caffeine for the treatment and for the prevention of PDPH, the major conclusion was that there was no valid pharmacologic reason for the use of caffeine. Furthermore, the number of trials is small, and the trials used weak or flawed methodology.[42] There is no scientific basis to recommend caffeine for the treatment or for the prevention of PDPH.

Another medication that has been proposed is neostigmine and atropine.[43] The study was based upon a patient who required neostigmine/atropine for management of an ileus prior to an epidural blood patch. After the medication, the patient noted relief of the headache. It was believed that the neostigmine was responsible for the relief given its ability to pass through the choroid plexus. Neostigmine and atropine were used with good results in patients who developed a PDPH from spinal anesthesia using a Quincke needle. It is unclear of the applicability of the results given that it was used in patients who received spinal anesthesia with a sharp beveled needle. Furthermore, there is the confounding of studying patients who delivered by cesarean section, who already are at low risk for developing a headache

INVASIVE MEANS ARE AVAILABLE FOR THE TREATMENT OF A POST-DURAL PUNCTURE HEADACHE

There are several options available when it comes to treating PDPH, which include conservative and invasive approaches. Conservative approaches have no proven efficacy and no benefit to the patient if the PDPH results from ADP with an epidural needle. Invasive treatments are effective, varying in degrees of risk and success. The two procedures that may be used in the management of PDPH include the sphenopalatine ganglion block and the epidural blood patch.

Sphenopalatine Ganglion Block

The sphenopalatine ganglion block (SPGB) is a minimally invasive procedure that is performed easily in almost any setting, including the emergency room, the bedside, the clinic, or even the comfort of the patient's home (when given the proper instructions).[11] The sphenopalatine ganglion is located in the pterygopalatine fossa and it targets parasympathetic and sympathetic ganglia, as well as sensory innervation of the maxillary distribution of the trigeminal nerve, lacrimal glands, glands of the nasal cavity, paranasal sinuses, palate, and upper pharynx.[44] The relief results from blocking the parasympathetic ganglia, which counteracts the vasodilation that results from the CSF leak caused by the dura puncture.[11] The block is simple to perform, involving a cotton swab soaked with 2%–4% viscous lidocaine inserted into the nasal cavity until it meets the posterior pharyngeal wall superior to the middle turbinate (Figure 36.1). After the application has been held in place for 5–10 minutes, it is then removed and repeated in the other nostril. The block is relatively safe with minimal associated side effects, which include bleeding and discomfort during application of the swab.[44]

Currently, the only reported literature regarding the effectiveness of the SPGB for treating PDPH are case reports and case series. One study demonstrated that the SPGB may be an effective first-line treatment for PDPH, but more studies are needed. Another publication reported on SPGB in obstetric patients with PDHD. This case series examined only 3 patients with PDPH, but all 3 did receive immediate relief with SPGB.[44] Another study compared sphenopalatine

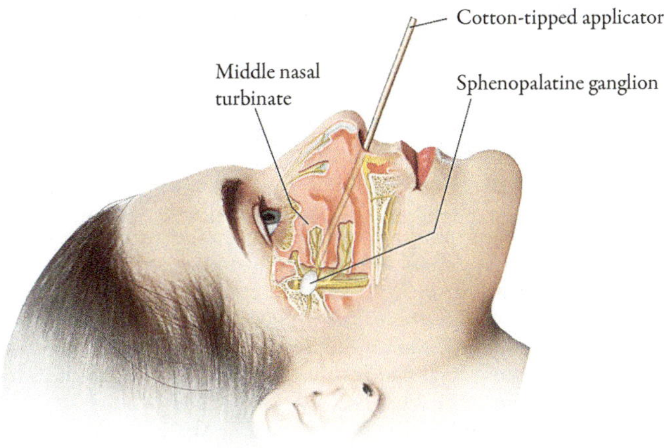

Figure 36.1. Transnasal sphenopalatine block.

block to epidural blood patch.[45] This study was retrospective; as such, patients were not randomized. A total of 39 patients received an epidural blood patch and 42 patients received an SPGB. The onset of relief was faster in the SPGB. Given that the study was not randomized, it is not possible to determine whether the patients in both groups had similar severity of headache. While reassuring, the study did not demonstrate the superiority of SPGB as compared to epidural blood patch. In short, with more prospective data, the SPGB could prove to be a beneficial first-line treatment for PDPH, reserving epidural blood patch for circumstances where symptoms are not relieved with this block.

Epidural Blood Patch

An epidural blood patch is a procedure in which autologous blood is injected into the epidural space to "patch" the hole where the dura was punctured. The benefit of an epidural blood patch for PDPH was established by Gormley.[46] While doing lumbar punctures, he noted that those individuals who had blood-contaminated fluid had a lower chance of developing a headache. He postulated that the blood was forming a seal at the hole and also that the injection of blood into the epidural space would treat the headache. Individuals were not able to repeat his results, most likely because he recommended 2–3 mL. The optimal amount of blood to use for an epidural blood patch is 20 mL.[13] The long-term benefit to an epidural blood patch is the "sealing" of the dural puncture; the immediate relief occurs from compression of the intrathecal space in the lumbar area, forcing cerebrospinal fluid cephalad. To perform an epidural blood patch, the patient is positioned either sitting or lateral. Once the epidural space is accessed, 10–20 mL of autologous blood is drawn in an aseptic fashion, and then slowly injected into the epidural space. While it is possible to perform this procedure with one person, a team of two or three individuals is helpful in order to aid in placing the intravenous catheter to retrieve the blood and to position the patient. Although epidural blood patch has been the gold standard of treatment for PDPH, it incurs risks such as bleeding, infection, neurologic complications, back pain, and repeat dural puncture.[47] A few things to consider prior to performing an epidural blood patch include headache and fever, which is concerning for meningitis, an infection at the site of the epidural puncture, a patient presenting with a headache that is not consistent with the symptoms of PDPH, a patient with a coagulopathy (including anticoagulation), and patient refusal. While the SPGB shows potential for becoming a first-line procedure for treating PDPH, not enough evidence is available to definitively recommend it as such. At this time, epidural blood patch remains the standard definite treatment.

An epidural blood patch is contraindicated in patients with fever because of concern of bacteremia. It is also contraindicated in patients with infection in the lumbar area and those who are taking anticoagulant medications. If the patient is taking anticoagulant medication, the epidural blood patch must be delayed until an appropriate time period in which the anticoagulant is held. The primary complication to an epidural blood patch is back pain which persists for approximately 48 hours. Other extremely rare complications include infection and neurologic injury.

CONCLUSION

Ms. RH developed a PDPH after an ADP during attempted epidural catheter placement for labor. Given her age, gender, and mode of delivery (vaginal), she was at a high risk for the development of PDPH. At the time of ADP, patients should be informed of the increased risk and of the need to contact the anesthesiologist if symptoms develop. Informing the patient of the risk does not increase the chance of developing a PDPH. At the time of the ADP, the anesthesiologist may have placed an intrathecal catheter. An intrathecal catheter would provide rapid onset of analgesia and decreased the chance of a second ADP; an intrathecal catheter does not decrease the chance of developing a PDPH. In this case, the epidural catheter was re-sited. While a prophylactic epidural blood patch may be injected through the catheter prior to its removal, there are infectious risks and the data supporting this practice are not universal. A sphenopalatine block relieved the symptoms and does not treat the underlying cause of the PDPH. An epidural blood patch relived her PDPH. She is still at risk for the development of a chronic headache; the reason that some individuals develop this chronic condition is unknown.

REFERENCES

1. Grobman WA, Rice MM, Reddy UM, et al. Labor induction versus expectant management in low-risk nulliparous women. *N Engl J Med.* 2018;379:513–523.
2. Stella CL, Jodicke CD, How HY, Harkness UF, Sibai BM. Postpartum headache: is your work-up complete? *Am J Obstet Gynecol.* 2007;196:318.
3. Sprigge JS, Haper SJ. Accidental dural puncture and post dural puncture headache in obstetric anaesthesia: presentation and management a 23-year survey in a district general hospital. *Anaesthesia.* 2008;63:36–43.

4. Choi PT, Galinski SE, Takeuchi L, Lucas S, Tamayo C, Jadad AR. PDPH is a common complication of neuraxial blockade in parturients: a meta-analysis of obstetrical studies. *Can J Anesth.* 2003;50:460–469.
5. Bolden N, Gebre E. Accidental dural puncture management: 10-year experience at an academic tertiary care center. *Reg Anesth Pain Med.* 2016;41:169–174.
6. Loures V, Savoldelli G, Kern K, Haller G. Atypical headache following dural puncture in obstetrics. *Int J Obstet Anesth.* 2014;23:246–252.
7. Angle P, Thompson D, Halpern S, Wilson DB. Second stage pushing correlates with headache after unintentional dural puncture in parturients. *Can J Anesth.* 1999;46:861–866.
8. Scavone BM, Wong CA, Sullivan JT, Yaghmour E, Sherwani SS, McCarthy RJ. Efficacy of a prophylactic epidural blood patch in preventing post-dural puncture headache in parturients after inadvertent dural puncture. *Anesthesiology.* 2004;101:1422–1427.
9. Russell IF. A prospective controlled study of continuous spinal analgesia versus repeat epidural analgesia after accidental dural puncture in labour. *Int J Obstet Anesth.* 2012;21:7–16.
10. Aida S, Taga K, Yamakura T, Endoh H, Shimoji K. Headache after attempted epidural block: the role of intrathecal air. *Anesthesiology.* 1998;88:76–81.
11. Kent S, Mehaffey G. Transnasal sphenopalatine ganglion block for the treatment of postdural puncture headache in obstetric patients. *J Clin Anesth.* 2016;34:194–196.
12. Webb CA, Weyker PD, Zhang L, et al. Unintentional dural puncture with a Tuohy needle increases risk of chronic headache. *Anesth Analg.* 2012;115:124–132.
13. Booth JL, Pan PH, Thomas JA, Harris LC, D'Angelo R. A retrospective review of an epidural blood patch database: the incidence of epidural blood patch associated with obstetric neuraxial anesthetic techniques and the effect of blood volume on efficacy. *Int J Obstet Anesth.* 2017;21:10–17.
14. Chambers DJ, Bhatia K. Cranial nerve palsy following central neuraxial block in obstetrics: a review of the literature and analysis of 43 case reports. *Int J Obstet Anesth.* 2017;31:13–26.
15. Pogodzinski MS, Shallop JK, Sprung J, Weingarten TN, Wong GY, McDonald TJ. Hearing loss and cerebrospinal fluid pressure: case report and review of the literature. *Ear Nose Throat J.* 2008;87:144–7.
16. Richman JM, Joe EM, Cohen SR, et al. Bevel direction and postdural puncture headache: a meta-analysis. *Neurologist.* 2006;12:224–228.
17. Zorrilla-Vacca A, Mathur V, Wu CL, Grant MC. The impact of spinal needle selection on postdural puncture headache: a meta-analysis and meta-regression of randomized studies. *Reg Anesth Pain Med.* 2018;43:502–508.
18. Sharma R, Panda A. Ondanseton-induced headache in a parturient mimicking postdural puncture headache. *Can J Anesth.* 2010;57:187–188.
19. Todorov L, Laurito CE, Schwartz DE. Postural headache in the presence of cerebral venous sinus thrombosis. *Anesth Analg.* 2005;101:1499–1500.
20. Guglielminotti J, Landau R, Li G. Major neurologic complications associated with postdural puncture headache in obstetrics: a retrospective study. *Anesth Analg.* 2019;129:1328–1336.
21. Mathers JD, Lo N, Leung P, Ho A, Das S. Large intracranial subdural haematoma with midline shift following accidental dural puncture for labour analgesia. *Int J Obstet Anesth.* 2015;24:391–393.
22. Baer ET. Post-dural puncture bacterial meningitis. *Anesthesiology.* 2006;105:381–393.
23. Wang YF, Fuh JL, Lirng JF, et al. Cerebrospinal fluid leakage and headache after lumbar puncture: a prospective non-invasive imaging study. *Brain.* 2015; 138:1492–1498.
24. Pannullo SC, Reich JB, Krol G, Deck MD, Posner JB. MRI changes in intracranial hypotension. *Neurology.* 1993; 43:919–926.
25. Nowaczewska M, Ksiazkiewicsa B. Cerebral blood flow characteristics in patients with post-lumbar puncture headache. *J Neurol.* 2012;259:665–669.
26. Lybecker H, MIdler JT, May O, Nielsen HK. Incidence and prediction of postdural puncture headache: a prospective study of 1021 spinal anesthesias. *Anesth Analg.* 1990;70:389–394.
27. Practice guidelines for obstetric anesthesia: an updated report by the American Society of Anesthesiologists Task Force on Obstetric Anesthesia and the Society for Obstetric Anesthesia and Perinatology. *Anesthesiology.* 2016;124:270–300.
28. Dripps RD, Vandam LD. Long-term follow-up of patients who received 10,098 spinal anesthetics: failure to discover major neurological sequelae. *JAMA.* 1954;156:1486–1491.
29. Wu CL, Rowlingson AJ, Cohen SR, et al. Gender and post-dural puncture headache. *Anesthesiology.* 2006;105:613–618.
30. Miu M, Paech MJ, Nathan E. The relationship between body mass index and post-dural puncture headache in obstetric patients. *Int J Obstet Anesth.* 2014; 23:371–375.
31. Peralta F, Higgins N, Lange E, Wong CA, McCarthy RJ. The relationship of body mass index with the incidence of postdural puncture headache in parturients. *Anesth Analg.* 2015;121:451–456.
32. Crane SS, Wojtowycz MA, Dye TD, Aubry RH, Artal A. Association between pre-pregnancy obesity and the risk of cesarean delivery. *Obstet Gynecol.* 1997;89:213–216.
33. Angle PJ, Kronberg JE, Thompson DE, et al. Dural tissue trauma and cerebrospinal fluid leak after epidural needle puncture: Effect of needle design, angle, and bevel orientation. *Anesthesiology.* 2003;99:1376–1382.
34. Ayad S, Demian Y, Narouze SN, Tetzlaff JE. Subarachnoid catheter placement after wet tap for analgesia in labor: Influence on the risk of headache in obstetric patients. *Reg Anesth Pain Med.* 2003;28:512–515.
35. Verstraete S, Walters MA, Devroe S, Roofhooft E, Van de Velde M. Lower incidence of post-dural puncture headache with spinal catheterization after accidental dural puncture in obstetric patients. *Acta Anaesthesiol Scand.* 2014;58:1233–1239.
36. Heesen M, Hilber N, Rijs K, et al. Intrathecal catheterization after observed accidental dural puncture in laboring women: up-date of a meta-analysis and a trial-sequential analysis. *Int J Obstet Anesth.* 2020; 41:71–82.
37. Tien M, Peacher DF, Franz AM, Jia SY, Habib AS. Failure rate and complications associated with the use of spinal catheters for the management of inadvertent dural puncture in the parturient: a retrospective comparison with re-sited epidural catheters. *Curr Med Res Opin.* 2016;32:841–846.
38. Stein MH, Cohen S, Mohiuddin MA, Dombrovskiy V, Lowenwirt I. Prophylactice vs therapeutic blood patch for obstetric patients with accidental dural puncture: a randomized controlled trial. *Anaesthesia.* 2014;69:320–326.
39. Hakim SM. Cosyntropin for prophylaxis against postdural puncture headache after accidental dural puncture. *Anesthesiology.* 2010;113:413–420.
40. Hanling SR, Lagrew JE, Colmenar DH, Quiko AS, Drastol CA. Intravenous cosyntropin versus epidural blood patch for treatment of postdural puncture headache. *Pain Med.* 2016;25:14.
41. Arevalo-Rodriguez I, Ciapponi A, Roque I, Figuls M, Munoz L, Bonfill Cosp X. Posture and fluids for preventing post-dural puncture headache. *Cochrane Database Syst Rev.* 2016 Mar 7;3(3):CD009199.
42. Halker RB, Demaerschalk BM, Wellik KE, et al. Caffeine for the prevention and treatment of postdural puncture headache: debunking the myth. *Neurologist.* 2007;13:323–7.
43. Mahmoud AAA, Mansour AZ, Yassin HM, et al. Addition of neostigmine and atropine to conventional management of postdural puncture headache: a randomized controlled trial. *Anesth Analg.* 2018;127:1434–1439.
44. Abhijit SN, Basanth KR. Sphenopalatine ganglion block for relieving postdural puncture headache: technique and mechanism of action of block with a narrative review of efficacy. *Korean J Pain.* 2017;30:93–97.
45. Cohen S, Levin D, Mellender S, et al. Topical sphenopalatine ganglion block compared with epidural blood patch for postdural

puncture headache management in postpartum patients: A retrospective review. *Reg Anesth Pain Med.* 2018;43:880–884.
46. Cullen S. Current concept. *Anesthesiology.* 1960;21:564–568.
47. Duffy PJ, Crosby ET. The epidural blood patch: resolving the controversies. *Can J Anesth.* 1999;46:878–886.

REVIEW QUESTIONS

(1) Which of the following factors is MOST likely to decrease the risk of a parturient from developing a PDPH following an accidental dural puncture (ADP)?

A. Age
B. Sex
C. Cesarean delivery
D. Intrathecal catheter

(2) Which of the following cranial nerves is MOST likely to be affected in a patient who has an ADP during epidural catheter placement?

A. II
B. VI
C. VII
D. IX

(3) A 24-year-old G2P1 woman at 39 weeks gestation requests labor analgesia. During epidural placement, she has an ADP. The following day, she develops a positional headache. She is febrile and has photophobia. Which of the following diagnoses is MOST likely?

A. Subdural hematoma
B. Post-dural puncture headache
C. Cortical vein thrombosis
D. Meningitis

(4) Which of the following occurrences is MOST likely responsible for the symptoms of a PDPH?

A. Loss of cerebrospinal fluid
B. Intrathecal air
C. Cerebral vasodilation
D. Intrathecal blood

(5) A 31-year-old female presents 3 days post-delivery complaining of a frontal headache that is worse with sitting up. She reports that she had an epidural catheter, which the anesthesiologist "took forever" to place. She reports that, in addition to her newborn, she has a toddler at home, so she is not able to lay around all day waiting for her headache to resolve. As the consultant, she asks you what can be done to help with her symptoms, expressly stating that she does not want to be "stabbed in the back" again. What is the MOST appropriate next step?

A. Administer a fluid bolus along with a dose of caffeine.
B. Persuade the patient that an epidural blood patch is the only way to definitively alleviate her symptoms.
C. Discuss the risks and benefits of a sphenopalatine ganglion block (SPGB).
D. Reassure her that with bed rest and time, the headache will resolve on its own.

(6) The sphenopalatine ganglion block works by which of the following mechanisms?

A. Aids in increased production of cerebral spinal fluid
B. Vasoconstriction via parasympathetic ganglia
C. Relieves tension on the meninges
D. Vasodilation via sympathetic ganglia

(7) What is the mechanism to the long-term effectiveness of an epidural blood patch?

a. Sealing the dural puncture site to prevent further leakage of CSF
b. Replacing the CSF that was lost during the accidental dural puncture
c. Relieving tension on the strained meninges
d. Increasing intracranial pressure by volume replacement

(8) A 24-year-old woman presents 3 days after lumbar puncture with a 22-gauge Quincke needle for the evaluation of lower extremity paresthesias and weakness. You are consulted for treatment of PDPH. The patient reports dioplopia, nausea, and a unilateral temporal headache that is unchanged with sitting upright. Which of the following is the appropriate course of action?

A. Proceed with an epidural blood patch
B. Recommend further noninvasive treatments
C. Recommend further workup for other etiologies
D. Proceed with a sphenopalatine ganglion block (SPGB)

ANSWERS

(1) **C.** There are certain patient characteristics that increase the risk of a patient developing a post-dural puncture headache (PDPH) following an accidental dural puncture (ADP). While young age and female sex have been implicated as risk factors, this increase has only been established for spinal anesthesia using a Quincke needle. The avoidance of pushing following ADP with an epidural needle has been shown to decrease the risk of developing a PDPH. The postulated mechanism is the variability of thickness of the dura. If an ADP occurs in a location of thin dura and arachnoid maters, bearing down may increase the dural rent. Although it was initially thought that an intrathecal catheter would decrease the probability of developing a PDPH, this supposition was not supported in a randomized study.

Reference

Angle P, Thompson D, Halpern S, Wilson DB. Second stage pushing correlates with headache after unintentional dural puncture in parturients. *Can J Anesth.* 1999;46:861–866.

(2) **B.** With an ADP, there is a loss of cerebrospinal fluid (CSF) into the epidural space. This decrease in CSF results in intracranial hypotension, affecting some of the cranial nerves. The nerves affected include CN III, IV, VI, and VIII. This effect explains the diplopia and the alteration in hearing that

may accompany an ADP. The cranial nerve most commonly affected is VI, due to its long intracranial course.

References

Chambers DJ, Bhatia K. Cranial nerve palsy following central neuraxial block in obstetrics: a review of the literature and analysis of 43 case reports. *Int J Obstet Anesth*. 2017;31:13–26.

Pogodzinski MS, Shallop JK, Sprung J, Weingarten TN, Wong GY, McDonald TJ. Hearing loss and cerebrospinal fluid pressure: case report and review of the literature. *Ear Nose Throat J*. 2008;87:144–147.

(3) **D.** Anytime the dura is punctured, the patient is at risk for the development of meningitis. Means to prevent meningitis involve maintaining aseptic technique and wearing a face mask. It is still possible to develop meningitis even if aseptic technique is maintained. A positional headache suggests a PDPH; fever is NOT a component of PDPH and merits workup for meningitis. Cortical vein thrombosis and subdural hematoma are increased in patients with ADP; these headaches tend to be constant and have accompanying neurologic symptoms.

Reference

Baer ET. Post-dural puncture bacterial meningitis. *Anesthesiology*. 2006;105:381–393.

(4) **A.** A PDPH results from a loss of cerebrospinal fluid (CSF) into the epidural space and cerebral venous dilation. The loss of CSF causes intracranial hypotension, placing traction on the meninges in the frontal and occipital areas. This traction results in a positional headache in the frontal-occipital area. While cerebral vasodilation does occur, the contribution to the headache is minimal. Intrathecal air, as occurs when loss of resistance to air is used to locate the epidural space, results in an immediate headache that is non-positional and resolves within 24 hours.

References

Wang YF, Fuh JL, Lirng JF, et al. Cerebrospinal fluid leakage and headache after lumbar puncture: a prospective non-invasive imaging study. *Brain*. 2015; 138:1492–1498.

Pannullo SC, Reich JB, Krol G, Deck MD, Posner JB. MRI changes in intracranial hypotension. *Neurology*. 1993; 43:919–926.

(5) **C.** The patient explicitly stated that she was not interested in an epidural blood patch but is seeking a therapy that will help to alleviate her symptoms so she can take care of her family. Patient refusal is an absolute contraindication for any procedure. Fluid bolus and caffeine have not been proven efficacious for alleviating the symptomatology of PDPH and would not be the best course of action. While PDPH is usually self-limited, the headache can sometimes progress to a chronic headache, subdural hematoma, or cortical vein thrombosis. Although more studies are needed to suggest SPGB as first-line treatment of PDPH, it has been shown to be effective at relieving symptoms.

Reference

Abhijit SN, Basanth KR. Sphenopalatine ganglion block for relieving postdural puncture headache: technique and mechanism of action of block with a narrative review of efficacy. *Korean J Pain*. 2017;30:93–97.

(6) **B.** The SPG has postsynaptic parasympathetic ganglion fibers from multiple locations, including lacrimal glands, glands of the nasal cavity, paranasal sinuses, palate, and upper pharynx. Blockade of this ganglion results in vasoconstriction of blood flow to these multiple sites, providing symptomatic relief to a variety of headache etiologies, including PDPH.

Reference

Kent S, Mehaffey G. Transnasal sphenopalatine ganglion block for the treatment of postdural puncture headache in obstetric patients. *J Clin Anesth*. 2016; 34:194–196.

(7) **A.** The blood patch acts as a seal of the dura to prevent further drainage. CSF forms at a rate of 500–700 mL/day. Sealing the source of the CSF leak provides long-term benefit. The initial relief comes from the compression of the intrathecal space in the lumbar area, displacing the CSF cephalad. This displacement relieves the intracranial hypotension. The long-term benefit is proposed sealing of the dural puncture.

Reference

Duffy PJ, Crosby ET. The epidural blood patch: resolving the controversies. *Can J Anesth*. 1999;46:878–886.

(8) **C.** This patient does not have symptomatology consistent with PDPH and would warrant further workup. The unilateral headache and lack of positionality suggests that the headache is not due to the dural puncture. Further imaging is required for a diagnosis. Although an SPGB may help alleviate some of her symptoms, it may not aid in a true diagnosis of her current pathology.

References

Todorov L, Laurito CE, Schwartz DE. Postural headache in the presence of cerebral venous sinus thrombosis. *Anesth Analg*. 2005;101:1499–400.

Guglielminotti J, Landau R, Li G. Major neurologic complications associated with postdural puncture headache in obstetrics: a retrospective study. *Anesth Analg*. 2019;129:1328–1336.

Mathers JD, Lo N, Leung P, Ho A, Das S. Large intracranial subdural haematoma with midline shift following accidental dural puncture for labour analgesia. *Int J Obstet Anesth*. 2015;24:391–393.

Baer ET. Post-dural puncture bacterial meningitis. *Anesthesiology*. 2006;105:381–393.

SECTION 9

PEDIATRICS

Kamen V. Vlassakov

37.

REGIONAL ANESTHESIA TECHNIQUES FOR CIRCUMCISION AND CONGENITAL INGUINAL HERNIA REPAIR

Leah Margalit Winters Webb and Melissa Brooks Peterson

STEM CASE 1 AND KEY QUESTIONS

A 2-year-old male child presents for circumcision under general anesthesia due to phimosis. His medical history is significant for uncomplicated delivery at 39 weeks gestational age and recurrent acute otitis media; he is otherwise healthy and has met all developmental milestones on time. Surgical history is significant for bilateral myringotomy and pressure equalizing tubes at age 12 months. His prior anesthetic was uneventful. The parents request an opioid-free anesthetic, are concerned for any type of neuraxial procedure, and would like to discuss options.

(1) WHAT ARE THE CHOICES FOR ANESTHETIC MANAGEMENT OF THIS CHILD? WHAT ARE THE POTENTIAL REGIONAL TECHNIQUES?

Anesthetic options for this child include general anesthesia (GA) alone, GA combined with regional anesthesia (RA), or RA alone. Conventionally, general anesthesia is employed outside of the newborn period. General anesthesia with supplemental nerve blockade for postoperative analgesia is another option for this patient, particularly in an effort to avoid opioids.

Several regional techniques are commonly used to provide analgesia for circumcision. Due to the parents' refusal, neuraxial anesthesia is contraindicated; otherwise, options would include spinal anesthetic block (SAB) and caudal epidural (CE) block. Peripheral nerve blockade techniques that can provide appropriate coverage include dorsal penile nerve block (DPN Block), pudendal nerve block (PN Block), and less commonly a ring block (Ring Block) of the penis. Topical anesthesia with eutectic mixture of local anesthetic (EMLA) can also be used. Dorsal penile nerve block (DPNB) has historically been the most frequently used peripheral nerve block for circumcision.[1–4]

(2) AFTER DISCUSSION OF THE ABOVE, THE PARENTS OPT FOR GENERAL ANESTHESIA WITH A BLOCK. THEY REQUEST MORE INFORMATION ABOUT THE OPTIONS FOR PERIPHERAL NERVE BLOCKADE AND ANY PROS AND CONS. DESCRIBE, IN DETAIL, HOW EACH OF THE FOLLOWING BLOCKS ARE PERFORMED: DORSAL PENILE NERVE BLOCK (DPNB), PUDENDAL NERVE BLOCK (PNB), AND RING BLOCK OF THE PENIS (RB).

DPN Block, first described in the 1970s, is commonly performed by urologic surgeons for patients undergoing circumcision.[3] Dalens landmark technique describes needle placement by starting at a point about halfway between the symphysis pubis and base of the penis and advancing into the sub-pubic space for injection, indicated by a pop which is consistent with penetration of Scarpa's fascia[5] (Figure 37.1). Then, injection of local anesthetic, after negative aspiration, is made on either side of the base of the penis.[5] DPNB can also be performed with ultrasound guidance. One method, described by Teunkens et al.,[6] uses a linear ultrasound probe placed between the symphysis pubis and penile base in a transverse orientation. Visualizing both sides of the sub-pubic space, and using an out-of-plane technique, local anesthetic is deposited below Scarpa's fascia and into the sub-pubic space.[6]

An alternative method for DPNB is the ultrasound-guided perineal approach, described by Qian et al.[7] For this approach, the patient is supine with the legs flexed to 90 degrees at the hips and knees to expose the perineum. Then, a linear probe is placed in a coronal parallel position beneath the skin of the scrotum and ultrasound scanning is used to identify the paired penile neurovascular sheaths.[7] Each neurovascular sheath contains the deep dorsal penile vein, the dorsal penile artery, and other branches of the internal pudendal vessels, and the distal branches of the pudendal nerves.[7] Using an in-plane approach, a 22-gauge echogenic nerve block needle is advanced until it lies next to the neurovascular sheath, at which point negative aspiration confirms absence of intravascular needle tip

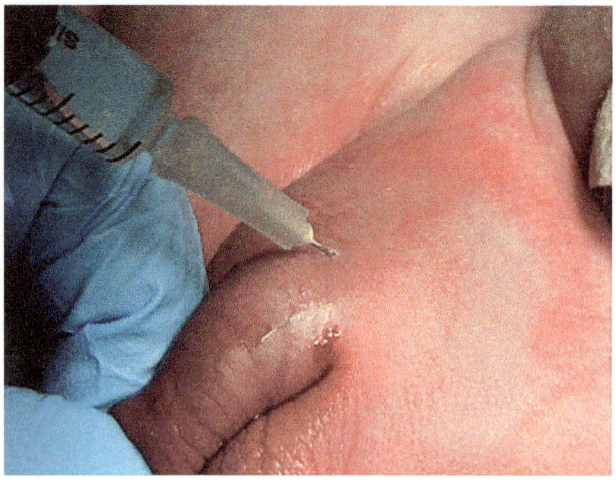

Figure 37.1. Dorsal penile nerve block (landmark technique). From Wikimedia Commons. Retrieved February 19, 2021, from https://commons.wikimedia.org/wiki/File:Dorsal_penile_nerve_block.jpg.

location, and local anesthetic is injected.[7] Ultrasound visualization confirms local anesthetic spread from one neurovascular sheath and across to the other[7] (Figure 37.2A, B).

PNB for circumcision is a newer technique that has been well-described in the literature and can be performed with landmark-nerve stimulator combination or with ultrasound guidance. As described by Tutuncu et al.,[8] the ischial tuberosities are identified by palpation, usually lying around the 3 and 9 o'clock position in relation to the anus; a stimulating needle is advanced at this point until the appropriate motor response (perineal muscle contraction as identified by up-down penile movements) is detected, at which point local anesthetic is injected.[8] The ultrasound-guided approach first identifies the ischial tuberosity by placing a linear ultrasound probe at the 3 or 9 o'clock position, as relates to the anus, in the coronal position; the needle is directed out-of-plane just medial to the tuberosity and local anesthetic is injected, with repetition on the contralateral side.[9]

RB of the penis, first described in the 1990s, is another regional technique that has been used to treat circumcision pain. The technique is a field block whereby local anesthetic is deposited subcutaneously and circumferentially around the base of the penis.[10]

(3) BASED ON YOUR DISCUSSION, THE PARENTS OPT FOR PUDENDAL NERVE BLOCKS (PNBS).

Anesthesia is induced uneventfully via inhalation in the operating room, and intravenous line is placed, and the airway is secured with an laryngeal mask airway (LMA). You perform bilateral ultrasound-guided PNBs uneventfully. (These authors prefer a 2-inch 22-gauge B bevel echogenic needle, with at least 2, and up to 5 mL, per side of 0.2% ropivacaine or 0.25% bupivacaine without epinephrine.) The surgeon enters the OR and asks you to draw up antibiotics. You turn around to reconstitute the antibiotics and notice that the surgeon is just completing a DPNB; you immediately inform him that you have already performed bilateral PNBs. He shrugs, says, "Well, fine," and gruffly demands the nurse to prep and drape the patient. Over the next 4–5 minutes the patient becomes progressively bradycardic (pulse 47 beats per minute), hypotensive (46/25 mmHg), and the ECG shows ST depression and inverted T waves. You immediately suspect local anesthetic systemic toxicity (LAST). **Explain the mechanism of LAST and the differences in presentation in children versus adults.**

Local anesthetic (LA) circulates in plasma as "bound" (to α1-acid glycoprotein) and "unbound" or free form. LAST occurs when unbound fraction LA then binds to fast sodium channels. Infants, particularly under age 6 months, have a higher risk of LA toxicity due to higher plasma concentrations of unbound LA (and therefore free to bind fast sodium channels). Adults tend to have progressive onset of symptoms (CNS → cardiac → CV collapse), whereas infants and small children have a more rapid progression of CNS → CV symptoms or even co-presentation.

(4) AFTER TREATING LAST, THE PATIENT STABILIZES WITH VITAL SIGNS RETURNING TO BASELINE. SURGERY IS CANCELED AND THE PATIENT EMERGES AND RECOVERS WITHOUT SEQUELAE. THE PARENTS ARE INFORMED OF THE MEDICAL ERROR. NOW, YOU ARE TASKED WITH ADDRESSING THE SURGEON'S DISRUPTIVE BEHAVIOR. DEFINE AND DESCRIBE "DISRUPTIVE BEHAVIOR" AND DISCUSS WAYS TO MANAGE IT.

Disruptive behavior, which can be defined as "any behavior that is: interpersonal (i.e. directed towards others or occurring in the presence of others); results in perceived threat to victims and/or witnesses; and violates a reasonable person's standard of respectful behavior."[11] Managing disruptive behavior includes (1) setting behavioral standards, (2) creating a plan to prevent causes of disruptive behavior, and (3) avoiding hiring people who are likely to behave disruptively.

STEM CASE 2 AND KEY QUESTIONS

A 6-week-old 2.3 kg male infant born at 32 weeks gestational age presents for left inguinal herniorrhaphy with laparoscopic look on the right. His history is significant for premature delivery due to maternal pre-eclampsia, induction of labor and failure to progress, necessitating cesearean section. He was admitted to the neonatal intensive care unit (NICU) for hypoglycemia and continuous positive airway pressure (CPAP) requirement for 2 weeks. The patient has a history of apnea and bradycardia but has not had any episodes in the past 1 week and is on 1/4 L/min O_2 via nasal canula. He is otherwise ready to discharge from NICU after his herniorrhaphy. He is appropriately NPO and was on maintenance intravenous fluid (MIVF) overnight.

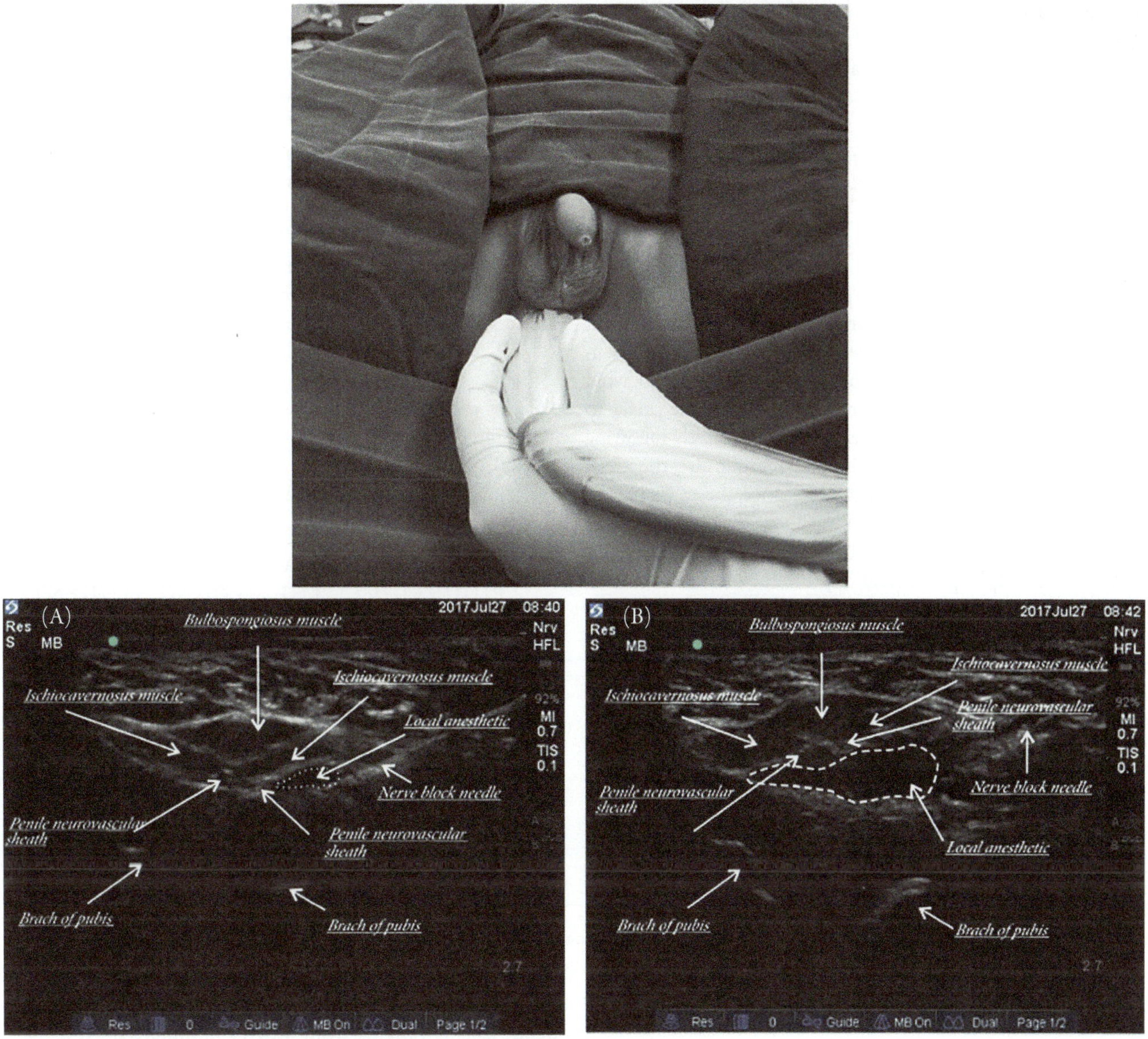

Figure 37.2 Ultrasound-guided dorsal penile nerve block via perineal approach.

(A) An ultrasound image of a penile neurovascular sheath before a complete nerve block injection; (B) an ultrasound image of a penile neurovascular sheath after a complete DPNB injection. On the ultrasound image, injected local anesthetics were shown as a black hypoechoic area, first filled in one side of the neurovascular sheath and then spread to the opposite side.

Wang X, Dong C, Beekoo D, et al. Dorsal penile nerve block via perineal approach, an alternative to a caudal block for pediatric circumcision: a randomized controlled trial. *BioMed Res Int*. 2019, Article ID 6875756, https://doi.org/10.1155/2019/6875756.

(1) WHAT ARE YOUR OPTIONS FOR ANESTHESIA AND ANALGESIA FOR THIS INFANT? WHAT ARE THE BENEFITS TO AVOIDANCE OF GENERAL ANESTHESIA (GA) IN THIS PATIENT? DESCRIBE THE BENEFITS AND RISKS OF REGIONAL ANESTHESIA (RA) IN THIS PATIENT.

Anesthetic options for this neonate include general anesthesia (GA) and/or regional anesthesia (RA). RA options include subarachnoid block (SAB), caudal epidural (CE) with/without catheter, ilioinguinal/iliohypogastric nerve block (IINB), or field block by the surgeon.

RA confers several potential benefits to this patient. First, RA in awake and anesthetized patients has been shown to be safe and effective.[12] Also, avoidance of general anesthesia may decrease the risk of postoperative apnea in the neonate. The risks of RA in this patient are low and include block failure, local anesthetic systemic toxicity (LAST), postoperative neurologic symptoms, and block site infection.

(2) YOU DECIDE TO PROCEED WITH SAB. DESCRIBE USEFUL LANDMARKS IN THE NEONATE FOR NEURAXIAL BLOCKADE.

The main landmarks that are useful for neuraxial blockade in the infant are the inferior angle of the scapula at the thoracic region, Tuffier's (or the "intercristal") line at the lumbar spine, and the sacral cornua and hiatus of the sacrum. Ideal placement of a neonatal spinal is at L4–L5 or L5–S1, due to the termination of the spinal cord at L2–L3 and the dural sac at S3. The spinal cord and dural sac reach adult position (L1 and S2, respectively) by age 2.[13]

(3) WHAT ARE THE CONSIDERATIONS FOR PLACEMENT OF SAB IN THIS NEONATE, INCLUDING BLOCK PLACEMENT, DOSING, POSITIONING, AND DURATION?

Conventionally, neonatal SAB is placed either at the L4–L5 or L5–S1 interspace. Positioning during and after block placement is critical. The patient can be placed either sitting or lateral decubitus for block placement. After placement, it is crucial to avoid a "head down" position to prevent high spinal. Some prefer to place the patient in reverse Trendelenburg immediately following SAB. If access to the patient's back is necessary soon after the spinal injection, to place a grounding pad for instance, the entire patient should be lifted, avoiding lifting the legs above the patient's head.

Average duration of SAB is significantly shorter in neonates. Tetracaine with epinephrine and bupivacaine have similar durations of approximately 90 to 120 minutes.[14] Increased cerebrospinal fuid (CSF) volume and more rapid turnover of CSF are likely mechanisms contributing to shorter duration of blockade.[14] Once the spinal is placed, time must be efficiently managed to provide adequate duration of blockade for the surgical procedure.

(4) YOU SUCCESSFULLY PLACE THE SAB ON YOUR FIRST ATTEMPT, CONFIRMED BY FREE CSF FLOW. AT 25 MINUTES AFTER THE SAB, INCISION IS MADE, BUT THE ATTENDING SURGEON IS CALLED TO AN EMERGENCY. AFTER 15 MINUTES, THE SURGEON RETURNS AND THE SURGERY CONTINUES UNEVENTFULLY, WITH THE INFANT SLEEPING. WHY HAS THE INFANT FALLEN ASLEEP WITHOUT ANY SEDATION?

A study by Antognini et al. found that spinal anesthesia "indirectly depresses cortical activity associated with electrical stimulation of the reticular formation."[15] As such, most infants are naturally sedated with the loss of afferent nociceptive input that occurs under SAB and will often fall asleep on their own.

(5) ONCE THE LAPAROSCOPIC LOOK IS PERFORMED, THE INFANT BEGINS SQUIRMING AND APPEARS UNCOMFORTABLE. A RIGHT-SIDED HERNIA REQUIRING REPAIR IS FOUND. WITH REMOVAL OF THE SCOPE, THE INFANT SETTLES, AND THE LEFT SIDE IS CLOSED. HOWEVER, UPON INCISION OF THE RIGHT SIDE, NOW 75 MINUTES AFTER THE SAB INJECTION, THE INFANT BEGINS TO SQUIRM AND CRY. THERE IS VISIBLE MOVEMENT OF THE LOWER EXTREMITIES. DESCRIBE YOUR ASSESSMENT AND OPTIONS FOR PROCEEDING.

The SAB is likely receding based on the patient's discomfort and return of motor function. Options for supplementation include non-pharmacologic and pharmacologic, including intravenous or inhalational anesthetics, to be used at the discretion of the provider. Facilitated tucking, non-nutritive sucking, sucrose, and other sweeteners are non-pharmacologic options for reducing pain.[16] Dexmedetomidine, ketamine, opioids, and benzodiazepines have all been used safely in neonates.[16] Additionally or alternatively, volatile anesthetics may be used, including nitrous oxide, either via mask, supraglottic device, or endotracheal tube. Though the use of sedating medications will negate the decreased risk of postoperative apnea with SAB,[17] they are likely necessary for the safe and comfortable completion of the surgical procedure in this patient.

(6) YOU DECIDE TO CONVERT TO A GENERAL ENDOTRACHEAL ANESTHETIC WITH SEVOFLURANE IN OXYGEN AND AIR. AFTER AN ADDITIONAL 45 MINUTES, NOW 120 MINUTES SINCE SAB PLACEMENT, THE SURGERY IS COMPLETE. FOR POSTOPERATIVE ANALGESIA, YOU WILL PERFORM A SINGLE-SHOT CAUDAL EPIDURAL (CE). THE MEDICAL STUDENT WORKING WITH YOU ASKS WHAT THAT IS. DESCRIBE THE LANDMARKS, APPROACH, DOSING, AND DURATION FOR SINGLE-SHOT CE.

The sacral canal is continuous with the lumbar epidural space, allowing for excellent analgesia via this approach. With the patient in the lateral decubitus position, landmarks for single-shot CE can be palpated as described above, with the target site for needle entry being the sacral hiatus. After locating the sacral cornua and indentation of the sacral hiatus, the needle approach is at a 45–60-degree angle.[18] A slight loss of resistance or "pop" may be felt as the needle pierces the sacrococcygeal ligament. At this point, the angle of the needle is flattened and advanced a few more millimeters, with the appropriate depth usually ranging from 5 to 15 millimeters.[18] If using an angiocath, the needle is removed, leaving the catheter in place. Then, the needle or catheter should be examined for CSF or blood; a negative aspiration will confirm their absence. An LA test dose containing 0.5 mcg/kg epinephrine should be injected while monitoring for T-wave conformation, heart rate, and blood pressure changes.[18]

CE can be dosed with a combination of local anesthetic and/or adjuvants. Concentration of LA affects the duration and degree of blockade, with more dilute solutions having shorter duration with less motor blockade. A general guideline for coverage based on volume of local anesthetic injected is: 0.5 cc/kg for sacral coverage; 0.75 cc/kg for inguinal coverage; 1 cc/kg for low thoracic (T10) coverage; and 1.25 cc/kg for mid-thoracic coverage.[18] Analgesia with 0.25% bupivacaine typically lasts 4–6 hours.[18] Additives to CE local anesthetic can prolong analgesia for up to several hours and include opioids (fentanyl 1–2 mcg/kg, morphine 12–50 mcg/kg), preservative-free ketamine (0.5-–1 mg/kg), tramadol (2 mg/kg), clonidine (1–2 mcg/kg), dexmedetomidine (1 mcg/kg), midazolam (50 mcg/kg), and neostigmine (1–4 mcg/kg).[19]

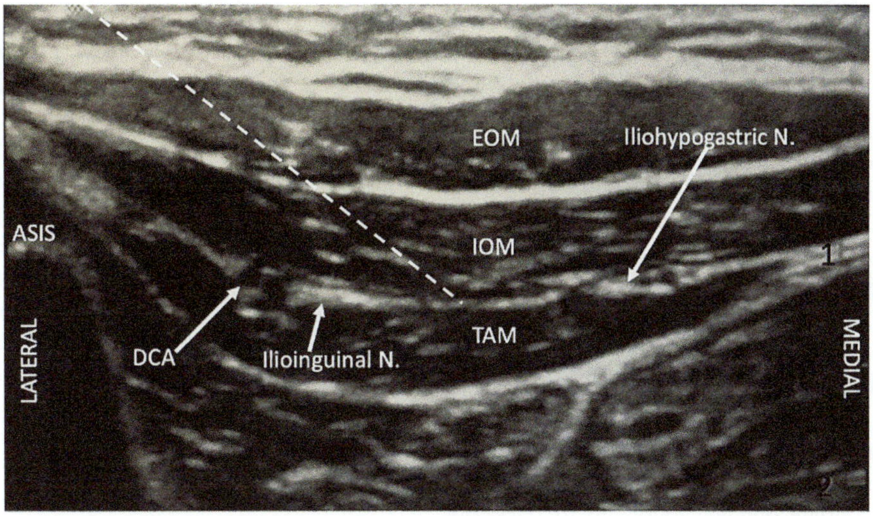

Figure 37.3. Image of ultrasound landmarks and needle trajectory for performing ilioinguinal/iliohypogastric peripheral nerve blockade. Local anesthetic is injected in the fascial plane between the internal oblique and transversus abdominis muscles.

(7) AT COMPLETION OF THE SURGERY, YOU PLACE THE PATIENT IN THE LATERAL DECUBITUS POSITION IN PREPARATION FOR THE CAUDAL. UPON INSPECTION OF THE BLOCK SITE, YOU NOTICE A SACRAL DIMPLE. HOW DOES THIS FINDING AFFECT YOUR PLANS FOR CAUDAL EPIDURAL PLACEMENT?

Sacral dimples occur at a rate of about 2%–7% in newborns and can be associated with a tethered cord, spina bifida, or spinal dysraphism.[20] Magnetic resonance imaging (MRI) has been used in the past to rule out associated anomalies, but ultrasound, in experienced hands, may be a useful diagnostic tool.[20] Potential tethering may lead to a spinal cord termination lower than expected. Thus, without further imaging, it is probably best to a avoid CE placement in this patient.

(8) BECAUSE CE MAY BE UNSAFE IN THIS PATIENT, YOU DECIDE TO PROCEED WITH ILIOINGUINAL/ILIOHYPOGASTRIC NERVE BLOCKS (IINB/IHNB). COMPARE THE LANDMARK AND ULTRASOUND TECHNIQUES FOR THE IINB/IHNB. HOW DOES THIS BLOCK DIFFER FROM A TRANSVERSUS ABDOMINUS PLANE (TAP) BLOCK?

Before the advent of ultrasound, the IINB/IHNB was commonly performed with a landmark technique (with a failure rate of about 20%–30%) and had been shown to be as effective as caudal epidural analgesia for inguinal herniorrhaphy.[21] To perform the technique, the anterior superior iliac crest (ASIS) is located and the needle is inserted about 1–2 cm medial and 1–2 cm inferior to the bone, advancing until a fascial "pop" is felt; at this point, LA is injected.[21] Complications included bowel puncture and hematoma.[21]

Using ultrasound, the probe is placed between the ASIS (laterally) and the umbilicus (medially) and the image examined to find the nerves located between the internal oblique abdominal muscle and the transversus abdominis muscle.[21] The needle is inserted and advanced until it is sufficiently near to the nerves and LA is injected and observed to surround the nerves[21] (Figure 37.3). Willschke et al. found that ultrasound-guidance improved IINB success rate and decreased the amount of LA needed for effective blockade.[21]

The transversus abdominis plane (TAP) block and IINB/IHNB differ mostly in performance of the block and area of coverage. To perform the TAP block, a linear ultrasound transducer is placed, with axial orientation, between the subcostal margin and ASIS in the midaxillary line; the three layers of abdominal muscle (external oblique, internal oblique, and transversus abdominis) and their separating fascial layers are identified.[22] An echogenic needle is advanced in-plane, from the medial side, until the tip lies between the internal oblique and transversus abdominis fascial plane, at which point LA is injected and can be seen separating the fascial layers.[22] The TAP block provides variable coverage from about T6–T12/L1 dermatomes, with T10–L1 being most reliably blocked.[22] Distribution of blockade from IINB/IHNB usually includes the following areas: hypogastric region, inguinal crease, upper medial thigh, mons pubis, partial labia, root of the penis, and anterior scrotum; however, coverage varies among individuals.[22]

(9) YOU, UNEVENTFULLY, PERFORM BILATERAL IINB WITH ULTRASOUND. YOU AWAKEN THE PATIENT, EXTUBATE HIM, AND SEND HIM TO THE NICU FOR RECOVERY. HE APPEARS COMFORTABLE AND HIS PARENTS ARE GRATEFUL FOR THE CARE YOU PROVIDED. HOWEVER, 2 DAYS LATER, IT IS NOTED THAT THE INFANT HAS AN ABSENT CREMASTERIC MUSCLE REFLEX. THE SURGEON TELLS THE FAMILY HE IS CERTAIN THIS IS NOT A SURGICAL COMPLICATION AND SAYS IT MUST BE FROM THE BLOCK YOU PERFORMED. WHAT

ARE THE MOST COMMON COMPLICATIONS AFTER IINB? WHAT DO YOU SAY TO THE FAMILY AND HOW CAN YOU REASSURE THEM?

While there is no right answer on how and when to apologize in the case of a medical error or adverse outcome, studies have found that patients/guardians desire full disclosure with an apology, and that doing so can minimize the risks of litigation.[23–25] You can reassure the family that, while it is possible that the injury resulted from your block, the Pediatric Regional Anesthesia Network (PRAN) found that in >100,000 cases there were zero incidences of permanent nerve injury after regional anesthesia.[26] Therefore, in the low likelihood this weakness is due to the nerve block, it is likely to be a time-limited event. Additionally, because the block was performed with ultrasound, you can confirm that the nerves were visualized with appropriate local anesthetic spread. Offering appropriate ongoing follow-up to track the resolution of the injury can also be helpful.

DISCUSSION

REGIONAL ANESTHESIA FOR CIRCUMCISION

Regional anesthesia (RA) for circumcision is a well-described approach. Studies have been done in newborns and older children showing varying degrees of effectiveness of topical and/or injectable local anesthetics for performing circumcision without the use of general anesthesia (GA).[1–4]

Upon analysis, DPN Block has a failure rate of about 4%–6.5%.[27] Common complications include hematoma, minor bleeding, and bruising at the injection site.[3] No difference in effectiveness of blockade was shown by Teunkens comparing landmark versus ultrasound-guided DPNB.[6] Faroni et al. found that failure rate remained the same between ultrasound and landmark guided groups; however, in the ultrasound group pain scores were reduced at 0 and 30 minutes postoperatively, time to rescue analgesia was increased, and procedural time was increased by 10 minutes.[28] The ultrasound-guided perineal approach DPNB provides equal postoperative pain scores to caudal blockade, with no significant adverse effects in either group, but with time to first micturition significantly shorter and time to first rescue analgesic significantly longer in the penile nerve block group.[29]

When comparing pudendal nerve block (PNB) (either landmark and nerve stimulator technique) to dorsal penile nerve block (DPNB) (landmark technique) Tutuncu et al.[8] found significantly higher pain scores in the DPNB group postoperatively; also, systemic analgesics were required by ~60% of patients 12 hours post-procedure in the DPNB group, while those receiving PNB did not require rescue analgesia until 24 hours postoperatively.[8] Naja et al.[27] compared PNB versus caudal block (CB) for circumcision and found that postoperative analgesia lasted significantly longer in the PNB group (18th postoperative hour in pudendal group versus 6th postoperative hour in the caudal group).[27] They also noted a significantly higher post-anesthesia care unit (PACU) rescue analgesia rate in the caudal group (25% of patients requiring rescue analgesia versus 0% of pudendal block patients).[27] Administration of oral analgesics in the first 24 hours postoperatively was also significantly higher in the caudal group with 100% of CB patients requiring oral analgesic medications compared to only 7.5% of patients in the pudendal group.[27] In comparing ultrasound-guided PNB to CB for hypospadias repair (a more extensive penile surgery than circumcision), Hecht et al.[9] found no difference in intra- and post-operative opioid use and non-opioid analgesic requirements, but did find that length of stay was significantly shorter in the PNB group.[9] In this same analysis, PNB patients had the benefit of avoiding urinary retention, maintaining lower extremity motor function, and utilizing effective regional anesthetic techniques even in patients with spinal abnormalities that may preclude caudal injection.[9]

Sharara-Chami et al.[3] compared different techniques for analgesia for neonatal circumcision, comparing EMLA alone to EMLA plus sucrose, EMLA plus sucrose plus DPNB, and EMLA plus sucrose plus ring block (RB).[3] All combination groups were more effective than EMLA alone, but the RB combination group was found to be more effective than other interventions for lysis of adhesions, which was felt to be the most painful part of the procedure.[3] The RB is less technically challenging than the other blocks described, with the main risks being hematoma and injection site bleeding, making it a viable option for those performing circumcision outside of the operating room.[2]

LAST IN PEDIATRIC PATIENTS

As described briefly above, infants have a higher risk of LAST due to lower plasma concentration of α1-acid glycoprotein conducive to higher concentrations of unbound LA. Additionally, α1-acid glycoprotein is an acute phase reactant; its concentration is lower in infants undergoing elective procedures (as opposed to urgent or emergent procedures). For these reasons, it is reasonable to consider reducing the bolus dose of LA by 30% for children <6 months old, compared to the adult dose.[30]

LA easily crosses the blood-brain barrier, so adults who can effectively communicate their symptoms usually manifest with central nervous system (CNS) changes prior to cardiovascular (CV) dysfunction. Adults typically present with the following CNS progression: perioral paresthesia → lightheadedness/dizziness → visual and auditory disturbances (difficulty focusing, tinnitus) → CNS excitation (generalized seizures) → CNS depression (respiratory arrest) → CV toxicity.[30] Shivering, slurred speech, and muscle twitching may be observed during this progression. Cardiovascular changes progress from peripheral vasodilation and myocardial depression to decreased blood pressure and bradycardia to cardiac arrest. ECG changes including ventricular dysrhythmias, peaked T waves, and ST-segment changes can be seen.[30]

In comparison to the adult onset of signs and symptoms of LAST, pediatric patients tend to progress more rapidly from CNS to CV dysfunction, may have both CNS and CV dysfunction present simultaneously, or may manifest CV dysfunction before CNS changes. Under general anesthesia with inhalational anesthetics, bupivacaine cardiotoxicity may be enhanced, while CNS effects are masked. Cardiovascular collapse, presenting similarly to adults as above, may be the first sign of LAST. This may occur even in the non-anesthetized child.[30]

Generally, treatment of LAST mandates stopping the LA, securing the airway and establishing IV access, giving intralipid (start with a bolus of intralipid 20% 1.5 mL/kg over 1 minute and then an infusion of 0.25 mL/kg/min), and continuously monitoring vital signs.[31] Midazolam (0.05–0.1 mg/kg IV) can be given for seizure and only low-dose epinephrine (1 μg/kg/dose) should be given for hemodynamic support.[31] For a detailed algorithm for treating pediatric LAST, and other pediatric emergencies, refer to the PediCrisis App.[31]

DISRUPTIVE BEHAVIOR AND ITS MANAGEMENT

Disruptive behavior has been well described in the workplace, particularly in operating room (OR) environments. Villafranca et al.[11] found that 98% of OR workers witnessed or experienced disruptive behavior in the past 1 year and that the average number of exposures was 64 events. Ubiquity (the proportion of clinicians behaving disruptively) was found to range from 6% ro 18%, based on disciplinary records.[11] Disruptive behavior affects patient care by interfering with communication, teamwork, and clinical performance, and reduces clinical decision-making.[11] It can lead to myriad problems, from an increase in clinician levels of stress to burnout.[11] Students are affected by an altered sense of acceptable behavior and avoidance of surgical, and even anesthesiology, residencies.[11] Institutionally, disruptive behavior can cause decreased productivity and increased staff turnover.[11]

Prevention and management of disruptive behaviors in the healthcare setting are critical. Prevention involves three steps: (1) setting behavioral standards with clearly defined disruptive behaviors and stated behavioral standards; (2) creating a comprehensive plan to prevent causes (workplace logistics, intrapersonal issues, broader context, and workplace relationships) of disruptive behavior; and (3) not hiring clinicians who are predisposed to acting disruptively.[11] Managing disruptive behavior involves macro- and micro-level intervention.[11] On a macro level, intervention can be staged based on the degree of the offense, ranging from an informal meeting with a supervisor for minor single occurrences to more intensive documentation and intervention (revoking of OR privileges, job termination, and/or referral to the licensing board) for more heinous offenses. Micro-level management depends on the victim/witness clinician tempering his/her response, with a focus on being assertive, without further contributing to the deleterious effects of disruptive behavior.[11]

REGIONAL AND GENERAL ANESTHESIA IN THE FORMER PRETERM INFANT

Risk factors for apnea after general anesthesia in an infant include prematurity, history of apnea/bradycardia, anemia with hematocrit <30%, chronic lung disease, and post-conceptual age <46–60 weeks.[32] A recent Cochrane Review found spinal anesthetic alone, when compared to a GA in preterm infants, reduces postoperative apnea, with relative risk 0.53.[17] Spinal anesthetic is also a reasonable choice when a portion of the procedure is performed laparoscopically.[33,34] Additionally, RA may provide superior analgesia, allowing both the avoidance of opioid medication and minimizing pain. Avoiding opioid analgesics prevents side effects of respiratory depression and gastrointestinal upset (nausea, vomiting, constipation). Further, because premature infants have an intact nociceptive system with limited inhibitory pathways[35] and are often subjected to repeated painful procedures (heel sticks, line placements, injections, etc.), they are predisposed to central sensitization, neurodevelopmental and behavioral problems, and increased stress response, all of which can be mitigated with adequate pain relief.[35] Use of RA can prevent the pain and stress of the surgery itself, as well as postoperative pain, thus avoiding an additional painful insult to this vulnerable patient.

Regarding the risks of RA in pediatric patients, a Cochrane Review found a significantly increased risk of anesthetic failure (relative risk 7.83) with SAB used alone.[17] LAST is another concern with the use of RA in pediatric patients, particularly infants under the age of 6 months. Severe LAST occurs at an incidence of 0.76/10,000 blocks, according to the Pediatric Regional Anesthesia Network (PRAN), with a higher incidence in younger infants.[26] Neurologic complications occur at a rate of 2.4/10,000, with no permanent complications in more than 100,000 blocks, while cutaneous infection occurs at a rate of 0.5% or 53/10,000.[26]

IMPORTANT LANDMARKS FOR NEURAXIAL ANESTHESIA

Landmarks for neuraxial blockade in infants are predictable. Similar to adults, the inferior angle of the scapula is at the level of the T7 spinous process. The T7 spinous process typically aligns with the T8 vertebral body and the T9–T10 spinal cord segments. This landmark can be used to locate other thoracic spinous processes, as well as cervical and lumbar processes, by counting above or below.

Tuffier's line connects the superior-most aspect of the iliac crests. In children, the line typically crosses the midline at the level of the L5 spinous process. In a study by van Schoor et al.,[36] 39 neonatal cadavers were examined in the prone and flexed position to assess the vertebral level of Tuffier's line. The study found that in the prone position, Tuffier's line crosses the L4–L5 interspace.[36] When the spine is flexed, the line shifts to the upper one-third of L5.[36] SAB can be safely performed at the level L4–L5 or L5–S1 in neonates, whose spinal cord and dural sac terminate lower at L3 and S3, respectively. The spinal cord and dural sac reach the adult position of L1 and S2, respectively, around the age of 2 years.[13]

Ultrasound guidance for performing neuraxial blockade has been reported in the literature. Using a linear probe in the longitudinal (or sagittal) view, one can visualize the hyperechoic bony structures and determine the interspace level by either counting down from the last rib or up from the junction of L5–S1.[37] The neuraxial structures are seen deep to the bony structures with the spinal cord appearing hypoechoic, surrounded by hyperechoic pia matter.[37] Tracing the cord in a caudal direction, the conus medullaris is visualized as the tapered end.[37] Cristiani et al.[37] found that using ultrasound guidance to perform lumbar puncture for SAB, they had a first-pass success rate of 64% and an overall (limited to 3 attempts) success rate of 86% in 14 infants.[37]

The sacral hiatus is the entry point for a caudal epidural (CE), whether single-shot or catheter. The landmark method for locating the sacral hiatus uses the posterior superior iliac spines (PSIS) as the base of an ipsilateral triangle, with the tip pointing inferiorly and overlying the sacral hiatus at the peak of the intergluteal cleft. The sacral cornua can be palpated 0.5–1 cm lateral to the apex of the intergluteal cleft, with the indentation between the cornua revealing the sacral hiatus. Ultrasound guidance can be also be used to localize the sacral hiatus. After positioning the patient, either lateral

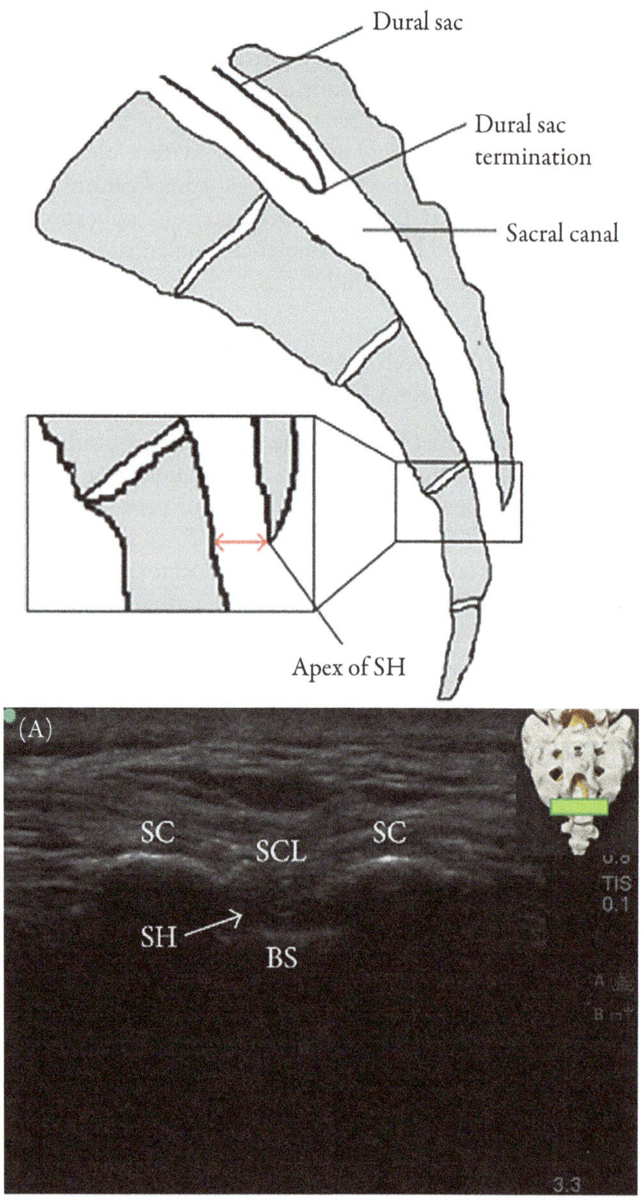

Figure 37.4A. Transverse ultrasound view of the sacral hiatus. The inset shows the position of the ultrasound transducer.
BS = base of sacrum; SC = sacral cornua; SCL = sacrococcygeal ligament; SH = sacral hiatus.

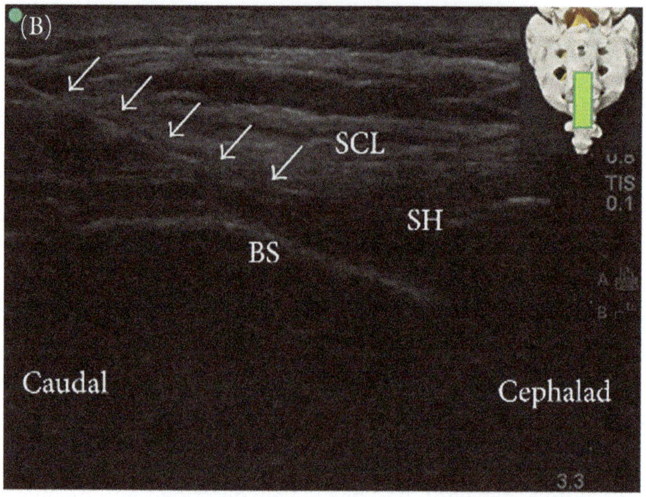

Figure 37.4B. Longitudinal ultrasound view of sacral hiatus. The inset shows the position of the ultrasound transducer.
BS = base of sacrum; SCL = sacrococcygeal ligament; SH = sacral hiatus; arrows = needle.
Figure 37.4A, B: License: Creative Common Attribution. Kao S-C, Lin C-S, Caudal epidural block: an updated review of anatomy and techniques. *BioMed Res Int*. 2017, Article ID 9217145, https://doi.org/10.1155/2017/9217145.

decubitus or prone, the linear probe is placed transversely in the midline overlying the hiatus.[38] The two sacral cornua will appear as hyperechoic structures on either side laterally.[38] The sacrococcygeal ligament and sacral bone, both hyperechoic structures, will appear between the cornua, with the sacrococcygeal ligament superficial to the dorsal surface of the sacral bone; the hypoechoic sacral hiatus lies between these structures.[38] Once visualized, the probe is rotated to the longitudinal view, wherein the needle can be advanced in an "in-plane" technique and visualized piercing the sacrococcygeal ligament[38] (Figure 37.4A, B).

SUBARACHNOID BLOCK (SAB) IN INFANTS

Cadaveric studies, such as the one by van Schoor, which found infant spinal cord termination most frequently at the L2–L3 vertebral level and conus medullaris termination at/above the L3 vertebral body,[39] support the safety of this approach for needle insertion in neonates. Needle depth, from skin to subarachnoid space, averages about 1.4 cm in neonates;[14] however, in infants >6 months age, epidural space depth is estimated to be about 1 mm per kg body weight.[40]

Local anesthetic (LA) choice and dosing depend on availability. Hyperbaric tetracaine and bupivacaine are the most common and useful choices for neonatal SAB, with dosing ranging from 0.5 to 1 mg/kg, usually with epinephrine 1:1000 added.[41,42]

COMPLICATIONS OF ILIOINGUINAL/ILIOHYPOGASTRIC NERVE BLOCK

There are some known complications, mostly minor, associated with the IINB. Transient femoral nerve paralysis is reported in the literature.[43] Other complications include puncture of or damage to surrounding structures (including vasculature, bladder, bowel), pelvic hematoma, urinary retention, local anesthetic systemic toxicity, and failed block. Using the landmark technique, the block failure rate may be as high as 50%–60%.[3] By comparison, in the pediatric population, the incidence of nerve injury directly from herniorrhaphy itself is not known.

REFERENCES

1. Awori Q, Li PS, Lee RK, et al. Use of topical versus injectable anaesthesia for ShangRing circumcisions in men and boys in Kenya: results from a randomized controlled trial. *PLoS One.* 2019;14(8):e0218066.
2. Rosen DA, Broadman LM. Ring block of the penis: a proven addition to multimodal pain relief for newborn circumcision. *Pediatrics.* 2017 Dec;140(6):e20172678.
3. Sharara-Chami R, Lakissian Z, Charafeddine L, Milad N, El-Hout Y. Combination analgesia for neonatal circumcision: a randomized controlled trial. *Pediatrics.* 2017 Dec;140(6):e20171935.
4. Wang J, Zhao S, Luo L, et al. Dorsal penile nerve block versus eutectic mixture of local anesthetics cream for pain relief in infants during circumcision: a meta-analysis. *PLoS One.* 2018;13(9):e0203439.
5. Dalens B, Vanneuville G, Dechelotte P. Penile block via the subpubic space in 100 children. *Anesth Analg.* 1989;69(1):41–45.
6. Teunkens A, Van de Velde M, Vermeulen K, et al. Dorsal penile nerve block for circumcision in pediatric patients: a prospective, observer-blinded, randomized controlled clinical trial for the comparison of ultrasound-guided vs landmark technique. *Paediatr Anaesth.* 2018;28(8):703–709.
7. Qian X, Jin X, Chen L, Pan Y, Wu B, Li J. A new ultrasound-guided dorsal penile nerve block technique for circumcision in children. *Anaesth Intensive Care.* 2015;43(5):662–663.
8. Tutuncu AC, Kendigelen P, Ashyyeralyeva G, et al. Pudendal nerve block versus penile nerve block in children undergoing circumcision. *Urol J.* 2018;15(3):109–115.
9. Hecht S, Piñeda J, Bayne A. Ultrasound-guided pudendal block is a viable alternative to caudal block for hypospadias surgery: a single-surgeon pilot study. *Urology.* 2018;113:192–196.
10. Hardwick-Smith S, Mastrobattista JM, Wallace PA, Ritchey ML. Ring block for neonatal circumcision. *Obstet Gynecol.* 1998;91(6):930–934.
11. Villafranca A, Fast I, Jacobsohn E. Disruptive behavior in the operating room: prevalence, consequences, prevention, and management. *Curr Opin Anaesthesiol.* 2018;31(3):366–374.
12. Taenzer AH, Walker BJ, Bosenberg AT, et al. Asleep versus awake: does it matter?: Pediatric regional block complications by patient state: a report from the Pediatric Regional Anesthesia Network. *Reg Anesth Pain Med.* 2014;39(4):279–283.
13. Gupta A, Saha U. Spinal anesthesia in children: a review. *J Anaesthesiol Clin Pharmacol.* 2014;30(1):10–18.
14. Suresh S, Polaner D, Cote C. Regional anesthesia. In: Cote' Charles J, Lerman J, Anderson BJ, eds. *A Practice of Anesthesia for Infants and Children.* 5th ed. Philadelphia: Elsevier; 2013.
15. Antognini JF, Jinks SL, Atherley R, Clayton C, Carstens E. Spinal anaesthesia indirectly depresses cortical activity associated with electrical stimulation of the reticular formation. *Br J Anaesth.* 2003;91(2):233–238.
16. Hall RW, Anand KJ. Pain management in newborns. *Clin Perinatol.* 2014;41(4):895–924.
17. Jones LJ, Craven PD, Lakkundi A, Foster JP, Badawi N. Regional (spinal, epidural, caudal) versus general anaesthesia in preterm infants undergoing inguinal herniorrhaphy in early infancy. *Cochrane Database Syst Rev.* 2015;6:CD003669.
18. Raux O, Dadure C, Carr J, Rochette A, Capdevila X. Paediatric caudal anaesthesia. *Update in Anesthesia.* 2010; 26:32–36.
19. Walker SM, Yaksh TL. Neuraxial analgesia in neonates and infants: a review of clinical and preclinical strategies for the development of safety and efficacy data. *Anesth Analg.* 2012;115(3):638–662.
20. Choi JH, Lee T, Kwon HH, You SK, Kang JW. Outcome of ultrasonographic imaging in infants with sacral dimple. *Korean J Pediatr.* 2018;61(6):194–199.
21. Willschke H, Marhofer P, Bösenberg A, et al. Ultrasonography for ilioinguinal/iliohypogastric nerve blocks in children. *Br J Anaesth.* 2005;95(2):226–230.
22. Chapter 42. Common ultrasound-guided truncal and cutaneous blocks. In: Hadzic A, eds. Hadzic's *peripheral nerve blocks* and *anatomy for ultrasound-guided regional anesth*esia, 2e. McGraw Hill; 2012.
23. Witman AB, Park DM, Hardin SB. How do patients want physicians to handle mistakes? A survey of internal medicine patients in an academic setting. *Arch Intern Med.* 1996;156(22):2565–2569.
24. Gallagher TH, Levinson W. Disclosing harmful medical errors to patients: a time for professional action. *Arch Intern Med.* 2005;165(16):1819–1824.
25. Pelt JL, Faldmo LP. Physician error and disclosure. *Clin Obstet Gynecol.* 2008;51(4):700–708.
26. Walker BJ, Long JB, Sathyamoorthy M, et al. Complications in pediatric regional anesthesia: an analysis of more than 100,000 blocks from the Pediatric Regional Anesthesia Network. *Anesthesiology.* 2018;129(4):721–732.
27. Naja Z, Al-Tannir MA, Faysal W, Daoud N, Ziade F, El-Rajab M. A comparison of pudendal block vs dorsal penile nerve block for circumcision in children: a randomised controlled trial. *Anaesthesia.* 2011;66(9):802–807.
28. Faraoni D, Gilbeau A, Lingier P, Barvais L, Engelman E, Hennart D. Does ultrasound guidance improve the efficacy of dorsal penile nerve block in children? *Paediatr Anaesth.* 2010;20(10):931–936.
29. Wang X, Dong C, Beekoo D, et al. Dorsal penile nerve block via perineal approach, an alternative to a caudal block for pediatric circumcision: a randomized controlled trial. *Biomed Res Int.* 2019;2019:6875756.
30. Suresh S, Polaner D, Coté CJ. Regional anesthesia. In: Cote' Charles J, Lerman J, Anderson BJ, eds. *A Practice of Anesthesia for Infants and Children.* 6th ed. Philadelphia, PA: Elsevier; 2019:42, 941–987.e9
31. Anesthesia SPA. Pedi Crisis 2.0. In: https://apps.apple.com/us/app/pedi-crisis-2-0/id1409734476; 2018.
32. Cote CJ, Zaslavsky A, Downes JJ, et al. Postoperative apnea in former preterm infants after inguinal herniorrhaphy: a combined analysis. *Anesthesiology.* 1995;82(4):809–822.
33. Sinha R, Gurwara AK, Gupta SC. Laparoscopic surgery using spinal anesthesia. *JSLS.* 2008;12(2):133–138.
34. Eizaga Rebollar R, García Palacios MV, Morales Guerrero J, Torres Morera LM. Spinal anesthesia for pediatric laparoscopic hernia repair: a case report. *A A Pract.* 2018;11(11):293–295.
35. Vinall J, Grunau RE. Impact of repeated procedural pain-related stress in infants born very preterm. *Pediatr Res.* 2014;75(5):584–587.
36. van Schoor A, Bosman MC, Bosenberg AT. The value of Tuffier's line for neonatal neuraxial procedures. *Clin Anat.* 2014;27(3):370–375.
37. Cristiani F, Henderson R, Lauber C, Boretsky K. Success of bedside ultrasound to identify puncture site for spinal anesthesia in neonates and infants. *Reg Anesth Pain Med.* 2019;44:893–895.
38. Kao SC, Lin CS. Caudal epidural block: an updated review of anatomy and techniques. *Biomed Res Int.* 2017;2017:9217145.
39. Van Schoor AN, Bosman MC, Bosenberg AT. Descriptive study of the differences in the level of the conus medullaris in four different age groups. *Clin Anat.* 2015;28(5):638–644.
40. Bosenberg A, Gouws E. Skin–epidural distance in children. *Anesthesia.* 1995;50(10):895–897.
41. Shenkman Z, Shorer S, Litmanowitz I, et al. [Spinal anesthesia in premature infants--indications, technical aspects and results]. *Harefuah.* 2002;141(9):770–774, 860, 859.

42. Shenkman Z, Hoppenstein D, Litmanowitz I, et al. Spinal anesthesia in 62 premature, former-premature or young infants: technical aspects and pitfalls. *Can J Anaesth.* 2002;49(3):262–269.
43. Mellert L, Cheung M, Gemma R. Femoral nerve palsy following landmark based ilioinguinal-iliohypogastric nerve block: case report and safety review. *J Med Cases.* 2017;8(5):155–158.

REVIEW QUESTIONS

(1) Which of the following is true about analgesia for newborn circumcision?

A. There are no long-term consequences of inadequate analgesia because newborns will not remember the procedure.
B. Inadequate analgesia is rare because circumcision is not a painful procedure.
C. Newborns do not have a mature system for pain perception, so they feel less pain.
D. Both behavioral and physiologic changes occur in response to inadequate analgesia in newborns.

(2) Which of the following is true regarding dorsal penile nerve block?

A. Effectiveness is improved with using ultrasound guidance compared to landmark technique.
B. It has a low failure rate of <2%.
C. It can be performed with an ultrasound-guided perineal approach.
D. It is as effective as caudal epidural blockade, regardless of technique.

(3) Pudendal nerve blockade may be superior to caudal epidural blockade for circumcision based on which of the following:

A. Length of blockade
B. Rate of urinary retention
C. Time to first use of rescue analgesia
D. All of the above

(4) Local anesthetic systemic toxicity (LAST) may present differently in children than adults in each of the following ways EXCEPT:

A. Neonates are more susceptible to LAST due to decreased plasma protein concentrations.
B. Cardiovascular collapse may present before central nervous system changes.
C. Seizures usually precede ventricular arrhythmias, hypotension, and bradycardia.
D. General anesthesia may mask warning signs of LAST in children.

(5) Disruptive behavior is a commonplace problem for operating room (OR) workers. Disruptive behavior can affect which of the following:

A. Patient care
B. Physician burnou
C. Medical student residency choice
D. All of the above

(6) What are the risks factors for apnea of prematurity after general anesthesia?

A. Prematurity, low birth weight, anemia with hematocrit <30%, chronic lung disease, and post-conceptual age <46–60 weeks
B. Prematurity, history of apnea/bradycardia, anemia with hematocrit <20%, chronic lung disease, and post-conceptual age <46–60 weeks
C. Prematurity, history of apnea/bradycardia, anemia with hematocrit <30%, current oxygen requirement, and post-conceptual age <46–60 weeks
D. Prematurity, history of apnea/bradycardia, anemia with hematocrit <30%, chronic lung disease, and post-conceptual age <46–60 weeks

(7) Premature infants undergo repeated painful procedures (heel sticks, line placements, injections), which predispose them to which of the following?

A. Central sensitization of pain
B. Neurodevelopmental and behavioral problems
C. Increased stress response
D. All of the above

(8) In neonates, placed in the flexed position, where does Tuffier's line most often cross?

A. L4 vertebral body
B. L4–L5 interspace
C. Upper 1/3 of L5 vertebral body
D. Lower 1/3 of L5 vertebral body

(9) A neonate is undergoing inguinal herniorrhaphy. What volume of injected local anesthetic will typically provide coverage up the T10 dermatome?

A. 0.5 cc/kg
B. 0.75 cc/kg
C. 1 cc/kg
D. 1.25 cc/kg

(10) A 12-kg infant requires epidural placement. What is the estimated depth from skin to epidural space in this patient?

A. 1.2 mm
B. 12 mm
C. 0.12 cm
D. 1 cm

ANSWERS

(1) **D.** Newborns do have mature capabilities of pain perception. The response to pain can be observed in both physiological and behavioral changes; one might observe changes in vital signs (increased heart rate and blood pressure and decreased oxygen saturation) as well as behaviors, including grimace, prolonged crying time, and irritability.[1] Neonatal circumcision is painful and acute, and long-term consequences of inadequate analgesia include altered response to painful stimuli, altered sensory processing, and

even psychological trauma.[1] Therefore, providing adequate analgesia for circumcision, while balancing the risks of side effects, is important, making regional anesthesia ideal for the procedure.

Reference

Sharara-Chami R, Lakissian Z, Charafeddine L, Milad N, El-Hout Y. Combination analgesia for neonatal circumcision: a randomized controlled trial. *Pediatrics*. 2017;140(6):e20171935.

(2) **C.** Dorsal penile blockade is a commonly performed regional anesthesia technique for circumcision and can be performed with either landmark or ultrasound-guided techniques. The failure rate is relatively high (>4%) regardless of technique, unless the ultrasound-guided perineal approach is used, which was found to be as effective as caudal blockade for circumcision in regard to postoperative pain scores.

References

Teunkens A, Van de Velde M, Vermeulen K, et al. Dorsal penile nerve block for circumcision in pediatric patients: a prospective, observer-blinded, randomized controlled clinical trial for the comparison of ultrasound-guided vs landmark technique. *Paediatr Anaesth*. 2018;28(8):703–709.

Wang X, Dong C, Beekoo D, et al. Dorsal penile nerve block via perineal approach, an alternative to a caudal block for pediatric circumcision: a randomized controlled trial. *Biomed Res Int*. 2019;2019:6875756.

(3) **D.** When comparing pudendal nerve blockade (PNB) to caudal epidural (CE) analgesia, several advantages have been identified. Analgesic duration is increased with PNB compared to CE (18 hours vs. 6 hours, respectively) and need for rescue analgesia is significantly decreased in the first 24 hours postoperatively with PNB (7.5% required vs. 100% required, in the pudendal versus caudal groups, respectively). Urinary retention and lower extremity weakness are avoided with PNB, and length of stay is significantly shorter, by about 25%, compared to CE in hypospadias surgery.

References

Naja Z, Al-Tannir MA, Faysal W, Daoud N, Ziade F, El-Rajab M. A comparison of pudendal block vs dorsal penile nerve block for circumcision in children: a randomised controlled trial. *Anaesthesia*. 2011;66(9):802–807.

Hecht S, Piñeda J, Bayne A. Ultrasound-guided pudendal block is a viable alternative to caudal block for hypospadias surgery: a single-surgeon pilot Study. *Urology*. 2018;113:192–196.

(4) **C.** LAST occurs in both children and adults, but the presentation in children can differ significantly from that of adults. Those with decreased plasma protein concentrations, such as infants <6 months of age who have decreased levels of α1-acid glycoprotein, are more susceptible to LAST due to a higher unbound fraction of local anesthetic, which is responsible for toxicity. Unlike adults, children may have cardiovascular (CV) and central nervous system (CNS) signs/symptoms present simultaneously, or even have CV effects occur first. General anesthesia may obscure earlier warning signs of LAST in children (and adults) such that CV collapse (hypotension, bradycardia, and ECG changes including ventricular dysrhythmias, T wave inversion, and ST-segment depression) is the first presenting sign.

Reference

Suresh S, Polaner D, Coté CJ. Regional anesthesia. In: Cote' Charles J, Lerman J, Anderson BJ, eds. *A Practice of Anesthesia for Infants and Children*. 6th ed. Philadelphia, PA: Elsevier; 2019:42, 941–987.e9

(5) **D.** Disruptive behavior, defined as "any behavior that is: interpersonal (i.e. directed towards others or occurring in the presence of others); results in perceived threat to victims and/or witnesses; and violates a reasonable person's standard of respectful behavior" is pervasive in the operating room (OR). Disruptive behavior affects patient care by interfering with communication, teamwork, and clinical performance, and reducing clinical decision-making. Clinicians are affected with stress, decreased well-being, career satisfaction, and self-esteem, and burnout. Disruptive behavior affects institutions by causing decreased productivity and increased staff turnover. An impact is even made on students by affecting their sense of acceptable behavior and decreasing their pursuit of surgical, and even anesthesiology, residencies.

Reference

Villafranca A, Fast I, Jacobsohn E. Disruptive behavior in the operating room: prevalence, consequences, prevention, and management. *Curr Opin Anaesthesiol*. 2018;31(3):366–374.

(6) **D.** There are several factors that increase the risk of postoperative apnea in the preterm neonate. Cote et al. found post-conceptual age (PCA) to be the most important factor, followed by gestational age (GA), in predicting postoperative apnea. As both PCA and GA increase, the rate of postoperative apnea decreases; however, each additional week of GA has a larger impact on the decrease risk of apnea than each week of PCA. Their findings indicate that, excluding infants with anemia and recovery room apnea, risk of postoperative apnea does not drop to <1% until GA 35 weeks and PCA 54 weeks and GA 32 weeks and PCA 56. When comparing small for gestational age (SGA), appropriate for gestational age (AGA), and large for gestational age (LGA) neonates, the SGA infants had a lower rate of postoperative apnea than the AGA and LGA infants, which were equivalent. Anemia (hematocrit <30%) independently increased risk of postoperative apnea, despite GA or PCA.

Reference

Coté CJ, Zaslavsky A, Downes JJ, et al. Postoperative apnea in former preterm infants after inguinal herniorrhaphy: a combined analysis. *Anesthesiology*. 1995;82(4):809–822.

(7) **D.** The sensory systems of preterm infants (<35 weeks gestational age; GA) are primed for the development of central sensitization of pain with repeated painful procedures given the fact that nociceptive circuitry is developed, but there is an imbalance in excitatory versus inhibitory signaling. Increased stress response is evident in preterm and extremely preterm (GA 24–28 weeks) infants with repeated painful procedures based on lower than expected cortisol levels at age 32 weeks GA (suggesting "exhaustion of resources") and above average cortisol levels at ages 8 and 18 months. Increased neonatal pain-related stress

has been linked to poor neurodevelopmental outcomes, showing decreased cognitive and motor function at corrected ages of 8 and 18 months and increased rates of anxiety and depression at corrected ages of 18 months and 7 years.

Reference

Vinall J, Grunau RE. Impact of repeated procedural pain-related stress in infants born very preterm. *Pediatr Res.* 2014;75(5):584–587.

(8) **C.** The intercristal, or Tuffier's, line connects the superior most aspect of the iliac crests. In a study by van Schoor et al., 39 neonatal cadavers were examined in the prone and flexed position to assess the vertebral level of Tuffier's line. The study found that in the prone position, Tuffier's line crosses the L4–L5 interspace, while the line shifts to the upper one-third of the L5 vertebral body when in the flexed position. This landmark is helpful for identifying a safe level for performing a spinal anesthetic block in the neonate given the lower termination of the spinal cord and thecal sac.

Reference

van Schoor A, Bosman MC, Bosenberg AT. The value of Tuffier's line for neonatal neuraxial procedures. *Clin Anat.* 2014;27(3):370–375.

(9) **C.** Approximate spread of local anesthetic injected into the caudal epidural space, as established by Armitage in 1986, is predicted by volume, as summarized in the Table 37.1. Subsequent studies have essentially agreed with these original findings.

Table 37.1 **VOLUME OF LOCAL ANESTHETIC INJECTED INTO THE CAUDAL EPIDURAL SPACE AND EXPECTED SPREAD**

VOLUME (CC/KG)	COVERAGE
0.5	Sacral
0.75	Inguinal
1	Low thoracic (T10)
1.25	Mid-thoracic

Reference

Armitage EN. Local anaesthetic techniques for prevention of postoperative pain. *Br J Anaesth.* 1986;58(7):790–800.

(10) B A rough estimate of epidural space depth is 1 mm of depth per kilogram body weight for children ages 6 months to 10 years. Hasan et al. suggest that depth to epidural space can be calculated using age or weight using the following formulas:

$$\text{depth (cm)} = 1 + 0.15 \times \text{age (years)}$$
$$\text{depth (cm)} = 0.8 + 0.05 \times \text{weight (kg)}.$$

References

Bosenberg A, Gouws E. Skin–epidural distance in children. *Anesthesia.* 1995;50(10):895–897.
Hasan MA, Howard RF, Lloyd-Thomas AR. Depth of epidural space in children. *Anaesthesia.* 1994;49(12):1085–1087. doi: 10.1111/j.1365-2044.1994.tb04361.x.

38.

EPIDURAL AND NEURAXIAL TECHNIQUES IN NEWBORNS AND CHILDREN

Balazs Horvath and Benjamin Kloesel

STEM CASE AND KEY QUESTIONS

PART A

A 1-day old premature male infant born at 34 weeks gestational age is diagnosed with type A esophageal atresia and presents for repair. There is no evidence for presence of VACTERL association (Vertebral defects, Anal atresia, Cardiac defects, Tracheo-Esophageal fistula, Renal anomalies, Limb abnormalities), and cardiac evaluation has not identified any abnormalities other than a patent foramen ovale and presence of a ductus arteriosus. The surgeon plans for a primary anastomosis and asks whether it is feasible to extubate the patient after the procedure.

(1A) WHAT REGIONAL ANESTHESIA TECHNIQUES CAN BE CONSIDERED TO SUPPORT EARLY EXTUBATION?

After uneventful induction of anesthesia, the patient is positioned in lateral decubitus position in preparation for a caudally threaded thoracic epidural catheter. Upon inspection of the patient's back, a sacral dimple is noted.

(2A) WHAT ARE THE IMPLICATIONS OF A SACRAL DIMPLE IN REGARD TO REGIONAL ANESTHESIA?

A caudal ultrasound had been performed earlier which ruled out a spina bifida or a tethered cord. Placement of a caudal block in absence of spinal imaging risks damaging an abnormally positioned part of the spinal cord.

(3A) WHAT TECHNIQUES ARE USED TO CONFIRM THE CORRECT EPIDURAL CATHETER POSITION?

To confirm catheter position, real-time ultrasound imaging is chosen, which avoids contrast and radiation exposure. Once the predetermined final catheter level is reached, a test injection of sterile saline can confirm tip location and epidural spread. Following negative aspiration for blood and cerebrospinal fluid, a test dose of 0.1 mL/kg lidocaine 1.5% with epinephrine 1:200,000 is administered to rule out inadvertent intravascular catheter placement.

(4A) WHAT TECHNIQUE CAN BE USED TO INCREASE THE STABILITY AND LONGEVITY OF A CAUDALLY INSERTED EPIDURAL CATHETER?

The anesthesiologist decides to tunnel the caudal catheter to place the skin exit site away from the diaper area, thereby decreasing the chances of soiling the site with bowel movements.

(5A) WHAT LOCAL ANESTHETIC AGENTS CAN BE USED FOR THIS PATIENT AND WHAT ARE THE RECOMMENDED DOSES?

The attending anesthesiologist decides to use a continuous infusion of 2-chloroprocaine 1.5% at a starting rate of 0.2 mL/kg/h.

PART B

The infant's postoperative course is complicated by new onset urosepsis. His condition requires endotracheal intubation, ventilation, and cardiovascular support. He improves and is later successfully extubated, but continues to require monitoring for recurrent episodes of apnea. After removal of the bladder catheter, the infant is diagnosed with posterior urethral valves and is scheduled for surgical ablation.

(1B) WHAT ARE THE ANESTHETIC CONCERNS IN THIS SCENARIO?

The neonatologist is wondering if this patient needs to remain intubated and ventilated after this surgery. He is concerned about the recurrent episodes of apnea, and also about the recent sepsis.

(2B) WHAT ARE THE ADVANTAGES OF THE SUBARACHNOID BLOCK (SAB) COMPARED WITH CAUDAL EPIDURAL BLOCK AND GENERAL ANESTHESIA (GA)?

Avoiding a technique that may increase both the incidence of apnea episodes and the need to keep the patient intubated after surgery is preferred. SAB is chosen as the primary anesthetic plan as the parents would like an attempt to avoid general anesthesia due to the potential long-term neurocognitive consequences for the developing brain. SAB decreases the risk of early, but not late, apnea episodes.

(3B) WHAT CIRCUMSTANCES ARE REQUIRED TO MANAGE THE CASE SUCCESSFULLY UNDER INTRATHECAL ANESTHESIA?

The anesthesiologist discusses this plan with the surgeon, who estimates his operative time to be approximately 40–45 minutes. The surgery is scheduled at the time when the infant is usually resting, while the NPO guidelines are followed. The operating room temperature is set at 80°F, the arms are swaddled following SAB, and a pacifier dipped in sucrose is offered to the patient.

(4B) WHAT LOCAL ANESTHETIC CHOICES ARE AVAILABLE?

Due to its long-standing safety record in children, 0.5% tetracaine with dextrose is chosen as local anesthetic. The tetracaine solution is mixed with 10% dextrose solution in 1:1 ratio, and the calculated 0.5 mg/kg dose is drawn into a 1 mL syringe.

(5B) WHAT ARE THE POTENTIAL COMPLICATIONS OF AN SAB?

The fellow is concerned about hemodynamic changes, infection, and post-dural puncture headache (PDPH), whereas the anesthesiologist is more concerned about the possibility of high or total spinal, local anesthetic toxicity, and transient neurological deficiencies.

DISCUSSION

ANATOMICAL CONSIDERATIONS FOR PEDIATRIC NEURAXIAL ANESTHESIA

The important differences between adults and neonates and infants are highlighted in this section. In neonates and infants, the spinal cord terminates at the L2–L3 level as opposed to L1–L2 in adults. The adult level is reached around 1 year of age. Therefore, it is common to choose L4–L5 or L5–S1 intervertebral spaces for needle placement to avoid spinal cord injury. The dural sac terminates at the S3 level in newborns, whereas it reaches only the S2 level in adults. Vertebral bodies are not fully calcified, and the ligamenta flava are thinner and softer, making needle engagement and approaches that use the "walk-off" technique more difficult. Vertebral arches do not ossify to allow fusion until late childhood, making the sacral hiatus accessible until a later age.

The caudal space is the distal extension of the epidural space located between the termination of the dural sac (proximal) and the sacral canal (distal). It contains the filum terminale, the extradural portion of the sacral spinal nerves, epidural fat, and sacral epidural vein plexus. The sacral hiatus is located at the end of the sacral canal. This structure is present due to lack of fusion of lamina and spinous process of the lower sacral vertebrae and can be located by palpation of two sacral cornua (remnants of the nonfused vertebral laminae) that border the sacral hiatus laterally. It is covered by the sacrococcygeal ligament, subcutaneous fat, and skin. By advancing a needle through those structures, the caudal epidural space can be accessed. The distance between the apex of the sacral hiatus (= upper margin of the sacrococcygeal membrane) and the termination of the dural sac measured by magnetic resonance imaging (MRI) shows significant variations, ranging from 3 mm to 13 mm in stillborn fetuses (gestational age 7–9 months) and 13 mm to 57 mm in children aged 10 months to 17 years.

PHYSIOLOGY OF NEURAXIAL ANESTHESIA

Cardiovascular System

The development and maturation stage of the autonomic nervous system is variable in term, and even more so in preterm neonates. Cardiac output is the major determinant of blood pressure and tissue perfusion, and it is dependent on heart rate since stroke volume cannot be increased by increasing preload due to the myocardial tissue structure at this age.[1] Systemic vascular resistance and vasomotor tone contribute to blood pressure and perfusion to a lesser extent due to the incomplete development of the sympathetic nervous system. To maintain the adaptability of the cardiovascular system, the parasympathetic tone is reduced initially. The peripheral blood volume is small.[2] Due to all of these factors, clinically significant hemodynamic compromise is uncommon in neonates and infants following a neuraxial block.

There is no compelling need for pre-block intravenous hydration; however, around the age of 5–8 years, children start to exhibit the same hemodynamic changes as those of adults following neuraxial blocks.[2,3] Despite the occasional modest and transient decrease in mean arterial pressure, the cerebral oxygen saturation remains stable within normal range in this patient population.[4]

Respiratory System

The primary respiratory muscle is the diaphragm. Accessory respiratory muscles play an insignificant role during tidal volume breathing in the resting state; therefore blocking their innervation does not interfere with normal breathing.[2,5] High level block (T2–T4) may result in paradoxical respiratory pattern without respiratory compromise due to the compensatory diaphragmatic contractions.[2] The temporary loss of proprioception of the thoracic muscles due to the block of those fibers contributes to a calm infant, in addition to swaddling.[6,7] On the other hand, bronchospasm has been reported with high block spread. Since the bronchial smooth muscle has minimal sympathetic nervous system control, it has been suggested that the reason for that adverse event is decreased activity of the adrenal glands, resulting in decreased catecholamine levels in the circulation.[5]

Central Nervous System (CNS)

The incomplete myelination of the infant neural tissue allows a fast diffusion of local anesthetics with fast onset and resolution of the block,[2] and neural tissues are also more sensitive to the neurotoxic effect of local anesthetics and adjuvants.[8,9] Therefore, care must be taken not to increase the intrathecal dose, and it is prudent to document the full recovery of sensory and motor function in the patient's chart.

Higher cerebrospinal fluid (CSF) volume as compared to adult patients results in higher local anesthetic volume requirement. The high cardiac output and dense vascular supply of the meninges shortens the duration of blocks in pediatric patients by causing a rapid local anesthetic drug absorption.[2]

Sedation is commonly observed after a successful SAB in neonates and infants without administration of any systemic sedative drugs. It is stipulated that there is a decreased afferent input from the peripheral receptors to the reticulo-thalamo-cortical projection pathways, and that results in decreased arousal.[10] This theory has been supported by both bispectral index (BIS) and SEF95 patterns suggesting decreased cortical activity following SAB.[6,7]

Gastrointestinal System

Effective pain control helps restore or preserve physiological gastrointestinal motility by attenuating the sympathetic surge of the autonomous nervous system. In addition, neuraxial anesthesia and analgesia decrease, or even eliminate intra- and postoperative systemic opioid requirements. That results in decreased incidence of both postoperative nausea and vomiting (PONV) and postoperative ileus.[3]

Genitourinary System

Postoperative urinary retention (POUR) is rare in infants and children due to the incomplete function of the autonomic innervation of the urinary bladder. S2–S4 sacral nerves block and addition of opioids to the local anesthetic solution increase the incidence of POUR, whereas it is less common with epidural analgesia at the thoracic level. Careful monitoring of urine output and emptying the bladder if needed should be part of the postoperative assessment.

Neuroendocrine Response

There is a marked and sustained attenuation of stress response to surgical stimulation and tissue damage based on the measured levels of stress hormones (e.g., catecholamines, cortisol, insulin) following neuraxial anesthesia with or without general anesthesia and compared with general anesthesia alone.[8,11]

PHARMACOLOGY OF NEURAXIAL ANESTHESIA

Both amide and ester types of local anesthetics are used for neuraxial anesthesia in newborns, infants, and children. The recommended doses for local anesthetic drugs that are commonly used in pediatric patients are listed in Table 38.1.

AMIDES

In newborns, the clinical use of continuous epidural administration of the amide local anesthetics is restricted by the increased susceptibility to their CNS and cardiac toxicity profile.[2,9] Amide local anesthetics are predominantly bound to plasma alpha-1-acid glycoprotein (AAG). Because of low AAG levels, the concentration of unbound local anesthetics, which is responsible for their systemic toxic effect, is higher in newborns and young infants.[9,12] Additionally, only the unbound fraction of local anesthetics can be metabolized. It is noteworthy that the S-—enantiomers of both bupivacaine (levobupivacaine) and ropivacaine (the commercially available form) have both better protein binding and lesser toxicity profile compared to that of the racemic mixture bupivacaine.[12] Surgical stress induces an increase in AAG concentration and thereby exerts some protective effect against local anesthetic toxicity in the perioperative period. However, binding of local anesthetics to AAG with subsequent slow release results in prolonged exposure of the newborn CNS and heart.[9] The risk of toxicity is further augmented by a decreased first-pass elimination of these drugs by the immature liver. In addition, hypoxemia, hypothermia, fluid-electrolyte imbalance, and acidosis increase the risk of cardiac toxicity.[9,12]

Epidural administration results in a more rapid rise of serum concentration, and toxic levels can be achieved more frequently compared to intrathecal administration.[9,10] The difference is likely related to both the significantly higher epidural/caudal doses and the higher vascularization of the epidural space compared with that of the pia mater and the spinal cord. The role of the rate of blood flow in the epidural pharmacokinetics of local anesthetics is supported by the slower rise and more sustained plasma concentration of ropivacaine that is a potent vasoconstrictor.

ESTERS

Tetracaine is used for SAB, whereas 2-chloroprocaine is used predominantly as continuous epidural infusion in neonates and small infants (<6 months).[5,13,14] Since these local anesthetics are not highly protein-bound, and are metabolized by plasma pseudocholinesterase and nonspecific esterases, their metabolism and clearance are not dependent on the liver.[14,15] The rare pseudocholinesterase deficiency puts affected infants at risk for toxic levels, although this risk is more theoretical since hydrolysis by nonspecific esterases still occurs.[16] Yet, it is recommended to ask the family about pertinent history of anesthesia complication (i.e.,

Table 38.1 LOCAL ANESTHETIC AGENTS AND DOSING FOR NEURAXIAL TECHNIQUES

LOCAL ANESTHETIC	DOSE	NOTES
SPINAL ANESTHESIA		
Tetracaine 0.5% in 5% dextrose	1 mg/kg (infants <4 kg BW) 0.5 mg/kg (infants >4 kg BW)	Most common local anesthetic used for spinal anesthesia
Hyperbaric Bupivacaine 0.5%	1 mg/k (<5 kg BW) 0.4 mg/kg (5–15 kg BW) 0.3 mg/kg (>15 kg BW)	
Tetracaine 1% in 10% dextrose	1 mg/year of age	Used for older children
Ropivacaine	0.5 mg/kg	
Levobupivacaine 0.5%	1 mg/kg	
Bupivacaine 0.5%	0.3–0.5 mg/kg	Children age 2 months to 12 years
CAUDAL ANESTHESIA		
Bupivacaine 0.25%	2.5 mg/kg	Modify volume to achieve desired block height: Sacral dermatomes: 0.5 mg/kg Lumbar dermatomes: 1 mL/kg Lower thoracic dermatomes: 1.25 mL/kg
Levobupivacaine 0.25%	2.5 mg/kg	
Ropivacaine 0.2%	2 mg/kg (practitioners have safely used 2.5 mg/kg)	
EPIDURAL ANESTHESIA: LOADING DOSE		
Bupivacaine 0.25%	Lumbar: 0.5 mL/kg	
Levobupivacaine 0.25%	Thoracic: 0.3 mL/kg	
Ropivacaine 0.2%	Subsequent top-up: 0.25 mL/kg	
EPIDURAL ANESTHESIA: CONTINUOUS INFUSION		
Bupivacaine 0.125% or 0.25%	0.2 mg/kg/h (age <3 months)	
Levobupivacaine 0.125% or 0.25%	0.3 mg/kg/h (age 3 months–1 year)	
Ropivacaine 0.1% or 0.2%	0.4 mg/kg/h (age >1 year)	
2-Chloroprocaine 1.5%	0.2 mg/kg/h (age <3 months) 0.3 mg/kg/h (age 3 months–1 year) 0.5 mg/kg/h (age >1 year)	
2-Chloroprocaine 1.5%	0.25–1.5 ml/kg/h (= 3.75–22.5 mg/kg/j)	Derived from cohort of 21 patients (ages 1 day to 3 years); all catheters positioned at thoracic level
2-Chloroprocaine 1.5%	0.45 ml/kg/h (= 6.75 mg/kg/h)	Derived from cohort of 26 patients (ages 42 to 80 days); all catheters positioned at thoracic level
2-Chloroprocaine 1%	Initial dose: 0.14–0.51 mL/kg/h (= 1.4–5.1 mg/kg/h) Maximal dose: 0.22–0.61 mL/kg/h (= 2.2–6.1 mg/kg/h)	Derived from cohort of 18 patients (ages 0.03 to 6.3 months); 15 catheters were positioned at thoracic level, the remainder at lumbar level
2-Chloroprocaine 1.5%	1 ml/kg/h (= 15 mg/kg/h)	Postoperative pain control for 6-week-old infant born at 34 weeks GA who underwent epicardial pacemaker placement

prolonged intubation and ventilation following succinylcholine), since severe cardiac toxicity following cocaine and seizure following epidural 2-chloroprocaine administration in patients with severe forms of pseudocholinesterase deficiency have been reported in the literature.

ADJUVANTS

Adjuvant drugs must be preservative-free to avoid direct neurotoxicity. The most commonly used drugs are listed in Table 38.2.

Table 38.2 ADJUVANT AGENTS AND DOSING FOR NEURAXIAL TECHNIQUES

ADJUVANT	EFFECT AND MECHANISM	INTRATHECAL DOSE	EPIDURAL DOSE	SIDE EFFECTS AND COMMENTS
Clonidine	Increases the efficacy of local anesthetics	1 mcg/kg	Single dose 1 mcg/kg Continuous infusion 0.1–0.2 mcg/kg/hr	Bradycardia Hypotension Hypoxemia Apnea
Dexmedetomidine	Prolongs the duration of caudal epidural analgesia	No data	Caudal 1 mcg/kg	No clinically significant observed

DEVELOPMENTAL AND BEHAVIORAL CONSIDERATIONS

Infants over 6 months of age and children before adolescence have a high level of anxiety and lack the ability to cooperate with the inconvenience and pain of needle placement.[2] Any movement during needle placement not only interferes with the success of the technique but can also result in injury to the patient. Furthermore, children cannot reliably differentiate between surgical pain and pressure or tugging, making a successful surgical anesthesia an intolerable experience. Prolonged inactivity and separation from the child's family are additional barriers. Therefore, epidural and caudal blocks are usually combined with general anesthesia or less frequently with deep sedation.[11,17] This practice is supported by evidence from large case numbers that report low complication rates for neuraxial blocks in anesthetized pediatric patients.[17,20] The theoretical risk of not recognizing early signs of CNS toxicity is offset by the anxious and erratic behavior that can be expected from a pediatric patient who is not mature enough to cooperate with the procedure; such behavior may be misinterpreted as early signs of CNS toxicity.[21]

However, when SAB is performed in newborns and young infants, sedation is rarely needed. That is a great advantage, since studies have shown that added sedation or general anesthesia might mitigate the advantage of SAB as single anesthetic technique by predisposing these patients to early postoperative apnea.[18] At this age there are no signs of apparent separation anxiety, and immobility is well tolerated. The decreased afferent input to the reticulo-thalamo-cortico projections, warm environment, and a pacifier with sucrose solution provide adequate immobility during surgery in the majority of cases. It is prudent to anesthetize the skin prior to needle placement. Noninvasive forms of anesthetizing the skin are preferred, such as using a pressurized lidocaine injector (J-Tip™) or preparing the skin with a topical anesthetic such as LMX4 topical anesthetic™ or EMLA® cream. However, the latter may cause methemoglobinemia in these patients, and attention must be paid to avoid applying excess amounts[19].

SPINAL ANESTHESIA

The safety and feasibility of SAB in pediatric patients are well documented.[22,23] SAB has the benefit of better postoperative recovery, including transitioning to effective analgesia, and better cognitive function.[5,22] Avoiding general anesthesia with endotracheal intubation minimizes the risk for prolonged intubation in patients with minimal respiratory reserve and muscle strength.[11] It was suggested by earlier clinical reports that in newborns, ex-premature and young infants, one of the primary benefits of SAB is a decreased incidence of postoperative apnea.[10,22] However, more recent data show that only the incidence of early apnea is decreased when regional anesthetic as sole anesthesia technique is compared with general anesthesia. There is no apparent difference in the occurrence of delayed apnea episodes between the two techniques.[24] That necessitates close extended postoperative respiratory monitoring of premature and term newborns who are prone to develop apnea following surgery regardless of what anesthetic method was used. In light of the concerns of the long-term impact of general anesthetic agents on the developing brain, the appropriate choice of regional techniques, including SAB, is probably a more appealing method than it has been historically.[14,23,24]

INDICATIONS/SURGICAL PROCEDURES

A wide variety of general surgery, urology, and orthopedic interventions can be managed under SAB,[5,10] the most common indication being inguinal hernia repair and short urogenital procedures. Procedures that last less than an hour are suitable for SAB in infants.[2]

TECHNIQUE

Since there is a limited number of patients and procedures where SAB can be considered as the first choice of anesthetic, it is prudent to identify an adequate number of pediatric anesthesiologists within a group who perform these blocks frequently enough to develop and maintain the necessary skills.[10] It is important to assess the normal anatomical development of the spine. Ultrasound is a valuable tool to identify the vertebral levels, midline, and the depth of the intrathecal space from the skin at the planned needle insertion point.

The patient can be held and stabilized either in sitting or lateral decubitus position with flexed hip. In newborns and infants, attention must be paid to avoid the anteflexion of the head since it can cause complete airway obstruction.[10,13] The assistant who is in charge of maintaining the optimal position has to hold the patient in a way that minimizes movement in any direction. The operating room needs to be warmed to provide comfort and to prevent hypothermia. A pacifier dipped in sucrose solution for infants, or other distracting devices for older children, must be readily available to calm and comfort them. The skin at the L4–L5 and L5–S1 levels can be anesthetized by either eutectic mixture of local anesthetics (EMLA) or 4% LMX ointments 30–45 minutes prior to needle placement; 22-, 25- and 27-gauge cutting-edge (short and long bevel) or pencil-point needles have been used successfully in newborns and infants.[2,25] Using a pencil-point needle in the narrow intrathecal space may result in a partial intrathecal local anesthetic delivery and a failed block due to the position of the distal orifice of the needle channel on the side wall instead of the needle tip. Recommended needle length is 25 to 38 mm in infants and 50 mm in small children.[25] The shorter the needle the easier to direct it, and CSF can be detected faster due to the smaller "dead space" of the needle. A needle with stylet is preferred to prevent introducing skin and other tissue fragments into the epidural and intrathecal spaces. Spinal dermoid tumor has been described as a consequence of dermal tissue inadvertently entering the vertebral canal. When a needle with stylet is used, the stylet must be removed frequently to check for CSF flow. The ligaments are weak, and there is frequently no characteristic "pop," even when piercing through the ligamentum flavum. Unlike in adult patients, there is no clear evidence in newborns and infants whether cutting-edge needles increase the incidence of post-dural puncture headache (PDPH). Because of both the low incidence of PDPH and the narrow subarachnoid space, short bevel cutting-edge needle with stylet seems to be the best choice for newborns and infants younger than 1 year.[2,25]

A 1 mL tuberculin syringe is a good choice to deliver the small volume of calculated dose.[2,13] The "dead space" volume of the needle needs to be added to the volume of local anesthetic in the syringe to ensure that the desired dose reaches the subarachnoid space. The volume of the needle can be measured by filling it with saline from a tuberculin syringe and measuring the amount of saline going into the needle until the first drop is seen at the needle tip.

The most commonly used local anesthetics for SAB are 0.5% isobaric or hyperbaric tetracaine and bupivacaine.[2] The hyperbaric solution can be made with 5% or 10% dextrose solution (1:1 local anesthetic: dextrose volume ratio if 1% tetracaine, and 2:1 local anesthetic: dextrose volume ratio if 0.75% isobaric bupivacaine is chosen). The dose for both local anesthetics is 0.5 mg/kg in newborns and infants. In older children weighing more than 20 kg, 0.3 mg/kg, up to the usual adult dose (10–15 mg), can be used.[2,25] The use of levobupivacaine and ropivacaine for SAB in pediatric patients has also been described.[25]

The onset of the block is virtually immediate; however, the local anesthetic can still spread cephalad, resulting in a rapidly developing high or total spinal block, especially in infants. Therefore, the patient must be kept in a strictly supine position, including when lifted to apply the electrocautery pad on the back.[25] The block level can be assessed by systematic application of noxious stimulation or ice from distal to cephalad direction; alternatively, transcutaneous electrical stimulation can be used in infants.[2]

The SAB-induced deafferentation results in sedation in these patients. In order to further comfort an infant, the arms should be swaddled at the side, and a pacifier dipped in sucrose solution is offered. A tape may carefully be placed across the distal thighs with the ends attached to the edge of the operating room table. The surgical team must be scrubbed, gowned, and ready to prep and drape the skin. The goal is to start the procedure as soon as possible after the block is placed since its duration is limited.

It is important to schedule the surgery with the feeding cycle of the infant in mind. If the time of the surgery is at the usual feeding time, hunger will likely make the child restless and inconsolable. This may be confused with an unsuccessful block and can even make an inguinal hernia repair difficult due to periodically increased intra-abdominal pressure secondary to forceful crying.

EPIDURAL/CAUDAL ANESTHESIA

Epidural and caudal blocks are versatile and can be used for intraoperative and postoperative analgesia for thoracic, abdominal, pelvic, and lower extremity procedures.

Caudal blocks have an excellent safety profile as the caudal space does not contain spinal cord, but they are more limited in utility. It is performed primarily in neonates and infants, and a reliable block can be achieved up to the inguinal/subumbilical area by a single-shot injection. Use of larger injection volumes may extend the block to the mid-abdominal and thoracic level, but this spread is unpredictable and should not be relied upon during procedures that require good pain control. Caudal catheters may be placed and threaded upward to be situated at a desired lumbar or thoracic level. Real-time ultrasound imaging is a useful method to assess both the threading and the final positioning of the catheter tip. Caudal blocks have been successfully performed in children up to 50 kg of body weight;[26] however, older children may be uncomfortable with residual motor or sensory blockade.

TECHNIQUE: LUMBAR AND THORACIC EPIDURAL

Epidural blocks can be performed with the patient either in sitting or lateral decubitus position. Most of the pediatric epidural blocks are performed in anesthetized patients. Depending on the planned catheter tip location, an entry point in the lumbar or thoracic area is identified. If a thoracic tip location is desired, some practitioners prefer to access the epidural space from a lumbar location and accept that the catheter needs to be threaded a longer distance. The needle entry point is midline; theoretically, a paramedian approach may be used, but in the pediatric population, this is often unnecessary as even high thoracic epidural spaces can easily be accessed using the midline technique. Furthermore, a paramedian approach has its risks, as lack of ossification renders the lamina very soft, making the distinction of needle engagement in the lamina versus the epidural space difficult. For neonates and infants, the use of a shorter epidural needle is recommended to improve stability and handling. The needle should be advanced through the skin and engaged in the ligamentum flavum. After removal of the stylet, a syringe with sterile, preservative-free saline is attached and the needle is slowly advanced to locate the epidural space via loss-of-resistance technique. Using air may cause pneumocephalus, venous air embolism, and spinal cord/nerve root compression. The "hanging-drop technique" is rarely used. Needle advancement can be in slow increments or in a continuous fashion—we recommend the incremental approach, especially in neonates, as the distance from skin to epidural space can be very short. The approximate skin-to-epidural space distance in children weighing more than 10 kg can be calculated as 1 mm per kg of body weight. Magnetic resonance imaging suggested that the distance from skin to epidural space in mm can be calculated using the formula of 9.00 mm + 0.62 mm × weight in kilograms.[27] Local anesthetic or an opioid can be administered for a single-shot technique or, more commonly, an epidural catheter is inserted. For the latter, it is often helpful to inject a small amount of preservative-free sterile saline (0.5–1 cc) to open the epidural space and facilitate catheter advancement. The catheter should thread without significant resistance. Catheter position can be confirmed by ultrasound, fluoroscopy, transesophageal echocardiography (TEE), or the use of an electrical epidural stimulation catheter. Since the needle entry point is chosen close to the planned surgical incision site, many practitioners forgo imaging of the exact epidural tip location. The catheter is secured and a local anesthetic test dose of 0.1 cc/kg body weight lidocaine 1.5% with 1:200,000 epinephrine is injected.

TECHNIQUE: CAUDAL EPIDURAL

Caudal blocks can be performed with the patient in lateral decubitus position with both legs flexed toward the chest, or with the patient in frog-legged prone position. Identification of the correct entry point is frequently feasible using the landmark technique, although ultrasound guidance is increasingly being used. The needle entry point is midline and just slightly distal to an imaginary line between the sacral cornua. To aid identification of the sacral cornua, both upper posterior iliac spines can be palpated, and an equilateral triangle can be drawn whose third edge will often overlay the area of the sacral cornua. Contemporary ultrasound studies have questioned the value of this approach given that in a significant number of cases, the sacral hiatus was located more cephalad than determined by the equilateral triangle method. A needle is then inserted at an angle of about 45–60 degrees; often, perforation of the sacrococcygeal membrane can be felt. If the needle encounters bone, it can be slightly withdrawn and moved cranial or caudal to allow another approach. After perforation of the sacrococcygeal membrane, the needle angle should be decreased to 20–30 degrees and the needle advanced another 1–2 mm. If a peripheral intravenous catheter is used, the plastic part can now be threaded off into the caudal space from the steel cannula. At this point, either a test dose or the local anesthetic can be injected incrementally, after confirming that aspiration does not yield blood or CSF. If the procedure takes multiple hours, some anesthesia providers repeat a single-shot caudal block at the end of surgery. Others prefer to leave the plastic intravenous cannula in place for repeat injection. This requires strictly sterile placement and dressing, as well as meticulous padding of the hub to prevent skin lesions (Figure 38.1A, B). No clear

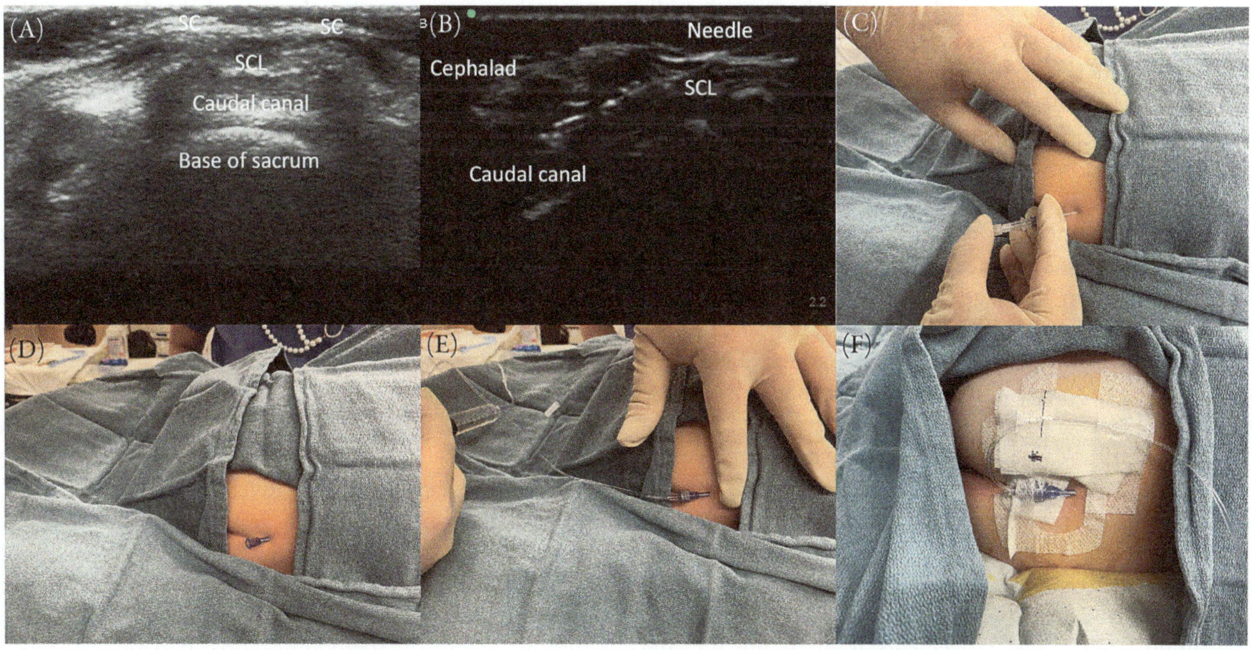

Figure 38.1. (A–B) Coronal and sagittal ultrasound image of the caudal canal (SC = sacral cornua; SCL = sacrococcygeal ligament); (C–F) 22 Ga intravenous catheter insertion. The intravenous catheter is left in the caudal space for repeat local anesthetic administration if the duration of the procedure necessitates, and/or for a repeat injection at the conclusion of surgery. The catheter and the extension tubing are padded, and an occlusive dressing is applied to prevent contamination of the insertion site. The catheter is removed at the end of the procedure.

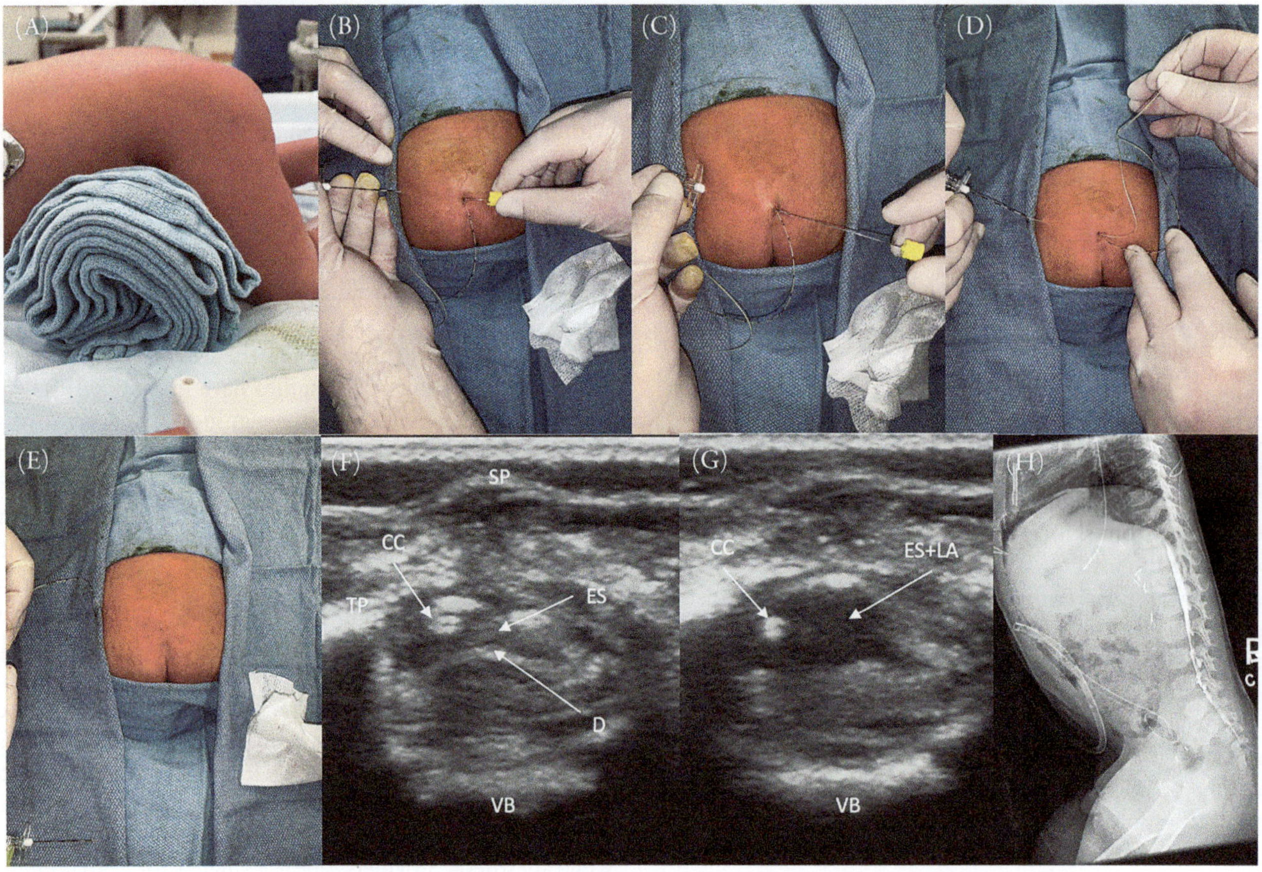

Figure 38.2. (A–E) Prone position and tunneling of a caudally inserted epidural catheter. (F–G) Ultrasound image of the caudal catheter (CC) in the thoracic epidural space (ES) before and after local anesthetic injection (ES + LA) at the T-10 (thoracic 10) intervertebral space.

(SP = spinous process; TP = transverse process; VB = vertebral body). (H) Epidurogram of a caudally inserted catheter showing proper height and extent of injectate.

guidelines exist that provide guidance about how much additional local anesthetic may be given; however, a conservative way is to calculate the hourly infusion dose as if a continuous catheter would have been used and to administer a dose up to the calculated dose times the hours that have passed since injection of the initial dose.

A caudal catheter can be advanced through the block needle or a peripheral intravenous catheter (a 20-gauge or larger peripheral intravenous catheter is needed to thread a 24-gague epidural catheter; an 18-gauge IV catheter is used for threading a 20-gauge epidural catheter). Preferably, the caudal space can be expanded by injection of a small amount (1–3 cc) of preservative-free sterile saline. The catheter should advance with minimal resistance. The distance of the needle insertion site to the intended catheter placement site can be measured. This method is inaccurate, and many catheters end up cranial or caudal of the intended level. More accurate methods to confirm placement include ultrasound, fluoroscopy, TEE imaging, and electric epidural stimulation catheters.

While caudal catheters may be left in place for multiple days, soiling from bowel movements is often the limiting factor. No clear guidelines exist regarding the management of this situation: some practitioners remove the caudal catheter as soon as the first bowel movement occurs, while other approaches involve careful cleaning of the dressing, followed by its removal and inspection of the caudal catheter entry site to determine whether penetration around the site has occurred (in which case the catheter is removed). If no penetration is detected, the site can be cleaned with a disinfectant and a new dressing can be applied. A way to increase the longevity of caudal catheters is to tunnel the distal end away from the initial needle insertion to exit more cranially (Figure 38.2A–H). No studies to date have documented a reduction of infectious complications, but bacterial colonization rates were found to be lower in tunneled caudal catheters.

TEST DOSE IN PEDIATRIC EPIDURAL/CAUDAL BLOCKS

The needle or catheter may inadvertently be placed into the cerebrospinal fluid or a blood vessel. Injection of the local anesthetic may subsequently lead to a total spinal block or local anesthetic systemic toxicity, respectively. Aspiration should be performed prior to local anesthetic injection, and return of cerebrospinal fluid or blood can identify needle malposition. Blood vessels can collapse upon aspiration, resulting in no blood return and the false sense of safety of correct position. A test dose can serve as a second safety measure, although its use to identify subarachnoid needle placement in pediatric patients under general anesthesia is not helpful, as signs of a spinal block may not be picked up. For identification of needle malposition into a blood vessel, test dosing is more effective but still fraught with problems.

During injection of 0.5 mcg/kg epinephrine (before or with the local anesthetic), the operator should watch for an increase in heart rate (≥10 beats per minute), systolic blood pressure (≥15 mmHg) and/ or changes of 25% in T-wave amplitude. During total intravenous anesthesia a positive test dose is best detected by an increase in systolic blood pressure.

CONTRAINDICATIONS TO NEURAXIAL TECHNIQUES

Contraindications to neuraxial anesthesia in infants and children are similar to those in adults. We consider patient and parental autonomy an important factor, and we do not perform neuraxial anesthesia when parents do not give consent, or when a child with appropriate understanding does not assent to the procedure. Local tissue infection at the planned needle insertion site and documented allergy to a given local anesthetic or adjunct are absolute contraindications as well.

Coagulopathy and ongoing anticoagulant therapy are considered relative contraindications. The most up-to-date guidelines of the American Society of Regional Anesthesia and Pain Medicine (ASRA)[28] state the role of appropriate clinical judgment for the individual patient who is anticoagulated and needs to undergo anesthetic management. We recommend to consider utilizing functional coagulation assays, such as thromboelastography, or measurement of specific coagulation factor activity when there are no clinical signs of impaired hemostasis but the conventional laboratory values suggest mild impairment (e.g., INR 1.2–1.4, thrombocyte number <150,000/microliter).[29] This approach assumes that there is sufficient time before performing the planned anesthetic, and general anesthesia carries above-average risk for the given patient.

Increased intracranial pressure, presence of ventriculoperitoneal shunt, intracranial mass with no, or minimal and stable, signs of neurological deficit may not prevent the use of neuraxial technique. Spinal dysraphism (spina bifida, tethered cord) and history of spinal instrumentation may impair the success of needle placement and local anesthetic spread and increase the risk of neural injury. Sacral dimple may indicate spina bifida occulta; prior to consideration of neuraxial technique, the patient should have an evaluation of the spine (ultrasound, MRI). History of recurrent urinary retention or urinary retention after neuraxial blockade may be considered relative contraindication as well.

COMPLICATIONS AND ADVERSE EFFECTS

Complications and adverse effects that apply to all neuraxial techniques include local infection at the needle/catheter insertion site, local hematoma, back pain, block failure, neural tissue injury, and local anesthetic systemic toxicity (LAST). Neonates and infants have increased susceptibility to the CNS and cardiac toxicity profile of local anesthetics. Given that the majority of neuraxial blocks in children are placed under general anesthesia, signs of CNS toxicity can often not be appreciated. Therefore, continuous cardiac monitoring, including electrocardiogram (EKG), during local anesthetic administration is warranted.

Epidural anesthesia carries the potential for spinal cord injury. The risk of spinal cord injury in caudal anesthesia is extremely low, but needle placement in the presence of spinal dysraphism such as a tethered cord may result in neural damage. Inadvertent epidural needle advancement into the spinal space can produce post-dural puncture headaches (PDPHs), and injection of a local anesthetic may lead to high or total spinal anesthesia.

Infants and children have a lower sympathetic tone and therefore a blunted hemodynamic response to sympathetic blockade achieved by a neuraxial block, but concomitant use of modifying factors such as general anesthesia, opioids, etc., may result in profound hypotension.

The most comprehensive evaluation of complications in pediatric neuraxial blocks comes from the Pediatric Regional Anesthesia Network. In 2018, Walker et al. published data from a prospective observational study that evaluated 2034 spinal blocks, 38,116 single-shot caudal blocks, 838 single-shot epidural blocks, 3166 caudal continuous catheters, and 9940 epidural continuous catheters.[20] Incidence of complications was reported as follows: 2:10,000 (neurologic, with no cases of permanent neurologic deficit); 0.92:10,000 (severe local anesthetic systemic toxicity); and 60:10,000 (local cutaneous infection). In addition, 1 patient developed an epidural abscess after lumbar epidural catheter placement, and 1 patient had a caudal continuous catheter unintentionally placed into the abdominal cavity. Long et al. analyzed complications during neuraxial catheter use in the neonatal population and reported an overall incidence of 13.3%; the majority of adverse effects were mild and included catheter malfunction (kinking, dislodgement), catheter contamination, vascular puncture, and block failure.[30] None of the patients experienced persistent neurologic problems, deep infection, spinal cord injury, or epidural hematoma.

REFERENCES

1. Hines MH. Neonatal cardiovascular physiology. *Semin Pediatr Surg.* 2013;22:174–178.
2. Gupta A, Saha U. Spinal anesthesia in children: a review. *J Anaesthesiol Clin Pharmacol.* 2014;30:10–18.
3. Tirmizi H. Spinal anesthesia in infants: recent developments. *Curr Opin Anaesthesiol.* 2015;28:333–338.
4. Sola C, Hertz L, Bringuier S, et al. Spinal anaesthesia in neonates and infants: what about the cerebral oxygen saturation? *Br J Anaesth.* 2017;119:964–971.
5. Tobias JD. Spinal anaesthesia in infants and children. *Paediatr Anaesth.* 2000;10:5–16.
6. Doufas AG, Wadhwa A, Shah YM, Lin CM, Haugh GS, Sessler DI. Block-dependent sedation during epidural anaesthesia is associated with delayed brainstem conduction. *Br J Anaesth.* 2004;93:228–234.

7. Hermanns H, Stevens MF, Werdehausen R, Braun S, Lipfert P, Jetzek-Zader M. Sedation during spinal anaesthesia in infants. *Br J Anaesth*. 2006;97:380–384.
8. Walker SM, Yaksh TL. Neuraxial analgesia in neonates and infants: a review of clinical and preclinical strategies for the development of safety and efficacy data. *Anesth Analg*. 2012;115:638–662.
9. Oda Y. Pharmacokinetics and systemic toxicity of local anesthetics in children. *J Anesth*. 2016;30:547–550.
10. Frawley G, Ingelmo P. Spinal anaesthesia in the neonate. *Best Pract Res Clin Anaesthesiol*. 2010;24:337–351.
11. Bosenberg A. Benefits of regional anesthesia in children. *Paediatr Anaesth*. 2012;22:10–18.
12. Mazoit JX, Dalens BJ. Pharmacokinetics of local anaesthetics in infants and children. *Clin Pharmacokinet*. 2004;43:17–32.
13. Abajian JC, Mellish RW, Browne AF, Perkins FM, Lambert DH, Mazuzan JE Jr. Spinal anesthesia for surgery in the high-risk infant. *Anesth Analg*. 1984;63:359–362.
14. Boretsky K. Pediatric regional anesthesia advances. *Curr Anesthesiol Rep*. 2019;9:100–109.
15. Veneziano G, Tobias JD. Chloroprocaine for epidural anesthesia in infants and children. *Paediatr Anaesth*. 2017;27:581–590.
16. Wilder RT. Local anesthetics for the pediatric patient. *Pediatr Clin North Am*. 2000;47:545558.
17. Polaner DM, Drescher J. Pediatric regional anesthesia: what is the current safety record? *Paediatr Anaesth*. 2011;21:737–742.
18. Walther-Larsen S, Rasmussen LS. The former preterm infant and risk of post-operative apnoea: recommendations for management. *Acta Anaesthesiol Scand*. 2006;50:888–893.
19. Brisman M, Ljung BM, Otterbom I, Larsson LE, Andreasson SE. Methaemoglobin formation after the use of EMLA cream in term neonates. *Acta Paediatr*. 1998;87:1191–1194.
20. Walker BJ, Long JB, Sathyamoorthy M, et al., Pediatric Regional Anesthesia Network. Complications in pediatric regional anesthesia: an analysis of more than 100,000 blocks from the Pediatric Regional Anesthesia Network. *Anesthesiology*. 2018;129:721–732.
21. Mossetti V, Ivani G. Controversial issues in pediatric regional anesthesia. *Paediatr Anaesth*. 2012;22:109–114.
22. Sartorelli KH, Abajian JC, Kreutz JM, Vane DW. Improved outcome utilizing spinal anesthesia in high-risk infants. *J Pediatr Surg*. 1992;27:1022–1025.
23. Whitaker EE, Wiemann BZ, DaJusta DG, et al. Spinal anesthesia for pediatric urological surgery: Reducing the theoretic neurotoxic effects of general anesthesia. *J Pediatr Urol*. 2017;13:396–400.
24. Davidson AJ, Morton NS, Arnup SJ, et al. Apnea after awake regional and general anesthesia in infants: the general anesthesia compared to spinal anesthesia study—comparing apnea and neurodevelopmental outcomes, a randomized controlled trial. *Anesthesiology*. 2015;123:38–54.
25. Kokki H. Spinal blocks. *Paediatr Anaesth*. 2012;22:56–64.
26. Keplinger M, Marhofer P, Klug W, et al. Feasibility and pharmacokinetics of caudal blockade in children and adolescents with 30–50 kg of body weight. *Paediatr Anaesth*. 2016;26:1053–1059.
27. Franklin AD, Lorinc AN, Shotwell MS, Greene EB, Wushensky CA. Evaluation of the skin to epidural and subarachnoid space distance in young children using magnetic resonance imaging. *Reg Anesth Pain* Med. 2015;40:245–248.
28. Horlocker TT, Vandermeulen E, Kopp SL, Gogarten W, Leffert LR, Benzon HT. Regional anesthesia in the patient receiving antithrombotic or thrombolytic therapy: American Society of Regional Anesthesia and Pain Medicine evidence-based guidelines (fourth edition). *Reg Anesth Pain Med*. 2018;43:263–309.
29. Forest DJ, Segal S. Update on thrombocytopenia in pregnancy and neuraxial anesthesia. *Curr Anesthesiol Rep*. 2017;7:111–118.
30. Long JB, Joselyn AS, Bhalla T, et al. The use of neuraxial catheters for postoperative analgesia in neonates: a multicenter safety analysis from the pediatric regional anesthesia network. *Anesth Analg*. 2016;122:1965–1970.

REVIEW QUESTIONS

(1) The duration of surgical anesthesia following a subarachnoid block (SAB) in neonates is limited to 60–80 minutes because:

A. They metabolize local anesthetics faster than adults.
B. Their body has a proportionally higher water content, resulting in a higher volume of distribution.
C. High cardiac output and vascularization of the meninges rapidly reduces the local anesthetic concentration at the spinal cord by enhanced systemic absorption.
D. Their serum alpha-1-acid glycoprotein concentration is low.

(2) What additive can most efficiently prolong the analgesia duration of a single-shot caudal epidural block in an infant?

A. Sodium bicarbonate
B. Epinephrine
C. Fentanyl
D. Clonidine

(3) SAB without sedation and general anesthesia reduces the risk of which of the following complications?

A. Early postoperative apnea
B. Delayed or late postoperative apnea
C. Postoperative hypotension
D. Hypothermia

(4) What is the most appropriate local anesthetic solution for postoperative continuous epidural analgesia in a 2-day-old neonate?

A. Ropivacaine
B. 2-chloroprocaine+clonidine
C. 2-chloroprocaine
D. Bupivacaine

(5) Tunneling caudal epidural catheters decrease the incidence of:

A. Meningitis
B. Sepsis
C. Bacterial colonization of the catheter tip
D. Bacteremia

(6) Ultrasound imaging of the spine in neonates and infants is beneficial for improving which of the following circumstances?

A. Assessing the depth of the epidural space from the skin
B. Verifying the location of the tip of the epidural catheter
C. Verifying the correct spread of the local anesthetic solution in the epidural space
D. All of the above

(7) Neonates and infants are more susceptible to the systemic neuro- and cardiotoxic effect of amide local anesthetics compared to adults because of:

A. Incomplete axonal myelinization
B. Decreased serum protein binding
C. Immature liver function
D. All of the above

(8) What is an absolute contraindication to epidural catheter placement in a 3-year-old boy?

A. INR 1.4
B. Parental refusal
C. Patient refusal
D. Contact precautions due to positive methicillin-resistant staphylococcus aureus nasal swab

(9) Neuraxial anesthesia with or without general anesthesia improves postoperative recovery in pediatric patients because:

A. It makes placement of an endotracheal tube unnecessary.
B. It eliminates the risk for urinary retention.
C. It blunts the neuroendocrine response to surgical stress.
D. It decreases the incidence of late apnea.

(10) Which of the following is the most practical technique to ensure catheter placement in the desired dermatomal level?

A. Transesophageal echocardiography (TEE)
B. Measuring distance between catheter insertion site and desired dermatomal level
C. Assessment of clinical response to surgical stimulation
D. Real-time ultrasound guidance

ANSWERS

(1) **C.** SAB using tetracaine or bupivacaine provides short duration of surgical anesthesia in neonates and infants due to quick removal of local anesthetics by systemic absorption that is related to high cardiac output and dense vascularization of the meningeal membranes. Metabolism is slower (A) compared to adults. The higher total water content (B) and lower alpha$_1$-acid glycoprotein concentration (D) do not have measurable impact on block duration in neonates and infants.

Reference

Gupta A, Saha U. Spinal anesthesia in children: a review. *J Anaesthesiol Clin Pharmacol*. 2014 Jan;30(1):10–18.

(2) **D.** Clonidine addition to local anesthetic agents provides improved analgesia and prolongs duration of action. Sodium bicarbonate (A) may shorten the onset of an epidural block but does not prolong the duration. Epinephrine (B) can also prolong block duration due to local vasoconstriction, but the effect is not consistent and typically is shorter compared to clonidine. The lipophilic fentanyl (C) contributes to a denser block but does not extend duration significantly.

Reference

Rowney DA, Doyle E. Epidural and subarachnoid blockade in children. *Anaesthesia*. 1998 Oct;53(10):980–1001.

(3) **A.** The incidence of early postoperative apnea is reduced in patients receiving a SAB without general anesthesia. (B) is not affected. While general anesthesia is more frequently associated with (C), it may also occur in subarachnoid blocks. (D) Subarachnoid blocks inhibit vasomotor and shivering responses and thereby increase the risk of hypothermia.

Reference

Davidson AJ, Morton NS, Arnup SJ, et al. Apnea after awake regional and general anesthesia in infants: the general anesthesia compared to spinal anesthesia study—comparing apnea and neurodevelopmental outcomes, a randomized controlled trial. *Anesthesiology*. 2015 Jul;123(1):38–54.

(4) **B.** In newborns, 2-choloroprocaine is metabolized by plasma pseudocholinesterase sufficiently fast to prevent cardiac or neurotoxicity. Clonidine improves the quality of the block and the risk of its potential cardiovascular and respiratory side effects is relatively low in an otherwise stable neonate. (A) and (D) are metabolized to a lesser rate by the immature liver and thereby the risk of their cardiotoxic and neurotoxic effects are increased. (C) provides lesser quality analgesia than the combination under (B).

Reference

Veneziano G, Tobias JD. Chloroprocaine for epidural anesthesia in infants and children. *Paediatr Anaesth*. 2017 Jun;27(6):581–590.

(5) **C.** Tunneling caudal catheters has been shown to reduce the bacterial colonization of the catheter tip but did not influence outcomes like meningitis and bacteremia.

Reference

Bubeck J, Boos K, Krause H, et al. Subcutaneous tunneling of caudal catheters reduces the rate of bacterial colonization to that of lumbar epidural catheters. *Anesth Analg*. 2004 Sep;99(3):689–693.

(6) **D.** Ultrasound can provide valuable information by assessing the anatomy as well as following the needle pathway and the spread of injected local anesthetics in real time.

Reference

Tsui BC, Suresh S. Ultrasound imaging for regional anesthesia in infants, children, and adolescents: a review of current literature and its application in the practice of neuraxial blocks. *Anesthesiology*. 2010 Mar;112(3):719–728.

(7) **D.** Incomplete axonal myelinization increases neuronal susceptibility to the direct toxic effects of local anesthetics.[10] Levels of alpha-1-glycoprotein (AAG), which binds amide local anesthetics, are 20%–50% of the adult concentration; consequently, less AAG is available to bind local anesthetics, hence increasing the free local anesthetic fraction, leading to an increased potential for toxicity. Lastly, immaturity of liver enzymes reduces the capacity to metabolize local anesthetics.

Reference

Oda Y. Pharmacokinetics and systemic toxicity of local anesthetics in children. *J Anesth*. 2016 Aug;30(4):547–550.

(8) **B.** Parental refusal is considered an absolute contraindication for the performance of neuraxial anesthesia. (A) should be considered a relative indication, but after weighing the risk/benefit ratio, many practitioners would proceed given the relatively mild elevation of the INR. (C) depends on the age and developmental level of the child. Around the age of 7 years, children may be able to provide assent, but prior to this age, the child is usually unable to participate in the consent process. (D) signifies colonization but no active infection at the needle entry site; therefore the neuraxial technique can be performed.

Reference

Marcelino R, Sawardekar A, Suresh S. Neuraxial anaesthesia in paediatrics. *Anaesth Intens Care Med.* 2019;20(6):338–343.

(9) **C.** It inhibits sensory input from the surgical incision and thereby blunts the neuroendocrine stress response. In some cases, (A) may be correct but many procedures still require a secured airway. (B): while uncommonly encountered in pediatric patients, neuraxial anesthesia carries a small risk of precipitating postoperative urinary retention. (D) is incorrect as studies have shown that while neuraxial anesthesia reduces the incidence of early apnea, late apnea is not affected.

Reference

Bosenberg A. Benefits of regional anesthesia in children. *Paediatr Anaesth.* 2012 Jan;22(1):10–18.

(10) **D.** Ultrasound provides real-time images of the catheter tip and can visualize adequate local anesthetic spread in the epidural space. (A) is also able to provide that information, but placement of a TEE probe is not without risk, and interpretation requires a skilled operator. (B) is unreliable as the catheter can take unexpected routes when threaded up in the epidural space. (C) provides information from which correct placement can be inferred, but it precludes further adjustments of the catheter in case of inadequate positioning.

Reference

Ponde VC, Bedekar VV, Desai AP, et al. Does ultrasound guidance add accuracy to continuous caudal-epidural catheter placements in neonates and infants? *Paediatr Anaesth.* 2017 Oct;27(10):1010–1014.

39.

REGIONAL ANESTHESIA FOR MAJOR ABDOMINAL SURGERY IN PEDIATRIC PATIENTS

Alina Lazar

STEM CASE AND KEY QUESTIONS

A 7-year-old boy with neurogenic bladder is scheduled for bladder augmentation. He has a past medical history of myelomeningocele, which was repaired at birth, hydrocephalus managed with a ventriculo-peritoneal (VP) shunt, and mild developmental delay. He has had numerous surgical interventions to reconstruct his urinary bladder, including appendicovesicostomy, and bladder neck reconstruction. His previous procedures were complicated by postoperative nausea and vomiting (PONV).

He has no drug allergies and weighs 20 kg. The planned incision is midline from above the umbilicus to the pubic symphysis. The bladder will be augmented with an ileal loop. A portion of the posterior rectus sheath will be harvested to create a bladder neck sling wrap, and a suprapubic vesicostomy will be placed. Extensive peritoneal adhesions and scarring of the bladder neck are anticipated.

(1) WHAT ARE THE ANESTHETIC CONCERNS FOR THIS CHILD? WHAT ARE THE OPTIONS FOR PERIOPERATIVE PAIN MANAGEMENT?

The anesthesiologist decides to avoid instrumenting the neuraxial space because of concerns related to anatomical changes caused by previous myelomeningocele repair. In anticipation of extensive surgery, with significant visceral involvement and adhesions from previous surgeries, and in light of prior history of PONV, a truncal block is proposed. The anesthesiologist discusses with parents the options of a single-shot block with adjuvants to extend its duration, and multimodal analgesia to minimize the possibility of rebound pain upon resolution of the block, versus continuous administration of local anesthetic (LA) via block catheters. To further minimize the risk of PONV, and reliably extend the effect of the block beyond the first 24 hours, continuous administration of LA is selected.

(2) HOW WOULD YOU DECIDE BETWEEN A PARAVERTEBRAL BLOCK (PVB), ERECTOR SPINAE PLANE (ESP) BLOCK, TRANSVERSUS ABDOMINIS PLANE (TAP) BLOCK, QUADRATUS LUMBORUM (QL) BLOCK, OR RECTUS SHEATH (RS) BLOCK?

Either QL or ESP blocks is considered, for their larger dermatomal spread, potential visceral analgesia, and longer duration of action, compared to TAP block. The anesthesiologist decides to place bilateral ESP catheters, because, as opposed to the QL block, the ESP block is in a more superficial location, less technically challenging, and the prepping/draping can be done in a single setup for both sides. In addition, the presence of a ventricular-peritoneal shunt may complicate QL catheters placement, although this concern can be addressed by bedside abdominal ultrasound scanning to map out and avoid puncturing the shunt during block placement. Consent is obtained from parents, and the patient is brought to the operating room. The child is anesthetized, intubated, and prepared for the block placement.

(3) HOW WOULD YOU POSITION THE PATIENT FOR THIS PROCEDURE? WHERE SHOULD THE TIP OF THE CATHETER BE OPTIMALLY LOCATED? AT WHAT DERMATOMAL LEVEL WOULD YOU INSERT THE NEEDLE? WHAT TYPE, DOSE, AND CONCENTRATION OF LA WOULD YOU USE? WOULD YOU ADMINISTER LA VIA THE NERVE CATHETER DURING THE PROCEDURE? WOULD YOU BOLUS THE CATHETERS PERIODICALLY, OR USE A CONTINUOUS INFUSION? WHAT ARE THE ADVANTAGES AND DISADVANTAGES OF EACH APPROACH?

With the patient in the left lateral decubitus, and under ultrasound visualization, the needle is advanced in a craniocaudal direction, aiming for the T10 transverse process.

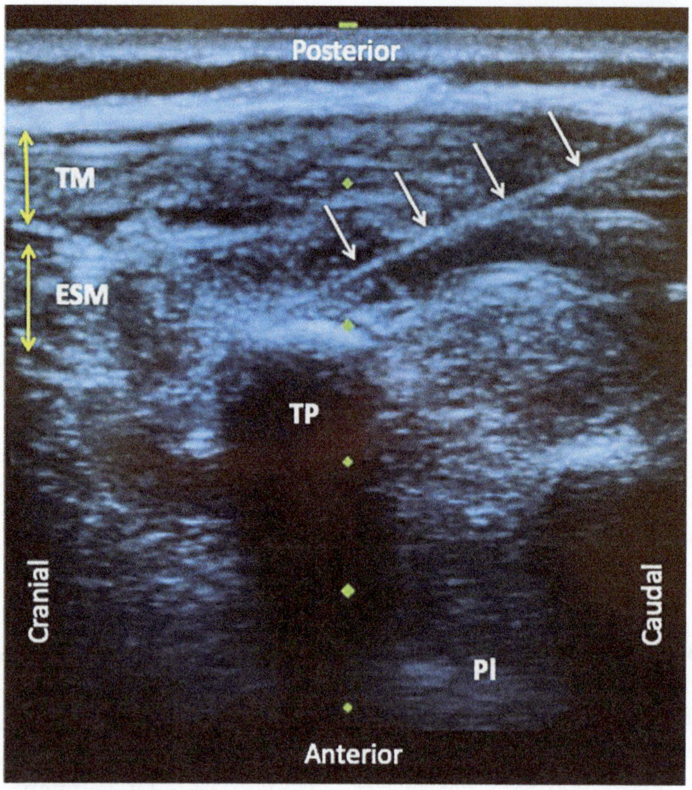

Figure 39.1. Ultrasound image of lateral QLB. Solid arrow indicates needle trajectory.
QL = quadratus lumborum muscle; LD = latissimus dorsi muscle; EO = external oblique muscle; IO = internal oblique muscle.

The ESP is identified using hydrodissection. Bilateral catheters are inserted, and following a negative test dose, each catheter is bolused with 8 mL bupivacaine 0.25% with epinephrine 1:200,000. There is minimal hemodynamic response to incision. One hour after incision, the O_2 saturation decreases gradually to 96% and the peak inspiratory pressure rises progressively from 16 to 25 cm H_2O (Figure 39.1).

(4) HOW WOULD YOU EVALUATE THE PATIENT? WHAT IS YOUR DIFFERENTIAL DIAGNOSIS? ARE YOU CONCERNED ABOUT A POSSIBLE PNEUMOTHORAX GIVEN THE RECENT PLACEMENT OF ESP BLOCKS? WHAT WOULD YOU DO NEXT?

Although pneumothorax is a concern with needle insertion at T10 and above, the breath sounds are equal bilaterally, and coarse. The capnogram shows a delayed rise. After suctioning the endotracheal tube, and lung recruitment, the peak airway pressure returns to baseline, and breath sounds become clear to auscultation. Surgery proceeds uneventfully. During the 5 hours of surgery, a total dose of 50 mcg fentanyl is administered, and the catheters are each bolused hourly with 6 mL bupivacaine 0.25% with epinephrine.

(5) HOW WOULD YOU CONTINUE TO ADMINISTER LA IN THE POSTOPERATIVE PERIOD? WHAT DOSE AND CONCENTRATION WOULD YOU USE? WHAT PRECAUTIONS WOULD YOU TAKE WHEN BOLUSING THE CATHETERS TO AVOID LOCAL ANESTHETIC SYSTEMIC TOXICITY (LAST)?

At the end of procedure, the ESP catheters are connected to infusion pumps. Hourly LA bolusing is chosen to allow for larger LA volumes and wider, more uniform spread along the fascial plane. The pumps are programmed to alternatively deliver boluses of 0.1% ropivacaine 5 mL per hour, staggered by 30 min to moderate peak LA concentration. Intravenous ketorolac and rectal acetaminophen are administered, and the child is transported to the post-anesthesia care unit (PACU), where he recovers from anesthesia uneventfully. However, he is not able to extend his knees.

WHAT IS THE EXPLANATION FOR THE LOWER EXTREMITY WEAKNESS? WHAT WOULD YOU TELL THE PARENTS ABOUT THE EXPECTED TIMING FOR THE RESOLUTION OF WEAKNESS?

The child is transferred to floor with plans in place to monitor the lower extremity strength. Two hours later, he becomes uncomfortable, and the on-call anesthesiologist is asked to evaluate him.

(6) HOW WOULD YOU EVALUATE THE CHILD'S PAIN, AND FUNCTIONALITY OF HIS ESPB? HOW WOULD YOU TEST THE SENSORY BLOCK? WHAT WOULD BE YOUR MANAGEMENT PLAN?

When asked about pain, the child is pointing toward the groin and abdomen area but is unwilling to provide further detail. His heart rate and blood pressure are elevated, and he appears to be in distress. The child is unable to cooperate with sensory block assessment with an ice cube. Light pressure on the incision site does not trigger a significant response, but deeper palpation causes distress. A dose of 2 mL 0.1% ropivacaine is administered through each of the ESP catheters, and subsequently the patient falls asleep. The ESP catheter boluses are increased to 6 mL every hour.

(7) SIX HOURS LATER, THE NURSE CALLS TO REPORT THAT THE PATIENT LOOKS COMFORTABLE, BUT IS VERY SLEEPY, GROGGY, AND IRRITABLE WHEN SHE ATTEMPTS TO WAKE HIM UP. THE CHILD'S MOTHER ALSO REPORTS OCCASIONAL MUSCLE TWITCHING.

(8) WHAT IS YOUR DIFFERENTIAL DIAGNOSIS? CAN THESE BE MANIFESTATIONS OF SYSTEMIC LAST? IS HIS SOMNOLENCE A RESIDUAL EFFECT OF ANESTHESIA OR A SIDE EFFECT OF OTHER MEDICATIONS? ARE YOU CONCERNED ABOUT A VP SHUNT MALFUNCTION? HOW WOULD YOU FURTHER EVALUATE THE PATIENT?

Physical examination is normal, but the child is unable to cooperate with evaluation of muscle strength. Vital signs, blood glucose, and electrolytes are within normal limits. Chart review shows that the VP shunt has recently been evaluated and is functioning normally. No other sedative medications have been administered after emergence from anesthesia. Telemetry shows no abnormalities. No changes in electrocardiogram, heart rate, or blood pressure occur after administration of 2 mL epinephrine 1:200,000 subsequently in each of the catheters.

(9) WHAT WOULD YOU DO NEXT?

Although the catheters have not migrated intravascularly, concerns for LAST from systemic absorption remain. The ropivacaine infusions are held for 1 hour, then restarted at 6 mL every 90 minutes. Later, he becomes more awake and interactive, and the twitching resolves. Fourteen hours after block placement, the quadriceps muscle strength returns to normal.

He remains comfortable, requiring only 2 doses of ibuprofen and no opioids during the first 2 postoperative days. The catheters are removed uneventfully on postoperative day 3. He is discharged home 1 day later.

DISCUSSION

A comprehensive approach to pain management for children undergoing major abdominal surgery is required to optimize analgesia and minimize side effects. Multimodal analgesia comprising regional blocks and/or systemic analgesia is essential in protecting against intense postoperative pain.

DIFFERENCES IN REGIONAL ANESTHESIA IN CHILDREN

Regional anesthesia (RA) has been increasingly used for major surgery in pediatric patients in part because of concern for the effects of general anesthetics and opioids on development, but also in an effort to optimize children's postoperative experience.

The safety of pediatric RA has been established by several large databases.[1] Neurologic risks are very low, although possibly higher for epidural anesthesia, especially in infants younger than 6 months. In general, it is safer to perform nerve blocks in an anesthetized rather than a struggling child, and there is a long record of safety with this approach. There is more controversy over direct needle placement of thoracic epidurals in anesthetized children, particularly in infants. The risk of LAST is higher in infants because of their lower levels of plasma alpha-1-acid glycoprotein and albumin and decreased hepatic metabolism. The maximum doses of LA should be calculated based on lean rather than actual body weight, and not exceeded (Table 39.1). LA dosing guidelines have been recently formulated by both the American and European Societies of Regional Anesthesia (ASRA/ESRA),[2] but have been critiqued as being too conservative.[3] Addition of epinephrine to LA decreases peak plasma LA concentration, and prolongs the time until such concentrations are reached.

Severe pain anticipated to persist beyond 24 hours can be managed by continuous infusion of LA, or by prolonging the duration of a single-shot block with adjuvants. Clonidine extends caudal analgesia duration by a factor of 2.5–3 compared to LA alone. Dexmedetomidine is at least as effective as clonidine and has less cardiovascular side effects. Addition of dexmedetomidine (1 mcg/kg) to caudal bupivacaine in pediatric major abdominal cancer surgery provided postoperative analgesia for up to 19 hours, with less use of analgesics, and prolonged duration of arousable sedation.[4] Addition of alpha-2-adrenoreceptor agonists in peripheral nerve blocks prolonged the time to first request for supplemental analgesia by 2.6 times compared to LA alone.[5] More than 60% of patients who received dexmedetomidine did not require rescue analgesia in the first 24 hours. The mechanism of action is not completely understood, but likely involves a primarily peripheral neural effect. A dose of 1 mcg/kg of dexmedetomidine is considered safe. Postoperative sedation is a common side effect, but clinically significant bradycardia and hypotension are rare in children. In adults, dexamethasone has been proved to prolong the duration of analgesia and decrease rebound pain when used as an adjunct to peripheral nerve blocks.

The equipment for RA needs to be adapted to the age and size of the patients. The use of linear array high-frequency

Table 39.1 MAXIMUM DOSES OF LA RECOMMENDED BY ASRA/ESRA IN CHILDREN[3]

	EPIDURAL (SINGLE INJECTION) (MG/KG)	EPIDURAL (CONTINUOUS INFUSION) (MG/KG/H)	FASCIAL PLANE BLOCKS (SINGLE INJECTION) (MG/KG)	FASCIAL PLANE BLOCKS (CONTINUOUS INFUSION) (MG/KG/H)
Bupivacaine	1.7	0.2 (<3 months old) 0.3 (3 months–1 year old) 0.4 (>1 year old)	0.25–0.75	0.1–0.3
Ropivacaine	1.7	0.2 (<3 months old) 0.3 (3 months–1 year old) 0.4 (>1 year old)	0.25–0.75	0.1–0.3
Chloroprocaine		0.2 (< 3 months old) 0.3 (3 months–1 year old) 0.5 (>1 year old)	No recommendation	No recommendation

ultrasound transducer for deep blocks is possible in children and has the advantage of sharper images. Lifting the skin or making a nick in the skin with a sharp beveled needle facilitates needle insertion. It is important to use non-LA solution when hydrodissecting tissue planes to maximize the amount of LA that can be injected at the desired location.

Thoracic epidural analgesia (TEA) provides significant pain relief (especially the dynamic pain component) with improved gastrointestinal function after laparotomy. Because children's ligaments are softer and easier to penetrate, a slow, deliberate approach should be exercised to avoid dural puncture. Loss of resistance to saline is preferred. In small children, it is critical to place the epidural catheter with its tip in immediate proximity to the surgical dermatomes. The position of the catheter can be confirmed fluoroscopically, via stimulating epidural catheters, or in young infants with ultrasonography. In infants a styletted catheter can be inserted caudally and advanced up to the thoracic level.

Typical loading volumes are 0.3 mL/kg for thoracic epidural. The dose of LA infusions is 0.03 mL/kg/h/spinal segment for mid-thoracic and 0.06 mL/kg/h/spinal segment for low-thoracic epidural. Typical infusions are a combination of LA and opioid and/or clonidine (Tables 39.1 and 39.2). Patient-controlled epidural anesthesia (PCEA) can be used in children as young as 5 years old. A common PCEA regimen is a basal rate of 0.2 mg/kg/h, bolus of 0.1 mg/kg/h, a lockout interval 15 minutes, and a maximum hourly rate of 0.4 mg/kg/h.

The contraindications to epidural analgesia are similar to those in adults. In the absence of hypovolemia, TEA in children younger than 8 years is associated with remarkable cardiovascular stability. If hypotension in a child with an epidural occurs in the absence of surgical bleeding, subarachnoid or subdural catheter placement should be suspected.

Post-dural puncture headache is rarely seen in children younger than 8 years of age. Epidural hematoma and neurologic injury are exceedingly rare complications in children; however, case reports from institutions where pediatric epidurals are placed regularly highlight this potential risk.[6] Catheter tip colonization is common in caudally threaded epidurals, but no serious neuraxial infections have been reported. In small children, the catheter can migrate cephalad, therefore its position should be checked after placement and postoperatively. Leakage around the catheter is common and may lead to catheter dislodgement.

Table 39.2 RECOMMENDED RATES OF ADJUVANTS FOR CONTINUOUS EPIDURAL INFUSION IN PEDIATRIC PATIENTS

DRUG	DOSE* (MCG/KG/HOUR)	TYPICAL CONCENTRATION (MCG/ML)		
		NEONATES (0–2 MONTHS)	INFANTS	CHILDREN
Fentanyl	0.1–0.5	1–2	2 (2–5)	5 (2–5)
Hydromorphone	1.5–2.5	NR	NR	10–20**
Morphine	3–5	NR	NR	25–50**
Clonidine §	0.1–0.2	NR	0.4	0.4–1 (lumbar epidural tip) 0.4–0.6 (thoracic epidural tip)

NR = not recommended.

* Larger doses of opioids are indicated for opioid-tolerant patients.

** Administration of hydrophilic opioids through a thoracic epidural is not recommended.

§ When clonidine is added to an epidural solution, the epidural opioid dose should be reduced by 50%.

Intrathecal morphine provides early relief from the visceral pain, alone in laparoscopic major surgery, or in addition to nerve blocks or wound infusion catheters in open surgery. An intrathecal morphine dose of 5–10 mcg/kg provides 12–24 hours postoperative analgesia but may cause delayed respiratory depression. Patients who receive neuraxial opioids require postoperative respiratory monitoring for 24 hours. If rescue opioids are needed, a mixed agonist-antagonist such as nalbuphine is preferred. Pruritus is a common side effect and may be treated with diphenhydramine or a low-dose naloxone infusion.

PARAVERTEBRAL BLOCK (PVB)

Continuous paravertebral blocks (PVBs) have been successfully used in children and provides somatic and visceral analgesia over 4–6 dermatomes. Its advantages include the ability to provide unilateral analgesia, thus avoiding potential hypotension as a result of bilateral sympathectomy, and similar efficacy to epidural anesthesia with lower risk of neuraxial injury.

TECHNIQUE

The ultrasound-guided approach has been described in children.[7] With the ultrasound probe in a transverse paraspinal position, a Tuohy needle is advanced in-plane from lateral to medial into the space posterior to the transverse process and lateral to pleura.

DOSES

A total of 0.5 mL/kg per side (maximum dose 15 mL per side) of ropivacaine 0.2% can be injected for a single-shot block. For continuous infusions, doses of ropivacaine 0.1% or 0.2% totaling 0.5 mg/kg/h (max 12 mL/h per side) can be used.

EFFICACY

The role of PVB is well established in major abdominal surgery involving large subcostal or transverse incisions such are hepatic or urological surgery.[7]

RISKS

In a series from a large tertiary institution, the most common complications were catheter leakage (5.9%) and dislodgement (4.9%).[8] There was only one case of LAST in an infant in whom a large dose of chloroprocaine was injected rapidly. The risk of amide LA systemic toxicity may preclude their use via bilateral catheters in young infants. Alternatively, an ester LA may be used.[9] Pneumothorax and vascular injury are very rare.

FASCIAL PLANE BLOCKS

Truncal blocks have been described as easy and safe alternatives to TEA and PVB. They are less potent than neuraxial blocks and are used as a component to multimodal analgesia (opioid-sparing, rather than opioid-eliminating effects). Their effects depend on LA spread (large boluses are required to "flood" the fascial plane), direction and speed of injection, respiratory movements, and gravity. The extent of analgesia does not necessarily correlate with the presence of a sensory block, which makes it difficult to assess the block by testing the response to cold or pinprick. This may be explained by the concept of differential blockade in which very low concentrations of LA preferentially block unmyelinated C fibers (responsible for the majority of nociception) over the larger A fibers (involved in touch and motor function). Because the block requires large volumes of LA, it is imperative to limit the dose to less than maximum recommended limits, add epinephrine, monitor patients, and be prepared to treat systemic toxicity. Table 39.3 summarizes the clinical indications of truncal blocks.

TRANSVERSUS ABDOMINIS PLANE (TAP) BLOCK

The transversus abdominis plane (TAP) is a potential anatomical space between transversus abdominis and internal oblique or rectus abdominis muscles which contains the abdominal branches of the thoracolumbar nerves. A good understanding of the anatomy and classification of TAP blocks[10,11] is important for the optimal block type selection. Injecting LA in the TAP at or anterior to the midaxillary line (lateral TAP block) often misses the lateral cutaneous branches, and thus provide analgesia between midline and midclavicular line and inferior to the umbilicus. LA administration posterior to the midaxillary line (posterior TAP block) produces a more complete blockade of the abdominal wall.

The iliohypogastric and ilioinguinal nerves (L1) run initially deep to the TAP, and only enter it close to the anterior superior iliac spine. The anatomic variability in their course contributes to the high failure rates for blockade of these nerves with the TAP block.[12] These nerves can be blocked by a direct approach (iliohypogastric/ilioinguinal nerve block, (IINB), quadratus lumborum block (QLB), or transversalis fascia plane block (TFPB). In the latter one, LA is injected deep to the tapered tip of the transversus abdominus muscle (TAM) and superficial to transversalis fascia, a thin membrane separating the transversus abdominis, quadratus lumborum, and psoas muscles from the peritoneum-covered viscera.[13] Abdominal analgesia will be restricted to the T12–L1 dermatomes but can be extended to cover a larger abdominal area if additional LA is injected in the TAP space on needle withdrawal.

Cutaneous innervation to the supraumbilical abdominal area is provided by the anterior branches of the T6–T9 intercostal nerves. After emerging from the anterior costal margin, these nerves pass between the TAM and the rectus sheath, then between the posterior layer of the rectus sheath and the rectus muscle itself, before penetrating anteriorly into the muscle.

In the subcostal TAP block, LA is deposited between the rectus abdominis and TAM, or underneath the posterior rectus

Table 39.3 TRUNCAL BLOCKS: CLINICAL INDICATIONS AND DOSES OF LOCAL ANESTHETICS

BLOCK	INDICATION	DOSE OF LOCAL ANESTHETIC (ML/KG/BLOCK)	COMMENTS
Lateral TAP (midaxillary)	Somatic analgesia for incisions in lower (T10 to T12–L1) anterior abdominal wall.	0.2–0.3	Will not cover incisions lateral to anterior axillary line. T12 and L1 are not consistently covered (they can be blocked by ilioinguinal/iliohypogastric, QL, or transversalis fascia blocks).
Posterior TAP (posterior to the midaxillary line)	Somatic analgesia for incisions in lower (T10 to T12–L1) anterior and lateral abdominal wall.	0.2–0.3	May share some similarities with the QL1 block.
Oblique subcostal TAP	Somatic analgesia for incisions in upper (T6–T7 to T9–T10) anterior abdominal wall.	0.2–0.3	Technically challenging. Will not cover incisions lateral to anterior axillary line.
Bilateral dual TAP	Somatic analgesia for extensive (T7-T12) incisions in anterior abdominal wall	0.15–0.2	Will not cover incisions lateral to anterior axillary line.
Rectus sheath (RS) block	Somatic analgesia -midline or paramedian laparotomy	0.1–0.2	Will not cover the area from symphysis pubis to the midpoint between umbilicus and pubic bone. Multiple injections will provide better coverage.
Quadratus lumborum (QL) block	Somatic and visceral analgesia for mid-lower (T8–T12) incisions in anterior abdominal wall	0.2-0.3	Lumbar plexus block may occur. Extent of block variable (up to T5–L2) depending on technique.
Transversalis fascia block	Analgesia for incisions over the anterior iliac crest, the anterior iliac crest itself, and L1 dermatome of the anterior abdominal wall	0.–0.3	Site of LA deposition is more inferior and anterior/lateral to that of the QL block. Lumbar plexus block may occur.
Erector spinae plane (ESP) block	Somatic and possible visceral analgesia to the entire abdomen (T6–T12 with needle tip at T7)	0.3–0.5	

sheath when the needle insertion point is close to the xiphoid where the TAM does not extend under the rectus abdominis. This block provides analgesia in the anterior portion of the upper abdomen. A curved needle can be used to hydrodissect in the TAP plane along the oblique subcostal line, thus blocking all nerves supplying the anterior abdomen.[14]

A dual TAP block combines a subcostal block with a posterior or lateral TAP block. Bilateral dual (four-quadrant) TAP blocks can provide analgesia to the entire abdominal wall. A catheter can be inserted to provide continuous analgesia. This approach may not be practical in children because large, potentially toxic doses of LA would be needed. Appropriate dilution of the initial bolus and subsequent infusions are critical to avoid systemic toxicity.

EFFICACY

The TAP block has been used in children for a variety of superficial abdominal wall procedures, but also in major abdominal surgery as part of a multimodal approach, particularly in children with contraindications to neuraxial anesthesia.

TECHNIQUE

TAP blocks (single-shot and continuous infusion), although technically more challenging in infants, have been described in all age groups.[15,16] Masters described the subcostal approach to the TAP block in infants undergoing major abdominal surgery via a transverse supraumbilical incision.[17]

DOSES

A volume of 0.2 mL/kg/side of LA (maximum 20 mL) is recommended in children. The total maximum dose of bupivacaine recommended to avoid toxicity is 2 mg/kg in the neonate, 3 mg/kg in children, and 4 mg/kg in adolescents.[15] A dose of 2.5 mg/kg bupivacaine was more effective than 1.25 mg/kg in reducing the 24-hour total analgesic consumption.[18]

RISKS

The risks of TAP block are low, and include intravascular injection, infection, perforation of the peritoneum, and liver damage.[19] In adults, LAST has been reported after TAP blocks with doses normally considered standard and safe.[20]

RECTUS SHEATH (RS) BLOCK

The anterior cutaneous branches of the spinal/intercostal nerves penetrate the posterior RS at the lateral edge of the rectus abdominis muscle (linea semilunaris), and after traveling a short distance through the muscle, emerge ventrally to innervate the overlaying skin. Posterior RS extends from the xyphoid process to the midpoint between the umbilicus and symphysis pubis (arcuate line). Deep to the posterior RS is fascia transversalis, and together they create the ultrasound appearance of tramlines. LA injected between the rectus muscle and its posterior sheath (above the tramlines) at the lateral border of the muscle spreads craniocaudally and provides analgesia for midline laparotomy. Caudal to the arcuate line, the only layers posterior to the rectus muscle are the transversalis fascia and peritoneum, which explains why blocks performed in this area are less effective.[21] In 10%–30% of the population, the nerves directly pierce the lateral edge of the rectus abdominis muscle or run anterior to the rectus muscle in the subcutaneous tissue and thus may be missed by an RSB. Injecting additional LA in the subcutaneous plane above the muscle, or alternatively, placing the block in the TAP plane just lateral to the linea semilunaris, may compensate for such variations.

Compared to the TAP block, the RSB appears to provide denser analgesia of a shorter duration. Thus, it can be used for prolonged postoperative analgesia only if continuous catheters are placed.

DOSES

The absorption kinetics of LA are slower after an RSB than after other compartment blocks or wound infiltration, likely a result of lesser vascularity in the posterior RS compartment. Flack found that 0.2 mL/kg/side of 0.25% bupivacaine was effective and yielded less than toxic systemic anesthetic concentrations, but warned against injecting larger volumes.[22] Ropivacaine 0.2 mL/kg injected at the lateral edge of the posterior RS compartment at the level of the umbilicus spread close to the subcostal margin (T8) superiorly in only less than half of the cases, and inferiorly to only approximately 1.5 cm below the lower margin of umbilicus.[23] If analgesia of the subcostal area (T6–T8) is desired, additional injections are needed. Alternatively, the oblique subcostal TAP block (between rectus and transverse abdominis muscle) with the needle inserted close to the xyphoid process may be used. Even then, it appears difficult to achieve spread to T6 and T7. Analgesia to the infraumbilical portion of the incision may be supplemented with additional blocks, such as a lateral TAP block. RS catheters can be bolused with 0.4 mL/kg/side of LA (up to a total of 20 mL) every 6 hours.

EFFICACY

In children, single-injection RS block is marginally more effective than wound infiltration, with the chief benefit being reduction of intraoperative opioids.[23] Because RSB provides only somatic analgesia, supplementary opiates are needed for the management of visceral pain.

QUADRATUS LUMBORUM (QL) BLOCK

The quadratus lumborum (QL) block was first described as an extension of the ultrasound-guided "posterior" transversus abdominis plane (TAP) block. However, QL and TAP blocks are essentially different because a posterior TAP block is, by definition, superficial to the transversus abdominis muscle and its aponeurosis, whereas the lateral QL block is deep to the transversus abdominis aponeurosis.[24] The pattern of LA spread and mechanism of action of the block are not fully understood. LA appears to spread to the thoracic paravertebral space along the thoracolumbar fascia (TLF), spinal nerve roots, and paravertebral sympathetic chain.[25] The TLF contains a high-density network of sympathetic fibers and mechanoreceptors, which are believed to contribute to the robust analgesic effect of the QLB. Because of widespread somatic (potentially T4–L1) and likely visceral blockade, this block may provide superior analgesia for abdominal surgery.

The lateral QLB (QLB1) involves injecting LA at the junction of QL and the aponeurosis of TAM, between the aponeurosis and transversalis fascia (Figure 39.1). The pattern of spread is similar to the transversalis fascia plane block (TFPB) but more posteriorly, along the ventral surface of the QL muscle. Some authors deliberately advance the needle tip into this location. Depending on the exact location of the needle tip at the lateral border of the QL muscle, LA could also spread posterior to the muscle.

In the posterior QL block, LA is injected just superficial to the middle layer of the TLF (seen as a bright hyperechogenic line) covering the QL muscle, and just distal to the attachment site of the internal and external oblique abdominal muscles to the TLF.[26] This space where the middle TLF joins the posterior TLF on the lateral border of the erector spinae is named the lumbar interfascial triangle. The advantages of using a posterior approach for the QL block when compared to the lateral or the anterior approach is a more superficial point of injection, better ultrasonographic resolution, and a potentially safer injection.

The anterior QL block involves injecting LA at the anterior aspect of the QL muscle, promoting consistent spread to the thoracolumbar paravertebral space.

TECHNIQUE

The most frequently used approach in children is the lateral QL block. The linear array high-frequency ultrasound transducer is often sufficient in children because less penetration is needed to visualize anatomical structures. The block can be done in the supine position, with a rolled towel placed under the hip to facilitate probe manipulation, or in lateral decubitus.

DOSES

The typical volume used is 0.2–0.3 mL/kg per block, with the LA concentration adjusted to keep within the maximum recommended dose range. The QL block is associated with lower plasma ropivacaine levels than TAP blocks, potentially making it safer in that regard.[27]

EFFICACY

Compared to the TAP block, the QL block covers a topographically broader area (T7–L1 vs. T10–T12), and yields longer analgesia (24–48 h vs. 8–12 h). The analgesic efficacy of the QL block has been described in pediatrics. The first continuous QL block reported in the literature was in a child undergoing colostomy closure.[28] Baidya et al. reported successful postoperative analgesia in children undergoing pyeloplasty.[29] The posterior QL block demonstrated a more sustained and effective analgesic effect compared to TAP blocks in pediatric patients undergoing low abdominal surgery.[26]

RISKS

Few adverse effects and complications have been reported. Visoiu described two cases of lumbar hematoma after QL block in children and recommends adjusting the needle path based on the location of lumbar arteries that travel posterior to the QL muscle.[30] Caution should be exercised when performing this block in coagulopathic patients. Lower extremity weakness has been reported with all approaches and is explained by inadvertent LA spread to the lumbar plexus.

ERECTOR SPINAE PLANE (ESP) BLOCK

The recently described ESP block is performed in the fascial plane between the erector spinae muscles and the transverse process.[31] This block is a simpler, safer alternative to thoracic epidural or paravertebral block. The block primarily targets the dorsal and lateral branches of the spinal nerves. Other suggested mechanisms include epidural, paravertebral, intercostal, and extensive lateral and longitudinal spread.[32] Both somatic and visceral analgesia have been reported. The ESP block was superior to the ilioinguinal/ iliohypogastric blocks for inguinal hernia repair, suggesting that a more proximal LA injection with spread into the paravertebral space may have a longer duration of action.[33] Cadaver studies have shown more extensive spread to the paravertebral space with ESP compared to the QL block.[34]

TECHNIQUE

Precise needle targeting is more challenging in children because of their thinner muscle layers, loose connective tissues, and sliding fascial planes. The transverse processes are recognized by their square appearance with a hint of pleura in between each 2 adjacent transverse processes (Figure 39.2).

DOSES

Relatively high volumes of LA are needed to ensure sufficient spread and analgesic effect; therefore LA concentration should be adjusted to not exceed the maximum recommended doses. The typical LA volume for a single-shot block is 0.5 mL/kg, with a maximum of 20 mL. The extent of analgesia after a single injection is usually 3 dermatomes above and below the block site, respectively. At least 0.1 mL/kg of local

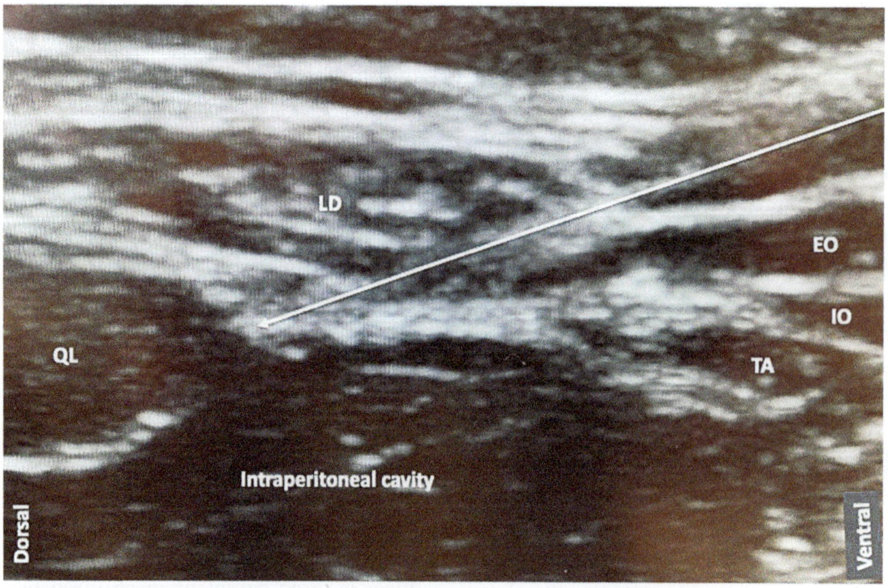

Figure 39.2. Ultrasound image of the erector spinae plane block (ESPB). White arrows indicate the needle.
TM = trapezius muscle; ESM = erector spinae muscle; TP = transversus process; Pl = pleura.

anesthetic is required per dermatome in infants and toddlers.[35] A single-injection ESPB provides effective analgesia for at least 8–12 hours.

EFFICACY

The block's opioid-sparing effectiveness in children has been described for a variety of procedures.[36] After pediatric cardiac surgery, the block significantly reduced pain scores and opioid consumption over the initial 12 hours, and was associated with lower sedation scores and shorter intensive care unit stay compared to patients who did not receive a block.[37] In a series of 22 children, after a median loading dose of 0.4 mL/kg ropivacaine 0.5%, intraoperative bolus of 0.3 mL/kg/h ropivacaine 0.2%, and a postoperative programmed intermittent bolus regimen of maximum 0.6 mg/kg/h, the authors reported excellent postoperative analgesia and a median dose of 0.16 mg/kg/day morphine equivalents. Of note, none of the patients in this study reported a sensory block.[38] These results are similar to those reported with the use of paravertebral catheters in children.[8] ESPB catheters were successfully used in neonates undergoing major abdominal surgery.[39]

RISKS

Motor weakness following lumbar or low thoracic ESPB with a high volume of LA is rare but possible due to spread to the lumbar plexus. Pneumothorax has also been reported, likely related to suboptimal technique.

CONTINUOUS WOUND INFILTRATION

Infiltration of LA around a surgical wound provides analgesia for 4–8 hours. Placement of wound catheters in the intra- or pre-peritoneal plane is simple and avoids the risks of RA. A continuous infusion of ropivacaine 0.2% 0.1–0.2 mL/kg/h up to a maximum of 0.5 mL/h can be infused, typically via epidural infusion pumps. Subcutaneous infected seroma has been reported as a complication of this technique. Children with spina bifida undergoing major reconstruction of the lower urinary tract managed with continuous incisional LA infusions had postoperative opioid requirements 3 times lower compared to systemic analgesia.[40]

OPIOIDS

Intravenous patient-controlled analgesia (PCA) with opioids is the preferred method for the management of moderate and severe acute pain in children older than 5–6 years of age in the absence of, or as an adjunct to, RA. Younger patients typically receive continuous infusions or intermittent boluses of opioids. Surrogate control of PCA by parents or nurses increases the risk of respiratory depression, and is allowed only in special circumstances, such as extensive surgery, and only with clear institutional protocols in place. In patients who received single-shot RA, provisions should be made to allow timely administration of systemic opioids as the block is wearing off.

A basal infusion rate may be used to replace a patient's baseline opioid requirement in patients who are taking opioids regularly. Morphine is the most common opioid administered via PCA. Hydromorphone induces less itching and nausea than morphine. Fentanyl may be associated with a higher incidence of apnea and hypoxemia.

Intravenous non-steroidal anti-inflammatory drugs (NSAIDs) and cyclooxygenase COX-2 inhibitors have opioid-sparing effects. When acetaminophen and an NSAID are combined, the benefit is synergistic. Ibuprofen is administered orally in a dose of 5–10 mg/kg with a maximum dose of 40 mg/kg/day in patients weighing less than 50 kg, and 200–800 mg every 6 hours in patients weighing more than 50 kg. The dose of ketorolac is 0.5 mg/kg every 6 hours intravenously or intramuscularly for up to maximum of 72 hours. Ketorolac is contraindicated in renal insufficiency. ASRA guidelines state that NSAIDs alone add no significant risk for spinal hematoma in patients undergoing neuraxial blocks. There is controversy regarding the risk of anastomotic leakage after colorectal surgery in patients who receive NSAIDs perioperatively. The risk appears to be higher in patients who undergo emergent colonic resection and have other risk factors.

Acetaminophen, especially if administered before surgery, has opioid-sparing effects, and reduces PONV. Plasma and effect site concentrations after intravenous administration of acetaminophen are approximately double the plasma concentration following oral or rectal administration, resulting in greater CNS penetration, which in turn results in better analgesia compared to oral acetaminophen.

Gabapentinoids have been extensively used for the management of acute postoperative pain in adults, but the literature is sparse in children. Gabapentin is associated with modest reductions in pain scores 5% to 15%, and a 35%–60% decrease in opioid consumption.[41] Gabapentinoids are indicated in patients who are receiving high doses of opioids preoperatively, and those at risk for severe and prolonged postoperative pain, especially when there is a neuropathic component. Their main side effect is sedation, which may be beneficial in patients with high anxiety levels.

Ketamine and lidocaine are important pain management adjuvants after major abdominal surgery. They are used in patients who have contraindications to, failed, or refused epidural analgesia, and in difficult-to-treat patients (chronic pain; opioid use, abuse, tolerance, or dependence; acute hyperalgesia; poorly controlled pain in the past; neuropathic pain). Ketamine improves the analgesic effect of co-administered opioids via a synergistic effect and by preventing central sensitization. It prevents and treats opioid hyperalgesia and opioid tolerance. A ketamine bolus of 0.5 mg/kg, followed by a 0.12 mg/kg/h infusion, is effective in major abdominal surgery.[42]

Intravenous lidocaine is used after major abdominal surgery as an analgesic, anti-inflammatory and anti-hyperalgesic.[43] It enhances the gut function recovery by a direct excitatory effect on gut smooth muscle, reduced opioid requirements, blockade of sympathetic reflexes, and decreased inflammation. A 1.5 mg/kg bolus, followed by 1.5 mg/kg/h for 6 hours, administered to children undergoing abdominal surgery has been associated with decreased opioid consumption and reduced hospital stay.[44]

CONCLUSIONS

- Major abdominal surgery in children can be managed with a variety of pain interventions. While thoracic epidural analgesia remains a gold standard, it is labor intensive, requires special expertise, has significant risks, and may be contraindicated in certain patients. It is particularly indicated for patients anticipated to have prolonged and/or severe postoperative pain, patients with chronic pain, or those who experience significant side effects from opioids.
- Ultrasound-guided truncal blocks represent a viable and ever-expanding alternative, especially within the context of multimodal analgesia. The selection of optimal truncal block technique depends on the location and type of abdominal incision, anticipated extent and duration of pain (especially its visceral component), and local expertise.
- Pediatric RA is safe but requires knowledge of particularities of the techniques in children and advanced training, as well as increased vigilance to avoid LAST. The literature on what constitutes maximum allowable doses of LA in children is still evolving, therefore awareness of current pediatric RA literature and guidelines from RA societies is strongly advised.

References

1. Walker BJ, Long JB, Sathyamoorthy M, et al. Complications in pediatric regional anesthesia: an analysis of more than 100,000 blocks from the Pediatric Regional Anesthesia Network. *Anesthesiology.* 2018;129:721–732.
2. Suresh S, Ecoffey C, Bosenberg A, et al. The European Society of Regional Anaesthesia and Pain Therapy/American Society of Regional Anesthesia and Pain Medicine Recommendations on local anesthetics and adjuvants dosage in pediatric regional anesthesia. *Reg Anesth Pain Med.* 2018;43:211–216.
3. Tsui BCH, Boretsky K, Berde C. Maximum recommended dosage of ropivacaine and bupivacaine for pediatric regional anesthesia. *Reg Anesth Pain Med.* 2018;43(8):895–896.
4. Fares KM, Othman AH, Alieldin NH. Efficacy and safety of dexmedetomidine added to caudal bupivacaine in pediatric major abdominal cancer surgery. *Pain Physician.* 2014;17:393–400.
5. Lundblad M, Trifa M, Kaabachi O, et al. Alpha-2 adrenoceptor agonists as adjuncts to peripheral nerve blocks in children: a meta-analysis. *Ped Anesth.* 2016;26:232–238.
6. Meyer MJ, Krane EJ, Goldschneider KR, et al. Case report: neurological complications associated with epidural analgesia in children: a report of 4 cases of ambiguous etiologies. *Anesth Analg.* 2012;115:1365–1370.
7. Boretsky K, Visoiu M, Bigeleisen P. Ultrasound-guided approach to the paravertebral space for catheter insertion in infants and children. *Ped Anesth.* 2013;23:1193–1198.
8. Vecchione T, Zurakowski D, Boretsky KR. Thoracic paravertebral nerve blocks in pediatric patients: safety and clinical experience. *Anesth Analg.* 2016;123:1588–1590.
9. Bardain S, Dodson B, Zurakowski D, Waisel DB, Jennings RS, Boretsky KR. Paravertebral nerve block catheters using chloroprocaine in infants with prolonged mechanical ventilation for treatment of long-gap esophageal atresia. *Ped Anesth.* 2015;25:1151–1157.
10. Tsai HC, Yoshida T, Chung TY, et al. Transversus abdominis plane block: an updated review of anatomy and technique. *Biomed Res Int.* 2017:1–12.
11. Tran DQ, Bravo D, Leurcharusmee P, Neal JM. Transversus abdominis plane block: a narrative review. *Anesthesiol* 2019;131(5):1166–1190.
12. Chin KJ, McDonnell JG, Carvalho B, et al. Essentials of our current understanding: abdominal wall blocks. *Reg Anesth Pain Med.* 2017;42:133–183.
13. Hebbard PD. Transversalis fascia plane block, a novel ultrasound-guided abdominal wall nerve block. *Can J Anaesth.* 2009;56(8):618–620.
14. Hebbard PD, Barrington MJ, Vasey C. Ultrasound-guided continuous oblique subcostal transversus abdominis plane blockade: description of anatomy and clinical technique. *Reg Anesth Pain Med.* 2010;35(5):436–441.
15. Suresh S, Chan VW. Ultrasound guided transversus abdominis plane block in infants, children and adolescents: a simple procedural guidance for their performance. *Ped Anesth.* 2009;19(4):296–299.
16. Visoiu M, Boretsky KR, Goyal G, et al. Postoperative analgesia via transversus abdominis plane (TAP) catheter for small weight children: our initial experience. *Ped Anesth.* 2012;22:281–284.
17. Masters OW, Thies KC. TAP block and low-dose NCA for major upper abdominal surgery. *Ped Anesth.* 2011;21(1):87–88.
18. Suresh S, Taylor LJ, de Oliveira GS. Dose effect of local anesthetics on analgesic outcomes for the transversus abdominis plane (TAP) block in children: a randomized, double-blinded, clinical trial. *Ped Anesth.* 2015;25(5):506–510.
19. Long JB, Birmingham PK, De Oliveira Jr GS, Schaldenbrand KM, Suresh S. Transversus abdominis plane block in children: a multicenter safety analysis of 1994 cases from the PRAN (Paediatric Regional Anesthesia Network) database. *Anesth Analg.* 2014;119(2):395–399.
20. Torup H, Mitchell AU, Breindahl T, Hansen EG, Rosenberg J, Moller AM. Potentially toxic concentrations in blood of total ropivacaine after bilateral transversus ab dominis plane blocks; a pharmacokinetic study. *Eur J Anaesthesiol.* 2012;29:235–238.
21. Visoiu M, Hauber J, Scholz S. Single injection ultrasound-guided rectus sheath blocks for children: distribution of injected anesthetic. *Ped Anesth.* 2019;29:280–285.
22. Flack SH, Martin LD, Walker BJ, et al. Ultrasound-guided rectus sheath block or wound infiltration in children: a randomized blinded study of analgesia and bupivacaine absorption. *Ped Anesth.* 2014;24:968–973.
23. Gurnaney HG, MaxwellL G, Kraemer FW, Goebel T, Nance ML, Ganesh A. Prospective randomized observer-blinded study comparing the analgesic efficacy of ultrasound-guided rectus sheath block and local anesthetic infiltration for umbilical hernia repair. *Br J Anaesth.* 2011;107:790–795.
24. Ueshima H, Otake H, Lin JA. Ultrasound-guided quadratus lumborum block: an updated review of anatomy and techniques. *Biomed Res Int.* 2017;2017:2752876.
25. Elsharkawy H, El-Boghdadly K, Barrington M. Quadratus lumborum block: anatomical concepts, mechanisms, and techniques. *Anesthesiol.* 2019;130(2):322–335.
26. Oksuz G, Bilal B, Gurkan Y, et al. Quadratus lumborum block versus transversus abdominis plane block in children undergoing low abdominal surgery: a randomized controlled trial. *Reg Anesth Pain Med.* 2017;42:674–679.
27. Murouchi T, Iwasaki S, Yamakage M. Quadratus lumborum block: analgesic effects and chronological ropivacaine concentrations after laparoscopic surgery. *Reg Anesth Pain Med.* 2016;41(2):146–150.
28. Visoiu M, Yakovleva N. Continuous postoperative analgesia via quadratus lumborum block: an alternative to transversus abdominis plane block. *Ped Anesth.* 2013;23:959–961.
29. Baidya DK, Maitra S, Arora MK, Agarwal A. Quadratus lumborum block: an elective method of perioperative analgesia in children undergoing pyeloplasty. *J Clin Anesth.* 2015;27:694–696.

30. Visoiu M, Pan S. Quadratus lumborum blocks: two cases of associated hematoma. *Ped Anaesth*. 2019;29:286–288.
31. Forero M, Adhikary SD, Lopez H, Tsui C, Chin KJ. The erector spinae plane block: a novel analgesic technique in thoracic neuropathic pain. *Reg Anesth Pain Med*. 2016;41:621–627.
32. De Cassai A, Bonvicini D, Correale C, Sandei L, Tulgar S, Tonetti T. Erector spinae plane block: a systematic qualitative review. *Minerva Anesthesiol*. 2019;85:308–319.
33. El-Emam E-SM, Abd El Motlb EA. Ultrasound-guided erector spinae versus ilioinguinal/iliohypogastric block for postoperative analgesia in children undergoing inguinal surgeries. *Anesth Essays Res*. 2019;13(2):274–279.
34. Elsharkawy H, Bajracharya GR, El–Boghdadly K, et al. Comparing two posterior quadratus lumborum block approaches with low thoracic erector spinae plane block: an anatomic study. *Reg Anesth Pain Med*. 2019;44:549–555.
35. Holland EL, Bosenberg AT. Early experience with erector spinae plane blocks in children. *Ped Anesth*. 2020;30(2):96–107.
36. Aksu C, Gürkan Y. Defining the indications and levels of erector spinae plane block in pediatric patients: a retrospective study of our current experience. *Cureus*. 2019;11(8): e5348.
37. Kaushal B Chauhan S, Magoon R, et al. Efficacy of bilateral erector spinae plane block in management of acute postoperative surgical pain after pediatric cardiac surgeries through a midline sternotomy. *J Cardiothorac Vasc Anesth*. 2020;34(4):981–986.
38. Munshey F, Caruso TJ, Wang EY, Tsui BCH. Programmed intermittent bolus regimen for erector spinae plane blocks in children: a retrospective review of a single-institution experience. *Anesth Analg*. 2018;130(3):e63–e66.
39. Moore R, Kaplan I, Jiao Y, Oster A. The use of continuous erector spinae plane blockade for analgesia following major abdominal surgery in a one-day old neonate. *J Clin Anesth*. 2018;49:17–18.
40. Chalmers DJ, Bielsky A, Wild TT, Siparsky GL, Wilcox DT. Continuous local anesthetic infusion for children with spina bifida undergoing major reconstruction of the lower urinary tract. *J Ped Urol*. 2015;11(2):72.e1–e5.
41. Dolemnan B, Heinink TP, Read DJ, Faleiro J, Lund JN, Williams JP. A systematic review and a meta-regression analysis of prophylactic gabapentin for postoperative pain. *Anesthesia*. 2015;70:1186–1204.
42. Zakine J, Samarcq D, Lorne E, et al. Postoperative ketamine administration decreases morphine consumption in major abdominal surgery: a prospective, randomized, double-blind, controlled study. *Anesth Analg*. 2008;106:1856–1861.
43. Sun Y, Li T, Wang N, et al. Perioperative systemic lidocaine for postoperative analgesia and recovery after abdominal surgery: a meta-analysis of randomized controlled trials. *Dis Colon Rectum*. 2012;55:1183–1194.
44. El-Deeb A, El-Morsy GZ, Ghanem AAA, Elsharkawy AA, Elmetwally AS. The effects of intravenous lidocaine infusion on hospital stay after major abdominal pediatric surgery: a randomized double-blinded study. *Egyptian J Anaes* 2013;29(3):225–230.

REVIEW QUESTIONS

(1) A 6-year-old is scheduled for repair of inguinal hernia. Which of the following regional anesthetic techniques is the most appropriate for postoperative analgesia?

A. Posterior transversus abdominis block (TAP) block
B. Ultrasound guided ilioinguinal/iliohypogastric nerve block
C. Paravertebral nerve block
D. Caudal block

(2) A 3-year old boy is scheduled to undergo ureteral reimplantation via a low abdominal transverse incision. Which of the following blocks is likely to be most effective for postoperative pain management?

A. Rectus sheath block (RSB)
B. Single-shot caudal block
C. TAP block
D. Quadratus lumborum block (QLB)

(3) When discussing the QLB for postoperative pain management after an open left orchiopexy in a 6-year-old boy, which of the following side effects should be considered?

A. Pneumothorax
B. Bradycardia
C. Leg weakness
D. Urinary incontinence

(4) Which of the following statements regarding the QLB is true?

A. One of the possible complications of posterior QLB is kidney injury.
B. The risk of local anesthetic systemic toxicity is higher with the QLB than with TAP block.
C. A potential mechanism of action of QLB is ipsilateral paravertebral spread.
D. The pattern of local anesthetic spread of the lateral QLB is identical to the transversalis fascia plane block (TFPB).

(5) The advantages of the QLB compared to the ESPB in children include which of the following?

A. May be performed when vertebral abnormalities preclude thoracic epidural analgesia
B. May be associated with more extensive paravertebral spread
C. Can cover all dermatomes, from cervical to sacral
D. May be performed with the patient in the supine position

(6) An 8-month-old 7-kg infant undergoes exploratory laparotomy for recurrent congenital diaphragmatic hernia. In the neonatal intensive care unit (NICU), his pain is managed postoperatively with bupivacaine 0.1% and fentanyl 2 mcg/mL, at a rate of 2 mL/hour administered via a thoracic epidural catheter inserted caudally and threaded to the T8–T9 level. His nurse reports fussiness, tachycardia, and increased blood pressure. What is your next step of action?

A. Do nothing, NICU babies are always fussy.
B. Order a chest radiograph to check the position of epidural catheter tip.
C. Increase epidural rate to 2.5 mL/hour.
D. Administer incremental boluses of chloroprocaine 2% via the epidural catheter.

(7) A possible side effect of an erector spinae plane block (ESPB) placed at the level of T6 transverse process is:

A. Nausea
B. Hypoxia
C. Lower extremity weakness
D. Upper extremity weakness

(8) A 13-year-old boy with severe Crohn's disease exacerbation and pain unresponsive to management with fentanyl patient-controlled analgesia is scheduled for laparoscopic colectomy and ileal pouch creation. He experiences severe nausea in response to opioids. Which of the following is the best perioperative pain management plan?

A. Thoracic epidural analgesia
B. Bilateral QLBs with ropivacaine and dexmedetomidine
C. Intravenous opioids and low-dose ketamine infusion
D. Bilateral TAP blocks

ANSWERS

(1) **B.** Ultrasound guided ilioinguinal/iliohypogastric nerve block is commonly used in children for inguinal hernia, hydrocelectomy, or orchidopexy. Because the anterior branch of the iliohypogastric nerve supplying the inguinal and suprapubic area travels deep to the transversus muscle and penetrates it in the proximity of the anterior superior iliac spine, it is not consistently blocked by a posterior TAP block (option A). The literature is equivocal regarding the comparison between the ilioinguinal/iliohypogastric nerve block and lateral TAP block. Some studies suggest that when performed with ultrasound guidance, ilioinguinal/iliohypogastric nerve block results in superior and longer duration of analgesia, and lower analgesic consumption compared to the lateral TAP block. This is explained by the variable point of entry of these nerves into the TAP, usually close to the anterior superior iliac spine. Answer D is not correct because caudal block has a shorter duration of action compared to ilioinguinal/inliohypogastric nerve blocks. In addition, it may cause reversible lower extremity weakness. Answer C is not correct because, although effective for inguinal hernia, PVB is more technically challenging and more likely to cause complications than ilioinguinal/iliohypogastric nerve blocks. QL, transversalis fascia plane, and erector spinae blocks are also effective for inguinal hernia repair.

Reference

Chin KJ, McDonnell JG, Carvalho B, et al. Essentials of our current understanding: abdominal wall blocks. *Reg Anesth Pain Med.* 2017;42:133–183.

(2) **D.** Postoperative analgesic management in children undergoing this type of surgery should address both somatic pain from a Pfannenstiel incision (T11–L1) and visceral bladder spasm pain. The exact mechanism of postoperative bladder spasm is not completely understood. Autonomic afferent nerves arise from the bladder and travel with sacral parasympathetic fibers to S2–S4 segments and with sympathetic fibers to T11–L2 spinal segments. Regional anesthesia options include epidural catheter, caudal block, or a truncal block including TAP block, QLB, or ESPB. The QLB (option D) is superior to the TAP block (option C) as it provides both somatic and visceral analgesia, and longer, more effective postoperative analgesia. Option B is not correct because although a single-shot caudal block (option B) provides a more complete coverage, it has a shorter duration (4–6 hours) than truncal blocks. In order to prolong the duration of caudal block analgesia, adjuncts such as morphine or clonidine are used; however, nausea, urinary retention, pruritus, are common. A continuous epidural technique would be preferable to a single-shot caudal. Option A is not correct because rectus sheath block does not reliably cover a Pfannenstiel incision. This is due to the fact that caudal to the arcuate line, the only layers posterior to the rectus muscle are the transversalis fascia and peritoneum.

Reference

Oksuz G, Bilal B, Gurkan Y, et al. Quadratus lumborum block versus transversus abdominis plane block in children undergoing low abdominal surgery: a randomized controlled trial. *Reg Anesth Pain Med.* 2017;42:674–679.

(3) **C.** Lower extremity weakness (option C) is a recognized complication of the QLB and may occur with all but the intramuscular approaches. Quadriceps muscle weakness is particularly common with the anterior QLB, and it is explained by the local anesthetic spread to the lumbar plexus. QLB may not be appropriate for day case surgeries due to the concern over residual weakness. Pneumothorax (option A) has been reported as a potential complication of ESP and paravertebral blocks, but does not occur with the QLB. High volumes and concentrations of LA, or the bilateral use of the QLB, could potentially cause sympatholysis, including bradycardia (option B) if local anesthetic reached the cardioaccelerator fibers at T4 level, although this has not been reported in children. Option D is not correct, because urinary incontinence is not a side effect of the QLB. The striated muscles of the external urethral sphincter receive their primary innervation from somatic nerves (S2–S4), which are not affected by a QLB.

Reference

Elsharkawy H, El-Boghdadly K, Barrington M. Quadratus lumborum block: anatomical concepts, mechanisms, and techniques. *Anesthesiol.* 2019;130(2):322–335.

(4) **C.** LA injected anterior to the QL muscle and posterior to the transversalis fascia will spread to the thoracic paravertebral space, along the endothoracic fascia to block the somatic nerves and thoracic sympathetic trunk of the lower thoracic levels (option C). Option B is not correct because the QL block is associated with lower, not higher plasma LA levels compared to the TAP blocks. Although the pattern of spread of the lateral QL block is similar to the transversalis fascia plane block, it is not identical (option D). In the lateral QL block, the injection point is more posterior, at the junction of the QL muscle and the distal end of the transversus abdominis aponeurosis. The LA spreads along the ventral surface of the QL muscle, and sometimes posterior to the muscle. Injury of retro- and intraperitoneal organs is possible with the QL block, but unlikely with the posterior approach, which is more superficial, and thus safer.

Reference

Elsharkawy H, El-Boghdadly K, Barrington M. Quadratus lumborum block: Anatomical concepts, mechanisms, and techniques. *Anesthesiol.* 2019;130(2):322–335.

(5) **D.** As opposed to the ESPB, which can only be placed in the lateral decubitus, sitting, or prone position, in children the QLB can be done in the supine position, with a rolled towel placed under the hip to facilitate visualization (option D). Both QL and ESP blocks can be performed when vertebral abnormalities contraindicate neuraxial analgesia (option A). The ESPB may be associated with more extensive spread to the paravertebral space compared to the QLB. The ESPB can be placed anywhere from cervical to sacral level, thus being effective for a large variety of procedures. The QLB provides coverage from T4 to L2–L3, depending on the level of needle placement, direction of needle, and location of needle tip along the thoracolumbar fascia (option C).

Reference

Elsharkawy H, El-Boghdadly K, Barrington M. Quadratus lumborum block: anatomical concepts, mechanisms, and techniques. *Anesthesiol.* 2019;130(2):322–335.

(6) **D.** Answer A is not correct because, although postoperative fussiness is commonly caused by other discomforts, the infant should be carefully evaluated to rule out surgical pain. The evaluation includes gentle palpation at the incision site, observation of behavioral and physiologic indicators of pain, how fast the patient relaxes after being manipulated, ascertaining the position of the epidural catheter tip with radiography or ultrasound, and testing the catheter with a short acting LA. Chloroprocaine administration (option D) results in rapid and dense numbness, analgesia, and motor block (within 3–5 minutes) along the expected dermatome, and allows for comparison of the patient before and after injection. Chloroprocaine has the advantages of both lower toxicity profile and short duration of action in the event of toxicity. Chest radiography (option B) exposes the infant to radiation, and is not the first line of intervention to evaluate epidural functionality in an infant. Option C is not correct because the infant is already receiving the maximum recommended dose of epidural bupivacaine for his age group, and further increasing the dose could cause systemic toxicity.

Reference

Suresh S, Ecoffey C, Bosenberg A, et al. The European Society of Regional Anaesthesia and Pain Therapy/American Society of Regional Anesthesia and Pain Medicine recommendations on local anesthetics and adjuvants dosage in pediatric regional anesthesia. *Reg Anesth Pain Med.* 2018;43:211–216.

(7) **B.** Pneumothorax resulting in hypoxia (option B) is a rare but possible complication of the ESPB placed at or above T10 and is related to suboptimal technique. Upper or lower extremity weakness is unlikely to be caused by an ESPB placed at a mid-thoracic level (options C and D). Motor weakness following lumbar or low thoracic ESPB with a high volume of LA has been reported and is due to spread to the lumbar plexus. Nausea (option A) has not been reported as a complication of the ESPB.

Reference

Holland EL, Bosenberg AT. Early experience with erector spinae plane blocks in children. *Ped Anesth.* 2020;30(2):96–107.

(8) **B.** Although epidural anesthesia is strongly recommended for open colorectal procedures, its risks are generally considered to outweigh its benefits in laparoscopic procedures. In the laparoscopic setting, alternatives such as TAP block, or QLB, which provides analgesia to the anterior abdominal wall, may be favored over epidural techniques. Compared to the TAP block, the QLB (option B) has the advantage of additional visceral analgesia, lower LA systemic absorption, and longer duration of analgesia. The addition of dexmedetomidine to LA significantly prolongs the duration of the block. A pain management strategy centered on intravenous opioids and low-dose ketamine infusion (option C) can be used if regional anesthesia is contraindicated or refused by the patient.

Reference

Murouchi T, Iwasaki S, Yamakage M. Quadratus lumborum block: analgesic effects and chronological ropivacaine concentrations after laparoscopic surgery. *Reg Anesth Pain Med.* 2016;41(2):146–150.

SECTION 10

COMPLEX ACUTE PAIN PATIENTS

Nabil Elkassabany

40.

ORTHOPEDIC TRAUMA IN A PATIENT WITH COMPLEX REGIONAL PAIN SYNDROME

Reda Tolba and Mohamed Fayed

STEM CASE AND KEY QUESTIONS

A 36-year-old male is sent to you by an orthopedic surgeon with a swollen painful left wrist that is not responsive to analgesics including opioids. Past medical history is unremarkable except for a left wrist fracture that was surgically treated 6 weeks ago. He also smokes a pack of cigarettes daily and marijuana occasionally.

You interview the patient, and he describes a constant burning agonizing pain involving the entire arm. Pain worsens when anything touches his skin. Examination showed soft compartments with a good radial pulse. Capillary refill time is less than 2 seconds, and the neurological exam of 3 major nerves is intact. However, the hand feels colder, edematous, and with a decreased range of motion than his other one.

(1) WHAT IS COMPLEX REGIONAL PAIN SYNDROME (CRPS)?

CRPS is a disorder of a body region, usually of the distal limbs, which is characterized by pain, swelling, limited range of motion, vasomotor instability, skin changes, and patchy bone demineralization.

(2) WHAT ARE THE CLINICAL DIAGNOSTIC CRITERIA FOR CRPS?

Meet all 4 criteria:

1. Pain: ongoing pain disproportionate to any inciting events
2. Symptoms: the patient must report at least 1 symptom in 3 of the following 4 categories (Sensory, Vasomotor, Sudomotor/Edema, and/or Motor/Trophic).
3. Signs: the patient must display at least 1 sign at the time of evaluation in 2 of the following 4 categories (Sensory, Vasomotor, Sudomotor/Edema, and/or Motor/Trophic).
4. No other cause of pain

(3) WHAT ARE ALLODYNIA, HYPERALGESIA, AND HYPERESTHESIA?

Allodynia is pain due to a stimulus which does not normally provoke pain.

Hyperalgesia is an increased response to a stimulus which is normally painful.

Hyperesthesia is an increased sensitivity to stimulation, excluding the special senses.

(4) WHAT ARE THE TYPES OF CRPS?

Types of CRPS:

- Type I (reflex sympathetic dystrophy, RSD): no evidence of peripheral nerve injury. It represents approximately 90% of clinical presentations.
- Type II (causalgia): associated with peripheral nerve injury.
- Author's insight: Type I: 1 issue (pain only); Type II: 2 issues (pain and peripheral nerve injury)

(5) WHAT ARE DIAGNOSTIC TESTS FOR CRPS?

CRPS is diagnosed clinically, it is a clinical diagnosis of exclusion. Several diagnostic studies may aid in the diagnosis of CRPS but are seldom pathognomonic.

(6) YOU MADE A DIAGNOSIS OF POSSIBLE CRPS AS THE CAUSE OF HIS PAIN. HOW WILL YOU TREAT THIS PATIENT?

A multimodal approach, involving multiple disciplinary teams, is the treatment of choice. Early diagnosis, aggressive physical therapy, and pharmacologic control of pain are the main elements. Treatment of CRPS will differ depending on whether the pain is sympathetically maintained pain (SMP) or sympathetically independent pain (SIP). A series of sympathetic blocks has been shown to be effective in treating SMP or CRPS. Many patients have a component of both SMP and SIP.

(7) WHAT IS THE STELLATE GANGLION AND WHAT IS ITS ROLE IN CRPS?

The stellate ganglion is a sympathetic ganglion that is formed by the fusion of the inferior cervical and the first thoracic ganglia. It helps to differentiate between SMP and SIP.

(8) DESCRIBE THE ANATOMY OF THE STELLATE GANGLION.

The stellate ganglion lies between the base of the transverse process of the seventh cervical vertebra and the neck of the first rib. It is bounded anteriorly by the carotid sheath; posteriorly by longus colli muscle, vertebral artery; and medially by the body of the vertebra.

The vertebral, subclavian, inferior thyroid, and the first intercostal arteries are in close proximity to the ganglion, and so is the recurrent laryngeal nerve. The pleura is located 1 to 2 cm inferior to it.

(9) HOW DO YOU PERFORM A STELLATE GANGLION BLOCK?

Techniques to block the stellate ganglion are:

- Landmark (blind) technique
- Ultrasound-guided technique
- Fluoroscopic-guided technique
- CT-guided block

Landmark (blind) technique: At the level of the cricoid cartilage, Chassaignac tubercle is identified and a needle is inserted perpendicularly between the trachea and the carotid pulse until it contacts the bony surface; then local anesthetic is injected.

Ultrasound-guided technique: A high frequency ultrasound transducer is used perpendicular to the tracheal axis at the cricoid cartilage and is moved inferiorly until the superior aspect of the thyroid gland is visualized. With an in-plane approach, the needle is placed beside the trachea with a lateral to medial direction. After negative aspiration, 5 ml of a local anesthetic is injected until the fluid spreads along the paravertebral fascia to the stellate ganglion.

(10) AFTER A STELLATE GANGLION BLOCK, THE PATIENT REPORTS NO SIGNIFICANT CHANGE IN THE DEGREE OF PAIN DESPITE HORNER SYNDROME. IS THE PAIN PSYCHOGENIC IN THIS PATIENT?

Not necessarily; Horner syndrome indicates only the interruption of sympathetic supply to the head and neck, i.e., that sympathetic block might not be effectively covering sympathetic supply of upper limb. In addition, SMP will respond to sympathectomy, whereas SIP will not. Block success can be confirmed by an increase in skin temperature, measured over the palmar aspect of the hand or fingers on the blocked side. The increase should begin within 2–3 minutes.

(11) HOW EFFECTIVE IS THE INTERVENTIONAL TREATMENT OF PAIN IN CRPS?

Sympathectomy produces short-term pain relief, but long-term results are poor and inconsistent. Spinal cord stimulator (SCS) is an effective treatment for CRPS pain, including recurrent pain after surgical or radiofrequency sympatholysis.

(12) NOW THE PATIENT NEEDS A REVISION OF HIS ARM. WHEN SHOULD THE SURGERY BE DONE?

Elective surgery should be performed when features of previous episodes of CRPS have improved and when the patient is stable; surgery should be avoided during exacerbations.

(13) WHAT ARE THE PERIOPERATIVE INTERVENTIONS TO PREVENT RECURRENCE OF CRPS OR FLARE-UPS?

- Maintenance of optimal perfusion
- Avoidance of tourniquet hemostasis
- Intensive rehabilitation
- Sympathetic block before surgery, e.g., stellate blocks
- Regional anesthesia/analgesia techniques
- Intraoperative use of ketamine
- Peripheral nerve stimulation if available

DISCUSSION

Complex regional pain syndrome (CRPS) is a disorder of a body region, usually of the distal limbs, which is characterized by pain, swelling, limited range of motion, vasomotor instability, skin changes, and patchy bone demineralization. It frequently starts following a fracture, soft tissue injury, or surgery. The pain is disproportionate in time or degree to the initial injury.[1]

EPIDEMIOLOGY

Incidence is between 5–26 per 100,000 per year. It occurs more commonly in women, especially in postmenopausal women.[2–6]

It is more common in the upper limbs; involvement of both upper and lower limbs in the same patient is unusual. However, the symptoms of CRPS may spread over time to involve adjacent areas of the affected limb or, occasionally, other ipsilateral or contralateral limbs.[2–4,7–9]

TYPES OF CRPS

CRPS has two types:

Type I (reflex sympathetic dystrophy, RSD): no evidence of peripheral nerve injury; represents approximately 90% of clinical presentations;

Type II (causalgia): associated with peripheral nerve injury.[1,10]

CRPS is also classified based on the temperature of the affected limb:[11]

Warm CRPS: skin temperature is increased at the onset of symptoms suggesting this as an inflammatory type;

Cold CRPS: skin temperature is decreased at the onset of symptoms.

Several inciting events are found to cause it:[2–4]

- Peripheral musculoskeletal: fractures 45%, sprains 18%, elective surgery 12%, e.g., carpal tunnel release, knee arthroplasty, knee arthroscopic. Dislocations, immobilization, fasciitis, tendonitis, arthritis can also cause it.
- Peripheral nerves and dorsal roots: trauma and injury to brachial plexus and other peripheral nerves
- Central nervous system (CNS): stroke, tumors, traumatic injuries to the CNS and spinal cord
- Viscera: can follow myocardial infarction
- Idiopathic: spontaneous <10%.

DIAGNOSTIC OF CRPS

CRPS is diagnosed clinically, and it is a clinical diagnosis of exclusion. Several diagnostic studies may aid in the diagnosis of CRPS but are of low sensitivity and specificity:

- Radiologic testing: Plain radiography often demonstrates patchy osteoporosis. Triple-phase bone scan using technetium Tc 99m may show increased periarticular uptake in the affected extremity.[12,13]
- Autonomic testing: Quantitative sweat test may show excessive sweating, and thermography may demonstrate abnormal heat regulation and disparity in temperature between affected and normal regions; it is not practical as a routine clinical test.[14]

PATHOPHYSIOLOGY

Several mechanisms contribute to the pathophysiology of CRPS. These mechanisms include:

1. Neurogenic inflammation[15]
2. Central sensitization: It is also hypothesized that elevated CNS glutamate levels promote wind-up and CNS sensitization. In addition, there is some evidence of NMDA receptor antagonist efficacy in treating CRPS.[16,17]
3. Sympathetic nervous system: Autonomic manifestations previously described to cause sympathetic over-activity could be due to catecholamine hypersensitivity and may involve the formation of a reflex arc after an inciting event. The pain sensation in response to injury may lead to increased sensitivity of injured axons to epinephrine and other substances released by local sympathetic nerves. The enhanced sensitivity can be blocked by the intravenous administration of sympatholytic agents.[18,19]
4. Brain plasticity: Some studies suggest cortical reorganization in sensory and motor regions of the brain, which could result from persistent activity of primary nociceptive neurons. These alterations are associated with greater pain intensity, hyperalgesia, impaired tactile discrimination, and perception of sensation outside the nerve distribution stimulated.[20–23]
5. Genetic factors some studies suggested that there is association with HLA and genetic component.[4,25]

CLINICAL PICTURE

Generally, symptoms and signs occur within 4–6 weeks of the inciting event. Initial symptoms include: pain, erythema, and swelling of the affected limb. In most cases, the limb is warm initially, though some are cold at presentation or evolve from warm to cold.[13,26]

SENSORY MANIFESTATIONS

- **Pain**: The most prominent and debilitating symptom
  - Character: burning, stinging, or tearing sensation
  - Site: felt deep inside the limb in most cases, though it can be superficial
  - Course: most often continuous and undulating but can be paroxysmal
  - Exacerbated by limb movement, contact, temperature variation, or stress.[4,13,27]
- **Other sensory symptoms**: Some patients may have hyperalgesia, allodynia, or hypesthesia, usually distal in the limb, sometimes in a stocking/glove pattern.[27]

MOTOR/TROPHIC CHANGES

- **Motor impairment**: occurs in approximately 2/3 of patients[4,13,27]
  - Reduction of complex muscle strength in handgrip or during tiptoe-standing
  - Some patients develop central motor manifestations, e.g., tremor, myoclonus, or dystonic postures.

- **Trophic**:
  - Increased hair growth, increased or decreased nail growth
  - Contraction and fibrosis of joints and fascia, and skin atrophy.[13]

AUTONOMIC

- Difference compared to the unaffected limb[10]
  - Vasomotor: temperature and color changes, mostly livedo or hyperemia
  - Sudomotor: edema in 70% of the patients and sweating.

DIAGNOSIS

CRPS is a clinical diagnosis; there is no "gold-standard" test or method for confirming the diagnosis. CRPS should be suspected when symptoms:

- Develop after limb trauma, usually within 4-6 weeks
- Are no longer fully explained by the initial trauma
- Affect the distal limb, go beyond the region of trauma or nerve territory.[13]

DIAGNOSTIC CRITERIA: THE BUDAPEST CONSENSUS CLINICAL DIAGNOSTIC CRITERIA[28]

i. **Pain**: continuing pain, which is disproportionate to any inciting event

ii. **Other symptoms**: the patient must report at least 1 symptom in 3 of the following 4 categories:

1. Sensory: hyperesthesia and/or allodynia
2. Vasomotor: temperature asymmetry, skin color changes and/or skin color asymmetry
3. Sudomotor/edema: edema, sweating changes and/or sweating asymmetry
4. Motor/trophic: decreased range of motion, motor dysfunction (weakness, tremor, dystonia) and/or trophic changes (hair, nail, skin)

iii. **Signs**: the patient must display at least 1 sign at the time of evaluation in 2 of the 4 following categories:

1. Sensory: hyperalgesia (to pinprick) and/or allodynia (to light touch, temperature sensation, deep somatic pressure and/or joint movement)
2. Vasomotor: temperature asymmetry (>1°C), skin color changes and/or asymmetry
3. Sudomotor/edema: edema, sweating changes and/or sweating asymmetry
4. Motor/trophic: decreased range of motion, motor dysfunction (weakness, tremor, dystonia) and/or trophic changes (hair, nail, skin)

iv. **No other cause**: There is no other diagnosis that better explains the signs and symptoms.

DIFFERENTIAL DIAGNOSIS

The following conditions may look like CRPS and need to be differentiated from it:

- Infection
- Compartment syndrome
- Peripheral vascular disease

Table 40.1 **BUDAPEST DIAGNOSTIC CRITERIA FOR CRPS**[28]

NO.	CRITERIA	CATEGORIES			
		SENSORY	VASOMOTOR	SUDOMOTOR/ EDEMA	MOTOR/ TROPHIC
i	Pain: constant pain, disproportionate to any inciting event				
ii	Symptom: ≥1 symptom in 3 out of 4 categories	Hyperesthesia Allodynia	Temperature asymmetry Skin color asymmetry	Edema Sweating changes Sweating asymmetry	Decreased range of motion Motor dysfunction (weakness, tremor, dystonia) Trophic changes (hair, nails)
iii	Sign: ≥1 sign in 2 out of 4 categories	Hyperalgesia (pinprick); Allodynia	Evidence of the above	Evidence of the above	Evidence of the above
iv	No other cause/diagnosis of pain				

- Deep vein thrombosis
- Peripheral neuropathy
- Vascular thoracic outlet syndrome
- Rheumatoid arthritis
- Raynaud phenomenon
- Conversion disorder
- Factitious disorder.

PREVENTION

PRIMARY PREVENTION

Vitamin C

Vitamin C is useful in CRPS in high-risk groups, such as older patients with distal radius fractures with poor baseline nutritional status. It helps to accelerate fracture healing and limit excessive soft tissue injury via antioxidant mechanisms. A 500 mg daily dose is used for 6–8 weeks. Two randomized trials showed that CRPS was less prevalent in those who received vitamin C.[29,30] However, a meta-analysis of 3 trials (n = 890) found a nonsignificant trend toward benefit of vitamin C.[31]

SECONDARY PREVENTION

Elective surgery should be performed when features of previous episodes of CRPS have improved and when the patient is stable; surgery should be avoided during exacerbations.

Perioperative and surgical strategies include:

a. Maintenance of optimal perfusion of the affected limb
b. Avoidance of tourniquet hemostasis
c. Perioperative intravenous infusion of mannitol reduces the recurrence and when it happens it is mild and temporary.[32]

Other measures that have been proposed include:[33–36]

d. Intensive rehabilitation
e. Sympathetic block before surgery
f. The use of continuous regional anesthesia/analgesia techniques
g. Other proposed treatments: pretreatment with calcitonin, intrathecal baclofen, hyperbaric oxygen
h. Post-surgery neuromodulation.

MANAGEMENT OF CRPS

- A multidisciplinary approach is suggested for the management of CRPS.[37] Treatment is more effective when it starts early in the course of the disease, ideally as soon as the diagnosis is established, and before radiographic changes appear.
- Early referral to an interventional pain specialist for appropriate intervention may reduce pain and enable patients with CRPS to tolerate aggressive physical therapy (PT).

Main lines of treatments include:

1. **Rehabilitation program**:
   - Patient education: help participation in physical and occupational therapy (OT)
   - Psychosocial and behavioral management.

   Rehabilitation techniques that have been developed in centers with CRPS expertise include:

   - Graded motor imagery[38]
   - Pain-exposure PT and graded exposure in vivo to reduce pain avoidance behaviors[39]
   - Self-administered tactile and thermal desensitization with the aim of normalizing touch perception.[40]
2. **Pharmacologic treatment**
3. **Interventional procedures**: utilized in an escalating fashion, especially in patients with progressive disease and an unsatisfactory response to the simple measures
   - Interventions such as continuous regional anesthesia using tunneled epidural or peripheral nerve catheter infusions can be helpful.
   - Sympathetic blocks such as stellate ganglion blocks and lumbar sympathetic blocks are useful.
   - Peripheral nerve stimulation, dorsal column spinal cord stimulation, and dorsal root ganglion DRG stimulation are all options.
4. **Alternative approaches**: suitable for patients with progressive CRPS who are unwilling to consider interventional procedures. It includes adding calcitonin and oral glucocorticoids to the initial treatment regimen.

PHARMACOLOGIC TREATMENT

- Nonsteroidal anti-inflammatory drugs (NSAIDs):

  Depending on the stage and severity of CRPS, NSAIDs are generally combined with any of the other medications.
- Anticonvulsants: Gabapentinoids are usually used; however, there is little data regarding efficacy in CRPS.

- Antidepressants, e.g., tricyclic antidepressants (TCA) or serotonin norepinephrine reuptake inhibitors (SSNRI): Often effective in reducing neuropathic pain, e.g., amitriptyline is a TCA used in a 10–25 mg dose at bedtime, which is increased as tolerated. Duloxetine is an SSNRI, its dose is started at 60 mg daily and increased gradually.
- Bisphosphonates: They may be effective for reducing pain in patients with early CRPS who have abnormal uptake on bone scan.[41]
- Topical lidocaine and capsaicin: A treatment trial of 3–5 days may suffice to assess effectiveness and tolerability of these agents. However, limited data suggest efficacy in CRPS. Local burning and skin irritation can occur with capsaicin, but this may become less of a problem with continued use.[42]
- Glucocorticoids: Reserved for use for early CRPS patients who do not respond to NSAIDs. However, the evidence is weak. The findings of one small trial suggests that oral glucocorticoids are more effective than NSAIDs.[43]
- Ketamine infusion: Low-dose ketamine infusions have been used successfully in treating refractory CRPS case. However, the duration of analgesia varies; some studies report potent analgesia of transient duration, while others reported longer analgesia up to 3 months when using longer infusions (4–14 days). A randomized placebo-controlled trial showed that intravenous ketamine (0.35 mg/kg/hr, up to 25 mg/hr over 4 hours for 10 days) resulted in significant reductions in pain.[37,44–47]
- Opioids: The use of opioids for neuropathic pain continues to be controversial. There is not strong evidence for their efficacy in CRPS. They can be used in select cases when other approaches have failed.[48,49]

INTERVENTIONAL PROCEDURES

Interventional procedures are indicated when conservative management is not effective. Sympathetic nerve blocks, or regional anesthesia techniques, are tried first, while more invasive measures such as spinal cord stimulation are offered for those who do not respond to sympathetic nerve blocks. It is recommended to wait for 2 weeks and watch for improvement before moving on to the next type of treatment.

In some tertiary centers, spinal cord stimulation would be considered by 12–16 weeks from the time therapy for CRPS is initiated.[50]

Peripheral nerve stimulation can be used early on, especially in the presence of specific peripheral nerve injury in CRPS type II.

PHARMACOLOGICAL INTERVENTIONS

- Pharmacologic sympathectomy: SMP may respond to the addition of an α-1 adrenoceptor antagonist as Prazosin or phenoxybenzamine.[51]
- Alpha-2 agonist: Clonidine patch (0.1 mg) every 7 days. Side effects are hypotension and bradycardia; these are less likely with the patch.
- Intravenous regional anesthesia (IVRA) Bier block: There is no strong evidence to support the use of IVRA for sympatholytic in CRPS. Several agents are used in IVRA, including guanethidine, reserpine, droperidol, ketanserin, atropine, and lidocaine. Combining local anesthetics with bretylium improved the analgesic duration of IVRA. When prilocaine and guanethidine were compared to placebo, no difference was shown after 4 blocks.[52]

ANATOMIC/REGIONAL LOCAL ANESTHETIC BLOCK

Stellate ganglion block and lumbar sympathetic block are used. Sympatholysis is associated with prolonged pain relief in some patients and helps to differentiate between SMP and SIP. Ultimately, the clinical benefit of sympathetic blocks arises from the analgesia provided that allows for participation in physical therapy to help in functional restoration in the affected limb.[48,53]

Stellate Ganglion Block

Landmark (Blind) Technique

Done at the level of the cricoid cartilage, the Chassaignac tubercle is identified—the C6 transverse process—and a needle is inserted perpendicularly between the trachea and the carotid pulse until it contacts the bony surface. The needle is then withdrawn 1–5 mm, and the local anesthetic is injected. Withdrawing the needle a few millimeters is supposed to bring the needle outside the longus colli muscle, where the stellate ganglion is thought to be situated (Figure 40.1).

The blind technique has been associated with unreliable results, side effects, and complications, including intravascular injection, bleeding, temporary paralysis of the recurrent laryngeal nerve, discitis, and esophageal injury.[54]

Ultrasound-Guided Technique

A high-frequency ultrasound transducer is placed perpendicular to the trachea at the level of cricoid cartilage and is moved inferiorly until the superior aspect of the thyroid gland is visualized. Then it is moved laterally to visualize the anterior aspect of the Chassaignac's tubercle on the C6 transverse process. The following structures are identified: the carotid artery, internal jugular vein, thyroid gland, trachea, longus colli, longus capitis muscle, prevertebral fascia, the root of C6 spinal nerve, and transverse process of C6. Then, using an in-plane approach, the needle is placed beside the trachea with a lateral to medial direction. The tip of the needle is advanced through the prevertebral fascia of the longus colli muscle. After negative aspiration, 5 ml of a local anesthetic is injected until the fluid spreads along the paravertebral fascia to the stellate ganglion (Figure 40.2).

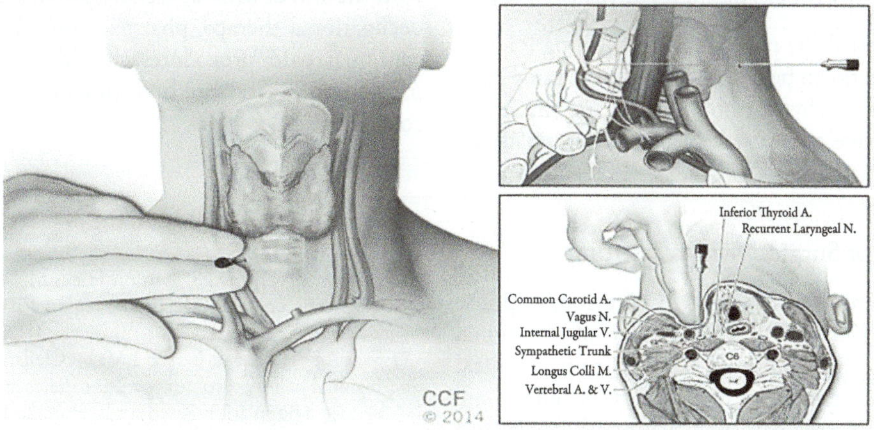

Figure 40.1. Stellate ganglion anatomy and block using the landmark technique.
From: Guirguis M, Abdelmalak J, Jusino E, Hansen MR, Girgis GE. Stellate ganglion block for the treatment of hot flashes in patients with breast cancer: a literature review. *Ochsner J.* 2015;15(2):162–169. License Creative Common Attribution License (CC BY).

Fluoroscopic Technique

The anterior approach is the same as the landmark technique.

The oblique approach involves obtaining a 25–30-degree oblique view on the ipsilateral side of the block to obtain a foraminal view of the lower cervical foramen. The needle is directed to the junction of the vertebral body and the transverse process at either the C6 or C7 level. Then with fluoroscopy, contrast is injected to confirm appropriate needle placement and to rule out intravascular or neuraxial injection.

If the needle is located subfascially, one will see local spread of contrast between the tissue planes cephalad and caudad; on the other hand, intra-arterial injection will result in immediate dissipation of contrast dye.[55]

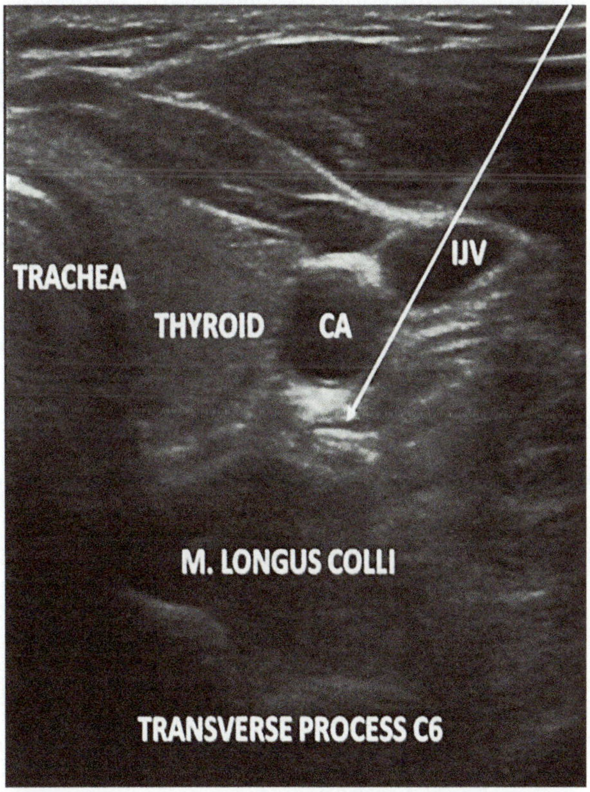

Figure 40.2. Ultrasound image of stellate ganglion with arrow trajectory for in-plane technique for stellate ganglion block.
CA = carotid artery; C6 = sixth cervical vertebra; IJV = internal jugular vein; M = musculus.
Figure courtesy of Dmitri Souzdalnitski, MD, PhD.
Guirguis M, Abdelmalak J, Jusino E, Hansen MR, Girgis GE. Stellate ganglion block for the treatment of hot flashes in patients with breast cancer: a literature review. *Ochsner J.* 2015;15(2):162–169. License Creative Common Attribution License (CC BY).

CT-Guided Technique

The development of ipsilateral Horner syndrome does not guarantee a successful stellate ganglion block to treat upper extremity CRPS. It only indicates only the interruption of sympathetic supply to the head and neck. Unless it is accompanied by objective changes in the arm like temperature changes, it does not indicate sympathetic nerve block of the upper extremity.[56]

Sympathectomy Outcome

Surgical, chemical, or radiofrequency sympathectomy produces short-term pain relief, but long-term results are poor and inconsistent. Delayed failure of sympathectomy may be due to regeneration of ipsilateral nerves or reinnervation from the contralateral sympathetic nerves.[33]

Epidural Infusion

Epidural infusion is used for patients refractory to other approaches. Local anesthetic agents or clonidine may reduce the pain of CRPS, but side effects such as hypotension and sedation can occur depending upon the dose. In one trial, 26 patients with severe chronic CRPS that was unresponsive to sympathetic blocks were randomly assigned to epidural clonidine (300 or 700 microgram bolus injection) or to placebo and were assessed for up to 6 hours. Epidural clonidine provided significantly greater pain relief than placebo injections. Pain relief was similar with both doses of epidural clonidine.[57]

Brachial Plexus Block/Catheter Infusion

These are used to control the pain while performing PT and OT. Perineural catheters can be kept in place in the same position for as long as 3 weeks. Sympatholytic local anesthetic and clonidine infusions have been used. Neurolytic sympathetic block.[58]

Chemical or Surgical Sympathectomy

These are used in patients who have shown a previous response to sympathectomy (i.e., SMP). Low-quality observational evidence suggests the possibility of benefit from chemical or surgical sympathectomy. High rates of adverse effects are reported, including increased pain, new neuropathic pain, and bothersome sweating.[48]

Neurostimulation

Neurostimulation has been used when traditional therapeutic modalities fail, particularly in patients with disease limited to one extremity. Spinal cord stimulation (SCS) plus PT reduced pain and improved health-related quality of life more than PT alone for up to 2 years but did not improve functional outcome measures.[13,59] In a systematic review of the clinical and cost-effectiveness literature, SCS appears to be an efficacious and cost-effective treatment for CRPS type I (level of evidence A) and type II.[60]

A study followed up 27 CRPS patients who had a spinal cord stimulator for a median of 8 years, and found that 30% of SCS devices were explanted, of which 7 were because of inefficient pain relief. Complications leading to revision occurred in 63% patients due to electrode migration or stimulation to the wrong area, 1 case of deep infection, 9 hardware malfunctions, 2 pulse generator discomforts, and 2 SCS replacements were reported. None of the 6 patients using strong opioids discontinued their use during the 2-year follow-up. Despite the fact that CRPS patients were not able to discontinue or reduce their strong opioid or neuropathic pain medication use, 70% continued to use their SCS device during a median 8-year follow-up.[7,59,61]

A retrospective review of 260 chronic pain patients who received an SCS for over 20 years found that 40 of the patients had complex regional pain syndrome type I (CRPS I). The study reported that 5% had no pain relief, 40% had poor pain relief, 47.5% had good pain relief, and 7.5% had excellent pain relief.[56]

Dorsal column stimulation dorsal root ganglion (DRG) and peripheral nerve stimulation have been adopted and approved for management of chronic refractory CRPS. Dorsal column stimulation has shown promising results.[62]

CONCLUSION

Complex regional pain syndrome (CRPS) is a disorder characterized by pain as well as a myriad of sensory, autonomic, and motor disturbances. Management should be multidisciplinary with the aim of early aggressive physical therapy. Physical and occupational therapy, pharmacological treatment, and interventional pain procedures should be considered for rapid pain control to restore limb function and prevent long-term complications.

REFERENCES

1. Harden RN, Bruehl S, Stanton-Hicks M, Wilson PR. Proposed new diagnostic criteria for complex regional pain syndrome. *Pain Med.* 2007;8(4):326–331.
2. Sandroni P, Benrud-Larson LM, McClelland RL, Low PA. Complex regional pain syndrome type I: incidence and prevalence in Olmsted county, a population-based study. *Pain.* 2003;103(1–2):199–207.
3. de Mos M, de Bruijn AG, Huygen FJ, Dieleman JP, Stricker BH, Sturkenboom MC. The incidence of complex regional pain syndrome: a population-based study. *Pain.* 2007;129(1–2):12–20.
4. Ott S, Maihofner C. Signs and symptoms in 1,043 patients with complex regional pain syndrome. *J Pain.* 2018;19(6):599–611.
5. Allen G, Galer BS, Schwartz L. Epidemiology of complex regional pain syndrome: a retrospective chart review of 134 patients. *Pain.* 1999;80(3):539–544.
6. Schwartzman RJ, Erwin KL, Alexander GM. The natural history of complex regional pain syndrome. *Clin J Pain.* 2009;25(4):273–280.
7. Kemler MA, Barendse GA, van Kleef M, et al. Spinal cord stimulation in patients with chronic reflex sympathetic dystrophy. *N Engl J Med.* 2000;343(9):618–624.
8. Maleki J, LeBel AA, Bennett GJ, Schwartzman RJ. Patterns of spread in complex regional pain syndrome, type I (reflex sympathetic dystrophy). *Pain.* 2000;88(3):259–266.
9. Barrera P, van Riel PL, de Jong AJ, Boerbooms AM, Van de Putte LB. Recurrent and migratory reflex sympathetic dystrophy syndrome. *Clin Rheumatol.* 1992;11(3):416–421.
10. Stanton-Hicks M, Janig W, Hassenbusch S, Haddox JD, Boas R, Wilson P. Reflex sympathetic dystrophy: changing concepts and taxonomy. *Pain.* 1995;63(1):127–133.
11. Eberle T, Doganci B, Kramer HH, et al. Warm and cold complex regional pain syndromes: differences beyond skin temperature? *Neurology.* 2009;72(6):505–512.
12. Wuppenhorst N, Maier C, Frettloh J, Pennekamp W, Nicolas V. Sensitivity and specificity of 3-phase bone scintigraphy in the diagnosis of complex regional pain syndrome of the upper extremity. *Clin J Pain.* 2010;26(3):182–189.
13. Birklein F, O'Neill D, Schlereth T. Complex regional pain syndrome: an optimistic perspective. *Neurology.* 2015;84(1):89–96.
14. Cohen SP, Raja SN. Does prolonged skin temperature measurement improve the diagnosis of complex regional pain syndrome? *Nat Clin Pract Neurol.* 2009;5(1):14–15.
15. Parkitny L, McAuley JH, Di Pietro F, et al. Inflammation in complex regional pain syndrome: a systematic review and meta-analysis. *Neurology.* 2013;80(1):106–117.
16. Correll GE, Maleki J, Gracely EJ, Muir JJ, Harbut RE. Subanesthetic ketamine infusion therapy: a retrospective analysis of a novel therapeutic approach to complex regional pain syndrome. *Pain Med.* 2004;5(3):263–275.
17. Kiefer RT, Rohr P, Ploppa A, et al. A pilot open-label study of the efficacy of subanesthetic isomeric S(+)-ketamine in refractory CRPS patients. *Pain Med.* 2008;9(1):44–54.
18. Wasner G, Schattschneider J, Heckmann K, Maier C, Baron R. Vascular abnormalities in reflex sympathetic dystrophy (CRPS I): mechanisms and diagnostic value. *Brain.* 2001;124(Pt 3):587–599.
19. Bruehl S. An update on the pathophysiology of complex regional pain syndrome. *Anesthesiology.* 2010;113(3):713–725.
20. Maihofner C, Handwerker HO, Neundorfer B, Birklein F. Cortical reorganization during recovery from complex regional pain syndrome. *Neurology.* 2004;63(4):693–701.

21. Pleger B, Tegenthoff M, Ragert P, et al. Sensorimotor retuning [corrected] in complex regional pain syndrome parallels pain reduction. *Ann Neurol.* 2005;57(3):425–429.
22. Freund W, Wunderlich AP, Stuber G, et al. Different activation of opercular and posterior cingulate cortex (PCC) in patients with complex regional pain syndrome (CRPS I) compared with healthy controls during perception of electrically induced pain: a functional MRI study. *Clin J Pain.* 2010;26(4):339–347.
23. Bussa M, Guttilla D, Lucia M, Mascaro A, Rinaldi S. Complex regional pain syndrome type I: a comprehensive review. *Acta Anaesthesiol Scand.* 2015;59(6):685–697.
24. Kemler MA, van de Vusse AC, van den Berg-Loonen EM, Barendse GA, van Kleef M, Weber WE. HLA-DQ1 associated with reflex sympathetic dystrophy. *Neurology.* 1999;53(6):1350–1351.
25. van de Beek WJ, Roep BO, van der Slik AR, Giphart MJ, van Hilten BJ. Susceptibility loci for complex regional pain syndrome. *Pain.* 2003;103(1-2):93–97.
26. Marinus J, Moseley GL, Birklein F, et al. Clinical features and pathophysiology of complex regional pain syndrome. *Lancet Neurol.* 2011;10(7):637–648.
27. Birklein F, Riedl B, Sieweke N, Weber M, Neundorfer B. Neurological findings in complex regional pain syndromes: analysis of 145 cases. *Acta Neurol Scand.* 2000;101(4):262–269.
28. Harden NR, Bruehl S, Perez R, et al. Validation of proposed diagnostic criteria (the "Budapest Criteria") for complex regional pain syndrome. *Pain.* 2010;150(2):268–274.
29. Zollinger PE, Tuinebreijer WE, Breederveld RS, Kreis RW. Can vitamin C prevent complex regional pain syndrome in patients with wrist fractures? A randomized, controlled, multicenter dose-response study. *J Bone Joint Surg Am.* 2007;89(7):1424–1431.
30. Zollinger PE, Tuinebreijer WE, Kreis RW, Breederveld RS. Effect of vitamin C on frequency of reflex sympathetic dystrophy in wrist fractures: a randomised trial. *Lancet.* 1999;354(9195):2025–2028.
31. Evaniew N, McCarthy C, Kleinlugtenbelt YV, Ghert M, Bhandari M. Vitamin C to prevent complex regional pain syndrome in patients with distal radius fractures: a meta-analysis of randomized controlled trials. *J Orthop Trauma.* 2015;29(8):e235–241.
32. Veldman PH, Goris RJ. Surgery on extremities with reflex sympathetic dystrophy. *Unfallchirurg.* 1995;98(1):45–48.
33. Furlan AD, Mailis A, Papagapiou M. Are we paying a high price for surgical sympathectomy? A systematic literature review of late complications. *J Pain.* 2000;1(4):245–257.
34. van Hilten BJ, van de Beek WJ, Hoff JI, Voormolen JH, Delhaas EM. Intrathecal baclofen for the treatment of dystonia in patients with reflex sympathetic dystrophy. *N Engl J Med.* 2000;343(9):625–630.
35. Kiralp MZ, Yildiz S, Vural D, Keskin I, Ay H, Dursun H. Effectiveness of hyperbaric oxygen therapy in the treatment of complex regional pain syndrome. *J Int Med Res.* 2004;32(3):258–262.
36. de Mos M, Huygen FJ, van der Hoeven-Borgman M, Dieleman JP, Ch Stricker BH, Sturkenboom MC. Outcome of the complex regional pain syndrome. *Clin J Pain.* 2009;25(7):590–597.
37. O'Connell NE, Wand BM, McAuley J, Marston L, Moseley GL. Interventions for treating pain and disability in adults with complex regional pain syndrome. *Cochrane Database Syst Rev.* 2013;4:CD009416.
38. Borchers AT, Gershwin ME. Complex regional pain syndrome: a comprehensive and critical review. *Autoimmun Rev.* 2014;13(3):242–265.
39. McCabe CS, Blake DR. An embarrassment of pain perceptions? Towards an understanding of and explanation for the clinical presentation of CRPS type 1. *Rheumatology (Oxford).* 2008;47(11):1612–1616.
40. Moseley LG, Zalucki NM, Wiech K. Tactile discrimination, but not tactile stimulation alone, reduces chronic limb pain. *Pain.* 2008;137(3):600–608.
41. Yanow J, Pappagallo M, Pillai L. Complex regional pain syndrome (CRPS/RSD) and neuropathic pain: role of intravenous bisphosphonates as analgesics. *Scientific World J.* 2008;8:229–236.
42. Hanlan AK, Mah-Jones D, Mills PB. Early adjunct treatment with topical lidocaine results in improved pain and function in a patient with complex regional pain syndrome. *Pain Physician.* 2014;17(5):E629–635.
43. Kalita J, Vajpayee A, Misra UK. Comparison of prednisolone with piroxicam in complex regional pain syndrome following stroke: a randomized controlled trial. *QJM.* 2006;99(2):89–95.
44. Duong S, Bravo D, Todd KJ, Finlayson RJ, Tran Q. Treatment of complex regional pain syndrome: an updated systematic review and narrative synthesis. *Can J Anaesth.* 2018;65(6):658–684.
45. Connolly SB, Prager JP, Harden RN. A systematic review of ketamine for complex regional pain syndrome. *Pain Med.* 2015;16(5):943–969.
46. Cohen SP, Bhatia A, Buvanendran A, et al. Consensus guidelines on the use of intravenous ketamine infusions for chronic pain from the American Society of Regional Anesthesia and Pain Medicine, the American Academy of Pain Medicine, and the American Society of Anesthesiologists. *Reg Anesth Pain Med.* 2018;43(5):521–546.
47. Xu J, Herndon C, Anderson S, et al. Intravenous ketamine infusion for complex regional pain syndrome: survey, consensus, and a reference protocol. *Pain Med.* 2019;20(2):323–334.
48. Perez RS, Zollinger PE, Dijkstra PU, et al. Evidence based guidelines for complex regional pain syndrome type 1. *BMC Neurol.* 2010;10:20.
49. Harke H, Gretenkort P, Ladleif HU, Rahman S, Harke O. The response of neuropathic pain and pain in complex regional pain syndrome I to carbamazepine and sustained-release morphine in patients pretreated with spinal cord stimulation: a double-blinded randomized study. *Anesth Analg.* 2001;92(2):488–495.
50. Stanton-Hicks M. Complex regional pain syndrome: manifestations and the role of neurostimulation in its management. *J Pain Symptom Manage.* 2006;31(4 Suppl):S20–24.
51. Raja SN, Treede RD. Testing the link between sympathetic efferent and sensory afferent fibers in neuropathic pain. *Anesthesiology.* 2012;117(1):173–177.
52. Tran DQ, Duong S, Bertini P, Finlayson RJ. Treatment of complex regional pain syndrome: a review of the evidence. *Can J Anaesth.* 2010;57(2):149–166.
53. O'Connell NE, Wand BM, Gibson W, Carr DB, Birklein F, Stanton TR. Local anaesthetic sympathetic blockade for complex regional pain syndrome. *Cochrane Database Syst Rev.* 2016;7:CD004598.
54. Gofeld M, Shankar H, Benzon B. Fluoroscopy and ultrasound-guided sympathetic blocks: stellate ganglion, lumbar sympathetic blocks, and visceral sympathetic blocks. In: Benzon HT, Raja S, Liu SS, Fishman S, Cohen SP, eds. *Essentials of Pain Medicine.* 4th ed. Philadelphia: Elseiver; 2018:789–804; e782.
55. Jadon A. Revalidation of a modified and safe approach of stellate ganglion block. *Indian J Anaesth.* 2011;55(1):52–56.
56. Reig E, Abejon D. Spinal cord stimulation: a 20-year retrospective analysis in 260 patients. *Neuromodulation.* 2009;12(3):232–239.
57. Rauck RL, Eisenach JC, Jackson K, Young LD, Southern J. Epidural clonidine treatment for refractory reflex sympathetic dystrophy. *Anesthesiology.* 1993;79(6):1163–1169; discussion 1127A.
58. Harden RN, Oaklander AL, Burton AW, et al. Complex regional pain syndrome: practical diagnostic and treatment guidelines, 4th edition. *Pain Med.* 2013;14(2):180–229.
59. Kemler MA, De Vet HC, Barendse GA, Van Den Wildenberg FA, Van Kleef M. The effect of spinal cord stimulation in patients with chronic reflex sympathetic dystrophy: two years' follow-up of the randomized controlled trial. *Ann Neurol.* 2004;55(1):13–18.
60. Taylor RS, Van Buyten JP, Buchser E. Spinal cord stimulation for complex regional pain syndrome: a systematic review of the clinical and cost-effectiveness literature and assessment of prognostic factors. *Eur J Pain.* 2006;10(2):91–101.
61. Hoikkanen T, Nissen M, Ikaheimo TM, Jyrkkanen HK, Huttunen J, von Und Zu Fraunberg M. Long-term outcome of spinal cord stimulation in complex regional pain syndrome. *Neurosurgery.* 2021;89(4):597–609.

62. Deer TR, Levy RM, Kramer J, et al. Dorsal root ganglion stimulation yielded higher treatment success rate for complex regional pain syndrome and causalgia at 3 and 12 months: a randomized comparative trial. *Pain.* 2017;158(4):669–681.

REVIEW QUESTIONS

(1) What is the basis of the diagnosis of CRPS?

A. X-ray of the affected extremity
B. Bone scan of the affected extremity
C. Diagnosis is made clinically based on Budapest Criteria.
D. Cold Stress Test

(2) How can you differentiate between CRPS type I and CRPS type II?

A. Presence of allodynia for CRPS type I but not for type II
B. Presence of x-ray changes over affected bone in CRPS type I but not for type II
C. Presence of specific peripheral nerve injury in CRPS type I but not in type II
D. Presence of specific peripheral nerve injury in CRPS type II but not in type I

(3) Stellate ganglion block was performed on the right side for right upper extremity CRPS. How can you confirm that the block was successful?

A. Skin temperature, measured over the palmar aspect of the hand or fingers on the blocked side, should begin to rise within 2–3 minutes.
B. Ptosis of the right eye lid
C. Miosis of the right pupil
D. Conjunctival injection

(4) A 45-year-old female sustained a right radius fracture following a fall. Conservative treatment was elected. Four weeks later, she develops severe pain along the ulnar aspect of the dorsum of the right thumb, the dorsum of the index and middle fingers, and the radial aspect of the fourth finger. The distal arm and mentioned fingers are cold to touch. Exam reveals allodynia and hyperalgesia over the affected fingers. The distal forearm and right thumb, index and middle fingers appear swollen and excessive sweating is noted. There is decrease range of motion of the affected fingers, but pulses are intact. Diagnosis of CRPS is made. What is your specific diagnosis?

A. CRPS type I of the right upper extremity
B. CRPS type II affecting the right superficial radial nerve
C. CRPS type I affecting of the right median nerve
D. CRPS type II affecting the right ulnar nerve

(5) A 55-year-old male developed severe right foot pain after sustaining a severe ankle sprain. He developed CRPS of the right foot that was resistant to medical management and other modalities. Dorsal root ganglion (DRG) stimulation has been approved for treatment of refractory CRPS. What is a contraindication for DRG placement?

A. Severe foraminal stenosis at the target level
B. Presence of allodynia and hyperalgesia on examination
C. Lack of response to lumbar sympathetic block
D, Lack of response to physical therapy

(6) A 24-year-old male is undergoing right lumbar sympathetic block for treatment of CRPS type I of the right foot. He described good relief after the block and was able to participate in physical therapy. However, he has developed persistent right groin and testis burning pain since the block. What is the likely diagnosis?

A. Incarcerated inguinal hernia
B. Hydrocele of the testis
C. Ilioinguinal neuralgia
D. Genitofemoral neuralgia

(7) A 50-year-old male with history of diabetes, peripheral vascular disease, L3–L5 laminectomy and fusion, and spinal stenosis presents with refractory CRPS of the lower extremity. He failed conservative management. Dorsal column stimulation was offered by the treating pain physician. What is a relative contraindication for dorsal column stimulation for this patient?

A. Moderate L2 central spinal stenosis
B. Moderate T10 central spinal stenosis
C. Severe foraminal stenosis at L3 level.
D. Fusion from L3–L5

(8) A 45-year-old female with CRPS type I of the upper extremity following wrist fracture is scheduled for right hand surgery. A supraclavicular brachial plexus block and catheter bupivacaine 0.5% infusion were performed. Shortly afterward, the patient started to complain of tinnitus, tongue and perioral numbness, paraesthesia, and restlessness, followed by suspected tonic clonic seizures. In addition to ACLS measures, epinephrine benzodiazepines, and oxygen, what else could be considered for management of this patient?

A. Propofol
B. Lipid emulsion
C. Ketamine
D. Amiodarone

ANSWERS

(1) **C.** CRPS is diagnosed clinically and is a diagnosis of exclusion. Tests such as x-ray, bone scan, and cold stress test can aid in the diagnosis of CRPS but have low sensitivity and specificity. The Budapest Consensus Clinical Diagnostic Criteria:

Meet all 4 criteria:

i. Pain: ongoing pain disproportionate to any inciting events

ii. Symptoms: the patient must report at least 1 symptom in 3 of the following 4 categories (Sensory, Vasomotor, Sudomotor/Edema, and/or Motor/Trophic).
iii. Signs: the patient must display at least 1 sign at the time of evaluation in 2 of the following 4 categories (Sensory, Vasomotor, Sudomotor/Edema and/or Motor/Trophic).
iv. No other cause of pain.

Reference

Harden NR, Bruehl S, Perez R, Birklein F, Marinus J, Maihofner C, et al. Validation of proposed diagnostic criteria (the "Budapest Criteria") for complex regional pain syndrome. *Pain*. 2010;150(2):268–274.

(2) **C.** CRPS type II (causalgia) is characterized by the presence of specific peripheral nerve injury, while CRPS type I does not present with a specific peripheral nerve injury.

Reference

Harden RN, Bruehl S, Stanton-Hicks M, Wilson PR. Proposed new diagnostic criteria for complex regional pain syndrome. *Pain Med.* 2007;8(4):326–331.

(3) **A.** Despite the development of ipsilateral Horner syndrome (answers B, C, and D), this does not confirm a successful stellate ganglion block to treat upper extremity CRPS. Horner syndrome indicates only the interruption of sympathetic supply to the head and neck. Unless it is accompanied by objective changes in the arm, it does not indicate sympathetic nerve block of the upper extremity.

Reference

Ackerman WE 3rd, Ahmad M. The relative increase in skin temperature after stellate ganglion block is predictive of a complete sympathectomy of the hand. *Reg Anesth Pain Med.* 1999 May-Jun;24(3):275–276. doi: 10.1016/s1098-7339(99)90148-7. PMID: 10338185.

(4) **B.** The clinical picture consists of CRPS type II or causalgia since it is affecting a specific peripheral nerve. The case describes the pain along the superficial radial nerve distribution, which can happen due to nerve injury following radius fracture.

Reference

Harden RN, Bruehl S, Stanton-Hicks M, Wilson PR. Proposed new diagnostic criteria for complex regional pain syndrome. *Pain Med.* 2007;8(4):326–331.

(5) **A.** DRG stimulation has been approved by the FDA for treatment of refractory CRPS. When patients fail conservative management such as physical therapy, medication management, and other interventional therapies, DRG can be a valid option. Severe narrowing of the neural foramen at the target level is a contraindication to proceed.

Reference

Deer TR, Levy RM, Kramer J, Poree L, Amirdelfan K, Grigsby E, et al. Dorsal root ganglion stimulation yielded higher treatment success rate for complex regional pain syndrome and causalgia at 3 and 12 months: a randomized comparative trial. *Pain*. 2017;158(4):669–681.

(6) **D.** Genitofemoral neuralgia is a possible side effect following lumbar sympathetic block. It is characterized by burning pain in the inguinal region radiating to the testis.

Reference

Feigl GC, Dreu M, Ulz H, Breschan C, Maier C, Likar R. Susceptibility of the genitofemoral and lateral femoral cutaneous nerves to complications from lumbar sympathetic blocks: is there a morphological reason? *Br J Anaesth*. 2014;112(6):1098–1104.

(7) **B.** Dorsal column stimulation can be a valid treatment options for patients with refractory CRPS of the lower extremity. Typically, the leads are placed around T8–T9 level to target back pain and leg pain, and possibly lower around T10–T11 levels to target foot pain. In the presence of moderate to advanced T10 central stenosis, putting a space occupying lead in the epidural space can trigger cord compression at this level. It is advised to obtain a thoracic MRI prior to lead placement.

Reference

Kreis PG, Fischman SA. *Spinal Cord Stimulation: Percutaneous Implantation Techniques*. New York: Oxford University Press; 2009.

(8) **B.** Local anesthetic systemic toxicity (LAST) due to inadvertent intravascular injection of bupivacaine should be recognized immediately and ACLS measures should be started. Lipid emulsion (20% intralipid) should be administered while continuing CPR to circulate the drug.

Reference

Neal JM. The American Society of Regional Anesthesia and Pain Medicine checklist for managing local anesthetic systemic toxicity: 2017 version. *RAPM Journal*. 2018;43:150–153.

41.

SURGERY IN THE PRESENCE OF ACTIVE ADDICTION OR MEDICATION ASSISTED ADDICTION TREATMENT

Neil Batta, Nabil Elkassabany, and Ignacio Badiola

STEM CASE AND KEY QUESTIONS

A 61-year-old male, with a history of active heroin and prescription opioid abuse, was involved in a motor vehicle accident and presents with multiple trauma, including clavicular, femoral, tibial, and ulnar fractures. The patient undergoes multiple orthopedic procedures with severe uncontrolled postoperative pain. He is ultimately discharged and the patient is started on Buprenorphine for medication assisted treatment (MAT) of his substance abuse and is titrated to 8 mg once a day. He is now scheduled for elective surgery to repair a malunion of his left ulna in 2 weeks.

(1) WHAT IS OPIOID ADDICTION/OPIOID USE DISORDER?

It is estimated that 5–8 million Americans take daily opioids to treat chronic pain.[1] In 2015 an estimated 20.5 million Americans older than 12 years of age had a substance use disorder, including 2 million to prescription analgesics and heroin.[2]

The terms *opioid dependence* and *addiction* were replaced by Opioid Use Disorder (OUD) in the *Diagnostic and Statistical Manual of Mental Disorders*, fifth edition (DSM-5). OUD is a problematic pattern of opioid use that leads to impairment and distress and reflects a compulsive self-administration of opioids that are not used for legitimate medical reasons. There are various criteria (total of 11) used in diagnosing OUD, such as use of opioid substances in larger amounts or a longer time frame than originally intended, craving opioid substances, and recurrent opioid use resulting in a failure to fulfill major role obligations in school, work, or at home. The diagnosis should also specify if the patient is in early or sustained remission, on maintenance therapy, and whether the individual is in an environment where there is restriction to opioid access. Severity is also considered (mild, moderate, severe) based on the number of criteria met.

(2) WHAT IS OPIOID TOLERANCE?

Opioid tolerance is defined as the need for increased opioid doses to achieve the same level of analgesia.[3] It implies that a patient is less susceptible to the opioid analgesic effect due to prior exposure. The US Food and Drug Administration (FDA) has defined a patient as being opioid tolerant if they take more than 60 mg oral morphine, 30 mg of oxycodone, or 8 mg of oral hydromorphone a day.[4] However, physiologically, exact doses vary per patient. Opioid tolerance can develop in a very short time frame, even within hours of exposure to high doses of opioids.[3] The mechanism of tolerance is very complex and includes changes in metabolizing enzyme expression, transporter function, and alterations in signaling pathways.[5] Pain management in patients who have developed opioid tolerance may be very difficult. These patients benefit from optimizing a multimodal approach to pain management, using medications and techniques that rely less on opioid therapy as the key component to pain management.

(3) WHAT ARE OTHER OPTIONS TO MANAGE PAIN IN PATIENTS WITH A HISTORY OF OPIOID USE OR AN OPIOID USE DISORDER?

A multimodal approach to perioperative pain management is ideal for patients who have developed tolerance to opioids. It relies on targeting various pathways in pain transmission, not just on the opioidergic pathway. There are 5 generally recognized types of pain: nociceptive pain, neuropathic pain, mixed pain (nociceptive and neuropathic), psychogenic pain, and idiopathic pain.[6] Various adjuncts have been shown to be of benefit in patients with these various causes of acute and perioperative pain, including gabapentanoids, nonsteroidal anti-inflammatory drugs (NSAIDs), acetaminophen, N-methyl-D-aspartate (NMDA) antagonists, and intravenous lidocaine. Depending on the cause of pain, muscle relaxants may also be used. Regional anesthetic techniques and neuraxial analgesia can also produce significant analgesia in opioid tolerant patients.

(4) HOW DO OPIOID REQUIREMENTS IN PATIENTS WITH ACUTE PAIN DIFFER IN PATIENTS WITH OPIOID TOLERANCE COMPARED TO THOSE WITHOUT?

Opioid tolerance can occur in individuals prescribed opioids for long-term management of chronic pain, or in cases of addiction/abuse. Effective pain management can be challenging when compared to those who are opioid naïve. Various pharmacological approaches for acute pain management in opioid-tolerant patients include continuation of an equivalent opioid medication or short-term use of a higher than average opioid dose. Additionally, analgesic drugs may be required for longer periods of time with more frequent prescription changes.[7] The primary goals of acute pain management in this setting are to promote adequate analgesia and prevent withdrawal. It is always appropriate to continue to assess and monitor so that analgesia can be individualized while differentiating new acute pain from the usual discomfort. Awareness of opioid-related side effects is recommended. Even though tolerance to side effects such as sedation, nausea, and respiratory depression can occur if opioid doses are significantly increased above baseline, respiratory status should be closely monitored.[8]

(5) WHEN SHOULD AN ADDICTIONOLOGIST BE CONSULTED IN PATIENTS WITH A HISTORY OF OPIOID USE DISORDER WHO ARE ADMITTED WITH ACUTE PAIN?

Inpatient care of patients with opioid use disorder (OUD) admitted with acute pain poses unique challenges from a medical, social, and psychological standpoint.[8] An acute hospital admission provides an opportunity to discuss addiction treatment. Seeking consultation from an addictionologist or addiction consult service is recommended to provide a framework to improve care for this patient population.[9] Initial consultation can help assure patients that their acute pain will be addressed, opioid agonist therapy can be continued or substituted, medication schedules can be reviewed, and provider and patient expectations can be outlined. Engaging patients about their opioid use can help to determine optimal strategies for transition to long-term outpatient treatment programs, non-opioid strategies for managing pain, and to help prevent discharges against medical advice. An addictionologist can further discuss harm-reduction strategies and prescribe new medications or short-term analgesics with close follow-up.[9]

(6) WHAT IS BUPRENORPHINE AND HOW IS IT USED IN PATIENTS WITH A HISTORY OF AN OPIOID USE DISORDER?

Buprenorphine is used as medication assisted treatment (MAT) for opioid use disorder as well as the treatment of pain disorders. There are currently three medications available for use in the treatment of OUD in MAT. They include methadone, naltrexone, and buprenorphine. Methadone and buprenorphine are the most commonly used. Buprenorphine is a semisynthetic opioid that acts as a partial agonist with high affinity for the mu receptor subtype while also acting as an antagonist at the kappa opioid receptor.[10] It is the activation of the kappa receptor that is thought to suppresses and decrease the cravings for opioids.[11,12] It is available in multiple formulations for the treatment of pain and is available in sublingual, injectable, and implantable formulations for the treatment of opioid use disorder. Some of these formulations also include naloxone (i.e., Suboxone) to help mitigate aberrant intravenous use of buprenorphine.

(7) SHOULD THIS PATIENT HAVE HIS BUPRENORPHINE HELD BEFORE THIS ELECTIVE PROCEDURE?

"To stop or not, that is the question."[13] There are three options available in managing buprenorphine in a patient presenting for elective surgery. The first is discontinuation in advance of the procedure long enough so that it is completely eliminated. The second option is to stop it and proceed with the planned procedure before it has been completely eliminated. The third option is to not discontinue it and proceed with surgery with the patient on buprenorphine. Each option has its own set of challenges. Stopping buprenorphine with enough time for elimination results in questions about substituting it with another opioid (i.e., methadone), while discontinuation without providing enough time may lead to unpredictable perioperative pain management. Continuation throughout the perioperative period may lead to higher opioid needs. Due to lack of adequate studies, it is still unknown which option leads to the best outcomes. However, current evidence is shifting toward the continuation of buprenorphine perioperatively. This is especially true if buprenorphine is maintained at lower doses (i.e., 8 mg). Due to the ubiquitous use of buprenorphine, most hospital systems have developed institutional pathways to help guide perioperative management of these patients; however, until high-quality evidence becomes available, these recommendations are based on low-quality evidence.

(8) WHAT IS A COMPREHENSIVE PERIOPERATIVE PAIN MANAGEMENT PLAN FOR THIS PATIENT?

This patient is undergoing surgery on his distal upper extremity. There are various options for postoperative pain. Unless there is a contraindication, regional anesthesia should be the cornerstone for perioperative pain management (i.e., infraclavicular brachial plexus block). This has the potential to provide dense analgesia for this type of procedure. This can be accomplished using a single-shot approach with a long-acting local anesthetic, in addition to one or more adjuncts (i.e., dexamethasone or clonidine) to prolong analgesia. A peripheral nerve catheter can also be left in place and a continuous local anesthetic infusion can be used after surgery to provide prolonged analgesia. Technology is available to allow patients to be discharged home with an infusion device that can provide local anesthetic through the catheter for 2–5 days. For many patients, analgesia from a peripheral nerve local anesthetic infusion may be adequate in providing analgesia. For others, it may not be, and adjunctive medications should also be provided, including acetaminophen and possibly gabapentinoids. If not contraindicated, nonsteroidal anti-inflammatory drugs (NSAIDs) are a great option.[14] For example, intraoperative ketorolac followed by 3 days of IV ketorolac (if inpatient) or oral NSAIDs (if outpatient) are great choices.

DISCUSSION

The opioid epidemic is challenging in many ways and has medical, psychological, and economic consequences. Both rural and urban communities have been devastated and are struggling to contain open market dealing. It has been reported that more United States citizens have died in the opioid epidemic than from the HIV crisis in the 1980s.[15] Annually there are more deaths related to opioid exposure than to both motor vehicle accidents and acquired immune deficiency syndrome (AIDS).[16] The death toll from drug overdose in the United States was more than 700,000 from 1999 to 2017, with the majority of these deaths related to opioid use.[17] Opioid-related deaths are increasing most rapidly from ages 25–44, accounting for 1 in 5 deaths. Data also predicted that opioid misuse would double in those 55 or older from 2004 to 2020. In 2016, 18.4% of all opioid-related deaths occurred in people 55 years or older.[18] As per the CDC, the rise in opioid-related death can be outlined in 3 distinct waves, beginning in the early 1990s with overdose deaths involving prescription opioids, around 2010 involving heroin, and in 2013 involving synthetic opioids such as prescription manufactured fentanyl. It has been reported that the rate of drug overdose deaths has increased significantly in recent years for both sexes, persons aged 25–44 years and over 55 years of age, non-Hispanic whites and non-Hispanic blacks in the United States.[2] As the opioid epidemic has come to the forefront of national attention, it can be expected that more patients will seek addiction treatment. The rate of surgical procedures continues to increase as well. Thus, it has and will continue to become more common for acute pain and perioperative pain physicians to be asked to consult on the pain management of these patients.[19]

Although terms such as *opioid addiction*, *abuse*, and *dependence* are on occasion used interchangeably, problematic opioid use terms have precise definitions. Opioid dependence and addiction were replaced by Opioid Use Disorder (OUD) in the DSM-5 in 2013. Opioid misuse is opioid use contrary to the prescribed pattern of use, regardless of the presence of harm or adverse effects.[20] An opioid use disorder is multifactorial, involving physiological, cognitive, and behavioral aspects, including social issues, risky behavior, and dependence. The DSM-5 lists specific criteria to make a diagnosis of opioid use disorder (see below). It includes signs and symptoms that reflect a compulsive and prolonged self-administration of opioids that are no longer being used for legitimate medical purposes. Risk factors for OUD include younger age, male, lower education and income, prior substance disorder, psychiatric disease, and genetics.[21]

Between 21% and 29% of patients prescribed opioids misuse them, and approximately 8%–12% develop an OUD.[20] Importantly, there is evidence suggesting that non-opioid-dependent users of oral opioid products have an almost 3% per year transition to heroin.[22] As healthcare providers adhere to the recent guidelines recommending decrease in opioid prescription, heroin use has increased from 373,000 users in 2007 to 828,000 in 2015, with 13,000 reported heroin-related deaths in 2013. Approximately 80% of heroin users misused prescription opioids first. The Midwestern region of the United States saw opioid overdoses increase by 70% from July 2016 to September 2017. Within this same time frame, opioid overdoses increased 30% in 52 areas in 45 states. The largest increase was noted in larger metropolitan areas with a population over 1 million. Although data from the 2016 National Drug Survey on Drug Use and Health indicated that heroin use and opioid misuse might be stabilizing, recent analysis by the Centers for Disease Control noted an increase in prevalence of opioid overdose attributed to the potency of illicit drug products.[23] The opioid epidemic continues to evolve and with this the need to alert communities to changes in prevalence of overdoses in order to help coordinate use of appropriate resources, such as naloxone supply or issuing health alerts and advisories. In certain states, post-overdose protocols can help prevent subsequent overdose by providing naloxone and connecting patients with syringe services or case management. For example, syringe services help facilitate the safe disposal of used needles and syringes. They also assist in providing testing, counseling, and sterile injection supplies as well.

There are various diagnostic criteria that fulfill the definition of OUD. This definition itself falls under the category of substance use disorders usually involving a level of tolerance or withdrawal. These are as listed in the DSM-5 to help providers determine if someone has a substance abuse problem:

An OUD is defined as a problematic pattern of opioid use that leads to serious impairment or distress. According to the American Psychiatric Association, for an individual to be diagnosed with opioid use disorder, he/she must have two or more of the following symptoms within a 12-month period of time:

1. Substance taken in larger amounts or for a longer time than intended
2. Persistent desire or unsuccessful effort to cut down or control use of a substance
3. Great deal of time spent obtaining, using, or recovering from substance use
4. Craving (a strong desire urge) to use opioids
5. Continued opioid use that causes failure to fulfill major obligations at work, school, or home
6. Continued opioid use despite causing recurrent social or personal problems
7. Important social, occupational, or recreational activities are reduced because of opioid use
8. Recurrent opioid use in dangerous situations
9. Continued opioid use despite related physical or psychological problems
10. Tolerance defined as the need to take higher doses of a drug to feel the same effects, or a reduced effect from the same amount
11. Withdrawal (which is defined as the experience of pain or other uncomfortable symptoms in the absence of a drug).

Furthermore, OUD can be classified as mild, moderate, and severe depending on the number of criteria the patient meets:

Mild: 2–3 symptoms

Moderate: 4–5 symptoms

Severe: 6 or more symptoms.

Opioid use disorder medication assisted treatment (MAT) consists of opioid agonists, partial agonists, or antagonists. There are three FDA-approved medications used to treat OUD: methadone, naltrexone, and buprenorphine preparations.

Methadone is a treatment option recommended for patients who are able to give informed consent and have no specific contraindications to agonist treatment in a plan that includes psychosocial intervention. It is a synthetic long-acting opioid working primarily as a μ-receptor agonist with pharmacologic actions similar to morphine. It is active in both oral and parenteral routes of administration and may mimic endogenous opioids, thus affecting the release of other neurotransmitters such as acetylcholine, substance P, dopamine, or norepinephrine. Given these properties, methadone can cause analgesia, respiratory depression, sedation, decreased bowel motility, miotic pupils, and increase in prolactin and growth hormone. Additionally, there can be withdrawal effects, such as nausea, fever, chills, tremors, and tachycardia, when stopped abruptly or if an opioid antagonist is administered. Maintenance therapy is the long-term administration of methadone to patients who are dependent on opiates.[24] The daily dosage of methadone for opioid use disorder ranges from 60 mg to 120 mg daily. Methadone should be titrated slowly (i.e., 5–10 mg every 7 days) to avoid over-sedation and other side effects due to its long half-life. The administration of methadone should be monitored in a supervised setting to avoid misuse. Even though methadone can be used, there should also be strategies directed at relapse prevention to ensure comprehensive addiction treatment.

Buprenorphine is an additional option for MAT. It is a μ-opioid receptor partial agonist. Unlike full agonists, increasing a partial agonist dose in an opioid-tolerant individual may not produce additional effect once they have reached maximal effect. This is one property that allows buprenorphine to be prescribed to treat opioid dependence. It is effective in retaining patients in addiction treatment compared to trials with placebo.[25] Lethal overdoses with buprenorphine are still possible in opioid-naïve individuals, especially if taken in combination with central nervous system depressants.

Naltrexone is a μ-opioid receptor antagonist that has been shown to reduce return to illicit drug use and reduce opioid craving compared with placebo in some research trials. An injectable extended-release formulation became available in 2010 for preventing relapse after medically supervised withdrawal.[26] Although naltrexone has no special regulatory requirements and no abuse liability, often it has low rates of acceptance because patients have difficulty achieving abstinence for the necessary time before initiation of treatment.[27] It does not exert any opioid effects, but taking it after recent use of opioids can precipitate withdrawal. Providers can use a naloxone challenge to assess opioid dependence appropriately. For administration, the XR-NTX IM formulation (an intramuscular injection of extended release formulation of naltrexone) can be used every 4 weeks. Patients can continue XR-NTX treatment for as long as they may benefit, although liver function should be assessed. Oral naltrexone is also available.

As the rates of patients using MAT increase—as does the rate of surgical procedures in the United States—it can be expected that acute pain physicians will be asked to consult on this patient population to help manage perioperative and acute pain. Pain in this patient population can be complex for various reasons, both physiological and psychological.

Tolerance and opioid-induced hyperalgesia (OIH) are neuroadaptive processes that must be considered in patients on chronic opioids including methadone (a full agonist) and buprenorphine (a partial agonist). Opioid tolerance is complex and involves pharmacokinetic and pharmacodynamics adaptations to opioid exposure. Metabolites of parent opioid compounds can also antagonize analgesia and even promote hyperalgesia.[28] Opioid binding to a μ receptor leads to chemical changes, often resulting in internalization of the receptor. The opioid receptor itself also undergoes changes, making it less responsive to opioid binding. These and other changes result in a need to escalate dose requirements to achieve the same level of analgesia. It must be noted that not all tolerance develops at the same rate. It is well known that tolerance to analgesia develops more rapidly than tolerance to some of the adverse effects of opioids, such as respiratory depression, thus necessitating very close observation for hypoventilation during dose escalation. Prolonged opioid exposure can also lead to adaptive responses due to the persistent downstream signaling resulting from opioid receptor stimulation. This includes activation of NMDA receptors and downregulation of glutamate transporters, as well as transmission of nociceptive signaling via other channels.[29]

OIH is a complex phenomenon. Hyperalgesia is defined as an increase in pain from a stimulus that would normally provoke pain. OIH is a state of enhanced pain sensitization in individuals who have been exposed to opioids. The pathophysiology of OIH is complex and has not been completely elucidated. Opioid-induced changes along both peripheral and central pain pathways have been proposed, including changes in the NMDA receptor and transmission, activation of descending pain pathways, and decreased reuptake of neurotransmitters enhancing aspects of the pain pathway.[30] Clinically, OIH can be confused with tolerance because of similar symptoms and complaints such as worsening pain. However, the pathophysiological mechanisms are very different between these phenomena, requiring completely polar therapies. While analgesic tolerance can be treated to some extent by increasing opioid dose, OIH treatment requires tapering doses of opioids. Increasing opioids in the setting of OIH may paradoxically worsen pain. Patients with OIH present with increases in pain over time, diffuse pain, or spreading of pain to locations apart from initial pain site, and an increase in pain sensation such as allodynia (pain to a nonpainful stimulus).[31] Management strategies in patients suspected of having OIH include reduction of opioid use, opioid rotation, and using adjuvants that target mechanisms implicated in the development of OIH. For example, ketamine may help reverse OIH by reducing NMDA activation. Perioperatively it is critical that OIH be recognized and treated, as there is evidence suggesting development of persistent postsurgical pain if untreated.[32]

The patient in our case stem has been placed on buprenorphine for MAT. He is scheduled for an elective orthopedic procedure. Patients presenting for surgery while using buprenorphine are becoming commonplace throughout the United States. From 2010 to 2016, annual prescriptions for products containing buprenorphine more than doubled. Thus, anesthesiologists and perioperative pain physicians are faced with the dilemma of what to do when patients on buprenorphine present for surgery.[33] Buprenorphine has unique pharmacologic properties, as it is a partial opioid agonist with a long half-life. It has a high affinity for the opioid receptor, blocking full opioid agonists from binding and staying bound to the receptor. Based on prior case reports of difficult to treat acute pain in patients using buprenorphine, prior recommendations included discontinuation of buprenorphine in patients who required opioid agonists. However, not all opioid receptors are occupied with whole brain opioid receptor availability of 59%, 20%, and 16% at 2, 16, and 32 mg of buprenorphine, respectively.[34] This suggests that even at high doses, opioid receptors are free and available for full agonist binding. Although the evidence is far from conclusive, there is evidence that patients maintained on perioperative buprenorphine have similar analgesia and outcomes following painful procedures such as total joint arthroplasties, albeit with significantly higher opioid requirements.[35]

Lembke and Ottstead note that discontinuation of buprenorphine before surgery introduces unnecessary risk, including addition of complexity such as surgery delay, more clinic visits to taper buprenorphine, and more preoperative instructions and tasks. There is also postoperative destabilization of patients, such as requiring patients to endure a period of opioid withdrawal before re-initiation of buprenorphine and the risk of relapse, as patients on buprenorphine for OUD experience an opioid deficit while receiving access to full opioid agonists.[33] Due to buprenorphine's high potency (up to 100 times that of morphine), buprenorphine cessation can leave a large opioid gap that is not filled when using standardized protocols meant for opioid-naïve patients.[36]

Historically, the cornerstone of perioperative analgesia has been opioids. However, there has been a shift in paradigm, especially as the opioid epidemic has come to the forefront in the United States. Importantly, there has been advancement in the science and pathophysiology of pain as new pain pathways have been discovered and new analgesics (as well as old ones) have been instituted to target these pathways. Current analgesia in the perioperative period should focus not only on opioids, but instead on multimodal therapy—the use of multiple classes of analgesics and modalities targeting various pain pathways, resulting in improvement of analgesia and a reduction in agent-specific adverse effects. One goal is to reduce reliance on opioids to manage perioperative pain. Various classes of agents are available (i.e., NSAIDs, acetaminophen, gabapentinoids). Regional anesthesia and neuroaxial anesthesia are also great options when indicated. It is extremely important that the regimen not be cookie cutter, but instead options should be tailored to specific patients and specific surgical procedures/acute pain processes. For the patient listed in this scenario, various options are available that can be used to maximize perioperative analgesia and minimize opioid use.

Acetaminophen is safe when used in suggested doses and is available in various formulations including oral, rectal, and intravenous. Oral and rectal formulations are inexpensive and should be administered around the clock for most patients. For patients that cannot tolerate oral or rectal formulations, an intravenous formulation is available, albeit at a much greater expense. Current evidence does not support IV use over oral acetaminophen solely for analgesia.[37]

Nonsteroidal anti-inflammatory drugs (NSAIDs) inhibit enzymes (i.e., cyclooxygenase) involved in the production of prostaglandins, helping reduce inflammation and pain. They can be used in combination with acetaminophen. A recent systematic review reported a number needed to treat of 1.5 to obtain a 50% reduction in pain when using a combination of ibuprofen with acetaminophen.[38] A commonly cited concern of using postoperative NSAIDs, especially ketorolac, is the increased risk of bleeding. However, a meta-analysis evaluating 2314 patients noted no increased risk of bleeding and improved analgesia in patients receiving ketorolac.[39]

Gabapentin and pregabalin have been used as analgesic adjuncts in patients with chronic pain, especially for patients with chronic neuropathic pain. As perioperative pain is usually multifactorial and mixed (nociceptive, inflammatory, and neuropathic pain) gabapentinoids have become commonplace in multimodal regimens. These medications are GABA analogues but do not bind to GABA receptors. They are thought to produce their clinical effect by inhibiting the alpha 2 delta subunit of voltage-gated calcium channels. Pregabalin has been shown to have mild to modest effects in reducing pain and analgesic consumption when used perioperatively.[40] A recent study of gabapentin suggested that its use perioperatively may promote opioid cessation and prevent chronic opioid use.[41] Gabapentinoids may also reduce central sensitization and thus have the potential to reduce the transition from acute to chronic pain, which theoretically may reduce the number of patients continuing opioids in the long term. However, further research is needed to find appropriate dosing and length of treatment.

Ketamine is an NMDA antagonist with other mechanisms of action, including decreasing tolerance to opioids, reducing central sensitization, and possibly modulating opioid receptors. Intraoperative use generates modest reductions in acute postoperative opioid consumption and pain intensity.[42] In one study, over 50 opioid-dependent patients undergoing major lumbar spine fusion surgery receiving intraoperative ketamine as a bolus and then infusion were noted to use less morphine at 24 and 48 hours as well as at 6 weeks. These patients also reported less pain intensity in the recovery room and at 6 weeks.[42] A more recent study confirmed these results with patients receiving intraoperative ketamine reducing morphine consumption for the first 24 hours.[43]

Regional anesthesia is also an excellent choice for this patient. This can be accomplished using a single-shot technique of blocking the brachial plexus with a long-acting local anesthetic with additional adjuncts such as dexamethasone or clonidine. This would provide excellent analgesia up to 12–24 hours. However, a perineural catheter with local anesthetic infusion would be a better option to provide a more prolonged block that may be titrated to achieve adequate analgesia.[44]

CONCLUSION

The patient on opioid maintenance therapy presenting for surgery or with an acute pain process poses a particular challenge for the pain physician. The opioid epidemic is now at the forefront of public health, making it more acceptable for patients with opioid use disorders to seek treatment. Along with the rising rates of surgical procedures, the pain physician can expect an increase in consultations on how to best manage pain in this patient population. Acute pain is not only a temporary inconvenience for these patients, but may have long-term consequences as severity of acute pain is one of the biggest risk factors in transitioning to chronic pain states. Exposing patients to opioid therapy perioperatively may also increase their risk of relapsing. Much research is still needed on how to best manage these patients, but multimodal analgesia with minimization of opioids and maximizing non-opioid therapies may be prudent.

REFERENCES

1. Reuben DB, Alvanzo AAH, Ashikaga T, et al. National Institutes of Health Pathways to Prevention Workshop: the role of opioids in the treatment of chronic pain. *Ann Intern Med.* 2015;162(4):295–300. doi: 10.7326/M14-2775.
2. Rudd RA, Aleshire N, Zibbell JE, Gladden RM. Increases in drug and opioid overdose deaths: United States, 2000–2014. *MMWR Morb Mortal Wkly Rep.* 2016;64(50–51):1378–1382. doi: 10.15585/mmwr.mm6450a3.
3. Hayhurst CJ, Durieux ME. Differential opioid tolerance and opioid-induced hyperalgesia: a clinical reality. *Anesthesiology.* 2016;124(2):483–488. doi: 10.1097/ALN.0000000000000963.
4. Heyward J, Olson L, Sharfstein JM, Stuart EA, Lurie P, Alexander GC. Evaluation of the Extended-Release/Long-Acting Opioid Prescribing Risk Evaluation and Mitigation Strategy Program by the US Food and Drug Administration: a review. *JAMA Intern Med.* 2020 Feb 1;180(2):301–309. doi: 10.1001/jamainternmed.2019.5459. PMID: 31886822.
5. Dumas EO, Pollack GM. Opioid tolerance development: a pharmacokinetic/pharmacodynamic perspective. *AAPS J.* 2008;10(4):537–551. doi: 10.1208/s12248-008-9056-1.
6. Wenzel JT, Schwenk ES, Baratta JL, Viscusi ER. Managing opioid-tolerant patients in the perioperative surgical home. *Anesthesiol Clin.* 2016;34(2):287–301. doi: 10.1016/j.anclin.2016.01.005.
7. Huxtable CA, Roberts LJ, Somogyi AA, MacIntyre PE. Acute pain management in opioid-tolerant patients: a growing challenge. *Anaesth Intensive Care.* 2011;39(5):804–823.
8. Kampman K, Jarvis M. American Society of Addiction Medicine (ASAM) national practice guideline for the use of medications in the treatment of addiction involving opioid use. *J Addict Med.* 2015;9(5):358–367. doi: 10.1097/ADM.0000000000000166.
9. Donroe JH, Holt SR, Tetrault JM. Caring for patients with opioid use disorder in the hospital. *Can Med Assoc J.* 2016;188(17–18):1232–1239. doi: 10.1503/cmaj.160290.
10. Quaye AN-A, Zhang Y. Perioperative management of buprenorphine: solving the conundrum. *Pain Med.* 2019 Jul 1;20(7):1395–1408. doi: 10.1093/pm/pny217.
11. Heit HA, Gourlay DL. Buprenorphine: new tricks with an old molecule for pain management. *Clin J Pain.* 2008;24(2):93–97. doi: 10.1097/AJP.0b013e31815ca2b4.
12. Kress HG. Clinical update on the pharmacology, efficacy and safety of transdermal buprenorphine. *Eur J Pain.* 2009;13(3):219–230. doi: 10.1016/j.ejpain.2008.04.011.
13. Anderson TA, Quaye ANA, Ward EN, Wilens TE, Hilliard PE, Brummett CM. To stop or not, that is the question: acute pain management for the patient on chronic buprenorphine. *Anesthesiology.* 2017;126(6):1180–1186. doi: 10.1097/ALN.0000000000001633.
14. Roberts M, Brodribb W, Mitchell G. Reducing the pain: a systematic review of postdischarge analgesia following elective orthopedic surgery. *Pain Med.* 2012;13(5):711–727. doi: 10.1111/j.1526-4637.2012.01359.x.
15. Theisen K, Jacobs B, Macleod L, Davies B. The United States opioid epidemic: a review of the surgeon's contribution to it and health policy initiatives. *BJU Int.* 2018;122(5):754–759. doi: 10.1111/bju.14446.
16. Zhao S, Chen F, Feng A, Han W, Zhang Y. Risk factors and prevention strategies for postoperative opioid abuse. *Pain Res Manag.* 2019;2019:Article ID 7490801, 12 pages. https://doi.org/10.1155/2019/7490801
17. Scholl L, Seth P, Kariisa M, Wilson N, Baldwin G. Drug and opioid-involved overdose deaths: United States, 2013–2017. *MMWR Morb Mortal Wkly Rep.* 2018;67(51–52):1419–1427. doi: 10.15585/mmwr.mm675152e1.
18. Gomes T, Tadrous M, Mamdani MM, Paterson JM, Juurlink DN. The burden of opioid-related mortality in the United States. *JAMA Netw Open.* 2018;1(2):e180217. doi: 10.1001/jamanetworkopen.2018.0217.
19. Soffin EM, Waldman SA, Stack RJ, Liguori GA. An evidence-based approach to the prescription opioid epidemic in orthopedic surgery. *Anesth Analg.* 2017 Nov;125(5):1704–1713. doi: 10.1213/ANE.0000000000002433. PMID: 29049115.
20. Vowles KE, McEntee ML, Julnes PS, Frohe T, Ney JP, van der Goes DN. Rates of opioid misuse, abuse, and addiction in chronic pain: a systematic review and data synthesis. *Pain.* 2015;156(4):569–576. doi: 10.1097/01.j.pain.0000460357.01998.f1.
21. Blanco C, Volkow ND. Management of opioid use disorder in the USA: present status and future directions. *Lancet.* 2019;393(10182):1760–1772. doi: 10.1016/S0140-6736(18)33078-2.
22. Carlson RG, Nahhas RW, Martins SS, Daniulaityte R. Predictors of transition to heroin use among initially non-opioid dependent illicit pharmaceutical opioid users: a natural history study. *Drug Alcohol Depend.* 2016;160:127–134. doi: 10.1016/j.drugalcdep.2015.12.026.
23. Vivolo-Kantor AM, Seth P, Gladden RM, et al. Vital signs: trends in emergency department visits for suspected opioid overdoses: United States, July 2016–September 2017. *MMWR Morb Mortal Wkly Rep.* 2018;67(9):279–285. doi: 10.15585/mmwr.mm6709e1.
24. Anderson IB, Kearney TE. Use of methadone. *West J Med.* 2000;172(1):43–46.
25. Mattick RP, Breen C, Kimber J, Davoli M. Buprenorphine maintenance versus placebo or methadone maintenance for opioid dependence. *Cochrane Database Syst Rev.* 2014;2:CD002207. doi: 10.1002/14651858.CD002207.pub4.
26. Krupitsky E, Nunes EV, Ling W, Illeperuma A, Gastfriend DR, Silverman BL. Injectable extended-release naltrexone for opioid dependence: a double-blind, placebo-controlled, multicentre

randomised trial. *Lancet*. 2011;377(9776):1506–1513. doi: 10.1016/S0140-6736(11)60358-9.
27. Sullivan MA, Garawi F, Bisaga A, et al. Management of relapse in naltrexone maintenance for heroin dependence. *Drug Alcohol Depend*. 2007;91(2–3):289–292. doi: 10.1016/j.drugalcdep.2007.06.013.
28. Smith MT. Neuroexcitatory effects of morphine and hydromorphone: evidence implicating the 3-glucuronide metabolites. *Clin Exp Pharmacol Physiol*. 2000;27(7):524–528. doi: 10.1046/j.1440-1681.2000.03290.x.
29. Martyn JAJ, Mao J, Bittner EA. Opioid tolerance in critical illness. *N Engl J Med*. 2019;380(4):365–378. doi: 10.1056/NEJMra1800222.
30. Yi P, Pryzbylkowski P. Opioid induced hyperalgesia. *Pain Med*. 2015;16 Suppl 1:S32–S36. doi: 10.1111/pme.12914.
31. Lavand'homme P, Steyaert A. Opioid-free anesthesia opioid side effects: tolerance and hyperalgesia. *Best Pract Res Clin Anaesthesiol*. 2017;31(4):487–498. doi: 10.1016/j.bpa.2017.05.003.
32. Colvin LA, Bull F, Hales TG. Perioperative opioid analgesia-when is enough too much? A review of opioid-induced tolerance and hyperalgesia. *Lancet*. 2019;393(10180):1558–1568. doi: 10.1016/S0140-6736(19)30430-1.
33. Lembke A, Ottestad E, Schmiesing C. Patients maintained on buprenorphine for opioid use disorder should continue buprenorphine through the perioperative period. *Pain Med*. 2019;20(3):425–428. doi: 10.1093/pm/pny019.
34. Greenwald MK, Johanson C-E, Moody DE, et al. Effects of buprenorphine maintenance dose on mu-opioid receptor availability, plasma concentrations, and antagonist blockade in heroin-dependent volunteers. *Neuropsychopharmacology*. 2003;28(11):2000–2009. doi: 10.1038/sj.npp.1300251.
35. Hansen LE, Stone GL, Matson CA, Tybor DJ, Pevear ME, Smith EL. Total joint arthroplasty in patients taking methadone or buprenorphine/naloxone preoperatively for prior heroin addiction: a prospective matched cohort study. *J Arthroplasty*. 2016;31(8):1698–1701. doi: 10.1016/j.arth.2016.01.032.
36. Silva MJ, Rubinstein A. Continuous perioperative sublingual buprenorphine. *J Pain Palliat Care Pharmacother*. 2016;30(4):289–293. doi: 10.1080/15360288.2016.1231734.
37. Jibril F, Sharaby S, Mohamed A, Wilby KJ. Intravenous versus oral acetaminophen for pain: systematic review of current evidence to support clinical decision-making. *Can J Hosp Pharm*. 2015;68(3):238–247. doi: 10.4212/cjhp.v68i3.1458.
38. Derry CJ, Derry S, Moore RA. Single dose oral ibuprofen plus paracetamol (acetaminophen) for acute postoperative pain. *Cochrane Database Syst Rev*. 2013;6:CD010210. doi: 10.1002/14651858.CD010210.pub2.
39. Gobble RM, Hoang HLT, Kachniarz B, Orgill DP. Ketorolac does not increase perioperative bleeding: a meta-analysis of randomized controlled trials. *Plast Reconstr Surg*. 2014;133(3):741–755. doi: 10.1097/01.prs.0000438459.60474.b5.
40. Eipe N, Penning J, Yazdi F, et al. Perioperative use of pregabalin for acute pain-a systematic review and meta-analysis. *Pain*. 2015;156(7):1284–1300. doi: 10.1097/j.pain.0000000000000173.
41. Hah J, Mackey SC, Schmidt P, et al. Effect of perioperative gabapentin on postoperative pain resolution and opioid cessation in a mixed surgical cohort: a randomized clinical trial. *JAMA Surg*. 2018;153(4):303–311. doi: 10.1001/jamasurg.2017.4915.
42. Loftus RW, Yeager MP, Clark JA, et al. Intraoperative ketamine reduces perioperative opiate consumption in opiate-dependent patients with chronic back pain undergoing back surgery. *Anesthesiology*. 2010;113(3):639–646. doi: 10.1097/ALN.0b013e3181e90914.
43. Nielsen RV, Fomsgaard JS, Siegel H, et al. Intraoperative ketamine reduces immediate postoperative opioid consumption after spinal fusion surgery in chronic pain patients with opioid dependency: a randomized, blinded trial. *Pain*. 2017;158(3):463–470. doi: 10.1097/j.pain.0000000000000782.
44. Ilfeld BM. Continuous peripheral nerve blocks: an update of the published evidence and comparison with novel, alternative analgesic modalities. *Anesth Analg*. 2017;124(1):308–335. doi: 10.1213/ANE.0000000000001581.

REVIEW QUESTIONS

(1) What is the mechanism of action of pregabalin?

A. Binding of sodium channels with reduction of transmission of nociceptive neurons
B. Increase in GABA release and thus reduction of transmission of nociceptive neurons
C. Binding of calcium channels
D. Binding to NMDA receptors

(2) Using local anesthetics as part of a multimodal approach to acute pain management leads to:

A. Increased risk of chronic post-surgical pain development
B. Higher risk of longer hospital stay due to potential for local anesthetic toxicity
C. Decreased opioid use
D. All of the above

(3) A 32-year-old female with a history of an L5–S1 fusion and post-laminectomy syndrome presents for left hip arthroscopic surgery. The procedure is done under total intravenous anesthesia using propofol and remifentanil. She is given hydromorphone prior to emergence. She is now complaining of severe pain in the recovery room. OIH is suspected. Which of the following is not an effective treatment for pain in a patient with OIH?

A. Ketorolac
B. Pregabalin
C. Ketamine
D. Fentanyl

(4) Which of the following is a sign of opioid dependence?

A. Withdrawal symptoms with dose reduction or cessation
B. Sacrificing hobbies with intent to obtain and use an opioid for non-medical reasons
C. Development of withdrawal symptoms, obsession with taking psychotropic drugs, and sacrificing hobbies for further opioid consumption
D. None of the above

(5) Mu opioid receptors are responsible for:

A. Nausea
B. Respiratory depression
C. Miosis
D. All of the above

(6) What are the main principles of multimodal analgesia?

A. Early enteral nutrition
B. Enable early mobilization
C. Decrease the stress response due to surgery
D. All of the above

(7) Which of the following are DSM-5 criteria for Opioid Use Disorder (OUD)?

A. Withdrawal after opioid cessation
B. Continued opioid use despite recurrent social or personal problems

C. Opioid use taken in larger amounts or for a longer time than intended
D. All of the above

ANSWERS

(1) **C.** Pregabalin and its related cousin—gabapentin—are gabapentinoids. These medications are GABA analogues but do not bind to GABA receptors. They are thought to produce their clinical effect by inhibiting the alpha 2 delta subunit of voltage-gated calcium channels. Local anesthetics bind to sodium channels and reduce transmission of nociceptive neurons. Ketamine binds to the NMDA receptor.

Reference

Eipe N, Penning J, Yazdi F, et al. Perioperative use of pregabalin for acute pain-a systematic review and meta-analysis. *Pain*. 2015;156(7):1284–1300. doi: 10.1097/j.pain.0000000000000173.

(2) **C.** Local anesthetics can be an important component of multimodal analgesia. They are usually used for regional anesthetics such as neuraxial anesthesia/analgesia as well as peripheral nerve blocks. They may decrease the amount of opioids needed to provide analgesia

Reference

Kumar K, Kirksey MA, Duong S, Wu CL. A review of opioid-sparing modalities in perioperative pain management: methods to decrease opioid use postoperatively. *Anesth Analg*. 2017 Nov;125(5):1749–1760. doi: 10.1213/ANE.0000000000002497. PMID: 29049119.

(3) **D.** All opioids have the potential to cause a reduction in pain threshold. Ketamine has the potential to decrease this effect. Pain is paradoxically worsened by opioids if due to opioid-induced hyperalgesia (OIH). Opioid-induced changes along both peripheral and central pain pathways have been proposed, including changes in the NMDA receptor and transmission, activation of descending pain pathways, and decreased reuptake of neurotransmitters enhancing aspects of the pain pathway.

References

Loftus RW, Yeager MP, Clark JA, et al. Intraoperative ketamine reduces perioperative opiate consumption in opiate-dependent patients with chronic back pain undergoing back surgery. *Anesthesiology*. 2010;113(3):639–646.

Nielsen RV, Fomsgaard JS, Siegel H, et al. Intraoperative ketamine reduces immediate postoperative opioid consumption after spinal fusion surgery in chronic pain patients with opioid dependency: a randomized, blinded trial. *Pain*. 2017;158(3):463–470.

(4) **C.** The ICD-10 (International Statistical Classification of Diseases and Related Health Problems) defines dependence as having at least 3 of the following over the last year: signs of tolerance, continued opioid use despite unwanted/negative consequences, development of withdrawal with dose cessation or reduction, an obsession with acquiring the substance.

Reference

American Psychiatric Association. *Diagnostic and Statistical Manual of Mental Disorders*. 5th ed. Arlington, VA: APA; 2013.

(5) **D.** Mu (μ) opioid receptors are also implicated in euphoria and dependence. There are other opioid receptors, including kappa receptors which mediate visceral and spinal analgesia. Delta opioid receptors may help facilitate mu receptor activity. Opioid receptors are G linked. Once bound, a cascade of reactions leads to activation of ion channels and gene transcription.

Reference

Machelska H, Celik MÖ. Advances in achieving opioid analgesia without side effects. *Front Pharmacol*. 2018 Nov 29;9:1388. doi: 10.3389/fphar.2018.01388. PMID: 30555325; PMCID: PMC6282113.

(6) **D.** Multimodal postoperative care and analgesia encompass not only pain management but address various dimensions of perioperative care. These include early mobilization and enteral nutrition. Pain management is a cornerstone of multimodal therapy. A key component is the use of various medications and techniques (i.e., peripheral nerve blocks) that act synergistically to improve analgesia while reducing adverse effects.

Reference

Kaye AD, Urman RD, Rappaport Y, et al. Multimodal analgesia as an essential part of enhanced recovery protocols in the ambulatory settings. *J Anaesthesiol Clin Pharmacol*. 2019;35(Suppl 1):S40–S45. doi: 10.4103/joacp.JOACP_51_18.

(7) **D.** The DSM-5 lists OUD under substance-related and addictive disorders. These include 10 various drug classes, including opioids, caffeine, cannabis, and alcohol. This group of disorders is a cluster that includes behavioral and physiological symptoms indicating that the individual continues using the substance even though the substance leads to substance-related problems.

Reference

American Psychiatric Association. *Diagnostic and Statistical Manual of Mental Disorders*. 5th ed. Arlington, VA: APA; 2013.

42.

THE PAINFUL VASO-OCCLUSIVE SICKLE CELL EPISODE

Amberly Orr, Dalia Elmofty, and Lynn Kohan

STEM CASE AND KEY QUESTIONS

A 25-year-old female with a history of sickle cell disease (SCD), asthma, depression, and adjustment disorder presents with a vaso-occlusive (VOC) episode. The patient was recently admitted to an outside hospital for 1 month and states that she was "kicked out without any pain medications." She left against medical advice when she was transitioned off her hydromorphone patient-controlled analgesia (PCA).

Prior to admission, the patient was taking morphine sulfate extended release 120 mg Q8h and oxycodone/acetaminophen 10/325 mg 1–2 tablets Q4h as needed for pain.

She reports having excruciating low back pain, bilateral hip pain, and leg pain. This is consistent with her usual VOC distribution. She also reports having chest pain, shortness of breath, and feeling febrile. The patient states that in the past year she has had 2 episodes of acute chest syndrome. She denies nausea, vomiting, diarrhea, constipation, and abdominal pain.

Physician examination is unremarkable. In the emergency department, the patient is hydrated with intravenous fluids and receives 2 doses of hydromorphone 1 mg intravenously. She refuses ketorolac and states it has never helped her in the past. She continues to report 20/10 pain and states that she has had long hospitalization stays with difficult pain control. She is admitted for further pain management.

Chest x-ray and a complete blood count are unremarkable except for a hemoglobin of 8.4, Her liver function tests, lactate dehydrogenase, creatinine, and coagulation profile are unremarkable, thus ruling out other complications.

The primary service discusses her prolonged hospitalization course and concerns for the likelihood of this being a chronic pain versus a VOC episode. They asked the patient questions about the severity and quality of her pain. Additional questions include timing of the pain (onset and duration), temporal relation of the pain to other activities, and aggravating and alleviating factors. Furthermore, past treatments, successful and unsuccessful, were queried. She is offered a trial of per os (PO) pain regimen with ketamine infusion but begins talking on the phone to her mother, avoiding eye contact with the medical team, and tells her mother that she is leaving because "nobody will treat her pain."

(1) WHAT ARE THE FEATURES ASSOCIATED WITH A VOC EPISODE THAT SUGGEST A GREATER LIKELIHOOD OF ADDITIONAL COMPLICATIONS OTHER THAN PAIN?

An acute VOC episode is an abrupt, intense pain that can last from hours to days, typically occurring in the chest, back, abdomen, and extremities. The most common sites involved include the long bones: tibia, femur, and the humerus. Infants may present with pain and swelling in the hands and feet, a condition known as dactylitis.

(2) WHAT IS THE INITIAL TREATMENT FOR A SUSPECTED VOC EPISODE?

Intravenous hydration reduces the sickling process for patients who are dehydrated or hypovolemic. Supplemental oxygen is warranted if saturations remain <92%. Blood transfusion is not recommended in an uncomplicated VOC episode; however, it is utilized for severe anemia causing physiologic compromise. Exchange transfusions are recommended for patients experiencing a cerebrovascular accident, treatment resistant acute coronary syndrome, or multi-organ failure. A multimodal approach for pain management that includes patient education, non-pharmacologic, pharmacologic, and interventional methods should be implemented.

(3) ARE THESE PATIENTS PAIN FREE BETWEEN THE VOC?

A large percentage of SCD patients who experience chronic pain between the VOC episodes have chronic pain in between the episodes. Chronic pain for SCD is defined as pain that is present on most days over the previous 6 months.

(4) WHAT IS OPIOID-INDUCED HYPERALGESIA (OIH), OPIOID-INDUCED TOLERANCE (OIT), OR IATROGENIC OPIOID WITHDRAWAL? HOW IS THAT RELATED TO SCD?

Frequent and increased administration of opioids can lead to opioid-induced tolerance (OIT) or opioid-induced hyperalgesia (OIH). OIT is a physiological process with a progressive lack of response to opioids that requires an increased dose to produce the same effect; there is a shift to the right of the dose-response curve. The lack of response is overcome by increasing the dose. OIH is a paradoxical response to opioids where patients experience a worsening of pain with the administration of opioids. Patients with SCD experiencing VOC pain are often viewed as drug-seeking. Medical professionals may view the increased use of opioids in this population as addiction, whereas it is most likely due to hyperalgesia and tolerance.

(5) WHAT IS THE ROLE OF PAIN INTERVENTIONS IN PAIN FROM SCD?

Several interventions can be helpful in treating pain from SCD; hip joint injections have been used successfully. The use of regional and neuraxial analgesia can reduce opioid consumption and help with vasodilation.

(6) WHAT IS THE VALUE OF EMPLOYING A PAIN MANAGEMENT ALGORITHM IN SCD?

Employing clinical algorithms to manage VOC pain results in faster delivery of analgesia, improved satisfaction, shorter hospital stays, and reduced costs. However, it increases use of primary care providers to manage pain.

(7) WHAT ARE OTHER ADVANCED LINES OF PAIN MANAGEMENT IN SEVERE SCD?

The use of intravenous lidocaine, low-dose ketamine, and methadone are advanced lines used to treat severe SCD pain.

DISCUSSION

Sickle cell disease (SCD) is the most common inherited blood disorder in the United States. The disease affects approximately 100,000 Americans and is most prevalent among African Americans.[1,2] SCD is an autosomal recessive disorder caused by mutations in *HBB*, a gene that encodes the β-globin chain of hemoglobin. The mutation, which is an amino acid substitution of a valine residue for glutamic acid in the β globin protein, results in sickle hemoglobin (HbS).[3] HbS can form rigid, unstable polymers when deoxygenated, leading red blood cells to assume a characteristic sickle shape. Erythrocyte sickling results in occlusion of microvasculature with subsequent ischemia of tissues. This vaso-occlusion is a hallmark of SCD and is characterized by acutely painful episodes.[4] Recent literature describes mechanisms that are more complex than attributing VOC episodes solely to acute cell sickling.

VOC episodes have historically been called "crises." Because this terminology has a negative connotation, the terms "vaso-occlusive episodes" or "vaso-occlusive pain" are used throughout this chapter. The word "crisis" infers that an individual with SCD is unable to self-manage their pain, yet individuals with SCD often manage their acute pain at home.[5] An epidemiology study demonstrates that pain episodes are managed at home more often than at healthcare facilities.[6]

PATHOPHYSIOLOGY

The pathophysiology of vaso-occlusion in SCD has evolved from a polymerization-based model to a multiple-pathway model that involves several complex events that underlie vaso-occlusion. In the polymerization-based model, hemoglobin polymerization is thought to be the primary event in VOC pain.[7] This is supported by clinical evidence that dehydration results in increased concentrations of HbS, resulting in symptoms of SCD.[8] Hydroxyurea, a common therapy used in SCD to decrease the frequency of painful episodes, increases levels of fetal hemoglobin (HbF), which does not sickle. This effectively leads to reduced HbS polymerization and fewer VOC episodes.[9]

Individuals with SCD and comorbidities associated with hypoxemia (e.g., obstructive sleep apnea) do not demonstrate increased frequencies of VOC episodes.[10] Cell sickling under hypoxic conditions is unlikely to be the sole factor in vaso-occlusion. The theory of sickling obstructing vasculature would lead to the assumption that smaller vessels are the most vulnerable to occlusion. Studies have shown occlusion of larger vessels.[11] It is possible that the mechanisms underlying occlusion vary with the anatomic site and various characteristics of the vascular bed.[12,13]

The multiple pathway model proposes that VOC pain is the result of a complex interplay among sickle erythrocytes, endothelial cells, leukocytes, and plasma proteins. Studies suggest that sickle erythrocytes activate adhesion receptors such as E-selectin, P-selectin, and ICAM-4, causing the sickle erythrocytes to have abnormal adhesive properties. Interactions among leukocytes, platelets, and endothelial cells result in aggregation, leading to vaso-occlusion.[14] This vaso-occlusion leads to ischemia and inflammation. An increase in inflammatory biomarkers such as IL-10, IL-6, TGF-alpha, and TNF-alpha sensitize nociceptors. Nociceptors translate the stimulus from inflammatory mediators into an electrical impulse (i.e., action potential) that is transmitted to the dorsal horn of the spinal cord via the dorsal root ganglion. A-delta fibers and C fibers activate second-order neurons in the dorsal horn of the spinal cord. The impulse then ascends to the contralateral spinothalamic tract and finally to the hypothalamus, thalamus, limbic system, and brain stem to cause the perception of pain. The excitatory neurotransmitter glutamate is involved in the transmission.[15,16] Chronic pain from SCD is likely caused by central and peripheral sensitization.

DIAGNOSIS

DNA-based testing can be done as part of prenatal testing. Newborn screening is currently performed in all states utilizing high-performance liquid chromatography (HPLC) or isoelectric focusing.[17] In premature babies, HbA levels may not be detected, thus causing a misdiagnosis.[18] DNA analysis can confirm the diagnosis. HPLC and isoelectric focusing are also commonly used in older, symptomatic individuals and allow for a definitive diagnosis.[19,20]

There are no laboratory tests or clinical findings that can diagnose a VOC episode. Most of the markers such as cytokines and other inflammatory molecules are indirect and are present in non-SCD pathogenesis. Laboratory tests and imaging are often ordered for SCD patients with VOC pain to rule out other serious conditions.

CLINICAL PRESENTATION

An acute VOC episode is distinguished by abrupt, intense pain that can last from hours to days, typically occurring in the chest, back, abdomen, and extremities. Some patients may experience a gradual onset of pain.[21] The most common sites involved include the long bones: tibia, femur, and the humerus. Infants may present with pain and swelling in the hands and feet, a condition known as dactylitis. Almost all patients with SCD will have an acute pain episode in their lifetimes. Episodes can begin as early as the first few months of life.[22] Infection, cold temperatures, dehydration, hypotension, menstruation, and hypoxia have been associated as precipitating factors. In many cases, no cause is identified.[23–26]

Because pain can occur in various sites, VOC episodes are often confused with or are a precursor to other medical emergencies, including stroke and acute coronary syndrome. It is crucial to promptly rule out other underlying causes of the pain. Low-grade fever can be an accompanying presentation in VOC pain. Patients with SCD are at increased risk for certain infections such as pneumonia and bone infections due to reduced or absent splenic function.[27] Infection must be ruled out in any patient with a fever.

Biliary tract dysfunction is common in patients with SCD and abdominal pain can be due to a number of conditions other than solely VOC pain, including cholecystitis and cholelithiasis, hepatic sequestration, and splenic sequestration.[28] Patients with SCD will experience infarction of the spleen before the end of their childhoods. The spleen is possibly affected due to its narrow vasculature, with entrapped erythrocytes leading to enlargement of the spleen and subsequent pain.[29]

Extremity pain in VOC episodes must be differentiated from deep vein thrombosis (DVT), osteomyelitis, gout, and avascular necrosis of a joint. Sickle cell patients are likely at increased risk for DVT, which further complicates the assessment.[30] Osteomyelitis will often present with fever, swelling of the joint, and leukocytosis. While imaging may reveal findings such as periosteal elevation, ultimately, imaging cannot be used to rule out a diagnosis.[22] Hyperuricemia and monoarticular pain that is unresponsive to typical therapy for VOC pain may raise suspicion for gout.[31] Avascular necrosis (AVN) is a relatively common complication of VOC episodes that is seen in up to 10% of sickle cell patients. It is most commonly found in the femoral head (i.e., hips); however, involvement in more than one joint is typical. History, physical exam, and imaging should involve the bilateral joints. Patients with SCD who experience hip or shoulder pain (the second most common site of AVN) should be evaluated for AVN.[32]

Acute chest syndrome (ACS) is terminology to describe a condition in SCD that presents with a constellation of symptoms that may include chest pain, cough, hypoxia, fever, and/or new lung infiltrates identified on imaging. ACS can occur as a complication of a VOC episode. It needs to be differentiated from other serious conditions such as a pulmonary embolism. ACS is a serious and potentially fatal condition. It is the leading cause of death in patients with SCD, accounting for approximately 25% of deaths.[27]

CLINICAL ASSESSMENT OF PAIN

One important aspect in assessing sickle cell pain is determining whether or not the pain is acute or chronic and discussing with the patient the potential differences. Determining the location and character of the pain may help the patient distinguish the etiology of the pain. Assessment of VOC pain relies mostly on the history obtained from the patient. A directed pain history should include the following: (1) medical record review, including review of prescription-monitoring programs; (2) patient interview to include symptomatology, current medications, and associated adverse effects; (3) preexisting pain conditions; (4) medical conditions that could influence a pain therapy; (5) history of opioid-induced tolerance or hyperalgesia and substance abuse; and (6) non-pharmacologic pain therapies, including alternative and complementary therapies tried in the past. A directed physical examination should be performed, and relevant imaging and labs reviewed. Collaboration with other healthcare providers (e.g., nurses, surgeons, internists, pain services, physical therapists, pharmacists, and psychologists) can facilitate a multidisciplinary care team model to manage VOC episodes.

Pain severity may be assessed by using patient self-report scales such as numeric ratings and visual analog scales. These tools do not allow for individual variability in pain tolerance. Behavior assessment tools can be used for patients who are unable to self-report; however, due to the subjective nature of pain, providers should use caution when using self-report scales. Adequate tools are lacking in appropriately measuring pain intensity in SCD, and tools to differentiate the types of pain (e.g., neuropathic versus nociceptive) are not fully developed.[33] Objective assessment of pain is encouraged. One way to obtain a better understanding of a patient's pain is to assess the impact that pain has on the patient's daily functioning and quality of life. The functional pain scale is a useful tool to facilitate the assessment of pain.[34] A comfort-function goal can be used to establish accountability for pain relief and a reference point when discussing pain and achieving satisfactory pain relief. The comfort-function goal is the pain score identified by the patient as the level of pain tolerance needed to participate in healing activities such as deep breathing, ambulation, and activities of daily living.[35] SCD-specific functional pain scales include the Adult Sickle Cell Quality of Life Measurement Information System (ASCQ-Me).[36] Further complicating the assessment of acute VOC pain is the large percentage of SCD patients who experience chronic pain. Chronic pain for SCD is currently defined as pain that is present on most days over the previous 6 months.[37] Chronic pain can contribute to the intensity of a VOC episode and make treatment more challenging. It is hypothesized that repeated stimulation of nociceptors during episodes of acute VOC pain leads to remodeling of neurons that cause chronic pain.

Frequent and increased administration of opioids can lead to opioid-induced tolerance (OIT) or opioid-induced hyperalgesia (OIH).[6] Determining the clinical differentiation between these two can be challenging. OIT is a physiological process with a progressive lack of response to opioids that requires an increased dose to produce the same effect; there is a shift to the right of the dose-response curve. The lack of response is overcome by increasing the dose. OIH is a paradoxical response to opioids where patients experience a worsening of pain with the administration of opioids. Inappropriate low dosing of opioids for patients on long-term therapy can lead to opioid withdrawal that presents as diffuse pain similar to VOC pain. If weaning of opioid therapy is indicated, a tapering program should be utilized based on oral morphine equivalents per day and chronicity of use.

Another challenging barrier in assessing patient pain is healthcare provider bias. Patients with SCD experiencing VOC pain are often viewed as drug-seeking.[38] Medical professionals may view the increased use of opioids in this population as addiction, whereas it is most likely due to hyperalgesia and tolerance. Providers are often reluctant and uncomfortable ordering high doses of opioids, leading to undertreatment of pain. The prevalence of opioid addiction in patients with SCD is estimated to be 0.5% to 8%, not significantly higher than in the general population.[39] Education on the complexity of VOC pain can help reduce the stigma and improve pain management.

PREVENTION

Interventions to reduce the frequency and/or severity of VOC episodes include patient education, psychological therapy, transfusion therapy, pharmacological management, and individualized home pain management plans (HPMP).[40,41]

Patient education involves devising strategies to prevent common triggers of VOC pain, such as maintaining adequate hydration. Transfusion therapy can play a role in reducing the frequency of painful episodes by decreasing the amount of sickle hemoglobin. Because transfusion therapy is not without risk, it is typically reserved for patients who have exhausted medical therapy without significant benefit.[41]

The 2 primary medications used in the prevention of VOC episodes are hydroxyurea and L-glutamine. Hydroxyurea is thought to reduce the frequency of VOC episodes by increasing the levels of HbF to prevent HbS polymerization. It has been suggested that its mechanism of action includes reduced adherence of erythrocytes via decreased receptor expression.[42] Hydroxyurea therapy is recommended for patients, starting at 6–12 months of age, with more than 2 severe VOC pain episodes within 1 year, with pain interfering with daily activities, or with recurrent episodes of ACS. L-glutamine was approved by the U.S. Federal Drug Administration (FDA) in 2017, for use in SCD patients 5 years and older.[43] L-glutamine is an essential amino acid that can have decreased production during stress.[44] It is the precursor of the antioxidant glutathione and helps neutralize the oxidative stress in sickle red blood cells, allowing them to be more flexible. FDA approval was based on a randomized trial that demonstrated fewer pain events, reduced hospitalizations, and decreased frequency of ACS in study patients receiving L-glutamine compared to placebo.[45] For uncomplicated VOC pain episodes, has been shown to reduce emergency room visits and overall healthcare costs.[46] The plan includes non-pharmacological and pharmacological management of pain based on a stepwise approach according to the intensity of pain. HPMPs allow patients to become active participants in managing their healthcare.

MANAGEMENT

Pain is the most common reason that patients with SCD are admitted to the hospital. Maintenance of intravenous hydration is warranted to reduce the sickling process for patients who are dehydrated or hypovolemic. Supplemental oxygen is warranted if saturations remain <92%. Blood transfusion is currently not recommended in an uncomplicated VOC episode; however, it is utilized for severe anemia causing physiologic compromise. Exchange transfusions are recommended for patients experiencing a cerebrovascular accident (CVA), treatment resistant ACS, or multi-organ failure.

The goals for managing acute VOC pain include early intervention, with prompt adjustments in the regimen for inadequately controlled pain. Reduction of pain to acceptable levels is necessary to facilitate recovery. Although opioids are currently the mainstay for treating acute VOC pain, a multimodal approach that includes patient education, nonpharmacologic, pharmacologic, and interventional methods should be implemented.

Important non-pharmacological strategies can be deployed to reduce the severity of pain, including: (1) physical rehabilitative approaches for reconditioning; (2) occupational therapy to facilitate proper body mechanics and resume normal levels of daily activities; (3) psychological approaches; and (4) other physical approaches.

Pharmacological agents include opioids and adjunct therapy such as nonsteroidal anti-inflammatory drugs (NSAIDs), acetaminophen, anticonvulsants, and antidepressants.

Opioids

Opioids remain the gold standard in reducing VOC pain. Opioids allow for rapid analgesia that is easy to titrate with different available routes of administration. Patients can be treated with a combination of long-acting in addition to short-acting opioids for breakthrough pain.[32] Every attempt should be made to taper opioid therapy to the lowest effective dose once the acute VOC episode has resolved. Hydromorphone and morphine are the most used intravenous opioids for SCD. The choice of intravenous opioid depends on several factors, including route availability, patient comorbidities, and past individual responses. Intranasal fentanyl has been used in children and those without intravenous access.[47] Methadone is an opioid that has some advantages over other opioids used for pain; as a mu receptor agonist that contains a unique N-methyl-D-aspartate (NMDA) antagonism property, methadone can counteract OIT and OIH.[48] It also inhibits reuptake of serotonin and norepinephrine (SNRI), which has additional analgesic benefits. Methadone is rapidly growing as a first-line treatment for acute pain in patients with a history of chronic pain. The potential benefits include its duration of action and incomplete cross-tolerance with opioid rotation. Methadone may be associated with respiratory depression, sedation, and QTc interval prolongation.

Tramadol is an opioid that has a serotonin-norepinephrine reuptake inhibitor (SNRI) property in addition to its action on mu receptors. There are conflicting studies regarding the efficacy of tramadol in VOC pain. A retrospective study of pediatric patients with VOC pain showed that the addition of tramadol to a morphine/ketorolac mixture failed to demonstrate a significant reduction in pain scores, consumption of other opiates, or length of hospital stay.[49] In contrast, a study that examined intravenous infusions of tramadol in combination with acetaminophen and ibuprofen in children resulted in resolution of acute VOC pain.[50] Another study in adults reported reduction in pain scores and opioid consumption with infusions of tramadol and ketorolac combined with exchange transfusions.[51] Larger, controlled studies are needed to determine the efficacy of tramadol in treatment of VOC pain.

The use of meperidine in sickle cell pain is controversial and should be avoided unless patients are intolerant of other opioids.[32] Accumulation of the metabolite normeperidine is associated with central nervous system toxicity and can lead to side effects ranging from dysphoria and irritability to clonus and seizures. Meperidine use is contraindicated in patients taking monoamine oxidase inhibitor antidepressants due to the risk of serotonin syndrome.[52] The recommendation is to limit use of meperidine to 48 hours or less with a maximum dose of 600 milligrams per 24 hours.[53]

PCA is shown to be more effective in the treatment of VOC pain compared to intermittent clinician administration of opioids.[54] Optimal PCA dosing is currently not determined. A randomized inpatient trial suggests that low infusions with higher-dose boluses result in faster pain control and decreased duration of hospital stays compared to low-bolus doses with high infusions; however, this study was terminated early due to poor accrual.[55] Records of previous dosing requirements, when available, can guide the decision.

Adjunct Therapy (NSAIDs, Acetaminophen)

For sickle cell patients with pain that is mild in intensity, NSAIDs and acetaminophen are considered a first-line therapy and should be considered adjunct therapy in patients with moderate to severe pain.[47] NSAIDs provide a significant anti-inflammatory effect. Both acetaminophen and NSAIDs have a ceiling effect in which increased doses do not provide further pain relief.[56] Caution must be taken prior to administering acetaminophen to patients with liver dysfunction or administering NSAIDs to individuals with renal disease or those at risk for gastrointestinal bleeding. NSAIDs should be avoided after 30 weeks gestation in pregnant women, as there is a risk of premature narrowing or closure of the ductus arteriosus.[57] NSAIDs reduce glomerular filtration rate and increase the risk for acute renal failure (ARF) in sickle cell patients. Due to a relative inability to maximally concentrate urine, those with SCD are particularly vulnerable to developing pre-renal ARF.[58] The parenteral NSAID, ketorolac, may be used as an adjunct in severe pain requiring hospitalization, but it should not be used longer than 5 days to avoid toxicity.[59]

Other Non-Opioid Adjuncts

Adjuvant medications such as anticonvulsants (e.g., gabapentin) and antidepressants are commonly used in multimodal analgesia and have been shown to reduce perioperative opioid use.[60] Studies on their use for VOC pain are currently lacking. Because neuropathic pain is thought to be a component of VOC pain, adjuvant medications may have a beneficial role in the treatment of acute sickle cell pain.[61]

Gabapentin is a common agent used in neuropathic pain. It binds to the alpha-2-delta subunit of voltage-dependent calcium ion channels. This subunit is upregulated in pain, and its blockade gives gabapentin its anti-hyperalgesic and anti-central sensitization effects.[62]

SNRIs and tricyclic antidepressants (TCAs) are effective in treating neuropathic pain. Duloxetine is a type of SNRI commonly used for the treatment of neuropathic pain. The mechanism underlying antidepressants' analgesic effect is complex, but studies suggest the reuptake inhibition of noradrenaline plays a crucial role. Noradrenaline inhibits pain signaling in the spinal cord.[63]

Ketamine

Ketamine is an n-methyl-D-aspartate (NMDA) receptor antagonist that may be useful for the treatment of refractory VOC pain. It has been proposed that patients with uncontrolled pain despite opioid therapy may have OIT or OIH.[47] Table 42.1 demonstrates a protocol for managing in-patient ketamine infusions, adapted from the University of Chicago Medical Center. Several published reports demonstrate the potential efficacy of low-dose ketamine infusion in sickle cell pain management. Of 17 sickle cell patients in case series, 14 (82%) of patients reported a significant reduction in opioid usage and pain severity. One patient developed side effects that required discontinuation of the infusion.[64] Further studies are needed to fully establish the role of ketamine in VOC pain.

Lidocaine

Lidocaine is an amide local anesthetic used to treat several different types of pain, including cancer pain, neuropathic pain, and post-surgical pain. Lidocaine blocks voltage-gated sodium channels, which are known for their role in nociception. In addition to nociceptive pain, lidocaine may contribute to the treatment of neuropathic pain common in patients

Table 42.1 **IN-PATIENT KETAMINE INFUSION PROTOCOL**

Consultation
Low-dose ketamine orders for pain management will be written by a member of the Pain Service or Palliative Care Team:

- Obtain baseline EKG and cardiac history
- Evaluate for arrhythmias
- Obtain consent

Common indications

- Opioid tolerance: typically for those requiring >100 mg of daily oral morphine equivalents
- Postoperative pain
- Severe intractable pain not controlled by escalating doses of opioids
- Opioid rotation fails to improve side effects
- Severe neuropathic pain
- Evidence of opioid-related hyperalgesia: when a painful stimulus is perceived as being out of proportion (unbearable) to the noxious stimulus under high-dose opioid therapies

Low-dose ketamine is contraindicated in patients with:

- Hypersensitivity to ketamine
- Uncontrolled/active seizures
- Uncontrolled/active psychotic disorder(s)
- Renal failure: oliguria
- Liver failure: AST/ALT ≥5 × ULN or evidence of impaired synthetic function (Child-Pugh class B score)

Low-dose ketamine may be used with caution in patients with:

- Elevated intracranial pressure (ICP) or intraocular pressure (IOP)
- Uncontrolled hypertension
- Severe ischemic heart disease or severe congestive heart failure
- Thyrotoxicosis
- Aneurysms
- Hemorrhagic cystitis

Dosing and monitoring
Dosing
Low-dose infusion is defined as 0.06–0.3 mg/kg/hr
Commonly: initial dose rate will be 0.12 mg/kg/hr

Low-dose oral is defined as 2–5 mg/kg/day (in divided doses)
Commonly: initial dose will be 0.5 mg/kg every 6 hours
Monitoring
Continuous pulse oximetry (CPO), routine VS; numeric pain rating scale (NPRS) and sedation scores every 2 hours × 2 then every 4 hours for the duration of the infusion
Document total drug amount infused every 12 hours

IF PATIENT IS HAVING SIDE EFFECTS NOT CONTROLLED WITH DOSE REDUCTION, CALL THE ORDERING PAIN SERVICE / PALLIATIVE CARE TEAM.

Table 42.2 **IN-PATIENT LIDOCAINE INFUSION PROTOCOL**

Consultation
Lidocaine infusion orders for pain management are written by a member of the Pain Service or Palliative Care Team:

- Obtain baseline EKG and cardiac history
- Evaluate patient for arrhythmias
- Obtain consent
- Assess for alertness
- Determine effects of previous infusion
  - Pain reduction
  - Duration of effects
  - Patient function
  - Decrease in use of pain medication

Common indications

- Opioid-induced tolerance: typically >100 mg of daily oral morphine equivalents
- Postoperative pain
- Severe neuropathic pain
- Pain caused by burn injuries
- Opioid-induced hyperalgesia: when a painful stimulus is perceived as being out of proportion (unbearable) to the noxious stimulus under high-dose opioid therapies

Intravenous lidocaine for pain is contraindicated in patients with:

- Hypersensitivity to lidocaine or any component of the formulation
- Adam-Stokes syndrome
- Wolff-Parkinson-White syndrome
- Severe degrees of SA, AV, or intraventricular heart block
- Allergies to corn or corn-related products; premixed injections may contain corn-derived dextrose

Intravenous lidocaine for pain may be used with caution in:

- Concurrent local anesthetic administration should be avoided
- Patients with hepatic dysfunction
- Elderly patients

Dosing and monitoring

Dosing intravenous lidocaine:
Three dosing strategies are utilized

1. **Low-dose continuous infusion**
   - Lidocaine for floor use
   - Patients ABW <70 kg: 0.5 mg/min
   - Patients ABW 70–100 kg: 0.75 mg/min
   - Patients ABW > 100 kg: 1 mg/min
2. **Moderate-dose continuous infusion**
   - Bolus: 1–1.5 mg/kg (IBW)
   - Continuous infusion: 0.5–3mg/kg/hr (IBW)
3. **Short duration, high-dose infusion with bolus**
   - A single bolus dose of 1 mg/kg over 3 minutes
   - Followed by a single 4 mg/kg dose infused over 30 minutes

Monitor

- Clinical response
- Therapeutic concentrations: 1.5–6 mcg/mL
- Document total drug amount infused every 12 hours

with sickle cell disease. A retrospective review examined studies performed during 2004–2014 on the use of lidocaine infusions in sickle cell adults with VOC pain. Patients received a lidocaine infusion for approximately 4.4 days. More than 50% of patients reported a significant reduction in pain scores. Patients had a mean reduction in opioid use of approximately 32%. Side effects, including disorientation and dizziness, were reported by 2 patients. Another recent retrospective study performed in sickle cell adolescents with VOC pain yielded similar results, demonstrating decreased opioid consumption in those receiving lidocaine infusions.[65] Table 42.2 illustrates a protocol for in-patient lidocaine infusions, adapted from the University of Chicago Medical Center.

Pain Interventions

VOC pain is challenging to manage. Pain interventions can reduce opioid consumption and improve functionality.

Long-term use of NSAIDs can have toxic side effects, and chronic opioid therapy often leads to OIT or OIH, with subsequent refractory pain. When conventional methods fail, interventional therapies can be an effective treatment option.

Joint Injections

Treatment for VOC pain and subsequent complications in affected joints depends on the extent of the disease. Patients in the early stages of AVN may require medical management, while patients in the later stages with severe symptoms will require surgical intervention (e.g., core decompression or hip arthroplasty). Disease progression involves the flattening and collapse of the femoral head, resulting in secondary degenerative arthritis (Figure 42.1).[66] Intra-articular hip injections with corticosteroids may provide temporary relief. Intra-articular hip injection can be performed under fluoroscopy or ultrasound guidance. Fluoroscopy allows confirmation of needle placement by visualization of contrast (Figure 42.2), while ultrasound shows neurovascular structures and avoids radiation exposure.[67]

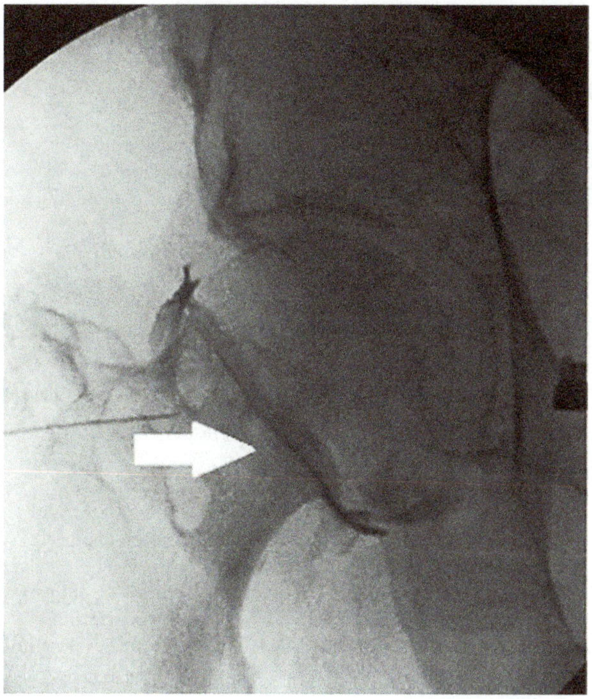

Figure 42.2. Intra-articular hip injection. Intra-articular hip joint injection under fluoroscopy with arthrography revealing the classic "halo" (white arrow) that forms as the contrasts circle the femoral head/neck junction.

Regional Anesthesia

Regional anesthesia, including neuraxial analgesia and peripheral nerve blocks, can offer certain benefits in the prevention and treatment of VOC pain. Neuraxial anesthesia is associated with vasodilation, theoretically decreasing the likelihood of a VOC episode. Local anesthetics decrease the adherence of leukocytes to endothelium, resulting in a systemic anti-inflammatory effect.[68] Neuraxial and regional anesthesia typically provide superior analgesia than opioids alone. Peripheral nerve blocks and epidurals are associated with less opioid consumption in the postoperative period and avoid the undesirable side effects of opioid therapy.[69] Intercostal nerve blocks can reduce chest wall pain and splinting.[70] The benefits of regional anesthesia must be weighed against the associated risks such as hypotension, bradycardia, and hypoxia (from high spinal levels of anesthesia), all of which will exacerbate an acute VOC episode.[71]

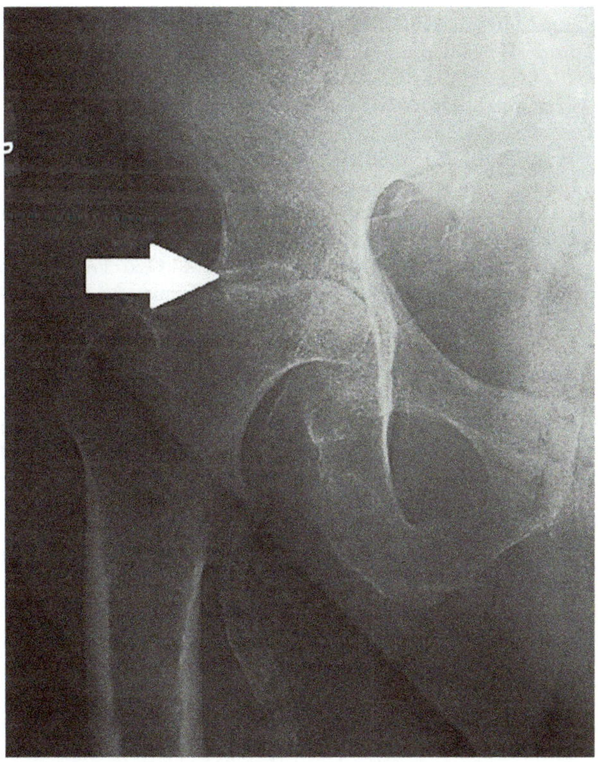

Figure 42.1. Avascular necrosis right hip. Deformity of the femoral head (white arrow) with diffuse flattening and depression of the superior articular surface perhaps representing sequela of avascular necrosis.

Current research is sparse on the use of regional anesthesia in VOC pain. One case report describes the successful use of a femoral nerve block to reduce refractory VOC lower extremity pain. The patient received a continuous infusion of ropivacaine via a femoral nerve catheter. The study did not report if there was a reduction in opioid consumption.[72] Regional anesthesia is a promising tool for the treatment of acute VOC pain that has not effectively been managed by medications.

Clinical Algorithms for Managing VOC Episodes

Multiple guidelines exist for the management of VOC pain episodes. Further studies are needed to evaluate the efficacy of varying opioid analgesics regimens in the treatment of VOC pain episodes. Employing clinical algorithms to manage VOC pain demonstrates faster delivery of analgesia, improved satisfaction, shorter hospital stays, reduced costs, and increased use of primary care providers to manage pain.[73] Table 42.3 is an example of a clinical algorithm for the treatment of acute

Table 42.3 **IN-PATIENT ACUTE VOC SICKLE CELL PAIN MANAGEMENT ALGORITHM**

Admission

- Review individualized HPMP
- Continue prior to admission (PTA) long-acting opioid
- Check Illinois prescription monitoring program
- Provide non-pharmacologic pain management patient education materials
- Initiate multimodal analgesia if not contraindicated:
  - o Acetaminophen 650 mg Q6h
  - o Ibuprofen 600 mg Q6h
    - Exclusion: acute kidney injury, cardiac disease
  - o Gabapentin 300 mg TID
  - o Hydromorphone PCA × 24 hours

24 hours from admission

- Discontinue PCA
- Continue acetaminophen, ibuprofen, and gabapentin
- *Pain is well-controlled*:
  - o Start oxycodone or hydromorphone "standard analgesic regimen"
    - Standing dose calculated by administering 50% of prior 24-hour consumption divided into Q4h administrations
    - Equivalent dose should be available as needed every 4 hours
- *Pain NOT controlled (at 24 hours)*:
  - o Start oxycodone or hydromorphone "standard analgesic regimen"
    - Standing dose calculated by administering 75%–100% of prior 24-hour consumption divided into Q4h administrations
    - Equivalent dose should be available as needed every 4 hours
  - o Start methadone

Methadone starting dose (mg)	Oral morphine equivalents (24-hour total)
2.5 mg TID	< 60 mg/day
5 mg TID	60–300 mg/day
Consider expert consultation	>300 mg/day

* Concurrent opioid dose should **not be escalated** while receiving methadone as a co-analgesic.

Titration:

- Patients started on 7.5 mg per day can be titrated to 15 mg per day after 24 hours of dosing (if no relief).
- Doses should not be titrated greater than 15 mg per day without expert consultation.

Pain still not relieved after 24 hours from above interventions

- Consult Acute Pain Service for consideration of ketamine, lidocaine, or interventional techniques.

Pain episode resolves

- Resume PTA medication and attempt to wean opioid therapy to lowest effective dose as tolerated.

VOC pain episode adapted from the University of Chicago Medical Center.

CONCLUSIONS AND KEY POINTS

- A thorough assessment is required given the range of pathophysiological manifestations of SCD.
- Incorporating patient education, psychological therapy, pharmacological agents, and individualized (HPMP) into treatment plans can reduce the frequency and/or severity of VOC episodes.
- Optimal management of a VOC pain episode should incorporate a multimodal approach that includes patient education and non-pharmacologic, pharmacologic, and interventional methods.
- Incorporating clinical algorithms for the treatment of acute VOC pain episodes can lead to improved overall pain control, decreased hospital stays, and increased utilization of provider services to manage pain.

REFERENCES

1. Yaster M, Kost-Byerly S, Maxwell LG. The management of pain in sickle cell disease. *Pediatr Clin North Am.* 2000;47(3):699–710.
2. Hassell KL. Population estimates of sickle cell disease in the U.S. *Am J Prev Med.* 2010;38(4 Suppl):S512–S521.
3. Ingram VM. A specific chemical difference between the globins of normal human and sickle-cell anaemia haemoglobin. *Nature.* 1956;178(4537):792–794.
4. Ballas SK, Lusardi M. Hospital readmission for adult acute sickle cell painful episodes: frequency, etiology, and prognostic significance. *Am J Hematol.* 2005;79(1):17–25.
5. Smith WR, Penberthy LT, Bovbjerg VE, et al. Daily assessment of pain in adults with sickle cell disease. *Ann Intern Med.* 2008;148(2):94–101.
6. Platt OS, Thorington BD, Brambilla DJ, et al. Pain in sickle cell disease: rates and risk factors. *N Engl J Med.* 1991;325(1):11–16.
7. Sundd P, Gladwin MT, Novelli EM. Pathophysiology of sickle cell disease. *Annu Rev Pathol.* 2019;14:263–292.
8. Bunn HF, Noguchi CT, Hofrichter J, Schechter GP, Schechter AN, Eaton WA. Molecular and cellular pathogenesis of hemoglobin SC disease. *Proc Natl Acad Sci U S A.* 1982;79(23):7527–7531.
9. Charache S, Dover GJ, Moore RD, et al. Hydroxyurea: effects on hemoglobin F production in patients with sickle cell anemia. *Blood.* 1992;79(10):2555–2565.
10. Brooks LJ, Koziol SM, Chiarucci KM, Berman BW. Does sleep-disordered breathing contribute to the clinical severity of sickle cell anemia? *J Pediatr Hematol Oncol.* 1996;18(2):135–139.
11. Stockman JA, Nigro MA, Mishkin MM, Oski FA. Occlusion of large cerebral vessels in sickle-cell anemia. *N Engl J Med.* 1972;287(17):846–849.
12. Kaul DK, Fabry ME, Nagel RL. Erythrocytic and vascular factors influencing the microcirculatory behavior of blood in sickle cell anemia. *Ann N Y Acad Sci.* 1989;565:316–326.
13. Wagner MC, Eckman JR, Wick TM. Sickle cell adhesion depends on hemodynamics and endothelial activation. *J Lab Clin Med.* 2004;144(5):260–267; discussion 227–268.
14. Telen MJ. Beyond hydroxyurea: new and old drugs in the pipeline for sickle cell disease. *Blood.* 2016;127(7):810–819.
15. Basbaum AI, Bautista DM, Scherrer G, Julius D. Cellular and molecular mechanisms of pain. *Cell.* 2009;139(2):267–284.
16. Ballas SK. Pathophysiology and principles of management of the many faces of the acute vaso-occlusive crisis in patients with sickle cell disease. *Eur J Haematol.* 2015;95(2):113–123.
17. Giordano P. Newborn screening for haemoglobinopathies. In: Old J, Angastiniotis M, Eleftheriou A, Galanello R, eds. *Prevention of Thalassaemias and Other Haemoglobin Disorders.* Vol 1. 2nd ed. Nicosia, Cyprus: Principles [Internet]; 2013.
18. Reed W, Lane PA, Lorey F, et al. Sickle-cell disease not identified by newborn screening because of prior transfusion. *J Pediatr.* 2000;136(2):248–250.

19. Michlitsch J, Azimi M, Hoppe C, et al. Newborn screening for hemoglobinopathies in California. *Pediatr Blood Cancer.* 2009;52(4):486–490.
20. Henthorn JS, Almeida AM, Davies SC. Neonatal screening for sickle cell disorders. *Br J Haematol.* 2004;124(3):259–263.
21. Ballas SK, Delengowski A. Pain measurement in hospitalized adults with sickle cell painful episodes. *Ann Clin Lab Sci.* 1993;23(5):358–361.
22. Almeida A, Roberts I. Bone involvement in sickle cell disease. *Br J Haematol.* 2005;129(4):482–490.
23. Smith WR, Bauserman RL, Ballas SK, et al. Climatic and geographic temporal patterns of pain in the Multicenter Study of Hydroxyurea. *Pain.* 2009;146(1–2):91–98.
24. Glassberg J, Spivey JF, Strunk R, Boslaugh S, DeBaun MR. Painful episodes in children with sickle cell disease and asthma are temporally associated with respiratory symptoms. *J Pediatr Hematol Oncol.* 2006;28(8):481–485.
25. Yoong WC, Tuck SM. Menstrual pattern in women with sickle cell anaemia and its association with sickling crises. *J Obstet Gynaecol.* 2002;22(4):399–401.
26. Resar LM, Oski FA. Cold water exposure and vaso-occlusive crises in sickle cell anemia. *J Pediatr.* 1991;118(3):407–409.
27. Borhade M, Kondamudi N. Sickle cell crisis. In. *StatPearls.* Treasure Island, FL: StatPearls [Internet]; 2021.
28. Ballas SK, Lieff S, Benjamin LJ, et al. Definitions of the phenotypic manifestations of sickle cell disease. *Am J Hematol.* 2010;85(1):6–13.
29. Hebbel RP, Boogaerts MA, Eaton JW, Steinberg MH. Erythrocyte adherence to endothelium in sickle-cell anemia: a possible determinant of disease severity. *N Engl J Med.* 1980;302(18):992–995.
30. Noubiap JJ, Temgoua MN, Tankeu R, Tochie JN, Wonkam A, Bigna JJ. Sickle cell disease, sickle trait and the risk for venous thromboembolism: a systematic review and meta-analysis. *Thromb J.* 2018;16:27.
31. Gupta S, Yui JC, Xu D, et al. Gout and sickle cell disease: not all pain is sickle cell pain. *Br J Haematol.* 2015;171(5):872–875.
32. Yawn BP, Buchanan GR, Afenyi-Annan AN, et al. Management of sickle cell disease: summary of the 2014 evidence-based report by expert panel members. *JAMA.* 2014;312(10):1033–1048.
33. Darbari DS, Brandow AM. Pain-measurement tools in sickle cell disease: where are we now? *Hematology Am Soc Hematol Educ Program.* 2017;2017(1):534–541.
34. Gloth FM, 3rd, Scheve AA, Stober CV, Chow S, Prosser J. The Functional Pain Scale: reliability, validity, and responsiveness in an elderly population. *J Am Med Dir Assoc.* 2001;2(3):110–114.
35. Pasero C, McCaffery M. Comfort-function goals: a way to establish accountability for pain relief. *Am J Nurs.* 2004;104(9):77–78, 81.
36. Keller SD, Yang M, Treadwell MJ, Werner EM, Hassell KL. Patient reports of health outcome for adults living with sickle cell disease: development and testing of the ASCQ-Me item banks. *Health Qual Life Outcomes.* 2014;12:125.
37. Dampier C, Palermo TM, Darbari DS, Hassell K, Smith W, Zempsky W. AAPT diagnostic criteria for chronic sickle cell disease pain. *J Pain.* 2017;18(5):490–498.
38. Shapiro BS, Benjamin LJ, Payne R, Heidrich G. Sickle cell-related pain: perceptions of medical practitioners. *J Pain Symptom Manage.* 1997;14(3):168–174.
39. Zempsky WT. Treatment of sickle cell pain: fostering trust and justice. *JAMA.* 2009;302(22):2479–2480.
40. Anie KA, Green J. Psychological therapies for sickle cell disease and pain. *Cochrane Database Syst Rev.* 2012;2:CD001916.
41. Miller ST, Wright E, Abboud M, et al. Impact of chronic transfusion on incidence of pain and acute chest syndrome during the Stroke Prevention Trial (STOP) in sickle-cell anemia. *J Pediatr.* 2001;139(6):785–789.
42. Bartolucci P, Chaar V, Picot J, et al. Decreased sickle red blood cell adhesion to laminin by hydroxyurea is associated with inhibition of Lu/BCAM protein phosphorylation. *Blood.* 2010;116(12):2152–2159.
43. FDA. https://www.fda.gov/NewsEvents/Newsroom/PressAnnouncements/ucm566084.htm. In: Accessed April 20, 2019.
44. Minniti CP. L-glutamine and the dawn of combination therapy for sickle cell disease. *N Engl J Med.* 2018;379(3):292–294.
45. Niihara Y, Smith WR, Stark CW. A phase 3 trial of l-glutamine in sickle cell disease. *N Engl J Med.* 2018;379(19):1880.
46. Crosby LE, Simmons K, Kaiser P, et al. Using quality improvement methods to implement an electronic medical record (EMR) supported individualized home pain management plan for children with sickle cell disease. *J Clin Outcomes Manag.* 2014;21(5):210–217.
47. Puri L, Nottage KA, Hankins JS, Anghelescu DL. State of the art management of acute vaso-occlusive pain in sickle cell disease. *Paediatr Drugs.* 2018;20(1):29–42.
48. Manfredi PL, Houde RW. Prescribing methadone, a unique analgesic. *J Support Oncol.* 2003;1(3):216–220.
49. Borgerding MP, Absher RK, So TY. Tramadol use in pediatric sickle cell disease patients with vaso-occlusive crisis. *World J Clin Pediatr.* 2013;2(4):65–69.
50. Erhan E, Inal MT, Aydinok Y, Balkan C, Yegul I. Tramadol infusion for the pain management in sickle cell disease: a case report. *Paediatr Anaesth.* 2007;17(1):84–86.
51. de Franceschi L, Finco G, Vassanelli A, Zaia B, Ischia S, Corrocher R. A pilot study on the efficacy of ketorolac plus tramadol infusion combined with erythrocytapheresis in the management of acute severe vaso-occlusive crises and sickle cell pain. *Haematologica.* 2004;89(11):1389–1391.
52. Latta KS, Ginsberg B, Barkin RL. Meperidine: a critical review. *Am J Ther.* 2002;9(1):53–68.
53. Friesen KJ, Falk J, Bugden S. The safety of meperidine prescribing in older adults: a longitudinal population-based study. *BMC Geriatr.* 2016;16:100.
54. Melzer-Lange MD, Walsh-Kelly CM, Lea G, Hillery CA, Scott JP. Patient-controlled analgesia for sickle cell pain crisis in a pediatric emergency department. *Pediatr Emerg Care.* 2004;20(1):2–4.
55. Dampier CD, Smith WR, Wager CG, et al. IMPROVE trial: a randomized controlled trial of patient-controlled analgesia for sickle cell painful episodes: rationale, design challenges, initial experience, and recommendations for future studies. *Clin Trials.* 2013;10(2):319–331.
56. Zempsky WT. Evaluation and treatment of sickle cell pain in the emergency department: paths to a better future. *Clin Pediatr Emerg Med.* 2010;11(4):265–273.
57. Parrish MR, Morrison JC. Sickle cell crisis and pregnancy. *Semin Perinatol.* 2013;37(4):274–279.
58. Allon M, Lawson L, Eckman JR, Delaney V, Bourke E. Effects of nonsteroidal antiinflammatory drugs on renal function in sickle cell anemia. *Kidney Int.* 1988;34(4):500–506.
59. Ketorolac. Ketorolac tromethamine injection, solution [product information]. Lake Forest IH, Inc; June 2011.
60. Amr YM, Yousef AA. Evaluation of efficacy of the perioperative administration of Venlafaxine or gabapentin on acute and chronic postmastectomy pain. *Clin J Pain.* 2010;26(5):381–385.
61. Wilkie DJ, Molokie R, Boyd-Seal D, et al. Patient-reported outcomes: descriptors of nociceptive and neuropathic pain and barriers to effective pain management in adult outpatients with sickle cell disease. *J Natl Med Assoc.* 2010;102(1):18–27.
62. Fink K, Dooley DJ, Meder WP, et al. Inhibition of neuronal Ca(2+) influx by gabapentin and pregabalin in the human neocortex. *Neuropharmacology.* 2002;42(2):229–236.
63. Obata H. Analgesic mechanisms of antidepressants for neuropathic pain. *Int J Mol Sci.* 2017;18(11).
64. Uprety D, Baber A, Foy M. Ketamine infusion for sickle cell pain crisis refractory to opioids: a case report and review of literature. *Ann Hematol.* 2014;93(5):769–771.
65. Puri L, Morgan KJ, Anghelescu DL. Ketamine and lidocaine infusions decrease opioid consumption during vaso-occlusive crisis in adolescents with sickle cell disease. *Curr Opin Support Palliat Care.* 2019;13(4):402–407.
66. Lespasio MJ, Sodhi N, Mont MA. Osteonecrosis of the hip: a primer. *Perm J.* 2019;23.

67. Benzon H, Raja S, Fishman S, Liu S, Cohen S. *Essentials of Pain Medicine*. Philadelphia: Elsevier Health Sciences; 2011 Jun 30.
68. Hollmann MW, Durieux ME. Local anesthetics and the inflammatory response: a new therapeutic indication? *Anesthesiology*. 2000;93(3):858–875.
69. Kettner SC, Willschke H, Marhofer P. Does regional anaesthesia really improve outcome? *Br J Anaesth*. 2011;107(Suppl 1):i90–i95.
70. Paul RN, Castro OL, Aggarwal A, Oneal PA. Acute chest syndrome: sickle cell disease. *Eur J Haematol*. 2011;87(3):191–207.
71. Khurmi N, Gorlin A, Misra L. Perioperative considerations for patients with sickle cell disease: a narrative review. *Can J Anaesth*. 2017;64(8):860–869.
72. Vuong J, Pilipovic M. Use of continuous regional anesthetic for management of pediatric sickle cell crisis. *Open J Anesthesiol*. 2012;2(5):228–229.
73. Kavanagh PL, Sprinz PG, Wolfgang TL, et al. Improving the management of vaso-occlusive episodes in the pediatric emergency department. *Pediatrics*. 2015;136(4):e1016–1025.

REVIEW QUESTIONS

(1) A 26-year-old female with a history of sickle cell anemia presents to the emergency department with complaints of severe dyspnea and pain in her extremities. She takes gabapentin 600 mg 3 times a day at home to treat chronic pain. She is afebrile with mildly elevated blood pressure, heart rate, and respiratory rate. Oxygen saturation is 94% on room air. Her lab values are within normal limits. She took ibuprofen 600 mg and acetaminophen 650 mg every 6 hours for the past 24 hours without benefit. What is the first step in management after initiation of intravenous hydration?

A. Erythrocyte transfusion
B. Intravenous (IV) hydromorphone
C. IV meperidine
D. Hydroxyurea

(2) Regional anesthesia may be beneficial in managing an acute vaso-occlusive crisis (VOC) pain episode for all of the following reasons, EXCEPT:

A. Decreased opioid consumption
B. Systemic vasoconstriction
C. Improved oxygenation
D. Good pain control

(3) A 32-year-old male with a history of SCD is taking hydroxyurea to aid in prevention of VOC episodes. He asks if there is anything else he can take. Which of the following medications would you recommend?

A. Acetylcysteine
B. L-carnitine
C. L-glutamine
D. Vitamin C

(4) In the majority of states, testing for sickle cell disease(SCD) is most commonly performed at what age?

A. In utero via blood sample
B. Newborn via blood sample
C. 6 months
D. 10 years

(5) A 26-year-old, 34-week pregnant patient with SCD is having a mild vaso-occlusive crisis episode (VOC). Which medicine should be avoided?

A. Nonsteroidal anti-inflammatory drugs (NSAIDs)
B. Acetaminophen
C. Gabapentin
D. Tramadol

(6) Methadone acts on all of the following, except:

A. A μ-receptor agonist
B. N-methyl D-aspartate receptor agonist
C. Reuptake inhibitor of serotonin and norepinephrine
D. Producer of incomplete cross-tolerance with opioid rotation

(7) Use of an individualized home pain management plans (HPMP) will result in all of the following, except:

A. Increased patient involvement in their healthcare
B. Increased hospital costs as a combination of different classes of analgesics can be expensive
C. Fewer emergency room (ER)visits
D. Decreased hospital costs

(8) Clinical algorithms for managing acute VOC pain episodes have demonstrated all of the following, except:

A. Decreased time to delivery of patient analgesia
B. Improved overall pain control
C. Reduced total days in the hospital
D. Decreased use of primary care providers

(9) A 21-year-old African American male with a history of SCD presents to the emergency department complaining of multiple joint pain and chest tightness occurring for 1 week. His vital signs and physical examination are unremarkable. His admission labs include hemoglobin of 7.4 g/dl, chest x-ray showing lower lobe opacity and interstitial thickening. He is treated for an acute VOC pain episode and community-acquired pneumonia with intravenous fluids, supplemental oxygen, and intravenous levofloxacin. He is placed on hydromorphone patient-controlled analgesia (PCA), oxycodone, ketorolac, and methadone with gabapentin and venlafaxine. Over the course of hospitalization, his chest pain resolves, but his joint pain continues. He has now been hospitalized for more than 4 weeks. What is your next step in managing his pain?

A. Increase his PCA dosage and frequency
B. Increase his oxycodone dosage and frequency
C. Add more opioids to his regimen
D. Add a ketamine infusion

(10) A 27-year-old female with SCD presents with an acute VOC pain episode. Tissue injury in SCD generates multiple pain mediators. All of the following are considered catalysts in pain transmission, except:

A. Serotonin
B. Bradykinin
C. IL-10
D. TGF-alpha

ANSWERS

(1) B In addition to hydration, the first step in managing an uncomplicated painful episode in patients with sickle cell disease (SCD) generally involves initiation of non-opioid and opioid medications. Meperidine is generally avoided in patients with SCD because it has a short half-life and may lower the seizure threshold. Blood transfusions are not recommended in the treatment of an uncomplicated VOC episode unless the patient has symptomatic anemia.

Reference

Puri, L, Nottage KA, Hankins JS, Anghelescu DL. State of the art management of acute vaso-occlusive pain in sickle cell disease. *Pediatric Drugs*. 2018;20(1):29–42.

(2) **B.** Local anesthetics cause vasodilation, which theoretically decreases the risk of VOC. Regional anesthesia has been shown to decrease opioid consumption and can decrease the risk of unwanted side effects from opioids, including hypoventilation.

Reference

Paul RN, Castro OL, Aggarwal A, Oneal, PA. Acute chest syndrome: sickle cell disease. *Eur J Haematol*. 2011;87(3):191–207.

(3) **C.** L-glutamine was approved by the FDA in 2017 to help prevent SCD complications in patients older than 5 years of age. The production of this essential amino acid is reduced during times of stress. A randomized controlled trial found fewer pain events, reduced hospitalizations, and decreased frequency of acute chest syndrome. The other medications listed are used to help with neuropathic pain.

Reference

Platt OS, Thorington BD, Brambilla DJ, et al. Pain in sickle cell disease: rates and risk factors. *N Engl J Med*. 1991;325(1):11–16.

(4) **B.** While diagnosis of SCD depends on a patient's age, a blood test to detect SCD is most commonly performed in newborns. Prenatal testing can also be performed, but amniotic fluid is used to make the diagnosis. Older patients can also be tested using high-performance liquid chromatography and isoelectric focused testing, but these occur less frequently than testing of newborns.

References

Giordano P. Newborn screening for haemoglobinopathies. In: Angastiniotis M, Eleftheriou A, Galanello R et al., eds. *Prevention of Thalassaemias and Other Haemoglobin Disorders*, Vol. 1: *Principles* [Internet]. 2nd ed. Nicosia, Cyprus: Thalassaemia International Federation; 2013. Chapter 10. Available from: https://www.ncbi.nlm.nih.gov/books/NBK190476/

Michlitsch J, Azimi M, Hoppe C, et al. Newborn screening for hemoglobinopathies in California. *Pediatr Blood Cancer*. 2009;52:486.

Henthorn JS, Almeida AM, Davies SC. Neonatal screening for sickle cell disorders. *Br J Haematol.* 2004;124:259.

(5) **A.** Nonsteroidal anti-inflammatory drugs (NSAIDs) should be avoided after the 30th week of pregnancy as they decrease glomerular filtration rate and increase the risk for ARF in patients with SCD.

References

Parrish MR, Morrison JC. Sickle cell crisis and pregnancy. *Semin Perinatol.* 2013;37:274–279.

Allon M, Lawson L, Eckman JR, et al. Effects of nonsteroidal anti-inflammatory drugs on renal function in sickle cell anemia. *Kidney Int.* 1988;34:500.

(6) **B.** Methadone is an N-methyl-D-aspartate receptor antagonist. Answers A, C, and D list the potential benefits of methadone over conventional opioids in counteracting opioid-induced hyperalgesia (OIH) and opioid induced tolerance (OIT).

Reference

Manfredi PL, Houde RW. Prescribing methadone, a unique analgesic. *J Support Oncol*. 2003; 1(3):2216–2220.

(7) **B.** Individualized HPMPs are being used more frequently in the sickle cell population as they have been shown to reduce the number of ED visits for SCD uncomplicated pain episodes by 84%. Patients and families feel empowered as they have more tools to manage uncomplicated pain episodes at home. Quality improvement studies have shown an overall decrease and not increase in healthcare costs.

Reference

Crosby LE, Simmons K, Kaiser P, et al. Using quality improvement methods to implement an electronic medical record (EMR) supported individualized home pain management plan for children with sickle cell disease. *J Clin Outcomes Manag*. 2014;21(5):210–217.

(8) **D.** Clinical algorithms for managing acute VOC pain episodes resulted in decreased time to delivery of analgesia, reduced total hospital days and costs, improved pain control, and increased use of primary providers to help patients manage pain.

Reference

Kavanagh P, Sprinz P, Wolfgang T, et al. Improving management of vaso-occlusive episodes in the pediatric emergency department. *Pediatrics*. 2015;136:1016–1025.

(9) **D.** Ketamine is a noncompetitive antagonist at NMDA receptor. This property has been shown to modulate OIT and OIH. There are very few published reports on the use of low-dose ketamine in sickle cell pain management. One study found that 14 of the 17 patients (82%) who received ketamine infusions showed improvement in self-reported pain intensity and significant reductions in opioid dosage.

Reference

Uprety D, Baber A, Foy M. Ketamine infusion for sickle cell pain crisis refractory to opioids: a case report and review of literature. *Ann Hematol*. 2014 May 1;93(5):769–771.

(10) **A.** VOC leads to ischemia and inflammation. An increase in inflammatory biomarkers such as bradykinin, substance P,

IL-10, IL-6, TGF-alpha, and TNF-alpha will sensitize nociceptors. Nociceptors translate the stimulus from inflammatory mediators. Serotonin does not sensitize nociceptors; in fact, it is an endogenous pain inhibitor.

Reference

Ballas SK. Pathophysiology and principles of management of the many faces of the acute vaso-occlusive crisis in patients with sickle cell disease. *Eur J Haematol.* 2015;95(2):113–123.

SECTION 11

ANTICOAGULATION AND REGIONAL ANESTHESIA

Jinlei Li

43.

EPIDURAL PLACEMENT AND ANTICOAGULATION

Maryam Nilforoshan, Veena Graff, and Taras Grosh

STEM CASE AND KEY QUESTIONS

A 55-year-old female presents to the emergency department with complaints of right chest pain, pain on inspiration, and dyspnea following a mechanical fall down half a flight of stairs approximately 1 hour ago. The patient's past medical history is notable for atrial fibrillation, for which she has been taking apixaban (Eliquis) 5 mg twice daily for the past 5 years. Anteroposterior and lateral chest films reveal multiple right-sided rib fractures. Despite treatment with escalating doses of acetaminophen, ketorolac, and intravenous hydromorphone, the patient continues to complain of severe chest pain, which is making inhalation difficult. An anesthesiologist is consulted for pain management recommendations.

(1) WHAT IS THE HALF-LIFE OF APIXABAN? FOR HOW LONG MUST APIXABAN BE HELD PRIOR TO EPIDURAL CATHETER PLACEMENT?

The anesthesiologist evaluates the patient and obtains a full history. The patient reports last taking apixaban 12 hours ago. The anesthesiologist explains that due to concerns for elevated risk of epidural hematoma in the setting of recent anticoagulation, an epidural cannot be done before 72 hours. The patient expresses interest in alternative regional anesthesia techniques.

(2) WHICH REGIONAL ANESTHESIA TECHNIQUES ARE ALTERNATIVES TO NEURAXIAL NERVE BLOCKS IN THE SETTING OF ANTICOAGULATION?

After explaining the risks and benefits and obtaining patient consent, the anesthesiologist places an erector spinae catheter. Following an initial bolus, a special pump is utilized to administer intermittent 8 mL boluses of ropivacaine 0.2% every 30 minutes. Within 15 minutes of catheter placement, the patient reports a marked reduction in pain. She is admitted to the floor and started on a multimodal analgesia regimen. She is doing well with stable vital signs until 4 hours later, when she is found to be acutely hypotensive (blood pressure 79/43), tachycardic (heart rate 131), and hypoxic. A chest tube is placed emergently and 1 liter of blood is evacuated, confirming hemothorax. The patient is scheduled for an emergent thoracotomy.

(3) WHAT REVERSAL AGENTS CAN BE USED TO REVERSE THE ANTICOAGULANT EFFECT OF DIRECT FACTOR XA INHIBITORS SUCH AS APIXABAN?

The patient receives a dose of Andexanet alfa (Andexxa). The patient successfully undergoes both a thoracotomy and exploratory laparotomy under general anesthesia. In the recovery room postoperatively, the patient complains of severe pain at the thoracotomy and laparotomy incision sites. The anesthesiologist removes the erector spinae catheter and places a thoracic epidural catheter. After an epidural bolus and initiation of a continuous infusion, the patient's pain greatly improves. The next morning, the anesthesiologist is consulted by the surgeon regarding starting the patient on twice-daily enoxaparin for deep vein thrombosis prophylaxis.

(4) WHAT ARE THROMBOPROPHYLAXIS OPTIONS FOR A PATIENT WITH AN INDWELLING EPIDURAL CATHETER? HOW LONG MUST ONE WAIT AFTER EPIDURAL PLACEMENT PRIOR TO INITIATION OF THROMBOPROPHYLAXIS?

You recommend starting the patient on once daily enoxaparin for deep vein thrombosis prophylaxis as well as intermittent pneumatic compression devices. The patient continues to progress well and reports feeling much improved. On postop day 5, her epidural is capped, and she is successfully transitioned to oral medications with adequate pain control.

(5) FOR HOW LONG MUST THROMBOPROPHYLAXIS BE HELD PRIOR TO EPIDURAL CATHETER REMOVAL?

The anesthesiologist examines the medication administration record and determines that the last dose of enoxaparin was 8 hours ago. He checks the patient's morning labs and notes that her platelet count has remained stable in the 200s throughout her admission. The epidural catheter is removed after 12 hours from the last enoxaparin dose.

(6) WHEN CAN ANTICOAGULANT MEDICATIONS BE RESUMED FOLLOWING EPIDURAL CATHETER REMOVAL?

The patient is discharged home with oral pain medications. She is instructed to take her first dose of home apixaban at least 6 hours after her epidural catheter was removed.

DISCUSSION

Epidural analgesia is a frequently used regional anesthesia technique for perioperative pain control. Use of epidural analgesia is associated with many benefits compared to traditional intravenous opioid-based analgesia, including superior analgesia, increased patient satisfaction, and reduced intensive care unit stay compared to intravenous analgesia alone.[1] However, epidural analgesia is not without risk, with potential for accidental dural puncture, neurovascular injury during catheter placement, epidural abscess, meningitis, and epidural hematoma. Although injury to spinal vasculature during epidural catheter placement occurs in 3%–12% of cases, the incidence of epidural hematoma is very low, at less than 1 in 150,000–220,000.[1] The main risk factor for epidural hematoma is anticoagulation.[2] As a result, anesthesiologists must exercise extreme caution when placing and removing epidural catheters in individuals on anticoagulation, as well as when starting thromboprophylaxis in patients with indwelling epidural catheters. The American Society of Regional Anesthesia (ASRA) has provided guidelines regarding administration of neuraxial anesthesia in the setting of anticoagulants and antiplatelets; these guidelines are based on the medication pharmacokinetics and pharmacodynamics, as well as published reports of neuraxial bleeding in patients receiving these medications.[3] In this chapter, we will discuss these guidelines in depth.

ALTERNATIVES TO NEURAXIAL NERVE BLOCKS IN THE PRESENCE OF ANTICOAGULATION

In instances where neuraxial nerve blocks are indicated for analgesia in patients on anticoagulation, one must carefully evaluate the patient's current anticoagulant medications, their dosages, and the timing of the most recent dose administration. Occasionally epidural placement may be contraindicated in these patients per ASRA recommendations. Although thoracic paravertebral blocks are often considered as an alternative to epidural catheters, the regional anesthesia community considers them deep non-compressible blocks, associated with potential for hemorrhagic complications. As such, ASRA recommends that when considering performance of deep peripheral blocks such as thoracic paravertebral blocks in a patient on anticoagulation, one applies the same guidelines as for neuraxial nerve blocks.[3] Fortunately, in the event that neuraxial nerve blocks and paravertebral nerve blocks are contraindicated due to anticoagulation, there are several alternative regional anesthesia techniques that can be used for effective analgesia, depending on the anatomic location requiring coverage.

INTERCOSTAL NERVE BLOCK (ICNB)

The block can be performed with a single injection; alternatively, continuous ICNBs entail threading an indwelling intercostal catheter Often, this technique will require multiple injections of local anesthetic, as it is recommended that one perform the block 2 dermatomes above and below the level of the surgical incision. Studies have shown that continuous ICNBs with indwelling intercostal catheters and thoracic epidurals provided postoperative analgesia of comparable efficacy.[4–6]

INTERPLEURAL BLOCK

The goal of the interpleural block is local anesthetic injection between the parietal and visceral pleura, resulting in ipsilateral sensory blockade of multiple thoracic dermatomes. It can be performed by needle insertion in the 8th intercostal space 10 cm lateral to the dorsal midline until a passive loss of resistance is identified, indicating negative pressure, and confirming the location of the needle in the interpleural space. The local anesthetic can be administered as either a bolus or as a continuous infusion via an indwelling interpleural catheter.[7]

The interpleural block can provide chest and upper abdominal analgesia for both chronic and acute pain. Acutely, it has been used for postoperative analgesia following thoracotomy, breast surgery, cholecystectomy, and renal surgery.[7] Although interpleural block has been shown to provide effective analgesia in the setting of unilateral subcostal and flank incisions, studies suggest that the interpleural block results in unreliable analgesia in the setting of thoracotomy.[8] A review evaluating regional techniques for post-thoracotomy analgesia identified thoracic epidural and paravertebral blocks as the most effective, followed by intercostal blocks and intrathecal techniques; however, interpleural blocks were found to provide ineffective analgesia for post-thoracotomy pain.[9] Possible reasons for this lack of efficacy include loss of local anesthetic through chest drains, dilution of local anesthetic in pleural effusions, and binding of local anesthetic with proteins.[8]

Contraindications to interpleural block include empyema, pleural effusions, pleural adhesions or history of pleurodesis, and contralateral phrenic nerve paralysis. The interpleural block is also associated with numerous possible side effects, including pneumothorax, local anesthetic systemic toxicity (LAST), catheter misplacement, Horner's syndrome, phrenic nerve paralysis, infection, and interbronchial injection. Of these potential complications, the primary concerns are pneumothorax, which has a 2% incidence, and LAST, which has a 1.3% incidence in patients undergoing interpleural blocks.[8]

THORACIC WALL BLOCKS

The Pectoralis nerve block (PEC) blocks and serratus anterior plane (SAP) Block provide analgesia for the anterior and lateral thoracic chest wall. These interfascial injections provide an alternative to epidurals in instances requiring analgesia of the thorax.[10]

Pectoralis Nerve (PEC) Blocks

The PEC blocks include the pectoral nerve block type I (PEC I) and pectoral nerve block type II (PEC II). PEC I blocks involve a local anesthetic injection in the fascial plane between the pectoralis major and pectoralis minor muscles, thereby blocking the medial and lateral pectoral nerves that innervate the pectoralis muscles.[10] Indications for the PEC I block include placement of breast expanders, shoulder surgery with deltopectoral groove involvement, and pacemaker insertion.[11]

Serratus Anterior Plane (SAP) Block

SAP Block provide effective analgesia for patients with multiple rib fractures and thoracic pain, leading to facilitation of weaning from mechanical ventilation, ambulation, and participation in chest physiotherapy.[12–14]

ERECTOR SPINAE PLANE BLOCK (ESPB)

Since the introduction of erector spinae plane block (ESPB), there have been many cases reported of ESPB being used to treat both chronic and acute pain, with the ESPB demonstrated as an effective alternative to epidural analgesia for chronic thoracic neuropathies, rib fractures + failed epidural analgesia, post-thoracotomy analgesia, and pediatric VATS, as well as lower abdominal surgeries.[15–21]

The goal of the ESPB is local anesthetic injection in the plane between the vertebral transverse process and the erector spinae muscle (ESM), which is composed of the spinalis, longissimus thoracis, and iliocostalis muscles. These muscles extend vertically through the cervical, thoracic, and lumbar regions. Deposition of local anesthetic here results in cranio-caudal distribution of local anesthetic along this fascial plane.[15] Cadaver studies have shown that a single injection at T5 can spread between the C7 and T8 levels.[19] Definitively, local anesthetic diffuses laterally to the intercostal space; but central coverage is controversial about whether or not local anesthetic reaches the paravertebral and epidural spaces anteriorly. Local anesthetic acts on the dorsal and possibly on the ventral ramus of the spinal nerves. The ventral ramus (the intercostal nerve) provides sensation to the anterolateral wall, while the dorsal ramus provides sensation to the posterior wall.[15]

Advantages of the ESPB include the extensive spread achieved with only a single injection. In addition, it is relatively easy to perform.[21]

RECTUS SHEATH CATHETER (RSC)

RSCs are indicated for procedures with midline abdominal incisions, as well as lower abdominal transverse incisions. The goal of rectus sheath analgesia is deposition of local anesthetic in the potential space between the rectus muscle and the posterior rectus sheath, either by bolus or continuous infusion of local anesthetic via a rectus sheath catheter (RSC).[22] This results in blockade of the ventral rami of the 7th through 12th intercostal nerves, leading to somatic analgesia of the anterior abdominal wall from the xiphoid process to the pubis.[22–24] RSCs do not provide visceral analgesia.[22,23]

TRANSVERSUS ABDOMINIS PLANE (TAP) BLOCK

The transversus abdominis plane (TAP) block provides postoperative analgesia after abdominal surgery. It does so by blocking the sensory afferents that innervate the abdominal wall.[26]

While not a direct replacement for the analgesia provided by a well-placed epidural catheter, when combined with multimodal analgesia, TAP blocks result in effective postoperative analgesia following surgeries involving abdominal incisions.[26] Indications for TAP block include postoperative analgesia after cesarean sections, hysterectomies, hernia repair, colectomy, cholecystectomy, and prostatectomy.[25–28] Posterior TAP blocks provide effective analgesia for lower abdominal incisions, while subcostal TAP blocks provide analgesia for supraumbilical incisions.[27] Additionally, TAP blocks can be performed in individuals on anticoagulant medications. Thus, TAP blocks can be considered as potential alternatives to epidurals for abdominal surgeries.[28]

QUADRATUS LUMBORUM BLOCK (QLB)

The quadratus lumborum block (QLB) provides both somatic and visceral analgesia of the abdomen, giving it an advantage over the TAP block, which only provides somatic anesthesia of the abdominal wall.[29] The QL muscle is covered by the transversals fascia (TF) and the thoracolumbar fascia (TLF).[30] There are several approaches to the QLB, differing in the specific site of local anesthetic injection. The transmuscular QLB involves local anesthetic injection anterior to the QL muscle, in the fascial plane between the QL and psoas muscles, resulting in local anesthetic spread extending to the thoracic paravertebral space. It results in somatic and visceral analgesia from T4–L1. The type 1 QLB (QLB1), also referred to as a fascia transversalis plane block, targets the space deep to the transversus abdominis aponeurosis and superficial to the TF, at the lateral aspect of the QL muscle. QLB1s result in anesthesia of the lateral cutaneous branches of the subcostal, iliohypogastric, and ilioinguinal nerves (T12–L1). The type 2 QLB (QLB2) involves local anesthetic injection posterior to the QL muscle and into the lumbar interfascial triangle (LIFT). The QLB can be used to treat chronic pain and has also been used for acute postoperative analgesia in the setting of abdominal surgery.[29–32] These studies support the potential use of the QLB as an alternative means of analgesia in cases where epidural placement is contraindicated.

ANTICOAGULANT AND ANTIPLATELET MEDICATION HALF-LIVES

Warfarin (Coumadin)

Warfarin has a variety of indications, including thromboembolism prophylaxis in patients with atrial fibrillation, use in patients with mechanical valves, and secondary prevention of venous thromboembolism.[33] Warfarin functions as a competitive inhibitor of vitamin K reductases, thus blocking the recycling of vitamin K and inhibiting vitamin K-dependent synthesis of both procoagulant proteins (factors II, VII, IX, and X) as well as anticoagulant proteins (protein C and S) in the liver.[34] Of these proteins, factor VII and protein C have the shortest plasma half-lives (6–8 h).[35] During initiation of warfarin therapy, the early anticoagulant effect due to reduction in factor VII is counteracted by the procoagulant effect of reduction in protein C.[36] In some instances, the relatively rapid decline in protein C levels during initiation of warfarin therapy can be accompanied by a paradoxical procoagulant effect. Thus, bridging therapy with heparin can be considered when initiating warfarin therapy.[37] Therapeutic warfarin anticoagulation requires an adequate decrease in factor II (half-life of 48–120 h) and factor X (half-life of 20–42 h) levels, which takes approximately 4–6 days.[35] Warfarin therapy is monitored using prothrombin time (PT) and the international normalized ratio (INR).[35]

One of the biggest disadvantages of warfarin therapy is the challenge of dosing warfarin. This challenge is due to the significant variability in response to warfarin therapy and at times unpredictable INR. Some of this variability is due to the fact that warfarin engages in many drug interactions, with many drugs either decreasing or increasing the intensity of warfarin anticoagulation. Some drugs such as amiodarone tend to increase INR, while others such as barbiturates tend to decrease INR. Meanwhile, co-administration of some drugs such as NSAIDs can lead to an increase in bleeding time without impacting INR. In addition, several patient variables such as age, gender, Asian ancestry, and comorbidities including liver, cardiac, and renal disease can also alter dose response to warfarin.[38] This unpredictability necessitates close serial INR monitoring for patients on warfarin therapy.

Warfarin is completely absorbed following oral administration with peak plasma concentrations occurring between 2 and 6 hours. Warfarin is metabolized by the cytochrome P-450 system, and has a half-life of 35 hours.[34]

Per ASRA guidelines, chronic warfarin therapy should be stopped 5 days before epidural placement; additionally, INR should be checked and confirmed to be within the reference range (INR ≤1.2) prior to epidural placement. It is recommended that warfarin therapy be discontinued for 5 days because during the first 1–3 days after stopping warfarin INR may be within normal limits due to a return in factor VII activity, but there may be inadequate hemostasis due to ongoing deficiency in factors II and X. ASRA also recommends against the concurrent use of medications such as aspirin, NSAIDs, and heparin, as these medications increase the patient's bleeding risk. In a patient not on chronic warfarin therapy, epidurals may be placed within 24 hours of an initial dose of warfarin. However, if the initial dose of warfarin was given more than 24 hours ago or a second dose of warfarin was administered, and INR should be checked prior to epidural placement.[3]

ANTI-FACTOR XA AGENTS

Fondaparinux (Arixtra)

Fondaparinux (Arixtra) is a synthetic pentasaccharide that results in factor Xa inhibition. It can be administered subcutaneously, with a peak effect 2–3 hours after administration. It has a half-life of 17–21 hours.[33] At the moment, there are no specific recommendations regarding the duration that fondaparinux should be held prior to epidural catheter placement. If an epidural catheter is being placed in a patient on fondaparinux, it is recommended that the catheter be placed under conditions similar to those of clinical trials (e.g., single needle pass).[3]

New Direct Oral Factor Xa Inhibitors

Direct factor Xa inhibitors function by noncovalent binding to free activated factor X, as well as activated factor X that is bound to the prothrombinase complex; as a result, they effectively disrupt both the intrinsic and the extrinsic coagulation pathways and prevent thrombin formation.[2] These new oral anticoagulants include apixaban (Eliquis), rivaroxaban (Xarelto), edoxaban (Savaysa), and betrixaban (Bevyxxa). These medications are used for stroke prophylaxis in patients with atrial fibrillation, prophylaxis and treatment of recurrent venous thromboembolism and pulmonary embolism, and primary prevention of venous thromboembolism in the setting of total hip arthroplasty.[3] They have demonstrated efficacy comparable to that of warfarin, but have several advantages, including rapid onset of action and short half-life, as well as no need for frequent lab monitoring.[3] Although routine monitoring of these anticoagulants is not required, if needed, their effects are best assessed using calibrated anti-factor Xa assays.[3]

- Apixaban has a rapid onset, with maximum plasma concentrations observed 3–4 hours after administration.[39] Apixaban has a half-life of approximately 12 hours; this half-life is slightly prolonged in patients with significant renal disease.[2]
- Rivaroxaban displays rapid inhibition of factor Xa, achieving maximum effect 2–3 hours after dosing.[40] The half-life of Rivaroxaban is 5.7–9.2 hours; however, half-life can be prolonged in patients with renal dysfunction.[2,40]
- Edoxaban quickly reaches maximum plasma concentrations 1–2 hours after ingestion. It is primarily metabolized through hydrolysis, with some CYP3A4 metabolism as well. It has an elimination half-life of 8–10 hours.[41] Unlike apixaban and rivaroxaban, compromised renal function does not have an effect on edoxaban half-life.[2]
- Betrixaban also has rapid absorption, with peak plasma concentrations occurring 3–4 hours after oral

administration.[42] Betrixaban is best suited for patients with renal impairment.[42,43] Additionally, it has a 20-hour half-life, which is significantly longer than the other drugs in the same family.[43]

ASRA guidelines suggest that for all direct factor Xa inhibitors (apixaban, rivaroxaban, edoxaban, and betrixaban), the medications be discontinued at least 72 hours prior to epidural placement. If considering epidural placement prior to 72 hours after the last medication dose, it is suggested that one check an anti-factor Xa activity level; however, there is no definitively identified acceptable level of residual medication activity for which it is recommended to proceed with epidural placement.[3]

DIRECT THROMBIN INHIBITORS

Argatroban (Acova), bivalirudin (Angiomax), lepirudin (Refludan), and desirudin (Revasc) are intravenous direct thrombin inhibitors. Desirudin can also be administered subcutaneously. The half-lives of argatroban, bivalirudin, lepirudin, and desirudin are 30–50 minutes, 25 minutes, 1 hour, and 1 hour, respectively. When administered subcutaneously, desirudin has a half-life of 2 hours.[33] These IV direct thrombin inhibitors are indicated as adjuncts to angioplasty procedures; they are also used for thrombosis prophylaxis and treatment in patients with HIT. IV direct thrombin inhibitors should not be administered in the setting of neuraxial anesthesia[3].

Dabigatran etexilate (Pradaxa) is the only FDA-approved oral direct thrombin inhibitor. It is approved for prevention of stroke in atrial fibrillation and for the prevention and treatment of venous thromboembolism.[33] Dabigatran rapidly binds to thrombin's active site and functions as a reversible competitive inhibitor of both free and clot-bound thrombin.[44] Although laboratory monitoring of dabigatran is not typically indicated, its anticoagulation effects can be assessed using thrombin clotting time (TT) and ecarin clotting time (ECT), the most sensitive clotting assays for dabigatran.[44] In emergency situations where these clotting assays are not available, one can also measure the activated partial thromboplastin time (aPTT), which is prolonged after dabigatran administration.[3] Prothrombin time is the least sensitive test.[45]

Following oral dabigatran etexilate ingestion, peak plasma concentrations occur after 1.5–3 hours. It has a half-life of 12–14 hours.[44] Renal insufficiency leads to significant half-life prolongation of up to 28 hours and results in increased dabigatran exposure.[46] Dabigatran is only 35% plasma protein bound, making it dialyzable. Yet, dabigatran is contraindicated in patients with severe renal insufficiency (creatinine clearance [CrCl] less than 30 mL/min).[44]

Given dabigatran's high reliance on renal excretion, for patients on dabigatran it is crucial to adequately assess renal function, as CrCl plays an important role in ASRA's epidural placement guidelines. Additionally, one must evaluate patients for other risk factors for bleeding, such as elderly age over 65 years and concurrent use of antiplatelet medications. Assuming no additional risk factors for bleeding, ASRA recommends holding dabigatran for 3–5 days prior to epidural placement, depending on CrCl. It should be held for:

- 5 days (120 hours) in patients with CrCl 30–49 mL/min
- 4 days (96 hours) in patients with CrCl 50–79 mL/min
- 3 days (72 hours) in patients with CrCl ≥ 80 mL/min.

In each scenario, if one is considering placing an epidural earlier than suggested by these recommendations, one may consider checking a dilute thrombin clotting time (dTT) or ECT. However, there is no specifically identified level of residual dabigatran activity for which it has been determined to be acceptable to proceed with epidural placement. Of note, ASRA recommends against epidural placement in patients with a CrCl of less than 30 mL/min.[3]

HEPARINS

Heparins are glycosaminoglycans, long linear polysaccharides.[33] Heparin binds to antithrombin III (ATIII), inducing a conformational change that converts ATIII into a more rapid inhibitor of coagulation factors. The heparin-ATIII complex primarily inactivates thrombin factor (IIa) and factor Xa, although it also inactivates factors IXa, XIa, and XIIa. Factor IIa inactivation requires that the heparin molecule be large enough to bind to both ATIII and to factor IIa.[47] Thus, while larger-weight heparin molecules will result in inhibition of both factors IIa and Xa, smaller-weight heparin molecules will only result in factor Xa inhibition.[3] Heparin exists as two preparations, unfractionated heparin (UFH) and low molecular weight heparin (LMWH).

Unfractionated Heparin (UFH)

UFH is a heterogeneous blend of heparins ranging in mass from 3000 to 30,000 daltons. UFH heparins have a mean molecular weight of 15,000 daltons, making UFH heparin molecules on average larger than LMWH heparin molecules (discussed in further detail, below).[47] The larger-sized heparin molecules in UFH result in equivalent anti-factor IIa and anti-factor Xa activity.[48] UFH effect is monitored by aPTT.[47] It can be administered either intravenously or subcutaneously.

Intravenous Unfractionated Heparin (IV UFH)

The peak effect of IV UFH occurs within 3 minutes of administration; it has a half-life of 1–1.5 hours.[33] Per ASRA guidelines, epidural placement should occur after IV heparin infusions have been discontinued for 4–6 hours and coagulation studies have been confirmed to be normal. Of note, given the potential for heparin-induced thrombocytopenia during heparin administration, platelet count should be assessed for patients receiving IV or SC UFH for more than 4 days prior to epidural placement or epidural catheter removal.[3]

SC Unfractionated Heparin (SC UFH)

The peak effect of SC UFH occurs 2–4 hours after administration, and its half-life is 1.5 hours.[33] Epidural management in patients receiving SC UFH depends on dose and frequency of dosing. For patients receiving low-dose SC UFH thromboprophylaxis (5000 U BID or TID), epidural placement should occur either 4–6 hours after the last heparin dose or after confirmation of normal coagulation studies. For patients receiving high-dose SC UFH thromboprophylaxis (7500–10,000 U BID or a daily dose of ≤20,000 U), epidural placement should occur at least 12 hours after the last heparin dose; additionally, normal coagulation studies should be confirmed prior to epidural placement. Finally, in patients receiving therapeutic SC UFH (individual heparin doses >10,000 U or daily dose >20,000 U) epidural placement should be delayed until 24 hours after the last heparin dose; additionally, normal coagulation studies should be confirmed prior to epidural placement.[3]

Low Molecular Weight Heparin (LMWH)

LMWHs include medications such as enoxaparin (Lovenox), dalteparin (Fragmin), and tinzaparin (Innohep). They are derived from heparin by depolymerization, resulting in heparin molecules ranging in mass from 1000 to 10,000 daltons, with a mean molecular weight of 4500–5000 daltons.[47] The smaller-sized heparin molecules in LMWH result in more specific factor Xa inhibition, with a ratio of anti-factor Xa activity to anti-factor IIa activity of about 4[48] LMWHs administered at lower dosages (such as enoxaparin 30 mg BID or 40 mg daily) can be used in the setting of venous thromboembolism prophylaxis. Higher dosages (such as enoxaparin 1 mg/kg BID or 1.5 mg/kg daily) can be used for the treatment of acute venous thromboembolism and pulmonary embolism. LMWHs have several advantages over UFH, including more predictable pharmacokinetics and lower risk of heparin-induced thrombocytopenia.[33] Although LMWH does not need to be routinely monitored, its effect can be assessed with anti-Xa levels.[47]

LMWHs are administered subcutaneously. After LMWH administration, peak effect is observed in 3–5 hours and half-life is approximately 3–6 hours. As LMWHs are primarily cleared renally, this half-life may be significantly prolonged (up to 16 hours) in patients with renal insufficiency.[3]

Epidural management in patients receiving LMWH depends on whether they are receiving prophylactic or therapeutic LMWH dosages, as well as dosing frequency. In patients receiving prophylactic LMWH, epidural placement should occur at least 12 hours after the last dose of LMWH. In patients being treated with therapeutic LMWH, epidural placement should be delayed at least 24 hours after the last LMWH dose. In the case of therapeutic LMWH, one may additionally consider assessing anti-factor Xa levels; however, there is no established acceptable level of residual anti-factor Xa at which point one should proceed with epidural placement. Of note, given the potential for heparin-induced thrombocytopenia during LMWH administration, platelet count should be assessed for patients receiving LMWH for more than 4 days prior to epidural placement or epidural catheter removal.[3]

NONSTEROIDAL ANTI-INFLAMMATORY DRUGS (NSAIDS)

Nonsteroidal anti-inflammatory drugs (NSAIDs) refer to a broad, diverse group of anti-inflammatory and analgesic medications. These medications have many routes of administration, including oral, intravenous, topical, and suppository. They include medications such as aspirin, diclofenac, ketorolac, indomethacin, ibuprofen, naproxen, and celecoxib. NSAIDs are used in the setting of arthritis, rheumatic disease, and treatment of musculoskeletal pain.[49] Aspirin offers the additional benefit of protection against stroke and thrombosis.[50] The half-lives of NSAIDs vary widely, ranging from 15 minutes to over 70 hours.[51]

NSAIDs' mechanism of action involves inhibition of cyclooxygenase (COX) activity, leading to a decrease in prostaglandin (PG) production. Most NSAIDs block both COX isoforms, COX-1 which is expressed under basal conditions, and COX-2 which has increased expression in the setting of inflammation. COX-1 inhibition leads to some of the adverse effects of NSAIDs, such as increased risk of bleeding and gastrointestinal ulceration. COX-2 inhibition inhibits PG production at the site of inflammation, thus leading to NSAIDs' anti-inflammatory and analgesic effects. A subset of NSAIDs, such as celecoxib (Celebrex), are COX-2 selective inhibitors; they offer the anti-inflammatory and analgesic benefits of COX-2 inhibition while avoiding the inhibition of platelet function and increased bleeding risk that comes with COX-1 inhibition.[49]

NSAIDs have not been shown to significantly increase the risk of spinal hematoma in patients undergoing neuraxial anesthesia. As such, NSAIDs (including aspirin) do not need to be held prior to epidural catheter placement. However, it is important to be cognizant of the increased bleeding risk that comes from concurrent administration of anticoagulant medications and NSAIDs. If patients on anticoagulation require anti-inflammatories, one may consider administration of COX-2 selective NSAIDs such as celecoxib.[3]

P2Y12 ADP RECEPTOR ANTAGONISTS

ADP antagonists include medications such as clopidogrel (Plavix), prasugrel (Effient), ticlodipine (Ticlid), ticagrelor (Brilinta), and cangrelor (Kengreal). These ADP antagonists inhibit platelet function by binding to platelet adenosine diphosphate (ADP) receptors of subtype P2Y12, thus preventing ADP binding, and leading to inhibition of downstream platelet aggregation. These medications are indicated in the setting of coronary artery disease with prior stenting, history of cerebrovascular accident, and peripheral vascular disease. They are usually administered concurrently with aspirin.[2] Clopidogrel, prasugrel, and ticlodipine are prodrugs that are activated by the hepatic CYP450 system prior to irreversibly binding the P2Y12 receptor.[3]

- **Clopidogrel (Plavix)** has a half-life of 7–8 hours;[52] it should be held for 5–7 days prior to epidural catheter placement[3].

- **Prasugrel (Effient)** has a half-life of 8 hours;[53] it should be held for 7–10 days prior to epidural catheter placement.[3]
- **Ticlodipine (Ticlid)** has a particularly long half-life of 20–50 hours;[54] it should be held for 10 days prior to epidural catheter placement.[3]
- **Ticagrelor (Brilinta)** is an orally active reversible P2Y12 receptor antagonist that does not require enzymatic activation prior to binding the P2Y12 receptor. It achieves peak effect 2–4 hours after administration and has a half-life of 7 hours.[2] Ticagrelor should be held for 5–7 days prior to epidural catheter placement.[3]
- **Cangrelor (Kengreal)** is an intravenous reversible P2Y12 receptor antagonist. It has a half-life of 3–6 minutes, and should be held for 3 hours prior to epidural catheter placement.[3]

PHOSPHODIESTERASE INHIBITORS

- **Cilostazol (Plctal)** is an anti-platelet agent and vasodilator that is indicated in the treatment of intermittent claudication in symptomatic peripheral vascular disease. It functions as a phosphodiesterase-III (PDE-III) inhibitor and as an adenosine reuptake inhibitor, leading to an elevation in intracellular cyclic adenosine monophosphate (cAMP).[55] Cilostazol has a half-life of 10.5 hours, and half-life is prolonged in patients with renal insufficiency.[3,55] Cilostazol should be held for 2 days prior to epidural catheter placement.[3]
- **Dipyridamole (Aggrenox)** is an anti-platelet agent and vasodilator. The combination of dipyridamole and aspirin has been shown to result in more effective protection in secondary prevention of stroke than aspirin alone. Although the mechanism of action of dipyridamole is not completely understood, it functions as a PDE-5 and PDE-6 inhibitor as well as an adenosine reuptake inhibitor.[56] Dipyridamole has a half-life of 10 hours and should be held for 24 hours prior to epidural catheter placement.[3]

THROMBOPROPHYLAXIS IN THE PRESENCE OF AN EPIDURAL CATHETER

WARFARIN (COUMADIN)

Following epidural placement, if warfarin therapy is indicated for a patient, they may immediately receive the first dose of warfarin without any delay. Patients with epidural catheters in place who are receiving low-dose warfarin therapy should have INRs monitored on a daily basis. For INRs greater than 3, it is recommended that warfarin doses be reduced or held. Additionally, patients should undergo frequent neurologic testing assessing sensory and motor function; epidural infusions using dilute local anesthetics are recommended in this setting in order to minimize the degree of epidural-related motor and sensory deficiency.[3]

ANTI-FACTOR XA AGENTS

Thromboprophylaxis with fondaparinux and the new direct oral factor Xa inhibitors should be avoided in the setting of indwelling catheters.[3]

DABIGATRAN (PRADAXA)

Thromboprophylaxis with dabigatran should be avoided in the setting of indwelling catheters.[3]

IV UNFRACTIONATED HEPARIN (IV UFH)

IV heparin infusions can be restarted 1 hour after epidural placement. However, these patients with indwelling epidural catheters receiving IV heparin should have their neurologic function closely monitored; epidural local anesthetic infusions should be tailored to minimize motor and sensory block, thus allowing for detection of pathologic neurologic deficits.[3]

SC UNFRACTIONATED HEPARIN (SC UFH)

After epidural placement, low-dose SC UFH thromboprophylaxis can be restarted immediately. However, high-dose SC UFH thromboprophylaxis should be approached with caution, as it poses an unknown risk. At the moment, we do not have sufficient data regarding the safety of administering SC UFH at greater than 5000 U/dose or at greater than 15,000 U daily. As such, the relative risks and benefits of high-dose SC UFH prophylaxis should be considered on a case-by-case basis. If the decision is made to proceed with high-dose SC UFH prophylaxis in a patient with an indwelling epidural catheter, the patient should be closely monitored for possible development or progression of new neurologic deficits. ASRA recommends against the administration of therapeutic SC UFH to patients with indwelling epidural catheters.[3]

LOW MOLECULAR WEIGHT HEPARIN (LMWH)

Once-daily prophylactic LMWH can be initiated 12 hours after epidural catheter placement; it is important to avoid giving a second prophylactic dose sooner than 24 hours after the first dose. Also concurrent administration of other antiplatelet and anticoagulation medications should be avoided. Twice-daily prophylactic LMWH and therapeutic LMWH should not be administered in the setting of indwelling epidural catheters.[3]

NONSTEROIDAL ANTI-INFLAMMATORY DRUGS (NSAIDS)

NSAIDs (including aspirin) can be restarted immediately following epidural placement.[3]

P2Y12 ADP RECEPTOR ANTAGONISTS

Prasugrel, ticagrelor, and cangrelor should not be administered in the setting of an indwelling epidural catheter. Clopidogrel and ticlodipine can be administered immediately following epidural catheter placement, as long as no loading dose is administered and the patient is at least 24 hours postop. If a patient is receiving clopidogrel or ticlodipine, the epidural catheter can be maintained for 1–2 days.[3]

PHOSPHODIESTERASE INHIBITORS

Cilostazol and dipyridamole should not be administered in the setting of an indwelling epidural catheter.[3]

HOLDING THROMBOPROPHYLAXIS BEFORE REMOVAL OF AN EPIDURAL CATHETER

WARFARIN (COUMADIN)

If thromboprophylaxis with warfarin has been initiated in a patient with an epidural catheter in place, the catheter can be removed within 24 hours of warfarin therapy. However, prior to epidural catheter removal, INR should be checked and confirmed to be less than 1.5. Of note, it is recommended that after catheter removal neurologic assessments continue for at least 24 hours.[3]

ANTI-FACTOR XA AGENTS

In the event that new direct oral factor Xa inhibitors are inadvertently administered to a patient with an indwelling epidural catheter, it is recommended that one wait a certain period of time following medication administration prior to catheter removal. In this case, epidural catheter removal should be delayed by 26–30 hours for apixaban, 22–36 hours for rivaroxaban, 20–28 hours for edoxaban, and 72 hours for betrixaban. Alternatively, it is also possible to make an assessment by performing an anti-factor Xa assay prior to catheter removal.[3]

DABIGATRAN (PRADAXA)

In the event that dabigatran is unintentionally administered to a patient with an indwelling epidural catheter, it is recommended that one wait 34–36 hours following medication administration prior to catheter removal. In this scenario, it may be prudent to also assess dTT or ECT.[3]

IV UNFRACTIONATED HEPARIN (IV UFH)

IV heparin infusions should be held for at least 4–6 hours prior to epidural catheter removal. Additionally, normal coagulation studies should be confirmed before epidural catheter removal.[3]

SC UNFRACTIONATED HEPARIN (SC UFH)

If thromboprophylaxis with low-dose SC UFH has been initiated in a patient with an epidural catheter in place, it should be held for 4–6 hours prior to epidural catheter removal. If a patient is receiving high-dose SC UFH thromboprophylaxis in the setting of an indwelling epidural catheter, catheter removal should be approached with caution due to the lack of sufficient data regarding associated risks.

LOW MOLECULAR WEIGHT HEPARIN (LMWH)

If once-daily LMWH prophylaxis has been initiated in a patient with an epidural catheter in place, LMWH should be held for 12 hours prior to epidural catheter removal.[3]

NONSTEROIDAL ANTI-INFLAMMATORY DRUGS (NSAIDS)

NSAIDS (including aspirin) do not need to be held prior to epidural catheter removal.[3]

P2Y12 ADP RECEPTOR ANTAGONISTS

Prasugrel, ticagrelor, and cangrelor should not be administered in the setting of an indwelling epidural catheter. Clopidogrel and ticlopidine can be administered immediately following epidural catheter placement, as long as no loading dose is administered and the patient is at least 24 hours postop. If an epidural catheter is in place, patients receiving clopidogrel or ticlopidine can leave the epidural catheter maintained for up to 1–2 days and then pulled.[3]

RESTARTING ANTICOAGULANT AND ANTIPLATELET MEDICATIONS AFTER REMOVAL OF AN EPIDURAL CATHETER

WARFARIN (COUMADIN)

After epidural catheter removal, warfarin therapy can be initiated without any delay.

ANTI-FACTOR XA AGENTS

- **Fondaparinux (Arixtra)** can be restarted 6 hours after epidural catheter removal[3].
- **New Direct Oral Factor Xa Inhibitors**: Apixaban, rivaroxaban, and edoxaban can be restarted 6 hours after epidural catheter removal, or 6 hours after performance of spinal. Epidural catheters should be removed 5 hours before the first dose of betrixaban.[3]

DABIGATRAN (PRADAXA)

Dabigatran can be restarted 6 hours after epidural catheter removal, or 6 hours after performance of spinal.[3]

IV UNFRACTIONATED HEPARIN (IV UFH)

IV heparin infusions can be restarted 1 hour after epidural catheter removal.[3]

SC UNFRACTIONATED HEPARIN (SC UFH)

Following epidural catheter removal, low-dose SC UFH thromboprophylaxis can be restarted after a 1-hour delay.[3] High-dose SC UFH thromboprophylaxis and therapeutic SC UFH can be restarted immediately after epidural catheter removal.[3]

LOW MOLECULAR WEIGHT HEPARIN (LMWH)

Prophylactic LMWH can be restarted 4 hours after epidural catheter removal or 12 hours after epidural placement, whichever is greater. Prophylactic LMWH can be restarted 12 hours after spinal anesthesia. Therapeutic LMWH can be restarted 4 hours after epidural catheter removal or 24 hours after epidural placement, whichever is greater. Therapeutic LMWH can be restarted 24–72 hours after spinal, depending on surgical bleeding risk (24 hours after low bleeding risk surgery and 28–72 hours after high bleeding risk surgery).[3]

NONSTEROIDAL ANTI-INFLAMMATORY DRUGS (NSAIDS)

NSAIDS (including aspirin) can be restarted immediately following epidural catheter removal.[3]

P2Y12 ADP RECEPTOR ANTAGONISTS

The oral P2Y12 ADP receptor antagonists can be restarted immediately after epidural catheter removal, or immediately after performance of spinal, as long as no loading dose is administered and the patient is at least 24 hours postop. Loading dose can be administered 6 hours after catheter removal or 6 hours after performance of spinal. Cangrelor can be restarted 8 hours after epidural catheter removal.[3]

PHOSPHODIESTERASE INHIBITORS

Cilostazol and dipyridamole can be restarted 6 hours after epidural catheter removal.[3]

ANTICOAGULANT REVERSAL

WARFARIN (COUMADIN) REVERSAL

Due to the variability in response to warfarin and the high potential for supratherapeutic INR, warfarin reversal is important. Reversal options include vitamin K (phytonadione) administration, as well as replacement of functional clotting factors with either fresh frozen plasma (FFP) or prothrombin complex concentrate (PCC) administration.

Vitamin K administration is an appropriate treatment for patients with supratherapeutic INR who are either nonbleeding, or who only have minor bleeding.[57] Vitamin K can be administered either orally or IV, with an oral to IV dosing conversion of 5:1. However, subcutaneous dosing of vitamin K is not recommended due to variable absorption.[33] Lubetsky et al. demonstrated that among patients with baseline INR >10, patients treated with oral and IV vitamin K exhibited a comparable decline in INR; however, among patients with baseline INR 6–10, those receiving oral vitamin K demonstrated a slower rate of INR decline, as well as a fewer number of patients adequately responding to treatment during the first 12 hours of treatment. On the other hand, compared to oral vitamin K, IV vitamin K is associated with an increased risk of overcorrection of INR. These findings suggested that while oral vitamin K is preferable for INR reversal in non-urgent cases due to its predictability, IV vitamin K may be of benefit in urgent scenarios with more serious bleeding.[57] Response to vitamin K is dependent on INR at presentation, and studies have shown that dosing vitamin K according to baseline INR is important in effectively restoring INR while avoiding failure in response or overcorrection of INR.[57] Of note, vitamin K-based reversal may have limited efficacy in correcting INR in the setting of patients with hepatic insufficiency.[33]

In cases of severe, life-threatening hemorrhage, FFP or PCC can be used to reverse the effects of warfarin. Although FFP is inexpensive and commonly used, it comes with several disadvantages. There are usually delays in obtaining FFP due to ABO blood group specificity and the need for thawing. Additionally, the recommended dose of FFP for warfarin reversal is 15 mL/kg, meaning that patients may require an infusion of upward of one liter of FFP; depending on their comorbidities, some patients may not be able to tolerate such a high-volume infusion. Finally, FFP administration is associated with possible transmission of infections and a risk of transfusion-related acute lung injury (TRALI).[58] FFP also has a short clinical half-life, and often requires redosing.[33]

PCC contains a mix of purified clotting factors, and is usually supplemented with heparin. Three-factor PCCs contain factors II, IX, and X, four-factor PCCs (such as Kcentra) contain factors II, VII, IX, and X, and activated four-factor PCCs contain activated factor VIIa. Dosing of PCC is weight dependent.[33] One disadvantage of PCC is the risk of thrombotic events, occurring in 1.5% of patients receiving PCC.[58] However, PCC does not require ABO matching, can be immediately available, carries no risk of infection, and has been shown to reverse anticoagulation secondary to vitamin K antagonists within 30 minutes, with effects lasting up to 24 hours.[33] Retrospective studies comparing FFP versus PCC for warfarin reversal suggest that PCC provides more rapid and effective correction of INR than FFP. As a result, PCC is recommended as first-line therapy for vitamin K antagonist anticoagulation reversal in patients with severe hemorrhage.[58]

DIRECT FACTOR XA INHIBITOR REVERSAL

Despite the many advantages of direct factor Xa inhibitors, their reversal has historically posed a challenge; for many years, there were no FDA-approved medications for reversal, with limited options for treatment in the setting of overdose or hemorrhage secondary to direct factor Xa inhibitor use. Additionally, due to the high degree of protein binding exhibited by all direct factor Xa inhibitors, these medications are not dialyzable, making their removal from systemic circulation challenging.[3] In the setting of overdose, activated charcoal can be used to reduce absorption of apixaban and rivaroxaban; however, activated charcoal must be administered within 3 hours of apixaban ingestion and within 8 hours of rivaroxaban ingestion.[59] For patients requiring Xa inhibitor reversal beyond this window, evidence suggests that PCCs can be used. The proposed mechanism is that large quantities of clotting factors contained in PCC overcome the upstream inhibition of direct factor Xa inhibitors.[33] Studies show that PCC reverses the in vitro anticoagulant activity of rivaroxaban in healthy adults; PT values normalized to baseline immediately after PCC administration, and this effect was maintained for 24 hours. However, PCC administration was associated with risk of rebound thrombosis.[59]

The recent advent of the recombinant protein Andexanet alfa (Andexxa), which was approved by the FDA in 2018 for reversal of apixaban and rivaroxaban in patients with severe bleeding, marked an important development. Andexanet is the first FDA approved antidote for direct factor Xa inhibitors. Andexanet is a truncated Xa analog that sequesters anticoagulants through noncovalent and reversible binding, thus preventing them from binding to factor Xa.[33] Dose of andexanet depends on the agent being reversed. As this reversal effect is transient, continuous infusions of andexanet are necessary for maintenance of reversal.[33] In a study of patients with acute major bleeding associated with factor Xa inhibitors, andexanet administration led to substantial reduction in antifactor Xa activity, achieving effective hemostasis in 79%.[60]

Cirapirantag is an investigational drug that may offer benefits in reversal of direct factor Xa anticoagulation. Cirapirantag noncovalently binds to and sequesters heparin, LMWH, direct factor Xa inhibitors, and direct thrombin inhibitors, thus inhibiting their anticoagulant effect.[33] Although animal studies have shown promising results of anticoagulation reversal using cirapirantag, the medication continues to require further study.[33]

DABIGATRAN (PRADAXA) REVERSAL

Dabigatran's effects can be reversed by activated charcoal, which must be administered within 1–2 hours of dabigatran ingestion. Dabigatran can also be systematically eliminated via dialysis.[2] More recently, an effective antidote for dabigatran was developed. Idarucizumab is a monoclonal antibody fragment that binds free and thrombin-bound dabigatran with a high affinity, thus inhibiting dabigatran's anticoagulant effect.[61] Idarucizumab was approved by the FDA in 2015 for patients on dabigatran when severe bleeding or emergent surgical procedures necessitate rapid anticoagulation reversal.[3] Studies have shown that in 88%–98% of patients with elevated baseline clotting times, idarucizumab administration results in rapid and total reversal of dabigatran's anticoagulant effects.[61] Clinical studies demonstrated that administration of a 5 g idarucizumab dose to patients on dabigatran who either had severe hemorrhage or who presented for emergency surgery resulted in reversal of coagulation abnormalities and normal intraoperative hemostasis in the majority of patients.[33]

HEPARINS

Protamine sulfate is a protein derived from fish sperm that binds to heparin, neutralizing its anticoagulant effects. The primary advantage of UFH over LMWH is the ability of protamine to quickly and completely reverse UFH, lowering the aPTT. Protamine only partially reverses LMWH; although it inhibits LMWH's anti-IIa activity, it only inhibits a variable portion of LMWH's anti-Xa activity. Despite this incomplete reversal, given the current lack of approved methods for completely reversing LMWH, the American College of Chest Physicians recommends that LMWH be reversed with protamine.[62]

Protamine has the potential for several adverse reactions. It can result in hypotension and bradycardia when administered rapidly. Additionally, it carries a risk of allergic reactions including anaphylaxis, particularly among patients who have previously had a vasectomy, have a known fish sensitivity, or who have previously taken protamine sulfate-containing insulin.[62]

CONCLUSIONS

As newer anticoagulation agents flood the market, and a full safety profile is not yet available, it is important to have options for effective analgesia. While a well-placed epidural catheter is arguably the gold standard for perioperative analgesia, the ever-increasing requirement for anticoagulation of hospitalized patients creates an additional barrier. Fortunately, advances in ultrasound technology facilitate improved sonoanotomy visualization at lower costs, resulting in a greater adoption of fascial plane blocks. When combined with a vetted multimodal pain management protocol, hospital discharge and patient pain scores are comparable. The American Society of Regional Anesthesiologists provides a downloadable smart-phone application which will help guide practitioners on how to manage anticoagulated patients needing neuraxial interventions.

REFERENCES

1. Unic-Stojanovic D, Babic S, Jovic M. Benefits, risks and complications of perioperative use of epidural anesthesia. *Med Arch*. 2012;66(5):340–343.
2. Lemay A, Kaye AD, Urman RD. Novel anticoagulant agents in the perioperative setting. *Anesthesiol Clin*. 2017;35(2):305–313.
3. Horlocker TT, Vandermeulen E, Kopp SL, Gogarten W, Leffert LR, Benzon HT. Regional anesthesia in the patient receiving antithrombotic or thrombolytic therapy: American Society of Regional Anesthesia and Pain Medicine Evidence-Based Guidelines (fourth edition). *Reg Anesth Pain Med*. 2018;43(3):263–309.
4. Ho AH, Buck R, Latmore M, Levine M, Karmakar MK. Intercostal nerve block. In: Hadzic A, ed. *Hadzic's Textbook of Regional Anesthesia and Acute Pain Management*. 2nd ed. New York: McGraw-Hill; 2017. http://accessanesthesiology.mhmedical.com/content.aspx?bookid=2070&sectionid=157607494. Accessed September 24, 2019.
5. Luketich JD, Land SR, Sullivan EA, et al. Thoracic epidural versus intercostal nerve catheter plus patient-controlled analgesia: a randomized study. *Ann Thorac Surg*. 2005;79(6):1845–1850.

6. Pyati S, Lindsay DR, Buchheit T. Acute and chronic post-thoracotomy pain. In: Barbeito A, Shaw AD, Grichnik K, eds. *Thoracic Anesthesia*. New York: McGraw-Hill; 2012. http://accessanesthesiology.mhmedical.com/content.aspx?bookid=516&sectionid=40997843. Accessed September 24, 2019.
7. Dravid RM, Paul RE. Interpleural block: part 1. *Anaesthesia*. 2007;62(10):1039–1049.
8. Dravid RM, Paul RE. Interpleural block: part 2. *Anaesthesia*. 2007;62(11):1143–1153.
9. Joshi GP, Bonnet F, Shah R, et al. A systematic review of randomized trials evaluating regional techniques for postthoracotomy analgesia. *Anesth Analg*. 2008;107(3):1026–1040.
10. Blanco R, Barrington MJ. Pectoralis and serratus plane blocks. In: Hadzic A, ed. *Hadzic's Textbook of Regional Anesthesia and Acute Pain Management*. 2nd ed. New York: McGraw-Hill; 2017. http://accessanesthesiology.mhmedical.com/content.aspx? bookid=2070&sectionid=157602747. Accessed September 24, 2019.
11. Kulhari S, Bharti N, Bala I, Arora S, Singh G. Efficacy of pectoral nerve block *versus* thoracic paravertebral block for postoperative analgesia after radical mastectomy: a randomized controlled trial. *Br J Anaesth*. 2016;117(3):382–386.
12. Khalil AE, Abdallah NM, Bashandy GM, Kaddah TA. Ultrasound-guided serratus anterior plane block versus thoracic epidural analgesia for thoracotomy pain. *J Cardiothorac Vasc Anesth*. 2017;31(1):152–158.
13. Kunhabdulla NP, Agarwal A, Gaur A, Gautam SK, Gupta R, Agarwal A. Serratus anterior plane block for multiple rib fractures. *Pain Physician*. 2014;17(4):E553–E555.
14. Madabushi R, Tewari S, Gautam SK, Agarwal A, Agarwal A. Serratus anterior plane block: a new analgesic technique for post-thoracotomy pain. *Pain Physician*. 2015;18(3):E421–E424.
15. Kot P, Rodriguez P, Granell M, et al. The erector spinae plane block: a narrative review. *Korean J Anesthesiol*. 2019;72(3):209–220.
16. Forero M, Adhikary SD, Lopez H, Tsui C, Chin KJ. The erector spinae plane block: a novel analgesic technique in thoracic neuropathic pain. *Reg Anesth Pain Med*. 2016;41(5):621–627.
17. Hamilton DL, Manickam B. Erector spinae plane block for pain relief in rib fractures. *Br J Anaesth*. 2017;118(3):474–475.
18. Forero M, Rajarathinam M, Adhikary S, Chin KJ. Continuous erector spinae plane block for rescue analgesia in thoracotomy after epidural failure: a case report. *A&A Case Rep*. 2017;8(10):254–256.
19. Adhikary SD, Pruett A, Forero M, Thiruvenkatarajan V. Erector spinae plane block as an alternative to epidural analgesia for post-operative analgesia following video-assisted thoracoscopic surgery: a case study and a literature review on the spread of local anaesthetic in the erector spinae plane. *Indian J Anaesth*. 2018;62(1):75–78.
20. Jain K, Jaiswal V, Puri A. Erector spinae plane block: relatively new block on horizon with a wide spectrum of application: a case series. *Indian J Anaesth*. 2018;62(10):809–813.
21. Luis-Navarro JC, Seda-Guzmán M, Luis-Moreno C, Chin KJ. Erector spinae plane block in abdominal surgery: case series. *Indian J Anaesth*. 2018;62(7):549–554.
22. Wilkinson KM, Krige A, Brearley SG, et al. Thoracic Epidural analgesia versus Rectus Sheath Catheters for open midline incisions in major abdominal surgery within an enhanced recovery programme (TERSC): study protocol for a randomised controlled trial. *Trials*. 2014. doi: 10.1186/1745-6215-15-400.
23. Yassin HM, Abd Elmoneim AT, El Moutaz H. The analgesic efficiency of ultrasound-guided rectus sheath analgesia compared with low thoracic epidural analgesia after elective abdominal surgery with a midline incision: a prospective randomized controlled trial. *Anesth Pain Med*. 2017;7(3). doi: 10.5812/aapm.14244.
24. Rucklidge M, Beattie E. Rectus sheath catheter analgesia for patients undergoing laparotomy. *Br J Anaesth*. 2018;18(6):166–172.
25. Tsai HC, Yoshida T, Chuang TY, et al. Transversus abdominis plane block: an updated review of anatomy and techniques. *BioMed Res Int*. 2017;2017:8284363. doi: 10.1155/2017/8284363.
26. McDonnell JG, O'Donnell B, Curley G, Heffernan A, Power C, Laffey JG. The analgesic efficacy of transversus abdominis plane block after abdominal surgery: a prospective randomized controlled trial. *Anesth Analg*. 2007;104(1):193–197.
27. Niraj G, Kelkar A, Jeyapalan I, et al. Comparison of analgesic efficacy of subcostal transversus abdominis plane blocks with epidural analgesia following upper abdominal surgery. *Anaesthesia*. 2011;66(6):465–471.
28. Niraj G, Kelkar A, Hart E, et al. Comparison of analgesic efficacy of four-quadrant transversus abdominis plane (TAP) block and continuous posterior TAP analgesia with epidural analgesia in patients undergoing laparoscopic colorectal surgery: an open-label, randomised, non-inferiority trial. *Anaesthesia*. 2014;69(4):348–355.
29. Elsharkawy H, Bendtsen TF. Ultrasound-guided transversus abdominis plane and quadratus lumborum blocks. In: Hadzic A, ed. *Hadzic's Textbook of Regional Anesthesia and Acute Pain Management*. 2nd ed. New York: McGraw-Hill; 2017. http://accessanesthesiology.mhmedical.com/content.aspx? bookid=2070&sectionid=157602698. Accessed September 24, 2019.
30. Cardoso JM, Sá M, Reis H, et al. Type II quadratus lumborum block for a sub-total gastrectomy in a septic patient. *Braz J Anesthesiol*. 2018;68(2):186–189.
31. Ishio J, Komasawa N, Kido H, Minami T. Evaluation of ultrasound-guided posterior quadratus lumborum block for postoperative analgesia after laparoscopic gynecologic surgery. *J Clin Anesth*. 2017;41:1–4.
32. Aditianingsih D, Pryambodho, Anasy N, Rahendra, Tantri AR. Comparison of quadratus lumborum versus continuous epidural block for laparoscopic donor nephrectomy: analysis of postoperative analgesia and motoric ability. *J Physics: Conf Series*. 2019;1246. doi: 10.1088/1742-6596/1246/1/012001.
33. Meltzer J, Guenzer JR. Anticoagulant reversal and anesthetic considerations. *Anesthesiol Clin*. 2017; 35(2): 191–205.
34. Holford, NH. Clinical pharmacokinetics and pharmacodynamics of warfarin: understanding the dose-effect relationship. *Clin Pharmacokinet*. 1986;11(6):483–504.
35. Benzon HT, Avram MJ, Benzon HA, Kirby-Nolan M, Nader A. Factor VII levels and international normalized ratios in early phase of warfarin therapy. *Anesthesiology*. 2010;112:298–304.
36. Harrison L, Johnston M, Massicotte MP, Crowther M, Moffat K, Hirsh J. Comparison of 5-mg and 10-mg loading doses in initiation of warfarin therapy. *Ann Intern Med*. 1997;126(2):133–136.
37. Kim Y, Bang OY. Paradoxical procoagulant effect of early doses of warfarin: possible role of non-vitamin K oral anticoagulant in patients with atrial fibrillation-related stroke. *J Stroke*. 2015;17(2):216–218.
38. Enneking FK, Benzon H. Oral anticoagulants and regional anesthesia. *Reg Anesth Pain Med*. 1998;23(6):140–145.
39. Frost C, Nepal S, Wang J, et al. Safety, pharmacokinetics and pharmacodynamics of multiple oral doses of apixaban, a factor Xa inhibitor, in healthy subjects. *Br J Clin Pharmacol*. 2013;76(5):776–786.
40. Kubitza D, Becka M, Wensing G, Voith B, Zuehlsdorf M. Safety, pharmacodynamics, and pharmacokinetics of BAY 59-7939—and oral, direct Factor Xa inhibitor—after multiple dosing in healthy male subjects. *Clin Pharmacol Therap*. 2005;78(4):412–421.
41. Bathala MS, Masumoto H, Oguma T, He L, Lowrie C, Mendell J. Pharmacokinetics, biotransformation, and mass balance of edoxaban, a selective, direct factor Xa inhibitor, in humans. *Drug Metab Dispos*. 2012;40(12):2250–2255.
42. Chan NC, Bhagirath V, Eikelboom JW. Profile of betrixaban and its potential in the prevention and treatment of venous thromboembolism. *Vasc Health Risk Manage*. 2015;11:343–351.
43. Turpie AG, Bauer KA, Davidson BL, et al. A randomized evaluation of betrixaban, an oral factor Xa inhibitor, for prevention of thromboembolic events after total knee replacement (EXPERT). *Thrombos Haemostas*. 2009;101(1):68–76.
44. Stangier J, Clemens A. Pharmacology, pharmacokinetics, and pharmacodynamics of dabigatran etexilate, an oral direct thrombin inhibitor. *Clin Appl Thromb/Hemostas*. 2009;15:9S–16S.
45. Benzon HT, Jabri RS, Van Zundert TC. Neuraxial anesthesia & peripheral nerve blocks in patients on anticoagulants. In: Hadzic A, ed. *Hadzic's Textbook of Regional Anesthesia and Acute Pain*

Management, 2nd ed. New York: McGraw-Hill; 2017. http://accessanesthesiology.mhmedical.com/content.aspx? bookid=2070&sectionid=157604570. Accessed September 24, 2019.

46. Stangier J, Rathgen K, Stähle H, Mazur D. Influence of renal impairment on the pharmacokinetics and pharmacodynamics of oral dabigatran etexilate: an open-label, parallel-group, single-centre study. *Clin Pharmacokinet*. 2010;49(4):259–268.
47. Hirsh J, Warkentin TE, Shaughnessy SG, et al. Heparin and low-molecular-weight heparin: mechanisms of action, pharmacokinetics, dosing, monitoring, efficacy, and safety. *Chest*. 2001;119(1):64S–94S.
48. Verstraete M. Pharmacotherapeutic aspects of unfractionated and low molecular weight heparins. *Drugs*. 1990;40(4):498–530.
49. Crofford LJ. Use of NSAIDs in treating patients with arthritis. *Arthritis Res Ther*. 2013;15(Suppl 3):S2. doi: 10.1186/ar4174.
50. Mitchell JA, Warner TD. Cyclo-oxygenase-2: pharmacology, physiology, biochemistry and relevance to NSAID therapy. *Br J Pharmacol.* 1999;128(6):1121–1132.
51. Davies NM, Skjodt NM. Choosing the right nonsteroidal anti-inflammatory drug for the right patient: a pharmacokinetic approach. *Clin Pharmacokinet*. 2000;38(5):377–392.
52. Schrör K. Clinical pharmacology of the adenosine diphosphate (ADP) receptor antagonist, clopidogrel. *Vasc Med*. 1998;3(3):247–251.
53. Yeung J, Holinstat M. Newer agents in antiplatelet therapy: a review. *J Blood Med.* 2012;3:33–42.
54. Desager JP. Clinical pharmacokinetics of ticlopidine. *Clin Pharmacokinet*. 1994;26(5):347–355.
55. Chapman TM, Goa KL. Cilostazol: a review of its use in intermittent claudication. *Am J Cardiovasc Drugs*. 2003;3(2):117–138.
56. Gamboa A, Abraham R, Diedrich A, et al. Role of adenosine and nitric oxide on the mechanisms of action of dipyridamole. *Stroke*. 2005;36(10):2170–2175.
57. Lubetsky A, Yonath H, Olchovsky D, Loebstein R, Halkin H, Ezra D. Comparison of oral vs intravenous phytonadione (vitamin K1) in patients with excessive anticoagulation: a prospective randomized controlled study. *Arch Intern Med.* 2003;163(20):2469–2473.
58. Ageno W, Garcia D, Aguilar MI, et al. Prevention and treatment of bleeding complications in patients receiving vitamin K antagonists, part 2: treatment. *Am J Hematol*. 2009;84(9):584–588.
59. Miyares MA, Davis K. Newer oral anticoagulants: a review of laboratory monitoring options and reversal agents in the hemorrhagic patient. *Am J Health-System Pharm*. 2012;69(17):1473–1484.
60. Connolly SJ, Milling TJ, Eikelboom JW, et al. Andexanet alfa for acute major bleeding associated with factor Xa inhibitors. *N Engl J Med.* 2016; 375: 1131–1141.
61. Pollack CV Jr, Reilly PA, Eikelboom J, et al. Idarucizumab for dabigatran reversal. *N Engl J Med.* 2015; 373: 511–520.
62. Garcia DA, Baglin TP, Weitz JI, Samama MM. Parenteral anticoagulants: Antithrombotic Therapy and Prevention of Thrombosis, 9th ed: American College of Chest Physicians Evidence-Based Clinical Practice Guidelines. *Chest*. 2012;141(2):e24s–e43s.

REVIEW QUESTIONS

(1) A 78-year-old male with past medical history of mechanical prosthetic aortic valve replacement on chronic warfarin anticoagulation presents to the hospital with multiple left-sided rib fractures. He complains of pain and difficulty breathing. You are consulted regarding possible epidural placement for analgesia. Per ASRA guidelines, which of the following conditions must be met in order to proceed with epidural placement in this patient?

A. Last dose of warfarin at least 5 days ago
B. INR ≤1.2
C. INR ≤1.4
D. A and B
E. A and C

(2) A 57-year-old male with a past medical history of atrial fibrillation on apixaban and recently diagnosed colon cancer presents to the hospital for a scheduled open colon resection. During review of his home medications, he mentions that he forgot to hold his apixaban for 72 hours as he had been instructed; he took his last dose of apixaban 32 hours ago. Epidural is contraindicated in this patient based on ASRA guidelines. Which of the following is NOT an appropriate alternative regional technique for postoperative analgesia in this patient?

A. Erector spinae plane block (ESPB)
B. Transversus abdominis plane (TAP) block
C. Rectus sheath catheter (RSC)
D. Paravertebral block

(3) Which of the following potential side effects/complications are associated with performance of an interpleural block?

A. Local anesthetic systemic toxicity
B. Pneumothorax
C. Interbronchial injection
D. All of the above

4. What is the half-life of dabigatran?

A. 1–1.5 hours
B. 6–8 hours
C. 12–14 hours
D. 20 hours

(5) Which of the following pairings does not accurately pair an anticoagulant medication with its reversal?

A. Dabigatran—Prothrombin complex concentrate (PCC)
B. Rivaroxaban—Andexanet alfa
C. Warfarin—Prothrombin complex concentrate (PCC)
D. Unfractionated heparin—Protamine sulfate

(6) A 65-year-old female with recently diagnosed mesothelioma presents to the hospital for a scheduled radical pleurectomy. A thoracic epidural catheter is placed prior to induction of general anesthesia and remains in place until postop day 5, at which point the team plans to remove the catheter. Throughout her postop course, the patient receives once daily prophylactic enoxaparin. Prior to removing the patient's epidural catheter, which of the following MUST be performed?

A. Wait at least 12 hours after the last enoxaparin dose
B. Check a platelet level
C. Check an anti-Xa level
D. A and B
E. A, B, and C

(7) Per ASRA guidelines, which of the following forms of anticoagulation can safely be administered to a patient with an indwelling epidural catheter?

A. Twice-daily prophylactic enoxaparin
B. IV unfractionated heparin infusion
C. Apixaban
D. Dabigatran

(8) A 48-year-old female with metastatic ovarian cancer presents for scheduled open laparotomy, debulking, and total abdominal hysterectomy with bilateral salpingo-oophorectomy. An epidural catheter is placed, and the case proceeds under general anesthesia. On postop day 2, the patient is diagnosed with a pulmonary embolism; an IV unfractionated heparin infusion is initiated. On postop day 5, the heparin infusion is paused for 6 hours, normal coagulation studies are confirmed, and the epidural catheter is removed. The surgical team wants to start the patient on therapeutic enoxaparin. For how long following epidural catheter removal must therapeutic enoxaparin administration be delayed?

A. No delay—therapeutic enoxaparin can be started immediately
B. 4 hours
C. 6 hours
D. 24 hours

ANSWERS

(1) **D.** The American Society of Regional Anesthesia (ASRA) recommends that chronic warfarin therapy be stopped 5 days before epidural placement; additionally, INR should be checked and confirmed to be less than or equal to 1.2 prior to epidural placement, although an INR of 1.4 or less in patients who have not been on warfarin does not increase the risk of spinal bleeding. In the first 1 to 3 days after discontinuation of warfarin therapy, the coagulation status may not be adequate for hemostasis despite a decrease in the INR (indicating a return of factor VII activity). Adequate levels of II, VII, IX, and X may not be present until the INR is within normal limits.

Reference

Horlocker TT, Vandermeulen E, Kopp SL, Gogarten W, Leffert LR, Benzon HT. Regional anesthesia in the patient receiving antithrombotic or thrombolytic therapy: American Society of Regional Anesthesia and Pain Medicine Evidence-Based Guidelines (fourth edition). *Reg Anesth Pain Med.* 2018;43(3):263–309.

(2) **D.** Erector spinae plane block (ESPB), transversus abdominis plane (TAP) block, and rectus sheath catheter (RSC) are all alternative regional techniques that can be used for postoperative abdominal wall analgesia when epidural is contraindicated due to anticoagulation. A paravertebral block would not be a valid alternative to epidural in this case. In the setting of anticoagulation, paravertebral blocks are high risk for hemorrhagic complications; as such, ASRA recommends that these blocks be performed using the same anticoagulation guidelines as neuraxial blocks. In this case, a paravertebral block would be contraindicated as well.

Reference

Horlocker TT, Vandermeulen E, Kopp SL, Gogarten W, Leffert LR, Benzon HT. Regional anesthesia in the patient receiving antithrombotic or thrombolytic therapy: American Society of Regional Anesthesia and Pain Medicine Evidence-Based Guidelines (fourth edition). *Reg Anesth Pain Med.* 2018;43(3):263–309.

(3) **D.** The interpleural block is associated with numerous potential complications including pneumothorax (2% incidence), local anesthetic systemic toxicity (1.3% incidence), catheter misplacement, Horner's syndrome, phrenic nerve paralysis, infection, and interbronchial injection.

References

Dravid RM, Paul RE. Interpleural block: part 1. *Anaesthesia.* 2007;62(10):1039–1049.
Dravid RM, Paul RE. Interpleural block: part 2. *Anaesthesia.* 2007;62(11):1143–1153.

(4) **C.** The half-life of dabigatran is 12-14 hours. Dabigatran etexilate (Pradaxa) is the only FDA-approved oral direct thrombin inhibitor. Its anticoagulation effects can be assessed using thrombin clotting time (TT) and ecarin clotting time (ECT). In emergency situations where these clotting assays are not available, one can also measure the activated partial thromboplastin time (aPTT). Prothrombin time is the least sensitive test. Following oral dabigatran etexilate ingestion, peak plasma concentrations occur after 1.5–3 hours. It has a half-life of 12–14 hours. Renal insufficiency leads to significant half-life prolongation of up to 28 hours and results in increased dabigatran exposure. ASRA recommends against epidural placement in patients with a CrCl of less than 30 mL/min. Dabigatran's effects can be reversed by activated charcoal within 1–2 hours of its ingestion. It can also be systematically eliminated via dialysis or using idarucizumab, a monoclonal antibody fragment that binds free and thrombin-bound dabigatran with a high affinity, thus inhibiting dabigatran's anticoagulant effect.

ASRA recommends holding dabigatran for 3–5 days prior to epidural placement, depending on CrCl. It should be held for:

- 5 days (120 hours) in patients with CrCl 30–49 mL/min
- 4 days (96 hours) in patients with CrCl 50–79 mL/min
- 3 days (72 hours) in patients with CrCl ≥80 mL/min

In the event that dabigatran is unintentionally administered to a patient with an indwelling epidural catheter, it is recommended that one wait 34–36 hours following medication administration prior to catheter removal. In this scenario, it may be prudent to also assess dTT or ECT.

References

Lemay A, Kaye AD, Urman RD. Novel anticoagulant agents in the perioperative setting. *Anesthesiol Clin.* 2017;35(2):305–313.
Horlocker TT, Vandermeulen E, Kopp SL, Gogarten W, Leffert LR, Benzon HT. Regional anesthesia in the patient receiving antithrombotic or thrombolytic therapy: American Society of Regional Anesthesia and Pain Medicine Evidence-Based Guidelines (fourth edition). *Reg Anesth Pain Med.* 2018;43(3):263–309.

(5) **A.** Warfarin can be reversed with vitamin K, FFP, or PCC. Rivaroxaban, a direct factor Xa inhibitor, can be reversed with Andexanet alfa. Protamine sulfate provides complete reversal of unfractionated heparin. However, dabigatran is reversed by idarucizumab, not PCC.

Reference

Meltzer J, Guenzer JR. Anticoagulant reversal and anesthetic considerations. *Anesthesiol Clin.* 2017;35(2):191–205.

(6) **D.** For a patient receiving once-daily enoxaparin prophylaxis in the setting of indwelling epidural catheter, enoxaparin should be held for at least 12 hours prior to catheter removal. Additionally, platelet count should be assessed prior to catheter removal if the patient has received enoxaparin for more than 4 days in order to rule out development of heparin-induced thrombocytopenia. Checking anti-Xa levels is not necessary prior to epidural catheter removal.

Reference

Horlocker TT, Vandermeulen E, Kopp SL, Gogarten W, Leffert LR, Benzon HT. Regional anesthesia in the patient receiving antithrombotic or thrombolytic therapy: American Society of Regional Anesthesia and Pain Medicine Evidence-Based Guidelines (fourth edition). *Reg Anesth Pain Med.* 2018;43(3):263–309.

(7) **B.** Apixaban and dabigatran are contraindicated in the setting of indwelling epidural catheter. Although once-daily prophylactic enoxaparin can be administered, twice-daily prophylactic enoxaparin is contraindicated. IV unfractionated heparin infusions can be restarted 1 hour after epidural placement; these patients receiving IV heparin should be closely monitored for development of neurologic deficits.

Reference

Horlocker TT, Vandermeulen E, Kopp SL, Gogarten W, Leffert LR, Benzon HT. Regional anesthesia in the patient receiving antithrombotic or thrombolytic therapy: American Society of Regional Anesthesia and Pain Medicine Evidence-Based Guidelines (fourth edition). *Reg Anesth Pain Med.* 2018;43(3):263–309.

(8) **B.** Therapeutic enoxaparin administration can be restarted following a 4-hour delay after epidural catheter removal, or a 24-hour delay after epidural catheter placement, whichever is greater.

44.

ACUTE CORONARY SYNDROME IN A PATIENT WITH A THORACIC EPIDURAL CATHETER

Yan Lai and Samiat Jinadu

STEM CASE AND KEY QUESTIONS

A 65-year-old, ASA 3, body mass index (BMI) of 40kg/m^2 man with a past medical history of well-controlled hypertension and obstructive sleep apnea controlled with continuous positive airway pressure (CPAP) therapy presents for a Whipple procedure. Preoperative labs including complete blood count, comprehensive metabolic panel, and coagulation panel were within normal limits. Preoperatively, a thoracic epidural catheter at T6 level was placed uneventfully. Two large bore IVs and an arterial line were also placed. He undergoes an uneventful anesthetic induction and airway is secured for the procedure. During the procedure, the patient suddenly becomes hypotensive with blood pressure dropping to 70/30 and heart rate rising to 123. Almost immediately, the surgeon informs you that there has been an inadvertent injury to the hepatic artery. As the surgical team works expeditiously to control the bleeding, the massive transfusion protocol is initiated and the patient is started on various vasopressors to maintain systemic perfusion. The surgical team is eventually able to control the bleeding, repair the hepatic artery, and complete the surgical procedure. Near the end of surgery, the patient received 10 units of packed red blood cells (PRBC), 10 units of fresh frozen plasma (FFP), and 3 units of pooled platelets.

Due to concerns for massive fluid shifts during surgery with possible tracheal edema, possibility for further hemorrhage and return to the operating room (OR) with ongoing coagulopathy, and potential challenges in postoperative oxygenation and ventilation, the anesthesiology team decide to keep the patient intubated after surgery. Patient was transported to the intensive care unit (ICU) and remained hemodynamically stable. However, on postoperative day 1 he becomes progressively more hypotensive with high vasopressor medication requirements. A 12-lead electrocardiogram (EKG) is performed and reveals ST segment elevations in leads II, V4, V5 and V6. Troponins are elevated and international normalized ratio (INR) remains at 1.8 on subsequent laboratory results. The cardiology team is consulted for immediate percutaneous coronary intervention (PCI) in the setting of a myocardial ischemia with a thrombotic origin (STEMI). In the interim, the patient was started on a heparin infusion with a target activated clotting time (ACT) before planned PCI.

(1) WHY WAS AN EPIDURAL CATHETER PLACED? WHY AT T6 LEVEL?

Thoracic epidural catheters and neuraxial techniques in general are excellent supplements to general anesthesia for major thoracic and abdominal surgeries. These techniques are important centerpieces in providing multimodal analgesic therapy and contribute to an opioid-sparing anesthetic. In the current context of our opioid epidemic, with a large number of patients experiencing chronic pain syndromes after surgery, these techniques offer invaluable and immense benefits on postoperative outcomes. Thoracic epidural catheters are one of the most effective tools for managing acute pain after major thoracic, abdominal, urological, and gynecological surgeries. Thoracic epidural catheters have numerous proven benefits such as:[1]

- Decreasing postoperative stress response. An activated stress response during surgery leads to the increase of plasma stress hormones such as catecholamines. This sympathetic response can raise ventricular afterload and heart rate resulting in decreased coronary perfusion.[2] In addition, an increase in circulating pro-inflammatory cytokines can also lead to plaque instability. The combination of decreased coronary perfusion and plaque instability can potentially elevate the risk of myocardial ischemia and the occurrence of perioperative acute coronary syndrome (ACS).[3]
- Decreasing incidence of perioperative cardiac events, especially when the epidural analgesia is continued for more than 24 hours.[4] It may also decrease the 30-day mortality for patients with high cardiac risk, as suggested by some small studies.[5]
- Prompt recovery of intestinal function by decreasing sympathetic tone and decreasing opioid use. The decrease in opioid use will lessen the side effects that accompany opioid therapy, such as constipation.[6]
- Allows for fast-track and earlier extubation with shorter mechanical ventilation times and decreased incidence of ventilator-associated pneumonia.[7]

For a Whipple or any large abdominal procedure, an epidural placed at T6 will provide dermatomal coverage to areas with significant postoperative pain, namely T4 to T12. The extent and level of coverage perioperatively also depends on the subsequent continuous local anesthetic infusion and any intermittent boluses that are employed and managed by the acute pain medicine service.

(2) IN THE SETTING OF MASSIVE HEMORRHAGE, WHAT ARE YOUR CONCERNS AND CONSIDERATIONS WITH THE EPIDURAL CATHETER?

After massive hemorrhage, persistent hemodynamic disturbances and coagulopathy are the main concerns during the perioperative period. In the setting of hypotension due to hypovolemia or shock states, an activated epidural catheter may potentiate or worsen hemodynamic lability and can make further management challenging. The epidural infusion may have to be decreased or stopped in the acute postoperative period. Further bolus dosing of opioids and especially local anesthetics should be avoided through the epidural catheter.

Another concern is the implications of massive hemorrhage on the coagulation cascade pathway. Despite the fact that this patient has normal coagulation panel preoperatively, massive hemorrhage will lead to a consumption of coagulation factors which can further exacerbate bleeding. With an epidural, this increased risk of bleeding brings into consideration increased risks for a thoracic epidural hematoma. Plans for adequate neurologic monitoring should be considered after surgery.

(3) IS THE HEPARIN INFUSION CONTRAINDICATED WITH AN INDWELLING EPIDURAL CATHETER? SHOULD THE EPIDURAL CATHETER BE REMOVED NOW?

The decision to remove the epidural catheter at this moment is an extremely difficult one, given the ongoing coagulopathy (elevated INR) and concomitant administration of an anticoagulant as a treatment for ACS. The removal of the catheter might cause tissue trauma and disrupt existing fibrin clot formation around the catheter. This may potentially trigger epidural hematoma formation when tissue hemostasis around the catheter is disturbed in an environment where anticoagulants are administered. This is consistent with the literature on epidural use in cardiac surgery where patients are routinely heparinized.[8]

The American Society of Regional Anesthesia (ASRA) guidelines on regional anesthesia and anticoagulation recommends the following precautions for minimizing risks during the removal of existing indwelling epidural catheter when heparinization is necessary:[8]

- When normal coagulation profile is restored, epidural catheters should be removed. Patients should be closely monitored for symptoms of hematoma formation
- Heparin dosing and reversal should be meticulously measured such that the lowest dose of heparin compatible with therapeutic goals is employed.

In this scenario, we need to consider the "benefits" of leaving a stable epidural catheter in place versus the risks of current and future anticoagulation regimen after potential cardiac stent placement. A multidisciplinary discussion with a patient's family, anesthesiology, cardiology, surgery, acute pain medicine, and ICU team should be considered to clarify expectations and plans moving forward.

(4) COULD WE HAVE REMOVED THE EPIDURAL CATHETER BEFORE INITIATION OF HEPARIN INFUSION?

Arguably, a potential window to remove the catheter might have existed before the initiation of heparin, despite the already elevated INR. The elevated INR might be caused by injury to the hepatic artery, manipulation of the liver during the surgery, massive transfusion during the operation, or likely a combination of these factors. After ACS is diagnosed in the ICU, coagulation panel, platelet aggregometry, and thromboelastography (TEG) can be acquired to provide further insights and information on the patient's coagulation status before a decision is made to remove the epidural catheter. However, given the acuity of the ACS episode, this might be impractical, and waiting on point-of-care testing results may delay definitive care such as immediate cardiac catheterization. Thorough multidisciplinary discussion should be initiated with the surgical and cardiology team on the risk-benefit of delaying cardiac intervention versus the risk of keeping the epidural in place in an anticoagulated patient and the risk of removing the epidural and starting anticoagulation immediately after.

Regardless of what decision is made, the patient is now at an increased risk of acquiring a thoracic epidural hematoma. Close neurological monitoring should be strongly considered so as to ensure prompt intervention if a hematoma is developed.

The epidural is kept in place on the way to cardiac catheterization. The patient undergoes PCI and a drug-eluting stent is placed. He started on dual antiplatelet therapy (DAPT) with aspirin 81 mg and clopidogrel 75 mg after loading doses were given. The team decided to remove the epidural on postoperative day 2 since long-term DAPT is expected. The catheter is blood-tinged on removal. On postoperative day 3, the patient is found to be anemic without any obvious signs for abdominal bleeding. There is concern for acute occult bleeding such as the formation of an epidural hematoma. However, the patient remains intubated and cannot tolerate light sedation in order to perform an extensive neurological monitoring.

(5) SHOULD THE EPIDURAL CATHETER BE REMOVED AFTER CESSATION OF HEPARIN THERAPY AND INITIATION OF DAPT?

According to ASRA guidelines, after initiation of clopidogrel, the drug should be discontinued 1–2 days to allow for safe removal of a neuraxial catheter.[8] However, this suggestion is based on the assumption that a loading dose is not administered. Furthermore, this recommendation is based on the concept that it can take up to 7 days for a steady state to be achieved with a dose of 75 mg of clopidogrel. In contrast, a loading dose of 300–600 mg will reach steady state in a matter of hours.[8] However, this is impractical in an

ACS setting such as this patient, where a loading is likely required to ensure cardiac stent survival. In addition, early interruption of his DAPT regimen in order for epidural catheter removal puts him at risk of occluding the drug-eluting stent (in-stent thrombosis or stenosis) that can result in disastrous consequences and carries fatality rates of up to 80%.

To assist with decision-making about removing epidural catheters, additional monitoring modalities such as basic coagulation panel including prothrombin time, activated partial thromboplastin time, platelet assays, and thromboelastography can be employed. Platelet assays such as platelet aggregometry can be a useful qualitative measure of platelet function. However, this test is limited by lengthy calibration and standardization processes that often require a control sample.[9] Thromboelastography (TEG) can be used to give a global assessment of hemostasis, ensuring that there is an adequate balance between clotting factors.[10] On a TEG, the R time gives the speed of the formation of a clot as a reflection of coagulation factors, mA describes the clotting strength as a reflection of the platelet function, and the alpha angle describes the speed of clot buildup and reflects the function of fibrinogen.[11] Despite the fact that these tests can be highly informative to guide point-of-care decision-making, it is difficult to apply in a patient on DAPT since there is minimal literature on the correlations between coagulation test results and the rare incidences of epidural hematoma formation.

(6) HOW DO WE DIAGNOSE EPIDURAL HEMATOMA IN AN INTUBATED AND SEDATED PATIENT, AND HOW SHOULD WE MANAGE ONCE DIAGNOSIS IS CONFIRMED?

Epidural hematoma is a rare event and its true incidence is unknown. Estimated incidences for epidural hematoma for patients exposed to heparin ranges from 1:220,000 to 1:2000.[8] Prompt diagnosis depends on a high index of suspicion, combined with constellation of clinical symptoms and signs of neurologic deficits. The ideal situation would be to proceed with prompt extubation when possible and safe for the patient so as to ensure proper neurological monitoring. However, when this is not possible, the most sensitive tool to detect an epidural hematoma would be emergent magnetic resonance imaging (MRI) or, if contraindicated, a computed tomography (CT) myelogram. Once diagnosed, emergent surgical spinal decompression is indicated, and the best outcomes are obtained when decompression occurs within the first 8 hours of diagnosis.[8]

(7) HOW SHOULD WE MANAGE HIS ABDOMINAL PAIN ONCE THE EPIDURAL CATHETER IS REMOVED AND HE IS NOW NEUROLOGICALLY STABLE ON POD 5? THE PATIENT ASKS IF ANY OTHER REGIONAL ANESTHETIC OPTIONS MAY BE USEFUL AT THIS POINT, AS THEY WOULD LIKE TO AVOID THE USE OF OPIOIDS.

This patient remains on DAPT, and any neuraxial or deep plexus block is now contraindicated. More superficial truncal blocks that may be applicable in this setting include transverse abdominis plane (TAP) block, subcostal TAP block, erector spinae block (ESPB), serratus anterior plane block, and quadratus lumborum block (QLB). ASRA guidelines suggest that the decision on whether to perform the block should be based on site compressibility, vascularity, and consequences of bleeding.[8] It is significant to note that a single injection of a long-acting local anesthetic such as ropivacaine or bupivacaine would provide relief for a maximum of only 10–12 hours. Other adjuncts or additives, as well as a truncal block catheter, should be considered based on analgesic benefits and further hemorrhagic risks. Nevertheless, the use of multimodal analgesia would be the safest and most beneficial approach for this patient, taking into consideration his concerns, history of obstructive sleep apnea and obesity, and complicated surgical and perioperative courses.

DISCUSSION

Thoracic neuraxial techniques are effective methods for managing acute pain after major thoracic, abdominal, urological, and gynecological surgeries. However, thoracic epidural anesthesia (TEA) is not without its risks, which include neurological injury, serious spinal or epidural bleeding and hematoma, infection, and possible decreased organ perfusion from resulting hypotension.[1] Despite the lack of serious sequelae that are reported in the literature, some of the controversial and relative benefits of TEA are still being debated, with some studies showing no difference in the risk of myocardial infarction when compared with general anesthesia.[5,8]

This discussion will focus on hemorrhagic complications of epidural techniques, its consequences and implications, especially in the setting of ACS. Epidural hematoma is a rare but catastrophic complication if the diagnosis is delayed or missed. In addition, thoracic epidurals are thought to have a higher risk of nerve injury compared to lumbar epidurals because of the presence of a smaller canal. It is of great importance for physician anesthesiologists to have a thorough understanding of the management of thoracic epidural catheters, risk factors for hematoma formation, and adequate neurologic monitoring to ensure prompt diagnosis.

THORACIC EPIDURAL PLACEMENT: ANATOMY AND PATHOPHYSIOLOGY OF INJURY

The epidural catheter can be placed using a midline or paramedian approach. The epidural is placed ensuring proper sterile technique.[12]

Injury after a neuraxial block can occur from injury to the structures of the spinal cord from an inadvertent dural puncture or injury to the nerve roots and surrounding vasculature. Direct injury can also occur from variations or abnormalities in the patient's anatomy, such as incompletely fused ligamentum, ligamaentum flavum hypertrophy, epidural space narrowing, and lipomatosis.[13]

To avoid inadvertent injury to the spinal cord, some providers advocate for light sedation while performing the blocks so that paresthesia caused by contact with the spinal cord can be properly communicated by the patient. However, patient sensation can be nonspecific and often is unreliable as the spinal cord is more sensitive to pain secondary to pressure and it is only through the injection of solution that the patient may report pain.[14] Injury of a blood vessel or intravascular catheter placement will be seen by positive aspiration of blood through the catheter or with a positive test dose.

EPIDURAL HEMATOMA

Epidural hematomas can be caused by direct trauma or can also be spontaneous in nature. The latter is known as spontaneous spinal epidural hematoma (SSEH). The incidence of SSEH is estimated to be 1:1 million.[15] SSEH can be caused by bleeding diathesis, disc herniation, anticoagulation use, uncontrolled hypertension, tumor, or vascular abnormalities such as arteriovenous malformations, and usually occurs in the posterior aspect of the spine because of the extensive network of epidural veins.[16,17] Spontaneous bleeding can be prompted by raised intra-abdominal or intrathoracic pressure; some authors believe it is most likely caused by arterial rupture instead of venous bleeding. This is because intrathecal pressures is greater than vertebral venous pressure, which should theoretically prevent a venous bleed.[18]

With an epidural catheter in place, the risk factors for a thoracic epidural hematoma include patient factors such as vertebral abnormalities, coagulation disorders, traumatic placement with multiple attempts, and pharmacological factors such as the use of anticoagulation and/or antiplatelet therapy.[19] Careful patient selection, thorough history, and meticulous technique are necessary to decrease bleeding risks.

Symptoms

The symptoms of a spinal or epidural hematoma include:

- Neck/back pain with radiating paresthesia to extremities (which can interestingly in itself mimic ACS symptoms)[20]
- Severe tenderness at the site of the epidural catheter
- Cauda equina symptoms can be seen if there is compression of the nerve roots in which the patient has motor weakness, sensory loss, urinary incontinence, and loss of rectal tone leading to fecal incontinence.[21]

Diagnosis

The gold standard to confirm diagnosis of a spinal epidural hematoma is an MRI. In patients who are unable to participate appropriately in neurological tests, such as intubated patients or patients with altered mental status, if there is a high suspicion or concern for a hematoma, an MRI should be done immediately to confirm the diagnosis. If an MRI is unavailable or contraindicated, a CT myelogram can be used.

Treatment

If an MRI is positive for an epidural hematoma, emergent neurosurgical consultation should be obtained. Prompt surgical evacuation of the hematoma should be performed to possibly reverse neurological deficits. Some minor cases of hematoma formation are treated conservatively with steroids; however, surgical treatment before 12 hours has been shown to lead to better outcomes than if treatment was delayed.[22] It is important to be aware that since the thoracic spine has a narrower canal than the lumbar spine, the time to surgery to improve neurological function may in actuality be sooner than 12 hours.

ACUTE CORONARY SYNDROME

Acute coronary syndrome occurs when there is obstruction of coronary blood flow to the heart leading to myocardial ischemia.

Acute coronary syndrome is diagnosed by:[23]

- Clinical symptoms such as chest pain, hypotension, and dyspnea. Chest pain is usually nonspecific and unreliable if a patient is under anesthesia or post-anesthesia.
- EKG changes: ST segment changes, new bundle branch changes, pathological Q waves
- Increase in cardiac biomarkers
- Wall motion abnormalities on imaging such as echocardiography
- Evidence on coronary angiogram.

When a patient is suspected to have myocardial ischemia with a thrombotic origin (STEMI), the next step is to proceed with a form of reperfusion therapy. The options for reperfusion include percutaneous coronary intervention (PCI) or administering potent thrombolytic agents.[23] PCI is the recommended mode of reperfusion therapy. Thrombolysis is indicated with if the patient is at a facility in which PCI is not readily available. However, thrombolysis has multiple contraindications, including prior intracranial hemorrhage, neoplasm or vascular lesion, suspected aortic dissection, active bleeding, and severe uncontrolled hypertension. Relative contraindications include history of chronic and poorly controlled hypertension, history of ischemic stroke longer than 3 months ago, major surgery performed less than 3 weeks ago, and noncompressible vascular puncture. The patient in the stem case would not have qualified for fibrinolytic therapy. However, if a patient were to qualify, they would initially receive heparin, lovenox, or fondaparinux, followed by a fibrinolytic agent that is continued for up to 14 days to a year.[23]

With PCI, the cardiology team decides on whether to proceed with balloon angioplasty, bare metal stent, or a drug-eluting stent. The goal is to perform this procedure 12–24 hours after the ischemic events. Patients usually receive a loading dose of clopidogrel, 300–600 mg, before or during the procedure, and clopidogrel 75 mg is continued daily and for 4 weeks after ACS or up to a year after stent placement. Unfractionated heparin can also be an alternative for the clopidogrel loading dose. Other anticoagulants that may be used are bivalirudin, enoxaparin, prasugrel, and ticagrelor.[23]

Cardiac complications remain the most common cause of perioperative morbidity and mortality.[24] As highlighted in the case, anticoagulation or thrombolytic therapy to treat ACS can result in other hemorrhagic complications such as epidural hematomas. Anticoagulation therapy is also commonly used in other occlusive diseases, ischemic cerebrovascular disease and peripheral vascular disease.[9] The placement and management of patients on such therapy has become more common. As a result, ASRA has published guidelines for placement of neuraxial deep plexus, deep peripheral blocks, and superficial peripheral blocks in patients on antithrombotic or thrombolytic therapy.[8] It is therefore important to be aware of current guidelines so as to properly assess and navigate unique situations when they arise.

ANTICOAGULATION GUIDELINES

As discussed previously, other alternatives to clopidogrel include unfractionated heparin, bivalirudin, enoxaparin, prasugrel, and ticagrelor.[23]

ENOXAPARIN

Enoxaparin is a low molecular weight heparin (LMWH). It binds and potentiates the effect of antithrombin III, which leads to the formation of a complex that irreversibly inactivates factor Xa.[25] When compared to unfractioned heparin, enoxaparin has less activity against factor IIa.

Enoxaparin may be monitored clinically by monitoring signs of bleeding and especially paying attention to dosing in renally impaired patients and obese patients. Anti-factor Xa level may be measured and is the recommended test to monitor efficacy.[26] The standard dosing of enoxaparin, barring renal impairment, is 1 mg/kg twice daily, subcutaneously. In other indications, such as for venous thromboembolic precautions, the dosing is 30 or 40 mg daily, subcutaneously.[26] Enoxaparin may be reversed using protamine sulfate which binds to the LMWH to form an inactive complex.[27] This leads to a 60% reduction in the activity of enoxaparin. The recommended dosing for reversal is 1 mg protamine sulfate per 1 mg of enoxaparin.[28]

Per the ASRA guidelines, for prophylactic or therapeutic twice daily dosing, indwelling catheters should be removed prior to initiation of LMWH, and therefore there are no recommendations for removal as a catheter should be avoided. For daily dosing, catheters may be removed 12 hours after the last enoxaparin dose.

HEPARIN

Per ASRA guidelines, there is an unknown risk for the removal of catheters in a patient receiving high-dose subcutaneous heparin (7500–10,000 U) and the risk/benefit should be assessed on a case-per-case basis. For low-dose subcutaneous heparin (5000 U), an indwelling neuraxial catheter may be removed 4–6 hours after the last dose. If heparin is administered intravenously, the catheter may be removed 4–6 hours after discontinuation of the intravenous dose and with return of normal coagulations status. Heparin may be reversed by protamine, with a dosing of 1.0–1.5 mg of protamine per 100 U of unfractionated heparin.[29]

TICAGRELOR AND CANGELOR

Ticagrelor, a nonthienopyridine, is a direct-acting oral antagonist of P2Y12-adenosine diphosphate (ADP) receptor blocker. Platelet activation includes the interaction between ADP and P2Y12 receptor, which activates glycoprotein IIb/IIa and leads to platelet aggregation.[30] Ticagrelor has a maximum plasma concentration 1–3 hours after treatment and a plasma half-life of 6–13 hours.[31] Cangrelor, another nonthienipyridine with similar mechanism of action to ticagrelor, achieves maximum platelet inhibition within 15 minutes of initiation of an infusion, without a bolus dose. Cangrelor also has a short plasma half-life, with a half-life of less than 9 minutes.[32] In comparison to clopidogrel (a thienopyridienes), ticagrelor is reversible and has greater platelet inhibition activity.[33] ASRA recommends the avoidance of ticagrelor or cangrelor in a patient with an epidural catheter.

Table 44.1 provides a summary of the ASRA guidelines for the management of an indwelling epidural catheter in patients taking other common medications that may be encountered in a patient with acute coronary syndrome.[8]

HERBAL MEDICATIONS

When discussing anticoagulation, it is important to be aware of the possible effects of herbal medications, as some of these medications can have unpredictable effects on coagulation. Common herbal medications that have such anticoagulation effects are garlic, which causes inhibition of platelet aggregation; ginkgo, which inhibits platelet activating factor; and ginseng, which can increase bleeding risk and decrease anticoagulant effect of warfarin (Table 44.2).

The current ASRA recommendations state that herbal medications have a low risk and therefore do not interfere with the placement and management of neuraxial blocks. However, it is important to be aware of the effects that herbal medications can have on normal coagulation as they can have an increased effect, especially when combined with other platelet aggregation inhibitors.

PATIENT WITH AN EPIDURAL CATHETER WHO DEVELOPS ACS

Managing an epidural catheter in a patient with ACS now on anticoagulation is a unique and challenging problem that can occur clinically. Clearly, there are no official recommendations on such a situation. However, there are multiple published case reports that discussed steps that were taken to ensure a safe outcome for the patient. It cannot be overstated the need for an interdisciplinary discussion to consider the risk

Table 44.1 THE MANAGEMENT OF AN INDWELLING EPIDURAL CATHETER ON COMMON MEDICATIONS IN A PATIENT WITH ACUTE CORONARY SYNDROME

	MECHANISM OF ACTION	HOLD MEDICATION BEFORE PROCEDURE	RESTART MEDICATION AFTER PROCEDURE	HOLD MEDICATION BEFORE CATHETER REMOVAL	RESTART MEDICATION AFTER CATHETER REMOVAL
Aspirin	Cox inhibitor	No restrictions *	No restrictions	No restrictions	No restrictions
Clopidogrel	ADP receptor antagonist	5–7 days	Immediately if no loading dose provided	Catheter can be maintained 1–2 days if no loading dose provided	Immediately. 6 hours if loading dose is provided
IV heparin	Potentiates Antithrombin III effect	4–6 hours and normal labs	1 hour	4–6 hours	1 hour
Enoxaparin	Factor Xa inactivation	24 hours for doses of 1 mg/kg twice daily or 1.5 mg/kg daily	Restart medications 12 hours after needle catheter placement. The second dose should occur no sooner than 24 hours. Catheters should be removed before before initiation of therapeutic LMWH treatment.	Catheters should be removed 12 hours after the prophylactic dose.	4 hours
Fondaparinx	Factor Xa inhibitor	Not recommendation	Not recommended	Not recommended	6 hours
Bivaliridin	Thrombin inhibitor	Not recommended	Not recommended	Not recommended	Not recommended

* No restrictions, if no other antiplatelet or anticoagulant therapy is being used concomitantly.

of removing the epidural with anticoagulation therapy being continued, discontinuing anticoagulation therapy to remove the epidural safely, or maintaining the epidural catheter in place.

The main options if such a problem were to arise are:

1. **Keeping the epidural in place**: In the stem case, the epidural catheter being kept in place initially after the complicated surgical course of massive bleeding is a reasonable decision (before ACS is diagnosed). It is thought that keeping the epidural catheter in place can serve as a tamponade until adequate coagulation activity is achieved in the patient.[34] Then, the patient was started acutely on a heparin infusion for ACS in the ICU. ASRA recommends that heparin be discontinued 4–6 hours before removal of epidural catheters.[8] This is based on a published case series that reported that 50% of spinal hematomas were diagnosed at the time of catheter removal in patients receiving systemic heparin.[8] By far, cardiothoracic surgery with cardiopulmonary bypass (CPB) provides the best example to explore the relationship between systemic heparinization and thoracic epidural catheters. Based on published studies with small sample sizes (4583 epidural and 10,840 spinal anesthetics), there are surprisingly no major complications that are associated in this cohort.[8] According to 2018 ASRA guidelines, there is only one published case of spinal hematoma in a patient receiving intravenous heparin during CPB.[8] In addition, this sole case had multiple confounding risk factors that conformed to a significantly higher hemorrhagic risk for this patient.[8] Thus, this unanswered relationship between heparin and epidural catheter removal is still debatable. Nevertheless, most clinicians agree that it is prudent to leave epidural catheters in place until a plan for heparin cessation is confirmed. Furthermore, the 2018 ASRA guidelines also acknowledge that the inherent risks are too controversial and appear too great for the perceived analgesic benefits in high-risk patients.[8] The 2018 ASRA guidelines proposed the following to minimize risks:[8]

   (a) Neuraxial blocks should be avoided in a patient with known coagulopathy from any cause.

   (b) Surgery should be delayed 24 hours in the event of a traumatic tap.

   (c) Time from instrumentation to systemic heparinization should exceed 60 minutes.

   (d) Heparin effect and reversal should be tightly controlled (smallest amount of heparin for the shortest duration compatible with therapeutic objectives).

   (e) Epidural catheters should be removed when normal coagulation is restored, and patients should be closely monitored postoperatively for signs and symptoms of hematoma formation.

   Subsequently, this patient received a drug-eluted stent which requires DAPT for at least 6 months (new

Table 44.2 ANTICOAGULATION AND REGIONAL ANESTHESIA

DRUG	MECHANISM/ SITE OF ACTION	HALF-LIFE	HOLD BEFORE PROCEDURE	RESTART AFTER PROCEDURE	HOLD BEFORE CATHETER REMOVAL	RESTART AFTER CATHETER REMOVAL
Anticoagulants						
Warfarin (Coumadin)	Vitamin K antagonism	35 hours	5 days and INR ≤1.2	No Delay	INR <1.5, 12–24 hours after warfarin dose	No delay
Fondaparinux (Arixtra)	Anti-Factor Xa Agents	17–21 hours	No recommendations	Avoid with catheters	Avoid with catheters	6 hours
Apixaban (Eliquis)		12 hours	72 hours	6 hours Avoid with catheters	26–30 hours	6 hours
Rivaroxaban (Xarelto)		5.7–9.2 hours	72 hours	6 hours Avoid with catheters	22–26 hours	6 hours
Edoxaban (Savaysa)		8–10 hours	72 hours	6 hours Avoid with catheters	20–28 hours	6 hours
Betrixaban (Bevyxxa)		20 hours	72 hours	5 hours Avoid with catheters	72 hours	5 hours
Dabigatran (Pradaxa)	Direct Thrombin Inhibitor	12–14 hours	3–5 days (depending on CrCl)	6 hours Avoid with catheters	34–36 hours	6 hours
Argatroban (Acova)		30–50 minutes	Avoid	Avoid	Avoid	Avoid
Bivalirudin (Angiomax)		25 minutes				
Lepirudin (Refludan)		1 hour				
Desirudin (Revasc)		1 hour (IV) 2 hours (SC)				
IV Heparin	Antithrombin III activator (IIa/Xa inhibition)	1–1.5 hours	4-6 hours AND Normal coags	1 hour	4–6 hours AND Normal coags	1 hour
SC Heparin 5000 U BID/TID		1.5 hours	4–6 hours OR Normal coags	Immediately	4-6 hours	Immediately
SC Heparin 7500–1000 U BID (or ≤20,000 U qd)			12 hours AND Normal coags	Unknown Risk	Unknown Risk	Immediately
SC Heparin Dose >10,000 U (or >20,000 U qd)			24 hours AND Normal coags	Avoid with catheters (app)	(no app/no article)	Immediately
LMWH Prophylactic Enoxaparin (Lovenox) Dalteparin (Fragmin) Tinzaparin (Innohep)	Antithrombin III activator (Xa>>IIa inhibition)	3–6 hours	12 hours	12 hours	12 hours	4 hours (or 12 hours after epidural placement, whichever is greater)
LMWH Therapeutic Enoxaparin (Lovenox) Dalteparin (Fragmin) Tinzaparin (Innohep)			24 hours	24–72 hours (depending on surgical bleeding risk) Avoid with catheters	Avoid with catheters	4 hours (or 24 hours after epidural placement, whichever is greater)

(*continued*)

Table 44.2 CONTINUED

DRUG	MECHANISM/ SITE OF ACTION	HALF-LIFE	HOLD BEFORE PROCEDURE	RESTART AFTER PROCEDURE	HOLD BEFORE CATHETER REMOVAL	RESTART AFTER CATHETER REMOVAL
Antiplatelet Agents						
NSAIDs (including aspirin)	COX inhibitors	Variable	No restrictions	No restrictions	No restrictions	No restrictions
Clopidogrel (Plavix)	P2Y12 ADP Receptor Antagonist	7–8 hours	5–7 days	Immediately (if no bolus and 24 hours post-op)	Avoid with Catheters	Immediately (if no bolus and 24 hours postop) 6 hours for loading dose
Prasugrel (Effient)		8 hours	7–10 days	Immediately (if no bolus and 24 hours postop) Avoid with catheters	Avoid with catheters	Immediately (if no bolus and 24 hours postop) 6 hours for loading dose
Ticlodipine (Ticlid)		20–50 hours	10 days	Immediately (if no bolus and 24 hours postop)	Avoid with Catheters	Immediately (if no bolus and 24 hours postop) 6 hours for loading dose
Ticagrelor (Brilinta)		7 hours	5–7 days	Immediately (if no bolus and 24 hours postop) Avoid with catheters	Avoid with catheters	Immediately (if no bolus and 24 hours postop) 6 hours for loading dose
Cangrelor (Kengreal)		3–6 minutes	3 hours	Avoid with catheters	Avoid with catheters	8 hours
Cilostazol (Pletal)	Phosphodiesterase Inhibitor	10.5 hours	2 days	Avoid with catheters	Avoid with catheters	6 hours
Dipyridamole (Aggrenox)		10 hours	24 hours			

generation stents versus 1 year for traditional stents). Therefore, keeping the epidural indefinitely is not a viable option. Although most published data of epidural catheter infections pertain to catheters that are not tunneled, the risk of infection of the catheter increases after 4 days. By day 4 of an indwelling catheter, 99% of the catheters are reported to be free of an infection and colonization. This rate decreases to 96% by day 7 and 73% by day 15. Also, mild signs of epidural catheter infection will usually worsen and can progress to an abscess if the catheter is left in place for long periods of time.[35]

2. **Discontinue anticoagulation using the ASRA guidelines and safely remove catheter**: An interdisciplinary discussion should weigh the risk of coronary stent re-occlusion versus risks of an epidural hematoma. In a patient with a newly placed coronary stent and an indwelling epidural catheter, Noll et al. discussed an approach where clopidogrel was discontinued for 5 days that was bridged with intravenous unfractionated heparin, aspirin for 1 day, and then stopping heparin for 6 hours. After checking for heparin reversal with activated partial thromboplastin time and platelet count, the epidural was removed. In this case, discussions with the cardiologists and neurosurgeons led to the decision that the risk of an epidural hematoma was greater than re-occlusion of the stent as the patient could be rapidly returned to the interventional unit if an acute re-occlusion were to occur.[36] While this approach appears conservative and prudent, it is important to fully understand the implications of prematurely discontinuing antiplatelet therapy.

Studies indicate that up to half of postoperative myocardial infarctions are due to the disruption of unstable plaques and the increased thrombogenicity of blood, coupled with the increased thrombogenic risk brought about by the stress response of surgery. Arguably, this is a crucial period in which a patient's antiplatelet therapy should be continued. This increased risk is the reason behind the recommendations by the American Heart

Association (AHA) that elective surgery should be delayed 30 days after the placement of a bare metal stent and 6 months after DES implantation.[37] After ACS with or without intervention, aspirin is a lifelong medication that should never be discontinued. Aspirin has been shown to decrease the risk of re-infarction by 30%.[38] Secondly, the period immediately after PCI is a vulnerable time for the patient as the stenotic coronary lesion has been made more unstable due to the rupture of its endothelial covering. This is further illustrated by the increased rate of myocardial ischemia and mortality in patients who undergo surgery in this period.[39] The acute and premature discontinuation of antiplatelet therapy has deleterious effects as there is a rebound prothrombotic effect. With acute disruption of aspirin, excessive thromboxane A2 formation and decreased fibrinogen are seen.[40] In addition, a study demonstrated that premature clopidogrel discontinuation is a major predictor of stent thrombosis. It is implicated in increased mortality and also late thrombosis of the drug eluting stent.[41,42] Despite high confidence in the patient being able to urgently return to the intervention unit for repeat PCI, emergent PCI for revascularization in the early postoperative period is more difficult. Finally, although heparin protects high-risk patients who are undergoing ACS, it has not been shown to mimic the effect of antiplatelets and should not be used liberally as a substitute for aspirin and clopidogrel.[43]

3. **Remove epidural and continue with neurological monitoring**: The optimal time to remove the epidural would be before the initiation of PCI and before starting of any initial anticoagulant therapy. It may also be removed after PCI before a second antiplatelet therapy is started.[11] Late removal may also be optimized by switching to a short-acting reversible inhibitor such as Tirofiban infusion to facilitate removal while decreasing the risk of stent re-thrombosis.[44] Coagulation studies, platelet assays, and TEG can lend further information on the patient's exact coagulation status before removal of the epidural catheter. Patients should be closely monitored for neurological changes for 12–24 hours after catheter removal, and they should be kept in an ICU setting.[9] In addition, neurosurgical and interventional cardiology teams should be ready to intervene in a timely manner.

CONCLUSIONS

- Thoracic epidural analgesia is an important modality for acute perioperative pain management.
- An epidural hematoma is a rare but catastrophic risk that can occur when an epidural is placed, or afterward. The risk of bleeding is increased by the use of anticoagulation therapy. The occurrence of an ACS episode can complicate the management of an epidural catheter as anticoagulation therapy is a mainstay treatment of ACS.
- Premature and acute interruption of anticoagulation following percutaneous coronary intervention can have serious implications.
- A multidisciplinary discussion is important to navigate challenging cases in which a patient with thoracic epidural analgesia in place suffers from acute coronary disease. Every case is unique and should be managed on a case-by-case basis.
- In the case that an epidural hematoma forms, it should be surgically intervened on before 8 hours to prevent permanent neurological damage.

REFERENCES

1. Friese, H, Van Aken H. Risks and benefits of thoracic epidural anaesthesia. *Br J Anaesthes.* 2011;107(6):859–868.
2. Meissner A, Rolf N, Van Aken H. Thoracic epidural anesthesia and the patient with heart disease: benefits, risks, and controversies. *Anesth Analg.* 1997;85(3):517–528.
3. Gidron Y, Gilutz H, Berger R, Huleihel M. Molecular and cellular interface between behavior and acute coronary syndromes. *Cardiovasc Res.* 2002;56:15–21.
4. Beattie WS, Badner NH, Choi P. Epidural analgesia reduces postoperative myocardial infarction: a meta-analysis. *Anesth Analg.* 2001; 93: 853–858.
5. Schug S. The effect of neuraxial blockade on peri-operative mortality and major morbidity: an updated meta-analysis. *Anaesth Intens Care.* 2005;33:675.
6. Marret E, Remy C, Bonnet F. Meta-analysis of epidural analgesia versus parenteral opioid analgesia after colorectal surgery. *Br J Surg.* 2007;94:665–673.
7. Popping D, Elia N, Marret E, Remy C, Tramer MR. Protective effects of epidural analgesia on pulmonary complications after abdominal and thoracic surgery: a meta-analysis. *Arch Surg.* 2008; 143: 990–999.
8. Horlocker T, Vandermeulen E, Kopp S, Gogarten W, Leffert L, Benzon H. Regional anesthesia in the patient receiving antithrombotic or thrombolytic therapy: American Society of Regional Anesthesia and Pain Medicine Evidence-Based Guidelines (fourth edition). *Reg Anesth Pain Med.* 2018; 43: 263–309.
9. Osta W, Akbary H, Fuleihan S. Epidural analgesia in vascular surgery patients actively taking Clopidogrel. *Br J Anaesthes.* 2010; 104 (4): 429–432.
10. Glenn E, Mehl J, Rosinia FA, Henry Liu. Safe removal of an epidural catheter 72 hours after clopidogrel and aspirin administrations guided by platelet function analysis and thromboelastography. *J Anaesthesiol Clin Pharmacol.* 2013;29(1):99–101.
11. Wolf S, Kaisers U, Reske A, Strick M. Epidural catheter removal for initiation of emergency anticoagulant therapy in acute coronary syndrome: when is the time right? *Eur J Anaesthesiol.* 2015;32:581–589.
12. Manion S, Brennan T. Thoracic epidural analgesia and acute pain management. *Anesthesiology.* 2011; 115:181–188.
13. Neal J, Bernards C, Hadzic A et al. ASRA practice advisory on neurologic complications in regional anesthesia and pain medicine. *Reg Anesth Pain Med.* 2008;33(5):404–415.
14. Neal JM. Anatomy and pathophysiology of spinal cord injuries associated with regional anesthesia and pain medicine. *Reg Anesth Pain Med.* 2008;33:423–434.
15. Holtås S, Heiling M, Lönntoft M. Spontaneous spinal epidural hematoma: findings at imaging and clinical correlation. *Radiology.* 1996 May;199(2):409–413.
16. Groen RJ, Ponssen H. The spontaneous spinal epidural hematoma: a study of the etiology. *J Neurol Scie.* 1990;98:121–138.

17. Özyurtlu F, Çetin N, Pekel N, Özpelit, M. Spontaneous spinal hematoma developing after percutaneous coronary intervention: early diagnosis early intervention and good outcome. *Turk Kardiyol Dern Ars.* 2016;44(2):158–160.
18. Beatty R, Winston K. Spontaneous cervical epidural hematoma: a consideration of aetiology. *J Neurosurg.* 1984; 61:143–148.
19. Chan L, Bailin M. Spinal epidural hematoma following central neuraxial blockade and subcutaneous enoxaparin: a case report. *J Clin Anesthesiol.* 2004;16:382–385.
20. Mohammed N, Shahid M, Haque M, Qureshi M, Hoey E. Spontaneous spinal epidural haematoma mimicking acute coronary syndrome. *Quant Imaging Med Surg.* 2015;5(6):925–927.
21. Morse K, Weight M, Molinari R. Extensive postoperative epidural hematoma after full anticoagulation: case report and review of the literature. *J Spinal Cord Med.* 2007;30:3.
22. Lawton MT, Porter RW, Heiserman JE, Jacobowitz R, Sonntag VK, Dickman CA. Surgical management of spinal epidural hematoma: Relationship between surgical timing and neurological outcome. *J Neurosurg.* 1995;83:1–7.
23. Switaj T, Christensen S, Brewer D. Acute coronary syndrome: current treatment. *Am Fam Physician.* 2017;95:4.
24. Lee T, Marcantonio E, Mangione C, et al. Derivation and prospective validation of a simple index for prediction of cardiac risk of major non-cardiac surgery. *Circulation.* 1999;100:1043–1049.
25. Burnett A, Fanikos J, Spinler S, Wittkowsky A. Pharmacology of anticoagulants used in the treatment of venous thromboembolism. *J Thromb Thrombolysis.* 2016 Jan;41(1):15–31.
26. Merli GJ, Groce JB. Pharmacological and clinical differences between low-molecular-weight heparins: implications for prescribing practice and therapeutic interchange. *P T.* 2010;35(2):95–105.
27. Yamamoto S, Sakakura K, Taniguchi Y, et al. Safety of reversing anticoagulation by protamine following elective transfemoral percutaneous coronary intervention in the drug-eluting stent era. *Int Heart J.* 2018 May 30;59(3):482–488.
28. Tahaineh L, Edaily SM, Gharaibeh SF. Anti-factor Xa levels in obese patients receiving enoxaparin for treatment and prophylaxis indications. *Clin Pharmacol.* 2018;10:63–70.
29. Khandelwal A, Phua CW, Chaudhry HR, et al. Confounding effect of therapeutic protamine and heparin levels on routine and special coagulation testing. *Blood Coag Fibrinolysis.* 2020;31(1):60–64.
30. Davi G, Patrono C. Platelet activation and atherothrombosis. *N Engl J Med.* 2007;357(24):2482–2494.
31. Husted S, Van Giezen JJ. Ticagrelor: the first reversibly binding oral P2Y12 receptor antagonist. *Cardiovasc Ther.* 2009; 27(4):259–274.
32. Storey RF, Oldroyd KG, Wilcox RG. Open multicentre study of the P2T receptor antagonist AR-C69931MX assessing safety, tolerability and activity in patients with acute coronary syndromes. *Thromb Haemost.* 2001;85(3):401–407.
33. Wallentin L, Becker RC, Budaj A, et al. Ticagrelor versus clopidogrel in patients with acute coronary syndromes. *N Engl J Med.* 2009;361(11):1045–1057.
34. Han I, Chung E, Hahn Y. Spinal epidural hematoma after epidural anesthesia in a patient receiving enoxaparin: a case report. *Korean J Anesthesiol.* 2010; 59(2): 119–122.
35. Bomberg H, Bayer I, Wagenpfeil S, et al. Prolonged catheter use and infection in regional anesthesia: a retrospective registry analysis. *Anesthesiology.* 2018 Apr;128(4):764–773.
36. Noll E, Fischer F, Collange O, Ohlman P, Steib. Neuraxial catheter and antithrombotic therapy for myocardial infarction: Wwen can we remove it? *Anaesthesiol Crit Care Pain Med.* 2016;35:173–174.
37. Levine G, Battes E, Bittl J, et al. 2016 ACC/AHA guideline focused update on duration of dual antiplatelet therapy in patients with coronary artery disease. *J Am Coll Cardiol.* 2016 Sep6;68(10):1082–115.
38. Antithrombotic Trialist's Collaboration. Collaborative meta-analysis of randomized trials of antiplatelet therapy for prevention of death, myocardial infarction, and stroke in high risk patients. *Br Med J.* 2002;324:71–86.
39. Kaluza G, Joseph J, Lee J, Raizner M, Raizner A. Catastrophic outcomes of noncardiac surgery soon after coronary stenting. *J Am Coll Cardiol.* 2000;35:1288–1294.
40. Vial J, McLeod L, Roberts M. Rebound elevation in urinary thromboxane B2 and 6-keto-PFF1 alpha exacerbation after aspirin withdrawal. *Adv Prostaglandin Thromboxane Leukot Res.* 1991;21A:157–160.
41. Iakovou I, Schmidt T, Bonizzoni E, et al. Incidence, predictors, and outcome of thrombosis after successful implantation of drug-eluting stents. *JAMA.* 2005;293:2126–2130.
42. Ong A, McFadden E, Regar E, et al. Late angiographic stent thrombosis (LAST) events with drug-eluting stents. *J Am Coll Cardiol.* 2005;45:2088–2092.
43. Chassot P, Delabays A, Spahn D. Perioperative antiplatelet therapy: the case for continuing therapy in patients at risk for myocardial infarction. *Br J Anaesthes.* 2007;99(3):316–328.
44. Böhle H, Fröhlich J, Laufenberg-Feldmann R. Risk consideration for peridural catheter removal in acute coronary syndrome:epidural hematoma versus stent thrombosis. *Anaesthesist.* 2014;63:651–655.

REVIEW QUESTIONS

(1) A 30-year-old female received a labor epidural catheter 3 days ago that has since been removed. She now complains of back pain and paresthesia on her lower extremity. What is the gold standard to confirm the diagnosis of epidural hematoma?

A. Clinical exam and history
B. Labs including platelet count and coagulation panel
C. MRI
D. X-ray of lumbar spine

(2) A 63-year-old woman presents for elective procedure and neuraxial analgesia is discussed. She had a new generation drug-eluting stent placed 3 months ago and is on aspirin and clopidogrel (Plavix). The surgical team wants to postpone surgery with patient on DAPT and absolutely wants an epidural catheter for this procedure down the line. How much longer does patient need to be on clopidogrel before it can be discontinued for safe placement of the neuraxial block?

A. You can discontinue clopidogrel now.
B. 3 months
C. 9 months
D. 12 months

(3) A 63-year-old woman presents for a nephrectomy, and neuraxial analgesia is discussed. She had a drug-eluting stent placed 7 months ago and is on aspirin and clopidogrel (Plavix). Her cardiologist states that clopidogrel can be discontinued for the placement of her spinal. How many days should her clopidogrel be discontinued for?

A. 1 day
B. 7 days
C. Spinal cannot be placed in a patient on aspirin.
D. 14 days

(4) These are the associated reported advantages of thoracic epidural analgesia EXCEPT:

A. Better postoperative glucose control
B. Decreased opioid use
C. Decreased postoperative release of catecholamines
D. Shorter mechanical ventilation times.

(5) You are placing an epidural catheter with the midline approach while explaining the relevant anatomy of the procedure to the medical student. You are describing what layers are being passed; the correct order is:

A. Skin, subcutaneous fat, supraspinous ligament, ligamentum flavum
B. Skin, subcutaneous fat, supraspinous ligament, ligamentum flavum, dura
C. Skin, subcutaneous fat, supraspinous ligament, intraspinous ligament, ligamentum flavum
D. Skin, subcutaneous fat, intraspinous ligament, supraspinous ligamentous ligament, ligamentum flavum

(6) Which of the following symptoms is more indicative of a thoracic spinal hematoma in a patient with a T10 epidural?

A. Back pain
B. Decrease in rectal tone
C. Fever
D. Weakness in arms

(7) What is the mode of action of clopidogrel?

A. Cox inhibitor
B. Gp IIb/IIa inhibitor
C. Antithrombin III activator
D. ADP receptor antagonist

(8) What does the R time on a thromboelastogram describe?

A. Platelet number
B. Clotting time
C. The strength of the clot
D. The bleeding time

(9) A 54-year-old female with a history of hypertension is scheduled for a total abdominal hysterectomy. The anesthetic plan includes an epidural catheter for postoperative pain management. After a thorough history, she reports taking garlic supplements and aspirin 81 mg every day. What is your next step?

A. Avoid the placement of an epidural catheter because she is on garlic supplements and this can increase her bleeding risk.
B. Avoid the placement of an epidural catheter because she is on aspirin and this is a contraindication for a neuraxial procedure.
C. Proceed with the case.
D. Avoid the placement of an epidural catheter because the combination of aspirin and garlic can increase her bleeding risk even further.

ANSWERS

(1) **C.** An MRI is the confirmatory test for a spinal epidural hematoma. There are other causes of back pain and neurological complaints, such as paresthesia following labor delivery, nerve injury during positioning, and lumbosacral muscular strain; therefore A is incorrect. Labs are nonsensitive and also epidural hematoma can occur even with normal labs. D is incorrect as an x-ray is better for detecting bony deformity and not nerve damage or compression.

Reference

Horlocker T, Vandermeuelen E, Kopp S, Gogarten W, Leffert L, Benzon H. Regional anesthesia in the patient receiving antithrombotic or thrombolytic therapy: American Society of Regional Anesthesia and Pain Medicine Evidence-Based Guidelines (fourth edition). *Reg Anesth Pain Med.* 2018;43:263–309.

(2) **B.** Per the AHA recommendations, clopidogrel should be continued for 6 months before it can be held for an elective surgery after placement of the new generation of coronary stents. For traditional stents, the recommendation is 12 months. Verification with the interventional cardiologist who placed the stents should be undertaken. Therefore, if an epidural is absolutely desired for this procedure, then the patient will have to wait an additional 3 months. Hence, options A, B, and D are incorrect.

Reference

Horlocker T, Vandermeuelen E, Kopp S, Gogarten W, Leffert L, Benzon H. Regional anesthesia in the patient receiving antithrombotic or thrombolytic therapy: American Society of Regional Anesthesia and Pain Medicine Evidence-Based Guidelines (fourth edition). *Reg Anesth Pain Med.* 2018;43:263–309.

(3) **B.** The ASRA recommendations are that a neuraxial block can be placed after clopidogrel is discontinued for 5–7 days. Aspirin use (dose <300 mg daily) is not a contraindication for neuraxial placement, making option C incorrect.

Reference

Horlocker T, Vandermeuelen E, Kopp S, Gogarten W, Leffert L, Benzon H. Regional anesthesia in the patient receiving antithrombotic or thrombolytic therapy: American Society of Regional Anesthesia and Pain Medicine Evidence-Based Guidelines (fourth edition). *Reg Anesth Pain Med.* 2018;43:263–309.

(4) **A.** Epidural analgesia has not been shown to have any effects on glucose control; however, it has been shown to result in a decrease in stress response to surgery, hence a decrease in catecholamine release, shorter mechanical ventilation, and decreased opioid use.

Reference

Friese, H, Van Aken H. Risks and benefits of thoracic epidural anaesthesia. *Br J Anaesth.* 2011;107(6):859–868.

(5) **C.** The correct order of layers that an epidural needle transverses is: skin, subcutaneous fat, supraspinous ligament, intraspinous ligament, ligamentum flavum. Therefore the other options are incorrect.

Reference

Manion S, Brennan T. Thoracic epidural analgesia and acute pain management. *Anesthesiology.* 2011;115:181–188.

(6) **B.** Cauda equina which presents as fecal or urinary incontinence and decreased rectal tone on exam is more concerning

for a hematoma. Back pain is a nonsensitive symptom and can be attributed to musculoskeletal pain or infection. Fever is not a symptom of epidural hematoma; however, it can be seen with an epidural catheter infection. Loss of motor function in lower extremities can point toward an epidural hematoma; however, weakness in arms would require that the epidural catheter was placed at a higher level.

Reference

Mohammed N, Shahid M, Haque M, Qureshi M, Hoey E. Spontaneous spinal epidural haematoma mimicking acute coronary syndrome. *Quant Imaging Med Surg.* 2015;5(6):925–927.

(7) **D.** Clopidogrel selectively inhibits the binding of adenosine diphosphate (ADP) to its platelet receptor. The other options are incorrect for the following reasons: abciximab, tirofiban, and eftibatide are types of Gp IIb/IIa inhibitors; heparin is an antithrombin III activator, which potentiates its effect; aspirin is a Cox inhibitor.

Reference

Davi G, Patrono C. Platelet activation and atherothrombosis. *N Engl J Med.* 2007;357(24):2482–2494.

(8) **B.** The R time stands for the time it takes for a clot to form. MA describes the strength of the clot. The platelet number or bleeding time is not measured by the TEG.

Reference

Wolf S, Kaisers U, Reske A, Strick M. Epidural catheter removal for initiation of emergency anticoagulant therapy in acute coronary syndrome: when is the time right? *Eur J Anaesthesiol.* 2015;32:581–589.

(9) **C.** The recommendations state that regional anesthesia can be continued in a patient who is taking herbal medications and therefore there is no reason to cancel a procedure. If the patient is seen in pre-assessment clinic, discontinuation of herbal medication can be advised; however, this is not a mandatory recommendation. There are no contraindications on performing neuraxial anesthesia on a patient taking aspirin.

Reference

Horlocker T, Vandermeuelen E, Kopp S, Gogarten W, Leffert L, Benzon H. Regional anesthesia in the patient receiving antithrombotic or thrombolytic therapy: American Society of Regional Anesthesia and Pain Medicine Evidence-Based Guidelines (fourth edition). *Reg Anesth Pain Med.* 2018;43:263–309.

45.

ELECTIVE ABDOMINAL AORTIC ANEURYSM WITH EPIDURAL ANALGESIA

Michael Akerman, Ariel Anderson, and Ryan Norman

STEM CASE AND KEY QUESTIONS

A 57-year-old male patient is scheduled for elective abdominal aortic aneurysm repair. His past medical history is significant for diabetes mellitus, hypertension, hyperlipidemia, and chronic kidney disease. Preoperative laboratory results are unremarkable with platelets of 198k. You place a thoracic epidural for postoperative pain management. The surgery lasts for 7 hours and proceeds without apparent complication. During the course of the procedure, the patient receives a total of 7000 units of heparin and 50 mg of protamine at the end of the case. Postoperatively, the patient receives subcutaneous heparin 5000 units every 8 hours for prophylaxis against deep venous thromobosis (DVT). However, after the surgery and prior to epidural removal, the patient develops heparin induced thrombocytopenia (HIT) with a platelet count of 45k and needs to be transitioned to a non-heparin anticoagulant. As the patient is in the immediate postoperative period, a continuous infusion of argatroban. The patient is continued on the Xa inhibitor while the epidural remains in place.

HIT blood tests are pending and argatroban has been started. The epidural infusion has been held and the patient continues to have 5/5 motor strength in upper and lower extremities. His pain remains well controlled with oral and intravenous medication. The patient is advised to notify his nurse if he experiences a return of sensory or motor blockade, bowel or bladder incontinence, or worsening back pain. Frequent neurological checks are continued for 24 hours after removal of the epidural catheter, and the patient's strength and sensation in his bilateral lower extremities remains normal.

The patient's platelet count is followed and improves to 81k two days after the discontinuation of heparin and initiation of argatroban. Since his thrombocytopenia has improved and his pain is well controlled, the decision is made to remove his epidural catheter.

(1) WHAT IS HEPARIN INDUCED THROMBOCYTOPENIA (HIT)?

Heparin induced thrombocytopenia (HIT) is an immune-mediated, low blood platelet count as a result of the medication heparin. The clinical features, including the recovery of platelet count with discontinuation of heparin therapy and recurrent thrombocytopenia with repeat heparin challenge as well as the immune component.

(2) HOW IS THE DIAGNOSIS OF HIT MADE? HOW IS HIT MANAGED?

HIT most commonly presents as thrombocytopenia with a temporal association with heparin therapy. This thrombocytopenia can occur as either a 50% relative decrease in the number of platelets or as an absolute thrombocytopenia (platelet count <150,000) within 5–10 days of initiation of heparin therapy. Less commonly, the patient may present clinically with arterial or venous thrombosis, skin necrosis at medication injection site, or in rare cases anaphylaxis or adrenal hemorrhage secondary to adrenal vein thrombosis. The American Society of Hematology recommends the use of the 4Ts score to estimate the probability of HIT for patients with suspected HIT.[6] The 4Ts system takes into consideration the degree of thrombocytopenia (both relative and absolute), timing of onset, presence of thrombosis, and likelihood of other causes of thrombocytopenia. Therefore, in low probability patients, HIT is unlikely and heparin therapy can be continued. In patients with intermediate to high probability of HIT, immunoassay should be obtained, heparin should be discontinued, and non-heparin anticoagulation should be initiated.

(3) WHAT IS ARGATROBAN?

Argatroban is a reversible inhibitor of thrombin with a relatively short duration of action, which is a preferred medication characteristic in this setting due to the patient's increased risk of bleeding or further procedural intervention in the postoperative period. Parenteral and oral options are considered, including lepirudin, argatroban, bivalrudin, fondaparinux, and rivaroxaban.

(3) WHAT OTHER MEDICATIONS CAN BE USED IN THE SETTING OF HIT?

Oral, subcutaneous, and parenteral non-heparin anticoagulants are available. Parenteral therapy is often preferred. Options include lepirudin, argatroban, and bivalrudin, which are thrombin inhibitors. In clinically stable patients with average bleeding risk, direct oral anticoagulants (DOACs), fondaparinux, or warfarin can be considered for HIT therapy. Fondaparinux is a renally cleared, indirect factor Xa inhibitor. Rivaroxaban is an oral direct factor Xa inhibitor that has also been used in the management of acute HIT.

(4) IS DEEP VEIN THROMBOSIS (DVT) PROPHYLAXIS NECESSARY IN THE SETTING OF HIT AND THROMBOCYTOPENIA?

As many as 25% of patients develop life-threatening pulmonary embolism, and initiation of therapeutic anticoagulation with a non-heparin anticoagulant is recommended. Despite the thrombocytopenia of HIT, therapeutic anticoagulation is recommended to decrease the risk of thrombosis formation in patients with HIT.

(5) WHAT ARE THE RECOMMENDATIONS IN REMOVING A NEURAXIAL CATHETER IN A PATIENT RECEIVING ARGATROBAN? WHAT ARE THE RECOMMENDATIONS IN REMOVING A NEURAXIAL CATHETER IN A PATIENT WITH HIT?

Current recommendations from the American Society of Regional Anesthesia recommend against the placement or use of neuraxial in patients receiving direct thrombin inhibitors, such as argatroban. However, given the patient's clinical course, suspected HIT was identified early, treatment for HIT was started expeditiously, and we are confronted with a patient who is on a therapeutic direct thrombin inhibitor while having an epidural in place. Based on the European Society of Anaesthesiology's recommendation and that of expert colleagues, you recommend to hold argatroban for 4 hours and check an aPTT and a Direct Thrombin Inhibitor Assay, which return with normal values. You also recheck the platelet values and confirm that there is no further decline in his platelets.

(7) ONCE THE EPIDURAL IS REMOVED, WHAT ELSE SHOULD THE PATIENT AND THE PATIENTS' HEALTHCARE TEAM BE TOLD TO LOOK OUT FOR? HOW LONG SHOULD THE PATIENT BE INSTRUCTED TO REMAIN ON THERAPEUTIC ANTICOAGULATION? WHEN CAN THE PATIENT BE TRANSITIONED FROM PARENTERAL TO ORAL THERAPY?

The patient is advised to notify his nurse if he experiences a return of sensory or motor blockade, bowel or bladder incontinence, or worsening back pain. Frequent neurological checks are continued for 24 hours after removal of the epidural catheter, and the patient's strength and sensation in his bilateral lower extremities remain normal.

The argatroban infusion is resumed 2 hours after removal of the epidural catheter and ultimately the immunoassay and functional assay are positive, confirming the diagnosis of HIT. Therefore, after the resolution of thrombocytopenia, the decision is made to start warfarin for continued anticoagulation after discharge. To minimize the risk of thrombosis and limb gangrene, you recommend 5 days of overlap prior to stopping the argatroban infusion. Outpatient follow-up for warfarin is scheduled with duration of therapy planned for 4 weeks. Screening lower extremity Dopplers are negative for deep vein thrombosis. These are performed since the presence of thrombosis would increase the duration of therapy to 3 months.

DISCUSSION

Heparin induced thrombocytopenia (HIT) is an immune-mediated, potentially life-threatening process occurring in 0.2% to 3% of patients exposed to heparin. The paradoxical thrombosis in patients after receiving heparin was first described in 1958 by two surgeons, Weismann and Tobin, who reported 10 patients on heparin therapy with paradoxical thrombosis. The clinical features, including the recovery of platelet count with discontinuation of heparin therapy and recurrent thrombocytopenia with repeat heparin challenge, as well as the immune component, were outlined in 1973 by Rhodes et al.[1]

There are two forms of HIT described: HIT type I and HIT type II. Only HIT type II is clinically significant. HIT type I presents as a mild and transient drop in platelets and is not immunologically mediated. This typically occurs with the first day or two of heparin exposure. Unlike HIT type II, the platelet count often returns to normal even with continuation of heparin therapy. This is not considered to be an immune complex mediated reaction but rather a direct effect of heparin on platelets, causing platelet clumping and sequestration. This type of HIT does not result in thrombosis and patients can remain on heparin while being managed.

HIT type II occurs as a result of formation of autoantibodies directed to complexes of heparin and endogenous platelet factor 4 (PF4). The antibody complex can activate platelets and cause severe and life-threatening arterial and venous thrombosis. If untreated, HIT can have a mortality rate of up to 20%. However, with prompt recognition and treatment, mortality rates are as low as 2%. When thrombosis is present, the patient is considered to have acute HIT complicated by thrombosis, or HITT. Though antibody formation is common, occurring in 2%–17% of patients receiving unfractionated heparin (UFH) or low molecular weight heparin (LMWH) and as many as 50% of patients undergoing cardiac surgery, only a subset of patients develop HIT. HIT most commonly presents as thrombocytopenia with a temporal association with heparin therapy. This thrombocytopenia can occur as either a 50% relative decrease in the number of platelets or as an absolute thrombocytopenia (platelet count <150,000) within 5–10 days of initiation of heparin therapy. Less commonly, the patient may present clinically with arterial or venous thrombosis, skin necrosis at medication injection site, or in rare cases anaphylaxis or adrenal hemorrhage secondary to adrenal vein thrombosis. In HIT with thrombosis (HITT), the heparin-PF4 antibodies bind FcgRII (CD32) receptors on platelets and monocytes, leading to activation of platelets, thrombin generation, and resultant arterial and venous thrombosis.[1]

Venous thrombosis (DVT and/or PE) occurs more frequently than arterial thrombosis (limb artery thrombosis, thrombotic stroke, MI), with reported frequencies being 17%–55% and 3%–10%, respectively. If left untreated, HIT carries a 5%–10% daily risk of thromboembolism, amputation, and death.[6] Due to the risk for thrombosis, it is recommended that patients diagnosed with HIT be started on therapeutic anticoagulation with a non-heparin medication, as well as undergo venous ultrasounds of the legs to evaluate for asymptomatic DVT, as the presence of thrombosis impacts the duration of anticoagulation therapy.[2] Upper extremities do not require screening Dopplers unless a peripherally inserted central catheter (PICC) is in place.[6] HIT is associated with a high incidence of peri-catheter thrombosis and should be ruled out if a catheter is present.[1]

Studies have shown that risk factors for HIT include type of heparin, patient population, and gender. At prophylactic doses, LMWH has nearly a 10-fold lower risk of developing HIT than UFH.[3] At therapeutic doses, this difference is no longer present. Surgical patients have higher rates of HIT development than obstetric or medical patients. Females are at approximately twice the risk of HIT compared to males (OR 2.37, 95% CI 1.37–4.09; P = 0.001).[4]

A tertiary care hospital in Toronto demonstrated a reduction in suspected and diagnosed cases of HIT and HITT after implementing a program to minimize heparin exposures. The Avoid Heparin Initiative included the replacement of most prophylactic and therapeutic uses of UFH with LMWH, use of saline flushes rather than heparinized saline in arterial and venous lines, and decreased ease of access to ordering/administering UFH. In the years following implementation of this initiative, the hospital saw decreases in the annual rate of suspected HIT, positive HIT assays, patients treated for HIT, and cases of HITT.[5]

In addition to patients with asymptomatic seroconversion, variations of HIT are also described. Heparin-naïve patients may develop spontaneous HIT in which anti-PF4/heparin antibodies are present with no prior exposure to heparin. Although not completely understood, a proposed mechanism is due to platelet PF4 binding to bacterial walls in infected patients, thus priming the immune system to target PF4, leading to platelet activation and hypercoagulability.[1] Alternatively, surgical inflammation may play a role in immune sensitization. Delayed onset HIT refers to a delayed presentation of thrombocytopenia outside of the expected window of 5–14 days after first exposure to heparin. This abnormal presentation can lead to delayed diagnosis and treatment, resulting in increased risk of thrombosis and associated morbidity and mortality. Refractory HIT presents with thrombocytopenia even weeks after the discontinuation of heparin.

DIFFERENTIAL AND DIAGNOSIS

Thrombocytopenia has a broad differential, but HIT should be considered in any patient with recent exposure to heparin who develops thrombocytopenia due to the potential for serious morbidity and mortality. Other causes of thrombocytopenia include sepsis, recent surgery, chemotherapy, autoimmune thrombocytopenic purpura, drug-induced immune thrombocytopenia, or disseminated intravascular coagulation (DIC) from non-HIT cause.

As there are many causes of thrombocytopenia, the American Society of Hematology recommends the use of the 4Ts score to estimate the probability of HIT for patients with suspected HIT.[6] The 4Ts system takes into consideration the degree of thrombocytopenia (both relative and absolute), timing of onset, presence of thrombosis, and likelihood of other causes of thrombocytopenia. A score ranging from 0 to 8 is obtained and is used to stratify the patient as low (0–3), intermediate (4–5) or high risk (6–8). Metanalysis of the 4Ts score showed high negative predictive value (0.998; 95% confidence interval 0.970–1.000).[7] Therefore, in low probability patients, HIT is unlikely and heparin therapy can be continued. In patients with intermediate to high probability of HIT, immunoassay should be obtained, heparin should be discontinued, and non-heparin anticoagulation should be initiated. Typically the immunoassays take a couple of days to result. In patients with intermediate to high probability of HIT, non-heparin therapeutic anticoagulation should be started while awaiting the immunoassay results due to high risk of clot formation through immune-mediated platelet activation. Immunoassays identify the presence of anti-platelet factor 4 (PF4) antibodies. As discussed above, not all patients with anti-PF4 antibodies develop HIT. However, in the absence of antibodies, HIT can be ruled out (sensitivity >99%[1]). Therefore if the immunoassay is negative, heparin therapy can be resumed. If positive, a functional assay should be obtained to confirm diagnosis of HIT. Functional assays have a higher specificity (>95%[1]) than immunoassays, as functional assays detect platelet activation by anti-PF4 antibodies in the presence of heparin. Examples include serotonin release assay (SRA) and heparin-induced platelet activation (HIPA).

In 90% of cases of HIT, platelet count recovery occurs within 7 days of stopping heparin therapy. Clinically, patients do not need routine monitoring with functional or immunoassays. However, studies have shown that functional assays remain positive for a median of 50 days after heparin is suspended. Immunoassays become undetectable around 85 days after discontinuation of heparin. These time intervals become relevant for patients undergoing cardiovascular surgery. For patients who still have positive functional assays, the American Society of Hematology recommends using non-heparin anticoagulants intraoperatively. In patients with negative functional assays, heparin may be used intraoperatively with a plan for non-heparin anticoagulants pre- and postoperatively. These patients should be monitored closely for signs of HIT.[6]

MANAGEMENT

As outlined above, management first begins with discontinuation of heparin therapy at the time HIT is suspected. Since patients with isolated thrombocytopenia (isolated HIT) are at high risk for progression to HITT (up to 50% of patients) and as many as 25% of patients developing life-threatening pulmonary embolism,[8] initiation of therapeutic anticoagulation with a non-heparin anticoagulant is recommended.

In patients taking a vitamin K antagonist (VKA), such as warfarin, the VKA should also be discontinued and IV vitamin K should be administered in addition to a non-heparin anticoagulant to minimize the risk for warfarin-induced skin necrosis and venous limb gangrene.[2,6] It is important to note that in some patients, particularly those with protein C deficiency or any other hypercoagulable pathology, warfarin initiation may lead to a temporary prothrombotic state that can cause warfarin-induced skin necrosis. This is likely due to the short half-life of protein C relative to the other vitamin K-dependent coagulation factors. Since protein C functions to inhibit the conversion of prothrombin to thrombin, a decrease in protein C activity can lead to more thrombin activation and increased clot formation. Time to presentation of skin reactions is typically 3–5 days after initiation of warfarin.[15] In one retrospective study of 158 patients with HITT, 8 out of 8 patients that developed limb gangrene were being treated with warfarin for the heparin-associated DVT. Furthermore, 3 out of 10 patients with arterial thrombosis in HIT were being treated with warfarin.[16]

Oral, subcutaneous, and parenteral non-heparin anticoagulants are available. When choosing a non-heparin anticoagulant, one must take into consideration pharmacologic factors such as timing of onset and institutional availability, as well as patient factors such as renal or hepatic function and potential need for reversal of anticoagulation. Parenteral therapy is often preferred in patients with critical illness, increased bleeding risk, or increased likelihood of urgent procedure due to shorter duration of action. Options include lepirudin, argatroban, and bivalrudin, which are thrombin inhibitors. Lepirudin is a renally cleared recombinant hirudin that irreversibly binds thrombin. Argatroban is a hepatically cleared, synthetic reversible inhibitor of thrombin. Bivalrudin is a hirudin analog that reversibly inhibits thrombin and is cleared by plasma proteases with partial renal clearance. Lepirudin and argatroban are FDA approved for use in patients with HIT, whereas bilvalrudin carries an FDA approval for the treatment of patients with known or suspected HIT undergoing percutaneous intervention (PCI). Danaparoid is an indirect factor Xa inhibitor that can be administered IV or subcutaneously, but was withdrawn from the US market by the manufacturer in 2002. No head-to-head trials comparing these agents have been performed, though they have all been used to treat HIT and HITT, with studies showing decreased occurrence of thrombosis when compared to historical controls.

In clinically stable patients with average bleeding risk, direct oral anticoagulants (DOACs), fondaparinux, or warfarin can be considered for HIT therapy. Fondaparinux is a renally cleared, indirect factor Xa inhibitor. Rivaroxaban is an oral direct factor Xa inhibitor that has also been used in the management of acute HIT. Other DOACs have also been used; however, rivaroxaban is the most commonly described. Warfarin, an oral vitamin K antagonist, should not be started prior to platelet count recovery due to increased risk of thrombosis and limb gangrene. Additionally, when transitioning from parenteral anticoagulation to warfarin, a minimum of 5 days of overlap is indicated.[6]

Duration of anticoagulant therapy is determined by the presence of thrombosis. In isolated HIT, non-heparin anticoagulation should be continued for at least 4 weeks after platelet recovery,[2,6] whereas in HITT, the American College of Chest Physicians (ACCP) recommends 3 months of therapy.

CONSIDERATIONS FOR NEURAXIAL ANALGESIA

Neuraxial anesthesia is used in a variety of settings including, but not limited to, use as an intraoperative anesthetic, postoperative pain management and labor pain management. It is crucial to evaluate each patient for candidacy to receive a neuraxial technique. The evaluation begins with a history and physical, paying special attention to any history of unexplained bleeding. Inquire about a patient's current medications, with careful attention to coagulation modifiers, including anti-platelet agents, and the time of the last administration. One must also consider postoperative coagulation modifiers especially used as DVT thromboprophylaxis. Depending on which medications the patient is using and the time of the last dose, they may not be a candidate for a neuraxial procedure and are at risk for hemorrhagic complications, including spinal epidural hematoma, which has a varied reported incidence anywhere from 1:2700 to 1:190,000[9] and as little as zero related to spinal punctures.[10] In certain circumstances, one should also evaluate certain laboratory values, such as platelets count, international normalized ratio (INR), and partial thromboplastin time (PTT), before proceeding.

The decision to use a neuraxial technique is complex and should be evaluated on a patient-specific basis, especially those patients who are receiving antithrombotic therapy. After evaluating the patient's history, medications, physical and laboratory values, a discussion with the patient, including risks and benefits, will help guide the decision.

As mentioned previously, timing of administration of antithrombotics is an important factor. It is important for placing, as well as removing, a catheter, if one is placed for continued analgesic needs. Many postoperative patients receive DVT prophylaxis in the form of LMWH or subcutaneous unfractionated heparin. These medications impact the ability to safely perform neuraxial techniques, as well as impact the timing of catheter removal due to concerns for heightened risk of neuraxial bleeding and spinal hematoma formation.

As per the American Society of Regional Anesthesia guidelines, patients receiving heparin subcutaneously for DVT prophylaxis should wait 4–6 hours from the last dose before a neuraxial procedure is performed. However, once the neuraxial procedure has been performed, the medication can be administered or restarted immediately after. Low molecular weight heparins are another class of anticoagulants also commonly used for DVT prophylaxis and carry different recommendations when in use with neuraxial. For one example, enoxaparin, the American Society of Regional Anesthesia and

Pain Management (ASRA) recommends waiting a minimum of 12 hours since the last dose before performing a neuraxial block, and waiting 12 hours to resume medication after the block has been done. Additionally, they recommend that the second dose of prophylactic enoxaparin after the procedure should occur no sooner than 24 hours after the first dose. In patients receiving heparin or LMWH at therapeutic doses, the recommended interval prior to performing neuraxial block is increased. The ASRA recommends waiting a minimum of 8–12 hours in patients on subcutaneous UFH and 24 hours for patients receiving therapeutic LMWH. It is important to note that due to the risk of developing HIT in heparin-exposed patients, the ASRA recommends that a platelet count be obtained prior to neuraxial block or catheter removal in patients receiving LMWH, IV or subcutaneous heparin for more than 4 days to screen for thrombocytopenia and HIT.

Though it is not recommended that neuraxial techniques be performed on patients receiving direct thrombin inhibitors, some patients may be diagnosed with HIT and have non-heparin anticoagulation started after catheter placement. The European Society of Anesthesiology recommends holding argatroban for 4 hours and desirudin 8–10 hours prior to catheter manipulation or removal.

NEURAXIAL ANESTHESIA AND VON WILLEBRAND DISEASE

In addition to iatrogenic bleeding diatheses, anesthesiologists are likely to encounter patients with preexisting genetic bleeding disorders. Von Willebrand disease (VWD) is the most commonly inherited bleeding disorder, with a reported prevalence ranging from 1:100 to 1:10,000 patients depending on diagnostic criteria.[17] Von Willebrand factor (VWF) normally functions to assist platelet aggregation by binding to platelets and subendothelial collagen at sites of vascular injury. VWF also assists in coagulation by preventing breakdown of coagulation factor VIII.[18]

Von Willebrand disease can result from either quantitative or qualitative defects in the production of VWF. Type I VWD, accounting for about 80% of cases, is a heterozygous mutation that results in reduced production of VWF. Type II VWD produces dysfunctional VWF and is further subdivided based on the specific defect. Type III VWD is a homozygous defect resulting in the complete absence of VWF and is the most severe form of the disease (accounting for <5% of cases).[18] A basic understanding of the different types of VWD is important for appropriate patient selection for neuraxial anesthesia.

Type I VWD is caused by either a heterozygous nonsense or missense mutation leading to reduced VWF protein level and activity, as well as a secondary reduction in factor VIII activity. Genetic screening studies have reported a disease prevalence of 1%. However, due to incomplete penetrance and variable expression, roughly 1 in 10 of these patients experience medically significant bleeding.[17] Type I VWD presents as mucocutaneous bleeding and is more frequently diagnosed in females due to significant menorrhagia. Diagnosis is made through positive personal or family history plus laboratory testing revealing concordant reduction is both VWF antigen levels (VWF:Ag) and VWF activity of less than 30 IU/dL. These antigen and activity levels will be important for monitoring and treating von Willebrand patients undergoing neuraxial techniques.

While type I VWD has variable severity, ranging from asymptomatic to severe bleeding, types II and III VWD are more commonly moderate to severe. Type III disease results from homozygous nonsense mutations resulting in undetectable VWF levels and severe bleeding. Clinical presentation appears similar to hemophilia A with joint and soft tissue bleeding in addition to mucocutaneous hemorrhage. The various subtypes of type II VWD result from functional defects including: reduced platelet binding (with or without defects in formation of VWF multimers); increased platelet binding that results in platelet sequestration and reduced circulating levels of VWF; and reduced binding to factor VIII (VWF normally functions to prevent breakdown of factor VIII by protein C). Diagnosis is again made through history and lab findings. However, VWF activity is decreased out of proportion relative to VWF:Ag levels due to the functional defects listed above.[18]

In any patient with impaired coagulation, whether intentionally through therapeutic anticoagulation in the setting of HIT or due to inherited bleeding disorders such as VWD, the risk of spinal hematoma plays a role in the anesthetic considerations. While there are no official evidence-based guidelines for neuraxial anesthesia in patients with VWD or other inherited bleeding disorders, retrospective case studies and expert opinion can help to inform the anesthetic plan. Hematology guidelines recommend VWF activity and factor VIII levels of at least 50 IU/dL for minor procedures.[19]

In patients with mild cases of type I or II VWD, desmopressin may be used to transiently increase VWF and factor VIII levels. Patients with VWD type III are not responsive to desmopressin as they do not produce VWF. The use of desmopressin as maintenance treatment is limited by tachyphylaxis. For more severe cases or for longer treatment, VWF/factor VIII concentrate (e.g., Humate P) is the treatment of choice.[19] There are no data comparing different VWF activity levels while the epidural is in place. However, case reports of successful neuraxial techniques in von Willebrand patients maintain VWF activity levels and factor VIII levels sustained above 50 IU/dL.[12] Factor VIII levels must be monitored if VWF/factor VIII concentrate is administered and should not exceed 200 IU due to increased risk for venous thrombosis. For this reason, Humate P is the gold standard concentrate due to the high ratio of VFW to factor VIII.

A retrospective literature review of neuraxial anesthesia in patients with VWD revealed 74 obstetric cases, including patients with VWD type I, type IIA, and type III. Of these 74 patients, no spinal hematoma was reported. Of note, 64 of the 74 patients had normalization of their VWF levels without treatment through normal physiologic changes of pregnancy; 10 of the 74 patients received either desmopressin or VWF/factor VIII concentrate. While these results are reassuring, extrapolating this data from an obstetric population to a general surgical population is problematic. First of all, normal physiological changes of pregnancy lead to increased levels of VWF without any pharmacologic intervention. Furthermore, neuraxial technique for non-obstetric surgery carries up to an 18-fold increased risk of spinal hematoma compared to obstetric patients. Finally, the cases reported are limited to only 2 patients with type II VWD and 1 patient with type III VWD. For any patient with VWD, the decision to perform neuraxial anesthesia should be made with an interdisciplinary team including hematology.[20]

REFERENCES

1. Arepally GM. Heparin-induced thrombocytopenia. *Blood.* 2017; 129:2864.
2. Linkins L-A, Dans AL, Moores LK, Bona R, Davidson BL, Schulman S, Crowther M. Treatment and prevention of heparin-induced thrombocytopenia: antithrombotic therapy and prevention of thrombosis, 9th ed: American College of Chest Physicians evidence-based clinical practice guidelines. *Chest.* 2012;141(2 Suppl):e495S–e530S.
3. Martel N, Lee J, Wells PS. Risk for heparin-induced thrombocytopenia with unfractionated and low-molecular-weightheparin thromboprophylaxis: a meta-analysis. *Blood.* 2005;106(8):2710–2715.
4. Warkentin TE, Sheppard JA, Sigouin CS, Kohlmann T, Eichler P, Greinacher A. Gender imbalance and risk factor interactions in heparin-inducedthrombocytopenia. *Blood.* 2006;108(9):2937–2941.
5. McGowan KE, Makari J, Diamantouros A, et al. Reducing the hospital burden of heparin-inducedthrombocytopenia: impact of an avoid-heparinprogram. *Blood.* 2016;127(16):1954–1959.
6. Cuker A, Arepally GM, Chong BH, et al. American Society of Hematology 2018 guidelines for management of venous thromboembolism: heparin-induced thrombocytopenia. *Blood Adv.* 2018;2(22):3360–3392.
7. Cuker A, Gimotty PA, Crowther MA, Warkentin TE. Predictive value of the 4Ts scoring system for heparin-induced thrombocytopenia: a systematic review and meta-analysis. *Blood.* 2012;120(20):4160–4167.
8. Warkentin TE, Kelton JG. A 14-year study of heparin-induced thrombocytopenia. *Am J Med.* 1996;101(5):502–507.
9. Li S-L, Wang D-X, Ma D. Epidural hematoma after neuraxial blockade: a retrospective report from China. *Anesth Analg.* 2010 Nov;111(5):1322–1324.
10. Jian-xiong AN, Fang, Qi-wu; Sullivan EA, Williams JP. Spine surgery may cause more spinal epidural hematomas than spinal puncture. *Chinese Med J.* 2013 Jan 20;126(2):286–289.
11. American Society of Hematology. Quick reference: 2012 clinical practice guideline on the evaluation and management of von Willebrand Disease (VWD). 2012. Adapted from: The diagnosis, evaluation, and management of von Willebrand disease. National Heart, Lung, and Blood Institute, NIH Pub. no. 08–5832. Dec 2007.
12. Choi S, Brull R. Neuraxial techniques in obstetric and non-obstetric patients with common bleeding diatheses. Anesth Analg. 2009; 109:648–660.
13. Gonzalez-Fiol A, Eisenberger A. Anesthesia implications of coagulation and anticoagulation during pregnancy. *Semin Perinatol.* 2014;38:370–377.
14. Lawton MT, Porter RW, Heiserman JE, Jacobowitz R, Sonntag VK, Dickman CA. Surgical management of spinal epidural hematoma: relationship between surgical timing and neurological outcome. *J Neurosurg.* 1995 Jul; 83(1):1–7.
15. Kakagia DD, Papanas N, Karadimas E, Polychronidis A. Warfarin-induced skin necrosis. *Ann Dermatol.* 2014;26(1):96–98. doi: 10.5021/ad.2014.26.1.96.
16. Warkentin TE, Elavathil LJ, Hayward CP, Johnston MA, Russett JI, Kelton JG. The pathogenesis of venous limb gangrene associated with heparin-induced thrombocytopenia. *Ann Intern Med.* 1997;127(9):804–812. doi: 10.7326/0003-4819-127-9-199711010-00005.
17. Bowman M, Hopman WM, Rapson D, Lillicrap D, James P. The prevalence of symptomatic von Willebrand disease in primary care practice. *J Thromb Haemost.* 2010;8: 213–216. doi:10.1111/j.1538-7836.2009.03661.x
18. Leebeek FW, Eikenboom JCJ. Von Willebrand's disease. *N Engl J Med.* 2016;2067–2080. doi: 10.1056/NEJMra1601561.
19. Franchini M. Surgical prophylaxis in von Willebrand's disease: a difficult balance to manage. *Blood Transfus.* 2008;6(Suppl 2):s33–s38. doi: 10.2450/2008.0035-08.
20. Gonzalez-Fiol A, Eisenberger A. Anesthesia implications of coagulation and anticoagulation during pregnancy. *Semin Perinatol.* 2014;38:370–377.

REVIEW QUESTIONS

(1) A 45-year-old female is POD 7 from open total colectomy. She has been on subcutaneous heparin for DVT prophylaxis. On routine labs her platelets have decreased from 175,000 to 71,000. You are concerned the patient has heparin induced thrombocytopenia (HIT). Which of the following is the best first step in managing this patient?

A. Stop heparin
B. Start vitamin K antagonist
C. Send serotonin release assay
D. No change to treatment plan and continue daily labs

(2) A 27-year-old G1P0 female is referred for anesthesia evaluation prior to anticipated vaginal delivery due to a history of von Willebrand's disease. She was diagnosed with von Willebrand's disease after having prolonged bleeding following wisdom teeth extraction. She requests epidural placement for labor analgesia. Her pregnancy has been uneventful. She is otherwise healthy and denies symptoms of bleeding or easy bruising at home. How do you counsel her regarding her options for labor analgesia?

A. Neuraxial technique is contraindicated in all patients with bleeding disorders.
B. No further testing is necessary prior to epidural placement.
C. Patient is candidate for only remifentanil PCA.
D. Coagulation labs should be checked and discussion with patient prior to labor epidural placement.

(3) A 68-year-old male is POD 3 from exploratory laparotomy and resection of abdominal mass. Postoperatively his pain has been managed by an epidural PCA. He is tolerating a regular diet and the surgical team requests his epidural be removed. On chart review, you find that he just received a dose of 5000 units subcutaneous unfractionated heparin for DVT prophylaxis. How long should you wait prior to removing the epidural catheter?

A. Okay to remove catheter at anytime
B. 4 hours
C. 12 hours
D. 24 hours

(4) A 71-year-old female presents for elective total hip replacement. She has a mechanical mitral valve and is anticoagulated

with coumadin. Preoperatively she was prescribed a therapeutic dose of enoxaparin for anticoagulation bridging. Her last dose of coumadin was 5 days ago and she reports last administering enoxaparin yesterday morning. Your anesthetic plan is for combined spinal epidural (CSE). How soon after therapeutic enoxaparin dose can CSE be performed?

A. 6 hours
B. 12 hours
C. 24 hours
D. 36 hours

(5) A 65-year-old female is POD 1 from left hip hemiarthroplasty. The surgery was performed under a combined spinal epidural. She has an epidural PCA in place for postoperative pain management. You are called to evaluate the patient for new back pain and right leg weakness and bowel incontinence. The back pain is worse with coughing. On exam he has 3/5 strength in the proximal leg. What is the best first step in the management of this patient?

A. Obtain emergent MRI
B. Increase epidural infusion
C. Reassure and continue to observe
D. Stop epidural infusion

(6) A 32-year-old male is having a lower extremity removal of hardware performed under the spinal block with Mepivacaine. His PACU course is uneventful with resolution of the spinal in 3 hours and he is discharged home. The following day the patient calls and complains of mild aching pain in the lower back and buttock area with radiation to the posterior thighs. He reports no weakness, numbness, or bowel and bladder incontinence. What should you advise next?

A. Come immediately to the hospital for further evaluation
B. Reassurance and recommend NSAID use
C. Schedule outpatient pain physician follow-up
D. Consult with risk management

(7) A 52-year-old female is diagnosed with HIT after receiving prophylactic subcutaneous heparin and heparinized saline via an arterial line. Screening bilateral lower extremity ultrasound is negative for DVT. In addition to stopping the heparin, you plan to start a non-heparin anticoagulant. How long will she require therapy?

A. Until platelet counts return to baseline
B. 4 weeks
C. 3 months
D. 6 months

(8) A 77-year-old male with atrial fibrillation underwent elective total knee replacement. Postoperatively he was bridged to warfarin using low molecular weight heparin. On POD 7 he develops right lower extremity edema. Labs reveal new thrombocytopenia, an INR of 2.7, and ultrasound of the right lower extremity reveals a DVT. ELISA is positive for anti-PF4/heparin antibodies. How should this patient's anticoagulation regimen be managed?

A. Continue warfarin since the patient's INR is currently therapeutic.
B. Discontinue warfarin and start therapeutic heparin infusion.
C. Discontinue warfarin and start alternative non-heparin anticoagulant.
D. Discontinue warfarin, reverse INR with IV vitamin K, and start non-heparin anticoagulant.

ANSWERS

(1) **A.** The most important step in managing a patient with concern for heparin induced thrombocytopenia (HIT) is discontinuing any heparin exposure. This includes, but is not limited to, discontinuing any UFH or LMWH prescribed for DVT prophylaxis or therapeutic anticoagulation, as well as heparinized saline which may be used for arterial and venous lines. After stopping the heparin exposure, next steps in management would include starting a non-heparin anticoagulant, performing immunoassay and possibly a functional assay (C). Vitamin K antagonists, such as coumadin, should not be initiated (B) in a patient suspected of having HIT due to the risk of developing thombosis and venous limb gangrene.

Reference

Linkins L-A, Dans A, Moores LK, et al. Treatment and prevention of heparin-induced thrombocytopenia: antithrombotic therapy and prevention of thrombosis, 9th ed: American College of Chest Physicians evidence-based clinical practice guidelines. *Chest.* 2012;141(2 Suppl):e495S–e530S.

(2) **D.** Coagulation labs should be checked and discussion with the patient should occur prior to labor epidural placement. Von Willebrand's disease (VWD) can present as bleeding from mucosal surfaces and prolonged bleeding time with minor trauma. It is the most commonly inherited bleeding disorder and is classified as either type I, type II, or type III, characterized by a quantitative, qualitative, or complete absence of von Willebrand's factor (VWF), respectively. Use of neuraxial technique has been described for surgical anesthesia and labor analgesia in patients with type I von Willebrand's disease. Though there are case reports and series that describe the successful use of neuraxial anesthesia in these patients, no formal, evidence-based minimum "safe" guidelines regarding factor levels are available. In pregnancy, VWF increases and many women with type I von Willebrand's have normal levels at the time of delivery. If coagulation factors are normal, neuraxial can be considered in these patients, but it is imperative to discuss the possibility of epidural hematoma and they should be monitored for signs of neurologic impairment post-procedure. Coagulation factors including VWF and factor VIII should be monitored while the epidural catheter is in place.

References

American Society of Hematology. Quick reference: 2012 clinical practice guideline on the evaluation and management of von Willebrand Disease (VWD). 2012. Adapted from: The diagnosis, evaluation, and

management of von Willebrand disease. National Heart, Lung, and Blood Institute, NIH Pub no 08–5832. Dec 2007.
Choi S, Brull R. Neuraxial techniques in obstetric and non-obstetric patients with common bleeding diatheses. *Anesth Analg.* 2009; 109:648–660.
Gonzalez-Fiol A, Eisenberger A. Anesthesia implications of coagulation and anticoagulation during pregnancy. *Semin Perinatol.* 2014;38:370–377.

(3) **B.** The American Society of Regional Anesthesia guidelines recommend that patients receiving unfractionated heparin subcutaneously for DVT prophylaxis should wait 4–6 hours from the last dose before performing a neuraxial procedure. This includes spinal placement of an epidural catheter, and manipulation/removal of previously placed catheter. For therapeutic subcutaneous doses of UFH, ASRA recommends a time interval of 4–6 hours. For subcutaneous individual doses >10,000 per dose or >20.000 U total daily doses, 24 hours lapse are needed before placing a neuraxial block. After performing a neuraxial procedure, there should be at least a 1-hour interval prior to administration of heparin via the intravenous route and it can be started immediately after the subcutaneous route.

Reference

Horlocker TT, Vandermeulen E, Kopp SL, Gogarten W, Leffert LR, Benzon HT. Regional anesthesia in the patient receiving antithrombotic or thrombolytic therapy: American Society of Regional Anesthesia and Pain Medicine Evidence-Based Guidelines (fourth edition). *Reg Anesth Pain Med.* 2018 Apr;43(3):263–309.

(4) **C.** To minimize the risk of spinal hematoma, ASRA recommends that neuraxial procedure be performed no sooner than 24 hours after the last dose of any therapeutic LMWH. This recommended interval is decreased to 12 hours if the patient is receiving prophylactic doses of LMWH. Also, the patient should wait 4 hours after neuraxial procedure, including catheter placement, manipulation, or removal, prior to resuming LMWH. These recommendations apply to patients with normal renal function and are based on an elimination half-life of 3–6 hours when administered subcutaneously.

Reference

Horlocker TT, Vandermeulen E, Kopp SL, Gogarten W, Leffert LR, Benzon HT. Regional anesthesia in the patient receiving antithrombotic or thrombolytic therapy: American Society of Regional Anesthesia and Pain Medicine Evidence-Based Guidelines (fourth edition). *Reg Anesth Pain Med.* 2018 Apr;43(3):263–309.

(5) **A.** This patient has symptoms and physical exam findings concerning spinal epidural hematoma. New focal neurologic deficit, return of motor and/or sensory deficits after resolution of blockade, bowel and bladder incontinence, back pain worse with valsalva, and history of difficult neuraxial should all raise suspicion for spinal epidural hematoma. After confirming the epidural catheter is MRI compatible, an emergent MRI should be obtained. Epidural infusion should be stopped, not increased, to allow for any neurologic impact from the infusion itself to resolve. Early identification and surgical decompression are imperative as delayed treatment can result in permanent neurological sequelae. Therefore, given the red flag symptoms the patient is experiencing, it would be inappropriate to reassure and continue to observe.

Reference

Lawton MT, Porter RW, Heiserman JE, Jacobowitz R, Sonntag VK, Dickman CA. Surgical management of spinal epidural hematoma: relationship between surgical timing and neurological outcome. *J Neurosurg.* 1995 Jul;83(1):1–7.

(6) **B.** Transient neurologic symptoms (TNS) is a complication following intrathecal administration of local anesthetic. Often described using lidocaine, as it has a higher incidence, it can occur with all local anesthetics. It presents 1–24 hours after resolution of the spinal with pain in the lower back that radiates down the posterior thigh. There are no neurologic sequelae associated with TNS. Its course often resolves after 2 days. Reassurance to the patient and recommendation of NSAIDs is standard treatment. In contrast, presence of neurologic changes, such as lower extremity weakness, numbness, and bowel or bladder incontinence are concerning for spinal epidural hematoma and the patient should seek immediate care.

Reference

Forget P, Borovac JA, Thackeray EM, Pace NL. Transient neurological symptoms (TNS) following spinal anaesthesia with lidocaine versus other local anaesthetics in adult surgical patients: a network meta-analysis. *Cochrane Database Syst Rev.* 2019 Dec 1;12(12):CD003006.

(7) **B.** In this patient diagnosed with HIT without evidence of thrombosis, 4 weeks of anticoagulation therapy is recommended by the American Society of Hematology and the American College of Chest Physicians. If thrombosis is detected, the duration increases to 3 months.

Reference

Linkins L-A, Dans AL, Moores LK, et al. Treatment and prevention of heparin-induced thrombocytopenia: antithrombotic therapy and prevention of thrombosis, 9th ed: American College of Chest Physicians evidence-based clinical practice guidelines. *Chest.* 2012;141(2 Suppl):e495S–e530S.

(8) **D.** Discontinue warfarin, reverse INR with IV vitamin K, and start non-heparin anticoagulant. Reversal with IV vitamin K is recommended by the American Society for Hematology and the American College of Chest Physicians for patients taking a vitamin K antagonist at the time of HIT diagnosis. This is in addition to discontinuing the patient's warfarin and starting a non-heparin anticoagulant. Warfarin can be resumed after platelet counts have recovered. Continuing warfarin or failure to reverse with IV vitamin K places the patient at increased risk of developing venous limb gangrene and skin necrosis. This patient has clinical and laboratory findings concerning for HIT with thrombosis (HITT). Therefore all heparin should be discontinued. Though commonly used to treat acute DVTs in postoperative patients, initiation of a therapeutic heparin infusion would expose the patient to additional heparin.

Reference

Ahmed I, Majeed A, Powell R. Heparin induced thrombocytopenia: diagnosis and management update. *Postgrad Med J.* 2007;83(983):575–582. doi: 10.1136/pgmj.2007.059188.

46.

LOWER EXTREMITY WEAKNESS IN A PATIENT WITH EPIDURAL ANALGESIA

Erik Helander and Yury Zasimovich

STEM CASE AND KEY QUESTIONS

A 72-year-old woman presents an open colectomy for adenocarcinoma of the sigmoid colon. She is 5′2″ and 55 kg with a past medical history significant for hypertension, type 2 diabetes mellitus, lumbar spinal stenosis, osteoporosis, and a transient ischemic attack. She takes clopidogrel daily and her last dose was 7 days ago.

Her preoperative labs are as follows: hemoglobin, 9.6 g/dL; platelets, 146,000/uL; international normalized ratio, 1.1; and partial thromboplastin time, 34.5 seconds. Before surgery, a T10–T11 epidural is placed using loss of resistance (LOR) to air. Placement is difficult and requires multiple attempts. After a 3-mL negative test dose of 1.5% lidocaine with 1:200,000 epinephrine, an additional 5 mL of 0.2% ropivacaine is administered through the epidural catheter. Before the patient is taken to the operating room, an examination is performed with the patient reporting no perception to cold from T8 to L2 bilaterally and 5/5 strength in her bilateral lower extremities. A patient-controlled epidural anesthesia pump with 0.2% ropivacaine and 2 mcg/mL of fentanyl is set to run at 8 mL/hour with the option of a one-time 4-mL bolus every hour. The preoperative nurse asks if and when the 5000 units of subcutaneous heparin that was ordered by the surgical team can be administered.

The patient is given a prophylactic dose of 5000 units of subcutaneous heparin and is taken to the operating room. A continuous infusion of 0.2% ropivacaine is maintained for the duration of the case. During the case, the patient has significant blood loss, requiring 2 units of packed red cells. She also experiences hypotension that is treated with fluid administration and a phenylephrine infusion. The surgery is completed, and she is brought to the post-anesthesia care unit in stable condition, no longer requiring vasoactive support. On her postoperative examination, she has loss of sensation on her right side from T8 to L2 but no appreciable level on the left side. She reports her pain as 5/10 in severity with most of the pain on the left side of her abdomen. She also reports some minor back pain near the epidural insertion site.

On inspection, the epidural catheter is secured at 10 cm at the skin. During placement, LOR is achieved at 4.5 cm. The dressings around the catheter are removed and the catheter is pulled back 2 cm using a sterile technique. A hand bolus dose of 4 mL of 0.2% ropivacaine is given through the epidural. After 10 minutes, the patient reports her pain has subsided to 2/10. On examination, she has a level from T8 to L2 on the right and T9 to L2 on the left.

In the evening, you are called by the bedside nurse because the patient is experiencing complete leg weakness bilaterally.

You ask the nurse to discontinue the ropivacaine infusion and indicate that you will assess the patient. The patient reports complete leg weakness that started 2 hours ago. She said she administered a patient-controlled bolus dose about 30 minutes prior to the onset of leg weakness but has not experienced this with prior doses. She also reports urinary incontinence and worsening back pain. On physical examination, the patient's strength is 0/5 in the bilateral lower extremities, and she has loss of sensation just below the umbilicus to the back of her calves, as well as the dorsal and plantar aspects of both feet. The epidural site appears clean, with no evidence of erythema, purulence, or drainage. However, the patient reports tenderness to palpation surrounding the epidural site. She is receiving 5000 units of heparin 3 times daily.

The patient is sent for an immediate magnetic resonance imaging (MRI) of the thoracic and lumbar spines. Imaging reveals a spiculated mass that, compared to the spinal cord, is hypointense in T1-weighted images and hyperintense on T2-weighted images with a mosaic pattern resulting in compression of the spinal cord at T12 to L2. The patient's most recent laboratory values include a platelet count of 135,000/uL, an international normalized ratio of 1.2, a partial thromboplastin time of 36 seconds, and thromboelastography values with heparinase within normal limits.

An emergent consult with neurosurgery is placed and a decompressive laminectomy is performed. After the surgery, the patient reports return of sensation but has 3/5 strength in her bilateral lower extremities. On the fifth postoperative day after the laminectomy, the patient continues to experience urinary incontinence and weakness in both of her lower extremities. She is scheduled to begin intensive rehabilitation.

(1) WHAT IS THE DIFFERENTIAL DIAGNOSIS FOR LOWER EXTREMITY WEAKNESS WITH A NEURAXIAL BLOCKADE?

Spinal epidural hematomas (SEHs) should be high on the differential with sudden onset leg weakness or unexpected neurologic changes or deterioration. However, more commonly, this may be due to the motor effects of local anesthetic on the lumbar roots, or the inadvertent placement of a catheter in the intrathecal instead of intended epidural space.

(2) WHAT RISK FACTORS DOES THIS PATIENT HAVE FOR DEVELOPING AN EPIDURAL HEMATOMA?

Risk factors include spinal pathology, advanced age, traumatic tap, and coagulopathy. The use of anticoagulants is one of the biggest risk factors for SEH.

(3) WHAT ARE THE GUIDELINES REGARDING NEURAXIAL BLOCKADE AND ASPIRIN, CLOPIDOGREL, AND SUBCUTANEOUS HEPARIN? CAN ENOXAPARIN BE USED INSTEAD?

In patients taking aspirin, there are no restrictions to placing an epidural; however, there is an increased risk for bleeding, which is likely compounded by the use of other nonsteroidal anti-inflammatory drugs (NSAIDs). American Society of Regional Anesthesia and Pain Medicine guidelines recommend holding clopidogrel 5 to 7 days and prior to enoxaparin (once daily prophylaxis dosing) for 12 hours before placing an epidural. Enoxaparin can be restarted 4 hours after catheter removal. For subcutaneous heparin, the time to withhold prior to epidural placement is dependent on the dose and frequency of the drug. However, once an epidural is placed, the subcutaneous heparin can be given subcutaneously immediately after epidural placement.

(4) WHAT TESTS WOULD YOU ORDER? WHAT IS THE TREATMENT FOR A SYMPTOMATIC EPIDURAL HEMATOMA?

The gold standard for diagnosis is MRI, and many patients will need emergent decompressive laminectomy. If MRI is not immediately available, computed tomography (CT) of the spine should be performed, though this modality will not be as sensitive.

(5) WHAT FACTORS INFLUENCE LOCAL ANESTHETIC SPREAD?

Age, volume, and injection site and rate can influence the spread of local anesthetics within the epidural space. The hypotensive side effects from epidurals can be mitigated by the addition of opioids to the local anesthetic infusion within the epidural space.

DISCUSSION

The LOR technique to access the epidural space was first described in 1921 and remains the primary method used today. Despite the widespread use of epidurals, a significant failure rate of up to 32% for thoracic epidurals has been reported.[1] Correct placement of an epidural catheter is paramount for its success. The prevalence of difficult epidural placement has been cited as being approximately 5.6%. Difficulty when placing a block may be associated with neurologic complications, decreased patient satisfaction, and/or increased risk of bleeding.[2] The top risk factors associated with difficult epidural placement include elevated body mass index, abnormal anatomy, high American Society of Anesthesiologists score, increasing age, inability to palpate spinal landmarks, and history of prior difficulty.[2,3]

SUB EPIDURAL HEMATOMA (SEH)

SEH, defined as bleeding into the extradural space (between the bone and the dura) that results in neurologic deterioration, is a rare but potentially devastating consequence of neuraxial anesthesia.[4] Many SEHs likely go unnoticed because bleeding within the vertebral canal may not be significant enough to result in compression of neural structures. This is evidenced in the fact that therapeutic epidural blood patches are often performed in the management of post-dural puncture headaches and do not result in permanent neurologic injury. Only bleeding sufficient to cause compression will result in appreciable neurologic deficits requiring prompt diagnosis and treatment. Although they are rare, SEHs are the most common cause of neuraxial injury leading to litigation.[4]

INCIDENCE

Although the incidence of SEHs is low, it is likely underestimated and may be increasing due to the widespread use of anticoagulants.[5] In obstetric patients, the incidence has been estimated to be 1 in 200,000, compared to 1 in 22,000 in elderly females undergoing surgery for hip fractures and 1 in 3,600 in elderly females undergoing total knee arthroplasty.[5] This disparity between the obstetric population and others is likely due to the hypercoagulable state of pregnancy, as well as the fact that patients undergoing total joint surgery are older and have other risk factors for developing SEHs. SEHs are slightly more common after epidural anesthesia than spinal anesthesia.[5] Risk factors cited for the development of SEHs include pharmacological or pathological disorders of coagulation, spinal pathology, advanced age, bloody tap, and technically challenging placement.[5–7]

DIAGNOSIS

Prompt diagnosis is necessary to limit neurological deterioration and improve chances for recovery. The first step in diagnosis is a focused history and physical examination, with a review of current anticoagulant medications, as well as the doses and timing of administration. Laboratory evaluation for potential coagulopathy is also warranted, with a complete blood count that includes platelet count, international normalized ratio, prothrombin time, partial thromboplastin time, and thromboelastography. When there is suspicion for SEH or deteriorating neurologic symptoms, local anesthetic infusions should be stopped because they can obscure the clinical picture. Continued sensory and motor loss after cessation of the local anesthetic is highly suggestive of an SEH. Normal coagulation status does not exclude the possibility of SEH. Commonly, severe back pain may be the initial symptom.[5,8] Weakness of the lower extremities that is inconsistent with the level of the block, progressive, or more intense than expected can often be the first symptom that patients present with. Symptoms can range from signs of nerve root compression/agitation to full loss of neurologic function.[9]

Signs and symptoms of SEH include:

- Back pain
- Tenderness over the spine
- Exacerbation of back pain with coughing
- Sensory changes
- Paresthesias
- Radicular pain (unilateral or bilateral)
- Leg weakness or fatigue
- Paraplegia
- Bladder or bowel incontinence
- Saddle anesthesia.

Typically, symptoms are characteristic of lower motor neuron pathology with flaccid paralysis and hyporeflexia.[10] The time for presentation of symptoms can range from 6 hours to 3 days, but symptoms may appear up to 2 weeks after placement of a block.[5] However, in 95% of cases, symptoms developed within the first 48 hours after placement or removal of the catheter.[11]

Computed tomography (CT), MRI, and myelogram can aid in the diagnosis of an epidural hematoma, but MRI is the gold standard. MRI can identify the existence, size, and location of a hematoma, as well as differentiate between causes and severity of cord compression.[12] CT scans may identify bleeding into the epidural space, but they can result in false-negative results. Although MRI is the most sensitive test, it can lead to delayed diagnosis. The MRI scanner may not be immediately available, especially outside of normal working hours. Discussions with the radiologist are an option to determine if an immediate CT is appropriate.

Hematomas generally appear as spindle-shaped structures with a mosaic character due to the degradation of hemoglobin.[13] Epidural hematomas can have different characteristics on MRI based on the degradation of hemoglobin. In the hyperacute phase (<24 hours), a hematoma will appear isointense on T1-weighted images and hyperintense on T2-weighted images. During the acute phase (1–3 days), hemoglobin will appear hypointense on T1- and T2-weighted images.[14]

MANAGEMENT

Neuraxial anesthesia should not be performed in patients with coagulopathies. Knowledge of guidelines and awareness of risk factors can mitigate the risk of developing an SEH (Table 46.1). If neuraxial anesthesia is planned for patients receiving anticoagulants, the route, timing, and dosage of anticoagulant medication should be checked before block placement and catheter removal.

Discontinuation of the epidural infusion is the first step when an epidural hematoma is suspected. This will allow for proper neurologic assessment and can mitigate compression pressures within the epidural space. The primary management of symptomatic spinal hematomas is urgent decompression by laminectomy. Expeditious decompression may offer the best chance for neurological recovery; however, there are some reports of conservatively managed symptomatic spinal hematomas. The anesthesiologist should consult neurosurgical colleagues as soon as a diagnosis is made. It may be prudent to alert the neurosurgical team once a patient is suspected of having an SEH (even before a definitive diagnosis is made) to facilitate resources and determine operating room staff availability should surgery be needed. Providers should consider correcting any coagulopathies because this condition can worsen an evolving hematoma.

PROGNOSIS

Patients who undergo surgical decompression within 8 hours of symptom onset have the best outcomes; however, some reports indicate that within 72 hours of neurologic symptoms, outcomes can still be favorable.[15,16] In one large study from Sweden, only 18% (6/33) of patients had full neurologic recovery.[5] However, partial or full neurologic recovery may occur only in up to 38% of patients undergoing laminectomy within 8 hours.[17] Hematomas that result in more pressure on the spinal cord are more likely to result in ischemia. Thus, the extent of damage or possibility of recovery likely depend on the severity and duration of cord compression. Long-term neurologic complications can consist of sensory deficits, paraparesis, paraplegia, or cauda equina syndrome.[5]

OTHER CAUSES

Other pathologies that can present similarly to SEHs include spinal cord infarction, Guillain-Barré syndrome, anterior spinal artery syndrome, epidural abscess, and progression of underlying neurological disease.[18–20] Guillain-Barré syndrome is also a rare cause of lower extremity weakness. It can present in the same time frame as a hematoma but it is more likely to present within several days to 2 weeks postoperatively.[20] Anterior spinal artery syndrome should also be considered for surgeries involving a retroperitoneal dissection and vascular procedures, including open and endovascular repairs of thoracic aortic aneurysms, because there is a potential risk for damaging the artery of Adamkiewicz.[19] One case of spinal cord infarction after epidural anesthesia at the site of catheter insertion has been reported.[18]

Table 46.1 COMMON ANTICOAGULANTS AND RECOMMENDATIONS

ANTICOAGULANT	HOLD BEFORE BLOCK	RESTART AFTER BLOCK	HOLD BEFORE CATHETER REMOVAL	RESTART AFTER CATHETER REMOVAL
Aspirin	No	Immediately	No	Immediately
Apixaban	72 h	6 h	Not recommended with catheters	6 h
Clopidogrel	5–7 days	Immediately if no loading dose; if loading dose, wait 6 h	Can maintain catheter for 1–2 days because the effect is not immediate	Immediately if no loading dose
Enoxaparin 1) Therapeutic 2) BID (prophylaxis) 3) QD	1) 24 h 2) 12 h 3) 12 h	1) 24–72 h 2) 12 h 3) 12 h	1) Remove catheter before initiation 2) Remove catheter before initiation 3) 12 h	1) 4 h 2) 4 h 3) 4 h
Heparin 1) IV 2) SQ Dose >15,000 U/day 3) SQ Dose ≤15,000 U/day	1) 4–6 h + normal PTT 2) 12 h + assess PTT 3) 4–6 h	1) 1 h 2) Unknown 3) Immediately	1) 4–6 h + normal PTT 2) Unknown 3) 4–6 h	1) 1 h 2) Immediately 3) Immediately
Rivaroxaban	72 h	6 h	22–26 h or factor Xa assay	6 h
Warfarin	5 days + normal INR	Immediately	Remove with INR <1.5; removal within 12–24 h does not seem to increase risk	Immediately

BID = twice a day; QD = once a day; INR = international normalized ratio; IV = intravenous; PTT = partial thromboplastin time; SQ = subcutaneous.

Adapted from Horlocker TT, et al.[4]

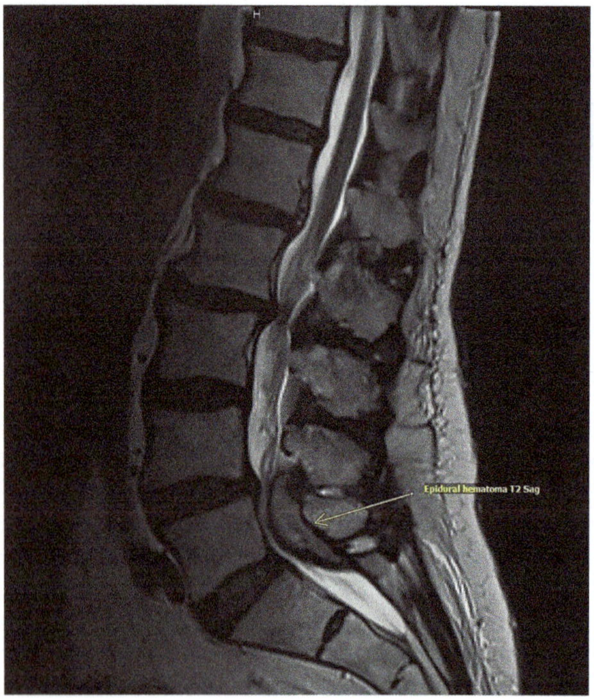

Figure 46.1. T2-weighted sagittal view of the lumbar spine showing an epidural hematoma.

POSITION OF EPIDURAL CATHETER TIP AND FLOW OF INJECTATE WITHIN THE EPIDURAL SPACE

The flow of injectate within the epidural space varies widely among patients, and unilateral epidural analgesia can occur in up to 21% of cases.[21] The epidural space potentially contains venous plexus and fatty tissue.[22] The extent of the spread of the injectate has been shown to correspond to the level of analgesia.[23] The spread of injectate within the epidural space is influenced by technical and patient factors, including the site and speed of injection, injection of air bubbles, fascia of the posterior longitudinal ligament, pregnancy, height, volume and concentration of the local anesthetic, and the location of the epidural catheter tip.[21,24,25] Age can also influence the spread of injectate within the epidural space, with dose requirements decreasing as age increases.[24,26–28] Dosing requirements in elderly patients (60–79 years) can be 40% lower than in young adults (20–39 years).[29] Unlike spinal anesthesia, patient position has no appreciable effect on the spread of injectate within the epidural space.[22] Injectate within the epidural space is often irregular; it can spread through many small conduits, as opposed to an advancing uniform column of local anesthetic. This flow is directed by tissue planes, and the preferential path of injectate is out of the intervertebral foramen.[30] Increasing the uniformity of the spread of the injectate can be improved with increasing volumes.[21,30] The spread of solution within the epidural space is more extensive with a bolus injection compared to continuous infusions.[31] Epidural catheter tips can reside in or near the posterior epidural space and the intervertebral foramina; lateral to the intervertebral foramina in the paravertebral tissues; and rarely in the posterior midline.[21] In a small cadaveric study, there was a strong association between bevel orientation and cephalad/caudad location of the epidural catheter.[32]

CONCLUSIONS

- SEH is a rare but devastating complication of epidural anesthesia.
- Risk factors include advanced age, spinal pathology, traumatic tap, and coagulopathy.
- MRI is the gold standard for diagnosis of SEH.
- In most cases, symptoms present within 48 hours of instrumentation; however, there have been cases with symptom onset days to even weeks after initial block placement.
- The prognosis is best when decompressive surgery is performed within 8 hours of symptom onset.

REFERENCES

1. Elsharkawy H, Sonny A, Chin KJ. Localization of epidural space: a review of available technologies. *J Anaesthesiol Clin Pharmacol*. 2017;33:16–27.
2. Sprung J, Bourke DL, Grass J, et al. Predicting the difficult neuraxial block: a prospective study. *Anesth Analg*. 1999;89:384–389.
3. Stendell L, Lundstrom LH, Wetterslev J, Itenov TS, Rosenstock CV. Risk factors for and prediction of a difficult neuraxial block: a cohort study of 73,579 patients from the Danish Anaesthesia Database. *Reg Anesth Pain Med*. 2015;40:545–552.
4. Horlocker TT, Vandermeulen E, Kopp SL, Gogarten W, Leffert LR, Benzon HT. Regional anesthesia in the patient receiving antithrombotic or thrombolytic therapy: American Society of Regional Anesthesia and Pain Medicine Evidence-Based Guidelines (fourth edition). *Reg Anesth Pain Med*. 2018;43:263–309.
5. Moen V, Dahlgren N, Irestedt L. Severe neurological complications after central neuraxial blockades in Sweden 1990–1999. Anesthesiology. 2004;101:950–959.
6. Renck H. Neurological complications of central nerve blocks. *Acta Anaesthesiol Scand*. 1995;39:859–868.
7. Wulf H. Epidural anaesthesia and spinal haematoma. *Can J Anaesth*. 1996;43:1260–1271.
8. Neal JM, Barrington MJ, Brull R, et al. The Second ASRA Practice Advisory on Neurologic Complications Associated With Regional Anesthesia and Pain Medicine: executive summary 2015. *Reg Anesth Pain Med*. 2015;40:401–430.
9. Gao X, Li L, Cao J, et al. Symptomatic postoperative spinal epidural hematoma after spine tumor surgery: incidence, clinical features, and risk factors. *Spinal Cord*. 2019;57:708–713.
10. Al-Mutair A, Bednar DA. Spinal epidural hematoma. *J Am Acad Orthop Surg*. 2010;18:494–502.
11. Bauer ME, Toledano RD, Houle T, et al. Lumbar neuraxial procedures in thrombocytopenic patients across populations: a systematic review and meta-analysis. *J Clin Anesth*. 2020;61:109666.
12. Moriarty HK, R OC, Moriarty PD, Stanley E, Lawler LP, Kavanagh EC. MR imaging of spinal haematoma: a pictorial review. *Br J Radiol*. 2019;92:20180532.
13. Tamburrelli FC, Meluzio MC, Masci G, Perna A, Burrofato A, Proietti L. Etiopathogenesis of traumatic spinal epidural hematoma. *Neurospine*. 2018;15:101–107.
14. Pierce JL, Donahue JH, Nacey NC, et al. Spinal hematomas: what a radiologist needs to know. *Radiographics*. 2018;38:1516–1535.
15. Persson J, Flisberg P, Lundberg J. Thoracic epidural anesthesia and epidural hematoma. *Acta Anaesthesiol Scand*. 2002;46:1171–1174.
16. Schmidt A, Nolte H. [Subdural and epidural hematomas following epidural anesthesia. A literature review]. *Anaesthesist*. 1992;41:276–284.
17. Horlocker TT. Complications of spinal and epidural anesthesia. *Anesthesiol Clin North Am*. 2000;18:461–485.
18. Kobayashi K, Narimatsu N, Oyoshi T, Ikeda T, Tohya T. Spinal cord infarction following epidural and general anesthesia: a case report. *JA Clin Rep*. 2017;3:42.
19. Linz SM, Charbonnet C, Mikhail MS, et al. Spinal artery syndrome masked by postoperative epidural analgesia. *Can J Anaesth*. 1997;44:1178–1181.
20. Mangar D, Sprenker C, Karlnoski R, Puri S, Decker D, Camporesi E. Rapid onset of Guillain-Barre syndrome after an obstetric epidural block. *A A Case Rep*. 2013;1:19–22.
21. Hogan Q. Epidural catheter tip position and distribution of injectate evaluated by computed tomography. *Anesthesiology*. 1999;90:964–970.
22. Park WY, Hagins FM, Massengale MD, Macnamara TE. The sitting position and anesthetic spread in the epidural space. *Anesth Analg*. 1984;63:863–864.
23. Yokoyama M, Hanazaki M, Fujii H, et al. Correlation between the distribution of contrast medium and the extent of blockade during epidural anesthesia. *Anesthesiology*. 2004;100:1504–1510.
24. Park WY, Massengale M, Kim SI, Poon KC, Macnamara TE. Age and the spread of local anesthetic solutions in the epidural space. *Anesth Analg*. 1980;59:768–771.
25. Omote K, Namiki A, Iwasaki H. Epidural administration and analgesic spread: comparison of injection with catheters and needles. *J Anesth*. 1992;6:289–293.
26. Bromage PR. Spread of analgesic solutions in the epidural space and their site of action: a statistical study. *Br J Anaesth*. 1962;34:161–178.
27. Bromage PR. Ageing and epidural dose requirements: segmental spread and predictability of epidural analgesia in youth and extreme age. *Br J Anaesth*. 1969;41:1016–1022.
28. Simon MJ, Veering BT, Stienstra R, van Kleef JW, Burm AG. The effects of age on neural blockade and hemodynamic changes after epidural anesthesia with ropivacaine. *Anesth Analg*. 2002;94:1325–1330.
29. Hirabayashi Y, Shimizu R. Effect of age on extradural dose requirement in thoracic extradural anaesthesia. *Br J Anaesth*. 1993;71:445–446.
30. Hogan Q. Distribution of solution in the epidural space: examination by cryomicrotome section. *Reg Anesth Pain Med*. 2002;27:150–156.
31. Mowat I, Tang R, Vaghadia H, Krebs C, Henderson WR, Sawka A. Epidural distribution of dye administered via an epidural catheter in a porcine model. *Br J Anaesth*. 2016;116:277–281.
32. Shaparin N, Bernstein J, White RS, Kaufman A. Bevel direction of epidural needles reliably predicts direction of catheter placement and contrast spread in human cadavers: results of a pilot study. *J Clin Anesth*. 2014;26:587–590.

REVIEW QUESTIONS

(1) A 56-year-old man with adenocarcinoma of the rectum presents for a low anterior resection. The patient has a history of myocardial infarction with stent placement 18 months ago and continues to take 81 mg of aspirin daily for secondary

prevention. What are the recommendations regarding timing of epidural placement in patients on aspirin?

A. Aspirin should be held for 7 days.
B. Aspirin should be held for 3 days.
C. There are no restrictions for epidural placement in patients on aspirin and there is no increased risk.
D. There are no restrictions for epidural placement in patients on aspirin, but there is an increased risk for spinal hematoma.

(2) A 53-year-old man with an 80-pack year smoking history, severe chronic obstructive pulmonary disease, chronic back pain, and prior opioid abuse is scheduled for a 3-vessel coronary artery bypass graft surgery with cardiopulmonary bypass. Due to his history of chronic obstructive pulmonary disease, chronic pain, and opioid abuse, you plan to place a preoperative thoracic epidural for postoperative analgesia. Placing the epidural proves to be difficult and at one point, dark blood is seen coming out of the Tuohy needle. What should you do for this patient regarding timing of systemic heparinization?

A. Proceed to surgery without waiting
B. Wait at least 60 minutes between epidural insertion and heparinization
C. Postpone surgery for 24 hours
D. Postpone surgery for 12 hours

(3) A 75-year-old male smoker with a history of hypertension, type 2 diabetes mellitus, atrial fibrillation, transient ischemic attack, and deep vein thrombosis undergoes esophagectomy for squamous cell carcinoma of the esophagus. The patient has a preoperative thoracic epidural placed at T6. After the surgery, the patient is started on 40 mg of enoxaparin daily. On postoperative day 4, the epidural catheter is removed with the tip intact. Per American Society of Regional Anesthesia and Pain Medicine recommendations, when can the next dose of enoxaparin be given after catheter removal?

A. Immediately
B. 4 hours
C. 6 hours
D. 8 hours

(4) A 69-year-old male former smoker with a history of hypertension and lumbar radiculopathy recently underwent a right open radical nephrectomy with thoracic epidural for analgesia. On postoperative day 2, the epidural catheter is removed, and the patient is discharged. The following day, the patient returns to the emergency room complaining of severe 10/10 back pain and pain that radiates down both of his legs. On examination, his strength is 5/5 in both lower extremities. What test, if any, should you order?

A. Computed tomography scan
B. Plain films of the lumbar spine
C. Magnetic resonance imaging
D. No test is needed as this is likely a recurrence of his lumbar radiculopathy.

(5) Which of these is NOT a known risk factor for a symptomatic spinal epidural hematoma?

A. Pregnancy
B. Spinal stenosis
C. Advanced age
D. Traumatic tap

(6) What variables influence the spread of local anesthetic?

A. Volume
B. Age
C. Rate and site of injection
D. All of the above

(7) Which of the following is not a potential side effect of neuraxial opioids?

A. Hypotension
B. Pruritus
C. Respiratory depression
D. Nausea and vomiting

(8) Which of the following is the most likely initial presenting symptom of a symptomatic spinal epidural hematoma?

A. Urinary incontinence
B. Saddle anesthesia
C. Unexpected leg weakness
D. Radicular pain

ANSWERS

(1) **D.** According to the 2018 guidelines from the American Society of Regional Anesthesia, there are no restrictions for patients taking aspirin for placement of neuraxial block and/or removal of an epidural catheter. However, the guidelines recommend exercising caution if other non-NSAID anticoagulants are planned to be administered in the early postoperative period due to an increased risk for bleeding complications. In addition, although there are no restrictions for patients taking aspirin, there is an increased risk of spinal hematoma for both epidural and spinal anesthetics. There is a relative risk of 2.54 compared to those not taking anticoagulants with an atraumatic block placement.

Reference

Horlocker TT, Vandermeuelen E, Kopp SL, Gogarten W, Leffert LR, Benzon HT. Regional anesthesia in the patient receiving antithrombotic or thrombolytic therapy: American Society of Regional Anesthesia and Pain Medicine Evidence-Based Guidelines (fourth edition). *Reg Anesth Pain Med.* 2018;43:263–309.

(2) **C.** In the event of a bloody tap, surgery should be postponed for 24 hours in patients undergoing systemic heparinization for cardiopulmonary bypass. Epidural catheter placement should occur no less than 1 hour before heparinization. In a study of 278 patients who underwent coronary artery bypass grafting with thoracic epidural placement, no clinically significant spinal epidural hematomas were identified when following these parameters.

Reference

Warters D, Koch SM, Luehr S, Knight W. Thoracic epidurals in coronary artery bypass surgery. *Anesth Analg.* 2000;90:767.

(3) **B.** Enoxaparin may be more effective than heparin at reducing the incidence of deep vein thrombosis and thus may be preferred in patients at high risk for thrombosis. For patients on once daily enoxaparin, an interval of 12 hours is recommended before epidural placement, restarting medication after instrumentation, and catheter removal. However, after catheter removal, an interval of 4 hours is recommended before the next dose.

Reference

Horlocker TT, Vandermeulen E, Kopp SL, Gogarten W, Leffert LR, Benzon HT. Regional anesthesia in the patient receiving antithrombotic or thrombolytic therapy: American Society of Regional Anesthesia and Pain Medicine Evidence-Based Guidelines (fourth edition). *Reg Anesth Pain Med.* 2018;43:263–309.

(4) **C.** In the majority of patients, symptom onset for epidural hematomas occurs within 48 hours of instrumentation or catheter removal. However, some documented cases became clinically significant several weeks later. Any time a patient has had neuraxial anesthesia, spinal epidural hematoma should be considered in the event of new or worsening neurological symptoms. Sometimes the clinical picture can be clouded with patients who already have preexisting neurological conditions, which can lead to delays in diagnosis. Also, symptoms of spinal epidural hematoma can range from back pain to leg pain, which can range from unilateral or bilateral to complete loss of function of the lower extremities, along with bladder and bowel dysfunction. When spinal epidural hematoma is suspected, the gold standard for diagnosis is MRI.

References

Moriarty HK, R OC, Moriarty PD, Stanley E, Lawler LP, Kavanagh EC. MR imaging of spinal haematoma: a pictorial review. *Br J Radiol.* 2019;92:20180532.

Tamburrelli FC, Meluzio MC, Masci G, Perna A, Burrofato A, Proietti L. Etiopathogenesis of traumatic spinal epidural hematoma. *Neurospine.* 2018;15:101–107.

Pierce JL, Donahue JH, Nacey NC, et al. Spinal hematomas: what a radiologist needs to know. *Radiographics.* 2018;38:1516–1535.

(5) **A.** Spinal pathology, advanced age, difficult placement, coagulopathy, and traumatic tap have been associated with in increased risk for spinal epidural hematoma. Pregnant patients are often hypercoagulable, and the cited incidence of spinal epidural hematoma is around 1 in 168,000.

References

Horlocker TT, Vandermeulen E, Kopp SL, Gogarten W, Leffert LR, Benzon HT. Regional anesthesia in the patient receiving antithrombotic or thrombolytic therapy: American Society of Regional Anesthesia and Pain Medicine Evidence-Based Guidelines (fourth edition). *Reg Anesth Pain Med.* 2018;43:263–309.

Moen V, Dahlgren N, Irestedt L. Severe neurological complications after central neuraxial blockades in Sweden 1990–1999. *Anesthesiology.* 2004;101:950–959.

Renck H. Neurological complications of central nerve blocks. *Acta Anaesthesiol Scand.* 1995;39:859–868.

Wulf H. Epidural anaesthesia and spinal haematoma. *Can J Anaesth.* 1996;43:1260–1271.

(6) **D.** Age, as well as volume, injection site, and rate, can influence the spread of local anesthetics within the epidural space. As age increases over 40, the dose of local anesthetic needed decreases. Intuitively, larger volumes can influence uniformity of spread as well as the number of dermatomes; however, the total mass of local anesthetic may be the most important factor influencing analgesic level as well as motor and sensory block. Faster injection has been associated with a larger dermatomal distribution in lumbar epidural anesthesia.

References

Hogan Q. Epidural catheter tip position and distribution of injectate evaluated by computed tomography. *Anesthesiology.* 1999;90:964–970.

Park WY, Hagins FM, Massengale MD, Macnamara TE. The sitting position and anesthetic spread in the epidural space. *Anesth Analg.* 1984;63:863–864.

Park WY, Massengale M, Kim SI, Poon KC, Macnamara TE. Age and the spread of local anesthetic solutions in the epidural space. *Anesth Analg.* 1980;59:768–771.

Bromage PR. Spread of analgesic solutions in the epidural space and their site of action: a statistical study. *Br J Anaesth.* 1962;34:161–178.

Simon MJ, Veering BT, Stienstra R, van Kleef JW, Burm AG. The effects of age on neural blockade and hemodynamic changes after epidural anesthesia with ropivacaine. *Anesth Analg.* 2002;94:1325–1330.

(7) **A.** The hypotensive effects of local anesthetics can be mitigated with the administration of opioids in the epidural space. This is because decreased doses of local anesthetics can be used to provide similar analgesia in combination with opioids. However, the administration of opioids within the neuraxiom can have side effects and are generally dose dependent. These include pruritus, respiratory depression, urinary retention, and nausea and vomiting. Pruritus is the most common side effect and is likely secondary to opioid actions on the brain stem rather than histamine release.

Reference

Armstrong S, Fernando R. Side effects and efficacy of neuraxial opioids in pregnant patients at delivery: a comprehensive review. *Drug Saf.* 2016;39:381–399.

(8) **C.** All of the above symptoms have been associated with spinal epidural hematoma; however, the most common presenting symptoms are unexpected leg weakness or back pain. In some cases, back pain is the lone presenting symptom. Leg weakness that progresses, recurs, or is different from the expected dermatomal distribution should raise suspicion. This is especially true when it is accompanied by other symptoms, including saddle anesthesia, bladder/bowel dysfunction, and radicular symptoms.

References

Moen V, Dahlgren N, Irestedt L. Severe neurological complications after central neuraxial blockades in Sweden 1990–1999. *Anesthesiology.* 2004;101:950–959.

Neal JM, Barrington MJ, Brull R, et al. The Second ASRA Practice Advisory on Neurologic Complications Associated With Regional Anesthesia and Pain Medicine: executive summary 2015. *Reg Anesth Pain Med.* 2015;40:401–430.

Gao X, Li L, Cao J, et al. Symptomatic postoperative spinal epidural hematoma after spine tumor surgery: incidence, clinical features, and risk factors. *Spinal Cord.* 2019;57:708–713.

Al-Mutair A, Bednar DA. Spinal epidural hematoma. *J Am Acad Orthop Surg.* 2010;18:494–502.

47.

BIG TOE AMPUTATION WITH DIABETIC PERIPHERAL NEUROPATHY

Eman Nada and Sandra L. Kopp

STEM CASE AND KEY QUESTIONS

A 70-year-old man presents for toe amputation due to infection as a complication of diabetes. His past medical history is significant for morbid obesity with a body mass index of 42, hypertension, smoking 50 pack-years, type II diabetes mellitus, and chronic kidney disease (glomerular filtration rate of 25 mL/min). His diabetes mellitus is complicated by peripheral neuropathy and retinopathy.

You are requested to place a surgical nerve block for the procedure. The patient receives an uneventful popliteal nerve block with 0.5% ropivacaine under ultrasound guidance. The surgery is performed successfully under the block with sedation, and the patient is discharged on the same day. Thirty hours later, you receive a call that the patient still cannot move his foot.

When you examine the patient at the surgery clinic, you find that his foot's dorsiflexion and eversion is 0/5, yet he can plantar flex with a strength of 4/5. He cannot feel the pinpricks on the dorsum of his foot, while he can feel them on his sole. You reassure the patient that this condition is usually temporary and continue to follow up with him by phone. The patient's motor and sensory function recover completely on the third postoperative day.

(1) WHAT IS DIABETIC PERIPHERAL NEUROPATHY (DPN)?

DPN is a chronic, symmetrical, length-dependent sensorimotor polyneuropathy. Early symptoms such as numbness, pain, and autonomic dysfunction are caused by damage to small nerve fibers.

(2) HOW DO YOU DIAGNOSE DPN?

Although DPN is diagnosed based on clinical signs and symptoms, nerve conduction studies are the most accurate diagnostic method.

(3) IS THIS PATIENT AT AN INCREASED RISK OF NERVE INJURY AFTER A PERIPHERAL NERVE BLOCK?

Yes. This patient has many of the risk factors for regional anesthesia-related nerve injury. He is diabetic with severe diabetic neuropathy, male, and elderly. In addition, he has a history of cigarette smoking, body mass index extremes, peripheral vascular disease, and hypertension.

(4) WHAT IS THE RISK OF NERVE INJURY DUE TO NERVE BLOCKS IN NORMAL AND DIABETIC PATIENTS WITH DPN?

The risk of nerve injury due to peripheral nerve blocks is estimated to be approximately 0.04%. Patients with preexisting DPN have an incidence of 0.3% to 1.1%, which is 10 times higher than the general population.[1,2]

(5) HOW DO PATIENTS WITH DPN RESPOND TO REGIONAL ANESTHESIA?

Diabetic nerves are more sensitive to the effects of local anesthetics (LAs); thus, nerve blocks have higher success rates, shorter onset times, and a longer duration. Patients generally require fewer postoperative oral or intravenous analgesics. However, it is unknown whether this is a result of baseline numbness or related to the block.

(6) WHAT IS THE BEST WAY TO LOCATE THE NERVE IN PATIENTS WITH DPN?

The usual methods of nerve stimulation and/or ultrasound can be used to locate nerves. However, eliciting a response to nerve stimulation can be challenging. Ultrasound guidance may provide better localization of the nerve compared to nerve stimulation as an endpoint. Ultrasound guidance allows the proceduralist to visualize the needle tip, which may decrease the likelihood of intraneural injection.

(7) HOW DO DPN NERVES APPEAR UNDER ULTRASOUND?

Using ultrasound, DPN nerves have increased cross-sectional areas and more hypoechoic areas. They appear obscure, with surface irregularity and heterogeneity.

(8) HOW SAFE ARE LAS IN PATIENTS WITH DPN?

Experimental studies on diabetic test animals have shown increased neurotoxicity from LAs. Clinically worsening neurologic function after nerve blocks has been noted in neuropathic nerves, even in cases of mild neuropathy.

(9) HOW SAFE ARE PERINEURAL ADJUVANTS IN PATIENTS WITH DPN?

There is not enough evidence of safety of perineural adjuvants in humans. However, animal studies showed some vasoconstrictive properties or neurotoxicities that make them unsafe in patients with DPN.

(10) WHAT ARE THE IMPORTANT CONSIDERATIONS WHEN PROVIDING REGIONAL ANESTHESIA IN A PATIENT WITH DIABETES?

The American Society of Regional Anesthesia and Pain Medicine (ASRA) has compiled an advisory on using regional anesthesia in patients with preexisting neurologic disease.[3] Physicians should consider the following:

- Evaluate the risk.
- Document any preoperative neurologic deficits.
- Discuss the risk-to-benefit with the patient and the surgeon.
- Use ultrasound imaging when possible to aid in nerve localization. If peripheral nerve stimulation is used, it should be used in combination with ultrasound to decrease the chance of intraneural injection.
- Use lower concentrations of LAs for neural blockade.

(11) WHAT ARE THE MINIMAL ANESTHETIC VOLUME (MEV) AND MINIMAL ANESTHETIC CONCENTRATION (MEC) IN PATIENTS WITH DPN?

It is difficult to know what is truly safe, but the goal should be to use the lowest concentration possible to minimize the risk of injury.

(12) WHAT IS THE CLINICAL PICTURE OF POPLITEAL NERVE INJURY?

Injury of the sciatic nerve at the popliteal fossa will depend on which branch is injured. Sciatic nerve injury is typically associated with a predilection for peroneal nerve injury. This may be due to the lateral position of the common peroneal nerve, which is tauter in its course and has fewer fascicles and less supportive tissue compared with the tibial nerve. Injury of the common peroneal nerve results in foot drop and loss of sensations to the dorsum of the foot, while injury of the tibial nerve results in inability to plantarflex the ankle with loss of sensations to the sole of the foot.

(13) WHAT COULD HAVE BEEN DONE DIFFERENTLY THAT MAY HAVE CHANGED THIS PATIENT'S OUTCOME?

An ankle block would be less disabling than a popliteal sciatic nerve block in the event of nerve injury because an ankle block can anesthetize the terminal branches of the sciatic block more distally. For big toe amputation, blockade of the deep peroneal, superficial peroneal, and posterior tibial nerves may be all that is required for surgical anesthesia.

Another option is a limited block known as the Mayo block, which is commonly used by podiatrists (Figure 47.1). This field block uses LA infiltration from medial to lateral, slightly distal to the flare of the first metatarsal base. However, a Mayo block can be inadequate for surgical anesthesia in the presence of local infection or when using a surgical tourniquet.[10]

(14) WHAT SHOULD BE DONE IN THIS CASE?

If the deficits are in the distribution of the nerve block, i.e., persisting beyond the duration of the LA, and the symptoms are purely sensory (as is the case in two-thirds of peripheral nerve injuries), observation is all that is required because most of these deficits will resolve over days to weeks. Early neurologic consultation is indicated in cases of functionally limiting deficits or severe weakness or sensory loss.[11]

DISCUSSION

Neurologic complications due to nerve blocks are rare. Understanding the pathophysiology and associated risk factors may allow anesthesiologists and patients to make better decisions related to these procedures. DPN is an important risk factor for nerve injury and the most common form of neuropathy in developed countries. Regional anesthesiologists will encounter increasingly more surgical patients with DPN. DPN occurs because of microvascular insufficiency, increased production of reactive oxygen species that trigger nitro-oxidative stress, defective neurotropism, and autoimmune-mediated nerve destruction.[12,13]

DIABETIC PERIPHERAL NEUROPATHY

DPN is a chronic, symmetrical, length-dependent sensorimotor polyneuropathy. Early symptoms including numbness, pain, and autonomic dysfunction are caused by damage to small nerve fibers.[14] It is characterized by a loss of myelinated and unmyelinated fibers, axonal degeneration, decreased

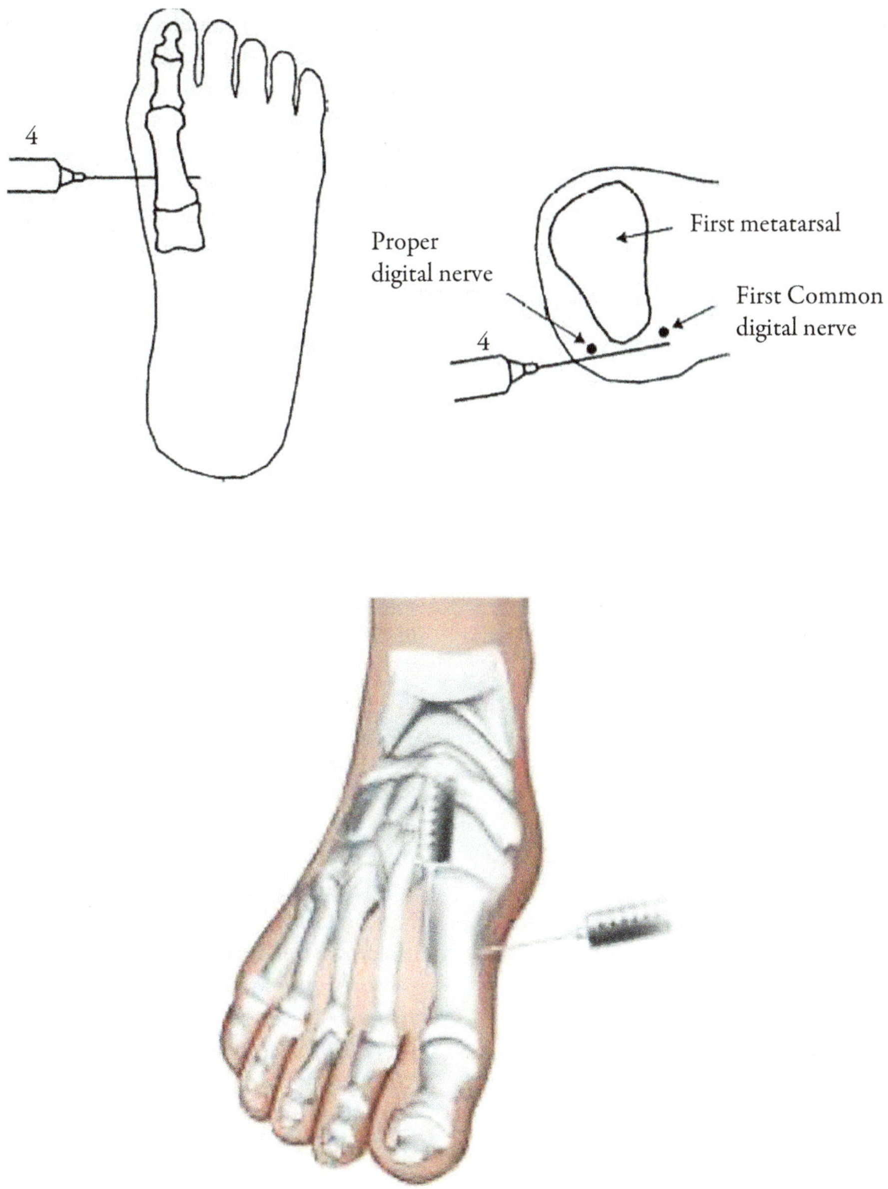

Figure 47.1. The Mayo block uses local anesthetic infiltration from medial to lateral, slightly distal to the flare of the first metatarsal base.

regenerative activity, and loss of Schwann cells and tubes. Schwann cells and tubes regenerate nerves, as well as insulate the axons and maintain their caliber.[15]

CLINICAL PICTURE AND DIAGNOSIS OF DPN

DPN may be challenging to diagnose given that up to 50% of patients may be asymptomatic. Although DPN is typically diagnosed based on clinical signs and symptoms, nerve conduction studies combined with needle electromyogram are the most sensitive methods for diagnosing the condition, even in the subclinical stage. These studies can also predict ulceration and mortality in patients with diabetes. They are, however, invasive and painful, and thus are typically not indicated for the routine diagnosis of DPN.[16–18] The Michigan Neuropathy Screening Instrument and the United Kingdom screening tests are common screening tools for DPN.[19,20] The Toronto Clinical Scoring System is used to diagnose severity.[21]

Sensory changes include positive (painful) or negative (nonpainful) symptoms. Pain and temperature fibers most often are affected first, which increases the risk of painless burns and persistent foot ulcers.[22,23] Neuropathy typically starts in the toes and feet and progresses proximally; when it reaches approximately mid-calf, it starts to appear in the hands, which is why it has been termed "stocking and glove" distribution.[24,25] The clinical examination should evaluate sensations of pinprick, temperature, vibration, pressure sense, and proprioception. The motor examination should evaluate the patellar and ankle reflexes as well as dorsiflexion and plantarflexion of the ankle and big toe. It should include the Romberg test.

High-frequency ultrasound has increasingly been used as an easy screening test. DPN nerves, when examined by ultrasound, have increased cross-sectional areas, more hypoechoic areas, increased thickness of the nerve fascicle, obscurity, surface irregularity, and heterogeneity. These findings have correlated with neuropathy severity.[26–28] Although DPN nerves have a progressive loss of myelinated nerve fibers, they appear larger by ultrasound because they are swollen due to thickening of the vasculature, accumulation of microfibrillar material in the vicinity of perineurial cells, and increased diameter of endoneurial collagen fibrils. These changes have even been noted to precede the development of DPN and are thought to be due to the higher hemoglobin A1c levels.[27,29,30] The demyelination and axonal loss might be the reason for the obscure, irregular surface appearances and the heterogeneity in the echogenicity of nerves on ultrasound imaging. On the other hand, the spinal cord area in imaging studies is smaller in patients with DPN compared to those who do not have diabetes and correlated with reduced electrophysiological function.[31,32]

SEVERITY OF DPN

DPN is commonly staged as follows:[33]

- N0: No neuropathy
- N1a: Signs but no symptoms of neuropathy
- N2a: Symptomatic mild DPN; sensory, motor, or autonomic symptoms; the patient is able to heel-walk
- N2b: Severe symptomatic DPN; the patient is unable to heel-walk
- N3: Disabling DPN

RISK OF NERVE INJURY AFTER NERVE BLOCK

Based on the double-crush phenomenon, patients with preexisting neuropathy who undergo a second insult are at a greater risk of subsequent nerve injury. This second insult can be mild and harmless to normal nerves. In patients with DPN, the metabolic derangement renders the nerves more susceptible to a second "hit" from regional anesthesia (e.g., needle injury or chemical toxicity of LAs). Other risk factors for regional anesthesia-related nerve injury are male gender, old age, extremes of body mass index, and history of cigarette smoking, peripheral vascular disease, and hypertension.[3,11,34–36]

NERVE LOCALIZATION IN PATIENTS WITH DPN USING NERVE STIMULATION

Localizing the peripheral nerves using nerve stimulation in patients with DPN can be difficult and may be unsuccessful. A higher threshold of stimulation and longer pulse wave duration are needed.[37] When using a low-threshold stimulation current for nerve blockade in a hyperglycemic dog model, all needle insertions resulted in intraneural injections.[38] One study found that 18% of brachial plexus supraclavicular blocks studied required a 2-fold increase in the electrical stimulation threshold in patients with diabetes who did not have symptoms of neuropathy.[39]

Some studies tried to quantify the current threshold increase in patients with DPN. In a study of lower limb procedures with a popliteal nerve block using both nerve stimulation and ultrasound, patients with DPN with decreased proprioception and decreased sensation required an average of 1.3- and 1.6-mA current thresholds, respectively, as opposed to a 0.5-mA current threshold in normal patients.[40] They started with a rising stimulation current from 0 mA, with a stimulus duration of 0.1 ms, and a frequency of 1 Hz. Another study of patients with DPN presenting for foot surgery needed a 7.2-fold increase in the stimulation threshold in patients with diabetes compared to patients who did not have diabetes (1.9 vs. 0.26 mA).[41] Similarly, Sites et al.[42] reported an unusually high threshold of stimulation of 2.4 mA to localize the popliteal nerve when the needle tip was seen by ultrasound close to the nerve in patients with diabetes.

RISK OF PERIOPERATIVE NERVE INJURY

Perioperative peripheral nerve injury is associated with several underlying factors related to the patient, the anesthetic, and surgical factors. Theoretically, patients with a preoperative neurologic deficit or neural compromise are at increased risk. Anesthetic risk factors related to nerve block include intrafascicular injection, mechanical damage to the perineurium, and neurotoxicity of LAs. Surgical factors include tourniquet neuropathy, certain surgical procedures, and inflammatory mechanisms related to surgery. The ulnar nerve at the elbow and the common peroneal nerve are usually at increased risk for peripheral nerve injury.[9]

RESPONSE OF PATIENTS WITH DPN TO REGIONAL ANESTHESIA

Diabetic nerves are sensitive to the LA effect, which can be seen in the form of the higher block success rate, rapid onset time, and longer duration of action in patients with DPN. One study reported that patients with diabetes were 3.3 times more likely to have a successful supraclavicular brachial plexus block.[43] The axillary brachial plexus block lasted 1.5 times longer,[44] while the popliteal nerve block was 59% faster in onset and lasted 1.57 times longer in patients with diabetes and DPN.[45] Even patients with minor clinical DPN had a longer duration of sensory block with sciatic nerve block (1.2 times longer) compared to nondiabetics.[46] Rapid onset and longer duration of sensory and motor block regression have been reported with spinal anesthesia as well.[47]

In particular, prolongation of nerve blocks has been noted in patients who have had diabetes for a longer period, had poorer glycemic control, and with a higher level of glycosylated hemoglobin A levels.[44,48] On the other hand, Cuvillon et al.[46] and Salviz et al.[44] reported no difference between patients with or without diabetes in onset time, and Sertoz et al.[48] reported a slightly longer onset time in patients with a higher hemoglobin A1C level.

EFFECT OF LAS ON DPN

LAs are neurotoxic in high doses; however, they may also be neurotoxic in normal doses in neuropathic nerves. In general, toxicity correlates with the concentration, dose, and duration of action of the LA.[4,49–51] Experimental studies in diabetic test animals have shown increased neurotoxicity from LAs. Clinically worsening neurologic function after nerve blocks has been noted in neuropathic nerves, even those exhibiting mild neuropathy.

The neurotoxicity of LAs results from the death of Schwann cells, infiltration by macrophages, and myelin damage. LAs also have a direct vasoconstrictive effect and decrease blood flow to nerves, potentially resulting in ischemic injury.[49,52]

It is thought that neurotoxicity is comparable between LAs at equipotent doses, but this remains controversial.[51,53] Lirk et al.[14] suggested using half of the concentration of the LA in the presence of DPN (e.g., using 0.25% bupivacaine instead of 0.5% bupivacaine or 0.375% ropivacaine instead of 0.75% ropivacaine). However, the severity of neuropathy varies, and there is not enough evidence to recommend the use of one concentration in all patients with DPN.

Extrapolating from nerve blocks in patients without diabetes might be a useful guide. Tables 47.1 and 47.2 show studies that used a step-up/step-down model—the Dixon and Massey method—to calculate the MEV or MEC for 90% of patients. All of the blocks were performed using ultrasound guidance to show the MEV and MEC for different types of nerve blocks.

The MEV and MEC in patients with diabetes are unknown. In a diabetic animal model, 1% lidocaine has been used successfully.[4] For femoral and sciatic blocks, 20 mL of 0.25% bupivacaine per block has been used successfully for diabetic foot surgery.[5,6] It is difficult to know what is truly safe, but the goal should be to try to use the lowest concentration possible to minimize the risk of worsening neurologic injury.

EFFECT OF PERINEURAL ADJUVANTS

Perineural adjuvants are usually used to prolong the duration of the block or to provide a dose-sparing effect. The nerve block duration is prolonged in patients with diabetes, and prolonged exposure of nerves to LAs is harmful. As a result, because of the harmful effect of prolonged exposure of the nerve to local anesthetics, the addition of adjuvants without a corresponding decrease in LA concentration is generally not recommended.[4,78] However, in limb-amputation cases in which the prolonged functional limitation may not be an issue, it may be beneficial to prolong the block for pain control. Perineural adjuvants differ markedly and DPN nerves respond to them differently.

Epinephrine's vasoconstriction in the presence of diabetic angiopathy further decreases LA uptake, prolongs its duration, and may increase its neurotoxicity. Epinephrine is not recommended as an adjunct to peripheral nerve block in patients with DPN because of its vasoconstrictive property in the presence of angiopathy. When epinephrine is mixed with LAs, LA neurotoxicity is increased and epinephrine's vasoconstrictive effect is increased; furthermore, epinephrine has no LA-sparing effect.[79,80] In animal studies, an epinephrine concentration of 5 mcg/mL with or without LA caused histologic evidence of axonal degeneration, while 2.5 mcg/mL of epinephrine was safer. However, 2.5 mcg /ml of epinephrine resulted in transient increase in the nerve blood flow, followed by return to base line after 2–3 minutes. Topical epinephrine decreased sciatic blood flow in rats in a dose-dependent manner. Administration of 5 and 10 mcg/mL of epinephrine resulted in a reduction in neural blood flow of approximately 20% and 35%, respectively.[81] When using 2% plain lidocaine, the blood flow reduction was 30%, compared to a 77.8% reduction with 2% lidocaine plus 5 mcg/mL epinephrine.[79,82]

A dose of 7.5 mcg/mL of clonidine with 1% lidocaine produced histologic evidence of axonal degeneration in sciatic nerves of diabetic rats.[4] However, that was a much higher dose than what is usually used clinically. No studies have evaluated the neurotoxicity of lower, clinically used concentrations of clonidine in patients with diabetes.

Dexmedetomidine's neurotoxic effect is controversial. Dexmedetomidine does not have LA properties by itself, although some evidence supports a LA-sparing effect.[83,84] It is neuroprotective in experimental animals.[85,86] When added to LAs, less perineural inflammation and nerve damage were noted than when using LAs alone.[87,88] However, experimental evidence found potential neurotoxicity using high-dose perineural dexmedetomidine with ropivacaine in a rodent model of type 1 diabetes mellitus with DPN. Neurotoxicity was also noted when used epidurally in experimental animals.[89,90]

Dexamethasone does not increase neurotoxicity except in high doses in experimental studies. However, its use is restricted in patients with diabetes due to its hyperglycemic effect.

POPLITEAL SCIATIC NERVE BLOCK DISTRIBUTION

The popliteal block is a nerve blockade of the sciatic nerve at the popliteal fossa; the sciatic nerve consists of the tibial and the common peroneal nerves, which physically separate 5 to 7 cm above the popliteal crease. The tibial nerve arises from the anterior division of the sacral plexus (L4–S3), whereas the common peroneal nerve arises from the posterior division of the sacral plexus (L4–S2). The tibial nerve innervates the posterior compartment of the leg and the sole and is responsible for plantarflexion of the foot and the sensory innervation of the plantar aspect of the foot. The common peroneal nerve, also known as the common fibular nerve, provides sensory innervation to the lateral aspect of the leg below the knee and

Table 47.1 MINIMUM EFFECTIVE VOLUME OF LOCAL ANESTHETICS IN 90% OF PATIENTS FOR VARIOUS TYPES OF BLOCKS

NERVE BLOCK	VOLUME (ML)	LA	TECHNIQUE	REFERENCE
Interscalene brachial plexus block	5	0.75% ropivacaine	NS and US. The needle was placed beside each trunk in succession, and the LA was injected in three equal aliquots. The study was stopped upon achieving the secondary stopping rule of 10 consecutive successful blocks using 5 mL of 0.75% ropivacaine.	Gautier P, Vandepitte C, et al., 2011[54]
	0.95 mL for the whole plexus when the pinprick sensations and thermal sensations were absent in three points and motor function ≤2. MEV 90 for each trunk: 15. 1.35 mL for the upper trunk 16. 1.64 mL for the middle trunk 17. 2 mL for the lower trunk The above criteria were sought in all of the regions and muscle groups that are innervated by the respective trunk. The estimated maximum volume for the non-occurrence of diaphragmatic paralysis in 95% of patients was 4.29 mL and the MEV for effective postoperative analgesia for 6 h was 2.34 mL	0.5% bupivacaine with 1:200,000 epinephrine	NS and US. The injection was given in two equal aliquots: one between the upper and middle trunk and one between the middle and lower trunk of the brachial plexus.	Falcao LF, Perez MV, et al., 2013[55]
	3.6	0.75% ropivacaine	US guidance. The transverse process of vertebra C7, subsequently root C7, the tip of the needle positioned just lateral and posterior to root C7. Sensation with pinprick testing in dermatomes C3 to T1 and dermatomes C5 and C6 with the same quantitative procedure as previously described. Block success was defined as the absence of sensation in dermatomes C5 and C6 30 min after performance.	Renes SH, van Geffen GJ, et al., 2010[56]
	8.64	0.75% ropivacaine	NS and US. The needle was placed beside each trunk in succession, and the LA was injected in three equal aliquots. Success was judged by motor and sensory blockade in the territory of C5 to C6 as assessed at 5-min intervals up to 30 min, after completion of the last injection.	Mittal K, Janweja S, et al. 2019[57]
	0.9 US 5.4 NS	0.5% ropivacaine	One group used US and the other used NS guidance. In the US group, the LA was injected so that spread was seen immediately posterior to or between the C5 and C6 nerve roots. In the NS group, successful block was defined by assessing the sensations in the upper extremity by pinprick from the C4 to T1 dermatomes, motor strength, and pain scores.	McNaught A, Shastri U, et al. 2011[58]

Supraclavicular brachial plexus block	17	1.5% mepivacaine	US guidance. LAs were injected near the lower trunk of the brachial plexus and as the needle was withdrawn.	Song JG, Jeon DG, et al., 2013[59]
	23 (middle age) 11.9 (elderly)	0.5% levobupivacaine, 2% lidocaine (equal volumes)	US guidance. The first half of the LA was injected in the corner pocket, then the other half was injected cranial to the neural cluster.	Pavicic Saric J, Vidjak V, et al., 2013[60]
	27	0.5% bupivacaine	US guidance. The LA was deposited at three locations: in the "corner pocket," adjacent to the middle of the neural plexus, and adjacent to the superficial aspect of the plexus.	Kant A, Gupta PK, et al., 2013[61]
	32	1.5% lidocaine with epinephrine	US guidance. Half of the volume was injected in the corner pocket and the other half was injected in the neural cluster of the brachial plexus.	Tran DQ, Dugani S, et al., 2011[62]
Axillary brachial plexus block	1 mL/nerve	2% lidocaine with epinephrine	US guidance. The needle was advanced adjacent to the median, ulnar, and radial nerves in this order. The injectate was administered slowly in 0.5 mL aliquots. Circumferential perineural injectate spread was ensured.	O'Donnell BD and Iohom G, 2009[63]
	23.5 mL for perivascular injection 5.5 mL/MCN	1.5% lidocaine, 5 μg/mL epinephrine	US guidance. Double injection technique of MCN and dorsal to the axillary artery.	Gonzalez AP, Bernucci F, et al., 2013[64]
	1.56 mL/nerve	0.5% bupivacaine with epinephrine	NS and US guidance. Deposited the medications close to the nerve.	Ferraro LH, Takeda A, et al., 2014[65]
Femoral nerve block	22	0.5% ropivacaine	NS group and US group. Direct visualization of the needle tip within the fascial space as close as possible to the femoral nerve.	Casati A, Baciarello M, et al., 2007[66]
Midfemoral sciatic nerve block	5.6	0.75% ropivacaine	US guidance. The block was performed with an in-plane and multi-injection needle guidance technique, injected epineurally with the aim of achieving maximum encirclement around the nerve.	Keplinger M, Marhofer P, et al., 2015[67]
Subgluteal sciatic nerve block	14	1.5% mepivacaine	NS guidance. Identification of the tibial nerve with a current intensity of >0.2 mA but <0.5 mA and a frequency of 2 Hz. LA was injected followed by perineural catheter placement.	Danelli G, Ghisi D, et al., 2009[68]
	17	1.5% mepivacaine	NS guidance. Identification of the tibial nerve with a stimulating intensity <0.5 mA, with the goal of positioning the stimulating catheter close to the tibial nerve.	Taboada M, Rodriguez J, et al., 2006[69]
Popliteal sciatic nerve block	13.3	1% lidocaine, 0.25% bupivacaine, epinephrine	US guidance. The needle tip was positioned between the tibial and peroneal nerves inside the paraneural sheath. Adequate tip placement was defined as the presence of circular expansion of the paraneural sheath.	Techasuk W, Bernucci F et al., 2014[70]
	30	1.5% mepivacaine	NS. Final catheter position was considered acceptable when the plantar flexion was elicited at a current output via the catheter <0.5 mA.	Taboada M, Rodriguez J, et al. 2006[69]

LA = local anesthetic; NS = nerve stimulator; US = ultrasound; MCN = musculocutaneous nerve; MEV = minimum effective volume.

Table 47.2 MINIMAL EFFECTIVE CONCENTRATION OF LOCAL ANESTHETICS IN 90% OF PATIENTS FOR VARIOUS TYPES OF BLOCKS

NERVE BLOCK	LA	VOLUME (ML)	TECHNIQUE	REFERENCE
Supraclavicular	0.257% ropivacaine	44	US guidance. The LA was injected in the corner pocket and center of the neural bundle.	Fang G, Wan L, et al.[71]
Axillary brachial plexus block	0.241% bupivacaine	5 mL for each nerve	NS was used to confirm the identification of the four nerves (median, ulnar, radial, and musculocutaneous) separately. A dose of 5 mL of bupivacaine without epinephrine was slowly injected around each nerve visualized with ultrasound for a total of 20 mL.	Takeda A, Ferraro LH, et al., 2015[72]
Femoral (surgical anesthesia)	0.93% lidocaine	15	NS and US. Placed 10 ml deep and 5 mL superficial to the nerve.	Taha AM and Abd-Elmaksoud AM, 2013[73]
	0.167% ropivacaine	15	NS and US. Placed 10 ml deep and 5 mL superficial to the nerve. Adequate local anesthetic spread around the nerve was confirmed.	Taha AM and Abd-Elmaksoud AM, 2014[74]
Femoral (postoperative analgesia)	0.271% bupivacaine	22	US guidance. LA was injected around the nerve.	Moura EC, de Oliveira Honda CA, et al., 2016[75]
Femoral/sciatic (postoperative analgesia)	0.2% ropivacaine	20 mL for each	US guidance. For the femoral nerve, perineural injection was assured. For the sciatic nerve, deep injection into the subgluteal space, and around the nerve.	Yao J, Zeng Z, et al., 2013[76]
Popliteal sciatic nerve block (postoperative analgesia)	1% lidocaine, 0.25% bupivacaine, epinephrine	13.3 mL	US guidance. The needle was advanced until its tip was positioned between the tibial and peroneal nerves inside the paraneural sheath. Circular expansion around the paraneural sheath.	Techasuk W, Bernucci F, et al., 2014[70]
Subgluteal sciatic nerve block (surgical block)	1.12% mepivacaine	30 mL	NS guidance. Current intensity of 0.3 to 0.4 mA for a tibial response. LA was injected incrementally with repeated aspirations.	Cappelleri G, Aldegheri G, et al. 2007[77]
Popliteal sciatic nerve block (surgical block)	1.98% mepivacaine	30 mL		

LA = local anesthetic; NS = nerve stimulator; US = ultrasound.

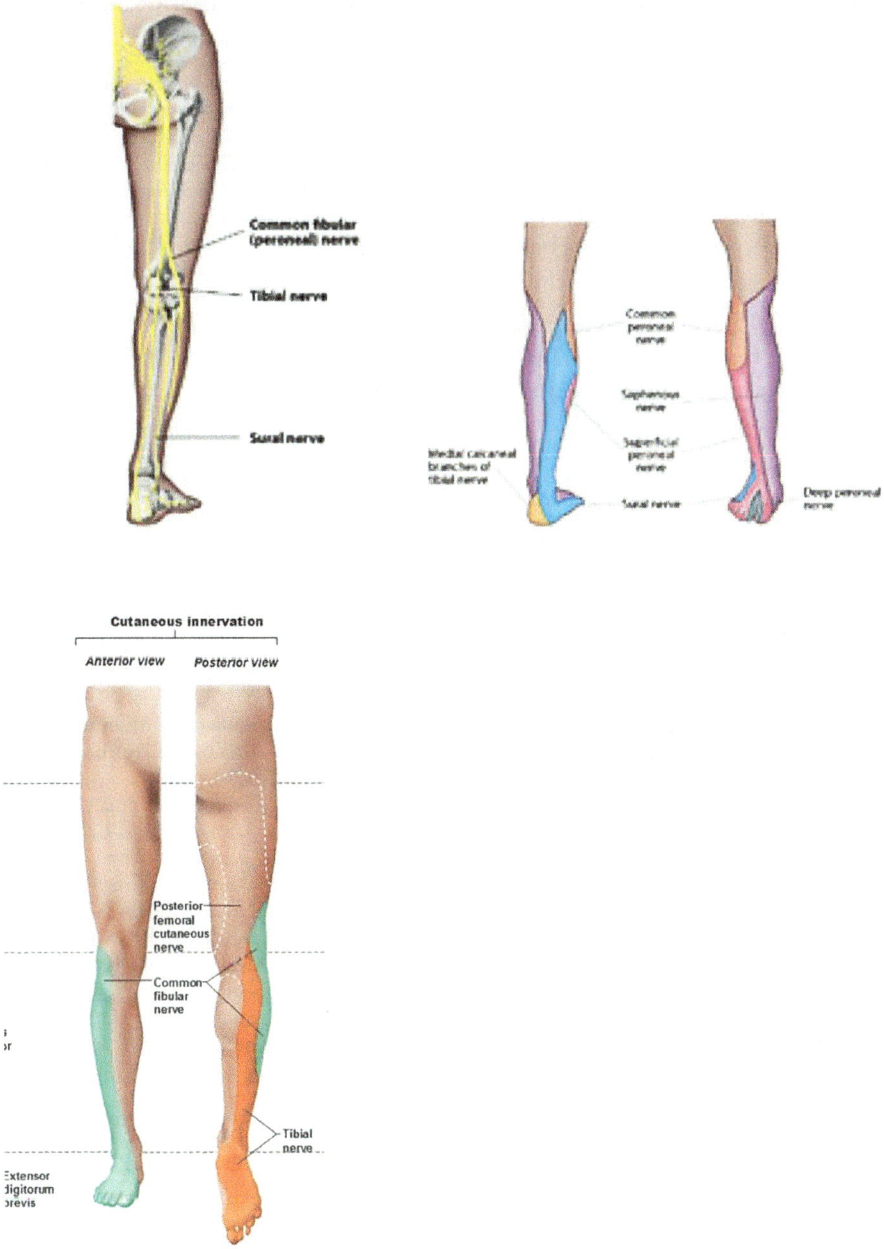

Figure 47.2. Sciatic innervation

dorsum of the foot and motor innervation to the muscles that dorsiflex and evert the foot (Figure 47.2).[91]

MANAGEMENT OF NEUROLOGIC DEFICIT FOLLOWING NERVE INJURY

A nerve block is considered prolonged if it extends beyond the anticipated duration of the LAs. When a nerve injury is suspected, the provider should perform a thorough neurologic examination to determine the distribution of nerve injury. Based on the anatomical deficit of the nerve injury, one may be able to differentiate anesthesia- or surgical-related peripheral nerve injury. If the deficits are in the distribution of the nerve block, persist beyond the anticipated duration of the LA, and the symptoms are purely sensory (two-thirds of peripheral nerve injuries), observation is all that is required because most of these will resolve over days to weeks. It may be prudent to rule out any ongoing and potentially reversible processes that may be causing the neurologic impairment, such as a hematoma or stretch or compression of the nerve due to a tight cast or dressing. These conditions need to be corrected immediately.

Early neurologic consultation is indicated in cases of functionally limiting deficits, severe weakness, sensory loss, progressive deficits, or difficult-to-localize neurologic impairment.[11]

CONCLUSIONS

- Nerves in patients with diabetes are sensitive to LAs. Because of that sensitivity, nerve blocks in this patient population have higher success rates, shorter onset times, and a longer duration of action. These patients generally require less postoperative analgesia.

- The incidence of neurologic injury related to nerve blocks in these patients is much higher than in patients without neuropathy. Because LAs are generally neurotoxic, the regional anesthesiologist should consider using lower volumes and concentrations of LA when performing blocks in patients with diabetes.
- Despite the risks of administering regional anesthesia to patients with DPN, there is no evidence to suggest that regional anesthesia should be withheld from patients when there is a good indication and after a thorough risk-benefit discussion.

REFERENCES

1. Hebl JR, Kopp SL, Schroeder DR, Horlocker TT. Neurologic complications after neuraxial anesthesia or analgesia in patients with preexisting peripheral sensorimotor neuropathy or diabetic polyneuropathy. *Anesth Analg*. 2006;103:1294–1299.
2. Hebl JR, Horlocker TT, Kopp SL, Schroeder DR. Neuraxial blockade in patients with preexisting spinal stenosis, lumbar disk disease, or prior spine surgery: efficacy and neurologic complications. *Anesth Analg*. 2010;111:1511–1519.
3. Neal JM, Barrington MJ, Brull R, et al. The Second ASRA Practice Advisory on Neurologic Complications Associated With Regional Anesthesia and Pain Medicine: executive summary 2015. *Reg Anesth Pain Med*. 2015;40:401–430.
4. Kroin JS, Buvanendran A, Williams DK, et al. Local anesthetic sciatic nerve block and nerve fiber damage in diabetic rats. *Reg Anesth Pain Med*. 2010;35:343–350.
5. Kocum A, Turkoz A, Bozdogan N, Caliskan E, Eker EH, Arslan G. Femoral and sciatic nerve block with 0.25% bupivacaine for surgical management of diabetic foot syndrome: an anesthetic technique for high-risk patients with diabetic nephropathy. *J Clin Anesth*. 2010;22:363–366.
6. Sun J, Feng X, Zhu Q, et al. Analgesic effect of perineural magnesium sulphate for sciatic nerve block for diabetic toe amputation: a randomized trial. *PLoS One*. 2017;12:e0176589.
7. Yuen EC, So YT, Olney RK. The electrophysiologic features of sciatic neuropathy in 100 patients. *Muscle Nerve*. 1995;18:414–420.
8. Aubuchon A, Arnold WD, Bracewell A, Hoyle JC. Sciatic neuropathy due to popliteal fossa nerve block. *Muscle Nerve*. 2017;56:822–824.
9. Brull R, Hadzic A, Reina MA, Barrington MJ. Pathophysiology and etiology of nerve injury following peripheral nerve blockade. *Reg Anesth Pain Med*. 2015;40:479–490.
10. Worrell JB, Barbour G. The Mayo block: an efficacious block for hallux and first metatarsal surgery. *AANA J*. 1996; 64:146–152.
11. Watson JC, Huntoon MA. Neurologic evaluation and management of perioperative nerve injury. *Reg Anesth Pain Med*. 2015;40:491–501.
12. Neal JM, Bernards CM, Hadzic A, et al. ASRA practice advisory on neurologic complications in regional anesthesia and pain medicine. *Reg Anesth Pain Med*. 2008;33:404–415.
13. Vinik A, Ullal J, Parson HK, Casellini CM. Diabetic neuropathies: clinical manifestations and current treatment options. *Nat Clin Pract Endocrinol Metab*. 2006;2:269–281.
14. Lirk P, Birmingham B, Hogan Q. Regional anesthesia in patients with preexisting neuropathy. *Int Anesthesiol Clin*. 2011; 49:144–165.
15. Dyck PJ, Giannini C. Pathologic alterations in the diabetic neuropathies of humans: a review. *J Neuropathol Exp Neurol*. 1996;55:1181–1193.
16. England JD, Gronseth GS, Franklin G, et al. Distal symmetric polyneuropathy: a definition for clinical research: report of the American Academy of Neurology, the American Association of Electrodiagnostic Medicine, and the American Academy of Physical Medicine and Rehabilitation. *Neurology*. 2005;64:199–207.
17. Dyck PJ, Albers JW, Andersen H, et al. Diabetic polyneuropathies: update on research definition, diagnostic criteria and estimation of severity. *Diabetes Metab Res Rev*. 2011;27:620–628.
18. Moon HI, Kwon HK, Kim L, Lee HJ, Lee HJ. Ultrasonography of palm to elbow segment of median nerve in different degrees of diabetic polyneuropathy. *Clin Neurophysiol*. 2014;125:844–848.
19. Young MJ, Boulton AJ, MacLeod AF, Williams DR, Sonksen PH. A multicentre study of the prevalence of diabetic peripheral neuropathy in the United Kingdom hospital clinic population. *Diabetologia*. 1993;36:150–154.
20. Feldman EL, Stevens MJ, Thomas PK, Brown MB, Canal N, Greene DA. A practical two-step quantitative clinical and electrophysiological assessment for the diagnosis and staging of diabetic neuropathy. *Diabetes Care*. 1994;17:1281–1289.
21. Liu F, Mao JP, Yan X. [Toronto clinical scoring system in diabetic peripheral neuropathy]. *Zhong Nan Da Xue Xue Bao Yi Xue Ban*. 2008;33:1137–1141.
22. Said G, Slama G, Selva J. Progressive centripetal degeneration of axons in small fibre diabetic polyneuropathy. *Brain*. 1983;106:791–807.
23. Shun CT, Chang YC, Wu HP, et al. Skin denervation in type 2 diabetes: correlations with diabetic duration and functional impairments. *Brain*. 2004;127:1593–1605.
24. Pop-Busui R, Boulton AJ, Feldman EL, et al. Diabetic neuropathy: a position statement by the American Diabetes Association. *Diabetes Care*. 2017;40:136–154.
25. Callaghan BC, Price RS, Feldman EL. Distal symmetric polyneuropathy: a review. *JAMA*. 2015;314:2172–2181.
26. Riazi S, Bril V, Perkins BA, et al. Can ultrasound of the tibial nerve detect diabetic peripheral neuropathy? A cross-sectional study. *Diabetes Care*. 2012;35:2575–2579.
27. Ishibashi F, Taniguchi M, Kojima R, Kawasaki A, Kosaka A, Uetake H. Morphological changes of the peripheral nerves evaluated by high-resolution ultrasonography are associated with the severity of diabetic neuropathy, but not corneal nerve fiber pathology in patients with type 2 diabetes. *J Diabetes Investig*. 2015;6:334–342.
28. Zheng Y, Wang L, Krupka TM, et al. The feasibility of using high frequency ultrasound to assess nerve ending neuropathy in patients with diabetic foot. *Eur J Radiol*. 2013; 82:512–517.
29. Yagihashi S, Yamagishi S, Wada R. Pathology and pathogenetic mechanisms of diabetic neuropathy: correlation with clinical signs and symptoms. *Diabetes Res Clin Pract*. 2007;77 Suppl 1:S184–S189.
30. Yasuda H, Terada M, Maeda K, et al. Diabetic neuropathy and nerve regeneration. *Prog Neurobiol*. 2003;69:229–285.
31. Eaton SE, Harris ND, Rajbhandari SM, et al. Spinal-cord involvement in diabetic peripheral neuropathy. *Lancet*. 2001;358:35–36.
32. Selvarajah D, Wilkinson ID, Emery CJ, et al. Early involvement of the spinal cord in diabetic peripheral neuropathy. *Diabetes Care*. 2006;29:2664–2669.
33. Llewyn JG, Tomlinson DR, Thomas PK. Diabetic neuropathies in peripheral neuropathy. In: Dyck PJ, Thomas PK, eds. *Peripheral Neuropathy*. 4th ed. Philadelphia: Elsevier; 2005:1951–1992.
34. Prielipp RC, Warner MA. Perioperative nerve injury: a silent scream? *Anesthesiology*. 2009;111:464–466.
35. Upton AR, McComas AJ. The double crush in nerve entrapment syndromes. *Lancet*. 1973;2:359–362.
36. Welch MB, Brummett CM, Welch TD, et al. Perioperative peripheral nerve injuries: a retrospective study of 380,680 cases during a 10-year period at a single institution. *Anesthesiology*. 2009;111:490–497.
37. Szerb J, Persaud D. Long current impulses may be required for nerve stimulation in patients with ischemic pain. *Can J Anaesth*. 2005;52:963–966.
38. Rigaud M, Filip P, Lirk P, Fuchs A, Gemes G, Hogan Q. Guidance of block needle insertion by electrical nerve stimulation: a pilot study of

the resulting distribution of injected solution in dogs. *Anesthesiology*. 2008;109:473–478.
39. Bigeleisen PE, Moayeri N, Groen GJ. Extraneural versus intraneural stimulation thresholds during ultrasound-guided supraclavicular block. *Anesthesiology*. 2009;110:1235–1243.
40. Heschl S, Hallmann B, Zilke T, et al. Diabetic neuropathy increases stimulation threshold during popliteal sciatic nerve block. *Br J Anaesth*. 2016;116:538–545.
41. Keyl C, Held T, Albiez G, Schmack A, Wiesenack C. Increased electrical nerve stimulation threshold of the sciatic nerve in patients with diabetic foot gangrene: a prospective parallel cohort study. *Eur J Anaesthesiol*. 2013;30:435–440.
42. Sites BD, Gallagher J, Sparks M. Ultrasound-guided popliteal block demonstrates an atypical motor response to nerve stimulation in 2 patients with diabetes mellitus. *Reg Anesth Pain Med*. 2003;28:479–482.
43. Gebhard RE, Nielsen KC, Pietrobon R, Missair A, Williams BA. Diabetes mellitus, independent of body mass index, is associated with a "higher success" rate for supraclavicular brachial plexus blocks. *Reg Anesth Pain Med*. 2009;34:404–407.
44. Salviz EA, Onbasi S, Ozonur A, Orhan-Sungur M, Berkoz O, Tugrul KM. Comparison of ultrasound-guided axillary brachial plexus block properties in diabetic and nondiabetic patients: a prospective observational study. *J Hand Surg Am*. 2017;42:190–197.
45. Baeriswyl M, Taffe P, Kirkham KR, et al. Comparison of peripheral nerve blockade characteristics between non-diabetic patients and patients suffering from diabetic neuropathy: a prospective cohort study. *Anaesthesia*. 2018;73:1110–1117.
46. Cuvillon P, Reubrecht V, Zoric L, et al. Comparison of subgluteal sciatic nerve block duration in type 2 diabetic and non-diabetic patients. *Br J Anaesth*. 2013;110:823–830.
47. Echevarria M, Hachero A, Martinez A, et al. Spinal anaesthesia with 0.5% isobaric bupivacaine in patients with diabetes mellitus: the influence of CSF composition on sensory and motor block. *Eur J Anaesthesiol*. 2008;25:1014–1019.
48. Sertoz N, Deniz MN, Ayanoglu HO. Relationship between glycosylated hemoglobin level and sciatic nerve block performance in diabetic patients. *Foot Ankle Int*. 2013;34:85–90.
49. Yang S, Abrahams MS, Hurn PD, Grafe MR, Kirsch JR. Local anesthetic Schwann cell toxicity is time and concentration dependent. *Reg Anesth Pain Med*. 2011;36:444–451.
50. Kalichman MW, Calcutt NA. Local anesthetic-induced conduction block and nerve fiber injury in streptozotocin-diabetic rats. *Anesthesiology*. 1992;77:941–947.
51. Werdehausen R, Fazeli S, Braun S, et al. Apoptosis induction by different local anaesthetics in a neuroblastoma cell line. *Br J Anaesth*. 2009;103:711–718.
52. Kalichman MW. Physiologic mechanisms by which local anesthetics may cause injury to nerve and spinal cord. *Reg Anesth*. 1993;18:448–452.
53. Lirk P, Haller I, Colvin HP, et al. In vitro, inhibition of mitogen-activated protein kinase pathways protects against bupivacaine- and ropivacaine-induced neurotoxicity. *Anesth Analg*. 2008;106:1456–1464.
54. Gautier P, Vandepitte C, Ramquet C, DeCoopman M, Xu D, Hadzic A. The minimum effective anesthetic volume of 0.75% ropivacaine in ultrasound-guided interscalene brachial plexus block. *Anesth Analg*. 2011;113:951–955.
55. Falcao LF, Perez MV, de Castro I, Yamashita AM, Tardelli MA, Amaral JL. Minimum effective volume of 0.5% bupivacaine with epinephrine in ultrasound-guided interscalene brachial plexus block. *Br J Anaesth*. 2013;110:450–455.
56. Renes SH, van Geffen GJ, Rettig HC, Gielen MJ, Scheffer GJ. Minimum effective volume of local anesthetic for shoulder analgesia by ultrasound-guided block at root C7 with assessment of pulmonary function. *Reg Anesth Pain Med*. 2010;35:529–534.
57. Mittal K, Janweja S, Prateek, Sangwan P, Agarwal D, Tak H. The estimation of minimum effective volume of 0.5% ropivacaine in ultrasound-guided interscalene brachial plexus nerve block: a clinical trial. *J Anaesthesiol Clin Pharmacol*. 2019;35:41–46.
58. McNaught A, Shastri U, Carmichael N, et al. Ultrasound reduces the minimum effective local anaesthetic volume compared with peripheral nerve stimulation for interscalene block. *Br J Anaesth*. 2011;106:124–130.
59. Song JG, Jeon DG, Kang BJ, Park KK. Minimum effective volume of mepivacaine for ultrasound-guided supraclavicular block. *Korean J Anesthesiol*. 2013;65:37–41.
60. Pavicic Saric J, Vidjak V, Tomulic K, Zenko J. Effects of age on minimum effective volume of local anesthetic for ultrasound-guided supraclavicular brachial plexus block. *Acta Anaesthesiol Scand*. 2013;57:761–766.
61. Kant A, Gupta PK, Zohar S, Chevret S, Hopkins PM. Application of the continual reassessment method to dose-finding studies in regional anesthesia: an estimate of the ED95 dose for 0.5% bupivacaine for ultrasound-guided supraclavicular block. *Anesthesiology*. 2013;119:29–35.
62. Tran DQ, Dugani S, Correa JA, Dyachenko A, Alsenosy N, Finlayson RJ. Minimum effective volume of lidocaine for ultrasound-guided supraclavicular block. *Reg Anesth Pain Med*. 2011;36:466–469.
63. O'Donnell BD, Iohom G. An estimation of the minimum effective anesthetic volume of 2% lidocaine in ultrasound-guided axillary brachial plexus block. *Anesthesiology*. 2009;111:25–29.
64. Gonzalez AP, Bernucci F, Pham K, Correa JA, Finlayson RJ, Tran DQ. Minimum effective volume of lidocaine for double-injection ultrasound-guided axillary block. *Reg Anesth Pain Med*. 2013;38:16–20.
65. Ferraro LH, Takeda A, dos Reis Falcao LF, Rezende AH, Sadatsune EJ, Tardelli MA. Determination of the minimum effective volume of 0.5% bupivacaine for ultrasound-guided axillary brachial plexus block. *Braz J Anesthesiol*. 2014;64:49–53.
66. Casati A, Baciarello M, Di Cianni S, et al. Effects of ultrasound guidance on the minimum effective anaesthetic volume required to block the femoral nerve. *Br J Anaesth*. 2007;98:823–827.
67. Keplinger M, Marhofer P, Marhofer D, et al. Effective local anaesthetic volumes for sciatic nerve blockade: a clinical evaluation of the ED99. *Anaesthesia*. 2015;70:585–590.
68. Danelli G, Ghisi D, Fanelli A, et al. The effects of ultrasound guidance and neurostimulation on the minimum effective anesthetic volume of mepivacaine 1.5% required to block the sciatic nerve using the subgluteal approach. *Anesth Analg*. 2009;109:1674–1678.
69. Taboada M, Rodriguez J, Valino C, et al. What is the minimum effective volume of local anesthetic required for sciatic nerve blockade? A prospective, randomized comparison between a popliteal and a subgluteal approach. *Anesth Analg*. 2006;102:593–597.
70. Techasuk W, Bernucci F, Cupido T, et al. Minimum effective volume of combined lidocaine-bupivacaine for analgesic subparaneural popliteal sciatic nerve block. *Reg Anesth Pain Med*. 2014;39:108–111.
71. Fang G, Wan L, Mei W, Yu HH, Luo AL. The minimum effective concentration (MEC90) of ropivacaine for ultrasound-guided supraclavicular brachial plexus block. *Anaesthesia*. 2016;71:700–705.
72. Takeda A, Ferraro LH, Rezende AH, Sadatsune EJ, Falcao LF, Tardelli MA. [Minimum effective concentration of bupivacaine for axillary brachial plexus block guided by ultrasound]. *Rev Bras Anestesiol*. 2015;65:163–169.
73. Taha AM, Abd-Elmaksoud AM. Lidocaine use in ultrasound-guided femoral nerve block: what is the minimum effective anaesthetic concentration (MEAC90)? *Br J Anaesth*. 2013;110:1040–1044.
74. Taha AM, Abd-Elmaksoud AM. Ropivacaine in ultrasound-guided femoral nerve block: what is the minimal effective anaesthetic concentration (EC90)? *Anaesthesia*. 2014;69:678–682.
75. Moura EC, de Oliveira Honda CA, Bringel RC, Leal Pda C, Filho Gde J, Sakata RK. Minimum effective concentration of bupivacaine in ultrasound-guided femoral nerve block after arthroscopic knee meniscectomy: a randomized, double-blind, controlled trial. *Pain Physician*. 2016;19:E79–E86.
76. Yao J, Zeng Z, Jiao ZH, Wang AZ, Wang J, Yu A. Optimal effective concentration of ropivacaine for postoperative analgesia by single-shot femoral-sciatic nerve block in outpatient knee arthroscopy. *J Int Med Res*. 2013;41:395–403.

77. Cappelleri G, Aldegheri G, Ruggieri F, Mamo D, Fanelli G, Casati A. Minimum effective anesthetic concentration (MEAC) for sciatic nerve block: subgluteus and popliteal approaches. *Can J Anaesth*. 2007;54:283–289.
78. Williams BA, Murinson BB, Grable BR, Orebaugh SL. Future considerations for pharmacologic adjuvants in single-injection peripheral nerve blocks for patients with diabetes mellitus. *Reg Anesth Pain Med*. 2009;34:445–457.
79. Neal JM. Effects of epinephrine in local anesthetics on the central and peripheral nervous systems: neurotoxicity and neural blood flow. *Reg Anesth Pain Med*. 2003;28:124–134.
80. Williams BA, Hough KA, Tsui BY, Ibinson JW, Gold MS, Gebhart GF. Neurotoxicity of adjuvants used in perineural anesthesia and analgesia in comparison with ropivacaine. *Reg Anesth Pain Med*. 2011;36:225–230.
81. Partridge BL. The effects of local anesthetics and epinephrine on rat sciatic nerve blood flow. *Anesthesiology*. 1991;75:243–250.
82. Myers RR, Heckman HM. Effects of local anesthesia on nerve blood flow: studies using lidocaine with and without epinephrine. *Anesthesiology*. 1989;71:757–762.
83. She YJ, Zhang ZY, Song XR. Caudal dexmedetomidine decreases the required concentration of levobupivacaine for caudal block in pediatric patients: a randomized trial. *Paediatr Anaesth*. 2013;23:1205–1212.
84. Lu Y, Sun J, Zhuang X, et al. Perineural dexmedetomidine as an adjuvant reduces the median effective concentration of lidocaine for obturator nerve blocking: a double-blinded randomized controlled trial. *PLoS One*. 2016;11:e0158226.
85. Tufek A, Kaya S, Tokgoz O, et al. The protective effect of dexmedetomidine on bupivacaine-induced sciatic nerve inflammation is mediated by mast cells. *Clin Invest Med*. 2013;36:E95–102.
86. Zhang H, Zhou F, Li C, et al. Molecular mechanisms underlying the analgesic property of intrathecal dexmedetomidine and its neurotoxicity evaluation: an in vivo and in vitro experimental study. *PLoS One*. 2013;8:e55556.
87. Brummett CM, Norat MA, Palmisano JM, Lydic R. Perineural administration of dexmedetomidine in combination with bupivacaine enhances sensory and motor blockade in sciatic nerve block without inducing neurotoxicity in rat. *Anesthesiology*. 2008;109:502–511.
88. Kim BS, Choi JH, Baek SH, Lee DH. Effects of intraneural injection of dexmedetomidine in combination with ropivacaine in rat sciatic nerve block. *Reg Anesth Pain Med*. 2018;43:378–384.
89. Yu ZY, Geng J, Li ZQ, et al. Dexmedetomidine enhances ropivacaine-induced sciatic nerve injury in diabetic rats. *Br J Anaesth*. 2019;122:141–149.
90. Konakci S, Adanir T, Yilmaz G, Rezanko T. The efficacy and neurotoxicity of dexmedetomidine administered via the epidural route. *Eur J Anaesthesiol*. 2008;25:403–409.
91. Morton DA, Foreman KB, Albertine KH. Chapter 37. Leg. In: *The Big Picture: Gross Anatomy*. New York: McGraw-Hill; 2011.
92. Dyck PJ, Kratz KM, Karnes JL, et al. The prevalence by staged severity of various types of diabetic neuropathy, retinopathy, and nephropathy in a population-based cohort: the Rochester Diabetic Neuropathy Study. *Neurology*. 1993;43:817–824.
93. Barr EL, Wong TY, Tapp RJ, et al. Is peripheral neuropathy associated with retinopathy and albuminuria in individuals with impaired glucose metabolism? The 1999-2000 AusDiab. *Diabetes Care*. 2006;29:1114–1116.

REVIEW QUESTIONS

(1) Patients with diabetic peripheral neuropathy exhibit:

A. Prolonged nerve block duration
B. Shorter nerve block duration
C. Increased failure rate
D. Need for more postoperative pain medications

(2) The incidence of regional anesthesia-related nerve injury in patients with diabetes compared to the normal population is:

A. 2 times higher
B. 10 times higher
C. 5 times lower
D. 5 times higher

(3) A 69-year-old man with a 23-year history of type II diabetes mellitus with no symptoms of neuropathy presents for right bunionectomy. He receives an uneventful ultrasound-guided popliteal nerve block. However, on his follow-up visit 1 week later with his podiatrist, he still complains of numbness on the lateral side of the leg and the dorsum of the foot. Which of the following would you do next?

A. Neurology consult
B. Nerve conduction study
C. Assurance that the condition is likely to be temporary and will resolve spontaneously
D. Electromyography

(4) Using ultrasound imaging, compared to normal nerves, the nerves in patients with diabetic peripheral neuropathy appear:

A. Smaller in diameter
B. Clear and well-delineated
C. Larger in diameter
D. Hyperechoic

(5) The prolongation of nerve block duration in patients with diabetic peripheral neuropathy correlates with all of the following EXCEPT:

A. The duration the patient had diabetes mellitus
B. Hemoglobin A1C level
C. The severity of the neuropathy
D. The acute control of hyperglycemia

(6) Which of the following is not recommended in cases of profoundly symptomatic diabetic peripheral neuropathy?

A. Limiting the local anesthetic dose
B. Limiting the local anesthetic concentration
C. Using the nerve stimulator only to localize the nerve
D. Avoiding the use of perineural epinephrine

(7) Which of the following does not strongly correlate with the presence of diabetic peripheral neuropathy in an asymptomatic patient?

A. Diabetes mellitus diagnosed for more than 5 years
B. Diabetic nephropathy
C. Diabetic retinopathy
D. Dyslipidemia

(8) The use of perineural adjuvants in diabetic peripheral neuropathy is indicated for which of the following reasons?

A. They result in a local anesthetic-sparing effect
B. Nerve blocks have a shorter duration than usual

C. The perineural vasoconstriction helps to prolong the block
D. They generally have neuroprotective effects

(9) The most definitive method to diagnose diabetic peripheral neuropathy is:

A. History
B. Physical examination
C. Screening tools
D. Nerve conduction studies

ANSWERS

1. **A.** Nerve blocks in patients with diabetic peripheral neuropathy (DPN) usually have a shorter onset time and longer duration of action. The axillary brachial plexus block in patients with type II diabetes has been reported to be 1.5 times longer in patients with DPN compared to controls without DPN. Popliteal nerve blocks in patients with DPN have been reported to have a 59% shorter onset time, prolonged median time to first opioid request of 1.57, and lower overall pain scores. Even patients with minor clinical DPN still have longer sciatic sensory block durations than those who are nondiabetic.

References

Salviz EA, Onbasi S, Ozonur A, Orhan-Sungur M, Berkoz O, Tugrul KM. Comparison of ultrasound-guided axillary brachial plexus block properties in diabetic and nondiabetic patients: a prospective observational study. *J Hand Surg Am*. 2017;42:190–197.

Baeriswyl M, Taffe P, Kirkham KR, et al. Comparison of peripheral nerve blockade characteristics between non-diabetic patients and patients suffering from diabetic neuropathy: a prospective cohort study. *Anaesthesia*. 2018;73:1110–1117.

Cuvillon P, Reubrecht V, Zoric L, et al. Comparison of subgluteal sciatic nerve block duration in type 2 diabetic and non-diabetic patients. *Br J Anaesth*. 2013;110:823–830.

(2) **B.** The risk of nerve injury due to peripheral nerve blocks is estimated to be approximately 0.04%. Patients with preexisting diabetic peripheral neuropathy have an incidence of 0.3% to 1.1%, which is 10 times higher than the general population.

References

Hebl JR, Kopp SL, Schroeder DR, Horlocker TT. Neurologic complications after neuraxial anesthesia or analgesia in patients with preexisting peripheral sensorimotor neuropathy or diabetic polyneuropathy. *Anesth Analg*. 2006;103:1294–1299.

Hebl JR, Horlocker TT, Kopp SL, Schroeder DR. Neuraxial blockade in patients with preexisting spinal stenosis, lumbar disk disease, or prior spine surgery: efficacy and neurologic complications. *Anesth Analg*. 2010;111:1511–1519.

(3) **C.** If the deficits are in the distribution of the nerve block, persisting beyond the duration of the local anesthetic, and purely sensory, only observation is required because most of these conditions will resolve over days to weeks. Neurologic consultation if indicated if sensory symptoms persist for a significant amount of time.

Reference

Watson JC, Huntoon MA. Neurologic evaluation and management of perioperative nerve injury. *Reg Anesth Pain Med*. 2015;40:491–501.

(4) **C.** Nerves in patients with diabetic peripheral neuropathy (DPN) show increased cross-sectional areas, more hypoechoic areas, increased thickness of the nerve fascicle, obscurity, surface irregularity, and heterogeneity on ultrasound imaging. These findings correlate with the severity of neuropathy. Although DPN is characterized by the progressive loss of myelinated nerve fibers, the condition results in nerves that appear larger by ultrasound due to swelling. The swelling happens due to the thickening of the vasculature, accumulation of microfibrillar material in the vicinity of perineurial cells, and an increase in the diameter of endoneurial collagen fibrils. It even precedes the development of DPN and is thought to be due to the higher hemoglobin A1C levels.

References

Riazi S, Bril V, Perkins BA, et al. Can ultrasound of the tibial nerve detect diabetic peripheral neuropathy? A cross-sectional study. *Diabetes Care*. 2012;35:2575–2579.

Ishibashi F, Taniguchi M, Kojima R, Kawasaki A, Kosaka A, Uetake H. Morphological changes of the peripheral nerves evaluated by high-resolution ultrasonography are associated with the severity of diabetic neuropathy, but not corneal nerve fiber pathology in patients with type 2 diabetes. *J Diabetes Investig*. 2015;6:334–342.

Zheng Y, Wang L, Krupka TM, et al. The feasibility of using high frequency ultrasound to assess nerve ending neuropathy in patients with diabetic foot. *Eur J Radiol*. 2013;82:512–517.

(5) **D.** Prolongation of the nerve blocks was especially noted in patients who had diabetes for a longer time, had poorer glycemic control, and had a higher level of glycosylated hemoglobin A1C.

References

Salviz EA, Onbasi S, Ozonur A, Orhan-Sungur M, Berkoz O, Tugrul KM. Comparison of ultrasound-guided axillary brachial plexus block properties in diabetic and nondiabetic patients: a prospective observational study. *J Hand Surg Am*. 2017;42:190–197.

Sertoz N, Deniz MN, Ayanoglu HO. Relationship between glycosylated hemoglobin level and sciatic nerve block performance in diabetic patients. *Foot Ankle Int*. 2013;34:85–90.

(6) **C.** Limiting local anesthetic volume and concentration and avoiding epinephrine are recommended. However, localizing the peripheral nerves using the nerve stimulator in patients with diabetic peripheral neuropathy can be difficult and may be unsuccessful. Usually, a higher threshold of stimulation and longer pulse wave duration are needed. When using a low-threshold stimulation current in a hyperglycemic dog model, all needle insertions resulted in intraneural injections.

Reference

Rigaud M, Filip P, Lirk P, Fuchs A, Gemes G, Hogan Q. Guidance of block needle insertion by electrical nerve stimulation: a pilot study of the resulting distribution of injected solution in dogs. *Anesthesiology*. 2008;109:473–478.

(7) **D.** A history of associated diabetes and organ dysfunction such as retinopathy and nephropathy increase the chances of neuropathy.

References

Dyck PJ, Kratz KM, Karnes JL, et al. The prevalence by staged severity of various types of diabetic neuropathy, retinopathy, and nephropathy in a population-based cohort: the Rochester Diabetic Neuropathy Study. *Neurology*. 1993;43:817–824.

Barr EL, Wong TY, Tapp RJ, et al. Is peripheral neuropathy associated with retinopathy and albuminuria in individuals with impaired glucose metabolism? The 1999–2000 AusDiab. *Diabetes Care*. 2006;29:1114–1116.

(8) **A.** Perineural adjuvants are usually used to prolong the duration of the block or to provide a dose-sparing effect. Block duration is prolonged in patients with diabetes, and because of the harmful effect of prolonged exposure of the nerve to local anesthetics (LAs), the addition of adjuvants without a corresponding decrease in LA concentration is generally not recommended.

References

Kroin JS, Buvanendran A, Williams DK, et al. Local anesthetic sciatic nerve block and nerve fiber damage in diabetic rats. *Reg Anesth Pain Med*. 2010;35:343–350.

Williams BA, Murinson BB, Grable BR, Orebaugh SL. Future considerations for pharmacologic adjuvants in single-injection peripheral nerve blocks for patients with diabetes mellitus. *Reg Anesth Pain Med*. 2009;34:445–457.

(9) **D.** Diabetic peripheral neuropathy (DPN) may not be easy to diagnose; up to 50% of patients may be asymptomatic. History, physical examination, screening methods, and ultrasound studies are helpful. However, nerve conduction studies combined with needle electromyogram are the most sensitive methods to diagnose DPN, even in the subclinical stage. They can also predict ulceration and mortality in patients with diabetes. However, because they are invasive and painful, they are not usually indicated for the routine diagnosis of DPN.

References

England JD, Gronseth GS, Franklin G, et al. Distal symmetric polyneuropathy: a definition for clinical research: report of the American Academy of Neurology, the American Association of Electrodiagnostic Medicine, and the American Academy of Physical Medicine and Rehabilitation. *Neurology*. 2005;64:199–207.

Dyck PJ, Albers JW, Andersen H, et al. Diabetic polyneuropathies: update on research definition, diagnostic criteria and estimation of severity. *Diabetes Metab Res Rev*. 2011;27:620–628.

48.

CAUDA EQUINA SYNDROME AFTER SPINAL ANESTHESIA

Lauren Steffel and Joseph M. Neal

STEM CASE AND KEY QUESTIONS

A 75-year-old woman receives an uneventful spinal anesthetic dosed with 12.5 mg of isobaric bupivacaine prior to undergoing right total knee arthroplasty. During her postoperative recovery, she is noted to have ongoing bilateral lower extremity motor weakness and urinary incontinence. She also experiences a sensory loss in the low sacral distribution. There is no interval improvement in her symptoms over several hours. Magnetic resonance imaging (MRI) reveals incidental moderate lumbar spinal stenosis, but there is no reversible etiology to explain her neurological deficits.

(1) WHAT IS CAUDA EQUINA SYNDROME (CES)? HOW DOES IT TYPICALLY PRESENT?

CES is a constellation of syndromes that result from lesions to the spinal nerve roots caudad to the conus medullaris (see anatomy of the cauda equina in Figure 48.1). Clinical presentation and physical exam in CES may be nonspecific. Most cases involve lower extremity weakness, lower extremity and sacral sensory changes, and bowel/bladder dysfunction. Back or lower extremity pain is a nonspecific finding.

(2) WHAT IS THE INCIDENCE OF CES?

The incidence of CES is estimated to be between 1.9–3.8/100,000 neuraxial anesthetics.[2,3]

(3) WHAT ARE THE POTENTIAL ETIOLOGIES OF CES?

Potential CES etiologies include inflammatory insults, neurotoxic insults, and surgical factors; they may also be multifactorial or idiopathic. Idiopathic etiologies for CES appear to be the most common. Mass lesions that may result in CES include intervertebral disc herniation, epidural abscess, epidural/intradural extramedullary tumor, lumbar spine spondylosis, and spinal-epidural hematoma. Inflammatory reactions of the arachnoid membrane can be secondary to infection, trauma (surgery or neuraxial procedures), or the presence of blood. Chemical neurotoxicity can occur due to local anesthetics or antiseptic agents.

(4) WHAT ARE RISK FACTORS OF CES?

Most CES cases occur following unremarkable neuraxial anesthesia. Known associated risk factors include mass lesions, local anesthetic neurotoxicity/neuroinflammation, patient risk factors, and surgical positioning.

(5) HOW IS CES DIAGNOSED AND TREATED?

Computerized tomography (CT) imaging may rule out a reversible cause such as a decompressible mass lesion. When the clinical syndrome suggests a localized process within the spinal canal, a more extensive imaging study, usually MRI of the relevant spinal cord section, may be required urgently or emergently. Unless there is a reversible mass lesion that may respond to surgical intervention, *there is no known treatment to alter the course of CES.* Steroids are generally not recommended and should be used at the discretion of neurological consultants.

(6) WHAT ARE THE ANTICIPATED OUTCOMES IN PATIENTS PRESENTING WITH CES?

Most patients with CES from non-reversible, non-mass lesion etiologies exhibit little if any improvement with time, and there is no treatment to alter the course of CES.

(7) WHAT ARE CURRENT RECOMMENDATIONS TO MINIMIZE RISK OF CES?

To prevent CES, it is recommended that proceduralists use appropriate doses of neuraxial local anesthetics, avoid redosing spinal anesthetics, allow for adequate drying time of topical antiseptic agents, and prevent cross-contamination with antiseptic agents.

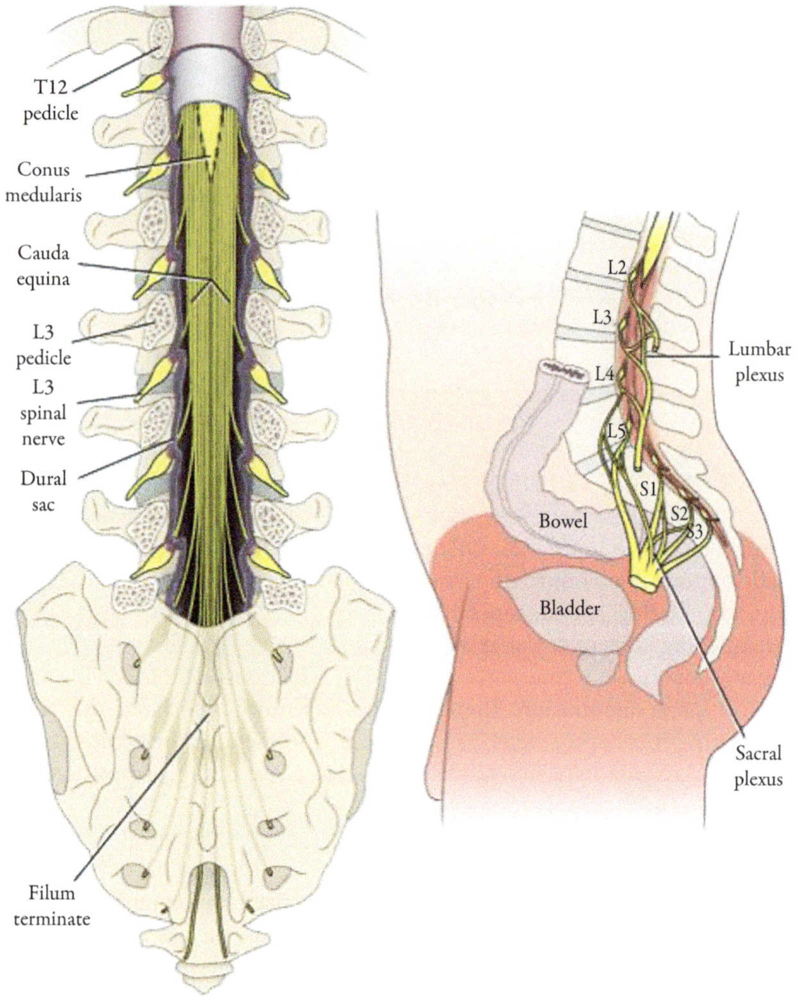

Figure 48.1. Anatomy of the cauda equina.
Used with permission from: Neal JM, Rathmell JP. *Complications of Regional Anesthesia and Pain Medicine*. 2nd edition. Philadelphia: Lippincott Williams & Wilkins; 2013.

DISCUSSION

PRESENTATION OF CES

CES describes a constellation of symptoms that can result from various lesions involving spinal nerve roots caudad to the conus medullaris. Although clinical presentation is variable, most cases involve lower extremity weakness, lower extremity and sacral sensory changes, and bowel/bladder dysfunction. Back or lower extremity pain is a nonspecific finding. CES can result from obvious, sometimes reversible, causes that involve space-occupying lesions within the spinal canal, such as blood, pus, or a herniated disc. However, many cases of CES do not involve a compressive etiology but rather less-understood conditions such as neurotoxicity or inflammation. Indeed, once mass lesions have been ruled out, many if not most cases of CES are of idiopathic etiology.

The spinal cord usually terminates as the conus medullaris near the lower margin of the first lumbar vertebral body (L1). Below that level, the spinal canal contains the lumbar, sacral, and coccygeal spinal nerve roots that comprise the cauda equina. CES is therefore caused by a variety of lesions affecting the lumbosacral nerve roots below the level of the conus medullaris.

The syndrome is caused by loss of function of 2 or more of the 18 nerve roots comprising the cauda equina, as depicted in Figure 48.1. Localizing symptoms include:[1]

1. Dorsal nerve root: low back pain accompanied by unilateral or bilateral radicular pain
2. S1, S2 nerve roots: weakness of foot plantar flexion, loss of ankle reflex
3. S3 to S5 nerve roots: bladder and rectal sphincter paralysis, particularly new urinary incontinence
4. All nerve roots: loss of all sensorimotor modalities.

INCIDENCE OF CES

Severe neurological complications following neuraxial blockade are extremely rare, but the incidence is likely underestimated. Contemporary estimates specific to CES can be derived from the following studies.

In a 1990–1999 Swedish retrospective population study of approximately 1,260,000 spinal anesthetics and 450,000 epidural anesthetics, including 200,000 labor epidural anesthetics, CES was a complication in 32 cases (1.9/100,000).[2] Of those cases, 8 occurred in the setting of epidural blockade, 4 in the setting of combined spinal-epidural blockade, 8 in the setting of spinal blockade, and 2 in the setting of continuous spinal blockade.

In a 10-month prospective survey based in France, 3 cases of CES after spinal, epidural, or combined spinal-epidural blockade were identified from a sample size of 78,104. All occurred in a non-obstetric population after spinal anesthesia (there were no cases of CES in the epidural or combined spinal-epidural groups), resulting in an incidence of 3.8/100,000.[3]

POTENTIAL ETIOLOGIES OF CES

To our best current understanding, potential CES etiologies include inflammatory insults, neurotoxic insults, and surgical factors; they may also be multifactorial or idiopathic.[1,4]

Idiopathic Etiologies

Idiopathic etiologies of CES appear to be the most common in large cohort studies.[2] A subset of patients developed CES in the absence of known risk factors and may have developed neurotoxicity in response to a clinically appropriate dose of local anesthetic or due to factors unrelated to the anesthetic. When no alternative risk factors are identified (normal local anesthetic dosing, normal spinal imaging, etc.), some neurologists speculate that the CES etiology is likely to involve incompletely elucidated mechanisms of neurotoxicity, inflammation, or as yet unknown patient/surgical/anesthetic factors. Most CES cases occur after unremarkable cases of neuraxial anesthesia with atraumatic neuraxial instrumentation and standard local anesthetic dosing.

Mass Lesions

Timely evaluation is needed to rule out decompressible lesions and thereby differentiate a reversible lesion from an irreversible one. Physical examination often cannot distinguish between reversible and non-reversible etiologies early in the clinical course.

Mass lesions that may result in CES include intervertebral disc herniation, epidural abscess, epidural/intradural extramedullary tumor, lumbar spine spondylosis, and spinal-epidural hematoma. A spinal-epidural hematoma is a rare complication of neuraxial anesthesia and has a higher incidence with epidural anesthesia than with spinal anesthesia.[2,3,5] In a 2004 retrospective study,[2] the incidence was 1 in 18,000 epidurals and 1 in 158,000 spinals. Risk factors for spinal-epidural hematoma include advanced age, coagulopathy, and difficult neuraxial anesthetic instrumentation.

However, this chapter focuses primarily on non-mass lesion causes of CES, such as local anesthetic toxicity and inflammatory conditions, which are discussed below in the context of their shared presumed etiology of neurotoxicity.

Inflammatory/Neurotoxic Etiologies

Most risk factors are unknown, but inflammatory reactions and chemical neurotoxicity are some conditions that have been correlated with CES.[6,7] Inflammatory reaction of the arachnoid membrane can be secondary to infection, surgical/procedural trauma, or the presence of blood.

Chemical neurotoxicity can occur due to local anesthetics or antiseptic agents. Local anesthetic-mediated neurotoxicity has been associated with:

a. supranormal doses of local anesthetics and/or

b. maldistribution of local anesthetic spread within the intrathecal space, such as in the setting of local anesthetic accumulation on the sacral side of the lumbar lordotic curve while in the supine position, and/or

c. spinal stenosis.[2,3]

Although all local anesthetics can cause neurotoxicity, lidocaine appears to have a higher potential for neurotoxicity compared to bupivacaine when intrathecally administered. More so than the type of local anesthetic, the most important causative component of CES in relation to local anesthetic toxicity is any use in higher than recommended doses (especially continuous spinal anesthesia). Most of the commonly used local anesthetic adjuvants and preservatives are not believed to cause neurotoxicity when used in routine clinical concentrations.

Spinal arachnoiditis due to antiseptics is somewhat speculative and limited to a narrow subset of patient cases.[8] This form of arachnoiditis, when it occurs, may or may not have the traditional components of CES in its presentation. For instance, it may present with severe back pain and progressive paresis that ascends to higher cerebrospinal levels.[8]

Two percent chlorhexidine gluconate and 10% povidone-iodine are cytotoxic to human neuronal and rat Schwann cells,[9] and at lower doses, chlorhexidine exhibits neurotoxic effects on peripheral adrenergic nerve terminals.[10] In comparing the effectiveness of these two methods of antisepsis, cultures of epidural catheter tips in patients for whom chlorhexidine antiseptic was used were significantly less likely to yield microorganisms upon removal compared to those for whom povidone-iodine was used.[11] In a study of over 11,000 patients receiving spinal anesthesia at Mayo Clinic Rochester from 2006 to 2010, there was no increased risk of neurologic complications associated with the use of chlorhexidine skin antisepsis (0.04%) compared to other previously used antiseptics. Therefore, it was concluded that chlorhexidine may be used for skin antisepsis prior to spinal placement without increasing the risk of neurologic complications attributed to the spinal anesthetic.[12]

The use of chlorhexidine-containing antiseptic solution for skin preparation prior to neuraxial block is recommended in a practice advisory from the American Society of Anesthesiologists Task Force on Infectious Complications Associated with Neuraxial Techniques and the American Society of Regional Anesthesia and Pain Medicine, with the stipulations that there be an adequate drying time of 2–3 minutes prior to neuraxial procedure and that there be a physical separation between the antiseptic agent and its applicator from other drugs and equipment.[13]

Spinal Stenosis

The presence of spinal stenosis is associated with CES.[2] The presumed mechanism involves the decreased vascular clearance of a neurotoxin such as a local anesthetic, as well as a predisposition to nerve root ischemia from compression of the spinal vasculature. CES is occasionally concurrent with degenerative and congenital spinal diseases.[14]

Surgical Positioning

There may be a higher risk for CES with certain surgical positions that presumably worsen spinal cord perfusion, especially in patients with preexisting spinal stenosis. Examples of such positions include extreme lateral flexion or hyperlordosis.

CES DIAGNOSIS AND TREATMENT

When there is concern for CES, its clinical presentation and physical examination may be nonspecific; therefore, timely evaluation and emergent neurologic consultation are paramount. Rapid and readily available CT imaging may rule out a reversible cause, such as a decompressible mass lesion, and is recommended in the practice advisory from the American Society of Anesthesiologists Task Force on Infectious Complications Associated with Neuraxial Techniques and the American Society of Regional Anesthesia and Pain Medicine.[13]

When the clinical syndrome suggests a localized process within the spinal canal, a more extensive imaging study, usually MRI of the relevant spinal cord section, may be required urgently or emergently.[15]

In the case of CES, imaging is typically normal unless associated with specific risk factors such as spinal stenosis. *There is no known treatment to alter the course of CES.* Steroids are generally not recommended and should be used at the discretion of neurological consultants.

Of note, CES may be confused with other neurologic phenomena such as transient neurologic symptoms (TNS). It is important to note that TNS has a delayed presentation compared with the sudden onset of CES, and, unlike the CES hallmark of multiple neurologic deficits, TNS presents exclusively as pain and/or dysesthesia, with normal neurologic examination and imaging. TNS resolves spontaneously over the course of several days. Most experts believe the etiology of TNS does not involve neurotoxicity. The features of CES and TNS are compared in Table 48.1.

PROGNOSIS

Most patients with CES from non-reversible causes exhibit limited if any improvement with time.[13,16]

RECOMMENDATIONS TO MINIMIZE RISK OF CES

1. Use appropriate doses and concentrations of neuraxial local anesthetics.
2. Avoid re-dosing failed spinal anesthetics, and if re-dosing occurs, never allow the total dose to exceed the maximum recommended dose specific to that local anesthetic.

Table 48.1 **DIFFERENTIAL DIAGNOSIS FOR NEUROLOGICAL DEFICITS**

DIFFERENTIAL DIAGNOSIS	TIMING	IMPROVEMENT	NEUROLOGIC DEFICIT	IMAGING
Cauda equina syndrome *non-mass lesion*	Patient emerges from anesthetic with symptoms	Irreversible symptoms	Commonly involves sensory loss, motor weakness, bowel/bladder dysfunction	Negative
Cauda equina syndrome (*mass lesion*)	Patient may emerge from anesthetic with symptoms, or they may worsen slowly over hours to days as mass lesion continues to expand	Reversible or partially reversible with decompression	Commonly involves sensory loss, motor weakness, bowel/bladder dysfunction with or without back pain	Mass lesion
Transient neurologic symptoms	Hours after resolution of neuraxial block	Spontaneously improves over several days	None; pain is the only symptom	Negative
Ischemic injury	May or may not be associated with severe, prolonged perioperative hypotension	May be reversible in rare cases (re-establish perfusion pressure)	Commonly involves sensory loss, motor weakness, bowel/bladder dysfunction	May be normal initially, but eventually signs of spinal cord ischemia/infarction

3. Perform a careful risk/benefit analysis when electing to use a neuraxial anesthetic in patients with abnormal spinal anatomy (e.g., severe spinal stenosis) or surgical positioning (extreme lateral flexion or hyperlordosis) that are risk factors for CES.
4. When using an antiseptic solution for skin preparation prior to neuraxial block, allow for adequate drying time (2–3 minutes) and physical separation of the antiseptic agent and its applicator from other drugs and equipment.[13]

SUMMARY

CES results from a variety of lesions involving spinal nerve roots caudad to the conus medullaris. Symptoms are due to the involvement of multiple nerve roots of the cauda equina and may include sensory loss in the distribution of one or more nerve roots, paresthesias, patchy and asymmetrical weakness, loss of lower extremity deep tendon reflexes, and bowel/bladder dysfunction. Back and radicular pain are inconsistent symptoms. Pain is likewise not always present with neuraxial mass lesions, but back and/or radicular pain radiating to one or both legs is a presentation that raises concern for CES stemming from a space-occupying, potentially decompressible lesion within the spinal canal.

The spinal cord terminates as the conus medullaris near L1, caudad to which is found the cauda equina, which contains lumbar, sacral, and coccygeal spinal nerve roots. CES is caused by lesions in these nerve roots, including low back pain (dorsal nerve root), loss of plantar foot flexion/ankle reflex (nerve S1–S2 roots), bowel/bladder incontinence (S3–S5 nerve roots), and sensorimotor loss.[1]

The incidence of CES is rare but likely underestimated. Contemporary population studies estimate an incidence of 1.9 to 3.8 per 100,000 neuraxial anesthetics.[2,3]

The most common etiology of CES is idiopathic; that is, most CES cases occur after an unremarkable neuraxial anesthetic in the absence of known risk factors. In this setting, some neurologists speculate that CES etiology involves neurotoxicity, neural inflammation, or unidentified patient, surgical, or anesthetic risk factors. Associated risk factors include mass lesions (decompressible and, therefore, potentially reversible), inflammatory/neurotoxic etiologies (blood, infection, trauma, supranormal doses of local anesthetic, and possibly neurotoxicity or arachnoiditis secondary to antiseptics), spinal stenosis, and surgical positioning (such as extreme lateral flexion or hyperlordosis) that limits spinal perfusion.

The clinical presentation and physical examination in CES may be nonspecific, and concern for the syndrome necessitates emergent neurological consultation and evaluation. CT imaging may rapidly rule out a reversible cause, and MRI can further evaluate a localized process within the spinal cord or canal. In patients with CES, neuroimaging will be normal (at least initially), and the syndrome typically presents as neurologic deficits occurring after the expected resolution of the neuraxial anesthetic. *Most patients with CES from non-reversible causes exhibit little if any improvement with time, and there is no known treatment to alter the course of CES.* Steroids are generally not recommended.

To minimize the risk of CES, we recommend the use of appropriate doses/concentrations of neuraxial local anesthetics, avoiding the practice of re-dosing failed spinal anesthetics, allowing for adequate drying time of skin antiseptic solutions, preventing cross-contamination of neuraxial drugs and equipment with antiseptic agents, and a careful risk/benefit analysis when electing to use a neuraxial anesthetic in patients with risk factors associated with CES.

CONCLUSIONS

- CES is a constellation of syndromes that result from lesions to the spinal nerve roots caudad to the conus medullaris.
- Clinical presentation and physical examination in CES may be nonspecific, and concern for the syndrome necessitates emergent neurological consultation and evaluation. CT or MRI imaging may rule out a reversible cause and evaluate a localized process within the spinal canal.[13]
- The incidence of CES is estimated to be between 1.9 and 3.8/100,000 neuraxial anesthetics.[2,3]
- CES is differentiated from TNS by the presence of neurologic deficit, earlier onset, and the lack of spontaneous resolution of symptoms.
- Most CES cases occur after unremarkable neuraxial anesthesia.
- Known associated risk factors include mass lesions, local anesthetic neurotoxicity/neuroinflammation, patient risk factors, and surgical positioning.
- Most patients with CES from non-reversible, non-mass lesion etiologies exhibit little if any improvement with time, and there is no treatment to alter the course of CES.
- To prevent CES, it is recommended that proceduralists use appropriate doses of neuraxial local anesthetics, avoid re-dosing spinal anesthetics, allow for adequate drying time of topical antiseptic agents, and prevent cross-contamination with antiseptic agents. Additionally, risk/benefit analysis should be used when using a neuraxial anesthetic in a patient with known risk factors for CES.

REFERENCES

1. Orendácová J, Cízková D, Kafka J, et al. Cauda equina syndrome. *Prog Neurobiol.* 2001;64:613–637.
2. Moen V, Dahlgren N, Irestedt L. Severe neurological complications after central neuraxial blockades in Sweden 1990–1999. *Anesthesiology.* 2004;101:950–959.
3. Auroy Y, Benhamou D, Bargues L, et al. Major complications of regional anesthesia in France: the SOS regional anesthesia hotline service. *Anesthesiology.* 2002;97:1274–1280.

4. Podnar, S. Epidemiology of cauda equina and conus medullaris lesions. *Muscle Nerve*. 2007;35:529–531.
5. Bos E, Haumann J, de Quelerij M, et al. Haematoma and abscess after neuraxial anaesthesia: a review of 647 cases. *Br J Anaesth*. 2018;120:693–704.
6. Aldrete J. Neurological deficits and arachnoiditis following neuroaxial anesthesia. *Acta Anaesthesiol Scand*. 2003;47:3–12.
7. Killeen T, Kamat A, Walsh D, Parker A, Aliashkevich A. Severe adhesive arachnoiditis resulting in progressive paraplegia following obstetric spinal anaesthesia: a case report and review. *Anaesthesia*. 2012;67:1386–1394.
8. Iqbal MI, Morris R, Hersch M. Adhesive arachnoiditis following inadvertent epidural injection of 2% chlorhexidine in 70% alcohol-partial recovery over the ensuing eight years. *Anesth Intensive Care*. 2018;6:572–574.
9. Doan L, Piskoun B, Rosenberg AD, Blanck TJ, Phillips MS, Xu F. In vitro antiseptic effects on viability of neuronal and Schwann cells. *Reg Anesth Pain Med*. 2012;37:131–138.
10. Henschen A, Olson L. Chlorhexidine-induced degeneration of adrenergic nerves. *Acta Neuropathol*. 1984;63:18–23.
11. Kinirons B, Mimoz O, Lafendi L, Naas T, Meunier J-F, Nordmann P. Chlorhexidine versus povidone iodine in preventing colonization of continuous epidural catheters in children: a randomized, controlled trial. *Anesthesiology*. 2001;94:239–244.
12. Sviggum HP, Jacob A, Arendt KW, Mauermann ML, Horlocker TT, Hebl JR. Neurologic complications after chlorhexidine antisepsis for spinal anesthesia. *Reg Anesth Pain Med*. 2012;37:139–144.
13. American Society of Anesthesiologists Committee on Standards and Practice Parameters. Practice advisory for the prevention, diagnosis, and management of infectious complications associated with neuraxial techniques: an updated report by the American Society of Anesthesiologists Task Force on Infectious Complications Associated with Neuraxial Techniques and the American Society of Regional Anesthesia and Pain Medicine. *Anesthesiology*. 2017;126:585–601.
14. Radcliff KE, Kepler CK, Delasotta LA, et al. Current management review of thoracolumbar cord syndromes. *Spine*. 2011; 11:884–892.
15. Offenbacher H. The diagnostic impact of magnetic resonance imaging on the evaluation of suspected spinal cord disease. *Wien Klin Wochenschr*. 1992;104:589–593.
16. Neal JM, Kopp SL, Pasternak JJ, Lanier WL, Rathmell JP. Anatomy and pathophysiology of spinal cord injury associated with regional anesthesia and pain medicine: 2015 update. *Reg Anesth Pain Med*. 2015;40:506–525.

REVIEW QUESTIONS

(1) What is the approximate incidence of cauda equina syndrome following neuraxial anesthetics?

A. 0.5 to 1/100,000 cases
B. 1 to 2/100,000 cases
C. 2 to 4/100,000 cases
D. 5 to 10/100,000 cases

(2) Select the correct corresponding nerve root and neurologic deficit:

A. S3–S5 nerve roots: bladder and rectal sphincter paralysis
B. S1–S3 nerve roots: saddle anesthesia
C. S3 nerve root: loss of ankle reflex
D. Dorsal nerve roots: weakness of foot plantar flexion

(3) A spinal-epidural hematoma is a rare complication of neuraxial anesthesia, and the enlarging hematoma may act as a mass lesion compressing the cauda equina, resulting in cauda equina syndrome. TRUE or FALSE: There is a higher incidence of hematoma with spinal anesthesia than with epidural anesthesia.

(4) Current strategies to minimize risk of cauda equina syndrome include all of the following EXCEPT:

A. Avoid re-dosing failed spinal anesthetics.
B. Use appropriate doses of neuraxial local anesthetics.
C. Allow for adequate drying time for antiseptic agents prior to neuraxial procedure.
D. Elect for spinal anesthetic in patients with severe spinal stenosis.

(5) Symptoms of cauda equina syndrome may be mistaken for transient neurologic symptoms. Which of the following is true about transient neurologic symptoms?

A. Neurologic deficits are seen on physical examination.
B. Its etiology is secondary to neurotoxicity.
C. It presents exclusively as pain and/or dysesthesia.
D. Patients exhibit limited clinical improvement once presenting with symptoms.

(6) Chemical neurotoxicity from intrathecally dosed local anesthetics is a known association of cauda equina syndrome. All of the following have been associated with cauda equina syndrome EXCEPT:

A. Supranormal doses of local anesthetic
B. Single doses of intrathecal anesthesia
C. Hyperlordosis or extreme lateral flexion during surgical positioning
D. Spinal stenosis

(7) Which of the following statements regarding chlorhexidine is FALSE?

A. It is the most efficacious antiseptic for neuraxial indications.
B. It is recommended by major anesthesiology society practice advisories for neuraxial antisepsis.
C. It should be allowed to dry prior to neuraxial procedure.
D. Its use is contraindicated when there is concern for cauda equina syndrome.

8. You perform a routine spinal anesthetic with a standard clinical dose of bupivacaine. Upon emergence from anesthesia, the patient never regains motor function of his right lower extremity and has bowel/bladder dysfunction. Neuroimaging is normal. TRUE or FALSE: You must have made a clinical error in this patient's care.

ANSWERS

(1) C The incidence of cauda equina syndrome is rare but likely underestimated. Contemporary population studies estimate an incidence of 1.9 to 3.8 per 100,000 neuraxial anesthetics.

References

Moen V, Dahlgren N, Irestedt L. Severe neurological complications after central neuraxial blockades in Sweden 1990–1999. *Anesthesiology.* 2004;101:950–959.

Auroy Y, Benhamou D, Bargues L, et al. Major complications of regional anesthesia in France: the SOS regional anesthesia hotline service. *Anesthesiology.* 2002;97:1274–1280.

(2) **A.** Common localizing symptoms of cauda equina syndrome include bladder and rectal sphincter paralysis, particularly new urinary incontinence, and localizing to the S3–S5 nerve roots. Deficits in the S3–S5 nerve roots also result in saddle anesthesia. The S1, S2 nerve roots are responsible for foot plantar flexion and the ankle reflex. Dorsal nerve roots localize to low back pain/radicular pain.

Reference

Orendácová J, Cízková D, Kafka J, et al. Cauda equina syndrome. *Prog Neurobiol.* 2001;64:613–637.

(3) **False**. There is a higher incidence of hematoma with epidural anesthesia (1 in 18,000 epidurals) than with spinal anesthesia (1 in 158,000 spinals). Risk factors include advanced age, coagulopathy, and difficult neuraxial anesthetic instrumentation

References

Moen V, Dahlgren N, Irestedt L. Severe neurological complications after central neuraxial blockades in Sweden 1990–1999. *Anesthesiology.* 2004;101:950–959.

Bos E, Haumann J, de Quelerij M, et al. Haematoma and abscess after neuraxial anaesthesia: a review of 647 cases. *Br J Anaesth.* 2018;120:693–704.

(4) **D.** Careful consideration of risks and benefits is useful when considering a neuraxial anesthetic in patients with known risk factors for cauda equina syndrome such as spinal stenosis. To minimize the risk of cauda equina syndrome, it is additionally recommended to use appropriate doses/concentrations of neuraxial local anesthetics, avoid re-dosing spinal anesthetics, and allow for adequate drying time and prevent cross-contamination with antiseptic agents.

Reference

Moen V, Dahlgren N, Irestedt L. Severe neurological complications after central neuraxial blockades in Sweden 1990–1999. *Anesthesiology.* 2004;101:950–959.

(5) **C.** Cauda equina syndrome (CES) may be confused for other neurologic phenomena such as transient neurologic symptoms (TNS). TNS, however, is not concentration related or secondary to neurotoxicity. Most importantly, TNS has a delayed presentation compared with the sudden onset of CES, and, unlike the CES hallmark of multiple neurologic deficits, TNS presents exclusively as pain and/or dysesthesia. TNS resolves spontaneously over the course of several days.

(6) **B.** To prevent cauda equina syndrome, there are recommendations to avoid re-dosing failed spinal anesthetics, and if re-dosing occurs, to never allow total local anesthetic dose to exceed the maximum recommended dose. Supranormal doses of local anesthetics and/or maldistribution of local anesthetic spread within the intrathecal space, such as in spinal stenosis or in the setting of local anesthetic accumulation on the sacral side of the lumbar lordotic curve in the supine position, are also known to be associations with cauda equina syndrome.

References

Moen V, Dahlgren N, Irestedt L. Severe neurological complications after central neuraxial blockades in Sweden 1990–1999. *Anesthesiology.* 2004;101:950–959.

Auroy Y, Benhamou D, Bargues L, et al. Major complications of regional anesthesia in France: the SOS regional anesthesia hotline service. *Anesthesiology.* 2002;97:1274–1280.

(7) **D.** Chlorhexidine is the most efficacious antiseptic for neuraxial indications, and its use is recommended by the American Society of Regional Anesthesia and Pain Medicine, provided that there is adequate drying time (2–3 minutes) prior to neuraxial procedure and physical separation of the antiseptic agent and its applicator from other equipment. The occurrence of cauda equina syndrome in association with chlorhexidine antisepsis is somewhat speculative and is limited to a narrow range of patient cases. It is not contraindicated, even in a patient with risk factors associated with cauda equina syndrome.

Reference

American Society of Anesthesiologists Committee on Standards and Practice Parameters. Practice advisory for the prevention, diagnosis, and management of infectious complications associated with neuraxial techniques: an updated report by the American Society of Anesthesiologists Task Force on Infectious Complications Associated with Neuraxial Techniques and the American Society of Regional Anesthesia and Pain Medicine. *Anesthesiology.* 2017;126:585–601.

(8) **False.** The clinical scenario describes a case of cauda equina syndrome (CES) with irreversible motor deficits and bowel/bladder dysfunction in the setting of normal neuroimaging. Although there are known risk factors associated with CES (mass lesions, local anesthetic neurotoxicity/neuroinflammation, patient risk factors, and surgical positioning), most CES cases occur after unremarkable neuraxial anesthesia.

49.

NERVE BLOCKS IN A PATIENT WITH MULTIPLE SCLEROSIS

Lisa L. Klesius and Shelly B. Borden

STEM CASE AND KEY QUESTIONS

A 56-year-old female with a past medical history significant for multiple sclerosis (MS) presents for an elective right total knee arthroplasty (TKA). She describes bilateral leg numbness associated with her diagnosis of MS. Additional past medical history is significant for obstructive sleep apnea (OSA) and mild pulmonary hypertension. She has been told that she is difficult to intubate and previously required a fiberoptic bronchoscope for intubation.

The patient was diagnosed 17 years ago with a relapsing-remitting subtype of MS when symptoms and magnetic resonance imaging (MRI) findings were consistent with central nervous system (CNS) demyelinating lesions. She currently has no significant leg weakness but uses a cane for support when walking. She also describes a decline in her respiratory status over the past year after her last relapse and is concerned that she may be advancing toward a secondary-progressive subtype of MS. She uses continuous positive airway pressure for her OSA due to pharyngeal muscle weakness. She is currently being treated with interferon-beta but was also prescribed high-dose methylprednisolone for her most recent relapse.

After an extensive discussion of the risks and benefits of potential anesthetic options for this patient, providers decide to proceed with neuraxial anesthesia given the patient's high risk for respiratory compromise and history of difficult intubation. In the event of a failed neuraxial technique, the patient agrees to proceed with general anesthesia with an awake fiberoptic intubation. Difficult airway equipment will be available in the event of a high neuraxial block.

The patient is very concerned about postoperative pain management with opioids given her pulmonary disease and OSA and would prefer to limit opioid consumption perioperatively. She is also concerned about the possibility of peripheral nerve blocks exacerbating her leg numbness.

The patient agrees to undergo placement of an adductor canal block in addition to a multimodal analgesia regimen including scheduled acetaminophen and ketorolac, with opioids only as needed for severe breakthrough pain. An intra-articular injection of local anesthetic will also be performed by the surgeon intraoperatively to help with postoperative pain control. The patient is satisfied with the anesthetic plan and perioperative analgesia regimen and agrees to proceed with the planned surgical operation.

(1) HOW WILL YOU ASSESS THE SEVERITY OF MS?

The severity of MS is determined by performing a thorough history and physical examination to assess current symptoms, severity of symptoms, and disability. In general, early disease onset and longer duration of illness correlate with higher disease severity. Cerebral atrophy and lesion load on MRI imaging can also help determine disease severity.

(2) WHAT ARE THE POTENTIAL ANESTHETIC IMPLICATIONS OF THE TREATMENTS FOR MS?

Treatment of MS involves several different immune-modulating medications, which can cause liver dysfunction and increase the risk of severe infections. Liver function tests should be performed preoperatively. Patients receiving corticosteroid therapy may require perioperative steroid replacement for secondary adrenal insufficiency.

(3) WHAT FACTORS COULD INCREASE THE RISK OF A RELAPSE OF MS DURING THE PERIOPERATIVE PERIOD?

Increased risk of relapse is primarily related to both physical and psychological stress in the perioperative period. There is no difference in risk between anesthetic types; both general and regional anesthesia are safe. Elevated body temperature can cause "pseudo-relapses," which can lead to temporary worsening of symptoms due to nerve conduction block but do not represent a true relapse.

(4) WHAT ARE THE RISKS AND BENEFITS OF GENERAL ANESTHESIA VERSUS NEURAXIAL ANESTHESIA FOR A PATIENT WITH MS?

Both general and neuraxial anesthesia are safe to perform, and decisions regarding which option is best should be made jointly between the patient and the anesthesiologist. Patients with severe muscular weakness or poor respiratory status may benefit from avoidance of general anesthesia and neuromuscular blocking medications, if possible. Current evidence suggests that both spinal and epidural anesthetics can be safely performed without symptom exacerbation.

(4) WHAT IS THE RISK OF SYMPTOM EXACERBATION FROM PERIPHERAL NERVE BLOCKS IN A PATIENT WITH MS?

Peripheral nerve blocks are safe to perform without increasing the risk of symptom exacerbation based on current evidence. However, there are reports of peripheral nervous system involvement in patients with MS, and the anesthesiologist must pay close attention to preexisting neurologic deficits before performing a block.

DISCUSSION

Multiple sclerosis (MS) is the most common immune-mediated inflammatory demyelinating disease of the CNS. The disease is more prevalent in women, and symptoms typically develop between the ages of 20 and 40 years.[1] The exact etiology of MS is unknown but likely involves genetic, environmental, and potentially infectious factors.[1] MS is a heterogenous disease characterized by variable clinical and pathologic features reflecting the lesions of inflammation, demyelination, and axonal injury across the CNS.[2,3] Several different clinical subtypes help delineate the disease course and severity; however, the most common presentation is characterized by relapses and remissions of neurologic dysfunction.[4,5] Given the heterogenous nature of the disease, anesthetic management of these patients can be challenging, highlighting the need for individualized perioperative care. Both general and regional anesthetic techniques have been successfully used in patients with MS, and decisions regarding perioperative care should be made jointly between the patient and the anesthesiologist and should be tailored to clinical symptoms and disease severity.

EPIDEMIOLOGY, ETIOLOGY, AND PATHOPHYSIOLOGY

The incidence and prevalence of MS varies geographically, with the highest prevalence found in Europe, southern Canada, the northern United States, New Zealand, and Australia.[6] While it was once thought that geographic variation was due to racial differences (higher in Caucasian women in Europe, for instance), studies in the United States have demonstrated that there is an increased incidence in black adults and children, which is a shift in previously held beliefs about the disease.[7] In addition, women are affected more frequently than men. The female-to-male incidence is approximately 2:1, with more recent epidemiologic data suggesting that the ratio is even higher.[8] The onset in women is typically years earlier than in men.[1]

Although the exact etiology of MS is unknown, the most widely accepted theory is that the disease begins as an immune-mediated inflammatory disorder characterized by autoreactive lymphocytes. Supporting evidence for the immunopathology of MS includes:[1,3,5]

- Evidence of inflammation and blood-brain barrier disruption on MRI
- Inflammatory T cells, B cells, and macrophages on histopathologic examination of MS lesions
- Presence of IgG and IgM oligoclonal bands in the cerebrospinal fluid (CSF) but not the serum of patients with MS.

Alternative theories for the etiology of MS include environmental and genetic susceptibilities. An immune etiology related to a chronic viral infection has been proposed; however, no individual virus has been consistently associated with MS.[9] In addition, a genetic predisposition has also been suggested, which involves a genetically determined neuroglial degenerative process. Over 100 different genetic polymorphisms have been associated with MS, and most involve the major histocompatibility complexes (MHC type I and II).[10] In addition, the risk for monozygotic twins is at least 20% and may reach as high as 39%, whereas the risk for dizygotic twins is similar to that of siblings (3%–5%).[11] Other environmental factors that have been implicated include geographic latitude and place of birth, sunlight exposure, vitamin D levels, and tobacco smoking.[6,12]

The neuropathology of MS is characterized by the presence of focal demyelinated plaques within the CNS with variable amounts of gliosis, inflammation, and relative axonal preservation. These plaques tend to be in the optic nerves, spinal cord, brainstem, cerebellum, and periventricular white matter.[13,14] However, lesions have been identified in disseminated regions through the CNS, including the cortical gray matter. In addition, gray matter lesions may be more indicative of disease severity, neurocognitive disability, and disease progression.[13,15] Overall, characterization of demyelinated lesions in the CNS remains challenging, with variable definitions of disease activity and severity seen in the acute and chronic phases of plaque progression. Clinical implications of the neuropathology of different stages of demyelinated plaques also remains controversial, particularly for determining the clinical subtypes of the disease.[13,14]

CLINICAL SUBTYPES

The phenotypic descriptions of the clinical subtypes of MS were updated in 2013 to improve communication, prognostication, and treatment. The core phenotypes are described as relapsing or progressive. However, several modifiers of these core phenotypes are used to further delineate the clinical subtypes to include descriptions of disease activity and progression of disability.[4] Disease activity is further defined by clinical relapses and new or enlarging lesions on CNS imaging.[4]

Table 49.1 **CHARACTERISTIC FEATURES OF CLINICAL SUBTYPES OF MULTIPLE SCLEROSIS, INCLUDING DISEASE ONSET AND PATTERN**[1,4,5,16–18]

CLINICAL SUBTYPES OF MS[a]	DISEASE ONSET AND PATTERN
Clinically isolated syndrome	Single episode with signs and symptoms reflecting a CNS inflammatory demyelinating event Represents the first clinical episode suggestive of MS Occurs in the absence of fever or infection Symptoms develop over hours to days and gradually remit over weeks to months Recovery may not be complete Occurs in a patient not known to have MS
Relapsing-remitting	Accounts for vast majority of cases at disease onset Characterized by attacks (relapses) and remissions Minimal disease progression during remissions Relapses peak in days to weeks followed by periods of remission with or without full recovery Minimum duration of a relapse is 24 hours Relapses tend to occur in the same locations early in the disease course Most cases eventually advance to secondary progressive subtype
Secondary progressive	Transition from relapsing-remitting subtype to gradual worsening of disease May still involve relapses, minor remissions, or plateaus Diagnosis is made retrospectively because no established diagnostic criteria exist Transition usually occurs 10 to 20 years after disease onset
Primary progressive	Progressive accumulation of disability from disease onset May still involve occasional plateaus, temporary minor improvements, or acute relapses Diagnosis is made exclusively on patient history More common when disease onset is after age 40 May have worse prognosis for disability and disease severity

[a] MS = multiple sclerosis; CNS = central nervous system.

The four main clinical subtypes are: clinically isolated syndrome, relapsing-remitting, secondary progressive, and primary progressive (Table 49.1).

DIAGNOSIS AND RADIOGRAPHIC FINDINGS

The diagnosis of MS is based on presentation of clinical symptoms and evidence of CNS lesions. Diagnosis requires dissemination of clinical attacks in time and evidence of multiple lesions across the CNS. MRI is the gold standard for diagnosing MS. After diagnosis, patients are categorized according to disease onset and pattern into subtypes, as outlined in Table 49.1. Understanding the onset and pattern of symptoms also helps properly prescribe therapeutic interventions.

The clinical manifestations of MS are highly variable, and no unique characteristics differentiate MS from other demyelinating diseases. However, several clinical signs and symptoms are frequently associated with the disease. The most common clinical symptoms include acute unilateral optic neuritis, double vision due to sixth nerve palsy, facial sensory loss, trigeminal neuralgia, cerebellar ataxia, partial myelopathy, sensory symptoms (typically reflecting spinothalamic, dorsal column, or dorsal root lesions), asymmetric limb weakness, and urge incontinence or erectile dysfunction.[1] Atypical clinical presentations include bilateral optic neuritis, complete gaze palsy, intractable nausea/vomiting or hiccups, encephalopathy, subacute cognitive decline, headache or meningism, isolated fatigue, and constitutional symptoms.[1]

Once patients present with symptoms suggestive of MS, an MRI is performed to confirm the diagnosis and exclude other diseases.[19] Pathognomonic findings on brain MRIs include multifocal T2-hyperdense white matter lesions in locations such as periventricular, juxtacortical (abutting cerebral cortex), and infratentorial areas.[1] Figures 49.1–49.3

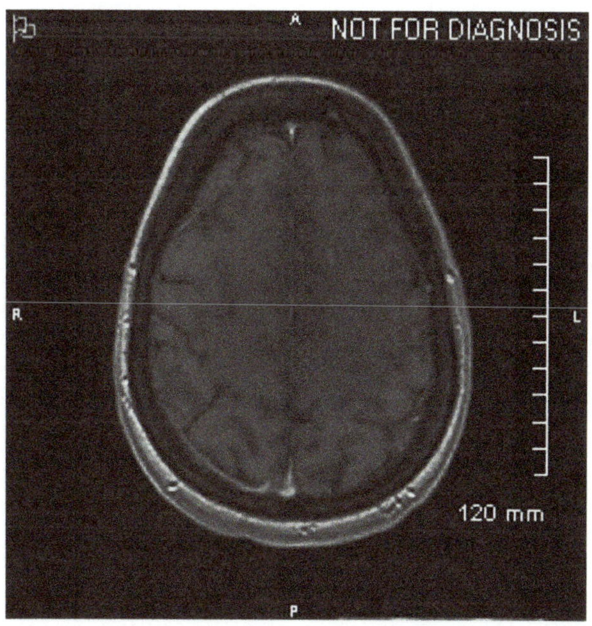

Figure 49.1 Post contrast Axial MR image show enhancement of active plaque.

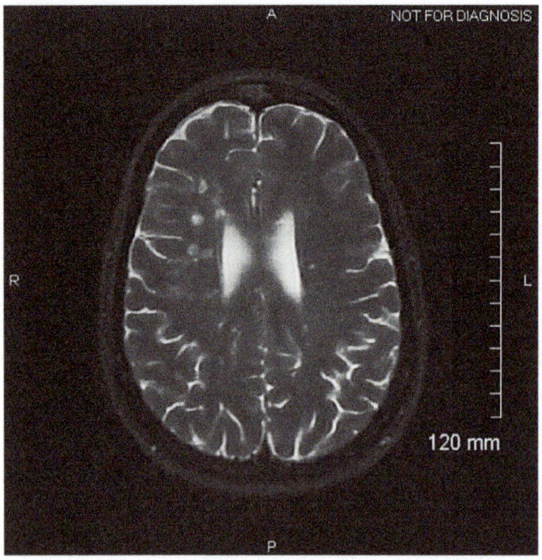

Figure 49.2 Axial T2 sequence showing T2 hyperintensities, which can be seen in demyelinating disease.

demonstrate lesions typically seen on brain MRIs in patients with MS.

Routine spinal cord imaging is controversial, but lesions occur in 80%–90% of patients with known MS. Lesions typically extend over 1 to 2 vertebral segments, and enhancement may occur after gadolinium administration.[1]

CSF examination and assessment are not required but can support the diagnosis. Mildly increased white blood cell count (>25 cells per cm^3), elevated protein (usually >1 g/L), and a raised IgG index are CSF findings seen in MS.[20] Routine lab assessment may reveal nonspecific antibodies such as low-titer antinuclear antibodies, but this may not be clinically relevant.[1]

An MS diagnosis can be challenging given the breadth of clinical symptoms, which can be either misdiagnosed or missed on initial presentation. In addition, the differential diagnosis is expansive, including inflammatory disease (e.g., systemic lupus erythematosus), infectious disease (e.g., Lyme disease and human immunodeficiency virus), granulomatous disease (e.g., sarcoidosis), and many others. All providers must keep MS on the differential diagnosis due to its variable presentation. New pathological, immunological, imaging, and clinical findings continue to emerge to help improve diagnosis.

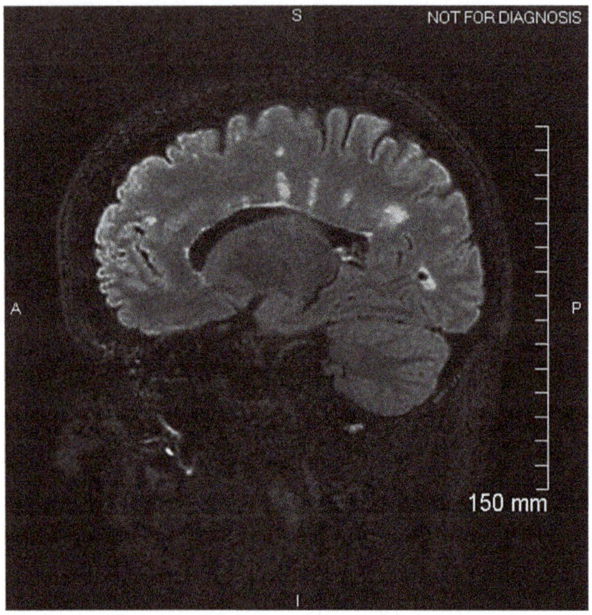

Figure 49.3 Sagittal sequence showing periventricular FLAIR hyperintensities (Dawson's Fingers) consistent with MS.

DISEASE SEVERITY, PROGNOSIS, AND DISABILITY

The prognostic factors of MS include relapsing versus remitting disease, early symptoms, MRI markers, pregnancy, and demographics. A systematic review of 27 studies revealed that patients with relapsing-remitting MS and bowel and/or urinary symptoms at onset and early accumulation of disability were consistent with long-term disability.[21] The MRI markers of disease severity include lesion load (assessed on T2-weighted, fluid-attenuated inversion recovery [FLAIR]) and cerebral atrophy (assessed on T1-weighted MRI sequences). While spinal atrophy can be associated with disability and worse prognosis, cranial MRI abnormalities do not consistently correlate with the degree of clinical symptoms.[22] In general, pregnancy appears to be protective against relapses, but there is an increased incidence of relapse in the early postpartum period. Breastfeeding is safe in mothers affected with MS and may even be protective.[23]

Therapeutic modalities can slow or stop the impairment caused by the progressive nature of MS. Symptoms causing disability include: mobility impairment (80%), balance impairment (75%), ataxia (80%), fatigue (80%), bladder dysfunction (58%–75%), spasticity (60%–90%), pain (55%–70%), cognitive dysfunction (60%–70%), depression (25%–50%), and pseudobulbar affect (10%).[24] Pain due to MS can be neurogenic (paroxysmal pain, persistent pain from dysesthesias, and episodic neuropathic pain) or musculoskeletal (caused by spasticity and immobility). In a meta-analysis including 28 studies and over 7,000 patients with MS, pain presented as headache (43%), neuropathic extremity pain (26%), back pain (20%), painful spasms (15%), and trigeminal neuralgia (4%).[25] While no specific symptoms or disabilities are unique to MS, the primary goal of treatment is to improve quality of life.

TREATMENT

MS treatment is aimed at improving either acute exacerbations or chronic symptoms in the progressive phase of MS. Acute exacerbations are defined as episodes of focal neurologic disturbances lasting longer than 24 hours in patients with previously stable symptoms. As noted, MRI is the imaging technique of choice to determine if the symptoms are the result of an exacerbation or a "pseudo-relapse," which is a temporary worsening of symptoms due to heat exposure or infection. Treatment of acute exacerbations includes glucocorticoids (oral or intravenous)[26] or plasma exchange for patients who do not respond to glucocorticoid therapy.[27]

Treatment for the progressive phase of MS is more challenging than treatment of relapsing-remitting subtypes of MS. More options for disease-modifying therapies are available for relapsing forms compared to progressive forms of MS. For all types of MS, immune-modulating treatment is individualized based on disease activity and progression as well as patient preference. While immunomodulators can aid in symptom management, they also have important side effects, including severe infections. Disease-modifying therapies include ocrelizumab,[28] siponimod,[29] and cladribine. Other immune-modulating treatments include glucocorticoids, azathioprine, cyclophosphamide, interferons, cyclosporine, methotrexate, plasma exchange, rituximab, and stem cell treatment. This continues to be an active area of study and development.

Additional pharmacologic treatment is directed toward symptom management and may include agents such as baclofen for spasticity, Botox injections for bladder spasms, and antidepressants for depression. In addition to pharmacotherapy, interventions such as balance exercises, physiotherapy exercises, aerobic exercise training, resistance training, and even surgical interventions (thalamotomy or deep brain stimulation) can be considered to manage MS symptoms.[24]

ANESTHETIC IMPLICATIONS OF MS

Perioperative management of patients with MS presents a challenge to the anesthesiologist given the heterogenous nature of the disease. Anesthetic decisions should be tailored to the patient's phenotypic presentation, including disease severity, symptoms, and comorbidities, in addition to patient preferences. A thorough history and physical examination, including current neurologic impairment, acute exacerbations, and medications, should be performed before making decisions regarding anesthetic techniques.[30]

PREOPERATIVE CONSIDERATIONS

Respiratory status should be carefully assessed in patients with MS. Demyelinating lesions involving the respiratory centers in the brainstem and the cervical and thoracic spinal cord may result in respiratory compromise.[31] In addition, respiratory disease is seen more frequently in severely impaired patients with MS but may be present in earlier stages, even in asymptomatic patients.[30] Development of restrictive lung disease due to poor expiratory muscle function can be seen with decreases in functional residual capacity and vital capacity, highlighting the need for adequate preoxygenation.[32] Diaphragmatic paralysis has also been reported due to lesions in the cervical spinal cord.[31] Although difficulty with intubation is rare, patients with pharyngeal muscle weakness and cough impairments due to cranial nerve involvement may be at a high risk of chronic aspiration. Patients with respiratory weakness are also more likely to have sleep apnea and may require noninvasive ventilatory support perioperatively.[30–32] Although preoperative clinical assessment of respiratory function is important, no specific tests (e.g., pulmonary function tests, arterial blood gas analysis) have reliably predicted respiratory outcomes in patients with MS.[30,33]

Neurologic status of the patient should be thoroughly assessed preoperatively with careful documentation of current symptoms, deficits, and severity of disease.[31] Patients with symptoms of syncope, orthostasis, cardiac dysrhythmias, or bowel and bladder dysfunction should alert the anesthesiologist to the potential for autonomic dysfunction. These patients may be more likely to develop autonomic instability in the perioperative period with marked hypotension and reduced response to intravenous fluids and vasopressors, particularly after sympathetic blockade with central regional anesthetic techniques and induction of general anesthesia.[30,31]

Current medications for MS treatment should be reviewed because they may complicate anesthetic techniques. Several medications used in MS treatment may cause liver dysfunction and alter the pharmacokinetics of hepatically metabolized anesthetic medications. A liver function test should be evaluated preoperatively to identify adverse effects of MS treatments.[30] Baclofen, used to treat spasticity, may result in increased muscle weakness and sensitivity to neuromuscular blocking agents.[30,31] Patients with recent exacerbations receiving treatment with high-dose corticosteroids or those on chronic steroid therapy should receive supplemental steroid replacement perioperatively, given the potential for adrenal insufficiency.[30,31]

One of the main perioperative concerns regarding anesthesia for surgery is the risk of disease exacerbation. Several studies have shown a consistent association between stressful life events, including both physical and psychological stressors, and acute exacerbations of MS.[34,35] In addition, other stressors, including infection, inflammation, fever, childbirth, and emotional stress, need to be considered and optimized in the perioperative period.

INTRAOPERATIVE CONSIDERATIONS

Both inhalational and intravenous anesthetic agents have been successfully used in patients with MS without evidence of disease exacerbation and no preference has been reported for any particular agent.[31,36–39] No complications have been reported with nitrous oxide or volatile anesthetics, including desflurane and sevoflurane.[30,39,40] Sedative-hypnotic agents including benzodiazepines have been used successfully in patients with MS, but should be given cautiously in those with respiratory compromise.[30,40] However, considering that the stress response has been implicated in the development of MS exacerbations, premedication with benzodiazepines may be helpful in reducing perioperative stress and anxiety and thus the risk of relapses.[30,34]

Special consideration should be given to neuromuscular blocking agents as patients with demyelinating neuromuscular disorders may develop upregulation of nicotinic acetylcholine receptors of skeletal muscle.[30,31] Although succinylcholine has been used successfully in patient with MS, hyperkalemic cardiac arrests have occurred,[41,42] and patients with acute MS exacerbations or evidence of progressive disease and baseline symptomatic motor weakness or spasticity are more likely to develop hyperkalemia with succinylcholine administration; succinylcholine is best avoided.[42] Regarding nondepolarizing neuromuscular blocking agents, both relative resistance (with upregulation of nicotinic acetylcholine receptors) and increased sensitivity (decreased muscle mass/muscular weakness implicated) have been described.[43,44] However, normal responses to these agents have also been described.[39,43,45] Thus, careful and appropriate titration of these medications should be employed given the unpredictable responses.

Elevated body temperature has been implicated in the development of "pseudo-relapses" in the perioperative period.[46] When exposed to excess heat, demyelinated neurons develop a conduction blockade, leading to temporary symptom exacerbation.[46,47] Continuous temperature monitoring should always be employed, with avoidance of intraoperative warming devices and careful regulation of operating room temperatures.

NEURAXIAL ANESTHESIA

The safety and use of neuraxial anesthetic techniques in patients with MS are controversial given the concern for local anesthetic-induced neurotoxicity of exposed, demyelinated axons.[44] A majority of anesthesiologists prefer to avoid spinal anesthetics in patients with MS due to fear of exacerbating symptoms. The theory for worsening neurologic impairment after spinal anesthetic involves exposure of the demyelinated, unprotected nerve roots to higher-than-expected concentrations of local anesthetics, resulting in neurotoxicity.[44] This aligns with the "double-crush" phenomenon, which describes worsening neurologic function in patients with preexisting neurologic disease who are exposed to a secondary insult, including mechanical (needle/catheter) trauma, ischemia from vasoconstrictor use, or chemical toxicity from local anesthetics.[48]

However, spinal anesthetics have been performed without evidence of symptom exacerbation.[49,50] A case report of a patient with advanced, progressive MS and severe respiratory dysfunction who preferred to avoid intubation underwent a total abdominal hysterectomy with a combined spinal-epidural anesthetic technique without evidence of disease exacerbation.[50] Another case described a patient who underwent an uneventful combined spinal and general anesthetic with a preinduction intrathecal injection of tetracaine and morphine.[49] In addition, a retrospective case series of 139 patients with preexisting CNS disorders (including 35 patients with MS) who underwent neuraxial techniques for surgical procedures including spinal, epidural, or combined spinal-epidural did not show evidence of new or worsening neurologic deficits postoperatively.[48] Importantly, 74% of the patients in this series reported active neurologic symptoms preoperatively, and standard dosing of local anesthetics were used.[48] In contrast, two separate case reports detailed new-onset neurologic dysfunction after intrathecal local anesthetic administration in patients who were subsequently diagnosed with MS.[51,52] Unanswered questions from these case reports include whether local anesthetics may have unmasked previously silent demyelinated lesions or prolonged the duration of nerve blockade.[53] In addition, the neurologic symptoms that have developed after spinal anesthetics are typically transient and reversible, implying no true relapse or worsening of the underlying condition.[30,53] The variability of these case reports highlights the fact that the etiology of postoperative neurologic dysfunction is often difficult to ascertain and likely involves many factors, including the patient, surgery, and anesthetic. Before performing a spinal anesthetic in a patient with MS, providers should thoroughly discuss the risks and benefits, including the potential for worsening or unmasking neurologic impairment, and consider the patient's level of disability and disease severity. However, the current evidence suggests that a diagnosis of MS is likely not a contraindication to performing a spinal anesthetic.

Contrary to spinal anesthetics, epidural anesthetics are generally considered safe to perform in patients with MS without a significantly increased risk of relapse.[30,31,44,48,53] With epidurally administered local anesthetics, a lower concentration reaches the intrathecal space, which may decrease the risk of local anesthetic-induced neurotoxicity compared to a spinal anesthetic.[30,31] Some research suggests that the risk of relapse may be increased with higher concentrations and longer durations of local anesthetics, but other case reviews have not shown the same association.[48,54] Although epidural anesthetics are generally considered safe to perform, there have been reports of worsening neurologic function and possible disease relapse.[55,56] Similar to spinal anesthetics, the etiology of these relapses is difficult to pinpoint and likely involves many factors.[30,31,53] Overall, the available data and case reports suggest that epidural anesthetics are likely safe to perform but still require a discussion of the risks and benefits specific to the patient and their disease process.

PERIPHERAL REGIONAL ANESTHESIA

While MS is described as a demyelinating disease limited to the CNS, the involvement of the peripheral nervous system (PNS) has not been fully clarified and remains controversial.[57,58] Postmortem analyses of patients with MS have described PNS lesions similar in appearance to those found in postinfectious inflammatory polyneuropathies.[58] However, despite case reports of subtle peripheral nerve abnormalities on electrophysiologic and neuropathologic examinations in patients with MS, no prospective studies examining the potential involvement of the PNS exist.[57] In addition, peripheral nerve conduction studies were performed on 60 patients with MS and only 3 patients (5%) had abnormalities suggestive of demyelination.[59] All 3 of the patients had documented diagnoses of MS that preceded development of demyelinating neuropathy by several years.[59] Another study, however, found peripheral nerve lesions involving more than one nerve on electrophysiologic studies in 30 out of 110 patients with MS (42.8%) with no correlation to disease severity or duration.[60] Thus, the frequency of peripheral demyelinating neuropathies in patients with MS remains unknown, and identifying patients that could be at higher risk for PNS involvement is challenging.

There is only one case report of a severe brachial plexopathy after an ultrasound-guided interscalene nerve block was performed in a patient with MS for a total shoulder arthroplasty.[61]

However, the final diagnosis of inflammatory brachial neuritis was confounded by several factors, including possible surgical trauma and an undiagnosed subclinical peripheral nerve pathology.[61,62] Currently, the American Society of Regional Anesthesia (ASRA) Practice Advisory on Neurologic Complications in Regional Anesthesia and Pain Medicine states that our limited data regarding the risk of nerve injury following regional anesthetic techniques in patients with MS cannot be confirmed or refuted; therefore, consideration may be given to avoiding more potent local anesthetics, reducing the local anesthetic dose and/or concentration, and avoiding or limiting vasoconstrictive additives (Class II level of evidence).[63,64] Given the overall lack of evidence documenting nerve injuries or worsening of neurologic function after peripheral nerve blocks in patients with MS, peripheral regional anesthetics are most likely safe. However, anesthesiologists must pay careful attention to any preexisting neurologic deficits and must be aware of the potential for nerve toxicity related to the "double-crush" phenomenon given the controversial and unknown frequency of PNS involvement in MS. Similar to neuraxial anesthetics, thorough discussions with patients regarding the risks and benefits of peripheral nerve blocks must occur. Patient-specific factors and preferences may play an important role in the decision-making process, particularly in patients with severe respiratory compromise for whom avoiding general anesthetics and potent opioids may be desirable.

ANESTHETIC CONSIDERATIONS FOR THE OBSTETRIC PATIENT

During pregnancy, MS symptoms tend to decrease. However, given the elevated physiologic and psychologic stress in the early postpartum period, gravid patients often experience increased symptom severity after delivery. Pre-pregnancy severity of MS also correlates with the postpartum severity of relapse.[55] However, neuraxial analgesia has not appeared to worsen MS severity in pregnancy. In 2004, a large prospective investigation from the Pregnancy in Multiple Sclerosis (PRIMS) study assessed the influence of pregnancy on the clinical course of MS. This study included patients who received labor epidurals, which did not correlate with relapse risk.[56] Furthermore, a prospective study published in 2019 that followed 389 gravid patients with MS (40% of whom received labor epidurals) until at least 3 months postpartum showed no association between neuraxial analgesia and postpartum relapse.[65] Importantly, no randomized controlled trials have studied epidural analgesia in parturients, and thus a selection bias may exist if epidural analgesia was offered only to patients with milder symptoms. In addition, epidural concentrations and rates of infusion have not been studied in this population, indicating that further research is needed to clarify the risk of epidural analgesia.

MULTIMODAL ANALGESIA FOR TKA: APPROACH IN A PATIENT WITH MS

In patients who undergo TKA, the goals of therapy are to relieve pain, ease transition from the hospital to home or rehabilitation center, decrease hospital length of stay, and achieve patient satisfaction. One of the most effective ways to do this is to employ multimodal analgesia for pain control. Multimodal analgesia involves addressing analgesia by administering medications that act on different parts of the pain pathway via various mechanisms of action. For patients undergoing TKA, multimodal analgesia regimens may include acetaminophen, nonsteroidal anti-inflammatory drugs (NSAIDs), gabapentinoids, opioids (for severe or breakthrough pain), ketamine, and regional anesthetics (including neuraxial and peripheral techniques) (see Chapter 5 for a more thorough review of multimodal analgesic options).

The prevalence of neuropathic pain, including headaches, back pain, extremity pain, and/or trigeminal neuralgia, in patients with MS is over 80%.[66] Because the pain pathways associated with MS are complex, multimodal analgesia including opioids, NSAIDs, and antiepileptics have often been employed in these patients before surgery. As a result, it is extremely important to perform a thorough pain history to ensure that preoperative multimodal analgesics are continued appropriately and that surgical pain is not the only focus in the perioperative period. To further support the need for a thorough multimodal analgesia plan, a study published in the *Journal of Arthroplasty* of a cohort of 10,000+ patients with MS compared with a 10:1 matched non-MS cohort concluded that patients with MS have a higher rate of medical complications, significantly higher costs, and longer lengths of hospital stays for joint arthroplasty.[67] There is a paucity of data investigating postoperative pain control in the MS patient population post-joint surgery, but multimodal analgesia is likely an important aspect in the care of these patients and should be further researched to help improve outcomes.

CONCLUSIONS

MS is a complex and heterogenous immune-mediated inflammatory demyelinating disease of the CNS. Successful anesthetic management of these patients requires careful considerations of all symptoms and disabilities with thoughtful perioperative planning, including a thorough discussion of risks and benefits of all anesthetic options. Key points are summarized below:

- Current therapies for symptom management of MS should be thoroughly reviewed and perioperative stress-dose steroid administration should be considered in patients who have recently received steroids for relapses.
- Although epidural anesthetics are generally considered safer than spinal anesthetics due to lower intrathecal concentrations of local anesthetics and thus lower risk of neurotoxicity, both techniques have been successfully used in patients with active neurologic symptoms without evidence of increased risk of MS relapse. The decision to proceed with neuraxial anesthetics should be made jointly between the patient and the anesthesiologist while weighing the risks and benefits of the different techniques.

- Hyperthermia results in decreased axonal transmission in patients with MS and causes "pseudo-relapses." Core body temperature should be closely monitored to avoid hyperthermia.
- Peripheral nerve blocks are most likely safe to perform in patients with MS, despite controversial involvement of MS in the PNS and a few case reports suggesting prolonged blockade following peripheral nerve blocks.

REFERENCES

1. Brownlee WJ, Hardy TA, Fazekas F, Miller DH. Diagnosis of multiple sclerosis: progress and challenges. *Lancet.* 2017;389(10076):1336–1346.
2. Dendrou CA, Fugger L, Friese MA. Immunopathology of multiple sclerosis. *Nat Rev Immunol.* 2015;15(9):545–558.
3. Lucchinetti C, Bruck W, Parisi J, Scheithauer B, Rodriguez M, Lassmann H. Heterogeneity of multiple sclerosis lesions: implications for the pathogenesis of demyelination. *Ann Neurol.* 2000;47(6):707–717.
4. Lublin FD, Reingold SC, Cohen JA, et al. Defining the clinical course of multiple sclerosis: the 2013 revisions. *Neurology.* 2014;83(3):278–286.
5. Thompson AJ, Banwell BL, Barkhof F, et al. Diagnosis of multiple sclerosis: 2017 revisions of the McDonald criteria. *Lancet Neurol.* 2018;17(2):162–173.
6. Simpson S Jr, Blizzard L, Otahal P, Van der Mei I, Taylor B. Latitude is significantly associated with the prevalence of multiple sclerosis: a meta-analysis. *J Neurol Neurosurg Psychiatry.* 2011;82(10):1132–1141.
7. Langer-Gould A, Brara SM, Beaber BE, Zhang JL. Incidence of multiple sclerosis in multiple racial and ethnic groups. *Neurology.* 2013;80(19):1734–1739.
8. Alonso A, Hernan MA. Temporal trends in the incidence of multiple sclerosis: a systematic review. *Neurology.* 2008;71(2):129–135.
9. Hernan MA, Zhang SM, Lipworth L, Olek MJ, Ascherio A. Multiple sclerosis and age at infection with common viruses. *Epidemiology.* 2001;12(3):301–306.
10. Sawcer S, Hellenthal G, Pirinen M, et al. Genetic risk and a primary role for cell-mediated immune mechanisms in multiple sclerosis. *Nature.* 2011;476(7359):214–219.
11. Sadovnick AD, Armstrong H, Rice GP, et al. A population-based study of multiple sclerosis in twins: update. *Ann Neurol.* 1993;33(3):281–285.
12. Franklin GM, Nelson L. Environmental risk factors in multiple sclerosis: causes, triggers, and patient autonomy. *Neurology.* 2003;61(8):1032–1034.
13. Frischer JM, Weigand SD, Guo Y, et al. Clinical and pathological insights into the dynamic nature of the white matter multiple sclerosis plaque. *Ann Neurol.* 2015;78(5):710–721.
14. Popescu BF, Lucchinetti CF. Pathology of demyelinating diseases. *Annu Rev Pathol.* 2012;7:185–217.
15. Calabrese M, Favaretto A, Martini V, Gallo P. Grey matter lesions in MS: from histology to clinical implications. *Prion.* 2013;7(1):20–27.
16. Eriksson M, Andersen O, Runmarker B. Long-term follow up of patients with clinically isolated syndromes, relapsing-remitting and secondary progressive multiple sclerosis. *Mult Scler.* 2003;9(3):260–274.
17. Mowry EM, Deen S, Malikova I, Pelletier J, Bacchetti P, Waubant E. The onset location of multiple sclerosis predicts the location of subsequent relapses. *J Neurol Neurosurg Psychiatry.* 2009;80(4):400–403.
18. Weinshenker BG. Natural history of multiple sclerosis. *Ann Neurol.* 1994;36(Suppl):S6–S11.
19. Offenbacher H, Fazekas F, Schmidt R, et al. Assessment of MRI criteria for a diagnosis of MS. *Neurology.* 1993;43(5):905–909.
20. Freedman MS, Thompson EJ, Deisenhammer F, et al. Recommended standard of cerebrospinal fluid analysis in the diagnosis of multiple sclerosis: a consensus statement. *Arch Neurol.* 2005;62(6):865–870.
21. Langer-Gould A, Popat RA, Huang SM, et al. Clinical and demographic predictors of long-term disability in patients with relapsing-remitting multiple sclerosis: a systematic review. *Arch Neurol.* 2006;63(12):1686–1691.
22. Schlaeger R, Papinutto N, Zhu AH, et al. Association between thoracic spinal cord gray matter atrophy and disability in multiple sclerosis. *JAMA Neurol.* 2015;72(8):897–904.
23. Langer-Gould A, Smith JB, Hellwig K, et al. Breastfeeding, ovulatory years, and risk of multiple sclerosis. *Neurology.* 2017;89(6):563–569.
24. Feinstein A, Freeman J, Lo AC. Treatment of progressive multiple sclerosis: what works, what does not, and what is needed. *Lancet Neurol.* 2015;14(2):194–207.
25. Foley PL, Vesterinen HM, Laird BJ, et al. Prevalence and natural history of pain in adults with multiple sclerosis: systematic review and meta-analysis. *Pain.* 2013;154(5):632–642.
26. Galea I, Ward-Abel N, Heesen C. Relapse in multiple sclerosis. *BMJ.* 2015;350:h1765.
27. Weinshenker BG, O'Brien PC, Petterson TM, et al. A randomized trial of plasma exchange in acute central nervous system inflammatory demyelinating disease. *Ann Neurol.* 1999;46(6):878–886.
28. Montalban X, Hauser SL, Kappos L, et al. Ocrelizumab versus placebo in primary progressive multiple sclerosis. *New Engl J Med.* 2017;376(3):209–220.
29. Kappos L, Bar-Or A, Cree BAC, et al. Siponimod versus placebo in secondary progressive multiple sclerosis (EXPAND): a double-blind, randomised, phase 3 study. *Lancet.* 2018;391(10127):1263–1273.
30. Makris A, Piperopoulos A, Karmaniolou I. Multiple sclerosis: basic knowledge and new insights in perioperative management. *J Anesth.* 2014;28(2):267–278.
31. Dorotta IR, Schubert A. Multiple sclerosis and anesthetic implications. *Curr Opin Anaesthesiol.* 2002;15(3):365–370.
32. Levy J, Bensmail D, Brotier-Chomienne A, et al. Respiratory impairment in multiple sclerosis: a study of respiratory function in wheelchair-bound patients. *Eur J Neurol.* 2017;24(3):497–502.
33. Fiorentino G, Esquinas AM. Respiratory function in multiple sclerosis: is there a reliable test? *Eur J Neurol.* 2017;24(6):e32–e33.
34. Buljevac D, Hop WC, Reedeker W, et al. Self reported stressful life events and exacerbations in multiple sclerosis: prospective study. *BMJ.* 2003;327(7416):646.
35. Mohr DC, Hart SL, Julian L, Cox D, Pelletier D. Association between stressful life events and exacerbation in multiple sclerosis: a meta-analysis. *BMJ.* 2004;328(7442):731.
36. Kono Y, Ueda N, Kano T. [Anesthetic management for a patient with multiple sclerosis]. *Masui.* 2005;54(8):906–908.
37. Lee KH, Park JS, Lee SI, et al. Anesthetic management of the emergency laparotomy for a patient with multiple sclerosis: a case report. *Korean J Anesthesiol.* 2010;59(5):359–362.
38. Zuccolotto EB, Nunes GC, Nogueira RS, Pagnussatt Neto E, Nociti JR. Anesthetic management of a patient with multiple sclerosis: case report. *Braz J Anesthesiol.* 2016;66(4):414–417.
39. Inoue S, Furuya H. Sevoflurane is safe for anesthetic management in patients with multiple sclerosis. *Acta Anaesthesiol Taiwan.* 2006;44(3):187–189.
40. Sahin L, Korkmaz HF, Sahin M, Aydin T, Toker S, Gulcan E. Desflurane anaesthesia in a patient with multiple sclerosis in total hip replacement. *Arch Med Sci.* 2010;6(6):984–986.
41. Kytta J, Rosenberg PH. Anaesthesia for patients with multiple sclerosis. *Ann Chir Gynaecol.* 1984;73(5):299–303.
42. Levine M, Brown DF. Succinylcholine-induced hyperkalemia in a patient with multiple sclerosis. *J Emerg Med.* 2012;43(2):279–282.
43. Brett RS, Schmidt JH, Gage JS, Schartel SA, Poppers PJ. Measurement of acetylcholine receptor concentration in skeletal muscle from a patient with multiple sclerosis and resistance to atracurium. *Anesthesiology.* 1987;66(6):837–839.
44. Briggs ED, Kirsch JR. Anesthetic implications of neuromuscular disease. *J Anesth.* 2003;17(3):177–185.

45. Ceyhan A, Uyar ET, Gencay IY, Gunal SE. Anesthesia in multiple sclerosis and obstructive sleep apnea: case report and literature review. *J Res Med Sci.* 2011;16(6):828–835.
46. Guthrie TC, Nelson DA. Influence of temperature changes on multiple sclerosis: critical review of mechanisms and research potential. *J Neurol Sci.* 1995;129(1):1–8.
47. Stutzer P, Kesselring J. Wilhelm Uhthoff: a phenomenon 1853 to 1927. *Int MS J.* 2008;15(3):90–93.
48. Hebl JR, Horlocker TT, Schroeder DR. Neuraxial anesthesia and analgesia in patients with preexisting central nervous system disorders. *Anesth Analg.* 2006;103(1):223–228, table of contents.
49. Berger JM, Ontell R. Intrathecal morphine in conjunction with a combined spinal and general anesthetic in a patient with multiple sclerosis. *Anesthesiology.* 1987;66(3):400–402.
50. Vadalouca A, Moka E, Sykiotis C. Combined spinal-epidural technique for total hysterectomy in a patient with advanced, progressive multiple sclerosis. *Reg Anesth Pain Med.* 2002;27(5):540–541.
51. Finucane BT, Terblanche OC. Prolonged duration of anesthesia in a patient with multiple sclerosis following paravertebral block. *Can J Anaesth.* 2005;52(5):493–497.
52. Levesque P, Marsepoil T, Ho P, Venutolo F, Lesouef JM. [Multiple sclerosis disclosed by spinal anesthesia]. *Ann Fr Anesth Reanim.* 1988;7(1):68–70.
53. Perlas A, Chan VW. Neuraxial anesthesia and multiple sclerosis. *Can J Anaesth.* 2005;52(5):454–458.
54. Bader AM, Hunt CO, Datta S, Naulty JS, Ostheimer GW. Anesthesia for the obstetric patient with multiple sclerosis. *J Clin Anesth.* 1988;1(1):21–24.
55. Confavreux C, Hutchinson M, Hours MM, Cortinovis-Tourniaire P, Moreau T. Rate of pregnancy-related relapse in multiple sclerosis: Pregnancy in Multiple Sclerosis Group. *New Engl J Med.* 1998;339(5):285–291.
56. Vukusic S, Hutchinson M, Hours M, et al. Pregnancy and multiple sclerosis (the PRIMS study): clinical predictors of post-partum relapse. *Brain.* 2004;127(Pt 6):1353–1360.
57. Couratier P, Boukhris S, Magy L, Traore H, Vallat JM. [Involvement of the peripheral nervous system in multiple sclerosis]. *Rev Neurol (Paris).* 2004;160(12):1159–1163.
58. Poser CM. The peripheral nervous system in multiple sclerosis: a review and pathogenetic hypothesis. *J Neurol Sci.* 1987;79(1–2):83–90.
59. Misawa S, Kuwabara S, Mori M, Hayakawa S, Sawai S, Hattori T. Peripheral nerve demyelination in multiple sclerosis. *Clin Neurophysiol.* 2008;119(8):1829–1833.
60. Pogorzelski R, Baniukiewicz E, Drozdowski W. [Subclinical lesions of peripheral nervous system in multiple sclerosis patients]. *Neurol Neurochir Pol.* 2004;38(4):257–264.
61. Koff MD, Cohen JA, McIntyre JJ, Carr CF, Sites BD. Severe brachial plexopathy after an ultrasound-guided single-injection nerve block for total shoulder arthroplasty in a patient with multiple sclerosis. *Anesthesiology.* 2008;108(2):325–328.
62. Sia S. Nerve blocks, ultrasounds, and multiple sclerosis. *Anesthesiology.* 2008;109(4):751–752; author reply 753.
63. Neal JM, Barrington MJ, Brull R, et al. The Second ASRA Practice Advisory on Neurologic Complications Associated With Regional Anesthesia and Pain Medicine: executive summary 2015. *Reg Anesth Pain Med.* 2015;40(5):401–430.
64. Neal JM, Bernards CM, Hadzic A, et al. ASRA Practice Advisory on Neurologic Complications in Regional Anesthesia and Pain Medicine. *Reg Anesth Pain Med.* 2008;33(5):404–415.
65. Lavie C, Rollot F, Durand-Dubief F, et al. Neuraxial analgesia is not associated with an increased risk of post-partum relapses in MS. *Mult Scler.* 2019;25(4):591–600.
66. Urits I, Adamian L, Fiocchi J, et al. Advances in the understanding and management of chronic pain in multiple sclerosis: a comprehensive review. *Curr Pain Headache Rep.* 2019;23(8):59.
67. Quinlan ND, Chen DQ, Werner BC, Barnes CL, Browne JA. Patients with multiple sclerosis are at increased risk for postoperative complications following total hip and knee arthroplasty. *J Arthroplasty.* 2019;34(8):1606–1610.

REVIEW QUESTIONS

(1) Which of the following symptoms causing disability is most commonly reported by patients with MS?

A. Depression
B. Mobility impairment
C. Memory impairment
D. Pseudobulbar affect

(2) Acute worsening of multiple sclerosis (MS) symptoms has been consistently described for which perioperative event?

A. Intraoperative hyperthermia
B. Exposure to volatile anesthetics
C. Intrathecal local anesthetic injections
D. Peripheral nerve blockade with local anesthetics

(3) Which of the following best describes the use of neuraxial anesthetics in patients with MS?

A. Spinal anesthetics are contraindicated in patients with MS.
B. Spinal anesthetics may unmask previously silent demyelinating lesions, but symptoms are typically transient and reversible.
C. Epidural anesthetics have not been associated with acute exacerbations of MS symptoms.
D. Patients with more severe and debilitating disease are at higher risk for developing worsening neurologic impairment after neuraxial anesthetics.

(4) Which factors have been implicated in the etiology of MS?

A. Immunopathology
B. Viral infections
C. Genetic predisposition
D. All of the above

(5) What characterizes the neuropathology of MS?

A. Degeneration of both upper and lower motor neurons with loss of axons
B. Focal demyelinated plaques in the central nervous system with associated gliosis and relative axonal preservation
C. Neurodegeneration and neuronal loss in the substantia nigra
D. Autoantibodies directed against the nicotinic acetylcholine receptors at the neuromuscular endplate with resultant loss of receptors

(6) Which of the following best describes the use of peripheral regional anesthetics in patients with MS?

A. Peripheral regional anesthetics are most likely safe to perform.
B. Peripheral nervous system involvement in MS is possible, and a thorough neurologic examination and history should be performed prior to performing a peripheral regional anesthetic.
C. To reduce the risk of neurotoxicity, the lowest volume and concentration of local anesthetics should be used,

and the use of vasoconstrictors should be minimized or avoided.

D. All of the above are true.

(7) During pregnancy and the postpartum period, what generally happens to MS symptoms? Does an epidural increase or decrease symptoms?

A. MS symptoms increase during pregnancy and increase in the postpartum period; epidural increases relapse rates.
B. MS symptoms decrease during pregnancy and decrease in the postpartum period; epidural increases relapse rates.
C. MS symptoms increase during pregnancy and decrease during the postpartum period; epidural does not affect relapse rates.
D. MS symptoms decrease during pregnancy and increase during the postpartum period; epidural does not affect relapse rates.

ANSWERS

(1) **B.** Symptoms most commonly causing disability include mobility impairment (80%), balance impairment (75%), ataxia (80%), fatigue (80%), bladder dysfunction (58%–75%), spasticity (60%–90%), pain (55%–70%), cognitive dysfunction (60%–70%), depression (25%–50%), and pseudobulbar affect (10%). No specific symptoms or disabilities are unique to MS, and primary treatment of MS is aimed at improving quality of life. Pain due to MS is very common; sources include headache, neuropathic extremity pain, back pain, painful spasms, and trigeminal neuralgia.

References

Feinstein A, Freeman J, Lo AC. Treatment of progressive multiple sclerosis: what works, what does not, and what is needed. *Lancet Neurol.* 2015;14(2):194–207.

Foley PL, Vesterinen HM, Laird BJ, et al. Prevalence and natural history of pain in adults with multiple sclerosis: systematic review and meta-analysis. *Pain.* 2013;154(5):632–642.

(2) **A.** Only hyperthermia has been consistently associated with acute worsening of MS symptoms in the perioperative period. These exacerbations or "pseudo relapses" are due to conduction blockade of nerves when exposed to increasing temperatures. While case reports of both intrathecal and peripheral nerve blockade with local anesthetics have been implicated in worsening MS symptoms, there is no consistent causality. In addition, spinal anesthetics have been performed successfully in patients with MS, but most anesthesiologists caution against this technique due to the concern for neurotoxicity associated with demyelinating lesions. Both IV and volatile anesthetics have been used safely.

References

Guthrie TC, Nelson DA. Influence of temperature changes on multiple sclerosis: critical review of mechanisms and research potential. *J Neurol Sci.* 1995;129(1):1–8.

Hebl JR, Horlocker TT, Schroeder DR. Neuraxial anesthesia and analgesia in patients with preexisting central nervous system disorders. *Anesth Analg.* 2006;103(1):223–228.

Berger JM, Ontell R. Intrathecal morphine in conjunction with a combined spinal and general anesthetic in a patient with multiple sclerosis. *Anesthesiology.* 1987;66(3):400–402.

Neal JM, Barrington MJ, Brull R, et al. The Second ASRA Practice Advisory on Neurologic Complications Associated With Regional Anesthesia and Pain Medicine: executive summary 2015. *Reg Anesth Pain Med.* 2015;40(5):401–430.

(3) **B.** Both spinal and epidural anesthetics have been successfully performed in patients with MS without evidence of worsening neurologic impairment, and neither anesthetic is absolutely contraindicated. However, most anesthesiologists agree that epidurals may be less likely to worsen neurologic function compared to spinals due to lower intrathecal concentrations of local anesthetics. However, both spinals and epidurals have also been associated with acute exacerbations of MS symptoms in case reports. There is no consistent association between disease severity and the risk of relapse; a retrospective case series showed no increase in neurologic impairment even in patients with active disease while using standard dosing of local anesthetics. Spinal anesthetics have been implicated in unmasking silent demyelinated lesions in patients with MS, but these symptoms are frequently transient and reversible.

References

Lavie C, Rollot F, Durand-Dubief F, et al. Neuraxial analgesia is not associated with an increased risk of post-partum relapses in MS. *Mult Scler.* 2019;25(4):591–600.

Makris A, Piperopoulos A, Karmaniolou I. Multiple sclerosis: basic knowledge and new insights in perioperative management. *J Anesth.* 2014;28(2):267–278.

Dorotta IR, Schubert A. Multiple sclerosis and anesthetic implications. *Curr Opin Anaesthesiol.* 2002;15(3):365–370.

Perlas A, Chan VW. Neuraxial anesthesia and multiple sclerosis. *Can J Anaesth.* 2005;52(5):454–458.

(4) **D.** All of the above have been implicated in MS etiology. The exact etiology is unknown and likely multifactorial. Geographic latitude and place of birth, smoking history, sunlight exposure, and vitamin D levels have also been implicated.

References

Brownlee WJ, Hardy TA, Fazekas F, Miller DH. Diagnosis of multiple sclerosis: progress and challenges. *Lancet.* 2017;389(10076):1336–1346.

Lucchinetti C, Bruck W, Parisi J, Scheithauer B, Rodriguez M, Lassmann H. Heterogeneity of multiple sclerosis lesions: implications for the pathogenesis of demyelination. *Ann Neurol.* 2000;47(6):707–717.

Thompson AJ, Banwell BL, Barkhof F, et al. Diagnosis of multiple sclerosis: 2017 revisions of the McDonald criteria. *Lancet Neurol.* 2018;17(2):162–173.

(5) **B.** MS is characterized by focal demyelinated plaques in the CNS with gliosis and relative axonal preservation. Neurodegeneration of both upper and lower motor neurons describes amyotrophic lateral sclerosis. Parkinson's disease is characterized by neurodegeneration in the substantia nigra. Autoantibodies directed against nicotinic receptors at the neuromuscular endplate with loss of receptors describe myasthenia gravis.

References

Frischer JM, Weigand SD, Guo Y, et al. Clinical and pathological insights into the dynamic nature of the white matter multiple sclerosis plaque. *Ann Neurol.* 2015;78(5):710–721.

Calabrese M, Favaretto A, Martini V, Gallo P. Grey matter lesions in MS: from histology to clinical implications. *Prion.* 2013;7(1):20–27.

(6) **D.** PNS involvement in patients with MS is possible, yet controversial, and the frequency of PNS involvement is unknown. Thus, precautions should be taken prior to performing a peripheral regional anesthetic, including performing a thorough neurologic history and physical exam, using the lowest volume and concentration of local anesthetics possible, and minimizing or avoiding the use of vasoconstrictors. However, the overall evidence for using peripheral regional anesthetics in patients with MS and the lack of documented reports of neurologic impairment following these procedures indicates that peripheral nerve blocks are most likely safe.

References

Koff MD, Cohen JA, McIntyre JJ, Carr CF, Sites BD. Severe brachial plexopathy after an ultrasound-guided single-injection nerve block for total shoulder arthroplasty in a patient with multiple sclerosis. *Anesthesiology.* 2008;108(2):325–328.

Neal JM, Barrington MJ, Brull R, et al. The Second ASRA Practice Advisory on Neurologic Complications Associated With Regional Anesthesia and Pain Medicine: executive summary 2015. *Reg Anesth Pain Med.* 2015;40(5):401–430.

(7) **D.** MS tends to be stable or decrease during pregnancy, although the stress physiologically and psychologically placed on the mother can increase symptoms in the postpartum period. Notably, pre-pregnancy severity of MS correlates with the postpartum severity of relapse. Studies have supported the use of labor epidurals and, to date, have shown no effect of epidurals on MS relapse rates.

References

Makris A, Piperopoulos A, Karmaniolou I. Multiple sclerosis: basic knowledge and new insights in perioperative management. *J Anesth.* 2014;28(2):267–278.

Dorotta IR, Schubert A. Multiple sclerosis and anesthetic implications. *Curr Opin Anaesthesiol.* 2002;15(3):365–370.

Bader AM, Hunt CO, Datta S, Naulty JS, Ostheimer GW. Anesthesia for the obstetric patient with multiple sclerosis. *J Clin Anesth.* 1988;1(1):21–24.

50.

NERVE INJURY AFTER PLEXUS AND PERIPHERAL NERVE BLOCKS FOR REGIONAL ANESTHESIA AND MEDICOLEGAL IMPLICATIONS

H. David Hardman

STEM CASE AND KEY QUESTIONS

A 56-year-old male is scheduled for a revision rotator cuff repair surgery. He injured his right shoulder in a motor vehicle accident 4 years earlier and previously underwent a right rotator cuff repair. His medical history is significant for sleep apnea, osteoarthritis, hypertension, tobacco use, and his body mass index is 40. He also reports chronic neck pain and stiffness since his motor vehicle accident. A recent magnetic resonance imaging (MRI) scan demonstrates a supraspinatus tear. His surgeon has booked the case, requesting an interscalene block (ISB) and general anesthesia.

The patient tells you he received an ISB as part of his previous anesthetic and although it provided good pain relief, he felt short of breath for several hours after he woke up and prefers not to have a nerve block again; however, his surgeon is insistent that he have a nerve block as part of his procedure.

The patient is moved into a block room, a peripheral intravenous line is placed, monitors are attached, and a preprocedure timeout is called.

After minimal sedation, an ultrasound-guided superior trunk block proceeds uneventfully, with 15 mL of bupivacaine 0.5% and 4 mg of perineural dexamethasone. After 90 minutes of surgery under general anesthesia, the patient is extubated and transported to the post-anesthesia care unit. He reports minimal pain at discharge. A member of the anesthesia team calls him the next day and the patient reports that he is doing well and not experiencing any breathing difficulties.

Ten days later, during his first postoperative office visit, the patient states that his right hand is numb and that he is having difficulty using eating utensils. He also claims he first noticed this after returning home. On examination, the surgeon notes decreased sensation over the palmar thenar aspect of the hand, including digits I through III, along with decreased grip strength. The patient is also having difficulty flexing all of his fingers.

On his subsequent clinic visit (24 days postoperatively), the patient is angry and upset that his hand is still numb and weak, and he is now experiencing severe pain in his right arm and right hand. On examination, the hand is discolored and exquisitely sensitive to touch. In contrast, the shoulder appears to be normal. The surgeon refers the patient to a neurologist for further workup.

Electrodiagnostic (EDX) study results obtained 4 weeks after surgery are summarized in Tables 50.1 through 50.3.

You receive notification that the patient has filed a civil suit alleging malpractice on your part in performing the PNB.

(1) HOW COMMON ARE NERVE INJURIES AFTER PLEXUS AND PERIPHERAL NERVE BLOCKS (PNB)?

Up to 19% of patients may report postoperative neurologic symptoms (PONS) on the first postoperative day, and this diminishes to 2.2% at 3 months, 0.8% at 6 months, and 0.2% at 1 year.[1–3] Permanent injury (PONS >1 year) is rare, with estimates ranging from a high of 9:10,000 to a low of 2:10,000 after PNB.[4–9]

(2) WHAT ARE THE RISK FACTORS FOR THE DEVELOPMENT OF PERIPHERAL NERVE INJURY?

PNB is not deemed to be an independent risk factor for developing PONS, though neurologic complications are more strongly associated with certain blocks (ISB, axillary, femoral, sciatic, popliteal) and the use of long, sharp bevel needles.[3,7,10,12] Orthopedic surgical procedures are associated with an elevated risk of developing PONS.[3,7,11] Specific surgical positions and techniques can lead to brachial plexus stretching, and direct injury to nerves can occur from surgical portal and anchor placements. Patient-specific risk factors for perioperative nerve injury (PNI) and PONS include diabetes, hypertension, and tobacco use, revision surgical joint procedures, and preexisting nervous system disorders.

Table 50.1 SENSORY NERVE STUDY RESULTS*

NERVE/ STIM. SITE: SENSORY	REC. SITE	ONSET MS	PEAK MS	NP AMP MV	PP AMP MV	DIST CM	VEL M/S
Right Median: Wrist	Dig III	NR					75.7
Left median: Wrist	Dig III	1.85	2.70	67.3	113.2	14	75.7
Right Ulnar: Wrist	Dig V	2.25	2.95	55.4	73.5	14	62.2
Left Ulnar: Wrist	Dig V	2.15	2.95	66.2	71.2	14	65.1
Right Radial: Forearm	Thumb	1.5	2.00	38.5	19.2	10	66.7
Right LABCN: Elbow	Forearm	2.6	4.9	66.3	67.0	12	46.1
Right MABCN: Elbow	Forearm	2.4	4.75	65.9	71.2	12	50.0

*SNAP = sensory nerve action potentials; NP = negative peak amplitude; PP = positive peak amplitude; LABCN = lateral antebrachial cutaneous nerve; MABCN = medial antebrachial cutaneous nerve.

(3) WHAT CONSTITUTES INFORMED CONSENT? HOW SHOULD THIS BE DOCUMENTED? IS A SEPARATE ANESTHESIA CONSENT NECESSARY?

Informed consent contains the following components: voluntary, competency, capacity, disclosure, authorization, and documentation. There is no requirement by the Centers for Medicare/Medicaid Services or The Joint Commission for a stand-alone anesthesia consent form, although local hospital policies may differ from federal requirements, but the American Society of Anesthesiologists recommends using a separate written anesthesia consent form to mitigate malpractice risk.[17] This form should be dated and timed, with name and signature of the patient, anesthesia provider, and witness, include an explanation of the type of anesthesia and monitoring being proposed and the material risks associated with these techniques, along with alternatives.

(4) IS THERE A PREFERRED TYPE OF NEEDLE LOCALIZATION GUIDANCE THAT WILL DECREASE THE RISK OF INTRANEURAL INJECTION AND/OR PNI?

There is no difference in the incidence of PONS when ultrasound guidance is used when compared to other needle localization techniques (paresthesia, nerve stimulation).[2,4,22] Although intraneural injection occurs more commonly than previously appreciated and does not invariably lead to functional nerve injury, the practice of intentionally seeking intraneural injection is not recommended.[3,12,42]

(5) WHAT ARE ELECTRODIAGNOSTIC (EDX) STUDIES, AND WHAT CAN THEY TELL YOU?

EDX studies can localize the site of injury in the peripheral nervous system and distinguish between demyelinating and axonal injury. EDX studies consist of nerve conduction studies

Table 50.2 COMPOUND MUSCLE ACTION POTENTIALS (CMAP) RESULTS

NERVE/STIM. SITE: MOTOR	REC. SITE	LATENCY MS	AMP MV	NORMAL AMP MV	DIST CM	VEL M/S	NORM VEL M/S
Right Median:							
Wrist	APB	3.7	0.2	>5.0	7.7	–	–
Elbow	APB	7.2	0.3	>5.0	18.6	47.2	>50
Left Median:							
Wrist	APB	3.6	7.4	>5.0	7.5	–	–
Elbow	APB	7.1	7.3	>5.0	18.5	52.8	>50
Right Radial:							
Proximal	EIP	1.8	5.1	>5.0	4	–	–
Elbow	EIP	5.1	5.3	>5.0	18	54.5	>50
Right Ulnar:							
Wrist	ADM	3.1	8.6	>5.0	7.5	–	>50
Below Elbow	ADM	5.8	9.1	>5.0	17.5	64.8	–
Above Elbow	ADM	7.3	8.9	>5.0	8.0	53.3	>50

APB = abductor pollicus brevis; EIP = extensor indicis proprius; ADM = abductor digiti minimi.

(NCS) and electromyography (EMG). NCS are subdivided into motor and sensory nerve studies. Compound motor action potentials (CMAP) are measurements taken in motor nerves, and sensory nerve action potentials (SNAP) are measurements taken in sensory nerves. NCS are not always helpful in distinguishing block-related from non-block-related causes, but needle electromyography (EMG) may help distinguish location of injury by sampling proximal and distal muscles, looking for pathologic denervation potentials and abnormal motor unit action potential (MUAP) activity.[55] EDX studies are typically obtained 3–4 weeks after injury, when the most information is obtainable from a single study.[52,53,55,56]

(6) WHAT KIND OF SURGICAL TREATMENT OPTIONS FOR NERVE INJURY ARE AVAILABLE, AND WHEN SHOULD THEY BE CONSIDERED?

Peripheral nerve reconstruction surgery (interposition autologous grafts, nerve transfer surgery) should be considered for any persistent serious motor nerve injury on clinical examination.

DISCUSSION

Permanent nerve injury is rare after PNB, although some form of transient injury is common. A review of the literature examining the upper limit of postoperative neurologic symptoms (PONS) reported in all studies since 1997 indicates that up to 19% of patients may report PONS on the first postoperative day. This rapidly diminishes to 2.2% at 3 months, 0.8% at 6 months, and 0.2% at 1 year.[1–3] Permanent injury (PONS >1 year) is rare, with estimates ranging from a high of 9:10,000 to a low of 2:10,000 after PNB.[4-9]

PNI is a multifactorial process, with a differential diagnosis that includes surgery-, patient-, and anesthesia-related factors. PNB is not deemed to be an independent risk factor for developing PONS, even in joint replacement surgeries involving the shoulder, hip, and knee.[3,7,10] Orthopedic surgical procedures are associated with an elevated risk of developing PONS, even in the absence of PNB.[3,7,11] A recent systematic review of factors associated with neurologic complications after PNB found the strongest associations with certain types of blocks (ISB, axillary, femoral, sciatic, popliteal) and the use of long, sharp bevel needles.[12]

PONS in arthroscopic shoulder surgery are reported to range between 0.1% and 10%, with most of these injuries being transient.[11] Mechanisms of injury include stretching the brachial plexus for surgical positioning and direct injury to nerves from surgical portal and anchor placements. The anterior shoulder portal may damage the lateral cord of the brachial plexus and musculocutaneous nerve, while the lateral portal can damage the axillary nerve. The suprascapular nerve can be injured secondary to mechanical compression forces exerted by anchors placed in the superior aspect of the glenoid during superior labrum repairs.[11]

Patient-specific risk factors for PNI and PONS include comorbidities such as diabetes, hypertension, and tobacco use, surgical joint revisions, and preexisting nervous system disorders, including subclinical entrapment neuropathies (carpal tunnel), cervical spondylosis, being post-chemotherapy (cisplatin, paclitaxel, vincristine), and alcohol-related polyneuropathy.[3,13]

These conditions may induce a subclinical ischemic neuropathy that can predispose a patient to developing clinical

Table 50.3 ELECTROMYOGRAPHY RESULTS

MUSCLE	NERVE	ROOT	SPONTANEOUS ACTIVITY			MUAP*				
			INS ACT	FIB	PSW	AMP	DUR	PPP	RECRUIT	INT PAT
R. deltoid	Axillary	C5–6	0	0	0	N	N	None	N	Complete
R. biceps	MSCT	C5–6	0	0	0	N	N	None	N	Complete
R. triceps	Radial	C6–8	0	0	0	N	N	None	N	Complete
R. abd. pol. brev.	Median	C8–T1	2+	4+	3+	N	Inc	2+	Rapid	25%
R. pronator teres	Median	C6–7	0	0	0	N	Inc	None	N	Complete
R. 1st D inteross	Ulnar	C7–8	0	0	0	N	N	None	N	Complete
R. abd. dig. min.	Ulnar	C8–T1	0	0	0	N	N	None	N	Complete
R. flex. carpi ulnaris	Ulnar	C8–T1	+2	3+	2+	N	N	None	Rapid	50%
R. flex. dig. prof. III–IV	Ulnar	C7–8, T1	1+	4+	3+	N	N	None	Rapid	25%
Paraspinal C5–T1		C5–T1	0	0	0					

*MUAP = Motor unit action potential; Ins Act = insertional activity; Fib = fibrillation potentials; PSW = positive sharp waves; Amp = amplitude; Dur = duration; PPP = polyphasia; Int Pat = interference pattern; MSCT = musculocutaneous nerve; 1st D inteross = 1st dorsal interosseous.

manifestation of PONS after surgery and anesthesia if additional damaging forces are exerted on the nerve. However, a recent systematic review did not find an association between preexisting neuropathy and the risk of developing PONS after PNB, although recovery from PONS was worse in this subset of patients.[12]

A patient with a history of osteoarthritis and a previous neck injury with pain may have an underlying subclinical injury, with possible compression of nerve roots and the spinal cord from degenerative changes in the intervertebral foramen and central spinal stenosis. This has the potential to cause further neural compromise related to surgical positioning and the administration of a PNB. Cervical spine disease may also be a risk factor for developing chronic phrenic nerve paralysis after ISB.[14]

ALTERNATIVES TO ISB FOR SHOULDER SURGERY

Alternatives to the ISB that provide noninferior analgesia while minimizing the risk of hemidiaphragmatic paralysis include the selective anterior suprascapular nerve block and the superior trunk block. Two recent studies have compared the adverse effects of ISB versus suprascapular nerve block with 15 mL of ropivacaine 0.5% in conjunction with general anesthesia, or selective superior trunk block versus ISB as the primary anesthetic utilizing 15 mL of bupivacaine 0.5%. These two alternatives decrease the risk of hemidiaphragmatic paralysis to 10% and 4.8%, respectively.[15,16]

There are many benefits associated with PNB in patients with a history of sleep apnea and elevated body mass. In addition to superior postoperative pain control, the potential for respiratory depression can be mitigated by avoiding or minimizing opioid analgesics.

INFORMED CONSENT

Informed consent must contain the following patient and physician components:

- Voluntary
- Competency
- Capacity
- Disclosure
- Authorization
- Documentation.

There is no requirement by the Centers for Medicare/Medicaid Services or The Joint Commission for a stand-alone anesthesia consent form, although local hospital policies may differ from federal requirements. The State of Texas requires a specific written anesthesia consent prior to epidural and spinal blocks, with mandated language describing risks in these forms. The American Society of Anesthesiologists recommends that its members use a separate written anesthesia consent form to mitigate malpractice risk.[17] This form should include an explanation of the type of anesthesia and monitoring being proposed and the material risks associated with these techniques, along with alternatives. The legal standard for disclosure of risk is a "reasonable person standard," i.e., what a reasonable person would want to know to make an informed decision. This is important in the setting of regional anesthesia, where offering a PNB is always a patient choice and is never the only option.[18] The consent form should be dated and timed, with the patient's name and signature authorizing the anesthesia plan; the name and signature of the anesthesia provider explaining the procedure and risks; and a witness signature from someone outside of the surgery–anesthesia team. For medicolegal purposes, this should be completed prior to any documentation of pre-procedural sedation.

STANDARD OF CARE, DOCUMENTATION, AND ANESTHETIC TECHNIQUE FOR PNB

The "standard of care" is a legal term broadly defined as requiring compliance with the generally recognized and accepted practices and procedures that would be followed by average competent practitioners in the physician's field of medicine under the same or similar circumstances. This definition recognizes flexibility in tailoring clinical decision-making to a variety of patient care scenarios.[19] Standard of care is not defined by clinical practice guidelines or advisories. For example, standard of care in regional anesthesia pertaining to administering a PNB would warrant informed consent prior to commencing the procedure, a medical record documenting the details of the procedure, placement of an intravenous fluid line, routine monitoring (electrocardiography, blood pressure, pulse oximetry), availability of resuscitation equipment, and not exceeding the maximal recommended dose of local anesthetics. Standard of care allows for a variety of PNB approaches and needle localization choices, block needle types, local anesthetic agents, volumes and concentrations, perineural adjuvants, and the decision to employ single-injection or continuous-catheter techniques.

A block note should be sufficiently granular to ensure that the documentation would allow a third party to review and understand the details of the block. The record could be essential in establishing standard of care practice and successfully defending against a future block-related medicolegal claim. In the real world, these notes vary based on individual practice settings and preferences; nonetheless, a comprehensive block note might include some or all the following data:

- Focused neurologic examination prior to the block
- Time-out (patient and block site identified, marked, and informed consent verified)
- Patient level of awareness during block (was meaningful verbal contact maintained during the procedure?)
- Aseptic skin preparation and drape

- Type of needle used (e.g., 22-gauge short bevel, 150 mm, manufacturer name)
- Skin depth to target prior to injection (if catheter, distance inserted after placement)
- Needle localization method (ultrasound, neurostimulation, paresthesia seeking, or combination)
- Initial and minimal current threshold prior to injection, and motor response observed with neurostimulation (e.g., deltoid muscle contraction)
- Presence or absence of paresthesia or pain with needle advancement prior to injection. If paresthesia occurred, did it immediately resolve prior to injection? Describe anatomic location of paresthesia.
- Presence or absence of paresthesia with onset of injection. If present, was the injection aborted, and did the paresthesia resolve with needle withdrawal prior to second injection?
- Presence or absence of resistance to onset of injection. If resistance was present, was the needle repositioned and the injection recommenced without further resistance?
- Was opening injection pressure (OIP) monitored or was a pressure injection-limiting device used? Was the pressure < 15 psi? How was the pressure measured (e.g., commercial device and name, or syringe with compressed air injection technique)?
- Test initial injection of 0.5 to 1.0 mL and absence of nerve diameter expansion (using ultrasound needle guidance)
- Negative or positive aspiration for blood prior to test injection
- Single-injection or multi-injection technique
- Local anesthetic type, concentration, and volume
- Perineural additives and dose (epinephrine, bicarbonate, dexamethasone, clonidine, buprenorphine, dexmedetomidine, preservative-free)
- Ultrasound pre- and post-injection image capture, or video loop of injection
- Block readiness for surgery (complete, partial, unable to assess, failure)
- Block supplementation (yes, no, local anesthetic concentration and volume, block supplementation site [e.g., axillary]).

The electronic medical record can create a customized PNB template with these data fields pre-populated and selected via check boxes, with the opportunity to input numerical values or free text entries where appropriate. A comprehensive block note can be quickly created with the help of an assistant entering information in real time.

A record of an inpatient follow-up visit, or phone call for an outpatient, should also be recorded in the medical record. Data collection can include the length of analgesia, the time of return to normal sensation and motor function, the presence and location of any sensory or motor deficits, the presence of paresthesia or dysesthesia, and patient satisfaction. When a continuous catheter is used, data collection can include the time of catheter removal and condition of the skin at the entry site to assess for inflammation or infection. If there is a persistent sensory or motor deficit, the patient should be called daily until the deficit resolves or the patient is assessed in the clinic.

Almost all upper extremity ultrasound-guided PNB can be performed with single-injection techniques; there is no advantage to multi-injection techniques in terms of block success rates, and the risk of procedural paresthesia increases with multiple injections.[20] In contrast, some lower extremity ultrasound-guided nerve blocks have demonstrated higher success rates with multi-needle pass injection techniques.[21]

NEEDLE-NERVE LOCALIZATION AND AVOIDING INTRANEURAL INJECTION

Although there are many advantages to ultrasound needle guidance, there is no difference in the incidence of PONS compared to other needle localization techniques.[2,4,22] Ultrasound probes do not have the lateral resolution to distinguish intraneural-intrafascicular needle placement from intraneural-extrafascicular needle placement[3,4,13,23] (Figure 50.1). Additionally, regional anesthesiologists do not always visualize their needle tip. Given these limitations, there may be a role for the selective use of additional needle localization monitoring technology, including neurostimulation and injection pressure monitoring.

Inadvertent intraneural needle entry and injection occur more commonly than previously appreciated—in up to 17% of PNB that use ultrasound.[24,25] In Hara et al. and Sala Blanch et al., none of the patients that sustained intraneural injections developed PONS. Using neurostimulation needle localization techniques, the incidence is even higher, with an intraneural injection rate of 66% when an evoked motor response (EMR) is elicited at less than 0.5 mA using a pulse width duration of 0.1 msec.[26] This is not surprising when other investigators have determined the sensitivity of needle-nerve contact associated with neurostimulation at 0.5 mA in the axillary brachial plexus to be only 74.5%.[27] In the same study, the sensitivity of paresthesia with needle-nerve contact was only 38.2%. This helps us interpret other evidence demonstrating that the elicitation of a paresthesia is not an independent risk factor to develop PONS and that PONS can occur without the presence of a paresthesia.

Forced needle entry into neural tissue triggers an inflammatory response, even without injection, although these inflammatory changes resolve without functional injury.[28] Intraneural injection of as little as 0.5 mL (85% sensitivity) can be detected by knowledgeable regional anesthesiologists with ultrasound experience.[29] Routinely using a test dose of 0.5 to 1.0 mL of local anesthetic can limit the volume of an

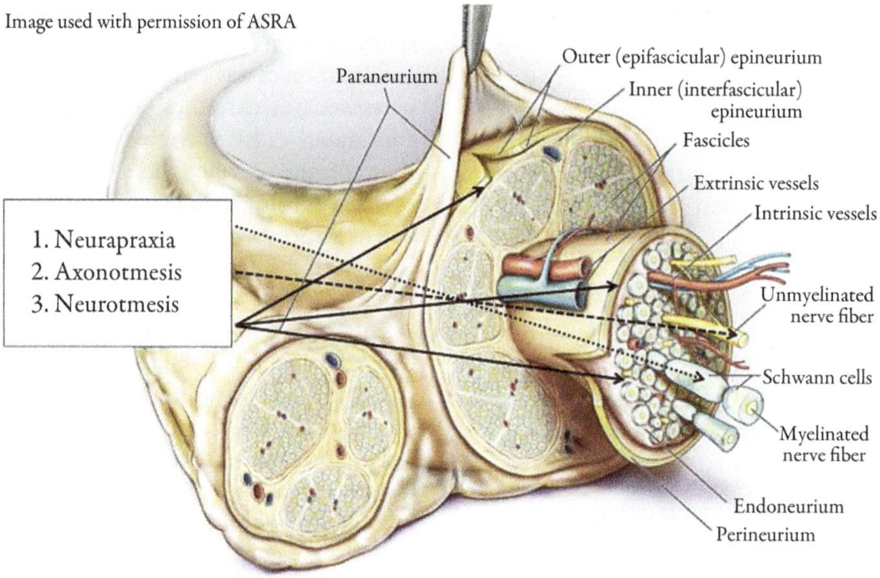

Figure 50.1. Peripheral nerve microanatomy and Seddon nerve injury classification.

inadvertent intraneural injection and allow time for needle repositioning prior to injecting larger volumes.

Several investigators have demonstrated that successful ISB can be performed in human patients without needle entry into the interscalene groove by depositing local anesthetic adjacent to the plexus and not between the nerve roots.[30,31] The maximum effective distance away from the plexus to deposit local anesthetic and provide block success in 95% of patients has been calculated to be 1.6 mm.[31]

Animal and human models demonstrate that neurostimulation is a specific but nonsensitive measure of needle-nerve contact. With needle-nerve contact or intraneural needle placement in animal models, EMR can occur with a stimulating current as low as 0.2 mA; however, in some cases, it may not occur unless the stimulating current is increased up to 1.8 mA.[32] The presence of an EMR at low stimulating currents <0.5 mA can only occur when the needle tip is very close to the nerve, in contact with the nerve, or inside the nerve.[3]

When neurostimulation is used as the primary needle localization method, the initial current may be set at 1.1 mA, and no attempt should be made to advance the needle, seeking an EMR below 0.5 mA. Neurostimulation can be an adjunct to ultrasound-guided needle localization in the setting of poor image quality and difficulty visualizing the needle tip. If an EMR is still present at <0.5 mA, the needle should be withdrawn until the EMR disappears prior to injecting a test dose of local anesthetic.

In contrast to neurostimulation, OIP monitoring is sensitive for needle-nerve contact and intraneural placement, but it is not specific. Contact with fascia, ligaments, cartilage, and bone can also elevate OIP. Several investigations in animal models link elevated OIP (>15 psi) to histologic and functional injury; other studies demonstrate histologic injury but not functional injury with OIP <15 psi despite evidence of intraneural injection as assessed by ultrasound.[33,34] Human models demonstrate elevated OIP with needle-nerve contact against the roots of the brachial plexus and the femoral nerve, as well as contact with the fascia iliaca.[35,36] A cadaver study has demonstrated elevated OIP with needle-nerve contact or intraneural placement in all lower extremity nerves. In contrast, extraneural needle placement was consistently associated with an OIP <15 psi.[37]

OIP monitoring is not used as a primary needle localization technology in clinical practice; however, it can supplement ultrasound and neurostimulation guidance. Animal data suggest the major benefit of OIP monitoring lies in confirming extraneural (or intraneural but extrafascicular) placement, as no functional injuries have ever been observed in animal models with low OIP. However, there are limited human data that confirm or refute the effectiveness of OIP in limiting PONS.[3,12,38]

Commercial pressure-monitoring devices can be inserted in the injection line to measure or limit pressure to <15 psi. The subjective feel of pressing on the syringe plunger and assessing OIP is unreliable.[39] A compressed air injection technique can be used to accurately assess OIP without having to purchase a commercial device.[40]

Other modalities to reduce the risk of needle-nerve contact and intraneural injection that are under investigation and development include electrical impedance monitoring and electromagnetic needle tracking guides that display current and projected future needle positions.[41]

In summary, although intraneural injection (as defined by the visible enlargement of nerve diameter under ultrasound imaging) occurs more commonly than previously appreciated and does not invariably lead to functional nerve injury, the practice of intentionally seeking intraneural injection is not recommended.[3,12,42] Targeted intracluster injections in the supraclavicular brachial plexus using India ink in cadavers remained subperineural in 24% of observed injections.[43] Recent studies by Cappelleri et al. involving intentional intraneural injection (defined as increase in nerve diameter during injection as visualized by ultrasound) of the popliteal nerve in humans supports the animal evidence.[38] Injection pressures were limited to <15 psi, implying intraneural-extrafascicular injection. Although no functional deficits were observed at 5 weeks and 6 months postinjection, the results of more sensitive EDX testing demonstrated a 40%–50% reduction in compound motor action potentials (CMAP) at 6 months, implying significant axonal damage. Accompanying editorials to these publications reiterated the advice that intentional intraneural injection should be avoided and not encouraged, as even small volumes of intraneural local anesthetics can cause long-term axonal damage.[44–47]

CONTINUOUS CATHETER TECHNIQUES, PERINEURAL ADJUVANTS, AND NERVE INJURY

There is limited evidence comparing the risk of developing PONS after single-injection PNB to continuous-catheter PNB, and a systematic review did not demonstrate any difference.[12] The most comprehensive data using ultrasound-guided procedures exist in the Dartmouth clinical registry, in a subset containing 2003 single-injection ISB and 230 continuous-catheter ISB blocks that did not show a statistical difference in the risk of developing long-term PONS between the two techniques, although there was a trend for a higher injury rate in patients with continuous catheters.[8]

All commonly used perineural adjuvants (dexamethasone, dexmedetomidine, clonidine, buprenorphine) demonstrate minimal neurotoxicity signals when tested in vitro under simulated clinical concentrations.[48] These adjuvants exhibit substantially lower neurotoxicity compared to ropivacaine. In other animal models, intrafascicular injection of dexamethasone did not injure axons, and intraneural injection of dexmedetomidine with ropivacaine demonstrates anti-inflammatory and neuroprotective effects.[44,49] Clinical data from the Dartmouth registry and a more recent case series did not show any statistically significant association between using adjuvants and developing PONS.[8,50]

All local anesthetics reduce neural blood flow, demonstrating a dose-dependent and concentration effect. The reduction in neural blood flow is greater with epinephrine than with local anesthetics, although the clinical consequences associated with perineural epinephrine are controversial.[51]

NERVE INJURY AND CLASSIFICATION

The fundamental mechanism of nerve injury is an ischemic injury to a metabolically active tissue, resulting in a loss of signaling function of the axons within the peripheral nerve. Mechanisms of injury can be attributed to mechanical, vascular, chemical, thermal, and/or inflammatory factors. Due to the multifactorial nature of these injuries (patient-, surgery-, and/or anesthesia-related), it can be difficult to determine causation, although imaging and EDX studies can be helpful in refining the differential diagnoses, as well as the prognosis for recovery.

All local anesthetics exhibit concentration-dependent cytotoxic, neurotoxic, and myotoxic effects in vitro. However, in vivo, connective tissue barriers between the axon and extraneural tissue where local anesthetics are deposited progressively dilute the concentration of local anesthetic to non-toxic levels before the local anesthetic reaches the axon. Most of the nerve diameter expansion visualized on ultrasound, when block needles inadvertently enter nerves, can be attributed to intraneural-extrafascicular injection. However, needle entry into the epineurium and subepineurium can damage the vasa nervorum (providing approximately 50% of neural blood flow) and lacerate blood vessels in the space between nerve fascicles, causing intraneural hematoma and compressive ischemic injury[11] (Figure 50.1).

The Seddon classification system of nerve injury is a structural, functional, and prognostic description of peripheral nerve injury (Figure 50.1). Three categories of injury are described: neurapraxia, axonotmesis, and neurotmesis.[52] Neurapraxia is the most commonly observed PNI, characterized by damage to the myelin layer around axons and resulting in the slowing of nerve conduction velocity. Although neurapraxia can result in severe motor and sensory impairment, the natural course is for complete recovery within weeks to months as the myelin layer spontaneously regenerates inside the intact endoneurial tube. Axonotmesis is a more serious injury, with damage to the axon that results in Wallerian degeneration. Although the axon has the potential to regenerate within the endoneurial tube, complete recovery does not always occur, and prognosis is guarded. Time to recovery is measured in months or years. Once regeneration begins, axons will extend at the rate of 1 mm per day, or 1 inch per month. Neurotmesis is the most serious injury, with damage to the axon and surrounding connective tissue. The least serious subcategory is damage limited to the axon and endoneurium, with potential to re-establish axonal continuity over months to years. More serious subcategories include disruption of the perineurium and epineurium that requires surgical intervention to restore continuity to these connective tissue layers.

EVALUATION AND TREATMENT OF PONS

A neurology consult should be obtained by any patient with significant motor loss that persists beyond the expected duration of the block. Early recognition and documentation of PONS is imperative to help establish causation and to diagnose and treat reversible lesions such as compressive hematoma.[53] A detailed examination of the plexus and peripheral nerves using ultrasound to scan along the length of the structure can assess for hematoma, discontinuity, and intraneural edema.[54] MRI can also reveal the presence of hematoma, discontinuity lesions, and evidence of inflammation and edema with hyperintense signals (Figure 50.2). Although MRI can detect inflammatory changes, these changes are not specific enough to determine causation. Interpretation requires clinical correlation with the patient history and physical, details of

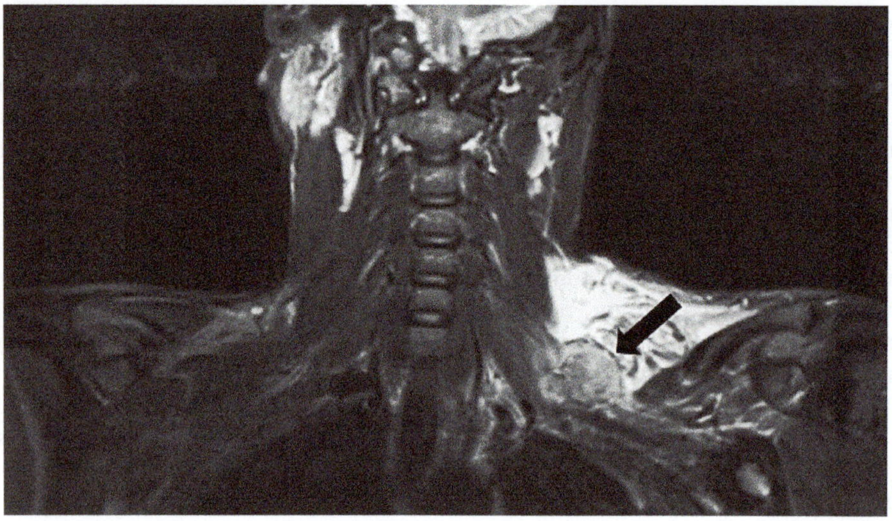

Figure 50.2. MRI image of brachial plexus hematoma (arrow) with inflammatory changes (bright signal).

the surgical procedure, and other diagnostic modalities such as EDX studies. EDX studies can localize the site of injury in the peripheral nervous system and distinguish between demyelinating and axonal injury.

Nerve conduction studies (NCS) are subdivided into motor and sensory nerve studies (Figure 50.3). CMAP are measurements taken in motor nerves, with a proximal supramaximal stimulus of the nerve and recording electrodes placed over a distal target muscle that records electrical signals generated as myofibrils depolarize. In contrast, sensory nerve action potentials (SNAP) are measurements taken in sensory nerves, with a proximal supramaximal stimulus of the nerve and recording electrodes placed over a distal part of the nerve that record electrical signals as the nerve depolarizes.

The hallmark of a focal demyelinating injury (neurapraxia) is a reduction in conduction velocity, increase in latency, and decrease in amplitude. Conduction velocities are <75% of normal values, and latencies are >130% of normal.[54] In contrast, axonal injuries (axonotmesis) appear as a reduction in amplitude without the associated decrease in conduction velocities and increases in latency. No signals are recorded with neurotmetic injuries.

NCS are not always helpful in distinguishing block-related from non-block-related causes. Most PNB are located at proximal sites in the upper and lower extremities, whereas NCS are located at distal sites in the extremities. Focal demyelinating injuries at proximal locations related to PNB will not be detected by stimulating distal to the site of injury because measured conduction velocities will be normal. It is technically difficult to stimulate proximal to the axilla, as nerves move away from the surface into deeper tissue and supramaximal stimulation is no longer possible. The opposite situation holds true with proximal axonal injuries: any stimulation of the nerve distal to the injury site will demonstrate abnormal signal amplitude. The site of injury cannot be determined by progressively "marching up" distal to proximal unless CMAP is

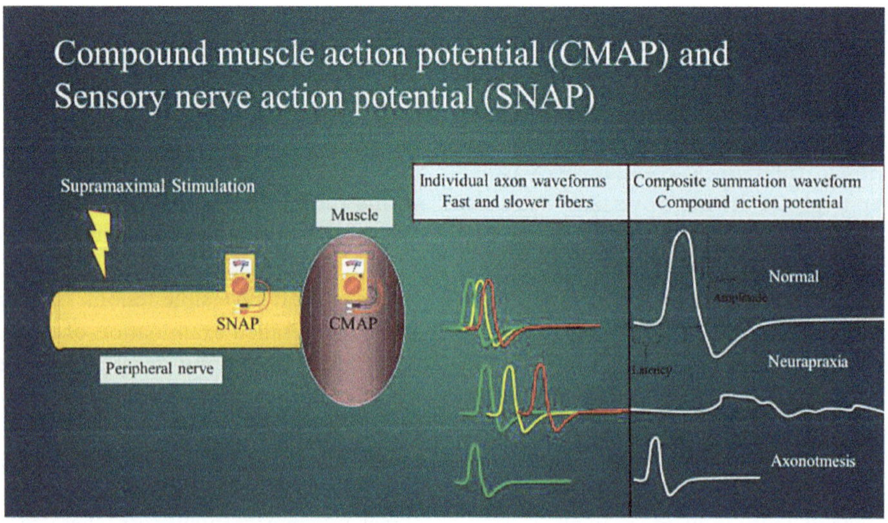

Figure 50.3. Example of nerve conduction study demonstrating features of a normal examination, neurapraxia (demyelination), and axonotmesis (axonal injury). Composite waveform is the algebraic sum of positive and negative wave amplitudes along the time axis.

measured in a new muscle that is proximal to the site of injury. In practice, this is done by using needle electromyography (EMG) instead of CMAP or SNAP, and sampling proximal muscles, looking for pathologic denervation potentials and abnormal motor unit action potential (MUAP) activity.[55,56]

The presence of denervation potentials imply injury to nerve axons at or proximal to the branch point of the most proximal muscles with denervation potentials. EMG studies also assess the number and type of MUAP and measure recruitment and activation of motor units.[55,56]

Morphologic changes in MUAP over time are used to follow the presence of reinnervation after axonal injury. With moderate injury, normal motor units adjacent to injured motor units will send out collateral neural branches to innervate adjacent muscle fibers denervated by damaged axons. This will increase the size of the motor unit (number of fibers innervated by a given axon) and increase the duration and number of phases of the MUAP.[55,56]

EDX studies are typically obtained 3 to 4 weeks after injury, when the most information is obtainable from a single study.[52,53,55,56] Pathologic denervation potentials associated with axonal injury are first detected in muscle 3 to 4 weeks after injury, allowing demyelinating injuries to be distinguished from axonal injuries. With evidence of moderate to severe axonal injury, EDX studies can be repeated at 3 and 6 months to assess the presence and degree of reinnervation, with referral to a reconstructive peripheral nerve surgeon for injuries not continuing to improve.[52,57]

INTERPRETATION OF EDX STUDY RESULTS

EDX study results obtained 4 weeks postinjury can be seen in Tables 50.1 through 50.3. They should be interpreted in context of the clinical examination that demonstrated injury to the median and ulnar nerves in the hand.

As illustrated in Table 50.1, no sensory nerve signal was obtained in the right median nerve supplying the abductor pollicus brevis (APB). This part of the median nerve originates in the medial cord, which contains the C8–T1 nerve roots. All other sensory nerve distributions displayed normal amplitudes and conduction velocities. The other medial cord-derived sensory nerve, the medial antebrachial cutaneous nerve (MABCN), was normal. This implies that the injury is distal to the takeoff of the MABCN from the medial cord. The type, location, and acuity of this injury cannot be determined from SNAP information alone.

Motor nerve studies illustrated in Table 50.2 provide further information about the type and severity of the injury. Conduction velocities for all nerves studied were within normal limits; however, the amplitude recorded in the right APB muscle was only 4% of the normal value. This signifies axonal injury, or axonotmesis. The percentage reduction in normal amplitude is a proxy for the number of axons injured within the nerve, and this represents a severe injury, with most of the axons being damaged. No additional information is available from this study to pinpoint the anatomic location of the median nerve injury.

EMG studies presented in Table 50.3 confirm axonal injury in the distribution of the median nerve branch supplying the right APB, with the presence of denervation potentials (0–4+ scale) in this muscle. These fibrillation potentials and positive sharp waves are not normally seen until 3 to 4 weeks after injury. There is also evidence of preexisting chronic injury, as demonstrated by the increased duration of MUAP and polyphasia in the APB. These signs of reinnervation do not occur until several months after injury, implying that there may have been some type of preexisting subclinical injury prior to the surgical procedure and nerve block. The EMG also demonstrates evidence of axonal injury in the branches of the ulnar nerve not tested in the motor examination. Selective injury in branches of the ulnar nerve derived from the C8–T1 roots of the medial cord, along with injury to medial cord-derived branches of the median nerve, are most likely localized to the forearm. Normal paraspinal EMG recordings indicate no pathology at the C5–T1 nerve root level, and muscles innervated with nerves derived from superior and middle trunk nerve roots (axillary, musculocutaneous, and radial) are all normal, excluding superior or middle trunk pathology. Denervation potentials in the flexor digitorum profundus muscle (which includes the C7 nerve root passing through the middle trunk) are most likely attributed to a distal injury, given that other muscles supplied from the lateral and posterior cord containing the C7 nerve root (pronator teres, triceps) are normal.

EDX study results confirm that the superior trunk nerve block was unlikely to have contributed to this patient's injury. Block-related axonal damage at the level of the superior trunk would manifest with denervation potentials in the deltoid, supraspinatus, and biceps muscle—with possible extension into middle trunk-innervated structures such as the pronator teres and triceps muscles. Arthroscopic shoulder surgery would most likely cause injuries to the axillary, musculocutaneous, and suprascapular nerves or diffuse brachial plexus injuries involving all trunks and cords secondary to a stretch injury associated with positioning.

The most likely explanation for this injury is a post-surgical inflammatory neuropathy (PSIN). These injuries can be multifocal and are often characterized by intense pain after a block wears off, followed by unexplained muscle weakness in multiple nerve locations. PSIN is underdiagnosed and frequently not considered in the differential diagnosis of PONS, with causation often erroneously attributed to PNB.[3,53,58]

SURGICAL TREATMENT OPTIONS

Peripheral nerve reconstruction surgery should be considered for any persistent serious motor nerve injury on clinical examination that affects shoulder, elbow, or hand function and minimal evidence of reinnervation on EDX studies at 6 months.[52,57] Irreversible functional changes in the neuromuscular junction and muscle of affected tissues will occur beyond 1 year after denervation, limiting the effectiveness of delayed reconstructive surgery restoring axonal continuity to target tissue. The emphasis has shifted from interposition autologous grafts to nerve transfer options.[57]

NEGLIGENCE AND MEDICAL MALPRACTICE RELATED TO PNB

Compared to other physician specialties, anesthesiologists face slightly below average risk of being named in a malpractice lawsuit.[59] With respect to anesthesiology-related claims, nerve injury is the second most common category of claim filed; however, most of these claims are associated with general anesthesia and neuraxial anesthesia, with only 2% of all anesthesia claims related to PNB.[60] ISB was the most frequently represented PNB in claims databases, although only 3.5% of these claims resulted in a payment.[61] Femoral and popliteal nerve blocks were the second and third most common PNB associated with claims in a recent analysis, with 50% of popliteal sciatic nerve block claims resulting in a payment.[61]

CONCLUSIONS

- PONS or PNI are frequently observed after PNB and orthopedic surgery.
- The incidence of long-term PONS following ultrasound-guided PNB is estimated to range between 2:10,000 and 9:10,000, which is not appreciably different from nerve stimulation needle localization techniques.
- Many instances of PNI are falsely attributed to PNB, and clinicians fail to consider other surgery- and patient-related causes, including inherent risks associated with orthopedic surgery and patient-related conditions, that predispose to subclinical peripheral neuropathy.
- PSIN may be responsible for many cases of PONS that have been incorrectly attributed to PNB.
- A separate anesthesia consent form and a comprehensive block note can establish standard of care practice for PNB and are encouraged for diagnostic and medicolegal reasons.
- Any serious motor nerve injury warrants a neurology consultation followed by either MRI or EDX studies. Together, these studies usually localize the site and severity of injury, although clinical correlation is required to assess causation.
- PNB blocks at the highest risk for a claim include ISB, femoral, sciatic, and popliteal sciatic.

REFERENCES

1. Brull R, McCartney CJ, Chan VW, El-Beheiry H. Neurological complications after regional anesthesia: contemporary estimates of risk. *Anesth Analg*. 2007;104:965–974.
2. Neal JM, Gerancher JC, Hebl JR, et al. Upper extremity regional anesthesia: essentials of our current understanding. *Reg Anesth Pain Med*. 2009;34:134–170.
3. Neal JM, Barrington MJ, Brull R, et al. The second ASRA practice advisory on neurologic complications associated with regional anesthesia and pain medicine: executive summary 2015. *Reg Anesth Pain Med*. 2015;40:401–430.
4. Neal JM. Ultrasound-guided regional anesthesia and patient safety: update of an evidence-based analysis. *Reg Anesth Pain Med*. 2016;41:195–204.
5. Auroy Y, Benhamou D, Bargues L, et al. Major complications of regional anesthesia in France: the SOS regional anesthesia hotline service. *Anesthesiology*. 2002;97:1274–1280.
6. Barrington MJ, Watts SA, Gledhill SR, et al. Preliminary results of the Australasian Regional Anaesthesia Collaboration: a prospective audit of over 7000 peripheral nerve and plexus blocks for neurological and other complications. *Reg Anesth Pain Med*. 2009;34:534–541.
7. Welch MB, Brummett CM, Welch TD, et al. Perioperative peripheral nerve injuries. A retrospective study of 380,680 cases during a 10-year period at a single institution. *Anesthesiology*. 2009;111:490–497.
8. Sites BD, Taenzer AH, Herrick MD, et al. Incidence of local anesthetic systemic toxicity and postoperative neurologic symptoms associated with 12,668 ultrasound-guided nerve blocks: an analysis from a prospective clinical registry. *Reg Anesth Pain Med*. 2012;37:478–482.
9. Orebaugh SL, Kentor ML, Williams BA. Adverse outcomes associated with nerve stimulator-guided and ultrasound-guided peripheral nerve blocks by supervised trainees: update of a single-site database. *Reg Anesth Pain Med*. 2012;37:577–582.
10. Yajnik M, Kou A, Mudumbai SC, et al. Peripheral nerve blocks are not associated with increased risk of perioperative peripheral nerve injury in a Veteran's Affairs inpatient surgical population. *Reg Anesth Pain Med*. 2019;44:81–85.
11. Dwyer T, Henry PD, Cholvisudhi P, Chan VW, Theodoropoulos JS, Brull R. Neurological complications related to elective orthopedic surgery: part 1: common shoulder and elbow procedures. *Reg Anesth Pain Med*. 2015;40:431–442.
12. Sondekoppam RV, Tsui B. Factors associated with risk of neurologic complications after peripheral nerve blocks: a systematic review. *Anesth Analg*. 2017;124:645–660.
13. Brull R, Hadzic A, Reina MA, Barrington MJ. Pathophysiology and etiology of nerve injury following peripheral nerve blockade. *Reg Anesth Pain Med*. 2015;40:479–490.
14. Swetha RP, Beckman JD, Lyman S, Zayas VM. Cervical spine disease is a risk factor for persistent phrenic nerve paresis following interscalene nerve block. *Reg Anesth Pain Med*. 2013;38:239–242.
15. Auyong DB, Hanson NA, Joseph RS, Schmidt BE, Slee AE, Yuan SC. Comparison of anterior suprascapular, supraclavicular, and interscalene nerve block approaches for major outpatient arthroscopic shoulder surgery: a randomized, double-blind, noninferiority trial. *Anesthesiology*. 2018;129:47–57.
16. Kim DH, Lin Y, Beathe JC, et al. Superior trunk block: a phrenic-sparing alternative to the interscalene block: a randomized controlled trial. *Anesthesiology*. 2019;131:521–533.
17. Bierstein K. Informed consent and the Medicare Interpretive Guidelines. *ASA Newsletter*. 2006;70:13–14.
18. Domino KB. Informed consent for regional anesthesia: what is necessary? *Reg Anesth Pain Med*. 2007;32:1–2.
19. Hardman HD, Smyth TW, Semo JJ, Rowan CC, D'Ercole FJ. Ultrasound-guided regional anesthesia (UGRA) and standard of care. *Reg Anesth Pain Med*. 2018;43:107.
20. Albrecht E, Mermoud J, Fournier N, Kern C, Kirkham KR. A systematic review of ultrasound-guided methods for brachial plexus blockade. *Anaesthesia*. 2016;71:213–227.
21. Yamamoto H, Sakura S, Wada M, Shido A. A prospective, randomized comparison between single and multiple injection techniques for ultrasound-guided subgluteal sciatic nerve block. *Anesth Analg*. 2014;119:1441–1448.

22. Liguori G, Zayas VM, YaDeau JT, et al. Nerve localization techniques for interscalene brachial plexus blockade: a prospective randomized comparison of mechanical paresthesia vs. electrical stimulation. *Anesth Analg*. 2006;103:761–767.
23. Neal JM, Wedel DJ. Ultrasound guidance and peripheral nerve injury: is our vision as sharp as we think it is? *Reg Anesth Pain Med*. 2010;335:335–337.
24. Liu SS, YaDeau JT, Shaw PM, Wilfred S, Shetty T, Gordon M. Incidence of unintentional intraneural injection and postoperative neurological complications with ultrasound-guided interscalene and supraclavicular nerve blocks. *Anaesthesia*. 2011;66:168–174.
25. Hara K, Sakura S, Yokokawa N, Tadenuma S. Incidence and effects of unintentional intraneural injection during ultrasound-guided subgluteal sciatic nerve block. *Reg Anesth Pain Med*. 2012;37:289–293.
26. Sala Blanch X, López AM, Carazo J, et al. Intraneural injection during nerve stimulator-guided sciatic nerve block at the popliteal fossa. *Br J Anaesth*. 2009;102:855–861.
27. Perlas A, Niazi A, McCartney C, Chan V, Xu D, Abbas S. The sensitivity of motor response to nerve stimulation and paresthesia for nerve localization as evaluated by ultrasound. *Reg Anesth Pain Med*. 2006;31:445–450.
28. Steinfeldt T, Poeschl S, Nimphius W, et al. Forced needle advancement during needle-nerve contact in a porcine model histological outcome. *Anesth Analg*. 2011;113:417–420.
29. Krediet AC, Moayeri N, Bleys RL, Groen GJ. Intraneural or extraneural: diagnostic accuracy of ultrasound assessment for localizing low-volume injection. *Reg Anesth Pain Med*. 2014;39:409–413.
30. Spence BC, Beach ML, Gallagher JD, Sites BD. Ultrasound-guided interscalene blocks: understanding where to inject the local anaesthetic. *Anaesthesia*. 2011;66:509–514.
31. Albrecht E, Kirkham KR, Taffé P, et al. The maximum effective needle-to-nerve distance for ultrasound-guided interscalene block: an exploratory study. *Reg Anesth Pain Med*. 2014;39:56–60.
32. Tsai TP, Vuckovic I, Dilberovic F, et al. Intensity of the stimulating current may not be a reliable indicator of intraneural needle placement. *Reg Anesth Pain Med*. 2008;33:207–210.
33. Kapur E, Vuckovic I, Dilberovic F, et al. Neurologic and histologic outcome after intraneural injections of lidocaine in canine sciatic nerves. *Acta Anaesthesiol Scand*. 2007;51:101–107.
34. Lupu CM, Kiehl TR, Chan VW, El-Beheiry H, Madden M, Brull R. Nerve expansion seen on ultrasound predicts histologic but not functional nerve injury after intraneural injection in pigs. *Reg Anesth Pain Med*. 2010;35:132–139.
35. Gadsden JC, Choi JJ, Lin E, Robinson A. Opening injection pressure consistently detects needle-nerve contact during ultrasound-guided interscalene brachial plexus block. *Anesthesiology*. 2014;120:1246–1253.
36. Gadsden JC, Latmore M, Levine DM, Robinson A. High opening injection pressure is associated with needle-nerve and needle-fascia contact during femoral nerve block. *Reg Anesth Pain Med*. 2016;41:50–55.
37. Vermeylen K, Hermans M, Soetens F, et al. Opening injection pressure is higher in intraneural compared with perineural injections during simulated nerve blocks of the lower limb in fresh human cadavers. *Reg Anesth Pain Med*. 2017;42:362–367.
38. Cappelleri G, Ambrosoli AL, Gemma M, Cedrati VLE, Bizzarri F, Danelli GF. Intraneural ultrasound-guided sciatic nerve block: minimum effective volume and electrophysiologic effects. *Anesthesiology*. 2018;129:241–248.
39. Theron PS, Mackay Z, Gonzalez JG, Donaldson N, Blanco R. An animal model of syringe feel during peripheral nerve block. *Reg Anesth Pain Med*. 2009;34:330–332.
40. Tsui BC, Li LX, Pillay JJ. Compressed air injection technique to standardize block injection pressures. *Can J Anesth*. 2006;53:1098–1102.
41. Johnson AN, Peiffer JS, Halmann N, Delaney L, Owen CA, Hersh J. Ultrasound-guided needle technique accuracy: prospective comparison of passive magnetic tracking versus unassisted echogenic needle localization. *Reg Anesth Pain Med*. 2017;42(2):223–232.
42. Bigeleisen P. Nerve puncture and apparent intraneural injection during ultrasound guided axillary block does not invariably result in neurologic injury. *Anesthesiology*. 2006;105:779–783.
43. Retter S, Szerb J, Kwofie K, Colp P, Sandeski R, Uppal V. Incidence of sub-perineural injection using a targeted intracluster supraclavicular ultrasound-guided approach in cadavers. *Br J Anaesth*. 2019;122:713–715.
44. Farber SJ, Saheb-Al-Zamani M, Zieske L, et al. Peripheral nerve injury after local anesthetic injection. *Anesth Analg*. 2013;117:731–739.
45. Short A, Chan VW, Perlas A. Is deliberate intraneural injection a case of "false economy?" *Reg Anesth Pain Med*. 2016;41:421–423.
46. Short A, Chan VW, Perlas A. A reply to Dr. Bigeleisen: safety and subepineural injections. *Reg Anesth Pain Med*. 2017;42:126–127.
47. Vlassakov K, Lirk P, Rathmell JP. Intraneural injection: is the jury still out? *Anesthesiology*. 2018;129:221–224.
48. Williams BA, Hough KA, Tsui BY, Ibinson JW, Gold MS, Gebhart GF. Neurotoxicity of adjuvants used in perineural anesthesia and analgesia in comparison with ropivacaine. *Reg Anesth Pain Med*. 2011;36:225–230.
49. Kim BS, Choi JH, Baek SH, Lee DH. Effects of intraneural injection of dexmedetomidine in combination with ropivacaine in rat sciatic nerve block. *Reg Anesth Pain Med*. 2018;43:378–384.
50. Williams BA, Ibinson JW, Gould AJ, Mangione MP. The incidence of peripheral nerve injury after multimodal perineural anesthesia/analgesia does not appear to differ from that following single drug nerve blocks. *Pain Med*. 2017;18:626–636.
51. Partridge BL. The effects of local anesthetics and epinephrine on rat sciatic nerve blood flow. *Anesthesiology*. 1991;75:243–250.
52. Simon NG, Spinner RJ, Kline DG, Kliot M. Advances in the neurological and neurosurgical management of peripheral nerve trauma. *J Neurol Neurosurg Psychiatry*. 2015:0:1–11.
53. Watson JC, Huntoon MA. Neurologic evaluation and management of perioperative nerve injury. *Reg Anesth Pain Med*. 2015;40:491–501.
54. Padua L, Di Pasquale A, Liotta G, et al. Ultrasound as a useful tool in the diagnosis and management of traumatic nerve lesions. *Clin Neurophysiol*. 2013;124:1237–1243.
55. Preston DC, Shapiro BE. *Electromyography and Neuromuscular Disorders: Clinical-Electrophysiologic Correlations (Expert Consult-Online)*. Philadelphia: Elsevier Health Sciences; 2013.
56. Perotto AO, et al. *Anatomical Guide for the Electromyographer: The Limbs and Trunk*. Springfield, IL: Charles C. Thomas; 2011.
57. Brown JM, Vivio N, Sheean GL. The clinical practice of reconstructive neurosurgery. *Clin Neurol Neurosurg*. 2012;114:506–514.
58. Staff NP, Engelstad J, Klein CJ, et al. Post-surgical inflammatory neuropathy. *Brain*. 2010;133:2866–2880.
59. Jena AB, Seabury S, Lakdawalla D, Chandra A. Malpractice risk according to physician specialty. *N Engl J Med*. 2011;365:629–636.
60. Lee LA, Posner KL, Kent CD, Domino KB. Complications associated with peripheral nerve blocks: lessons from the ASA closed claims project. *Int Anesth Clin*. 2011;49:56–67.
61. Saba R, Brovman EY, Kang D, Greenberg P, Kaye AD, Urman RD. A contemporary medicolegal analysis of injury related to peripheral nerve blocks. *Pain Physician*. 2019;22:389–399.

REVIEW QUESTIONS

(1) Which of the following statements is true regarding the incidence of postoperative neurologic symptoms (PONS) after peripheral nerve block (PNB) and surgery?

A. PNB is not a risk factor for developing PONS after total joint replacement surgery.
B. Diabetes is not a risk factor for developing PONS after surgery.

C. Hypertension is not a risk factor for developing PONS after surgery.
D. Tobacco use is not a risk factor for developing PONS after surgery.

(2) The risk of a neurologic injury after PNB that lasts for more than 1 year or is permanent is:

A. 1:10–1:100
B. 1:100–1:1000
C. 1:500–1:10,000
D. 2:10,000–9:10,000

(3) The incidence of inadvertent intraneural injection during ultrasound-guided PNB is approximately:

A. <1%
B. 10%
C. 20%
D. 75%

(4) Which of the following statements is true?

A. Ultrasound has 85% sensitivity in expert hands, detecting as little as a 0.5 mL volume of intraneural injection.
B. Intraneural injection invariably leads to functional nerve injury.
C. Ultrasound can discriminate between intraneural intrafascicular and intraneural extrafascicular injection.
D. Ultrasound can detect needle entry into the epineurium.

(5) Neurostimulation and injection pressure monitoring can assist ultrasound-guided PNB because:

A. Regional anesthesiologists do not consistently visualize the tip of the needle.
B. Neurostimulation is sensitive but not specific for needle tip distance from the nerve.
C. Elevated injection pressures (>15 psi) are specific for needle-nerve contact or intraneural position.
D. The subjective feeling of resistance at the onset of injection is a useful estimate of injection pressure.

(6) The most common type of nerve injury (PNI) observed after surgery and PNB is:

A. Neurotmesis
B. Axonotmesis
C. Neurapraxia
D. Motor nerve injuries

(7) Which of the following statements is true regarding the use of electrodiagnostic (EDX) studies?

A. Axonal injury is characterized by decreased amplitude and normal latency on NCS, with fibrillation potentials on needle EMG.
B. Neurapraxia is characterized by decreased conduction velocity on NCS, with normal amplitude.
C. Neurotmesis is characterized by decreased amplitude and increased latency on NCS.
D. EMG denervation potentials can be first detected 2 weeks after neurapraxia.

(8) Standard of care for PNB would require which of the following?

A. Use of ultrasound guidance during PNB.
B. Adherence to generally recognized and accepted practices that would be followed by an average, competent anesthesiologist performing PNB.
C. Fellowship training in regional anesthesia.
D. Avoiding local anesthetics with a higher potential for local anesthetic systemic toxicity.

ANSWERS

(1) **A.** B, C, and D are not correct because these are all risk factors for PONS.

References

Neal JM, Barrington MJ, Brull R, et al. The second ASRA practice advisory on neurologic complications associated with regional anesthesia and pain medicine: executive summary 2015. *Reg Anesth Pain Med.* 2015;40:401–430.
Welch MB, Brummett CM, Welch TD, et al. Perioperative peripheral nerve injuries: a retrospective study of 380,680 cases during a 10-year period at a single institution. *Anesthesiology.* 2009;111:490–497.

(2) **D.**

References

Neal JM, Barrington MJ, Brull R, et al. The second ASRA practice advisory on neurologic complications associated with regional anesthesia and pain medicine: executive summary 2015. *Reg Anesth Pain Med.* 2015;40:401–430.
Neal JM. Ultrasound-guided regional anesthesia and patient safety: update of an evidence-based analysis. *Reg Anesth Pain Med.* 2016;41:195–204.
Sites BD, Taenzer AH, Herrick MD, et al. Incidence of local anesthetic systemic toxicity and postoperative neurologic symptoms associated with 12,668 ultrasound-guided nerve blocks: an analysis from a prospective clinical registry. *Reg Anesth Pain Med.* 2012;37:478–482.

(3) **C.** The risk is 17% rate with the use of ultrasound PNB. D is correct for neurostimulation but incorrect for ultrasound PNB.

References

Liu SS, YaDeau JT, Shaw PM, Wilfred S, Shetty T, Gordon M. Incidence of unintentional intraneural injection and postoperative neurological complications with ultrasound-guided interscalene and supraclavicular nerve blocks. *Anaesthesia.* 2011;66:168–174.
Hara K, Sakura S, Yokokawa N, Tadenuma S. Incidence and effects of unintentional intraneural injection during ultrasound-guided subgluteal sciatic nerve block. *Reg Anesth Pain Med.* 2012;37:289–293.

(4) **A.** This is only true for experts (novices only 65%). B is incorrect. C is incorrect due to the limited resolution of current ultrasound technology visualizing fascicles, and D is incorrect for the same reason: limited resolution to define the epineurium.

References

Krediet AC, Moayeri N, Bleys RL, Groen GJ. Intraneural or extraneural; diagnostic accuracy of ultrasound assessment for localizing low-volume injection. *Reg Anesth Pain Med.* 2014;39:409–413.

Neal JM, Barrington MJ, Brull R, et al. The second ASRA practice advisory on neurologic complications associated with regional anesthesia and pain medicine: executive summary 2015. *Reg Anesth Pain Med.* 2015;40:401–430.

Sondekoppam RV, Tsui B. Factors associated with risk of neurologic complications after peripheral nerve blocks: a systematic review. *Anesth Analg.* 2017;124:645–660.

Bigeleisen P. Nerve puncture and apparent intraneural injection during ultrasound guided axillary block does not invariably result in neurologic injury. *Anesthesiology.* 2006;105:779–783.

(5) **A.** Neurostimulation and injection pressure monitoring can assist ultrasound-guided PNB because regional anesthesiologists do not consistently visualize the tip of the needle, particularly with non-experts. B is incorrect because neurostimulation is specific for needle-nerve contact but is not sensitive for needle-nerve distance. C is incorrect because elevated opening injection pressure (OIP) is sensitive but not specific for needle-nerve contact. D is incorrect.

References

Neal JM, Barrington MJ, Brull R, et al. The second ASRA practice advisory on neurologic complications associated with regional anesthesia and pain medicine: executive summary 2015. *Reg Anesth Pain Med.* 2015;40:401–430.

Theron PS, Mackay Z, Gonzalez JG, Donaldson N, Blanco R. An animal model of syringe feel during peripheral nerve block. *Reg Anesth Pain Med.* 2009;34:330–332.

Tsui BC, Li LX, Pillay JJ. Compressed air injection technique to standardize block injection pressures. *Can J Anesth.* 2006;53:1098–1102.

(6) **C.** B, C, and D occur less frequently since these are associated with long-term PONS, with an incidence of <0.2%.

References

Neal JM, Barrington MJ, Brull R, et al. The second ASRA practice advisory on neurologic complications associated with regional anesthesia and pain medicine: executive summary 2015. *Reg Anesth Pain Med.* 2015;40:401–430.

Neal JM. Ultrasound-guided regional anesthesia and patient safety: update of an evidence-based analysis. *Reg Anesth Pain Med.* 2016;41:195–204.

Watson JC, Huntoon MA. Neurologic evaluation and management of perioperative nerve injury. *Reg Anesth Pain Med.* 2015;40:491–501.

(7) **A.** Axonal injury is characterized by decreased amplitude and normal latency on NCS, with fibrillation potentials on needle EMG. B is incorrect since neurapraxia has decreased amplitude; C is incorrect because neurotmesis would have no signals; and D is incorrect because denervation potentials are not associated with neurapraxia.

References

Preston DC, Shapiro BE. *Electromyography and Neuromuscular Disorders: Clinical-Electrophysiologic Correlations (Expert Consult-Online).* Philadelphia: Elsevier Health Sciences; 2013.

(8) **B.** Adherence to generally recognized and accepted practices that would be followed by an average, competent anesthesiologist performing PNB. A is incorrect. C is incorrect because "fellowship-trained" does not meet the definition of "average, competent practitioner." D is incorrect because the standard of care allows multiple local anesthetic choice options, including bupivacaine.

References

Neal JM, Barrington MJ, Brull R, et al. The second ASRA practice advisory on neurologic complications associated with regional anesthesia and pain medicine: executive summary 2015. *Reg Anesth Pain Med.* 2015;40:401–430.

Hardman HD, Smyth TW, Semo JJ, Rowan CC, D'Ercole FJ. Ultrasound-guided regional anesthesia (UGRA) and standard of care. *Reg Anesth Pain Med.* 2018;43:107.

INDEX

For the benefit of digital users, indexed terms that span two pages (e.g., 52–53) may, on occasion, appear on only one of those pages.

Tables, figures, and boxes are indicated by *t*, *f*, and *b* following the page number